The A.S.P.E.N.
PEDIATRIC NUTRITION SUPPORT
CORE CURRICULUM, 2nd Edition

EDITOR-IN-CHIEF

Mark R. Corkins, MD, CNSP, SPR, FAAP
Division Chief of Pediatric Gastroenterology
University of Tennessee Health Science Center/Le Bonheur Children's Hospital
Memphis, TN

SECTION EDITORS

Jane Balint, MD
Co-Director Intestinal Support Service
Pediatric Gastroenterology, Hepatology, and Nutrition
Nationwide Children's Hospital
Columbus, OH

Elizabeth Bobo, MS, RD, LDN, CNSC
Clinical Dietitian
Nemours Children's Clinic
Jacksonville, FL

Steve Plogsted, PharmD, BCNSP, CNSC
Nutrition Support Pharmacist
Nationwide Children's Hospital
Columbus, OH

Jane Anne Yaworski, MSN, RN
Clinical Nurse Specialist for Nutrition Support and Intestinal Care
Children's Hospital of Pittsburgh of UPMC
Pittsburgh, PA

MANAGING EDITOR

Jennifer Kuhn, MPS
Director of Publications
American Society for Parenteral and Enteral Nutrition
Silver Spring, MD

AMERICAN SOCIETY FOR PARENTERAL AND ENTERAL NUTRITION

About A.S.P.E.N.

The American Society for Parenteral and Enteral Nutrition (A.S.P.E.N.) is a scientific society whose members are health care professionals; physicians, dietitians, nurses, pharmacists, other allied health professionals, and researchers; that envisions an environment in which every patient receives safe, efficacious, and high quality patient care.

A.S.P.E.N.'s mission is to improve patient care by advancing the science and practice of clinical nutrition and metabolism.

NOTE: This publication is designed to provide accurate authoritative information in regard to the subject matter covered. It is sold with the understanding that the publisher is not engaged in rendering medical or other professional advice. Trademarked commercial product names are used only for education purposes and do not constitute endorsement by A.S.P.E.N.

This publication does not constitute medical or professional advice, and should not be taken as such. Use of the information published herein is subject to the sole professional judgment of the attending health profes sional, whose judgment is the primary component of quality medical care. The information presented herein is not a substitute for the exercise of such judgment by the health professional.

Print ISBN: 978-1-889622-21-7
eBook ISBN: 978-1-889622-22-4

Printed in the United States of America.

Access Podcasts and Videos for This Book

The *A.S.P.E.N. Pediatric Nutrition Support Core Curriculum, 2nd Edition* features 13 podcasts and 4 videos hosted online as digital supplementary materials. Listen and watch as the authors of this text discuss the concepts presented in the chapter. Plug in for online content by visiting www.nutritioncare.org/PedCore2Extras to get started. Note, login is required to access podcasts and videos.

Look for these symbols to indicate which chapters include online components.

Podcast:

Video:

Need help?

For assistance with accessing these digital materials, please contact A.S.P.E.N. by email at aspen@nutritioncare.org.

Contents

Contributors

Alaa Al Nofal, MD
Pediatric Endocrinology Fellow
Mayo Clinic
Rochester, MN

Janice Antino, RD, MS, CNSC
Clinical Nutritionist
Stony Brook Children's Hospital
Stony Brook, NY

Jane Balint, MD
Co-Director, Intestinal Support Service, Pediatric
Gastroenterology, Hepatology, and Nutrition
Nationwide Children's Hospital
Columbus, OH

Allison Beck, MS, RD, LDN, CSP, CNSC
Clinical Dietitian II
Le Bonheur Children's Hospital
Memphis, TN

Michelle Beitzel, PharmD
Caseload Pharmacist
Indiana University Health Home Care
Indianapolis, IN

Elizabeth Bobo, MS, RD, LDN, CNSC
Clinical Dietitian, Division of Gastroenterology and Nutrition
Nemours Children's Clinic
Jacksonville, FL

Peggy R. Borum, PhD
Professor of Human Nutrition
University of Florida
Gainesville, FL

Jackie Buell, PhD, RD, ATC, CSSD
Assistant Professor - Clinical, Sports Nutrition
Division of Health Sciences and Medical Dietetics; Sports
Medicine, Sports Health and Performance Institute; Ohio State
University
Columbus, OH

Kristen Bunger, MS, RD, CNSC
Pediatric Dietitian
Phoenix Children's Hospital
Phoenix, AZ

Jessica Buschmann, MS, RD, LD
Clinical Dietitian for Sports Medicine
Nationwide Children's Hospital
Westerville, OH

Esther Castanys-Muñoz, PhD
Junior Scientist, University Science Park
Abbott Nutrition
Granada, Spain

Anupama Chawla, MD, DCH (UK), CNSC
Director of Pediatric Gastroenterology and Nutrition
Director of Celiac Disease and Gluten Sensitivity Center
Stony Brook Children's Hospital
Stony Brook, NY

Catherine Christie, PhD, RDN, LDN, FAND
Associate Dean and Professor
University of North Florida Brooks College of Health
Jacksonville, FL

Judith Christie, RN, MSN
Nutrition Support Nurse
Children's Hospital of Michigan
Detroit, MI

Mark R. Corkins, MD, CNSP, SPR, FAAP
Division Chief of Pediatric Gastroenterology
University of Tennessee Health Science Center/Le Bonheur
Children's Hospital
Memphis, TN

Catherine M. Crill, PharmD, FCCP, BCPS, BCNSP
Associate Professor of Clinical Pharmacy and Pediatrics, The
University of Tennessee Health Science Center
Director and Clinical Pharmacy Specialist, Parenteral Nutrition
Service, Le Bonheur Children's Hospital
Memphis, TN

Wendy Cruse, MMSc, CLS, RD
Pediatric Clinical Dietitian Specialist
Riley Hospital for Children at Indiana University Health
Indianapolis, IN

Molly Dienhart, MD
Co-Director, Intestinal Support Service, Pediatric
Gastroenterology, Hepatology, and Nutrition
Nationwide Children's Hospital
Columbus, OH

Jill Dorsey, MD, MS
Pediatric Gastroenterologist, Division of Gastroenterology and
Nutrition
Nemours Children's Clinic
Jacksonville, FL

Megan Dougherty, RD, CSP, LDN, CNSC
Clinical Pediatric Dietitian
Children's Hospital of Philadelphia
Philadelphia, PA

Kristi Drabouski, RD, CSP, LDN, CNSC
Clinical Pediatric Dietitian
Children's Hospital of Philadelphia
Philadelphia, PA

Mary Beth Feuling, MS, RD, CSP, CD
Advanced Practice Dietitian, Quality Improvement and
Research
Children's Hospital of Wisconsin
Milwaukee, WI

Mindy Freudenberg, RD, MS, CNSC
Clinical Nutritionist
Stony Brook Children's Hospital
Stony Brook, NY

Richard W. Gelling, PhD
Senior Lead Strategic Research
Abbott Nutrition and Department of Medicine, National
University of Singapore
Singapore

Donald George, MD
Chief, Division of Gastroenterology and Nutrition
Nemours Children's Clinic
Jacksonville, FL

Leslie M. Gimenez, MD
Assistant Professor, Division of Allergy and Clinical
Immunology
Medical College of Wisconsin
Milwaukee, WI

Praveen S. Goday, MBBS, CNSC
Professor, Division of Pediatric Gastroenterology and Nutrition
Medical College of Wisconsin
Milwaukee, WI

Monique L. Goldschmidt, MD
Staff Hepatologist, Division of Gastroenterology, Hepatology,
Nutrition
Cincinnati Children's Hospital Medical Center
Cincinnati, OH

Memorie M. Gosa, PhD, CCC-SLP, BCS-S
Assistant Professor
The University of Alabama, Department of Communicative
Disorders
Tuscaloosa, AL

Laura Grande, MS, RD, CSP, LDN
Clinical Dietitian
The Children's Hospital of Philadelphia
Philadelphia, PA

Kelly Green Corkins, MS, RD, LDN, CNSC
Clinical Dietitian III
Le Bonheur Children's Hospital
Memphis, TN

Sandeep K. Gupta, MD
Professor of Clinical Pediatrics and Internal Medicine
Riley Hospital for Children, Indiana University Health
Indianapolis, IN

Kathleen M. Gura, PharmD, BCNSP, FASHP, FPPAG
Clinical Pharmacy Specialist, Gastroenterology and Nutrition,
Center for Advanced Intestinal Rehabilitation (CAIR), Boston
Children's Hospital
Associate Professor Pharmacy Practice, MCPHS University
Boston, MA

Diane L. Habash, PhD, MS, RD, LD
Clinical Associate Professor, Division of Health Sciences and
Medical Dietetics
Associate Director of Education, Center for Integrative Health
and Wellness
Ohio State University, College of Medicine
Columbus, OH

Richard A. Helms, PharmD
Professor and Chair
Professor of Pediatrics
University of Tennessee Health Science Center, Department of
Clinical Pharmacy
Memphis, TN

David Henry, MS, BCOP, FASHP
Pediatric Hematology/Oncology Pharmacist, Associate
Professor and Chair Pharmacy Practice
University of Kansas Medical Center
Kansas City, KS

Oscar R. Herrera, PharmD
Assistant Professor
University of Tennessee Health Science Center, Department of
Clinical Pharmacy
Memphis, TN

Kyrie L. Hospodar, RN, MSN, CPNP
Pediatric Nurse Practitioner
Phoenix Children's Hospital/Mayo Clinic Arizona
Phoenix, AZ

Kishore R. Iyer, MBBS, FRCS (Eng), FACS
Associate Professor of Surgery & Pediatrics
Surgical Director, Intestinal Transplantation & Rehab Program
Mount Sinai Medical Center
New York, NY

Marisa Juarez, MPH, RD, LD
Sr. Pediatric Renal Dietitian
Texas Children's Hospital
Houston, TX

John A. Kerner, MD
Professor of Pediatrics
Stanford University Medical Center
Palo Alto, CA

Samuel A. Kocoshis, MD
Professor of Pediatrics, University of Cincinnati College of
Medicine
Medical Director, Intestinal Care Center and Intestinal
Transplantation, Cincinnati Children's Hospital Medical Center
Cincinnati, OH

Kelly Kolp, RD, CNSC
Pediatric Dietitian
Phoenix Children's Hospital
Phoenix, AZ

Kelly Cronin Komatz, MD, MPH, FAAP, FAAHPM
Medical Director, UF Center for the Medically Complex Child,
UF Pediatric Pain and Palliative Medicine Clinic, Community
PedsCare Program of Community Hospice of Northeast Florida
Program Director, UF Hospice and Palliative Medicine
Fellowship
Jacksonville, FL

Winston Koo, MBBS, FACN, CNS
Professor of Pediatrics
Louisiana State University
Shreveport, LA

Arlet G. Kurkchubasche, MD
Associate Professor of Surgery and Pediatrics
Alpert Medical School of Brown University
Providence, RI

Corinne Labyak, PhD, RDN
Assistant Professor
University of North Florida Brooks College of Health,
Department of Nutrition and Dietetics
Jacksonville, FL

José M. López-Pedrosa, PhD
Site Manager, University Science Park
Abbott Nutrition
Granada, Spain

Yen-Ling Low, PhD
Director, Clinical Research
Abbott Nutrition R&D, Asia-Pacific Center
Singapore

Mirjana Lulic-Botica, BSc, RPh, BCPS
Neonatal Clinical Pharmacy Specialist
Hutzel Women's Hospital
Detroit, MI

Beth Lyman, RN, MSN, CNSC
Senior Program Coordinator for the Nutrition Support Team
Children's Mercy Kansas City
Kansas City, MO

Allison Mallowe, MA, RD, LDN
Clinical Dietitian
The Children's Hospital of Philadelphia
Philadelphia, PA

Barbara Marriage, PhD, RD
Manager, Pediatric Clinical Research
Abbott Nutrition
Columbus, OH

Maria Mascarenhas, MBBS
Director of Nutrition Support and Service; Section Chief,
Nutrition, Division of Gastroenterology, Hepatology, and
Nutrition
The Children's Hospital of Philadelphia
Philadelphia, PA

Thaddaeus D. May, MD
Postdoctoral Fellow, Pediatric Gastroenterology, Hepatology,
and Nutrition
Baylor College of Medicine, Texas Children's Hospital
Houston, TX

Carol G. McKown, DDS, MS, PC
Owner/President, Carmel Pediatric Dentist
Volunteer Faculty, Riley Hospital Pediatric Dentistry
Department
Carmel, IN

Robin Meyers, MPH, RD, LDN
Outpatient Manager, Clinical Nutrition
The Children's Hospital of Philadelphia
Philadelphia, PA

Jessica Monczka, RD, LDN, CNSC
Registered Dietitian
Orlando Health
Orlando, FL

Christina L. Nelms, MS, RD, CSP, LMNT
Pediatric Renal Dietitian & Professor, Clarkson College
Owner/Operator, Peds Feeds LLC
Omaha, NE

Britt Olson, RN, MSN, CPNP
Hematology/Oncology Pediatric Nurse Practitioner
Phoenix Children's Hospital
Phoenix, AZ

Kalyan Ray Parashette, MD, MPH
Assistant Professor of Pediatrics
University of New Mexico Children's Hospital, UNM School of
Medicine
Albuquerque, NM

Susan R. Rheingold, MD
Associate Professor of Pediatrics
The Children's Hospital of Philadelphia
Philadelphia, PA

Judith C. Rodriguez, PhD, RDN, FAND
Chair and Professor
University of North Florida Brooks College of Health,
Department of Nutrition and Dietetics
Jacksonville, FL

Ricardo Rueda, MD, PhD
Research Fellow/Associate Director Strategic Research
Abbott Nutrition
Granada, Spain

May Saba, PharmD, BCNSP
Clinical Coordinator, Pharmacy Services
Children's Hospital of Michigan
Detroit, MI

Nancy Sacks, MS, RD, LDN
Pediatric Oncology Dietitian/Study Coordinator
The Children's Hospital of Philadelphia
Philadelphia, PA

Gerald L. Schmidt, PharmD, BCNSP
Pharmacy Nutrition Specialist
UF Health Jacksonville
Jacksonville, FL

W. Frederick Schwenk II, MD
Professor of Pediatrics
Mayo Clinic
Rochester, MN

Claudia Sealey-Potts, PhD, RDN, FAND
Assistant Professor
University of North Florida Brooks College of Health,
Department of Nutrition and Dietetics
Jacksonville, FL

Timothy Sentongo, MD, ABPNS
Associate Professor of Pediatrics; Director Pediatric Nutrition
Support; Director Pediatric Gastrointestinal Endoscopy
University of Chicago Medical Center
Chicago, IL

Wednesday Marie A. Sevilla, MD, MPH
Assistant Professor of Pediatrics
University of Tennessee Health Science Center/Le Bonheur
Children's Hospital
Memphis, TN

Sohail R. Shah, MD, MSHA, FAAP
Assistant Professor of Pediatric Surgery
Children's Mercy Kansas City
Kansas City, MO

Ala K. Shaikhkhalil, MD
Assistant Professor of Clinical Pediatrics
Nationwide Children's Hospital/Ohio State University
Columbus, OH

Christina Sherry, PhD, RD
Research Scientist
Abbott Nutrition
Columbus, OH

Robert J. Shulman, MD
Professor of Pediatrics
Baylor College of Medicine, Texas Children's Hospital
Houston, TX

Robert H. Squires, MD
Professor of Pediatrics
University of Pittsburgh School of Medicine
Pittsburgh, PA

Elaina Szeszycki, PharmD, BCNSP
Clinical Pharmacist - Nutrition Support and Pediatric
Gastroenterology
Riley Hospital for Children at Indiana University Health
Indianapolis, IN

Mary Pat Turon-Findley, MS, RD, LD
Registered Dietitian III
Cincinnati Children's Hospital Medical Center
Cincinnati, OH

Sandy Van Calcar, PhD, RD, LD
Assistant Professor
Oregon Health and Science University, Department of
Molecular and Medical Genetics, Graduate Programs in Human
Nutrition
Portland, OR

Cassandra L. S. Walia, MS, RD, CD, CNSC
Clinical Dietitian Specialist
Children's Hospital of Wisconsin
Milwaukee, WI

Bradley A. Warady, MD
Professor of Pediatrics, University of Missouri-Kansas City
School of Medicine
Senior Assoc. Chairman, Department of Pediatrics; Director,
Division of Pediatric Nephrology
Director, Dialysis and Transplantation
Children's Mercy Hospital
Kansas City, MO

Letitia Warren, RD, CSP
Pediatric Dietitian
Children's Hospital of Michigan
Detroit, MI

Jacqueline J. Wessel, MEd, RDN, CNSC, CSP, CLE
Neonatal Nutritionist
Cincinnati Children's Hospital
Cincinnati, OH

Renee A. Wieman, RD, LD, CNSC
Dietitian, Liver and Intestinal Transplantation
Cincinnati Children's Hospital Medical Center
Cincinnati, OH

Andrea White-Collins, RN, MS, CPNP
Hematology Oncology PNP, Center for Cancer and Blood
Disorders
Phoenix Children's Hospital
Phoenix, AZ

Elizabeth L. Wright, MS, RD, CSP, LDN
Clinical Pediatric Dietitian
Children's Hospital of Philadelphia
Philadelphia, PA

Desale Yacob, MD
Assistant Professor of Pediatrics, Pediatric Gastroenterology,
Hepatology, and Nutrition
Nationwide Children's Hospital
Columbus, OH

Reviewers

Roberta Anding, MS, RD/LD, CSSD, CDE
Director of Sports Nutrition
Texas Children's Hospital
Houston, TX

Edward M. Barksdale, Jr., MD
Robert J. Izant, Jr. Professor and Chief, Division of Pediatric
Surgery Surgeon in Chief
Rainbow Babies and Children's Hospital, University Hospitals,
Case Western School of Medicine
Cleveland, OH

Thomas G. Baumgartner, PharmD, MEd, FASHP
President and Chief Executive Officer
Consultant Pharmacists of America, Inc.
Gainesville, FL

Allison Beck, MS, RD, CSP, CNSC
Clinical Dietitian
Le Bonheur Children's Hospital
Memphis, TN

Jatinder Bhatia, MD, FAAP
Professor and Chief, Division of Neonatology
Georgia Regents University
Augusta, GA

Thomas A. Burrow, MD
Assistant Professor of Clinical Pediatrics
Cincinnati Children's Hospital Medical Center and Department
of Pediatrics, University of Cincinnati
Cincinnati, OH

Kirby-Rose Carpenito, RD, LD, BS
Clinical Dietitian (Cardiology and CTICU)
Nationwide Children's Hospital
Columbus, OH

Linda Casey, MD, FRCPC, MSc
Director, Complex Feeding & Nutrition Service
BC Children's Hospital
Vancouver, British Columbia, Canada

Paula Charuhas Macris, MS, RD, CSO, FAND, CD
Nutrition Education Coordinator and
Pediatric Nutrition Specialist
Medical Nutrition Therapy Services,
Seattle Cancer Care Alliance
Seattle, WA

Pamela Charney, PhD, RD, CHTS-CP
Program Chair, HCTM
Bellevue College
Bellevue, WA

Katherine Chessman, PharmD, FPPAG, FCCP, BCNSP, BCPS
Professor, Clinical Pharmacy and Outcome Sciences,
South Carolina College of Pharmacy,
Medical University of South Carolina (MUSC) Campus
Clinical Pharmacy Specialist, Pediatrics/Pediatric Surgery,
MUSC Children's Hospital
Charleston, SC

Michael Lloyd Christensen, PharmD
Professor
University of Tennessee Health Science Center and
Le Bonheur Children's Hospital
Memphis, TN

Mary Petrea Cober, PharmD, BCNSP
Clinical Pharmacy Coordinator, Neonatal Intensive Care Unit,
Akron Children's Hospital
Associate Professor, Pharmacy Practice, Northeast Ohio
Medical University College of Pharmacy
Akron, OH

Valeria Cohran, MD, MS
Assistant Professor of Pediatrics
The Ann and Robert H. Lurie Children's Hospital of Chicago
Chicago, IL

Conrad R. Cole, MD, MPH, MSc
Associate Professor
Cincinnati Children's Hospital Medical Center
Cincinnati, OH

Ann Condon Meyers, MS, LDN
Pediatric Dietitian – Generalist
Children's Hospital of Pittsburgh
Pittsburgh, PA

Cara Conti, MS, RD
Registered Research Dietitian
University of Pittsburgh and Children's Hospital of Pittsburgh of UPMC
Pittsburgh, PA

Laura C. Davis, MS, RD, LD, CNSC
Pediatric Clinical Nutrition Manager
Johns Hopkins Children's Center
Baltimore, MD

Donna Marie T. DiVito, RD, LDN, CNSC
Clinical Dietitian
The Children's Hospital of Philadelphia
Philadelphia, PA

Douglas Drenckpohl, MS, RD, CNSC, LDN
Advanced Practice Dietitian – Neonatal
Children's Hospital of Illinois at OSF-Saint Francis Medical Center
Peoria, IL

Megan M. Durham, MD
Physician
Emory University Department of Surgery
Atlanta, GA

Abimbola Farinde, PhD, PharmD
Professor
Columbia Southern University
Orange Beach, AL

Dianne M. Frazier, PhD, MPH, RD
Professor Emeritus
University of North Carolina
Chapel Hill, NC

Gretchen M. Garlow, MS, RD, LDN, CNSC
Senior Clinical Nutritionist
Massachusetts General Hospital
Boston, MA

Kathleen M. Gura, PharmD, BCNSP, FASHP, FPPAG
Clinical Pharmacist GI/Nutrition; Team Leader, Surgical Programs
Boston Children's Hospital
Boston, MA

Caroline Hartsell, MS, RD, CSR, CSP, LDN
Clinical Dietitian
St. Jude Children's Research Hospital
Memphis, TN

Sandra C. Hennessy, PharmD, CNSC, BCNSP
Clinical Pharmacy Specialist
Floating Hospital for Children at Tufts Medical Center
Boston, MA

Jonathan B. Hjelm, PharmD, BCPS, BCNSP, CGP
Director of Home Infusion Therapy
Banner Home Care
Gilbert, AZ

Susanna Huh, MD, MPH
Assistant Professor of Pediatrics, Harvard Medical School
Associate Director, Center for Nutrition, Boston Children's Hospital
Boston, MA

Doron Kahana, MD, CPNS
Medical Director
Center for Digestive Health and Nutritional Excellence
Torrance, CA

Ajay Kaul, MD
Professor of Clinical Pediatrics
Cincinatti Children's Hospital Medical Center
Cincinnati, OH

Donald F. Kirby, MD, FACP, FACN, FACG, AGAF, CNSC, CPNS
Director, Center for Human Nutrition
Cleveland Clinic
Cleveland, OH

Angela Kirkwood, RN, BSN, IBCLC, RLC
Lactation Clinician
Children's Hospital of Pittsburgh of UPMC and Children's Hospital of Pittsburgh General Academic Pediatric Primary Care Center
Pittsburgh, PA

Kimberly A. Klotz, RN, MSN, CRNI
Care Coordinator
Intestinal Care Center, Cincinnati Children's Hospital Medical
Center
Cincinnati, OH

Sue Konek, MA, RD, CSP, CNSC, FAND
Director of Clinical Nutrition
The Children's Hospital of Philadelphia
Philadelphia, PA

Joel Lim, MD
Associate Professor of Pediatrics
Children's Mercy Hospital, University of Missouri-Kansas City
School of Medicine
Kansas City, MO

Sheela N. Magge, MD, MSCE
Associate Professor of Pediatrics
Children's National Health System
Washington, DC

Allison Mallowe, MA, RD, LDN
Clinical Dietitian
The Children's Hospital of Philadelphia
Philadelphia, PA

Valerie Marchand, MD
Assistant Professor
Sainte-Justine UHC, University of Montreal
Montreal, Quebec, Canada

Melissa Meredith, MS, RD, LDN
Clinical Dietitian
Le Bonheur Children's Hospital
Memphis, TN

Cynthia Miller, RD, LDN
Clinical Dietitian
Children's Hospital of Pittsburgh
Pittsburgh, PA

Biren P. Modi, MD
Staff Surgeon, Boston Children's Hospital
Instructor in Surgery, Harvard Medical School
Boston, MA

Linda Muir, MD
Chief, Pediatric Gastroenterology
Oregon Health and Science University
Portland, OR

Joyce L. Owens, MS, RD, CD, CNSC
Clinical Dietitian Specialist
Medical College of Wisconsin/Children's Hospital of Wisconsin
Milwaukee, WI

Tavis Piattoly, MS, RD, LDN
Co-owner, My Sports Dietitian
Sports Dietitian, Tulane University/FFPLA Trust at Tulane
Institute of Sports Medicine and Fairchild Sports Performance
and Traction Center for Sports Excellence
New Orleans, LA

Megan Platz Reece, RD, CNSC
Kennett Square, PA

Barbara B. Robinson, MPH, RD, CNSC
Associate Professor, Johnson & Wales University
Adjunct Clinical Teaching Associate, Alpert Medical School of
Brown University
Clinical Nutrition Specialist, Hasbro Children's Hospital
Providence, RI

Jill Rockwell, RD, CSP, LD, CNSC
Clinical Dietitian
Children's Health Children's Medical Center Dallas
Dallas, TX

Carol Rollins, MS, RD, PharmD, CNSC, BCNSP, FASPEN
Coordinator, Nutrition Support Team, The University of
Arizona Medical Center
Clinical Professor, The University of Arizona College of
Pharmacy
Tucson, AZ

Denise Baird Schwartz, MS, RD, CNSC, FADA, FAND, FASPEN
Nutrition Support Coordinator
Providence Saint Joseph Medical Center
Burbank, CA

Laura Serke, RD, LD, IBCLC
NICU and Women's Care Dietitian
University of Louisville Hospital
Louisville, KY

Mary K. Sharrett, MS, RD, CNSC, LD
Clinical Dietitian
Nationwide Children's Hospital
Columbus, OH

Jonathan M. Spergel, MD, PhD
Professor of Pediatrics, The Children's Hospital of Philadelphia
Chief, Allergy Section, Perelman School of Medicine at
University of Pennsylvania
Philadelphia, PA

Brian Strang, PharmD, BCNSP, CNSC, CGP, BCPS, FASCP
Clinical Pharmacist
Tucson Medical Center
Tucson, AZ

Jill Taliaferro, RD, CNSC
Clinical Dietitian
ThriveRX Home Infusion
Attleboro, MA

Tina Tan, MS, CCC-SLP, BCS-S
Speech Language Pathologist
New York University Langone Medical Center
New York, NY

Kelly A. Tappenden, PhD, RD, FASPEN
Human Nutrition Endowed Professor
University of Illinois at Urbana-Champaign
Urbana, IL

Brandis Thornton, MS, RD, LD, CSP
Quality Improvement Service Line Coordinator
Nationwide Children's Hospital
Columbus, OH

Foreword

I am delighted to write the foreword for the second edition of *The A.S.P.E.N. Pediatric Nutrition Support Core Curriculum*. The first edition was published in 2010-- an outgrowth of the pediatric section concept that Russ Merritt, MD, PhD, Bill Byrne, MD, Walter Faubion, RN, and I started in the early 1980s. We recognized early on the need for programmatic recognition within A.S.P.E.N. of the special needs of infants and children. Dr Mark Corkins and his associate editors have met that need., representing the many disciplines that A.S.P.E.N. serves, and all having contributed to the evolution of pediatric nutrition science.

The first edition of the Pediatric Nutrition Support Core Curriculum has been well received, having been through several printings! Now, five years later, Dr Corkins and his able editorial staff have carefully updated the art and science of pediatric nutrition support in a second edition using the same multidisciplinary approach that has been the hallmark of success of the A.S.P.E.N. model. The format has been shaped by A.S.P.E.N.'s Standards of Practice, Clinical Guidelines, and interdisciplinary nutrition support competencies. In addition to providing a practical resource containing the core science of pediatric nutrition principles, it is designed to serve as (1) a companion resource to the *A.S.P.E.N. Adult Nutrition Support Core Curriculum, 2nd Edition;* (2) as an educational resource for those preparing for the specialization certification examination in nutrition support; (3) a valuable clinical resource for the generalist; and (4) an interdisciplinary document that recognizes both the common body of knowledge and the unique skills that each member of the multidisciplinary team possesses.

A wide range of specialties require a working knowledge of pediatric nutrition and form our target audience: dietetics, nursing, pharmacy, medicine, gastroenterology, surgery, and pediatrics. In addition to the expected comprehensive treatment of the basics of developmental physiology of the digestive process and the nutrition requirements of various organ systems, chapters include Evaluation and Monitoring, Nutrition Access, Obesity and Metabolic Disorders, Use of Fad and Popular Diets, Sports Nutrition, Implementation of the Plan, and Ethical Issues in the Provision of Nutrition. Each chapter contains evidence-based background information emphasizing core science, intended for the professional who already possesses a basic understanding of the principles of food biochemistry and nutrition in wellness and disease. The layout of each chapter includes a table of contents, learning objectives, and a concluding set of self-assessment questions to test the reader's understanding of the subject matter.

The second edition reflects new guidelines that have evolved in various disciplines, and benefits from a new formal definition of malnutrition, along with closure of several gaps pointed out by clinicians and reviewers. The flow of information has improved with two Nutritional Assessment chapters becoming one. And for the first time in A.S.P.E.N.'s publication history, electronic components have been added to include expository podcasts. Video content is also a click away for more effective presentation of vascular access issues, such as central venous catheter insertion and peripherally inserted central catheter placement.

It is my hope and expectation that this book will provide an effective learning experience and referenced resource for all health professionals caring for infants and children, leading to improved patient care.

John R. Wesley, MD, FACS, FAAP, FASPEN
Adjunct Professor of Surgery
Ann & Robert H. Lurie
Children's Hospital
Feinberg School of Medicine
Northwestern University

Preface

The first edition of *The A.S.P.E.N. Pediatric Nutrition Support Core Curriculum* was a labor of love. The editor group had a vision of how the book would flow and what it would cover. Since its publication in 2009, the editor team has been continuously pleased with how well the first edition has been received. The text is used in classrooms around the world to teach the basics of pediatric nutrition support, serves as a valuable resource to practicing clinicians, and is a popular study tool for individuals sitting for the Certified Nutrition Support Clinician exam administered by the NBNSC.

Then before I knew it, five years passed and it was time to think about updating the text for a second edition. This second edition provides valuable updates in the field of pediatric clinical nutrition, and includes research and information from newer published studies and clinical guidelines, particularly a new definition for pediatric malnutrition.

The editors learned a lot during the creation of the first edition to be able to better equip this updated text with the information readers care the most about. As a result, we expanded coverage in some areas and condensed others. Even as we prepared this second edition, I and the associate editors have made notes on ideas for potential improvements for the future.

I would also like to point out a new feature in this edition. For the first time in A.S.P.E.N.'s book publication history, we are offering digital components to accompany the text. Look for podcasts and video content in key chapters to expand your knowledge even more. These new features make for the perfect complement to classroom lectures and training.

This book is designed to start with the basic nutrition physiology before progressing through the principles for nutrition in specific disease states. It ends with the "nuts and bolts" for daily care. This curriculum is not intended to provide in-depth coverage of neonatal nutrition, although some of this is covered in the context of the physiology of development. This book is not designed to be exhaustive in its coverage of nutrition in the various disease states, but is rather meant to be the pediatric "core" curriculum—to be a disease-specific specialist will require study beyond this starting point. It is my hope that this book helps to create a firm foundation of pediatric nutrition support principles that anyone can build on in any way they wish.

Mark R. Corkins, MD, CNSP, SPR, FAAP
Editor-in-Chief

Acknowledgments & Dedication

Pulling together a text such as *The A.S.P.E.N. Pediatric Nutrition Support Core Curriculum, 2nd Edition* is team effort. I have to thank the associate editors, Jane Balint, Elizabeth Bobo, Steve Plogsted, and Jane Anne Yaworski, for returning contribute to the second edition. The job of updating the *Curriculum* for its second edition was a tremendous undertaking, requiring hours upon hours of dedication. Thank you all for volunteering your time to the pursuit of this revision and balancing this work in with your countless other obligations to family, careers, and other activities.

Thank you to the 87 authors who revised the text for the second edition, as well as to the authors of the first edition upon whose work this edition was built. Thank you to the 58 peer reviewers who contributed their expertise to ensure that this publication and the data contained within are as scientifically sound as possible. And of course we couldn't have done it without Jennifer Kuhn, Andrea Powers, and Megan White, A.S.P.E.N.'s publications staff.

This book is dedicated to all of the folks who taught me through the years—my mentors and faculty at every level, the nurses, pharmacists, and dietitians I worked with, and especially the patients. Last and most important, I have to dedicate this to the coauthor of my life, Kelly Green Corkins, who loaned me to A.S.P.E.N. for over a year to work on this revision.

Mark R. Corkins, MD, CNSP, SPR, FAAP
Editor-in-Chief

INTRODUCTORY AND BASIC PHYSIOLOGY

Mechanics of Nutrient Intake

Mark R. Corkins, MD, CNSP, SPR, FAAP; **Carol G. McKown,** DDS, MS, PC; and **Memorie M. Gosa,** PhD, CCC-SLP, BCS-S

CONTENTS

Learning Objectives

1. Understand how societal and behavioral influences guide food consumption.
2. Identify the psychological, mechanical, biochemical, and hormonal inputs that determine appetite and intake.
3. Describe the developmental stages in deglutition and corresponding changes in appropriate feedings in children.

Background

This chapter is a portion of a curriculum for nutrition in the pediatric age group. Thus, by necessity, it focuses on the biological and physiological needs of pediatric patients. Unlike other areas of medicine directed by genetic programming, a great deal of emotions and memories are associated with nutrition right from the start. The original source of nutrition is food, yet food is so much more than nutrition. It is symbolic, from the stalk of wheat in the A.S.P.E.N. logo to the traditional birthday cake. Marion Winkler, in her 2007 A.S.P.E.N. presidential address, related the story of the foods her mother requested when dying from cancer. Winkler realized that her requests were about more than just food, stating "It was always about the nostalgic stories that surrounded the food, the memories, the social aspects, and the companionship of the sharing of meals."[1]

Appetite

When we begin to explore the desire to eat, we realize that appetite has a cultural aspect.[2] Part of this derives from the environment; certain foods are more available in different geographic regions, and one culture's delicacy may be unacceptable in another. Children's memories and associations will thus influence their intake.[3] Also, human beings will eat some foods just because they taste good. The reward of taste stimulates feeding even in the absence of a true energy deficit.[4]

Critical periods of infant development hinge upon exposure to new tastes and textures. Genetic input affects the sense of taste itself, including the strength of response to sweet, salty, bitter, and sour.[5] Studies show that breastfed infants have greater willingness to try new tastes,[2,6] possibly because of their exposure to various flavors in breast milk. Early exposure to tastes determines taste and food preferences before a child develops neophobia.[2] Neophobia is the developmental stage at 18 months to 2 years of age when children resist trying new foods.[2,5] The more a child is exposed to a taste, the more likely he or she will accept it as a preferred taste.[5,6] Studies indicate that it may take 5–10 exposures before a food becomes an accepted taste.[6] Also, there appears to be a critical period for beginning solid foods, due to their texture, which is before 10 months of age. Northstone et al[7] reported on long-term feeding problems related to acceptance of the taste and texture of foods. Feeding difficulties identified by 9360 parents were found to occur more often among children for whom solid foods were delayed until after 10 months of age.[7]

Biological preferences are also altered by modeling that children observe in their parents and peers.[2,5] Eating with others influences the feeding behaviors and the food selections that children ultimately develop.[6]

Appetite control is centered in the hypothalamus of the brain and integrates information from multiple sources.[4,8] The general level of appetite is influenced by the amount of leptin, a hormone produced by the body's adipose tissue.[4,9] The liver also sends appetite-influencing signals to the brain, primarily through the energy products fat and glucose and the level of adenosine triphosphate in the liver cells.[8] The insulin level produced by the pancreas in response to serum glucose levels influences the general appetite level as well.[4,8] Leptin and insulin suppress inhibition, or drive the appetite, via the hypothalamus.[10]

The first stage in appetite is the cephalic phase, which is a biological response to feeding cues. This concept was first presented by Ivan Pavlov. Pavlov demonstrated that dogs could be conditioned to salivate at the ringing of a bell once they developed an association between the sound and feedings.[11] A variety of studies have shown that visual, olfactory, gustatory, tactile, and auditory inputs stimulate processes in the salivary glands, gastrointestinal tract, pancreas, and cardiovascular and renal systems.[12] These responses are quick and prepare the body to digest and absorb the anticipated meal.[12] The rest of the responses from the stomach and small intestine tend to decrease appetite.[9]

Following the cephalic phase, the appetite level is modified by inputs from the enteric nervous system (ie, from chemical and stretch receptors in the gastrointestinal tract) and hormonal and metabolic signals.[9] During the gastric phase, the brain receives signals concerning the volume of food ingested and data about its nutrient content.[9] Endocrine cells in the stomach produce ghrelin that stimulates appetite[4]; ghrelin levels are high when the stomach is empty and fall after eating.[4,10] Emptying of the stomach also influences the neural control of appetite with gastric distention signaling via the vagus nerve for appetite to decrease.[10]

The intestinal phase is communicated by a wide variety of signaling peptides that are released into the circulation. These peptides act to decrease appetite and are released in proportion to the amount of various nutrients ingested.[4] These include peptide YY, glucagon-like peptide 1, oxyntomodulin, cholecystokinin, and pancreatic polypeptide.[4] A variety of other peptides exist that may also influence appetite, but confirmatory studies are needed.

The hypothalamus integrates all these signals to regulate appetite. The heightened appetite drive that occurs in pediatric patients to increase the caloric intake for growth is not well understood. This drive may derive from programming within the hypothalamus itself or from signals indicating increased nutrient needs due to growth.

Mastication/Dentition

An important part of digestion is the initial homogenization of food that takes place in the mouth. Mastication, or the act of chewing, depends on the teeth to make foods a uniform consistency. Human beings are born toothless, which necessitates a reliance on liquid feedings. The muscles used in mastication are the temporalis, the masseter, and the medial and lateral pterygoids. The trigeminal nerve is the primary nerve involved in mastication. The act of chewing involves 2 sets of teeth, the anterior teeth (incisors and canines) and the posterior teeth (premolars and molars). The anatomy of the incisors and canines with their single cusps and their anterior position in the mouth allow them to tear food. The anatomy of the premolars and molars with multiple cusps and their posterior position in the mouth allow them to grind and chew food, preparing it for swallowing.[13]

The primary dentition, or development and eruption of teeth, consists of 20 teeth, all of which begin development at 13–20 weeks in utero. Teething, the act of tooth eruption, may cause infants malaise, with increased drooling plus stomach or bowel changes, but it is not associated with fevers. The mandibular central incisors are the first teeth to erupt at ages 6–10 months. The next teeth to erupt are the maxillary central incisors between ages 8 and 12 months. Over the next 2 years the other primary teeth come in as shown in Table 1-1.

Table 1-1. Primary Teeth by Age of Eruption

PRIMARY TEETH	AGE OF ERUPTION
Mandibular central incisors	6–10 mo
Maxillary central incisors	8–12 mo
Maxillary lateral incisors	9–13 mo
Mandibular lateral incisors	10–16 mo
Maxillary first molars	13–19 mo
Mandibular first molars	14–18 mo
Maxillary canines	16–22 mo
Mandibular canines	17–23 mo
Second molars	2–3 y

The primary dentition stays intact until ages 5–7 years when the permanent dentition begins to erupt. As the root end of the permanent tooth develops in the bone, it causes the crown of the tooth to emerge, which resorbs the root of the primary tooth leaving only the crown. The crown of the primary tooth is then shed, allowing the permanent tooth to erupt. The mandibular central incisors and mandibular and maxillary first molars are the first permanent teeth to erupt between ages 6 and 7 years. Their hard tissue formation begins shortly after birth. The subsequent progression of permanent tooth acquisition is shown in Table 1-2.

Table 1-2. Permanent Teeth by Age of Eruption

PERMANENT TEETH	AGE OF ERUPTION
Mandibular central incisors	6–7 y
Mandibular first molars	6–7 y
Maxillary first molars	6–7 y
Maxillary central incisors	7–8 y
Mandibular lateral incisors	7–8 y
Maxillary lateral incisors	8–9 y
Mandibular canines	9–10 y
Maxillary premolars	10–11 y
Mandibular premolars	10–12 y
Maxillary second premolars	10–12 y
Mandibular second premolars	11–12 y
Maxillary canines	11–12 y

The permanent third molars, or wisdom teeth, are the most commonly missing teeth and normally erupt between ages 17 and 21 years.[14]

Feeding Development

Swallowing

The process of swallowing is traditionally divided into 3 distinct physiological phases: the oral phase, the pharyngeal phase, and the esophageal phase. Each phase depends on the coordination of functional anatomy and neurophysiology of the muscles for feeding and respiration.

The oral phase consists of the preparatory stage and the transit stage with movement of food to the back of the mouth. Infants take liquids into the mouth by either breast or bottle and the liquids are deposited directly on the back third of the tongue. In infancy, this is an involuntary action as the infant reflexively suckles. As the infant grows and matures, the depository position of the liquid and food boluses changes to a more anterior position to allow for greater manipulation of the foods with greater texture. At this point, the oral preparatory stage transitions to a volitional process. The eruption of teeth and the downward forward growth of the mandible facilitate the transition from a purely liquid diet to a diet that includes purees and solids. Later in infant feeding development, the lips are used to assist with eating during the oral phase. Skills such as taking purees off a spoon and drinking through a straw will occur in the last half of the first year.[15,16]

The pharyngeal phase consists of the liquid or food moving through the pharynx towards esophagus. The soft palate and uvula lift so that liquid or food will not pass into the nasopharynx. The larynx closes by muscle contractions and the retroflexion of the epiglottis over the entrance to the larynx. Respiration ceases briefly (deglutition apnea) and, after the food has started its descent, expiration then inspiration will occur. In the infant, the swallow can occur at any part of the respiratory cycle, and it is variable.[17] The pharyngeal phase is involuntary, but the speed and strength of muscular action in this phase can be influenced by sensory characteristics of the bolus.

The esophageal phase is also involuntary but can be influenced by bolus characteristics such as volume. The upper esophageal sphincter opens by a combination of muscle relaxation and biomechanical forces (through hyolaryngeal excursion) so that the food can enter the esophagus in the beginning of the esophageal phase. Food travels to the stomach by esophageal peristalsis. Successful swallowing depends on all of these structures, muscles, and neurological and respiratory systems working in coordinated millisecond timing.[18,19] Anatomical or physiological abnormalities within these systems will affect feeding effectiveness and efficiency. Please see Figure 1-1 for an illustration of typical swallow sequencing in a bottle-feeding infant.

Feeding Skills in the First Year

The typical newborn is ready to feed shortly after birth. The reflexive root allows the infant to open the mouth, turn toward the food source, latch, and begin to suck. The newborn will suck, swallow, and breathe in a rhythmic sequence. This pattern is established through early reflexes and behaviors

Figure 1-1. Normal Swallow Sequence of Bottle Feeding Infant

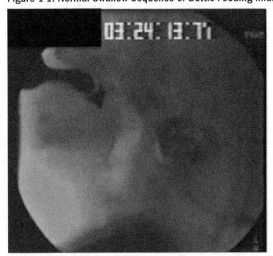

Oral Preparatory Stage
Bolus material is sucked from bottle
Bolus is collected on posterior 1/3 of tongue

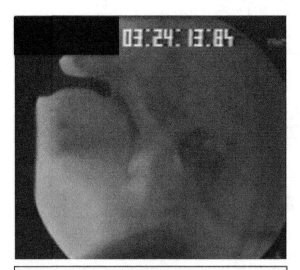

Oral Transit Stage
- Bolus is moved through the oral cavity towards the pharynx

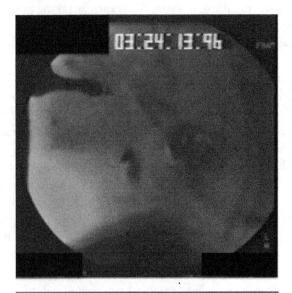

Pharyngeal Phase
Bolus is moved through the pharynx by sequential, peristaltic-like contraction of the superior, middle, and inferior pharyngeal constrictors
Larynx closes to prevent airway compromise

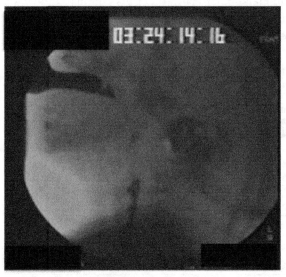

Esophageal Phase
- Upper esophageal sphincter is opened through relaxation of the cricopharyngeus and biomechanical forces
- Fluid is moved through esophagus towards the stomach via peristalsis

that develop in utero and improves by the third day of life.[20] The rooting reflex is among the most important and is activated by a light touch on or near the infant's mouth. Once latched onto the nipple, the infant's tongue and jaw work together to stroke the nipple and express milk.[21] The infant will feed in a burst-pause pattern that is usually quite regular, with the bursts being suck-swallow-and-breathe cycles and the pauses being brief and regular rest periods. Bursts of 8 sucks or more are seen in the typical newborn.[22] Sensing changes in the nipple, the infant can vary the suck pressure quite easily to control the flow of milk. During early infancy, the infant will increase the rate of expression per minute with age. Studies have varied on the changes in the volume of expression; however, it ranges from 0.26 to 0.4 mL per suck.[23,24] In a typical newborn, one suck-swallow-breathe cycle including all 3 phases lasts approximately 1 second.[23] As the infant's oromotor skills develop, the increase in control and efficiency of intake allows taking in more milk in less time.

Pacifier sucking differs from sucking for nutritional intake. In pacifier sucking (nonnutritive sucking), the suck rate is twice as fast as nutritive sucking.[22] The infant only has to balance breathing and swallowing when a critical volume of saliva has been collected to trigger a pharyngeal swallow response. Therefore, infants participating in nonnutritive sucking swallow with significantly less frequency as compared to swallowing frequency during nutritive sucking. This also means that infants sucking on a pacifier do not have to tolerate a swallow apnea with every suck, thus explaining why many nonfeeding infants can nonnutritively suck but have difficulty when a nipple introduces liquid.

Readiness for transitioning to spoon feeding has been debated, and recommendations have changed over the years. Brain growth, neural development, and anatomical changes in the upper oropharynx support development of a larger variety of oromotor movements. The tongue no longer moves in a forward-backward patterned response due to the expansion of the oral cavity with forward and downward growth of the mandible, reabsorption of fat pads, and eruption of primary teeth. The infant's tongue is able to stay in the mouth, not thrust out, and move side to side in response to stimulation, such as mouthing his or her fingers or hand. The infant no longer has a single oral response of suck-swallow-breathe or bursts of sucking without swallowing as in pacifier sucking. At 5–6 months of age an infant typically has some sitting balance and wants to feed in an upright position. The infant can anticipate the food and will open his or her mouth for the spoon. The lips will close on the spoon

to pull the food off.[25] The food is moved all around in the mouth, not strictly kept over the center of the tongue for propulsion back for swallowing. The tongue and the jaw no longer work only as a single unit. The gag is diminished to allow for nonliquids and will continue to be modulated as the experience with textures continues.[26] The critical period for introducing new tastes to promote an expansion in the flavors of food accepted by the infant is also between 4 and 6 months of age. It coordinates with the physiological changes in the infant that allow for greater variety of intake.[27]

When infants begin to pick up objects, at age 6–7 months, they naturally put them into their mouths. As the tongue can move in multiple directions and mouth objects, the parent introduces meltable solids and foods with greater texture (lumps) for the infant to handle. In late infancy, the infant begins to "munch" or use an up-down motion of the jaw to begin mastication of foods. These prechewing skills increase in efficiency with age.[28] Soft solid foods are then provided with small single bite-size pieces for the infant to move around in the mouth and eventually swallow. This feeding has less rhythm compared to nutritive sucking. The movements are volitional and no longer directed by reflex. Early reflexes are fading at 4–8 months and volitional patterns of oromotor skills are emerging.[29] The critical period for texture advancement coincides with the anatomical and physiological changes occurring between 6 and 7 months of age.[27]

By 9 months of age, with the development of the fine motor skills of reach, grasp, and release, self-feeding is established. Now the infant is skillful at watching others, communicating interests in foods, and eating. Cup and straw drinking begin as the infant is guided by a parent. The infant will not gum the cup, but opens his or her mouth to accept liquids from the cup that is guided by the parent. At this age, both breastfeeding and bottle-feeding begin to diminish as the infant takes in a greater proportion of liquids by cup and solids by spoon or hand.[26] Opportunities for oral exploration of various tastes and textures during these critical periods of feeding development are necessary to ensure appropriate feeding behavior. Please see Figure 1-2 for an outline summary of feeding development during the first year of life.[30]

Problems in Infant Feeding Skills
Neurological disorders, prematurity and its resulting sequelae, craniofacial anomalies, gastrointestinal disorders/diseases, aerodigestive anomalies, and pulmonary disorders/diseases may result in at least transient dysphagia in pediatric populations.[31] Dysphagia describes any difficulty

Figure 1-2. Typical Feeding Development in the First 12 Months of Life

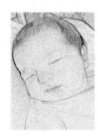

0-4 Months of Age
- Exclusive bottle/breast feeding
- Reflexive suckling pattern dominates intake of fluid from breast or bottle
- Newborns eat on demand every 1.5-2 hours
- 1-4 months of age, baby eats on demand every 2-3 hours

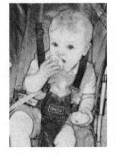

4-6 Months of Age
- Continue bottle or breast feeding on demand, usually every 3-4 hours
- Transitions from reflexive suckling to learned, mature sucking pattern between 4-6 months of age
- Introduction of baby cereal from a spoon when baby has:
  - Steady head control
  - Sits independently for 10-30 seconds
- Typical for baby to use suckling motion on spoon until they learn to use tongue and lips to clean bolus from spoon and swallow without losing the bolus out of the front of the mouth
- Learning to spoon feed is messy- it is not necessary or desirable to clean baby's mouth after every bite or to scoop the food from around the mouth and re-feed it to baby

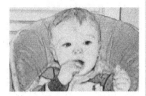

6-9 Months of Age
- Continue bottle or breast feeding on demand, usually every 3.5-4 hours
- Introduction of baby food- Stage 1 as baby uses mature spoon feeding skills
- Transition to Stage 2 foods around 8 months
- Transition to soft, mashed table foods at 9 months
- Baby begins hand to mouth play at ~6 months, sits independently for more than 3-5 minutes at 6-7 months, and has stable head control with no head bobbing by 6-7 months

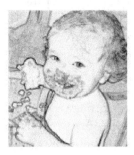

9-11 Months of Age
- Continue bottle or breast feeding on demand, usually every 4-6 hours
- Introduction of foods for oral play at 9 months of age; foods should be almost impossible for baby to bite through and should be administered with strict supervision
- Introduction of foods that dissolve easily at 10 months of age
- Introduction of foods that are easily chewed at 11 months of age
- Baby begins munching and moving food from side to side in mouth around 9 months of age as they are learning a mature chewing pattern

11-12 Months of Age
- Continue bottle or breast feeding on demand, usually every 6-8 hours
- Introduction of single ingredient soft foods at 11 months (like avocado)
- Introduction of multiple ingredient soft foods & Stage 3 foods at 12 months (like Mac & Cheese)
- Baby's chewing skills advance to a circular pattern, tongue actively moves food from side to side in mouth

moving liquid or food from the mouth to the stomach. This definition includes difficulty with oral preparation such as transferring liquid from a bottle to the mouth or chewing food sufficiently for safe pharyngeal transit. Craniofacial anomalies are congenital and may affect the structures and muscles of feeding and swallowing, as well as the physiolog-ical timing and efficiency of feeding, and lead to poor oral intake. In the extreme, dysphagia can be seen. Classically, cranial nerve abnormalities, such as those seen in Mobius syndrome, cause dysphagia. Neurodevelopmental problems in infants, such as muscle tone abnormalities, persistence of early reflexes, or abnormal oral reflexes, can also lead to dysphagia.[32] Infants with hypotonia (as may be seen in infants with Down's syndrome) may have significant oromotor dysfunction, dysphagia, and aspiration.[33] Even infants with normal development can have difficulty feeding if they have abnormal respirations, cardiac disorders, or gastroesophageal reflux. They may tire easily and self-limit their intake, or they may have difficulty with the suck-swallow-breathe sequence and self-limit due to aspiration, which is passage of liquid or solids into the airway during swallowing.[34]

Premature infants frequently have feeding difficulties because of respiratory problems, neurodevelopmental problems, or both. Early birth does not allow for the typical developmental sequence of oral skills. Poor growth, especially of the youngest gestational age infants, may not allow for maturation of neural pathways. Many premature infants have difficulty with "newborn" skills when they are at a "term-adjusted age" and may have significant feeding problems. Premature infants with bronchopulmonary dysplasia may have abnormal development of suck patterns.[35] Some infants, who had significant limitations in oral feeding attempts due to a high level of illness or respiratory disorders, can display aversion to attempts at oral feeding. In others, a persistent rapid breathing rate can interfere with establishing an efficient feeding rhythm. Lower gestational ages at birth and higher rates of neonatal morbidity are significantly correlated with longer transitions to full oral feeding in premature infants.[36] More preterm infants have respiratory complications than have neurologic complications in modern neonatal intensive care nurseries due to changes in neonatal medicine in the past 20 years.

Evaluation of the infant who is not feeding appropriately should be done through a multidisciplinary team consisting of a physician, nurse, occupational therapist, speech-language pathologist, dietitian, and/or psychologist trained in and experienced with the aspects of normal and abnormal infant feeding development. The evaluation will include a medical history, developmental history, and a neurological examination as well as an oromotor assessment including feeding or feeding attempt. Pediatric specialists in gastroenterology, neurology, rehabilitation, development, and others may be needed. The evaluation, under the direction of a physician, may include radiologic testing such as a feeding study (modified barium swallow study [MBS] and/or fiberoptic endoscopic evaluation of swallowing [FEES]), esophogram, or studies for reflux or gastric emptying. Neurological studies of the central nervous system may be needed for the diagnosis of neurodevelopmental abnormalities. Studies of respiratory function and sufficiency of ventilation may be needed to provide optimal respiratory support for feeding. It is important to determine the safety of feeding and ensure that the infant is not aspirating as a result of the underlying problems.[37]

Aspiration cannot be accurately diagnosed from bedside assessment. It requires objective evaluation from instrumental assessment. When evaluating for dysphagia, MBS and FEES are both commonly used with pediatric patients. The goal of instrumental assessment is not solely to confirm or deny the presence of dysphagia symptoms such as laryngeal penetration or aspiration, but instead to determine the cause of the symptoms and then identify the most appropriate treatment strategies to provide the safest and least invasive method of caloric intake for infants and children. When choosing which instrumental assessment to provide, the practitioner must consider the differences between the MBS and the FEES and hypothesize which stage of the swallow is the cause of the feeding problems. These considerations help the practitioner decide which test will provide the desired information about the patient's swallowing function.[38,39]

Sometimes, despite extensive evaluations, the etiology of the feeding difficulties is never discovered. In some situations the initiating organic cause may have resolved, but the resulting behavior has become established. Once the cause and extent of poor feeding is understood, a treatment plan can be undertaken to work on oral feedings and/or to provide supplemental feedings for the safety and growth of the infant. Supplemental feedings can consist of nasogastric or feedings into the jejunum. Such treatment plans should be drafted with the parents and a team of medical and therapy providers.

Feeding Skills in the Second Year

Toddlers typically need to expand their acceptance of foods and master self-feeding, including biting and chewing. This is a tall order as they are also developing independence and have the ability to make choices and affect their environment. The majority of toddlers (from 1 to 3 years of age) enter this stage eating "table foods." They have successfully transitioned to some of the foods their families eat by their first birthday.[40] Due to their immature oromotor skills, toddlers need their foods diced, chopped, or cut into small bite-sized pieces. This continues until their ability to bite a single mouthful of food becomes skillful. Only then can a parent rely on the toddler not to choke. During this period, chewing improves and changes from the up-down munching motion to the rotary chewing that allows the toddler to grind meat fibers by age 3 years. The toddler will increase chewing efficiency to 5 years of age.[41] Through careful trial and error, the parents will supply the toddler with small bites of their own foods and expand the toddler's diet. Meltable solids will be exchanged for nonmeltable solids that require biting off and chewing as the parent sees the child is ready for the single bite. Gradually, the diet will reach that of the preschooler.

The toddler may initially allow the parent to assist with providing bites, but this will diminish, and by 18 months, the child will insist on exclusive self-feeding. The use of utensils can start as early as 15 months but is generally not perfected until much later. Initially, sticky foods will be given to help with self-spoon feeding; later the child will learn to spear with a fork as well, particularly soft foods. Eating with his or her fingers to assist the utensil feeding will continue until the preschool age. Also, the child can now drink independently from an open cup.[26]

Behavior during mealtimes can be challenging as the toddler will seek to exert control over this environment as well. How the parents model and reinforce appropriate behavior to diminish unwanted behavior can affect not only eating but also sleeping habits and play interactions. Routine meals and snacks that are eaten with the child are the best times to teach appropriate mealtime behavior. As the toddler's ability to understand language increases, the parents need to demonstrate and explain appropriate behavior at mealtimes. Praise for sitting and eating with the family is necessary, as well as repetitive teaching of appropriate behaviors. Watching the toddler's cues is important, as throwing or playing with food may signal that the child is full. Ellyn Satter explains mealtime in a series of roles for parents and children.[42] She suggests that it is the child's job to decide what and how much to eat, and the parent's job is to decide when to eat and what to offer the child. Problems in mealtime behavior can often be traced back to crossing roles between parents and children. This is illustrated when the parent tries to force the child to eat beyond when he or she is finished or when the child tries to eat throughout the day (grazing) instead of eating when the parent offers food at a structured meal or snack time.[42] As with all behaviors, routine and consistency will teach both the easy as well as the difficult feeder.

Problems With the Toddler Feeder

Problems that affected an infant's feeding may still be present in toddlerhood. Problems such as anatomical anomalies, neurodevelopmental problems, gastrointestinal difficulties, and cardiorespiratory concerns require ongoing medical and therapeutic intervention. However, even toddlers who had normal feeding skills in their first year may have new behaviors affecting feedings or an aversion to advancing to a variety of flavors and textures. In one population study, parents described 20% of toddlers as having feeding problems.[43] At times a sentinel event can be recalled ("he had his tonsils out and couldn't eat"); other times, subtle problems with advancing textures in infancy were present but not well recognized. Still other issues include behavioral problems that become more evident at this age, such as short attention span, oppositionality, or slow learning. Sometimes the organic process that caused a feeding problem will resolve but the inappropriate feeding behavior persists.

Evaluating new feeding problems in the toddler begins with a thorough feeding history of who feeds the child and what, when, where, how, and how much he or she is fed. Often through this history, the initial therapeutic interventions can be determined. Review of the anthropometric measures since birth will identify growth failure, and a physical examination will determine the need for additional cardiac, respiratory, or gastrointestinal evaluation. The neurological and developmental examination can determine the need for feeding studies or further psychological or developmental evaluation.

Most therapeutic plans include a mealtime routine and appropriate modeling of eating behavior by parents and caregivers. Parents and practitioners need to keep in mind that "picky eating" can be part of typical feeding development. As toddlers strive for autonomy and independence between 24 and 36 months of age, their behaviors in relation to new foods may become increasingly frustrating to parents.[44] Choosing a variety of nutritious foods to serve at meals and as snacks will expand the feeding experience of the toddler and decrease pickiness with multiple offerings of new foods.[44–47] It is important to ascertain the toddler's baseline abilities with oromotor function, fine motor development, and cognitive function to determine the level at which to begin. Identification of the problem or problems as well as the parents' goals for feeding will direct the therapist's plans, dietary plans, and home intervention. For toddlers with medical comorbidities, weight loss, worsening feeding problems, or significant family stress, referral to a multidisciplinary feeding team can be helpful. The toddler with feeding problems may need such a team, including a psychologist, occupational and speech therapists, and dietitian, to provide behavioral plans, therapy, and dietary advice.

Dysphagia

As previously discussed, the definition of dysphagia includes any difficulty in moving liquid or food from the mouth to the stomach, and it includes difficulties with oral preparation such as sucking fluid from a bottle into the oral cavity or chewing textured foods to appropriate consistencies for safe swallowing. In the infant and young child, feeding proceeds in the developmental sequence mentioned, and abnormalities in feeding abilities need to be evaluated for their underlying physiologic cause. This diagnosis is made by history, a neurological examination by a physician, and a feeding observation. MBS or FEES, in which the infant or child is fed during video fluoroscopy or endoscopy observation, can identify problems of delayed swallow response, poor coordination for swallow, pharyngeal stasis, nasopharyngeal reflux, laryngeal penetration, or aspiration. During a swallowing study, the infant or child is fed liquids, purees, or solids laced with barium so that the ingested substance is visible under video fluoroscopy. During endoscopy, liquids, purees, or solids are colored with food dye so that the ingested substance is distinguishable from the soft tissue of the pharynx. At some institutions, swallowing studies can be done with pulse oximetry to see the effect of respiratory effort or deglutition apnea on the total saturation of oxygen. The real-time images are observed by the feeding/swallowing specialist (usually a speech-language pathologist), referring physician, and related specialist (such as the radiologist or otolaryngologist). When a child demonstrates abnormal feeding skills, the feeding plan is modified to avoid liquids or textures that the child is not able to safely eat. Further neurological diagnosis as to the cause of dysphagia should be investigated by the physician when warranted.

Therapeutic plans may include direct interventions to improve swallowing function and/or compensatory strategies to allow for safe oral intake despite deficient feeding skills. Direct interventions typically include combinations of motor, sensory, and behavioral approaches to improve feeding abilities. Therapeutic plans can include

- physical, occupational, and speech therapy to advance skills
- modifications of liquids or foods offered
- selection and/or adaptation of bottles/nipples, cups and utensils for feeding
- positioning assistance to obtain an optimal feeding position to facilitate safe and adequate oral intake
- dietitian adaptation of the diet to meet caloric, nutrition, and volume goals
- nutrition support through gastrostomy feedings
- diagnosis and treatment of gastroesophageal reflux
- medications
- referral to other medical specialists, additional instrumental assessments, or both

The goals of therapy will be to normalize tone and posture, particularly around head control and seating for feeding. Other goals will be to foster feeding development in the typical sequence as determined by the child's level of function and the safety of the feeding. For example, an infant who has had brain damage from meningitis may have dysphagia. Methods that lead to relaxation may need to be used on the infant to decrease hypertonicity and foster normal positioning. This infant may require a feeder seat for good positioning and may need to be offered purees only because liquids are aspirated. This infant may need dietary assistance with increased caloric density to decrease the volume of intake needed by tube feeding, or he or she may need to have small and frequent feedings if large gastrostomy feeding volumes are not tolerable. Once again, a team approach is needed in the feeding care of the infant or child who has dysphagia.[48]

Feeding Teams

Pediatric institutions that form feeding teams draw from the professional expertise at their organizations. With that in mind, each team will determine the problems they feel are appropriate in their setting and for their population. The usual team members include

- the child and his or her parents
- a physician, who may be a developmental pediatrician, gastroenterologist, general pediatrician, or pediatric physiatrist
- a coordinator, who may be in social work, psychology, or nursing
- a child psychologist
- a speech language pathologist and/or occupational therapist
- a dietitian
- a social worker

For the feeding team to be successful, the parents must clearly identify their goals and be willing to make changes and to work with the team members. Each professional must also be willing to work with team members and to support the parents and patient during the process. Setting clear goals with the team and reviewing those goals is an important part of a feeding team program. For example, "Abby" is a young toddler who has an aversion to eating because of severe respiratory problems caused by prematurity. Her respiratory status is significantly improved and she needs only occasional bronchodilators. She is gastrostomy fed and is very sensitive to the rate of feedings. Her mother has cut back on her feedings so Abby is also failing to thrive. The team members have many goals, and progress may vary between them. The family hopes to shorten feeding times and increase Abby's oral feedings so she can eventually stop gastrostomy feedings. These goals are appropriate for the child and the team members; however, they are long-term goals, and the progress is incremental and variable. The parents, with the team's help, determine the daily schedule for feeding and continue in the routine of feedings. The physician and dietitian may work on a short-term goal of improving Abby's weight gain while trying to shorten her feeding times. The therapists may start by improving her ability to stay at the table at mealtime and touch food for short time periods. The dietitian and therapists may use a "chaining" technique to select foods that are similar to foods Abby likes so as to slowly broaden her food choices. At each follow-up visit with the team, the goals are reassessed and the plan of care is revised based on the child's progress.[49] Referral to a feeding team is generally made by the child's primary care provider and reviewed by the coordinator for appropriateness to the team.

Test Your Knowledge Questions

1. Appetite is suppressed by
   A Sensory stimulus before eating
   B. Ghrelin release by the stomach
   C. Intestinal release of glucagon-like peptide 1
   D. Low leptin levels
2. An abnormal swallow contains
   A. Lift of the soft palate and uvula
   B. Continued respirations
   C. Closure of the epiglottis
   D. Opening of the upper esophageal sphincter
3. Chewing that allows the intake of higher texture foods requires
   A. Rotary chewing
   B. Forward-backward patterning
   C. Suck-swallow-breathe cycles
   D. Up-down motion of the jaw

Acknowledgments

The authors would like to acknowledge the contributions to this chapter by Dr. Anna Dusick who was a co-author in the first edition. She later lost a battle with cancer but is not forgotten for her input.

References

1. Winkler MF. American Society for Parenteral and Enteral Nutrition presidential address: food for thought: it's more than nutrition. *J Parenter Enteral Nutr.* 2007;31(4):334–340.
2. Harris G. Development of taste and food preferences in children. *Curr Opin Clin Nutr Metab Care.* 2008;11(3):315–319.
3. Lupton D. *Food, The Body and the Self.* Thousand Oaks, CA: Sage Publications; 1996.
4. Druce M, Bloom SR. The regulation of appetite. *Arch Dis Child.* 2006;91:183–187.
5. Scaglioni S, Salvioni M, Galimberti C. Influence of parental attitudes in the development of children eating behaviour. *Br J Nutr.* 2008;99(suppl 1):S22–S25.
6. Birch LL, Fisher JO. Development of eating behaviors among children and adolescents. *Pediatrics.* 1998;101(3 Pt 2):539–549.
7. Northstone K, Emmett P, Nethersole F. The effect of age of introduction to lumpy solids on foods eaten and reported difficulties at 6 and 15 months. *J Hum Nutr Diet.* 2001;14(1):43–54.
8. Erlanson-Albertsson C. Appetite regulation and energy balance. *Acta Paediatr Suppl.* 2005;94(448):40–41.
9. Blundell JE. The control of appetite: basic concepts and practical implications. *Schweiz Med Wochenschr.* 1999;129(5):182–188.
10. Inui A, Asakawa A, Bowers CY, et al. Ghrelin, appetite, and gastric motility: the emerging role of the stomach as an endocrine organ. *FASEB J.* 2004;18:439–456.
11. Pavlov IP. The centrifugal (efferent) nerves to the gastric glands and the pancreas. In: Thompson WH, ed. *The Work of the Digestive Glands.* Philadelphia, PA: Charles Griffin and Co; 1910:48–59.
12. Mattes RD. Physiologic responses to sensory stimulation by food: nutritional implications. *J Am Diet Assoc.* 1997;97(4):406–413.
13. McDonald RE, Avery DR, Dean JA. *Dentistry for the Child and Adolescent.* 8th ed. St. Louis, MO: Mosby; 2004:176–178.
14. Kronfeld R, Schour I. Chronology of the human dentition. *J Am Dent Assoc.* 1939;26:18–32.
15. Logemann JL. Anatomy and physiology of normal deglutition. In: Logemann JA, ed. *Evaluation and Treatment of Swallowing Disorders.* 2nd ed. Austin, TX: Pro-Ed; 1998:13–52.
16. Morris SE, Klein MD. *Pre-feeding Skills: A Comprehensive Resource for Feeding Development.* 2nd ed. Tucson, AZ: Therapy Skill Builders; 2000.
17. Kelly BN, Huckabee ML, Jones RD, Frampton CMA. The first year of human life: coordinating respiration and nutritive swallowing. *Dysphagia.* 2007;22(1):37–43.
18. Bosma JF. Development of feeding. *Clin Nutr.* 1986;5(5):210–218.
19. Derkay SD, Schechter GL. Anatomy and physiology of pediatric swallowing disorders. *Otolaryngol Clin North Am.* 1998;31(3):397–404.
20. Weber F, Wollridge MW, Baum JD. An ultrasonographic study of the organisation of sucking and swallowing by newborn infants. *Dev Med Child Neurol.* 1986;28(1):19–24.
21. Tamura Y, Horikawa Y, Yoshida S. Co-ordination of tongue movements and peri-oral muscle activities during nutritive sucking. *Dev Med Child Neurol.* 1996;38(6):503–510.
22. Wolff PH. The serial organization of sucking in the young infant. *Pediatrics.* 1968;42(6):943–956.
23. Qureshi MA, Vice FL, Taciak VL, Bosma JF, Gewolb IH. Changes in rhythmic suckle feeding patterns in term in-

fants in the first month of life. *Dev Med Child Neurol.* 2002;44(1):34–39.

24. McGowan JS, Marsh RR, Fowler SM, Levy SE, Stallings VA. Developmental patterns of normal nutritive sucking in infants. *Dev Med Child Neurol.* 1991;33(10):891–897.

25. Ayano R, Tamura F, Ohtsuka Y, Mukai Y. The development of normal feeding and swallowing: Showa University study of the feeding function. *Int J Orofacial Myology.* 2000:26:24–32.

26. Gesell A, Ilg FL. *Feeding Behavior in Infants. A Pediatric Approach to the Mental Hygiene of Early Life.* Philadelphia, PA: J.B. Lippincott Co; 1937.

27. Skuse D. Identification and management of problem eaters. *Arch Dis Childhood.* 1993;69:604–608.

28. Gisel EG. Effect of food texture on the development of chewing of children between six months and two years of age. *Dev Med Child Neurol.* 1991;33(1):69–79.

29. Sheppard JJ, Mysak ED. Ontogeny of infantile oral refluxes and emerging chewing. *Child Dev.* 1984;55(3):831–843.

30. Toomey K, Ross E. Picky eaters vs problem feeders. Sequential oral sensory approach to feeding therapy. Seminar Spring 2007; Naperville, IL.

31. Lefton-Greif MA. Pediatric dysphagia. *Phys Med Rehabil Clin N Am.* 2008;19(4):837–851.

32. Arvedson JC. Dysphagia in pediatric patients with neurologic damage. *Semin Neurol.* 1996;16(4):371–385.

33. Frazier JB, Friedman B. Swallow function in children with Down syndrome: a retrospective study. *Dev Med Child Neurol.* 1996;38(8):695–703.

34. Mercado-Deane MG, Burton EM, Harlow SA, et al. Swallowing dysfunction in infants less than 1 year of age. *Pediatr Radiol.* 2001;31(6):423–428.

35. Gewolb IH, Bosma JF, Taciak VL, Vice FL. Abnormal developmental patterns of suck and swallow rhythms during feeding in preterm infants with bronchopulmonary dysplasia. *Dev Med Child Neurol.* 2001;43(7):454–459.

36. Dodrill P, Donovan T, Cleghorn G, McMahon S, Davies PS. Attainment of early feeding milestones in preterm neonates. *J Perinatol* 2008;28(8):549–555.

37. Arvedson J, Rogers B, Buck G, Smart P, Msall M. Silent aspiration prominent in children with dysphagia. *Int J Pediatr Otorhinolaryngol.* 1994;28(2–3):173–181.

38. Benson J, Lefton-Greif MA. Videofluoroscopy of swallowing in pediatric patients: a component of the total feeding evaluation. In: Tuchman DN, Walter RS, eds. *Diagnosis of Feeding and Swallowing in Infants and Children: Pathophysiology, Diagnosis, and Treatment.* 1st ed. San Diego, CA: Singular Publishing Group; 1994:187–200.

39. Newman LA. Optimal care patterns in pediatric patients with dysphagia. Semin Speech Lang 2000;21(4):281–291.

40. Briefel RR, Reidy K, Karwe V, Jankowski L, Hendricks K. Toddlers' transition to table foods: impact on nutrient intakes and food patterns. *J Am Diet Assoc.* 2004;104(1)(suppl 1):S38–S44.

41. Gisel EG. Chewing cycles in 2- to 8-year-old normal children: a developmental profile. *Am J Occup Ther.* 1988;41(1):40–46.

42. Satter E. *Child of Mine: Feeding With Love and GOOD SENSE.* Boulder, CO: Bull Publishing Company; 2000.

43. Wright CM, Parkinson KN, Shipton D, Drewett RF. How do toddler eating problems relate to their eating behavior, food preferences, and growth? *Pediatrics.* 2007;120(4):e1069–e1075.

44. Carruth BR, Skinner J, Houck K, Moran J, Coletta F, Ott D. The phenomenon of "picky eater": a behavioral marker in eating patterns of toddlers. *J Am Coll Nutr.* 1998;17(2):180–186.

45. Gidding SS, Dennison BA, Birch LL, Daniels SR. Dietary recommendations for children and adolescents: a guide for practitioners. *Pediatrics.* 2006;17(2)544–559.

46. Satter E. *How to Get Your Kid to Eat: But Not Too Much.* Boulder, CO: Bull Publishing Co; 1987.

47. Jana L, Shu J. *Food Fights: Winning the Nutritional Challenges of Parenthood Armed With Insight, Humor, and a Bottle of Ketchup.* Washington, DC: American Academy of Pediatrics; 2008.

48. Dusick AM. Investigation and management of dysphagia. *Semin Pediatr Neurol.* 2003;10(4):255–264.

49. Fraker C, Fishbein M, Cox S, Walbert L. *Food Chaining: The Proven 6-Step Plan to Stop Picky Eating, Solve Feeding Problems, and Expand Your Child's Diet.* New York, NY: Marlowe & Co; 2007.

Test Your Knowledge Answers

1. The correct answer is **C**.
2. The correct answer is **B**.
3. The correct answer is **A**.

2

Gross Digestion Principles: Gastric Grinding and Gastrointestinal Motility

Molly Dienhart, MD; Desale Yacob, MD; and Jane Balint, MD

CONTENTS

Learning Objectives

1. Describe the normal response of the stomach to nutrient intake.
2. Explain the different motor patterns of the small intestine in the fasting and fed states.
3. Predict the response of the intestinal tract to different types of nutrients.
4. Develop management strategies for altered gastrointestinal motility.

Background

Gastrointestinal (GI) motility is necessary for the movement of nutrients from the stomach through the intestinal tract as well as for the breakdown and mixing of these nutrients with digestive enzymes, which in turn allows for digestion and absorption. An elementary understanding of these processes is helpful in planning and managing nutrition support.

The motor activity of the GI tract is regulated by the enteric nervous system (ENS), which consists of 2 nerve plexuses. The myenteric plexus (Auerbach's plexus) lies between the outer longitudinal muscle layer and the inner circular muscle layer. This plexus is key to the motility of the GI tract, including regulation of the normal motor patterns seen in the GI tract described in this chapter. The submucosal plexus (Meissner's plexus), found between the muscularis mucosa and the circular muscle layer, affects absorption, secretion, and blood flow. While the ENS can act independently, it receives input from the parasympathetic nervous system (primarily the vagus nerve), the sympathetic nervous system, and sensory nerves in the intestine, as well as from mast cells, paracrine signals, and endocrine signals. In addition, the ENS has multiple neurotransmitters for signaling, including acetylcholine, norepinephrine, serotonin, vasoactive intestinal peptide, nitric oxide, somatostatin, and tachykinins.[1–4]

Integral to the functioning of the GI tract are the interstitial cells of Cajal (ICC). Two types of these cells exist: those around the myenteric plexus that generate and propagate electrical slow waves (pacemakers), and those between neural fibers and smooth muscle cells providing communication between the two. The ICC help to coordinate peristaltic movement of the GI tract.[5,6] Slow waves have variable frequency in different parts of the GI tract. In the stomach, the slow-wave rhythm is 3 cycles per minute. In the proximal small bowel the rhythm is 11–12 cycles per minute, decreasing to 7–9 cycles per minute in the distal ileum. Slow waves do not generate contractions but dictate the frequency at which they can occur.[4,7]

Neuronal development of the ENS is not completed at birth. In fact, neurochemical maturation does not reach adult patterns until 1 month of postnatal life,[8] and it has been reported that the number and structure of cell bodies within the ganglia continue to change according to the age of the individual from the first day of life up to 15 years of age.[9]

Gastric Motility

The gastric fundus, which is the uppermost portion of the stomach, acts as a reservoir for ingested food. It lies in the antrum and body of the stomach where food is ground into small particles prior to passage into the small intestine. With swallowing at the onset of a feeding or meal, vagally mediated relaxation of the fundus occurs. As food enters the stomach, the proximal stomach further relaxes to provide a reservoir for nutrients. This receptive relaxation/gastric accommodation allows for an initial increase in the volume of the stomach without an increase in pressure. However, the pressure will ultimately increase, leading to a tonic contraction that then pushes the gastric contents toward the antrum. At the same time, regular phasic contractions (3 cycles per minute) start and both mix and grind (triturate) the gastric contents. During the churning process, the food bolus is first pushed toward the antrum where some grinding takes place. Distention of the antrum results in fundic relaxation and in turn retropulsion of contents back to the body of the stomach. Grinding is important for creating small particles, < 1–2 mm in size, that will pass into the duodenum through the pylorus. Mixing with gastric acid and pepsin begins the chemical digestion of food. This initial phase of mixing and

grinding is the lag phase in gastric emptying that occurs after ingestion of nutrients.[1,4,10–13]

Once the ingested nutrients are appropriately mixed and solid material is ground into small particles, antral contractions accompanied by pyloric relaxation allow small aliquots of this chyme to empty into the duodenum. This begins the second or linear gastric emptying phase. The time for gastric emptying varies and depends upon a variety of factors, but it is generally complete by 4 hours.[1,4,7,10,12,13]

The preterm infant has an immature pattern of GI motility, which affects both gastric emptying and small bowel motility, which in turn impact feeding. Gastric emptying is first seen at 13 weeks of gestation with the length of gastric slow waves increasing just prior to birth.[14] The normal electrical activity of the stomach, with a slow-wave frequency of 3 cycles per minute, does not develop until 32 weeks of gestation and does not become the dominant pattern until 35 weeks of gestation. This results in slower gastric emptying in these more premature infants in comparison to the term infant.[4,15,16] Additionally, extreme stress, such as the presence of systemic illness, which is not infrequently seen in premature neonates, can delay gastric emptying.[17]

Small Bowel Motility

Motor activity of the small intestine serves many important functions, including mixing chyme with intestinal secretions for further digestion, enhancing contact between enteric contents and the mucosa for absorption, moving ingested contents distally, and clearing the intestinal tract by powerful contractions that propagate in an aboral direction.[18]

In the fasting state, or interdigestive period, the migrating motor complex (MMC) has 3 phases. Phase I is a quiescent phase. In phase II intermittent, irregular contractions occur. Phase III is characterized by strong, propagating contractions that begin almost simultaneously in the stomach and duodenum and travel through the small bowel. Phase III of the MMC provides the housekeeping function of intestinal motility, sweeping material through the small bowel. It occurs at irregular intervals, ranging from 18 to 145 minutes, with an average occurrence of every 80 minutes, and lasts from 2 to 14 minutes (Figure 2-1).[1,4,18–20]

In the fed state, mixing and propulsion of intestinal contents are combined. In general, random bursts of activity occur that primarily result in mixing (Figure 2-2). When a contraction occurs, intestinal contents move. If the contraction in one region of the small intestine occurs in a coordinated manner with proximal and distal bowel, then the intestinal

Figure 2-1. Normal Gastric and Small Bowel Motility During a Fasting State With All 3 Phases of the Migration Motor Complex (MMC) Present

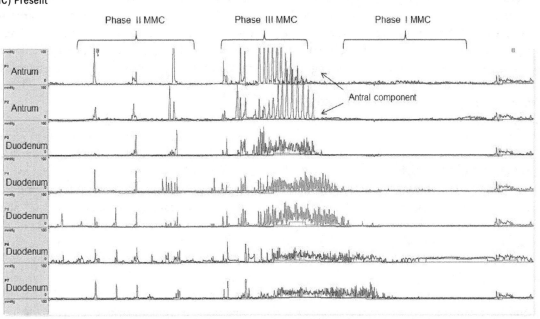

Figure 2-2. Increased Antroduodenal Motility in the Postprandial Period

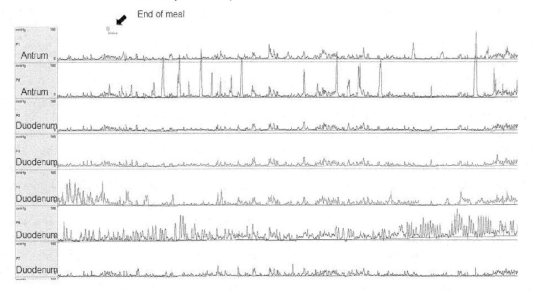

contents will be propelled downstream. If the contraction is not coordinated with activity of adjacent areas, then the intestinal contents move both retrograde and antegrade in the intestine, resulting in mixing.[3,19]

As noted above, the premature infant has not developed a normal pattern of intestinal motility. The fasting pattern of premature infants is characterized by short bursts of activity called clusters that do not progress aborally as a mature

phase III MMC does; the first motility patterns appear as spontaneous contractions that propagate both anally and orally and are generated by the muscle cells themselves, not the ENS.[21] The nature of the clusters differs depending upon the gestational age. The length of a cluster increases with gestational age from <90 seconds in the 27-week to 28-week gestation infant to 5–6 minutes at 36 weeks of gestation. At the same time, the frequency with which the clusters occur decreases. Preterm infants do not exhibit MMCs before 32 weeks of gestation,[22] and true, propagating, cyclical MMCs with clearly defined phases develop between 37 weeks of gestation and term.[23] The fed pattern also differs in the premature infant, with most demonstrating an abrupt cessation of intestinal contractions after a bolus feeding. Not surprisingly, intestinal transit is slower in the preterm infant. Some evidence exists that feeding premature infants, even small amounts, can promote maturation of intestinal motility.[15,24–26]

Effect of Intake on Motor Activity

Gastric emptying can be affected by a variety of characteristics of the ingested material as well as the rapidity of transit through the GI tract. With this, the time for gastric emptying can vary from 1 to 4 hours. The effect of nutrient composition on motor activity has been more clearly delineated for the stomach than the small bowel.

Consistency and Temperature

Liquids will empty from the stomach more quickly than solids. In turn, clear liquids will empty more rapidly than full liquids, with nonnutritive liquids emptying the fastest, leaving the stomach in about 20 minutes.[13,27] The viscosity of the feeds will also affect the speed of gastric emptying, with lower viscosity material emptying more rapidly. Thus, both soluble and insoluble fibers mixed with the feedings will slow emptying.[28,29] In addition to delaying gastric emptying, soluble fibers can prolong transit through the GI tract by prolonging the duration of the fed pattern of small bowel motor activity.[29] Meal temperature has also been shown to effect gastric emptying with warmer meals emptying faster[30] and cold liquids leaving the stomach more slowly.[31]

Nutrient Content

The response to the type of nutrient ingested is complex. Both hormonal and neural responses to food occur to regulate motor activity of the stomach and small intestine. These are interrelated in that neural activity can affect the release of some GI hormones. Once chyme starts to pass through the pylorus, there is feedback via vagal afferents from receptors in the duodenum that regulate gastric emptying. These receptors include those that detect fat, amino acids, glucose, pH, and osmolarity.[32] A component of the response is mediated by release of gastrin, cholecystokinin, pancreatic polypeptide, glucagon-like peptide 1, and peptide YY.[4,33,34] It has been demonstrated that carbohydrates will empty from the stomach before proteins, with fats emptying the most slowly.[4,35,36] Fats reaching the distal ileum inhibit both gastric emptying and small intestinal motility, a mechanism known as the ileal brake.[37] Complex carbohydrates that reach the distal small intestine can also stimulate the ileal brake.[1] In addition to the actual nutrient content, the pH will affect gastric emptying as well, with more acidic material emptying more slowly from the stomach.[38]

Caloric Density and Osmolarity

Increased caloric content of the ingested food or liquid will generally result in slower emptying from the stomach in the older child and adult.[28,39] For infant feeding this is less straightforward. A study in infants ranging from 32 to 39 weeks gestational age demonstrated that altering caloric density using different concentrations of infant formula below 20 kcal/oz (0 vs 6.5 kcal/oz; 6.5 vs 13 kcal/oz; and 13 vs 20 kcal/oz) impacted gastric emptying with the higher caloric density emptying more slowly in each case.[40] Even with this slower emptying, higher calorie feedings resulted in emptying of more calories over comparable time periods. Other researchers[41–43] looking at term (mean 36 weeks gestation) and preterm infants (mean gestational age 31 and 34 weeks) did not find differences in gastric emptying when the caloric density was increased above 20 kcal/oz both using formula as well as fortified breast milk. It has also been demonstrated, although somewhat inconclusively, that a meal with a higher calorie content will result in a longer fed pattern in the small bowel, leading to a longer transit time through the small intestine.[44,45]

Solutions that have a higher osmolarity will empty more slowly from the stomach than those that are lower in osmolarity.[34] In contrast, the small bowel motor response to chemically different liquid meals is similar with respect to both the length of the postprandial motor pattern as well as the contractile activity during the postprandial period.[43]

While each of these factors individually can influence gastric emptying in the older infant, child, and adult, the same does not always hold true in premature infants. In one study of infants of 25–30 weeks gestation, it was demonstrated that separately altering osmolality, caloric density, or the volume of the feeding did not change gastric emptying. However, when the volume of the feeding was increased in combination with decreasing the osmolality, gastric emptying was more rapid.[46] This further underscores that, across age groups in clinical practice, these factors can clearly overlap because nutrient content is closely tied to caloric density. For example, a meal or formula higher in fat will likely be higher in calories.

Altered Patterns of Motility and Potential Interventions

Disordered motility in any part of the GI tract can impact feeding tolerance.

Delayed Gastric Emptying

As already noted, slower gastric emptying occurs in the premature infant and may impair feeding advancement. Premature infants who require tube feedings due to immature suck and swallow may benefit from a slower intermittent infusion over as long as 2 hours, rather than a 15-minute bolus because this slower infusion has been demonstrated to result both in improved gastric emptying and a more mature duodenal motor pattern.[47,48] In the older infant or child, delayed emptying may occur during or following a viral illness, associated with a significant systemic illness or other stress, secondary to marked constipation as part of negative feedback via the intestino-intestinal reflex loop, as well as after surgery. This delayed emptying results in fullness, bloating, decreased appetite, and emesis.[49] Management strategies depend on the degree of the problem and how the child was being fed prior to the onset of the problem. If the child was eating a regular diet, smaller, more frequent meals that are lower in fat, fiber, and caloric density may empty better from the stomach.[50] Since liquids empty more readily than solids, increasing the liquid content of the meal may help. If the child is unable to tolerate any solids, a trial of liquid nutritional supplements is warranted. If the child was tube fed prior to the onset of the delayed gastric emptying, then adjusting the formula or the manner of delivery may be necessary. The osmolarity, caloric content, fat content, and fiber content of the formula should be evaluated and a determination made as to whether a change is possible because the higher each of these are, the slower emptying will be even under normal circumstances. Drip feedings, rather than bolus feedings, may need to be considered. Few pharmacologic options are currently available. Erythromycin, which acts as a motilin receptor agonist, can accelerate gastric emptying.[51] Safety of erythromycin in both preterm and term infants has been demonstrated; however, due to the lack of functional receptors, some debate exists regarding its effectiveness in infants of <32 weeks gestation.[21,22,52] If the problem is severe enough, continuous transpyloric or jejunal feedings may be necessary at least temporarily while awaiting response to treatment of the underlying problem or resolution of the illness.

Dumping

Very rapid gastric emptying, or dumping, is relatively uncommon in pediatrics.[49] It can occur as a result of surgery,

particularly involving the pylorus, or with damage to the vagal nerve such as during a fundoplication or cardiac surgery. Symptoms include nausea, abdominal distention, cramping, diarrhea, and vasomotor changes associated with swings in glucose. Some management strategies are the opposite of those suggested for use in delayed emptying. One can try to take advantage of normal physiology by increasing the fat and protein content of the diet and increasing the fiber content of the diet, including the addition of pectin and guar gum.[50] Rather than mixing liquids with the meal, liquids should be taken separately from solids. On the other hand, some of the same strategies recommended for treatment of delayed gastric emptying may also be helpful in too rapid emptying, specifically smaller, more frequent meals as well as continuous drip or postpyloric feedings. Pharmacologic therapeutic options are limited. Acarbose, an α-glucosidase inhibitor, has been used to treat dumping syndrome because it delays the hydrolysis of carbohydrates with resultant delayed absorption of glucose.[53,54] Octreotide, an analogue of somatostatin, can be beneficial because one of its specific actions is to delay gastric emptying.[55,56]

Slow Intestinal Transit

Slow intestinal transit may occur following surgery (postoperative ileus), following a viral illness or other systemic illness, as a side effect of many drugs, or as part of a significant motility disorder, ranging from disruptions in normal feedback loops to the most extreme circumstance of chronic intestinal pseudoobstruction. No clear evidence or consensus opinion exists to support recommendations in terms of nutrition interventions that may be beneficial in these circumstances. Currently, few drugs are available to help promote motility of the small bowel. Erythromycin has some augmenting effect on phase III MMCs in the small bowel.[57,58] Some data also indicate that amoxicillin-clavulanate may promote small bowel motility.[59] Recently, it has been shown that amoxicillin-clavulanate, when given preprandially, induces duodenal phase III MMCs within 10 minutes of enteral administration.[60] In more severe cases, octreotide may be beneficial. This somatostatin analogue has a wide range of effects on the GI tract, including induction of phase III MMC when given in small doses subcutaneously.[61]

Rapid Intestinal Transit

Rapid intestinal transit may occur following a systemic illness or due to surgery on the GI tract. This can result in malabsorption of nutrients and diarrhea. Feeding strategies will be discussed in detail in later chapters, including those on GI disease and intestinal failure. However, one approach that may be beneficial, regardless of the feeding selected or route of delivery, is the addition of soluble fiber such as pectin or guar gum to the feeding because these will prolong intestinal transit time.[29,62] Various drugs can be used in an effort to slow transit through the small bowel. Loperamide, a peripherally acting opioid analogue, inhibits both small bowel and colonic motility. Anticholinergic agents, such as hyoscyamine, can also help to slow intestinal transit.

While it is important to consider the impact of gastric and intestinal motility on feeding, it is only one of many factors that must be taken into account as will be discussed in subsequent chapters.

Test Your Knowledge Questions

1. Gastric emptying can be slowed by all of the following except:
    A. Soluble fibers
    B. Fats
    C. Liquids
    D. Protein

2. Strategies that can be effective in both rapid and delayed gastric emptying include all of the following except:
    A. Small frequent feeds
    B. Giving liquids with meals to increase the fluid content of the meal
    C. Continuous drip feeds
    D. Postpyloric feeds

3. Which of the following is true for the premature infant?
    A. Bolus feeds will promote normal small bowel motor activity.
    B. Transit through the small bowel is shorter than in the older infant.
    C. Gastric emptying is more rapid than in the older infant.
    D. Feeding can promote the development of intestinal motility.

References

1. Camilleri M. Integrated upper gastrointestinal response to food intake. *Gastroenterology.* 2006;131:640–658.
2. Costa M, Brookes SJH, Hennig GW. Anatomy and physiology of the enteric nervous system. *Gut.* 2000;47(Suppl IV):iv15–iv19.
3. Leger G. Basic physiology of motility, absorption and secretion. In: Langnas AN, Goulet O, Quigley EMM, Tappenden KA, eds. *Intestinal Failure: Diagnosis, Management and Transplantation.* Malden, MA: Blackwell Publishing; 2008:20–32.
4. Saps M, Di Lorenzo C. Gastric motility: normal motility and development of the gastric neuroenteric system. In: Kleinman RE, Sanderson IR, Goulet O, Sherman PM, Mieli-Vergani G, Shneider BL, eds. *Walker's Pediatric Gastrointestinal Disease.* Vol 1. 5th ed. Hamilton, Ontario: BC Decker, Inc; 2008:187–193.
5. Rolle U, Piaseczna-Piotrowska A, Puri P. Interstitial cells of Cajal in the normal gut and in intestinal motility disorders of childhood. *Pediatr Surg Int.* 2007;23:1139–1152.
6. Sanders KM, Koh SD, Ward SM. Interstitial cells of Cajal as pacemakers in the gastrointestinal tract. *Annu Rev Physiol.* 2006;68:307–343.
7. Altaf MA, Sood MR. The nervous system and gastrointestinal function. *Dev Disabil Res Rev.* 2008;14:87–95.
8. Thapar N, Faure C, Di Lorenzo C. Introduction to gut motility and sensitivity. In: Faure C, Di Lorenzo C, Thapar N, eds. *Pediatric Neurogastroenterology: Gastrointestinal Motility and Functional Disorders in Children.* New York, NY: Springer Science+Business Media; 2013:3–8.
9. Wester T, O'Briain DS, Puri P. Notable postnatal alterations in the myenteric plexus of normal human bowel. *Gut.* 1999;44:666–674.
10. Cuomo R, Sarnelli G. Food intake and gastrointestinal motility. A complex interplay. *Nutr Metab Cardiovasc Dis.* 2004;14:173–179.
11. Hennig GW, Brookes SJH, Costa M. Excitatory and inhibitory motor reflexes in the isolated guinea-pig stomach. *J Physiol.* 1997;501:197–212.
12. Lacy BE, Koch KL, Crowell MD. The stomach: normal function and clinical disorders. Manometry. In: Schuster MM, Crowell MD, Koch KL, eds. *Schuster Atlas of Gastrointestinal Motility in Health and Disease.* 2nd ed. Hamilton, ON, Canada: BC Decker, Inc; 2002:135–150.
13. Siegel JA, Urbain J-L, Adler LP, et al. Biphasic nature of gastric emptying. *Gut.* 1988;29:85–89.
14. Sase M, Miwa I, Sumie M, et al. Gastric emptying cycles in the human fetus. *Am J Obstet Gynecol.* 2005;193(3 Pt 2):1000–1004.
15. Berseth CL. Assessment in intestinal motility as a guide in the feeding management of the newborn. *Clin Perinatol.* 1999;26:1007–1015.
16. Riezzo G, Indrio F, Montagna O, et al. Gastric electrical activity and gastric emptying in term and preterm newborns. *Neurogastroenterol Motil.* 2000;12:223–229.
17. Berseth CL. Motor function in the stomach and small intestine in the neonate. *NeoReviews.* 2006;7:e28-33.
18. Kellow JE. Small intestine: normal function and clinical disorders. Manometry. In: Schuster MM, Crowell MD, Koch KL, eds. *Schuster Atlas of Gastrointestinal Motility in Health and Disease.* 2nd ed. Hamilton, ON, Canada: BC Decker, Inc; 2002:219–236.
19. Boccia G, Staiano A. Intestinal motility: normal motility and development of the intestinal neuroenteric system. In: Kleinman RE, Sanderson IR, Goulet O, Sherman PM, Mieli-Vergani G, Shneider BL, eds. *Walker's Pediatric Gastrointestinal Disease.* Vol 1. 5th ed. Hamilton, ON, Canada: BC Decker, Inc; 2008:665–674.

20. Scott SM, Knowles CH, Wang D, et al. The nocturnal jejunal migrating motor complex: defining normal ranges by study of 51 healthy adult volunteers and meta-analysis. *Neurogastroenterol Motil*. 2006;18:927–935.

21. Young HM, Beckett EA, Bornstein JC, Jadcherla SR. Development of gut motility. In: Faure C, Di Lorenzo C, Thapar N, eds. *Pediatric Neurogastroenterology: Gastrointestinal Motility and Functional Disorders in Children*. New York, NY: Springer Science+Business Media; 2013:23–35.

22. Jadcherla SR, Klee G, Berseth CL. Regulation of migrating motor complexes by motilin and pancreatic polypeptide in human infants. *Pediatr Res*. 1997;42(3):365–369.

23. Bisset WM, Watt JB, Rivers RP, Milla PJ. Ontongeny of fasting small intestinal motor activity in the human infant. *Gut*. 1988;29(4):483–488.

24. Berseth CL. Effect of early feeding on maturation of the preterm infant's small intestine. *J Pediatr*. 1992;120:947–953.

25. Commare CE, Tappenden KA. Development of the infant intestine: implications for nutrition support. *Nutr Clin Pract*. 2007;22:159–173.

26. McClure RJ, Newell SJ. Randomised controlled trial of trophic feeding and gut motility. *Arch Dis Child Fetal Neonatal Ed*. 1999;80:F54–F58.

27. Collins PJ, Houghton LA, Read NW, et al. Role of the proximal and distal stomach in a mixed solid and liquid meal emptying. *Gut*. 1991;32:615–619.

28. Marciani L, Gowland PA, Spiller RC, et al. Effect of meal viscosity and nutrients on satiety, intragastric dilution, and emptying assessed by MRI. *Am J Physiol Gastrointest Liver Physiol*. 2001;280:G1227–G1233.

29. Schönfeld J, Evans DF, Wingate DL. Effect of viscous fiber (guar) on postprandial motor activity in human small bowel. *Dig Dis Sci*. 1997;42:1613–1617.

30. Mishima Y, Amano Y, Takahashi Y, et al. Gastric emptying of liquid and solid meals at various temperatures. *J Gastroenterol*. 2009;44(5):412–418.

31. Sun WM, Houghton LA, Read NW, Grundy DG, Johnson AG. Effect of meal temperature on gastric emptying of liquids in man. *Gut*. 1988;29(3):302–305.

32. Schwartz GJ, Moran TH. Duodenal nutrient exposure elicits nutrient-specific gut motility and vagal afferent signals in rat. *Am J Physiol Regulatory Integrative Comp Physiol*. 1998;274:R1236–R1242.

33. MacIntosh CG, Andrews JM, Jones KL, et al. Effects of age on concentrations of plasma cholecystokinin, glucagon-like peptide 1, and peptide YY and their relation to appetite and pyloric motility. *Am J Clin Nutr*. 1999;69:999–1006.

34. Feinle C, O'Donovan D, Doran S, et al. Effects of fat digestion on appetite, APD motility, and gut hormones in response to duodenal fat infusions in humans. *Am J Physiol Gastrointest Liver Physiol*. 2003;284:G798–G807.

35. Houghton LA, Mangnall YF, Read NW. Effect of incorporating fat into a liquid test meal on the relation between intragastric distribution and gastric emptying in human volunteers. *Gut*. 1990;31:1226–1229.

36. Paraskevopoulos JA, Houghton LA, Eyre-Brooke I, Johnson AG, Read NW. Effect of composition of gastric contents on resistance to emptying of liquids from stomach in humans. *Dig Dis Sci*. 1988;33:914–918.

37. Ohtani N, Sasaki I, Naito H, Shibata C, Matsuno S. Mediators for fat-induced ileal brake are different between stomach and proximal small intestine in conscious dogs. *J Gastrointest Surg*. 2001;5:377–382.

38. Chaw CS, Yazaki E, Evans DF. The effect of pH change on the gastric emptying of liquids measured by electrical impedance tomography and pH-sensitive radiotelemetry capsule. *Int J Pharm*. 2001;227:167–175.

39. Boulby P, Moore R, Gowland P, Spiller RC. Fat delays emptying but increases forward and backward antral flow as assessed by flow-sensitive magnetic resonance imaging. *Neurogastroenterol Motil*. 1999;11:27–36.

40. Siegel M, Lebenthal E, Krantz B. Effect of caloric density on gastric emptying in premature infants. *J Pediatr*. 1984;104(1):118–122.

41. Siegel M, Lebenthal E, Topper W, Krantz B, Li PK. Gastric emptying in prematures of isocaloric feedings with differing osmolalities. *Pediatr Res*. 1982;16:141–147.

42. McClure RJ, Newell SJ. Effect of fortifying breastmilk on gastric emptying. *Arch Dis Child*. 1996;74:60–62.

43. Gathwala G, Shaw C, Shaw P, Yadav S, Sen J. Human milk fortification and gastric emptying in the preterm neonate. *Int J Clin Pract*. 2008;62(7):1039–1043.

44. Schönfeld J, Evans DF, Wingate DL. Daytime and night time motor activity of the small bowel after solid meals of different caloric value in humans. *Gut*. 1997;40:614–618.

45. Schönfeld JV, Evans DF, Renzing K, Castillo FD, Wingate DL. Human small bowel motor activity in response to liquid meals of different caloric value and different chemical composition. *Dig Dis Sciences*. 1998;43(2):265–269.

46. Ramirez A, Wong WW, Shulman RJ. Factors regulating gastric emptying in preterm infants. *J Pediatr*. 2006;149:475–479.

47. Baker JH, Berseth CL. Duodenal motor responses in preterm infants fed with formula with varying concentrations and rates of infusion. *Pediatr Res*. 1997;42:618–622.

48. De Ville K, Knapp E, Al-Tawil Y, Berseth CL. Slow infusion feedings enhance duodenal motor responses and gastric emptying in preterm infants. *Am J Clin Nutr*. 1998;68:103–108.

49. Di Lorenzo C, Ciamarra P. Pediatric gastrointestinal motility. In: Schuster MM, Crowell MD, Koch KL, eds. *Schuster Atlas of Gastrointestinal Motility in Health and Disease*. 2nd ed. Hamilton, ON, Canada: BC Decker, Inc; 2002:411–428.

50. Karamanolis G, Tack J. Nutrition and motility disorders. *Best Pract Res Clin Gastroenterol*. 2006;20:485–505.

51. Karamanolis G, Tack J. Promotility medications—now and in the future. *Dig Dis*. 2006;24:297–307.

52. Ng PC. Use of oral erythromycin for the treatment of gastrointestinal dysmotility in preterm infants. *Neonatology*. 2009;95:97–104.

53. Ng DD, Ferry RJ, Kelly A, et al. Acarbose treatment of postprandial hypoglycemia in children after Nissen fundoplication. *J Pediatr*. 2001;139:877–879.

54. Zung A, Zadik Z. Acarbose treatment of infant dumping syndrome: extensive study of glucose dynamics and long-term follow-up. *J Pediatr Endocrinol Metab*. 2003;16:905–915.

55. Lamers CB, Bijlstra AM, Harris AG. Octreotide, a long-acting somatostatin analog, in the management of post-operative dumping syndrome. An update. *Dig Dis Sci.* 1993;38:359–364.

56. Scarpignato C. The place of octreotide in the medical management of the dumping syndrome. *Digestion.* 1996;57(Suppl 1):114–118.

57. Costalos C, Gounaris A, Varhalama E, Kokori F, Alexiou N, Kolovou E. Erythromycin as a prokinetic agent in preterm infants. *J Pediatr Gastroenterol Nutr.* 2002;34(1):23–25.

58. Har AF, Croffie JMB. Drugs acting on the gut: prokinetics, antispasmodics, laxatives. In: Faure C, Di Lorenzo C, Thapar N, eds. *Pediatric Neurogastroenterology: Gastrointestinal Motility and Functional Disorders in Children.* New York, NY: Springer Science+Business Media; 2013:441–464.

59. Caron F, Ducrotte P, Lerebours E, et al. Effects of amoxicillin-clavulanate combination on the motility of the small intestine in human beings. *Antimicrob Agents Chemother.* 1991;35:1085–1088.

60. Gomez R, Fernandez S, Aspirot A, et al. Effect of amoxicillin/clavulanate on gastrointestinal motility in children. *J Pediatr Gastroenerol Nutr.* 2012;54(6):780–784.

61. Di Lorenzo C, Lucanto C, Flores AF, Idries S, Hyman PE. Effect of octreotide on gastrointestinal motility in children with functional gastrointestinal symptoms. *J Pediatr Gastroenterol Nutr.* 1998;27:508–512.

62. Finkel Y, Brown G, Smith HL, et al. The effects of a pectin-supplemented elemental diet in a boy with short bowel syndrome. *Acta Paediatr Scand.* 1990;79:983–986.

Test Your Knowledge Answers

1. The correct answer is **C.** Liquids empty from the stomach faster than solids; feeding higher in fiber, fat, and protein will empty more slowly.

2. The correct answer is **B.** Giving liquids with a meal increases gastric emptying, which is counterproductive in dumping syndrome.

3. The correct answer is **D.** It has been demonstrated that even small amounts of enteral feeding in the premature infant will encourage maturation of intestinal motility. Bolus feeds will actually cause a cessation of contractions in the proximal small bowel of the premature infant. Both gastric emptying and intestinal transit are slower in the premature infant.

Carbohydrates: Changes With Development

Thaddaeus D. May, MD; and **Robert J. Shulman,** MD

CONTENTS

Learning Objectives

1. Describe the structure and classification of carbohydrates.
2. Describe the process of carbohydrate digestion and absorption.
3. Discuss protein turnover, assessment of plasma amino acids, and nitrogen balance.

Carbohydrates Overview

Carbohydrates provide 4 kcal/g and typically supply 50% of the body's total energy requirement. Though carbohydrates are the fundamental energy substrate at the core of a multitude of processes related to cellular energetics, there is not a fundamental dietary carbohydrate. Human metabolic processes are instead exquisitely tuned to maintain the necessary level of carbohydrate in the bloodstream under a variety of circumstances. An example of this flexibility is in the use of ketogenic diets for the treatment of intractable epilepsy, demonstrating the feasibility of a "carbohydrate-free" diet. Recommended standards for the composition of infant formula (2005) allow for 36%–56% of calories to come from carbohydrates. With increasing age, dietary reference intake guidelines suggest that 45%–60% of calories be sourced from carbohydrates. Dietary carbohydrates consist of sugars and starches. The simplest carbohydrates are single molecules of sugar called *monosaccharides* (also known as simple sugars), such as glucose. Two single molecules of sugar can be connected together and are known as a *disaccharide*; an example is lactose (comprised of single molecules of glucose and galactose). Small-chain starches, generally 3–10 glucose units in length, are referred to as *oli-*

Figure 3-1. Classification of Carbohydrates

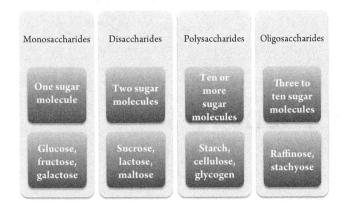

gosaccharides, whereas longer-chain starches are referred to as *polysaccharides* (Figure 3-1).

In general, carbohydrates exist as storage polysaccharides and structural polysaccharides known as starch and cellulose, respectively. Starches are abundant in normal diets and are found in many foods, such as rice, corn, and tapioca (used in infant formulas). In contrast, cellulose is an indigestible, insoluble fiber that occurs as a structural component in plant matter, such as celery. Both cellulose and starch consist of many glucose monomers joined by 1-4 linkages, but both have unique spatial arrangements. Starch is in the α configuration, while cellulose is in the β configuration.[1] Formula-fed infants are exposed to a variety of carbohydrates, including starches. *Complex carbohydrates* is a term commonly used to refer to starches used in infant formulas (ie, corn syrup solids, glucose polymers). Amylose, typically the simplest

Figure 3-2. Digestion and Absorption of Dietary Carbohydrates

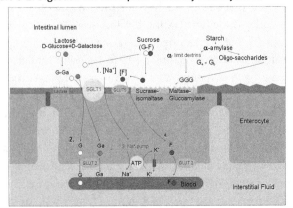

Modified with permission from *Textbook in Medical Physiology and Pathophysiology Essentials and Clinical Problems*, 2nd Edition. Chapter 22. http://www.zuniv.net/physiology/book/chapter22.html

starch consumed early in life, is a linear polymer of glucose molecules linked by α-1,4 glycosidic bonds.[1] However, amylopectin, a plant starch, is the major form of starch in the diet. Structurally it is similar to amylose, but α-1,6 branch points occur at every 20–30 glucose units.[1]

Digestion

Starch and Sucrose

Digestion of starch begins with digestion by salivary amylases and then subsequently pancreatic amylases. Amylase hydrolyzes starches at the internal α-1,4 bonds (Figure 3-2). Because it does not cleave bonds located next to α-1,6 bonds or those at the reducing end of the starch molecule, amylase breaks down amylose and amylopectin into maltotriose, maltose, and α-limit dextrins (a short-chain amylopectin that retains its 1-6 linkage) (Figure 3-2).[2] In older children and adults, sufficient intraluminal α-amylase activity exists to digest 10 times more starch than is typically consumed daily.[3]

Amylase, secreted by the salivary glands, is present in preterm infants (Figure 3-3). Although salivary amylase is inactivated at pH < 4, it tends to remain active in the stomachs of newborns because of poor acidification.[4] Pancreatic amylase activity is initially present at low levels in premature and term infants (Figure 3-3) and then increases at 4–6 months of age before finally reaching adult activity levels by 1–2 years of age.[5] Further digestion of the disaccharides and oligosaccharides occurs at the intestine's brush border (enterocyte surface) via maltase-glucoamylase and sucrase-isomaltase.

Maltase-glucoamylase is located in the brush border of the small intestine and is most active in the ileum. It cleaves α-1,4 bonds of nonbranching glucose polymers (ie, amylose) and nonreducing ends of polysaccharides (Figure

Figure 3-3. Development Profile of Pancreatic and Salivary Amylase

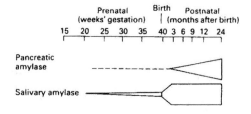

Little pancreatic amylase activity is present prior to birth, but salivary amylase demonstrates some activity prior to 40 weeks of gestation.[20]

Adapted from *Archives of Disease in Childhood*, McClean P and Weaver LT, vol. 68, pages 62-65, Copyright 1993 with permission from BMJ Publishing Group LTD.

3-2). Short chains (ie, < 10 glucose units) are more readily digested by glucoamylase than are longer-chain units.[6]

Glucoamylase activity is detectable early in gestation, and by 28 weeks of gestation, its activity appears to be comparable to that at term.[7,8] Infants < 1 year have glucoamylase activity similar to that of children and adults.[8,9] In preterm and term infants, glucoamylase is the primary enzyme for complex carbohydrate digestion since pancreatic amylase activity is low.[10] In adults, glucoamylase activity increases steadily throughout the small intestine, with greatest activity near the ileocecal valve.[9]

Sucrase-isomaltase, a disaccharidase also found in the brush border, has a high degree of activity in the proximal small intestine. Sucrase-isomaltase hydrolyzes 75%–80% of maltase, almost all dietary isomaltose, and 100% of sucrose. Sucrase-isomaltase is cleaved into 2 enzymes, sucrase and isomaltase, by pancreatic proteases.[1,2] Sucrase hydrolyzes sucrose into the monosaccharides glucose and fructose (Figure 3-2). Isomaltase cleaves the α-1,6 glycosidic bonds of amylopectin (Figure 3-2). By the beginning of the third trimester, sucrase-isomaltase activity is comparable to that of adults.[11] Activity remains high throughout life. Congenital sucrase-isomaltase deficiency is a relatively rare (1/5000) autosomal recessive disorder in which patients lack sucrase and have variable isomaltase activity.[12]

Lactose

Lactase is the enzyme responsible for digesting lactose, the primary carbohydrate present in human milk and most infant formulas. Lactase hydrolyzes lactose into the monosaccha-rides glucose and galactose (Figure 3-2).[1,2] Like maltase-glu-coamylase and sucrase-isomaltase, lactase is located along the brush border of the enterocytes lining the villi of the small intestine. Because the optimum pH for lactase activity is 6.0, its activity is highest in the jejunum and decreases toward the ileum.[9] This gradient is established by 11 weeks of gestation.[7] During gestation lactase activity increases until birth, with the greatest increase occurring during the third trimester. At the beginning of the third trimester, lactase activity is approximately 25% of that at term.[11,13]

In most individuals, lactase activity begins to decline with advancing age.[14] This genetically predetermined process, also known as primary lactase deficiency or primary hypolactasia, begins between 3 and 5 years of age and continues into adulthood.[15] The prevalence of hypolactasia varies among individuals according to ethnicity, ranging from 90% among Asians, 80% among blacks, 53% among Hispanics, and 15%–25% among non-Hispanic whites.[15] The role of variable digestive capacity for lactose among neonates is of uncertain significance for the development of illness. Studies conducted in preterm pigs suggest that incomplete digestion of carbohydrates may be linked to the pathogenesis of necrotizing enterocolitis.[16] Additionally, the time until full feeding tolerance is inversely related to lactase activity (Figure 3-4).[13,17] Among preterm infants who are receiving formula, the substitution of a combination of lactose and glucose polymers for lactose resulted in less feeding intolerance.[18] However, it also has been shown that early enteral feeding in preterm infants increases lactase activity (Figure 3-5).[13] Moreover, use of human breast milk has been shown

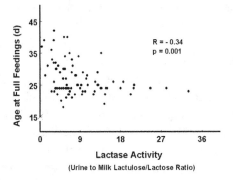

Figure 3-4. Age at Full Feedings vs Lactase Activity

A negative relationship exists between the time full enteral feedings are achieved and lactase activity.[2]

Reprinted from *The Journal of Pediatrics*, vol. 133(5), Shulman RJ, Schanler RJ, Lau C, Heitkemper M, Ou CN, Smith EO, Early feeding, feeding tolerance, and lactase activity in preterm infants, Pages 645-649, Copyright 1998, with permission from Elsevier.

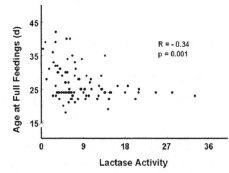

Figure 3-5. Lactase Development with Age and Type of Feeding

Lactase activity increases with age, but the increase is greater in the early fed group compared to the standard group (p < 0.01).[2] Lactase activity in the early fed group is greater than that in the standard group at 10 and 28 days of age (p = 0.004) but not at 50 days of age (p > 0.5).[2]

Reprinted from *The Journal of Pediatrics*, vol. 133(5), Shulman RJ, Schanler RJ, Lau C, Heitkemper M, Ou CN, Smith EO, Early feeding, feeding tolerance, and lactase activity in preterm infants, Pages 645-649, Copyright 1998, with permission from Elsevier.

to promote the development of lactase activity in preterm infants.[13] For instance, preterm infants fed human milk demonstrate greater lactase activity than those fed formula containing a combination of lactose and glucose polymers.[13] These observations further support the importance of human breast milk feeding.[19]

Congenital lactase deficiency is an autosomal recessive disorder characterized by a complete absence of lactase expression.[20] The incidence is unknown, but the disorder is so rare as to be reportable. Symptoms manifest at birth with the introduction of lactose in the diet. This newborn, genetic-type hypolactasia stands in stark contrast to secondary lactase deficiency, which results as a consequence of mucosal injury to the small intestine. Secondary lactase deficiency occurs most commonly following an acute infectious gastroenteritis and generally resolves with the resolution of the acute illness.[21] However, infants with a prolonged diarrheal illness resulting in severe dehydration may show clinical signs of lactose intolerance and temporarily benefit from a lactose-free formula until their symptoms resolve.[21,22]

Absorption

Dietary carbohydrates are absorbed in the form of glucose, galactose, and fructose.[22] Two categories of transporters, glucose transporters (GLUTs) and a sodium-glucose cotransporter (SGLT1), mediate absorption of glucose from the intestinal lumen into the interstitial space (Figure 3-2).[23,24] Active transport of glucose and galactose is present by 12 weeks of gestation and increases through gestation.[25,26] SGLT1 transports glucose along the sodium gradient maintained by the sodium-potassium ATPase pump located at the basolateral surface of the enterocyte (Figure 3-2).[23,24] SGLT1 is a high-affinity active transporter of glucose and galactose located at the intestinal villus brush border with binding sites for one glucose (or galactose) molecule and 2 sodium molecules. Once all sites are occupied, glucose and sodium are translocated across the enterocyte's apical membrane and released into the enterocyte.[23,24] This sodium-linked transport of glucose accentuates the osmotic absorption of water and accounts for the increased efficacy of oral rehydration solutions when glucose or starch are added to them.

Glucose-galactose malabsorption is a rare autosomal recessive disorder that results in watery diarrhea soon after birth.[27] Approximately 300 cases have been reported to date. Treatment is provided by substituting dietary glucose and galactose for fructose. Fructose is still absorbed effectively

Table 3-1. Selected Disorders Associated With Carbohydrate Malabsorption

CONGENITAL	HERITABLE	ACQUIRED
Sucrase-isomaltase deficiency	Adult-type hypolactasia	Postviral enteritis
Glucose-galactose malabsorption	Cystic fibrosis	Environmental enteropathy
Congenital lactase deficiency	Shwachman-Diamond syndrome	Short bowel syndrome
Congenital microvillus atrophy	Celiac disease	Autoimmune enteropathy
Tufting enteropathy		

in this disorder because it is transported into enterocytes via GLUT5 along its concentration gradient in a sodium-independent fashion (Figure 3-2).[23] GLUT2 has also been identified at the brush border (luminal surface), with evidence suggesting that ingestion of a carbohydrate load stimulates SGLT1, resulting in recruitment of GLUT2 receptors to the apical membrane of enterocytes.[28,29]

Short-Chain Fatty Acids

Up to 5%–20% of ingested starches resist digestion in the small intestine.[30] Upon reaching the colon, colonic fermentation of this *resistant starch* results in the production of short-chain fatty acids (SCFAs).[31] SCFAs are produced by fermentative modification of the carbon backbone structure of carbohydrates escaping digestion in the small bowel. In general, dietary fiber is approximately one-third soluble and two-thirds insoluble. The soluble components are fermented into SCFAs, while the insoluble components resist fermentation and contribute to fecal bulk.[23]

The total volume of SCFAs generated depends upon colonic microbial characteristics, amount of resistant starch ingested, and gut transit time.[31,32] Despite variability of these factors, the ratio of the SCFAs produced is fairly constant (acetate, propionate, and butyrate; 60:20:20, respectively).[32] This ratio is similar in both the proximal and distal colon, reflecting a relatively uniform absorptive capacity of the mucosa throughout the colon. The absorption of SCFAs by the colon is very efficient, and only 5%–10% of SCFAs produced are excreted in feces.[32] SCFAs play an essential role in maintenance of gut health, with important effects on colonic luminal pH, intracellular pH, cell volume, and ion transport as well as moderating effects on enterocyte proliferation, differentiation, and gene expression.[32]

Maldigestion/Malabsorption of Carbohydrates

Disorders of carbohydrate digestion/absorption are categorized in several ways (Table 3-1). These disorders are considered according to their pathogenesis[33]:

- Impairment of intrinsic digestive processes (usually congenital); examples include sucrase-isomaltase deficiency and glucose-galactose malabsorption.
- Malabsorption due to an associated disease state (may be acquired or heritable); examples include viral diarrhea, environmental enteropathy, celiac disease, and cystic fibrosis.
- Reduction of the gut's absorptive surface (usually acquired); examples include short bowel syndrome.

In all of these disorders, the volume of diarrhea is roughly proportional to the amount of ingested carbohydrate that is malabsorbed. The unabsorbed carbohydrate in the small intestine causes an increased osmotic gradient, which draws more water into the lumen and increases the volume of intestinal contents. This leads to increased peristalsis and decreased transit time, which further impairs digestion and absorption of the carbohydrates. On reaching the colon, fermentation of undigested carbohydrate results in an increased concentration of SCFAs, reducing the intestinal pH below 5.5. This increased acidity disrupts sodium absorption, leading to further increases of luminal water.[2] Once the rate of delivery of carbohydrates into the colon exceeds the fermentative capacity, the increased carbohydrate load in the colon, as in the small intestine, results in worsening of the osmotic diarrhea.[2]

Carbohydrate malabsorption can be detected by testing stool pH, testing for stool-reducing substances, and/or conducting a hydrogen breath test. Stool pH < 5.5 is indicative of excessive SCFA production in the stool, while reducing substances in stool indicate the presence of sugars (with the exception of intact sucrose), reflecting malabsorption from the small intestine. Fermentation of carbohydrate in the colon also produces hydrogen gas, a portion of which is absorbed into the systemic circulation and excreted in breath.[34] This forms the basis of the breath hydrogen test to detect carbohydrate malabsorption in the small intestine.[34]

Malabsorption of carbohydrates ranges from mild to severe depending on the cause. Similarly, treatment will vary depending on the entity causing malabsorption and may include special diets and formulas (eg, gluten-free diet for patients with celiac disease) or enzyme supplements (eg, sucrase for sucrase-isomaltase deficiency). In the future, gene therapy may become a viable therapeutic option for certain congenital enzyme defects.

Metabolism

In the general economy of the body's metabolism, glucose is the common currency and is used by nearly all cells in the body. Upon feeding after birth, dietary carbohydrates provide glucose in blood for uptake by cells throughout the body. Glucose that is not immediately utilized is stored in the form of glycogen (a storage carbohydrate).[1] Insulin is responsible for glycogenesis (glycogen synthesis), while glucagon effects glycogenolysis (glycogen degradation).

Case Study and Test Your Knowledge Questions

A baby girl is born at a gestational age of 27 weeks to a first time mother. The child weighs 1431 g and, despite significant respiratory distress at birth, is stabilized shortly thereafter with mechanical ventilator support. Following transfer to the neonatal intensive care unit at a regional children's hospital, an orogastric tube is placed and trophic feedings of expressed breast milk are started.

1. As enteral feedings are advanced, the supply of maternal breast milk is inadequate to meet the patient's nutritional requirements, and the patient receives formula. Which of the carbohydrates in the formula is a polysaccharide?
   A. Lactose
   B. Sucrose
   C. Maltose
   D. Amylose

2. When fed breast milk, which of the following types of enzymes is least important?
   A. Disaccharidases
   B. Lipases
   C. Amylases
   D. Proteases

3. The carbohydrate in the breast milk is hydrolyzed to which of the following by the action of lactase?
   A. Glucose and glucose
   B. Galactose and glucose
   C. Glucose and fructose
   D. Galactose and fructose

4. At the time of discharge from the hospital (at 39 weeks gestational age), which of the following enzymes will have exhibited the greatest increase in activity from the time of her admission?

A. Glucoamylase

B. Lactase

C. Sucrase

D. Salivary amylase

5. Because of gastroesophageal reflux, rice cereal is added to the infant's feeding, after which her stools become more frequent and watery. The stool pH is checked and found to be 4.5, suggesting which of the following?

A. Production of increased SCFAs

B. Increased osmotic drag

C. Increased colonic fermentation

D. All of the above

Acknowledgments

The authors of this chapter for the second edition of this text wish to thank Seema Mehta, MD, for her contributions to the first edition of this text.

References

1. Micronutrients and macronutrients. In: Kleinman RE, ed. *Pediatric Nutrition Handbook.* 6th ed. Elk Grove Village, IL: American Academy of Pediatrics, 2009:343–356.

2. Schmitz J. Maldigestion and malabsorption. In: Walker WA, Goulet O, Kleinman RE, Sherman PM, Shneider BL, Sanderson IR, eds. *Pediatric Gastrointestinal Disease.* 4th ed. Hamilton, ON, Canada: B.C. Decker Inc; 2004:8–9.

3. Fogel MR, Gray GM. Starch hydrolysis in man: an intraluminal process not requiring membrane digestion. *J Appl Physiol.* 1973;35:263–267.

4. Hodge C, Lebenthal E, Lee PC, Topper W. Amylase in the saliva and in the gastric aspirates of premature infants: its potential role in glucose polymer hydrolysis. *Pediatr Res.* 1983;17:998–1001.

5. McClean P, Weaver LT. Ontogeny of human pancreatic exocrine function. *Arch Dis Child.* 1993;68:62–65.

6. Eggermont E. The hydrolysis of the naturally occurring alpha-glucosides by the human intestinal mucosa. *Eur J Biochem.* 1969;9:483–487.

7. Raul F, Lacroix B, Aprahamian M. Longitudinal distribution of brush border hydrolases and morphological maturation in the intestine of the preterm infant. *Early Hum Dev.* 1986;13:225–234.

8. Lee PC, Werlin S, Trost B, Struve M. Glucoamylase activity in infants and children: normal values and relationship to symptoms and histological findings. *J Pediatr Gastroenterol Nutr.* 2004;39:161–165.

9. Triadou N, Bataille J, Schmitz J. Longitudinal study of the human intestinal brush border membrane proteins. Distribution of the main disaccharidases and peptidases. *Gastroenterology.* 1983;85:1326–1332.

10. Shulman RJ, Kerzner B, Sloan HR, et al. Absorption and oxidation of glucose polymers of different lengths in young infants. *Pediatr Res.* 1986;20:740–743.

11. Mobassaleh M, Montgomery RK, Biller JA, Grand RJ. Development of carbohydrate absorption in the fetus and neonate. *Pediatrics.* 1985;75:160–166.

12. Naim HY, Heine M, Zimmer KP. Congenital sucrase-isomaltase deficiency: heterogeneity of inheritance, trafficking, and function of an intestinal enzyme complex. *J Pediatr Gastroenterol Nutr.* 2012;55(suppl 2):S13–S20.

13. Shulman RJ, Schanler RJ, Lau C, Heitkemper M, Ou CN, Smith EO. Early feeding, feeding tolerance, and lactase activity in preterm infants. *J Pediatr.* 1998;133:645–649.

14. Lomer MC, Parkes GC, Sanderson JD. Review article: lactose intolerance in clinical practice—myths and realities. *Aliment Pharmacol Ther.* 2008;27:93–103.

15. Sahi T. Genetics and epidemiology of adult-type hypolactasia. *Scand J Gastroenterol Suppl.* 1994;202:7–20.

16. Thymann T, Møller HK, Stoll B, et al. Carbohydrate maldigestion induces necrotizing enterocolitis in preterm pigs. *Am J Physiol Gastrointest Liver Physiol.* 2009;297:G1115–G1125.

17. Shulman RJ, Ou CN, Smith EO. Evaluation of potential factors predicting attainment of full gavage feedings in preterm infants. *Neonatology.* 2011;99:38–44.

18. Griffin MP, Hansen JW. Can the elimination of lactose from formula improve feeding tolerance in premature infants? *J Pediatr.* 1999;135:587–592.

19. Kim JH, Froh EB. What nurses need to know regarding nutritional and immunobiological properties of human milk [published online ahead of print December 12, 2011]. *J Obstet Gynecol Neonatal Nurs.* doi:10.1111/j.1552-6909.2011.01314.x.

20. Torniainen S, Freddara R, Routi T, et al. Four novel mutations in the lactase gene (LCT) underlying congenital lactase deficiency (CLD). *BMC Gastroenterol.* 2009;9:8.

21. Brown KH. Dietary management of acute diarrheal disease: contemporary scientific issues. *J Nutr.* 1994;124:1455S–1460S.

22. Caballero B, Solomons NW. Lactose-reduced formulas for the treatment of persistent diarrhea. *Pediatrics.* 1990;86:645–646.

23. Karasov WH, Douglas AE. Comparative digestive physiology. *Compr Physiol.* 2013;3:741–783.

24. Wright EM, Hirayama BA, Loo DF. Active sugar transport in health and disease. *J Intern Med.* 2007;261:32–43.

25. Levin RJ, Koldovský O, Hosková J, Jirsová V, Uher J. Electrical activity across human foetal small intestine associated with absorption processes. *Gut.* 1968;9:206–213.

26. Rouwet EV, Heineman E, Buurman WA, ter Riet G, Ramsay G, Blanco CE. Intestinal permeability and carrier-mediated monosaccharide absorption in preterm neonates during the early postnatal period. *Pediatr Res.* 2002;51:64–70.

27. Wright EM, Turk E, Martin MG. Molecular basis for glucose-galactose malabsorption. *Cell Biochem Biophys.* 2002;36:115–121.

28. Kellett GL, Brot-Laroche E. Apical GLUT2: a major pathway of intestinal sugar absorption. *Diabetes.* 2005;54:3056–3062.

29. Roder PV, Geillinger KE, Zietek TS, Thorens B, Koepsell H, Daniel H. The role of SGLT1 and GLUT2 in intestinal glucose transport and sensing. *PLoS One.* 2014;9:e89977.

30. Cummings JH, Stephen AM. Carbohydrate terminology and classification. *Eur J Clin Nutr.* 2007;61(suppl 1):S5–S18.

31. Cummings JH, Macfarlane GT. Role of intestinal bacteria in nutrient metabolism. *JPEN J Parenter Enteral Nutr.* 1997;21:357–365.

32. Wong JM, de Souza R, Kendall CW, Emam A, Jenkins DJ. Colonic health: fermentation and short chain fatty acids. *J Clin Gastroenterol.* 2006;40:235–243.

33. Montalto M, Santoro L, D'Onofrio F, et al. Classification of malabsorption syndromes. *Dig Dis.* 2008;26:104–111.

34. Simren M, Stotzer PO. Use and abuse of hydrogen breath tests. *Gut.* 2006;55:297–303.

Test Your Knowledge Answers

1. **D**. Lactose, sucrose, and maltose are disaccharides. Amylose is a polysaccharide consisting of multiple glucose units.

2. **C**. Breast milk has very little complex carbohydrate.

3. **B**. Galactose and glucose.

4. **B**. Lactase activity at the start of the third trimester is < 25% of that at term.

5. **D**. Low amylase activity could result in malabsorption of the rice cereal, which is a starch, with a resultant increase in osmotic drag from the poorly absorbed carbohydrate and passage of the malabsorbed carbohydrate into the colon where it is fermented to SCFAs.

Fats

Peggy R. Borum, PhD

CONTENTS

Learning Objectives

1. Ability to list the different types of fatty acids.
2. Ability to contrast the different fatty acid oxidation pathways.
3. Ability to relate different pathological conditions to altered fat metabolism.

Introduction

Lipids are 1 of 3 macronutrients in the diet—the other 2 being carbohydrates and protein. Triglycerides (each containing 3 fatty acids) are one of the main storage forms of metabolic energy in the body. Since fatty acids are highly reduced hydrocarbons, they are calorically dense, providing more metabolic energy per gram than the other dietary macronutrients. This characteristic is advantageous when the patient has a limited stomach capacity, has fluid restrictions, and needs additional calories for growth or during critical illness. Fat is often viewed negatively by the public as a nutrient that should be reduced in the diet. However, the problem may not be excess fat, but rather excess calories. Once the diet provides appropriate calories, careful attention should be given to the types of fatty acid and amounts provided in the diet.

Different Types of Fat

Fats are diverse in structure, with uniformly poor solubility in water. Triglycerides are the major dietary form of lipid, but as already noted above, they consist of 3 fatty acids joined by a glycerol backbone. Typical fatty acids are carboxylic acids with hydrocarbon chains ranging from 4 to 24 carbons (see Figure 4-1). The chains are often unbranched but can contain a variety of substituents including rings, hydroxyl

Figure 4-1. The structure of typical fatty acids is a carboxylic acid with hydrocarbon chains ranging from 4 to 24 carbons. The image depicts the 18-carbon steric acid.

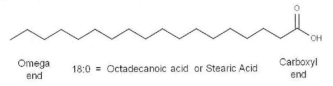

groups, and methyl groups. The chain can be saturated (no double bonds), monounsaturated (1 double bond), or polyunsaturated (2 or more double bonds).[1] As diagrammed in Figure 4-2, fatty acids can be classified according to the degree of chain saturation as well as their chain length. Though no consensus has been reached, fatty acids are frequently described in terms of their chain lengths: short (2–6 carbons), medium (8–12 carbons), and long (14 carbons or more). The chain lengths of the fatty acids contribute to both the physical characteristics of the food and the metabolism of the fat once it enters the body via ingestion, tube feeding, or parenteral nutrition (PN). The shorter and the more unsaturated the chain, the lower the melting point of the fat, making it liquid at room temperature. Thus, an animal product with a significant amount of stearic acid (18 carbons, no double bonds diagrammed in Figure 4-1) is solid at room temperature, whereas a medium-chain triglyceride oil (8–12 carbons) with a significant amount of saturated fatty acids can be liquid at room temperature, and olive oil with a higher

Figure 4-2. Fatty acids are classified based on the degree of chain saturation as well as their chain length.

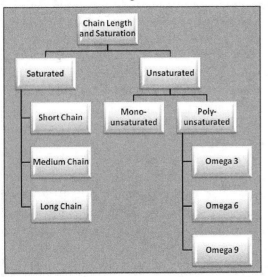

percentage of monounsaturated oleic acid (18 carbons, 1 double bond) is a liquid at room temperature.[1]

Membrane fluidity or viscosity is important in the function of many cell types and is greatly influenced by the degree of saturation of the fatty acids in the membrane phospholipids.[1] A 3-dimensional view of saturated fatty acids reveals that the hydrocarbon chains are straight and thus can be packed very tightly in membrane phospholipids. Most physiological unsaturated fatty acids have *cis* double bonds (ie, the chains on the same side of the double bond). Every *cis* double bond puts a "kink" or bend into the hydrocarbon chain. However, the fatty acid with *trans* double bonds is a straight hydrocarbon and can be packed very tightly in membranes, reducing membrane fluidity. Thus phospholipids containing *cis* unsaturated fatty acids cannot be packed as tightly, resulting in a membrane with increased fluidity. In the food industry, *trans* fatty acids (the chains are on the opposite side of the double bond) are made from unsaturated fatty acids both to change the consistency of the fat product and to make it less liquid-like at room temperature. Shelf life is increased by reducing the double bonds that make the fat product susceptible to rancidity. Increased concentration of polyunsaturated fatty acids in the membrane increases membrane susceptibility to oxidation and peroxidation. Because vitamin E is a major antioxidant in the membrane, an increase in dietary polyunsaturated fatty acids should always be accompanied by a careful evaluation of adequate vitamin E intake. Since the fatty acid composition of the membrane reflects the fatty acid composition of the diet, careful attention to the type of fatty acid in the diet is warranted.[2] Optimizing the dietary fatty acid profile can alter membrane structure provided to the body, which in turn can possibly alter cell signaling associated with clinical symptomatology.

Essential Fatty Acids

Two methods are used to number the carbons of a fatty acid. The chemist usually begins the numbering with the carboxylic acid carbon. In the field of nutrition, the numbering usually begins with the methyl carbon, or ω carbon, which is at the opposite end of the molecule from the carboxylic acid (see Figure 4-1). Using the ω system of numbering, an ω-3 fatty acid has its first double bond between C3 and C4 from the ω carbon, an ω-6 fatty acid has its first double bond between C6 and C7 from the ω carbon, and an ω-9 fatty acid has its first double bond between C9 and C10 from the ω carbon. Humans cannot synthesize ω-3 or ω-6 fatty acids, but many physiological processes are dependent on these fatty acids and their myriad products. Therefore, ω-3 and ω-6 fatty acids are required in the human diet and are termed "essential fatty acids."[1] The shortest chain ω-6 fatty acid is linoleic acid (LA). Humans can convert LA to arachidonic acid (ARA). The shortest chain ω-3 fatty acid is α-linolenic acid (αLA). Humans can convert αLA to eicosapentaeonic acid (EPA), and EPA very slowly to docosahexaenoic acid (DHA). The same enzyme pool is used to metabolize LA and αLA to their respective longer chain metabolites. The more prevalent fatty acid is preferentially metabolized. Thus, with a diet high in the ω-6 fatty acid LA, LA will be preferentially metabolized over the ω-3 fatty acid αLA. ARA (20-carbon polyunsaturated ω-6) and EPA (20-carbon polyunsaturated ω-3) are released from membranes and further metabolized to a cascade of eicosanoids. Although it is not quite so simple, eicosanoids from ω-6 fatty acids are generally considered proinflammatory and those from ω-3 fatty acids are considered weakly anti-inflammatory. The docosanoid products of DHA also have anti-inflammatory actions.[3] Transcription factors regulate gene expression. Fatty acids and eicosanoids can change the abundance of transcription factors, which in turn regulate gene expression. Thus, the fatty acid composition of the diet influences the composition of the cell membranes, which influences the availability of appropriate substrate to make either proinflammatory or anti-inflammatory fatty acid products. Three methods are available to diagnose essential fatty acid deficiency. Traditionally low intake of ω-3 and ω-6 fatty acids associated with an increase in an ω-9 fatty acid known as Mead acid in plasma has been used to diagnose essential fatty acid deficiency. A more recent method uses red blood cells and measures 2 additional parameters.[4] The emerging field of investigation known as of lipidomics measures all small molecular weight lipids in a sample and will likely provide the nutrition community with improved methods for specific essential fatty acid evaluation.

With the industrialization of Western society, dietary intake of the essential fatty acids has changed, reflecting the trend away from grains to more processed foods high in fat. Intake of LA relative to αLA has increased significantly. Currently the ratio of LA to αLA in the diet is 14:1 in contrast to the 2:1 or 1:1 ratio that is usually recommended.[2] Interestingly, the change in dietary fat intake follows a similar temporal pattern to the increase in inflammatory bowel disease incidence in the pediatric population.[5]

Different Functions of Adipose Tissue

Adipose tissue is not simply a place for the body to store fat. Adipose tissue is a complex organ with many different cell types containing receptors sensitive to inflammatory signals. Thus, changing the size of adipose tissue has far-reaching effects. When stimulated by signals accompanying changes in physiology, adipose tissue releases more than 20 diverse molecules known as adipokines that have a wide range of metabolic effects during both health and disease. Fat deposits in subcutaneous, intramuscular, and intrathoracic depots can differ in fatty acid composition, adipokine secretion, and storage capacity. Macrophage content of adipose tissue can increase from the usual 5%–10% to 60% during obesity and secrete an increasing amount of inflammatory cytokines. Taken together, obesity can have a striking effect not only on the size but also on the metabolism of the body.[2]

Storage of a metabolic fuel source and structural elements of membranes are the most generally recognized functions of fats. However, a long list of other functions for fat are now recognized as shown in Figure 4-3. Adipose tissue maintains a balance between clearance of plasma triglycerides and release of fatty acids. Excess dietary energy cannot be excreted. Diets with excess calories are frequently high in fat because dietary fat is highly palatable and calorically dense. Excess dietary energy from any of the macronutrients is converted to fatty acids and stored as triglycerides in adipocytes. Therefore, surplus dietary calories will increase adipose depots.

Importance of Dietary Fat in Infants

The percentage of total fetal body weight that is adipose tissue increases dramatically during human gestation. Fetal

Figure 4-3. Fat has multiple critical functions in the body.

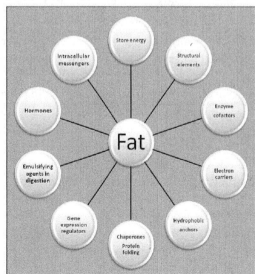

white adipose tissue increases at a rate of about 67 mg/d during the last trimester, and most of that is DHA. The brain also grows very rapidly during the last trimester and requires a large amount of DHA for the synthesis of myelin. At birth, the brain of the human is at about 50% of its adult size and continues to grow rapidly until reaching near-adult size at about 2 years of age. Thus, the extremely preterm infant born at 24 or 25 weeks of gestation requires a large amount of essential fatty acids, and ω-3 fatty acids in particular, to achieve the type of growth usually experienced by a fetus in utero during the same period post conception.[6,7]

Regulation of gene expression by nutrients is critically important in preterm neonates. Regulation of gene expression by ω-3 fatty acids involves multiple complex processes including regulation of the transcription factors sterol regulatory element–binding proteins and peroxisome proliferator-activated receptors that modulate many critical steps in metabolism.[8,9]

The 2 most abundant long-chain polyunsaturated fatty acids in the brain are DHA and ARA. DHA is concentrated in the prefrontal cortex and in some retinal cells.[10] Inadequate intake of ω-3 fatty acids not only results in decreased brain DHA but also increased brain ω-6 fatty acid concentration.[11,12] Worldwide, the various enteral products vary in their supply of ω-3 fatty acids and in DHA in particular. However, none of them provide the amount of essential fatty acids that would accumulate in the fetal brain during the last trimester of gestation without additional supplementation. Thus, the current diet provided to these infants appears to be deficient in DHA. Preterm infants fed increased amounts of DHA have been reported to have improved visual acuity and mental development.[13,14] A multicenter prospective, randomized, double-blind placebo-controlled trial in Italy compared 580 healthy term neonates receiving 20 mg of liquid DHA to 580 healthy term infants receiving placebo with a focus on developmental milestones. The infants receiving DHA were able to sit without support 1 week earlier, but the groups did not differ for hands-and-knees crawling, standing alone, and walking alone.[15] It is unclear how these data from healthy term neonates relate to preterm neonates. In infants being fed parenterally, the challenge to provide adequate DHA and ARA is even greater with the currently available lipid emulsions approved for use in this population.[16]

Digestion and Absorption

Since dietary lipids are hydrophobic, they must be hydrolyzed and emulsified to very small micelles before they can be absorbed by the intestine. Lingual and gastric lipases hydrolyze triglycerides to diglycerides and free fatty acids. After activation by colipase, pancreatic lipase hydrolyzes dietary fat to 2-monoglycerides, which are poor substrates for continued hydrolysis.[17] Gastric lipolysis is incomplete in adults, being responsible for 30% or less of dietary fat lipolysis.[18] Since neonates have limited expression of pancreatic enzymes needed for fat digestion in the intestine, gastric lipolysis has been assumed to have a more important role in neonates.[19] Supplementation of infant formula with medium-chain triglyceride has been reported to have conflicting effects on intragastric lipolysis in infants (no effect vs decreased lipolysis).[20] This finding may be related to differences in the medium-chain triglyceride concentration of the formula studied.[21]

The pH increases as the acidic stomach contents move to the intestine. The free fatty acid products of gastric lipase are ionized and become oriented to the outside of the oil droplets, which surrounds the oil droplet with charge and stabilizes the emulsion. Some of the free fatty acids dissociate from the droplet and interact with the intestinal epithelium. These fatty acids are potent stimuli of cholecystokinin release. Cholecystokinin stimulates an increase in pancreatic enzymes; relaxes the sphincter of Oddi, which allows the pancreatic juice to flow into the intestinal lumen; and contracts the gallbladder to provide a bolus of concentrated bile needed to form micelles (spheres of lipid that form in aqueous environments).[18] Secreted bile contains bile salts made in the liver that emulsify the products of lipid digestion. The resulting micelles transport the digested fat products through the aqueous intestinal lumen, making close contact with the brush border of the mucosal cells. Bile salts continue to the ileum where they are absorbed into the enterohepatic circulation.[17]

Phospholipase A_2 from the pancreas cleaves the fatty acid in the 2 position of dietary phospholipids. Pancreatic juice also contains cholesterol esterase, which hydrolyzes cholesterol esters; esters of vitamins A, D, and E; and all 3 fatty acids in triglycerides.[18] Cystic fibrosis affects many aspects of metabolism including adequate secretion of pancreatic enzymes for dietary fat absorption. Administration of pancreatic enzyme supplements can assist with the problem. Careful monitoring is required to ensure that children with cystic fibrosis do not develop essential fatty acid deficiency or deficiency in fat-soluble vitamins. Breast milk lipase produced by the mammary gland of lactating females is very similar to cholesterol esterase. Breast milk lipase also has broad specificity and may "predigest" the lipid components of breast milk and thus increase the efficiency of their uptake.[18,20]

Bile acids have an important role in solubilizing the products of luminal lipolysis and facilitating their transfer to the absorptive epithelium. Fatty acids and monoglycerides have enough solubility in the luminal contents that they can diffuse to the brush border and be absorbed.[17]

Role of Mucosal Cells During Enteral Nutrition

The intestinal epithelium is the site for some very important metabolic steps. The absorbed 2-monoglycerides are re-acylated to triglycerides. Several 1-monoglycerides in the emulsion are absorbed and hydrolyzed to fatty acids and glycerol. The glycerol released within the intestinal epithelium is reutilized for triglyceride synthesis. Long-chain fatty acids are esterified to triglycerides, secreted into the lymphatics as chylomicrons, and enter the blood via the thoracic duct. Free short-chain and medium-chain fatty acids are absorbed into the hepatic portal vein.[17]

Several different types of cells comprise the gastrointestinal mucosa. Each cell type has a separate role. The mucosal cells are intimately involved in not only digestion and absorption but also regulation of barrier function and immune homeostasis.[22] Many of these cells turn over rapidly, and their membranes contain components of cell signaling pathways. The mucosa is covered with mucus or a biofilm whose critical role in health is still under active investigation.[23] The role of dietary fatty acid profiles in the membrane health and optimal functioning of these cells is likely important in gastrointestinal health and the health of other organs.

Role of Gastrointestinal Microbiota During Enteral Nutrition

Nutritionists have long dealt with the deleterious effects of pathological gastrointestinal infections of different types of microbes, but they have also long recognized the benefit of gastrointestinal bacterial synthesis of such compounds as vitamin K. For many years, microbes in samples collected from humans could only be detected and studied if the laboratory could grow them using some culture technique. Development of nonculture techniques to identify and semiquantitate microbes has revealed that the gastrointestinal tract is actually an ecological niche for a huge number of bacteria, viruses, Archaea, and phages. The Human Microbiome Project has demonstrated that microbes on all surfaces of the human body impact human health.[24] The gastrointestinal bacterial community is probably the best studied, and this research has uncovered several surprising roles in promoting human health and disease, including malnutri-

tion in children.[25] As we continue to refine our assessment of malnutrition in the hospitalized patient and develop therapies, we need to consider the potential role of the gastrointestinal microbiome.[26]

Role of Mucosal Cells and Gastrointestinal Microbiota During PN

A naive approach would be to consider the gastrointestinal tract unimportant in the person receiving PN because it is not being used for digestion and absorption. However, it has been known for a long time that PN has dramatic effects on gastrointestinal structure and is associated with increased risks of infection. The gastrointestinal microbiome likely plays a role in both. The signaling of microbiota to host cells and the signaling of host cells to microbiota likely involves cellular membranes that can be altered by the fat metabolism. A 2014 American Society for Parenteral and Enteral Nutrition research workshop addressed the implications of these new microbiome data on the practice of nutritional support.[27]

Metabolism During Normal Physiology

Dietary fat can enter a diverse set of metabolic pathways that are intricately controlled and coordinated to meet the needs of the body. The cell can either oxidize fatty acids for immediate metabolic energy or synthesize fatty acids from other dietary components and store them for later use.

Synthesis of Fatty Acids

Excess calories in the form of protein, carbohydrate, or fat cannot be eliminated from the body once ingested or administered and must be stored in the form of fatty acids. Six cytosolic enzymes plus an acyl carrier protein are needed for fatty acid synthesis from acetyl-CoA. In the first step, malonyl-CoA is formed from acetyl-CoA, which has been shuttled out of the mitochondria. This reaction forming malonyl-CoA is the regulatory step for fatty acid synthesis. The sequence of subsequent reactions is a condensation, a reduction, a dehydration, and a second reduction. Both reduction reactions use nicotinamide adenine dinucleotide phosphate (NADPH) as the electron donor. The sequence of reactions adds 2 carbons at a time and is repeated until a chain length of about 16 carbons is made and released from the acyl carrier protein.[1]

As discussed in the Essential Fatty Acids section, humans cannot synthesize LA or αLA. Although humans have the necessary enzymes to make EPA from αLA and DHA from EPA, the capacity to do so is very low.[28] Only about 5% of αLA can be converted to EPA and < 0.5% of αLA can be converted to DHA. The capacity to convert LA to ARA is also low. Thus, although only LA and αLA are termed essential fatty acids, the administration of only LA or αLA often has only a negligible effect on plasma ARA, EPA, and DHA.[28,29] The optimal ratio of preformed EPA and DHA has not been established, but ratios of 1:2 to 2:1 are expected to be effective.[30]

β-Oxidation of Long-Chain Fatty Acids in Mitochondria

Lipoprotein lipase in the capillary endothelium releases free fatty acids, which are delivered to tissues by chylomicrons. Hormone-sensitive lipase mobilizes triglycerides from adipose tissue when needed. The fatty acids are carried in the blood bound to albumin and delivered to the tissues to use for fuel. When fatty acids are to be used for fuel, they are activated to the fatty acyl-CoA at the outer mitochondrial membrane. Fatty acyl-CoA is the correct high-energy state for β-oxidation, but the enzymes for β-oxidation are located within the mitochondrial matrix (see Figure 4-3), and the fatty acyl-CoA cannot cross the inner membrane of the mitochondria to reach these enzymes. In order to use long-chain fatty acids for metabolic energy, fatty acyl-CoA is converted to fatty acyl-carnitine via carnitine palmitoyltransferase 1, transported across the inner mitochondrial membrane via carnitine acylcarnitine translocase in exchange for free carnitine, and reconverted to fatty acyl-CoA in the matrix of the mitochondria via carnitine palmitoyltransferase 2. The end result is that the high-energy fatty acyl-CoA is now in the same location as the metabolic machinery for β-oxidation. Fatty acid oxidation and fatty acid synthesis do not occur at the same time because malonyl-CoA (an early intermediate in fatty acid synthesis) inhibits carnitine palmitoyltransferase1 and thus prevents the fatty acyl-CoA from reaching the site of β-oxidation.[1,31]

Patients with high plasma levels of triglycerides are sometimes given heparin (assuming that it will stimulate lipolysis of triglycerides) and carnitine (assuming it will stimulate β-oxidation of the released fatty acids). Definitive data to confirm these assumptions in patients on special nutrition support are yet to be obtained. In addition, it should be remembered that supplemented heparin and carnitine each have a variety of effects on the body's metabolism.

β-Oxidation of Medium-Chain Fatty Acids in Mitochondria

In liver cells, medium-chain fatty acids are transported into mitochondria (see Figure 4-4) as free fatty acids and then activated to medium-chain fatty acyl-CoA. Therefore, oxidation of medium-chain fatty acids is carnitine independent in the liver. However, other tissues activate medium-chain fatty acids to medium-chain fatty acyl-CoA on the cytoplasmic side of the inner mitochondrial membrane and require the carnitine shuttle for β-oxidation.[32,33] Thus, if dietary medium-chain fatty acids are provided in quantities in which they are expected to be a fuel substrate for skeletal muscle, carnitine will be required for their oxidation.

Steps of β-Oxidation

In mitochondria, 4 repeating reactions (dehydrogenation requiring flavin adenine dinucleotide, hydration, dehydrogenation requiring nicotinamide adenine dinucleotide, and cleavage requiring coenzyme A or CoA) produce a fatty acyl-CoA shortened by 2 carbons and acetyl-CoA. The shortened fatty acyl-CoA reenters the sequence, and the acetyl-CoA is oxidized to carbon dioxide in the citric acid cycle. The citric acid cycle coupled to the oxidative phosphorylation pathway yields metabolic energy as adenosine triphosphate. Oxidation of unsaturated fatty acids requires 2 additional enzymes in the mitochondria to deal with the double bonds.[1]

β-Oxidation of Very Long-Chain Fatty Acids in Peroxisomes

Peroxisomes are subcellular organelles in the cytoplasm that carry out β-oxidation in 4 repeating steps similar to those in the mitochondria. The difference is that the first reaction transfers electrons directly to oxygen, producing hydrogen peroxide. Peroxisomes oxidize very long-chain fatty acids (see Figure 4-4) and branched fatty acids. Fatty acids enter the peroxisome before they are esterified to fatty

Figure 4-4. Oxidation of medium-chain, long-chain, and very long-chain fatty acids in mitochondria.

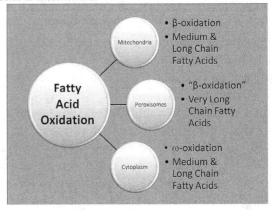

acyl-CoA, so the carnitine shuttle is not needed to deliver the fatty acids to the peroxisomes. The very long-chain fatty acids are shortened by 2 carbons during each reaction sequence producing the shortened fatty acyl-CoA and acetyl CoA. When the fatty acyl-CoA is a medium-chain fatty acyl-CoA, the oxidation sequence stops. Acetyl-CoA and the medium-chain fatty acyl-CoA must be transported out of the peroxisome via a carnitine shuttle. The medium-chain fatty acylcarnitine is transported into mitochondria to complete the oxidation to acetyl-CoA.[1]

ω-Oxidation of Fatty Acids

ω-Oxidation of fatty acids occurs in the endoplasmic reticulum in the cytoplasm (see Figure 4-4). The ω carbon is first converted to an alcohol by a cytochrome P450 mixed function oxidase, which requires both oxygen and NADPH. Alcohol dehydrogenase and aldehyde dehydrogenase convert the alcohol to a carboxylic acid on the ω carbon. Thus, the fatty acid is converted to a dicarboxylic acid, which can be esterified to carnitine and transported to the mitochondrial matrix. There it can enter the β-oxidation pathway to be shortened at both ends of the molecule at the same time. ω-Oxidation of fatty acids is normally a minor pathway. Dysfunctional β-oxidation in the mitochondria will increase ω-oxidation.[34]

Long-Chain Fatty Acids as Substrates for Cascades

In addition to providing substrates to make important cell structures and substrates to produce metabolic fuel, fatty acids are often used in signaling pathways. The 2 essential fatty acids and their elongated metabolites are the beginning of 2 enormous cascades controlling many aspects of physiology.[3] If the dietary supply is inadequate in either essential fatty acid or if the dietary ratio of the 2 essential fatty acids is inappropriate, one would expect pathophysiology. Both of these situations frequently occur in patients.

Metabolism During Pathophysiologies

Many chronic pathological conditions, including type 2 diabetes, hypertension, atherosclerosis, and obesity, are associated with altered fat metabolism. In some situations, inappropriate dietary fat quantity and/or composition contribute to the observed pathology.

Fat as Fuel for Preterm Infants

Early introduction of lipid emulsions to preterm neonates has not been shown to increase complications,[35] but it also has not been shown to improve short-term growth or prevent morbidity and mortality.[36] An emulsion with a mixture of medium-chain and long-chain fatty acids appears to be superior to an emulsion containing only long-chain fatty acids in terms of incorporation of essential fatty acids and long-chain polyunsaturated fatty acids into circulating lipids.[37] Adequate energy intake during the first days of life is associated with improved brain function. A recent study of 148 extremely low birth weight survivors showed that every 42 kJ/kg/d (10 kcal/kg/d) provided during the first postnatal week was associated with a 4.6-point increase in the Mental Development Index.[38]

Fat as Fuel for Home PN in Pediatrics

As previously discussed, ω-3 fatty acids including EPA and DHA, sometimes called fish oils, have several important functions in the body both during health and disease. Twelve children with pediatric short bowel syndrome who developed PN-associated liver disease received parenteral ω-3 fatty acids while awaiting liver transplant. They showed restoration of liver function to the point that 9 of the children were no longer considered for liver transplant. The remaining 3 children received a liver transplant with no complications attributable to the ω-3 emulsion.[39] In another study, 18 infants who developed cholestasis while receiving a parenteral emulsion high in ω-6 fatty acids were switched to an emulsion high in ω-3 fatty acids and compared to 21 historical controls who had similar symptoms and had been maintained on the ω-6 fatty acid emulsion. Patients receiving the ω-3 fatty acids experienced a reversal of cholestasis 6.8 times faster when the data were adjusted for baseline bilirubin concentration, gestational age, and diagnosis of necrotizing enterocolitis. The ω-3 fatty acid cohort had 2 deaths and no liver transplants, and the historical control cohort had 7 deaths and 2 liver transplantations.[40]

Parenteral lipid emulsions containing fish oil are still not approved for use in children, nor are they available in the United States.

To Esterify or to Oxidize—That Is the Cell's Question

The ability to synthesize or to oxidize fatty acids allows the cell to store excess calories as fat and to mobilize the stored fatty acids for metabolic fuel, which is a lifesaving adaptation during times of starvation. When products of digested macronutrients enter the cell during normal physiological situations, the cell responds to metabolic signals indicating the metabolic fuel status of the cell and either uses the fuel substrates to produce needed metabolic energy or stores the fuel substrate as fatty acids in triglycerides. However, if excess calories are chronically delivered to the cell, the ability of adipose tissue to serve as a "sink" and protect nonadipose tissues from fatty acid "spillover" appears to become saturated. As diagrammed in Figure 4-5, the result is lipid overload, or lipotoxicity, that overwhelms the abilities of both the endoplasmic reticulum and mitochondria to maintain cellular homeostasis and results in systemic release of both free fatty acids and inflammatory cytokines. Accumulation of fatty acids in skeletal muscle, heart, liver, and pancreas is likely the underlying factor in the development of insulin resistance, cardiomyopathy, liver steatosis, and type 2 diabetes. During normal physiological conditions, the use of fatty acids for energy and the use of glucose for energy are intricately coordinated. Likewise, during chronic intake of excess calories, excess lipids inhibit the utilization of glucose, and hyperglycemia interferes with fatty acid catabolism resulting in a situation some have termed "glucolipotoxicity."[41] Intake of excess carbohydrate increases cellular malonyl-CoA concentrations, which in turn inhibits carnitine palmitoyltransferase 1 activity, impairing β-oxidation of fatty acids. Insulin resistance is associated not only with the intake of excess calories but also with high intakes of saturated fat. Substituting saturated fat with unsaturated fat seems to improve insulin sensitivity.[42]

Metabolism of dietary fat is altered in overweight patients. For example, overweight patients with a fatty liver have a higher postprandial triglyceride response and an increased production of large very low-density lipoproteins after a fat load compared to control subjects.[43] When providing nutrition support, it is important to not only provide appropriate calories for the specific patient but also carefully evaluate how the patient's current metabolic status may impact the body's metabolism of the nutritional fat substrate provided.

Figure 4-5. Schematic of the steps leading to lipotoxicity.

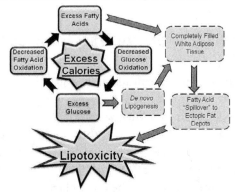

Test Your Knowledge Questions

1. In order to maintain health and prevent a patient receiving home PN from becoming overweight, the optimal nutrition support prescription
   A. restricts fat to an absolute minimum, while providing a generous amount of glucose.
   B. provides adequate calories including a fatty acid blend with appropriate chain length, chain saturation, and ratios of LA, αLA, ARA, EPA, and DHA.
   C. provides 80% of the calories recommended for oral intake.
   D. provides all the fat calories as the essential fatty acids LA and αLA.

2. The cellular site(s) for fatty acid oxidation in the body is (are)
   A. mitochondria.
   B. peroxisomes.
   C. cytoplasm.
   D. mitochondria, peroxisomes, and cytoplasm.

3. The essential fatty acid needs of a critically ill 24-week neonate in the neonatal intensive care unit requires dietary
   A. LA and αLA.
   B. αLA and DHA.
   C. LA and ARA.
   D. LA, αLA, ARA, and DHA.

References

1. Nelson DL, Cox MM. *Lehniger Principles of Biochemistry*. 6th ed. New York, NY: W.H. Freeman and Company; 2013.
2. Innis SM. Dietary lipids in early development: relevance to obesity, immune and inflammatory disorders. *Curr Opin Endocrinol Diabetes Obes*. 2007;14(5):359–364.
3. Maskrey BH, Megson IL, Rossi AG, Whitfield PD. Emerging importance of omega-3 fatty acids in the innate immune response: molecular mechanisms and lipidomic strategies for their analysis. *Mol Nutr Food Res*. 2013;57(8):1390–400.
4. Fokkema MR, Smit EN, Martini IA, Woltil HA, Boersma ER, Muskiet FAJ. Assessment of essential fatty acid and omega 3-fatty acid status by measurement of erythrocyte 20:3ω9 (Mead acid), 22:5ω6/20:4ω6 and 22:5ω6/22:6ω3. *Prostaglandins Leukot Essent Fatty Acids*. 2002;67(5):345–356.
5. Innis SM, Jacobson K. Dietary lipids in early development and intestinal inflammatory disease. *Nutr Rev*. 2007;65(12 Pt 2):S188–S193.
6. Marszalek JR, Lodish HF. Docosahexaenoic acid, fatty acid-interacting proteins, and neuronal function: breastmilk and fish are good for you. *Annu Rev Cell Dev Biol*. 2005;21:633–657.
7. Heird WC, Lapillonne A. The role of essential fatty acids in development. *Annu Rev Nutr*. 2005;25:549–571.

8. Deckelbaum RJ, Worgall TS, Seo T. n-3 fatty acids and gene expression. *Am J Clin Nutr.* 2006;83(6):1520S–1525S.

9. Georgiadi A, Kersten S. Mechanisms of gene regulation by fatty acids. *Adv Nutr.* 2012;3(2):127–134.

10. Agostoni C. Role of long-chain polyunsaturated fatty acids in the first year of life. *J Pediatr Gastroenterol Nutr.* 2008;47(suppl 2):S41–S44.

11. Innis SM. Dietary omega 3 fatty acids and the developing brain. *Brain Res.* 2008;1237:35–43.

12. Novak EM, Dyer RA, Innis SM. High dietary omega-6 fatty acids contribute to reduced docosahexaenoic acid in the developing brain and inhibit secondary neurite growth. *Brain Res.* 2008;1237:136–145.

13. Hay WW Jr. Strategies for feeding the preterm infant. *Neonatology.* 2008;94(4):245–254.

14. Innis SM. Omega-3 Fatty acids and neural development to 2 years of age: do we know enough for dietary recommendations? *J Pediatr Gastroenterol Nutr.* 2009;48(suppl 1):S16–S24.

15. Agostoni C, Zuccotti GV, Radaelli G, et al. Docosahexaenoic acid supplementation and time at achievement of gross motor milestones in healthy infants: a randomized, prospective, double-blind, placebo-controlled trial. *Am J Clin Nutr.* 2009;89(1):64–70.

16. Vanek VW, Seidner DL, Allen P, et al; Novel Nutrient Task Force, Intravenous Fat Emulsions Workgroup; American Society for Parenteral and Enteral Nutrition (A.S.P.E.N.) Board of Directors. A.S.P.E.N. position paper: clinical role for alternative intravenous fat emulsions. *Nutr Clin Pract.* 2012;27(2):150–192.

17. Bender DA, Mayes PA. Nutrition, digestion, & absorption. In: Murray RK, Bender DA, Botham KM, Kennelly PJ, Rodwell VW, Weil PA, eds. *Harper's Illustrated Biochemistry.* 29th ed. New York, NY: McGraw-Hill; 2012. http://accesspharmacy.mhmedical.com/content.aspx?bookid=389&Sectionid=40142523. Accessed January 7, 2015.

18. Barrett KE. Lipid assimilation. In: Barrett KE, ed. *Gastrointestinal Physiology.* New York, NY: McGraw-Hill; 2006.

19. Hamosh M. Digestion in the newborn. *Clin Perinatol.* 1996;23(2):191–209.

20. Hernell O, Blackberg L. Human milk bile salt-stimulated lipase: functional and molecular aspects. *J Pediatr.* 1994;125(5 Pt 2):S56–S61.

21. Hamosh M, Bitman J, Liao TH, et al. Gastric lipolysis and fat absorption in preterm infants: effect of medium-chain triglyceride or long-chain triglyceride-containing formulas. *Pediatrics.* 1989;83(1):86–92.

22. Peterson LW, Artis D. Intestinal epithelial cells: regulators of barrier function and immune homeostasis. *Nat Rev Immunol.* 2014;14(3):141–153.

23. Johansson ME, Sjovall H, Hansson GC. The gastrointestinal mucus system in health and disease. *Nat Rev Gastroenterol Hepatol.* 2013;10(6):352–361.

24. Ursell LK, Metcalf JL, Parfrey LW, Knight R. Defining the human microbiome. *Nutr Rev.* 2012;70(suppl 1):S38–S44.

25. Fujimura KE, Slusher NA, Cabana MD, Lynch SV. Role of the gut microbiota in defining human health. *Expert Rev Anti Infect Ther.* 2010;8(4):435–454.

26. Mehta NM, Corkins MR, Lyman B, et al; American Society for Parenteral and Enteral Nutrition Board of Directors. Defining pediatric malnutrition: a paradigm shift toward etiology-related definitions. *JPEN J Parenter Enteral Nutr.* 2013;37(4):460–481.

27. Alverdy J, Gilbert J, DeFazio JR, et al. Proceedings of the 2014 A.S.P.E.N. Research workshop: the interface between nutrition and the gut microbiome: implications and applications for human health. *JPEN J Parenter Enteral Nutr.* 2014;38(2):167–178.

28. Russo GL. Dietary n-6 and n-3 polyunsaturated fatty acids: from biochemistry to clinical implications in cardiovascular prevention. *Biochem Pharmacol.* 2009;77(6):937–946.

29. Plourde M, Cunnane SC. Extremely limited synthesis of long chain polyunsaturates in adults: implications for their dietary essentiality and use as supplements. *Appl Physiol Nutr Metab.* 2007;32(4):619–634.

30. Harris WS, Mozaffarian D, Lefevre M, et al. Towards establishing dietary reference intakes for eicosapentaenoic and docosahexaenoic acids. *J Nutr.* 2009;139(4):804S–819S.

31. Rasmussen BB, Wolfe RR. Regulation of fatty acid oxidation in skeletal muscle. *Annu Rev Nutr.* 1999;19:463–484.

32. Groot PHE, Hulsmann WC. The activation and oxidation of octanoate and palmitate by rat skeletal muscle mitochondria. *Biochim Biophys Acta.* 1973;316:124–135.

33. Rössle C, Carpentier YA, Richelle M, et al. Medium-chain triglycerides induce alterations in carnitine metabolism. *Am J Physiol Endocrinol Metab.* 1990;258:E944–E947.

34. Croston G. Biocarta omega oxidation pathway. http://www.biocarta.com/pathfiles/omegaoxidationPathway.asp. Accessed May 31, 2014.

35. Drenckpohl D, McConnell C, Gaffney S, Niehaus M, Macwan KS. Randomized trial of very low birth weight infants receiving higher rates of infusion of intravenous fat emulsions during the first week of life. *Pediatrics.* 2008;122(4):743–751.

36. Simmer K, Rao SC. Early introduction of lipids to parenterally-fed preterm infants. *Cochrane Database Syst Rev.* 2005;(2):CD005256.

37. Krohn K, Koletzko B. Parenteral lipid emulsions in paediatrics. *Curr Opin Clin Nutr Metab Care.* 2006;9(3):319–323.

38. Stephens BE, Walden RV, Gargus RA, et al. First-week protein and energy intakes are associated with 18-month developmental outcomes in extremely low birth weight infants. *Pediatrics.* 2009;123(5):1337–1343.

39. Diamond IR, Sterescu A, Pencharz PB, Kim JH, Wales PW. Changing the paradigm: omegaven for the treatment of liver failure in pediatric short bowel syndrome. *J Pediatr Gastroenterol Nutr.* 2009;48(2):209–215.

40. Gura KM, Lee S, Valim C, et al. Safety and efficacy of a fish-oil-based fat emulsion in the treatment of parenteral nutrition-associated liver disease. *Pediatrics.* 2008;121(3):e678–e686.

41. Brenna JT, Salem N Jr, Sinclair AJ, Cunnane SC; International Society for the Study of Fatty Acids and Lipids, ISSFAL. alpha-Linolenic acid supplementation and conversion to n-3 long-chain polyunsaturated fatty acids in humans. *Prostaglandins Leukot Essent Fatty Acids.* 2009;80(2–3):85–91.

42. Riserus U. Fatty acids and insulin sensitivity. *Curr Opin Clin Nutr Metab Care.* 2008;11(2):100-105.

43. Assy N, Nassar F, Nasser G, Grosovski M. Olive oil consumption and non-alcoholic fatty liver disease. *World J Gastroenterol.* 2009;15(15):1809–1815.

Test Your Knowledge Answers

1. Correct answer is **B**. The problems of overweight and obesity are the result of excess calories and not simply too much fat. In addition to customizing the caloric intake to meet the individual patient's needs, the ideal nutrition support will provide appropriate ratios of pre-formed LA, αLA, ARA, EPA, and DHA that cannot be made in adequate amounts by the patient.

2. Correct answer is **D**. Medium-chain and long-chain fatty acids are oxidized in mitochondria. Very long-chain fatty acids are oxidized in peroxisomes and mitochondria. Although it is normally a minor pathway, ω-oxidation in the endoplasmic reticulum of the cytoplasm becomes important if mitochondrial dysfunction occurs.

3. Correct answer is **D**. The neonate cannot synthesize LA or αLA. Although the enzymes are present to convert LA to ARA and αLA to EPA and DHA, the capacity to do so is not adequate to meet the needs of the neonate.

5

Protein Digestion, Absorption, and Metabolism

Richard A. Helms, PharmD; Oscar R. Herrera, PharmD; and John A. Kerner, MD

CONTENTS

Learning Objectives

1. Explain how protein metabolism and physiology are profoundly affected by the ontogeny of the gastrointestinal tract.
2. Describe the roles of the liver and kidney in amino acid metabolism.
3. Understand the functions of amino acids and proteins, protein requirements for age, and protein energy ratios during growth.
4. Discuss protein turnover, assessment of plasma amino acids, and nitrogen balance.

Introduction

An extraordinary range of knowledge exists related to protein in human nutrition. The basics of protein in adult nutrition have been nicely reviewed in *The A.S.P.E.N. Nutrition Support Core Curriculum*, and materials covered in that publication will not be extensively revisited here.[1] Because this chapter is restricted to protein in pediatrics, it will focus particularly on the rapidly developing neonate and infant. Ontogenic events relating to protein metabolism and physiology render the small child much different from the older child and adult. This chapter will review aspects of digestion, absorption, and metabolism of protein focusing on these differences.

Ontogeny of the Gastrointestinal Tract in Relation to Protein

The gastrointestinal (GI) tract has been described as the largest endocrine organ. It produces numerous regulatory gut peptides that are involved in GI tract development, growth, absorption, secretion, and gut motility. They function in

Table 5-1. Gastrointestinal Regulatory Peptides[2]

REGULATORY PEPTIDE	SOURCES	MECHANISMS	ACTIONS
Epidermal growth factor	Salivary glands Brunner glands Paneth cells	Hormone Paracrine	– Stimulates mucosal proliferation and differentiation – Regulates gastrointestinal secretion – Has cytoprotective/ulcer-healing effects
Insulin-like growth factor	Gastrointestinal tract Liver	Hormone Autocrine Paracrine	– Stimulates crypt cell proliferation and enterocyte differentiation – Promotes intestinal adaptation
Enteroglucagon	Ileum Colon	Hormone	– Stimulates gut mucosal growth – Regulates gut motility
Neurotensin	Ileum Central nervous system	Hormone Neurocrine	– Inhibits gastric emptying and acid secretion
Vasoactive intestinal polypeptide	All tissues	Neurocrine	– Promotes secretomotor, vasodilatation, and smooth muscle relaxation
Pancreatic polypeptide	Pancreas	Hormone	– Inhibits pancreatic enzyme secretion and gallbladder contraction
Motilin	Proximal small intestine	Hormone	– Stimulates gastrointestinal motility
Peptide YY	Gastrointestinal tract Central nervous system	Hormone Paracrine Neurocrine	– Inhibits gastric acid secretion and gut motility

Reprinted from Gilger MA. Normal gastrointestinal function. Table 342-1. In: McMillan JA, Feigin RD, DeAngelis C, Jones MD, eds. *Oski's Pediatrics*. 4th ed. Copyright © 2006 with permission from Lippincott Williams & Wilkins.

classic endocrine, autocrine, paracrine, and neurocrine pathways.[2,3] Selected GI regulatory peptides involved with the ontogeny of the GI tract as it relates to proteins are outlined in Table 5-1. All of these peptides are present by the end of the first trimester in the fetus, but adult levels may not be present until term.[4] The peptides that function as hormones are released in response to feeding. The release of some of these hormones is limited in the newborn compared to the adult.[4,5]

Significant differences exist in the ontogeny of the two main enzymes secreted by the gastric mucosa. In the human, even though both pepsin and gastric lipase are located at the same site (ie, in the chief cells of the gastric mucosa), the enzymes have different developmental patterns.[6] Pepsin activity and output are much lower in infants than adults.[7,8] In contrast, gastric lipase activity and output are equal in infants and adults.[7,8]

The ontogeny of the brush border amino-oligopeptidases as well as the dipeptide and amino acid transport systems parallel that of the carbohydrate enzymes. Amino-oligopeptidases are first detected immunohistochemically by 10–16 weeks gestation and their activity progressively increases during development. By 28–30 weeks gestation, enzyme levels are approximately one-half of the values found in term infants. Proteolytic activity increases rapidly after birth in premature and full-term infants.[9]

Protein Digestion

Initial protein digestion occurs in the stomach, where proteins are exposed to hydrochloric acid (HCl) and pepsin. Gastric acid produces an acidic environment in the stomach and denatures protein.[10,11] Although protein digestive activity within the GI tract has been identified as early as 16 weeks gestation, gastric acid secretion is relatively low and consequently less protein denaturation occurs in both preterm and term infants. In fact, there is relatively minimal functional protein digestion in the stomach in the first few weeks of life. It is not until about 2 years of age that adult levels of gastric acid secretion are reached.[9]

Chief cells secrete proenzymes (pepsinogen 1 and 2) into the stomach, which undergo auto-activation to form pepsins in the acidic milieu.[12] This acidic environment is critical for pepsin function as evidenced by its inactivity in the duodenum, where the pH is neutral.[13] These pepsins function as endopeptidases; they hydrolyze internal bonds of the polypeptides to primarily form shorter polypeptides, oligopeptides, and some free amino acids.[9,11] Gastrin stimulates both gastric acid and pepsin production and secretion, which initiates protein digestion in the stomach.[10]

The protein denaturation within the stomach does not appear to be critical because patients with a more neutral gastric pH do not have impaired protein digestion. However, the amino acids that are produced from protein digestion in the stomach do assist in releasing cholecystokinin (CCK) or pancreozymin.[12] CCK has a role in protein digestion by helping to release pancreatic digestive enzymes, stimulate gallbladder contraction, and relax the sphincter of Oddi.[11,12] CCK is released by the I cells located in the mucosal epithelium of the small intestine (mostly in the duodenum and jejunum). In contrast, the hormone secretin promotes pancreatic secretion of bicarbonate-rich fluid to help establish a favorable pH.[10]

The pancreatic digestive enzymes are secreted in their inactive proenzyme form, similar to the secretion of pepsin as pepsinogen in the stomach. The pancreas secretes both endopeptidases (trypsinogen, chymotrypsinogen, and proelastase) and exopeptidases (procarboxypeptidase A and B) into the proximal small intestine.[11] The activated endopeptidases and exopeptidases hydrolyze the proteins at peptide bonds within the polypeptide chains to form oligopeptides and at the carboxyl terminal to form single amino acids, respectively.[9–11]

Bile acids and trypsinogen together cause the release of enterokinase, a brush border enzyme, which converts trypsinogen into its active form trypsin. Trypsin then converts the remaining pancreatic peptidases into their respective active forms (chymotrypsin, elastase, and carboxypeptidase A and B) and assists in forming more trypsin from trypsinogen (see Figure 5-1).[9,10,13] Overall, the products of luminal protein digestion are about 70% oligopeptides and 30% free amino acids.[9]

Figure 5-1. Pancreatic Enzyme Activation[10]

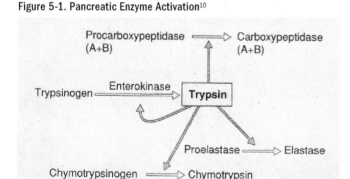

Reprinted from Wahbeh GT, Christie DL. Basic aspects of digestion and absorption. In: Wyllie R, Hyams JS, eds. *Pediatric Gastrointestinal and Liver Disease: Pathophysiology, Diagnosis, Management*. 3rd ed. Copyright © 2006 with permission from Elsevier.

Enterokinase and trypsin have been detected at 26 and 28 weeks gestation, respectively. Enterokinase levels at the time of birth are about 10% of adult levels except in those rare infants with congenital enterokinase deficiency.[9,14] Trypsin activity in duodenal juice of the premature infant is slightly less than in the full-term infant, but it does increase in response to food as in full-term infants. Infants have been found to have decreased trypsin activity in duodenal fluid compared with older children.[15] This reduced trypsin activity has been demonstrated to increase over the first 4 months of life, possibly resulting from the infants' relatively increased enteral protein intake.[9] However, the significance of these differences is unclear given that protein digestion and absorption are fairly efficient even in preterm infants. Term infants digest and absorb about 80%–85% of luminal proteins, while estimates for adults range from 95% to 98%.[9,11]

Protein Absorption

Normal protein absorption involves luminal processing, absorption into the intestinal mucosa, and transport into the circulation.[12] The brush border of enterocytes has different types of peptidases, including oligopeptidases, that further hydrolyze the partially digested proteins into amino acids, dipeptides, and tripeptides (see Figure 5-2).[9,10,12,16] Oligopeptidases have been detected as early as 10–16 weeks gestation, and they increase to nearly half of full-term levels by 28–30 weeks gestation.[9]

Absorption into the enterocyte involves both sodium-dependent and sodium-independent transport systems.[9] The sodium-dependent amino acid transporters are driven by a low intracellular sodium concentration and negative intracellular potential resulting from the sodium-potassium-adenosine triphosphatase (Na+-K+ ATPase) pump.[12] Many different transporters exist, including ones for neutral, acidic, and basic amino acids with narrow substrate specificity and for dipeptides and tripeptides with a broad substrate specificity (see Figure 5-3).[9,10,12,16]

Once the amino acids are transported into the cytoplasm, they undergo additional processing by cytoplasmic peptidases, mostly dipeptidases and tripeptidases, which convert the dipeptides and tripeptides into free amino acids.[10,12,13] Although most of these amino acids are transported into the blood stream, approximately 10% of amino acids, particularly glutamine and glutamic acid, are used directly by the enterocyte.[10,13] Luminal protein sources are more readily used than systemic protein, especially in apical

Figure 5-2. Overview of Protein Digestion and Absorption

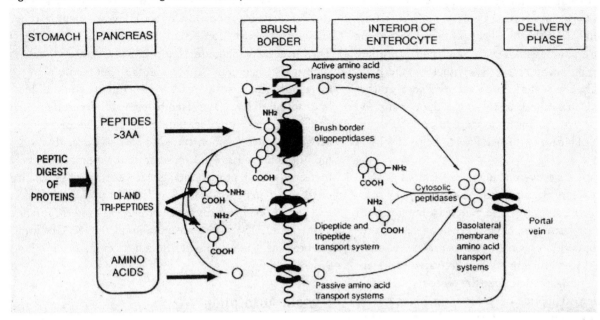

Reprinted from Roy CC, Silverman A, Alagille D. *Pediatric Clinical Gastroenterology.* Malabsorption syndrome. p. 307. (Modified and published with permission from Ahnen DJ. Protein digestion and assimilation. In: Yamada T, et al, eds. *Textbook of Gastroenterology.* Philadelphia, PA: Lippincott Williams & Wilkins; 1991.) Copyright © 1995 with permission from Elsevier.

Figure 5-3. The Transport of Amino Acids

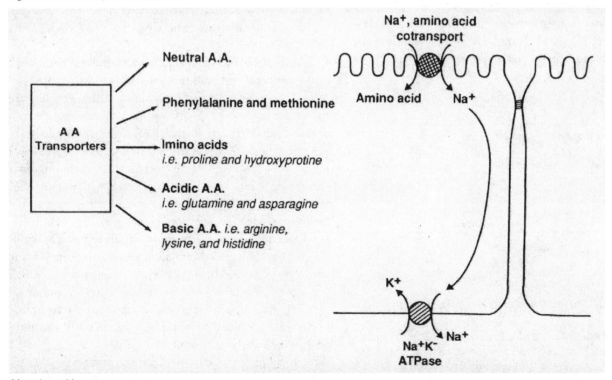

AA, amino acid.
Reprinted from Roy CC, Silverman A, Alagille D. *Pediatric Clinical Gastroenterology.* 4th ed. Copyright © 1995 with permission from Elsevier.

villous cells. Animals receiving parenteral nutrition (PN) without enteral feeds develop mucosal atrophy.[10]

Some of the sodium-independent amino acid transporters are located on the basolateral surface of the enterocyte and function to transport amino acids into the portal vein.[9] Although a significant majority of the protein that enters the portal circulation is in the form of free amino acids, small amounts of dipeptides and tripeptides enter the blood stream intact through normal transport systems.[10]

Studies have shown that an infant's intestine may have a higher capacity for absorption of macromolecules than the adult intestine.[17] Thus, among susceptible infants (eg, infants who sustain severe postinfectious villous injury and extensive injury from necrotizing enterocolitis), the early introduction of specific foods of increased antigenic potential may increase their risk of protein sensitization.[18,19]

Given the broad substrate specificity for dipeptidase and tripeptidase at the brush border, it is not surprising that clinically significant deficiencies resulting from specific amino acid transport abnormalities are uncommon. Two of the more well-known inherited defects of protein absorption include Hartnup syndrome and cystinuria. In Hartnup syndrome, neutral amino acid transport is defective and patients present with pellagra-like skin eruptions. In cystinuria (see Chapter 24), a defect in cystine reabsorption results in excessive cystine in the urine and subsequent renal stone formation. In contrast, acquired defects of protein absorption, including exocrine pancreatic insufficiency and transient brush border enzyme deficiency from gastroenteritis, are more common.[8]

Digestion and Absorption of Whey and Casein

The major proteins in milk are whey and casein. The protein content of unmodified cow's milk is approximately 18% whey and 82% casein. When this unheated casein-predominant substance enters the acidic environment of the stomach, it forms a relatively hard curd of casein and minerals that can be difficult to digest. In contrast, human milk protein is approximately 60%–70% whey and 30%–40% casein.[20,21] Human milk forms a very small, soft curd in acid. Some infant formula companies have developed whey-predominant formulas by combining equal amounts of demineralized whey protein and skim milk protein to yield a formula with 60% whey and 40% casein.

Other important differences exist between these 2 types of proteins. Whey results in a faster gastric emptying time, and is overall more easily digested. In contrast, casein is less soluble and has a slower rate of digestion, which results in an extended release of amino acids into the circulation. In human studies, casein-predominant formulas result in lower zinc bioavailability than whey-predominant formulas, presumably because of less complete digestion of casein.[22]

Other types of human whey proteins include secretory IgA and lactoferrin.[21] Secretory IgA attaches to the lining of the GI tract and prevents potential pathogenic microorganisms from adhering.[9] Lactoferrin is an iron-binding protein that limits the ability of bacteria to thrive in the intestines. Because this protein is biochemically similar to transferrin, it may have a significant role in iron absorption. However, in vivo studies do not definitively establish this role.[23] Also, some evidence suggests that lactoferrin has a role in stimulating intestinal mucosa growth.[24] These 2 proteins found in human milk, secretory IgA and lactoferrin, and the main protease inhibitors, α1-antitrypsin and α1-antichymotrypsin, are not well-digested in early infancy.[24,25] In fact, approximately 10% of intact milk proteins are found in infant stools prior to 1 month of age, decreasing to about 3% at 4 months of age.[24] In vitro studies suggest that α1-antitrypsin resists proteolysis by pepsin and pancreatic enzymes.[24,26] Alpha 1-antitrypsin has been found in considerable quantities in both human milk and in the stool of infants fed human milk; therefore, it should not be used to ascertain enteric protein loss in breastfed infants.[26]

Overall, infant formulas traditionally contain more protein than human milk due to the concern that proteins in infant formulas are less digestible. This concern is supported by the observation that formula-fed infants have higher blood urea nitrogen (BUN) levels due to the higher exposure to proteins. These infant formulas also have a higher proportion of whey, which should increase their digestibility. In addition, it is important to note that heat treatment of milk proteins does affect their digestibility. It has been observed that protein digestibility of powdered formulas is greater compared to identical liquid solutions. The heat treatment for powdered formulas is less intense than liquid formulas, with a lower maximum temperature and shorter duration. As a result, protein digestibility is increased with less intense heat treatment.[24]

Amino Acids

Literally hundreds of amino acids exist in nature, but only 20 are considered relevant in human nutrition. Lafayette B. Mendel (1872–1935) was the first to demonstrate that some amino acids cannot be synthesized in rats and subsequently defined them as essential amino acids required in their diet. In an amazing series of experiments completed in the 1940s

Table 5-2. Essential, Nonessential, and Conditionally Essential Amino Acids in Human Nutrition

ESSENTIAL	CONDITIONALLY ESSENTIAL	NONESSENTIAL
Histidine[a]	Cyst(e)ine[b]	Alanine
Isoleucine	Taurine	Aspartic acid
Leucine	Tyrosine	Asparagine
Lysine		Glutamic acid
Methionine		Glutamine
Phenylalanine		Glycine[c,d]
Threonine		Proline[d]
Tryptophan		Serine[c,d]
Valine		Arginine[c,d]

[a]Not initially identified by Rose[27] as being an essential amino acid.
[b]Cyst(e)ine is the sum of cysteine and cystine.
[c]Glycine and serine carbon skeletons can be readily synthesized by neonates and infants, but the rate of transamination is low.
[d]Laidlaw-Kopple classification as acquired indispensable (see Table 5-4).

and 1950s, William C. Rose (1887–1985, who completed his training under Mendel) and co-investigators determined the amino acid requirements of normal adults.[27] These experiments revealed 8 amino acids that resulted in negative nitrogen balance when excluded from the diet. Upon resumption of these amino acids in adequate amounts, negative nitrogen balance was completely reversed. These 8 amino acids are isoleucine, leucine, valine, lysine, methionine, phenylalanine, threonine, and tryptophan (Table 5-2). Other amino acids can be withheld without appreciable effect on nitrogen balance. Studies have confirmed these findings in infants and school-age children.

Amino acids can exist in 2 isomeric forms. The L-amino acids are utilized in humans and most animals. The stereoselectivity is related to enzymes that only recognize and utilize the L isomer. Amino acids do exist as D isomers, but only D-methionine can be converted to L-methionine by some animals, but not humans. For the rest of this chapter the authors will not identify amino acids as the L isomer; it should be assumed that the L isomer is being discussed.

Conditionally Essential Amino Acids

Investigations that followed Rose's extraordinary work generated questions as to whether other amino acids may be required in the diet under certain conditions of immaturity, metabolic imbalance, organ failure, disease, and highly defined diets such as PN.

Histidine is now considered essential in the human diet.[28] Histidine stores are particularly high in hemoglobin and in carnosine (found in large quantities in muscle).[29,30] It is widely accepted that histidine is the ninth essential amino acid in humans (Table 5-2). Snyderman et al[31] established histidine intake requirements in infants of 24 mg/kg/d, which is generally less than other essential amino acids. In studies by Heird et al,[32,33] the histidine requirements in neonates and infants on PN were greater than those demonstrated by these earlier studies and higher than predicted from older child and adult requirements (adjusted by kilogram of weight). The *Guidelines for the Use of Parenteral and Enteral Nutrition in Adult and Pediatric Patients*[34] states that histidine is a conditionally essential amino acid for neonates and infants up to 6 months of age.

Sulfur amino acid requirements of infants and children have been an area of intense research. The sulfur amino acids include methionine, cysteine, and taurine. Cysteine contains a free sulfhydryl group, and it is oxidized with another cysteine moiety to form the dimer cystine. After cysteine is incorporated into newly synthesized protein, the formation of cystine dimers aid in proper protein folding and stability. Cysteine is metabolized from methionine and can replace 50%–80% of methionine intake. Because it can reduce the required intake of an essential amino acid, it has been classified as a conditionally essential amino acid by Jackson.[35] Snyderman[36] defined intakes of cysteine in infants at 85 mg/kg/d, similar to many of the essential amino acids. Pohlandt[37] discovered that the requirement for cysteine in diet continues into infancy, perhaps to 5 months of age.

Most of the metabolic machinery for the metabolism of methionine and cysteine resides in liver parenchymal tissue near the portal vein. The transsulfuration pathway for methionine metabolism is a complex series of enzymatic steps leading to cysteine and taurine production (Figure 5-4). Many investigators have shown that multiple enzymes in this pathway have lower or no activity in the fetal liver or in the livers of infants of various gestational ages who died from non–liver-related causes.[38,39] λ-Cystathionase and cystathionine β-synthase were found to be absent or to have activity of less than half of the older child or adult. Zlotkin and Anderson[40] demonstrated that λ-cystathionase in liver of premature and term infants did not reach adult activity until 6–9 months postnatal age. This may be the reason that human milk is relatively rich in cysteine content. This renders cysteine as conditionally essential in neonates and infants.

Conflicting data on the essentiality of cysteine in neonates have been reported. In 2001 Lyons et al[41] showed that

Figure 5-4. Transsulfuration Pathway in the Metabolism of Methionine

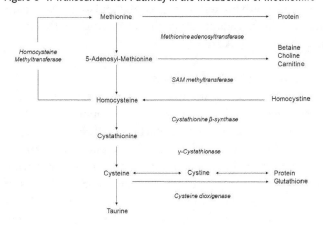

Table 5-3. Taurine Functions

Neurotransmitter
Bile acid conjugation
Brain and central nervous system development
Osmoregulation
Immunoregulation
Antioxidant
Retinal physiology
Platelet function
Mitochondrial function

pediatric septic patients receiving limited and variable protein intakes had higher plasma fluxes as well as increased oxidation rates for cysteine after a tracer (L-[1-13C] cysteine) infusion compared to healthy controls. In addition, septic patients were found to have lower whole-blood concentrations and lower absolute as well as fractional synthesis rates of glutathione. More recently, Courtney-Martin et al[42] observed no difference in glutathione concentrations and synthesis rates (absolute or fractional) in neonates who received cysteine supplementation (10 mg/kg/d) to their PN, in which the daily sulfur amino acid requirement was provided as methionine, compared to those who did not receive cysteine. The difference may lie in 2 factors: concurrent clinical conditions and provision of total sulfur amino acids. Sepsis can create enormous stress in the premature neonate and deplete essential amino acids stores despite adequate parenteral protein provision. While in the more clinically stable infant, as long as an adequate amount of sulfur amino acid substrate is provided, additional cysteine supplementation may not be required. As Shew et al[43] showed, very low birthweight (VLBW) neonates have the enzymatic ability to synthesize cysteine by transsulfuration pathways. Whether that production is sufficient to maintain appropriate levels of taurine and glutathione during disease or for further use in the body remains to be seen. These differences will need to be further addressed to establish a true essentiality of cysteine in vulnerable infants.

Cysteine is gradually oxidized to the dimer cystine in aqueous solution at neutral pH. Therefore, for PN solutions that contain it, cysteine is added at the time of preparation. The commonly used intravenous additive is provided as the cysteine hydrochloride salt. The pediatric daily requirement for cysteine has been studied by Helms et al.[44,45] These in-

vestigators found that a dose of 77.4 mg/kg/d, close to that of Snyderman,[36] appears to be required for ideal nitrogen retention, nitrogen balance, and growth in infants on PN. Problems of acidosis occasionally occur in VLBW infants and require acetate to be substituted for chloride in PN solutions. For every 160 mg of cysteine HCl that is infused as part of PN, 1 mmol of HCl is given to the pediatric patient. For the preterm infant and neonate, the prescriber should consider substitution of 1 mmol of acetate for 1 mmol of additional chloride given as part of cysteine HCl.

Taurine is one of the most abundant free "amino" acids in humans. It is not incorporated into protein in that no aminoacyl tRNA synthetase recognizing taurine has been identified. Taurine is actually a sulfonic acid (rare in nature) and does not contain a carboxyl group as do other amino acids. It has a host of important biological functions (Table 5-3). It is essential in the feline diet, and its absence results in retinal degeneration and blindness. In children on home PN with no added taurine, degenerative changes in electroretinograms were observed.[46] Cysteine sulfinic acid decarboxylase is key to production of taurine from cysteine (Figure 5-4). The enzyme has much lower overall activity in humans than in rats and cats, but its activity is even lower in human fetal liver.[47] Taurine is found in high concentrations in human milk when compared to cow's milk.[48] Formulas made from cow's milk protein require taurine supplementation, and taurine deficiency may occur with synthetic formulas not containing taurine. In neonates and premature infants, taurine continues to be renally wasted even in the presence of low serum taurine.[49]

Taurine is added to crystalline amino acid formulas designed for infants. Helms et al.[45,50] described plasma amino acid concentrations in preterm infants and in long-term home PN patients receiving a pediatric-designed amino acid formula as part of their PN. For infants, these investigators demonstrated that concentrations of the sulfur amino acids remain within age-related norms with the use of one of the commercially available formulas with L-cysteine HCl supplementation. Interestingly, even older children on home PN required cysteine supplementation to normalize plasma taurine concentrations.[50]

Tyrosine is exclusively metabolized from phenylalanine. Tyrosine, like cysteine for methionine, can reduce the dietary requirement for phenylalanine. Snyderman[36] demonstrated a dietary need for tyrosine of approximately 50 mg/kg/d in preterm infants. Classic phenylketonuria (PKU), the absence of the enzyme phenylalanine hydroxylase, results in extreme elevations in phenylalanine concentration and a requirement for tyrosine in the diet. PKU can lead to brain damage and possibly death if untreated. Tyrosine may be conditionally essential in patients with liver disease and is the precursor for the neurotransmitter dopamine.

Tyrosine content in parenteral amino acid solutions is restricted because of poor solubility. Christensen et al[51] found that N-acetyl-tyrosine (NAT), an aqueously soluble form of tyrosine with good stability in solution, was a reasonable intravenous source of tyrosine in older infants. However, clearance and nonrenal clearance was significantly decreased in younger infants of lower postconceptional age, suggesting NAT may not be the ideal tyrosine source in VLBW neonates. This investigative group was unable to normalize plasma tyrosine concentrations in most infants at a dose of approximately 50 mg/kg/d. Van Goudoever et al[52] were able to normalize plasma tyrosine levels with a NAT intake of 162 mg/kg/d.

Amino Acids of the Urea Cycle

The amino acids of the urea cycle are considered nonessential (Figure 5-5). Snyderman et al[53] found no evidence that arginine is essential in preterm infants. However, early amino acid solutions with relatively lower concentrations of arginine resulted in hyperammonemia in infants receiving these formulas as part of PN.[54] Higher concentrations of arginine reversed the finding of hyperammonemia.[55] Acute renal failure patients given large doses of protein with little supplemental arginine also present with hyperammonemia, which can be reversed with arginine supplementation.[56] Another intermediate of the urea cycle, citrulline, has entered the clinical research arena. Most of the citrulline produced in the liver is consumed in the next step of the cycle; however, enterocytes also synthesize citrulline and have been shown to contribute the majority of the circulating plasma citrulline.[57] It is this particular property that has gathered the interest of investigators for citrulline as a GI biomarker, which will be discussed in a later section. Other intermediates can sometimes become deficient due to abnormal enzymatic activity leading to urea cycle disorders. Treatment for these conditions generally involves the supplementation of low-dose essential amino acids and arginine.

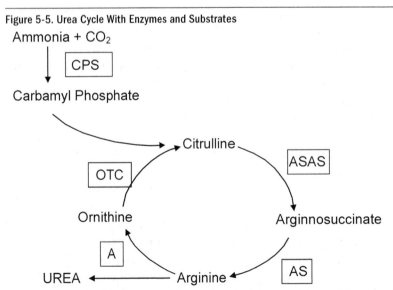

Figure 5-5. Urea Cycle With Enzymes and Substrates

A, arginase; AS, argininosuccinase; ASAS, argininosuccinic acid synthetase; CPS, carbamyl phosphate synthetase; OTC, ornithine transcarbamylase.

Useful Classification of Amino Acids for the Clinician

Laidlaw and Kopple[58] offer an alternative approach to the Jacksonian[35] classification of essential and nonessential amino acids. These 5 classifications enable the clinician to better understand the requirement of amino acids in the diet (Table 5-4).

Table 5-4. Modification of Amino Acid Classification in Humans[58]

CLASSIFICATION AND DESCRIPTION	EXAMPLE
1. Totally indispensable amino acids. No metabolic precursor or product can be substituted.	Lysine and threonine
2. Carbon-skeleton indispensable. Ketoacid analogue or hydroxyacid analogue can be substituted.	Histidine, isoleucine, leucine, methionine, phenylalanine, tryptophan, and valine
3. Conditionally indispensable. Reduce requirement for indispensable, and become indispensable in the absence of precursor in diet.	Tyrosine, cysteine, and taurine; possibly orthnithine and citrulline
4. Acquired indispensable. Become indispensable in states of metabolic disorders, immaturity, and severe stress.	Cysteine, taurine, tyrosine, arginine, citrulline, glycine, serine, and proline
5. Dispensable.	Alanine, glutamate, and aspartate

Liver and Kidney: Roles in Amino Acid Metabolism

The liver is important in the synthesis of transport and other constituent and functional proteins, metabolism of amino acids, gluconeogenesis, and urea formation.[59,60] Major plasma proteins derived from the liver, such as albumin, transthyretin (TTR) (also known as prealbumin for its migration pattern during electrophoresis), and retinol-binding protein (RBP) are present at early stages of development. Most liver-derived plasma proteins are at lower concentrations in premature infants. Lipoprotein concentrations rise rapidly after birth in response to high dietary fat intake, while albumin and TTR increase toward adult values in the first months to year of life. Acute phase proteins, such as C-reactive protein (CRP), appear to be inducible even in prematurity and are used to monitor inflammatory response to infection or metabolic stress. Reduction in visceral protein occurs in preterm infants, and response to protein and energy intake can be assessed through monitoring changes in serum concentrations of albumin, TTR, and RBP.[61]

The production of glutathione in the liver is essential; however, other tissues can produce it. Glutathione is an important sulfhydryl-reducing agent that protects cells from oxygen free radicals.[62] It is synthesized from glutamate, cysteine, and glycine, and cysteine is the rate-limiting substrate in production. Glutathione production depends on 2 distinct steps in cysteine production via the transsulfuration pathway (principally in the liver) or from dietary intake. The tripeptide also appears to be important in the transport of amino acids and in the synthesis of leukotrienes via the enzyme γ-glutamyl transpeptidase.[63,64]

The metabolism of amino acids is an important function of the liver. Several enzymes and enzyme systems, such as the transsulfuration pathway and phenylalanine hydroxylase, both predominantly located in the liver, are responsible for the metabolism of the essential amino acids methionine and phenylalanine, respectively. Enzyme activity is reduced in prematurity and early infancy, rendering the products of these enzyme systems as conditionally essential amino acids.

Approximately one-third of amino acids entering the liver from portal blood are used for protein synthesis.[65] The remainder may be used in energy production, or gluconeogenesis, with perhaps only a third of dietary amino acids entering the peripheral blood. This explains why plasma amino acids do not fluctuate substantially in the postprandial period. One group of amino acids that are released at higher relative concentrations from the liver in the postprandial period is the branched-chain amino acids,[66] that is, leucine, isoleucine, and valine. The branched-chain amino acids are preferentially metabolized in the periphery because they, as well as arginine, stimulate insulin release and muscle protein synthesis.[67] All stimulation is reversed in the postabsorptive period. As insulin concentrations fall, the muscle provides the principal gluconeogenic substrate, alanine, to the liver for production of glucose in the fasting period.

In parenterally fed neonates and infants, Heird et al[32,33] found that the branched-chain amino acid needs of infants were increased despite their relatively lower muscle mass. This would suggest that the shuttling of amino acids between the periphery and the small infant liver is actually higher than in the adult. Increased requirement of amino acids and energy for synthesis may be the likely explanation.

The urea cycle is the principal mechanism for nitrogen disposal (Figure 5-5). The catabolism of proteins and their component amino acids results in ammonia production. The liver will hydrolyze arginine to form urea and ornithine under the enzymatic control of arginase. Urea is then delivered to the kidney for excretion. In neonates and infants, the quantity of amino acids that enter into urea production is small, presumably due to a substantial need for amino acids for growth; therefore, BUN will be low.[68]

The kidney plays a minor role in amino acid and protein metabolism. Ninety percent of dietary protein nitrogen is incorporated into new tissue, and therefore it never requires formation of urea in the liver and excretion by the kidney. In premature infants and neonates, excretion of nitrogen is limited for the first months of life. Tubular reabsorption of amino acids is reduced in premature infants and neonates and may explain increased amino acid needs in these patients compared to older children or adults.[69,70]

Functions of Amino Acids and Proteins

Protein has multiple functions; it is essential for cell structure, maturation, remodeling, and growth. Besides being utilized for energy, amino acids and proteins serve as essential precursors for many biological processes.[71]

When protein is consumed, it is extensively broken down in the GI tract to amino acids, which can then enter cells or continue to circulate in plasma. Once in the cell, amino acids can be combined by peptide linkages to form small peptides (such as glutathione), they can be substrates for protein synthesis, or they can function as individual amino acids in the urea cycle. Specific amino acids can act as substrates, regulators, transporters, and precursors to neurotransmitters and hormones.[72]

In the cell, protein can be utilized for energy or it can be stored. Proteins are continuously being broken down. The carbon chain of the amino acids can be utilized for energy, and free amino acids can be released back into the plasma to maintain plasma amino acid concentrations.[71]

After synthesis within the cell, many proteins are released into the plasma. The 3 major types of plasma proteins are albumin, globulin, and fibrinogen. Albumin's role is to maintain osmotic pressure in the plasma. Globulins are involved in enzymatic activity in the plasma, as well as playing a vital role in natural and acquired immunity. Fibrinogen is essential for coagulation, both in blood clotting and repair of blood vessels.[71] For specific examples of the functions of amino acids and protein, refer to Table 5-5.

Protein Requirements and Protein-Energy Ratio During Growth

Protein is essential for growth, and its requirements (similar to total caloric requirements) are greater than usual for very low birth-weight neonates and gradually decrease with increasing age.[28] VLBW neonates have the highest protein requirements, often requiring 3 to 4 g/kg/d,[72,73] while term neonates require 2 to 2.5 g/kg/d. Two approaches to determine protein requirements in these infants have been discussed in the literature, including empirical and factorial methods.[74] Nitrogen balance, which will be discussed later, is an example of an empirical approach. The factorial method is based on the sum of estimates for replacement of inevitable nitrogen losses (urinary, stool, and dermal) plus the needs for lean body mass accretion.[74]

These and many other studies have demonstrated that adequate protein may be more critical for nutritional status and growth than total caloric requirements in preterm neonates and sick children.[18] Protein requirements can be increased by as much as 20%–50% in critical illness, thermal injury, and catch-up growth.[76]

Early initiation of protein has been shown to be beneficial in extremely low birth-weight infants. Poindexter et al[77] concluded that early amino acid administration was significant for better infant growth outcomes and neurodevelopment when evaluated at 36 weeks postmenstrual age and again at 18 months follow-up. Controversy still remains around whether increased protein intakes (3–4 g/kg/d) lead to increased growth or other markers of protein utilization in VLBW neonates. Several institutions have adopted these practices, but Vlaardingerbroek et al[73] recently showed that high-protein dose (3.6 g/kg/d) administration did not lead to improved nitrogen balance compared to controls receiving a conventional protein dosage (2.4 g/kg/d) in the short term (first week of life).

Protein requirements in term infants are based on studies in freely breastfed infants.[75] In infancy, 55% of daily protein is dedicated for growth while 45% is for maintenance. This ratio gradually decreases, and by 4 years of age only about 10% of total protein requirement is utilized for growth and the remaining 90% is used for daily maintenance.[78] Refer to Table 5-6 for age-based protein requirements.

Assessment of Protein Status

Besides the monitoring of visceral proteins (ie, albumin, TTR) and acute phase proteins (ie, CRP), nitrogen balance can be a useful tool in monitoring protein repletion and depletion in pediatric patients receiving specialized nutrition support. Nitrogen balance is an estimate of nitrogen intake minus nitrogen excretion. In adults, urinary urea nitrogen (in grams per liter multiplied by 1.2 to yield total urinary nitrogen [TUN]) multiplied by the urine volume (liters per

Table 5-5. Functions of Amino Acids and Protein[71]

FUNCTION	EXAMPLE
Amino acids	
Substrates for protein synthesis	Amino acids with a codon
Regulators of protein turnover	Leucine, arginine
Regulators of enzyme activity (allosteric)	Arginine and NAG synthetase, Phe and PAH activation
Precursor of signal transducer	Arginine and nitric oxide
Methylation reactions	Methionine
Neurotransmitters	Tryptophan (serotonin), glutamate, glycine, GABA
Ion fluxes	Taurine, glutamate
Precursor of physiologic molecules	Arginine (creatinine), glutamine
Nitrogen transport	Alanine, glutamine
Oxidation and reduction	Cystine, glutathione
Precursor of conditionally indispensable amino acids	Methionine (cys), phe (thy)
Gluconeogenic substrate and fuel	Alanine, serine, glutamine
Proteins	
Enzymatic catalysis	BCKADH
Transport	B12-binding proteins, ceruloplasmin, apolipoproteins
Messenger/signals	Insulin; growth hormones
Movement	Kinesin, actin
Structure	Collagens, elastin
Storage/sequestration	Ferritin, metallothionein
Immunity	Antibodies, TNF, interleukins
Growth, differentiation, and gene expression	EGF, IGFs, transcription factors

BCKADH, branched-chain alpha-keto acid dehydrogenase; EGF, epidermal growth factor; GABA, γ-aminobutyric acid; IGF, insulin-like growth factor; NAG, N-acetylglutamate; PAH, phenylalanine hydroxylase; Phe, phenylalanine; TNF, tumor necrosis factor.

day) plus 2–4 g nitrogen (to reflect all other unmeasured nitrogen lost) results in nitrogen balance. The method for collection and calculation of nitrogen balance is altered in pediatric patients.

Urine collections in neonates and infants are problematic, but not impossible. The use of urine bags with atten-

Table 5-6. Protein Requirements[75]

CATEGORY	PROTEIN (G/KG/D)
Very low birth weight (<1500 g)	3–4
Preterm	2.5–3
Infant/neonate	2–2.5
Infant	1.5–2
Preschool/school age	1–1.5
Adolescent	0.8–1.5

tive clinician support, or collection of diapers with elution of all urinary and stool nitrogen, has been used successfully in the clinical arena to assess nitrogen output in children.[79] While 24-hour urine collections have been considered the standard, use of 6-hour collection has been reported in pediatrics.[80] These authors are more comfortable using 24-hour urine collections to predict actual nitrogen balance over the period of observation.

A lower percentage of nitrogen is excreted as urea in neonates and infants, making use of adult correction factors inappropriate.[1] Several issues, such as the previous one described, should be considered when completing nitrogen balance studies in pediatrics. Helms et al[81] characterized nitrogen excretion in stressed pediatric intensive care unit patients and sick neonates. Urea as a percentage of total nitrogen output was in the range of 40%–60%, distinctly different from the 80% excretion as urea assumed in adults.

Because the percentage of nitrogen excreted as urea is substantially different than in adult patient and varies with clinical condition, use of TUN is recommended to increase accuracy and reliability for both children and adults.

With the advent of isotopic carbon oxidation studies, new methods have been established to determine amino acid intake requirements.[82] These methods include indicator amino acid oxidation (IAAO) and the 24-hour indicator amino acid oxidation and balance method (24h-IAAO/IAAB). They offer the advantage of being noninvasive, with the former being a little less time-consuming than the latter. IAAO consists of 2-day adaptation to fixed protein intakes followed by breath CO_2 measurement after 8 hourly meals enriched with [1-^{13}C]phenylalanine.[83] 24h-IAAO/IAAB encompasses 6-day adaptation to fixed protein intakes followed by assessment of oxidation during 12-hour fed state and 12-hour fasted state and assessment of balance by subtraction of [1-^{13}C]leucine oxidation from intake.[84] In particular, IAAO has been compared to the factorial method to determine amino acid requirements in children. The current Dietary Reference Intake report,[85] based on the latter, seems to underestimate mean protein requirements in healthy, school-aged children, 0.76 g/kg/d compared to the IAAO method, 1.3 g/kg/d.[86] Given the complexity of these assessments, they may be better suited for a stable, general-ward type of patient, rather than in a critically ill patient whose care is already challenging and demands more resources. As these techniques become more widely available, practitioners are advised that we could possibly see a change in protein intake standards for the different age populations in the future.

Monitoring Plasma Amino Acids

Plasma amino acids have been widely reported in pediatric patients. Storm and Helms[87] reviewed the hypothesis regarding normalization of plasma amino acids and its validation as a predictive tool in understanding outcomes in neonates and infants receiving PN. This review led to a number of investigations suggesting normalization results in improved growth, nitrogen balance, increased calcium and phosphorus intakes, and improved liver health.[88–92] It is likely that plasma amino acids will continue to be a benchmark for the efficacy of newly developed pediatric amino acid formulations. Concentrations of plasma citrulline, as introduced in a previous section, have been investigated in different GI insults and/or diseases such as mucosal injury after chemotherapy,[93] celiac disease,[94] short bowel syndrome,[95] and transplantation.[96] Recently, a couple of studies have evaluated plasma citrulline in patients with or without bowel resection as a marker of both intestinal mass and functionality,[97,98] identifying promising trends suggesting both properties. Most institutions can obtain whole profiles of amino acids with a considerably rapid turnaround time. The question for clinicians remains how to utilize that information. As new research arises, certain amino acids could be monitored and serve as descriptors of particular disease states or conditions. In order for individual assessment of plasma amino acids to more profoundly impact the clinical environment and outcomes in pediatric patients, less expensive, less time-consuming, and more accessible analytical technologies will have to be developed to replace those currently used for single amino acid detection in clinical research.

Case Presentation and Discussion

A 2-week-old male was transferred to the neonatal intensive care unit today. He was born at 32 weeks gestation with a birth weight of 1.6 kg. The mother could not produce enough breast milk, so he was started on preterm infant formula reaching full feedings about a week ago. Two days ago, the infant developed feeding intolerance and fever. This morning the nurse noted fever, abdominal distention, tachycardia, and specks of blood in the stool. Oxygen saturation dropped, requiring intubation; the infant was taken to the operating room for an exploratory laparotomy, and he was diagnosed with necrotizing enterocolitis. The nutrition team was consulted to evaluate the infant's nutrition needs.

Question: Explain how the infant's symptoms could be associated with the choice of enteral feeding.

Comment: Human milk contains IgA, which is important in host defense and can provide immunity to the infant, preventing bacterial overgrowth and possible infection. Human milk also has an increased whey content compared with formula. Whey is more easily digestible and promotes gastric emptying, which prevents feeding accumulation that can serve as energy source for bacteria.

Question: What would be your initial action and how would you monitor the effectiveness of your parenteral nutrition regimen?

Comment: This patient is anticipated to be nil per os (NPO) for an extended period. Parenteral nutrition should be started and L-cysteine supplementation should be considered. The best method for evaluation of protein and overall nutrition status in this patient would be daily weights and longitudinal assessment of visceral proteins such as transthyretin and albumin and nitrogen balance if feasible.

Question: What is the estimated protein requirement for this infant?

Comment: Because this infant is premature and critically ill due to necrotizing enterocolitis, 2.5–3 g/kg of protein should be provided. Protein should be dosed based on the birth weight of 1.6 kg. This corresponds to a total protein dose of approximately 4–4.5 g/d.

Question: What are your recommendations for this infant's nutrition once he is allowed to start enteral feedings?

Comment: Depending on whether bowel resection was necessary, this infant may need a specialized enteral feeding regimen. Breast milk, whether the mother's or a donor's, may confer advantages early on and is conventionally accepted as first line compared to formula (refer to particular chapters in this Core Curriculum); however, the latter may be more convenient in terms of discharge planning and mother's lack of production. If formula is chosen, it would be prudent to choose an infant formula that is easier to digest. A hydrolyzed or amino acid–based formula should be considered for this infant.

Test Your Knowledge Questions

1. Which amino acid will an infant who is diagnosed with phenylketonuria require?
   A. Phenylalanine
   B. Cysteine
   C. Histidine
   D. Tyrosine
   E. Methionine
2. Which of the following is an advantage of human milk over bovine milk?
   A. Human milk's pH is higher due to high bicarbonate concentration.
   B. Human milk has an increased whey content that promotes rapid gastric emptying.
   C. Human milk has an increased caloric density as compared to bovine milk.
   D. Human milk prevents children from developing colic.
   E. All of the above are advantages of human milk.
3. Protein digestion
   A. Occurs mostly in the small intestine.
   B. Is dependent on hydrochloric acid and pepsin to denature protein.
   C. Has been identified as early as 16 weeks gestation, but gastric acid secretion does not reach adult levels until 38 weeks gestation.
   D. Products include approximately 30% oligopeptides and 70% amino acids.

4. Which of the following is true regarding nitrogen balance?
   A. Nitrogen balance is not an accurate way to assess protein needs in a pediatric patient.
   B. In order to estimate a nitrogen balance, you must do a 24-hour urine collection.
   C. Total urinary nitrogen is a better estimate of urinary losses as compared to urinary urea nitrogen.
   D. Nitrogen balance is an estimate of nitrogen intake divided by nitrogen excreted.

Acknowledgments

The authors of this chapter for the second edition of this text wish to thank Emma M. Tillman, PharmD; and Anup J. Patel, MD, for their contributions to the first edition of this text.

References

1. Young LS, Kearns LR, Schoepfel SL. Protein. In: Gottschlich MM, DeLegge MH, Mattox T, Mueller C, Worthington P, eds. *The A.S.P.E.N. Nutrition Support Core Curriculum: A Case-Based Approach—The Adult Patient.* Silver Spring, MD: American Society for Parenteral and Enteral Nutrition; 2007:71–87.
2. Gilger MA. Normal gastrointestinal function. In: McMillan JA, Feigin RD, DeAngelis C, Jones MD, eds. *Oski's Pediatrics.* 4th ed. Philadelphia, PA: Lippincott Williams & Wilkins; 2006:1915–1921.
3. Berseth CL. Overview of the development of the gastrointestinal tract. UpToDate Web site. http://www.uptodate.com.ezproxy.uthsc.edu/contents/overview-of-the-development-of-the-gastrointestinal-tract?source=search_result&search=Overview+of+the+development+of+the+gastrointestinal+tract&selectedTitle=1~150. Updated October 11, 2005. Accessed December 19, 2008.
4. Lucas A, Bloom SR, Aynsley-Green A. Development of gut hormone responses to feeding in neonates. *Arch Dis Child.* 1980;55(9):678–682.
5. Berseth CL, Nordyke CK, Valdes MG, Furlow BL, Go VL. Responses of gastrointestinal peptides and motor activity to milk and water feedings in preterm and term infants. *Pediatr Res.* 1992;31(6):587–590.
6. Moreau H, Bernadac A, Gargouri Y, Benkouka F, Laugier R, Verger R. Immunocytolocalization of human gastric lipase in chief cells of the fundic mucosa. *Histochemistry.* 1989;91(5):419–423.
7. Armand M, Hamosh M, Mehta NR, et al. Effect of human milk or formula on gastric function and fat digestion in the premature infant. *Pediatr Res.* 1996;40(3):429–437.
8. Armand M, Hamosh M, DiPalma JS, et al. Dietary fat modulates gastric lipase activity in healthy humans. *Am J Clin Nutr.* 1995;62(1):74–80.
9. Rudolph CD. Structure and development of the gastrointestinal tract. In: Rudolph CD, Rudolph AM, Hostetter MK, Lister GE, Siegel NJ, eds. *Rudolph's Pediatrics.* 21st ed. New York, NY: McGraw-Hill; 2003.

10. Wahbeh GT, Christie DL. Basic aspects of digestion and absorption. In: Wyllie R, Hyams JS, eds. *Pediatric Gastrointestinal and Liver Disease: Pathophysiology, Diagnosis, Management.* 3rd ed. Netherlands: Saunders Elsevier; 2006:11–23.

11. Colaizzo-Anas T. Nutrient intake, digestion, absorption, and excretion. In: Gottschlich MM, DeLegge MH, Mattox T, Mueller C, Worthington P, eds. *The A.S.P.E.N. Nutrition Support Core Curriculum: A Case-Based Approach—The Adult Patient.* Silver Spring, MD: American Society for Parenteral and Enteral Nutrition; 2007:3–18.

12. Mason JB. Mechanisms of nutrient absorption and malabsorption. UpToDate Web site. http://www.uptodate.com.ezproxy.uthsc.edu/contents/mechanisms-of-nutrient-absorption-and-malabsorption?source=search_result&search=mechanisms+of+nutrient+absorption+and+malabsorption&selectedTitle=1~150. Updated October 18, 2007. Accessed December 19, 2008.

13. DeLegge MH, Ridley C. Nutrient digestion, absorption, and excretion. In: Gottschlich, MM, Fuhrman MP, Hammond KA, Holcombe BJ, Seidner DL, eds. *The Science and Practice of Nutrition Support: A Case-Based Core Curriculum.* Dubuque, IA: Kendall/Hunt Publishing Co; 2001:1–16.

14. Hadorn B, Tarlow MJ, Lloyd JK, Wolff OH. Intestinal enterokinase deficiency. *Lancet.* 1969;1(7599):812–813.

15. Johnson TR, Moore WM, Jeffries JE. *Developmental Physiology.* 2nd ed. Columbus, OH: Ross Laboratories; 1978: 150–152.

16. Roy CC, Silverman A, Alagille D. *Pediatric Clinical Gastroenterology.* 4th ed. St. Louis, MO: Mosby-Year Book, Inc; 1995:307–309.

17. Axelsson I, Jakobsson I, Lindberg T, Polberger S, Benediktsson B, Räihä NC. Macromolecular absorption in preterm and term infants. *Acta Paediatr Scand.* 1989;78(4):532–537.

18. Motil KJ. Meeting protein needs. In: Tsang RC, Zlotkin SH, Nichols BL, Hansen JW, eds. *Nutrition During Infancy: Principles and Practice.* 2nd ed. Cincinnati, OH: Digital Education Publishing, Inc; 1997:83–103.

19. Philipps AF, Sherman MP. Neonatal nutrition and gastrointestinal function. In: Rudolph CD, Rudolph AM, Hostetter MK, Lister GE, Siegel NJ, eds. *Rudolph's Pediatrics.* 21st ed. New York, NY: McGraw-Hill; 2003.

20. Hansen JW, Boettcher JA. Human milk substitutes. In: Tsang RC, Zlotkin SH, Nichols BL, Hansen JW, eds. *Nutrition During Infancy: Principles and Practice.* 2nd ed. Cincinnati, OH: Digital Education Publishing, Inc; 1997:441–466.

21. Schanler, RJ. Nutritional composition of human milk and preterm formula for the premature infant. UpToDate Web site. http://www.uptodate.com.ezproxy.uthsc.edu/contents/nutritional-composition-of-human-milk-and-preterm-formula-for-the-premature-infant?source=search_result&search=nutritional+composition+of+human+milk&selectedTitle=2~150. Updated September 7, 2007. Accessed December 19, 2008.

22. Lönnerdal B, Cederblad A, Davidsson L, Sandström B. The effect of individual components of soy formula and cow's milk formula on zinc bioavailability. *Am J Clin Nutr.* 1984;40(5):1064–1070.

23. Brock, JH. Lactoferrin in human milk: its role in iron absorption and protection against enteric infection in the newborn infant. *Arch Dis Child.* 1980;55(6):417–421.

24. Lönnerdal B. Digestibility and absorption of protein in infants. In: Räihä NC, ed. *Protein Metabolism During Infancy.* New York, NY: Raven Press; 1994:53–65.

25. Lindberg T, Ohlsson K, Weström B. Protease inhibitors and their relation to protease activity in human milk. *Pediatr Res.* 1982;16(6):479–483.

26. Davidson LA, Löonnerdal B. Fecal alpha 1-antitrypsin in breast-fed infants is derived from human milk and is not indicative of enteric protein loss. *Acta Paediatr Scand.* 1990;79(2):137–141.

27. Rose WC. The amino acid requirements of adult man. *Nutr Abstr Rev.* 1957;27:631–647.

28. Nasset ES, Gatewood VH. Nitrogen balance and hemoglobin of adult rats fed amino acid diets low in L- and D-histidine. *J Nutr.* 1956;53:163–176.

29. Kopple JD, Swendseid ME. Evidence that histidine is an essential amino acid in normal and chronically uremic man. *J Clin Invest.* 1975;55:881–891.

30. Kopple JD, Swendseid ME. Effect of histidine intake on plasma and urine histidine levels, nitrogen balance and N-methylhistidine excretion in normal and chronically uremic men. *J Nutr.* 1981;111:931–942.

31. Snyderman SE, Boyer A, Roitman E, Holt LE Jr, Prose PH. The histidine requirement of the infant. *Pediatrics.* 1963;31:786–801.

32. Heird WC, Dell RB, Helms RA, et al. Evaluation of an amino acid mixture designed to maintain normal plasma amino acid patterns in infants and children requiring parenteral nutrition. *Pediatrics.* 1987;80:401–408.

33. Heird WC, Hay W, Helms RA, Storm MC, Kashyap S, Dell, RB. Pediatric parenteral amino acid mixture in low birth weight infants. *Pediatrics.* 1988;81(1):41–50.

34. ASPEN Board of Directors and the Clinical Guidelines Task Force. Practice guidelines: protein requirements. In: Guidelines for the use of parenteral and enteral nutrition in adult and pediatric patients. *JPEN J Parenter Enteral Nutr.* 2002;26:27SA–28SA.

35. Jackson AA. Amino acids: essential and non-essential? *Lancet.* 1983;1:1034–1037.

36. Snyderman SE. The protein and amino acid requirements of the premature infant. In: Ionxix JHP, Visser HKA, Troelstra JD, eds. *Metabolic Processes in the Fetus and Newborn Infant.* Leiden, the Netherlands: HE Stenfert Kroesse NV; 1971:128–141.

37. Pohlandt F. Cystine: a semi-essential amino acid in the newborn infant. *Acta Pediatr Scand.* 1974;63:801–804.

38. Gaull G, Sturman JA, Raiha NCR. Development of mammalian sulfur metabolism: absence of cystathionase in human fetal tissues. *Pediatr Res.* 1972;6:538–547.

39. Sturman JA, Gaull G, Raiha NCR. Absence of cystathionase in human fetal liver: is cystine essential? *Science.* 1970;169:74–76.

40. Zlotkin SH, Anderson GH. Sulfur balances in intravenously fed infants: effects of cysteine supplementation. *Am J Clin Nutr.* 1982;36: 862–867.

41. Lyons J, Rauh-Pfeiffer A, Ming-Yu Y, et al. Cysteine metabolism and whole blood glutathione synthesis in septic pediatric patients. *Crit Care Med.* 2001;29(4):870–877.

42. Courtney-Martin G, Moore AM, Ball RO, Pencharz PB. The addition of cysteine to the total sulphur amino acid as methionine does not increase erythrocytes glutathione synthesis in the parenterally fed human neonate. *Pediatr Res.* 2010;67:320–324.

43. Shew SB, Keshen TH, Jahoor F, Jaksic T. Assessment of cysteine in very low-birth weight neonates using a [$^{13}C_6$] glucose tracer. *J Pediatr Surg.* 2005;40(1):52–56.

44. Helms RA, Chesney RW, Storm MC. Sulfur amino acid metabolism in infants on parenteral nutrition. *Clin Nutr.* 1995;14:381–387.

45. Helms RA, Christensen ML, Storm MC, Chesney RW. Adequacy of sulfur amino acid intake in infants receiving parenteral nutrition. *Nutr Biochem.* 1995;6:462–466.

46. Vinton NE, Heckenlively JR, Laidlaw SA et al. Visual function in patients undergoing long-term total parenteral nutrition. *Am J Clin Nutr.* 1990;52(5):895-902.

47. Sturman JA, Hayes KC. The biology of taurine in nutrition and development. In: Draper HH, ed. *Advances in Nutrition Research.* Vol. 3. New York, NY: Plenum Publishing Co; 1980:231–299.

48. Rassin DK, Sturman JA, Gaull GE. Taurine and other free amino acids in milk of man and other mammals. *Early Hum Dev.* 1978;2:1–13.

49. Zelikovic I, Chesney RW, Freidman AL, Ahlfors CE. Taurine depletion in very low birth weight infants receiving prolonged total parenteral nutrition: role of renal immaturity. *J Pediatr.* 1990;116:301–306.

50. Helms RA, Storm MC, Christensen ML, Hak EB, Chesney RW. Cysteine supplementation results in normalization of plasma taurine concentrations in children receiving home parenteral nutrition. *J Pediatr.* 1999; 134:358–361.

51. Christensen ML, Helms RA, Veal DF, Boehm KA, Storm MC. Clearance of N-acetyl-L-tyrosine in infants receiving a pediatric amino acid solution. *Clin Pharm.* 1993;12:606–609.

52. Van Goudoever JB, Sulkers EJ, Timmerman M, et al. Amino acid solutions for premature neonates during the first week of life: the role of N-acetyl-L-cysteine and N-acetyl-L-tyrosine. *JPEN J Parenter Enteral Nutr.* 1994;18:404–408.

53. Snyderman SE, Boyer A, Holt LE Jr. The arginine requirement of the infant. *AMA J Dis Child.* 1959;97:192–195.

54. Heird WC, Nicholson JF, Driscoll JM Jr, Schullinger JN, Winters RW. Hyperammonemia resulting from intravenous alimentation using a mixture of synthetic L-amino acids: a preliminary report. *J Pediatr.* 1972;81:162–167.

55. Thomas DW, Sinatra FR, Hack SL, Smith TM, Platzker ACG, Merritt RJ. Hyperammonemia in neonates receiving intravenous nutrition. *JPEN J Parenter Enteral Nutr.* 1982;6:503–506.

56. Motil KJ, Harmon WE, Grupe WE. Complications of essential amino acid hyperalimentation in children with acute renal failure. *JPEN J Parenter Enteral Nutr.* 1980;4:32–35.

57. Windmueller HG, Spaeth AE. Source and fate of circulating citrulline. *Am J Physiol.* 1981;241(6):E473–E480.

58. Laidlaw SA, Kopple JD. Newer concepts of the indispensable amino acids. *Am J Clin Nutr.* 1987;46:593–605.

59. Raiha NCR, Suihkonen J. Development of urea-synthesizing enzymes in human liver. *Acta Pediatr Scand.* 1968;57:121–124.

60. Raiha NCR, Lindros KO. Development of some enzymes involved in gluconeogenesis in human liver. *Ann Med Exp Biol.* 1969;47:146–150.

61. Helms RA, Dickerson RN, Ebbert ML, Christensen ML, Herrod HG. Retinol-binding protein and prealbumin: useful measures of protein repletion in critically ill, malnourished infants. *J Pediatr Gastroenteral Nutr.* 1986;5:586–592.

62. Beutler E. Nutritional and metabolic aspects of glutathione. *Annu Rev Nutr.* 1989;9:287–302.

63. Meister A. On the enzymology of amino acid transport. *Science.* 1973;180:33–39.

64. Svartz J, Hallin E, Soderstorm M, Hammarstrom S. Identification of regions of leukotriene C4 synthase which direct the enzyme to its nuclear envelope localization. *J Cell Biochem.* 2006;98;1517-1527.

65. Yamamoto H, Aikawa T, Matsutaka H, Okuda O, Ishikawa E. Interorganal relationships of amino acid metabolism in fed rats. *Am J Physiol.* 1974;226;1428–1433.

66. Munro HN. Fifth annual Jonathan E. Rhoads lecture. Metabolic integration of organs in health and disease. *J Parenter Enteral Nutr.* 1982;6:271.

67. Rocha DM, Falona GR, Unger RH. Glucagon-stimulating activity of 20 amino acids in dogs. *J Clin Invest.* 1972;51:2346.

68. Raiha NCR, Kekomaki MP. Studies on the development of ornithine-keto acid amino transferase activity in the liver. *Biochem J.* 1968;108:521–524.

69. Edelman CM, Wolfish NM. Dietary influence on renal maturation in premature infants. *Pediatr Res.* 1968;2:421–422.

70. Brodehl J, Gellissen K. Endogenous renal transport of free amino acids in infancy and childhood. *Pediatrics.* 1968;42:395–404.

71. Protein metabolism. In: Guyton AC, ed. *Textbook of Medical Physiology.* Philadelphia, PA: W.B. Saunders Co; 1991:765–770.

72. Radmacher PG, Lewis SL, Adamkin DH. Early amino acids and the metabolic response of ELBW infants (< or = 1000 g) in three time periods. *J Perinatol.* 2009;29(6):433–437.

73. Vlaardingerbroek H, Vermeulen MJ, Rook D, et al. Safety and efficacy of early parenteral lipid and high-dose amino acid administration to very low birth weight infants. *J Pediatr.* 2013;163(3):638–644.e1-5.

74. Ziegler EE. Protein requirements of very low birth weight infants. *J Pediatr Gastroenterol Nutr.* 2007;45(suppl 3):S170–S174.

75. Wu PYK, Edwards N, Storm MC. The plasma amino acid pattern of normal term breast-fed infants. *J Pediatr.* 1986;109:347–349.

76. Scrimshaw NS. Effect of infection on nutritional status. *Proc Natl Sci Counc Repub China B.* 1992;16:46–64.

77. Poindexter BB, Langer JC, Dusick AM, Ehrenkranz RA. Early provision of parenteral amino acids in extremely low

birth weight infants: relation to growth and neurodevelopmental outcome. *J Pediatr.* 2006;148:300–305.

78. American Academy of Pediatrics, Committee on Nutrition. Protein. In: Kleinman RE, ed. *Pediatric Nutrition Handbook.* 6th ed. Elk Grove Village, IL: American Academy of Pediatrics; 2009:325–341.

79. Boehm KA, Helms RA, Storm MC. Assessing the validity of adjusted urinary urea nitrogen as an estimate of total urinary nitrogen in three pediatric populations. *JPEN J Parenter Enteral Nutr.* 1994;18(2):172–176.

80. Lopez AM, Wolfsdorf J, Raszynski A, Contijoch-Serrano V. Estimation of nitrogen balance based on a six-hour urine collection in infants. *JPEN J Parenter Enteral Nutr.* 1986;10(5):517–518.

81. Helms RA, Mowatt-Larssen CA, Boehm KA, et al. Urinary nitrogen constituents in the postsurgical preterm neonate receiving parenteral nutrition. *JPEN J Parenter Enteral Nutr.* 1993;17:68–72.

82. Elango R, Ball RO, Pencharz. Recent advances in determining protein and amino acid requirements in humans. *Br J Nutr.* 2012;108(suppl 2):S22–S30.

83. Kriengsinyos W, Wykes LJ, Ball RO, Pencharz PB. Oral and intravenous tracer protocols of the indicator amino acid oxidation method provide the same estimate of the lysine requirement in healthy men. *J Nutr.* 2002;132(8):2251–2257.

84. Kurpad AV, Raj T, El-Khoury A, et al. Lysine requirements of healthy adult Indian subjects, measured by an indicator amino acid balance technique. *Am J Clin Nutr.* 2001;73(5):900–907.

85. Institute of Medicine, Food and Nutrition Board. *Dietary Reference Intakes: Energy, Carbohydrate, Fiber, Fat, Fatty Acids, Cholesterol, Protein and Amino Acids.* Washington, DC: The National Academies Press; 2005.

86. Elango R, Humayun MA, Ball RO, Pencharz PB. Protein requirement of healthy school-age children determined by the indicator amino acid oxidation method. *Am J Clin Nutr.* 2011;94(6):1545–1552.

87. Storm MC, Helms RA. Normalizing plasma amino acid levels in pediatric patients requiring parenteral nutrition. *Nutr Clin Pract.* 2007;22:194–203.

88. Helms RA, Christensen ML, Muer EC, Storm MC. Comparison of a pediatric versus standard amino acid formulation in preterm neonates requiring parenteral nutrition. *J Pediatr.* 1987;110:466–470.

89. Beck R. Use of a pediatric parenteral amino acid mixture in a population of extremely low birth weight neonates: fre-

quency and spectrum of direct bilirubinemia. *Am J Perinatol.* 1990;7(1):84–86.

90. Forchielli ML, Gura KM, Sandler R, Lo C. Aminosyn PF or TrophAmine: which provides more protection from cholestasis associated with total parenteral nutrition? *J Pediatr Gastroenterol Nutr.* 1995;21:374–382.

91. Pratt CA, Garcia MG, Poole RL, Kerner JA. Life-long total parenteral nutrition versus intestinal transplantation in children with microvillus inclusion disease. *J Pediatr Pharmacol Ther.* 2001;6:498–503.

92. Fitzgerald KA, MacKay MW. Calcium and phosphate solubility in neonatal parenteral nutrient solutions containing TrophAmine. *Am J Hosp Pharm.* 1986;43(1):88–93.

93. van Vliet MJ, Tissing WJ, Rings EH, et al. Citrulline as a marker for chemotherapy induced mucosal barrier injury in pediatric patients. *Pediatr Blood Cancer.* 2009;53(7):1188–1194.

94. Ioannou HP, Fotoulaki M, Pavlitou A, Efstratiou I, Augoustides-Savvopoulou P. Plasma citrulline levels in paediatric patients with celiac disease and the effect of a gluten-free diet. *Eur J Gastroenterol Hepatol.* 2011;23(3):245–249.

95. Bailly-Botuha C, Colomb V, Thioulouse E, et al. Plasma citrulline concentration reflects enterocyte mass in children with short bowel syndrome. *Pediatr Res.* 2009;65(5):559–563.

96. Hibi T, Nishida S, Garcia J, et al. Citrulline level is a potent indicator of acute rejection in the long term following pediatric intestinal/multivisceral transplantation. *Am J Transplant.* 2012;12(suppl 4):S27–S32.

97. Stultz J, Tillman EM, Helms RA. Plasma citrulline concentration as a biomarker for bowel loss and adaptation in hospitalized pediatric patients requiring parenteral nutrition. *Nutr Clin Pract.* 2011;26(6):681–687.

98. Herrera OR, Storm MC, Helms RA. Plasma citrulline concentrations in neonates/infants with or without gastrointestinal disease and bowel loss. In: *A.S.P.E.N. Clinical Nutrition Week 2014.* Silver Spring, MD: American Society for Parenteral and Enteral Nutrition. Abstract 1834574.

Test Your Knowledge Answers

1. The correct answer is **D**.
2. The correct answer is **B**.
3. The correct answer is **A**.
4. The correct answer is **C**.

6

Minerals

Winston Koo, MBBS, FACN, CNS; **Mirjana Lulic-Botica,** BSc, BCPS; **May Saba,** PharmD, BCNSP; and **Letitia Warren,** RD, CSP

CONTENTS

Learning Objectives

1. Review the biochemistry and physiology of calcium, phosphorus, and magnesium.
2. Define the common risk factors for the development of deficiency and manifestations of deficiency states for these nutrients.
3. Describe the potential risks with excessive intake of these nutrients.
4. Integrate the above information to understand the requirements and physiological regulation of these minerals.

Overview

Biochemistry and Physiology

Calcium (Ca) is the most abundant mineral in the body and together with phosphorus (P) accounts for the major inorganic content of bone. Magnesium (Mg) is the fourth most abundant cation and the second most common intracellular electrolyte in the body. The total body content of Ca, P, and Mg in the skeleton is approximately 99%, 85%, and 60%, respectively.

Less than 1% of the total body content of Ca, P, and Mg is in the circulation. However, disturbances in the serum concentrations of these minerals are associated with disturbances in numerous biological functions with and without clinical symptoms and signs. Acute changes in the serum concentrations likely reflect adaptive changes but not tissue storage status, although chronic and severely lowered serum concentrations of these minerals usually suggest a deficiency state.

From a clinical perspective, the skeleton has the dual function of providing structural and mechanical support and being a reservoir to maintain mineral homeostasis. Deficiency of Ca, vitamin D, or both, and in the case of small preterm infants, deficiency of P, can result in osteopenia and rickets in infants and children. Thus, circulating concentrations of Ca, P, and Mg within normal limits and the integrity of the skeleton are generally used as proxy for mineral homeostasis.[1,2]

Sources

Natural foods and various foods and beverages fortified with Ca are good sources for these minerals. Any food that provides 20% or more of the daily recommended intake per serving for a specific nutrient is considered to be "high" in that nutrient.[3] Dietary sources of minerals, including Ca-fortified foods and beverages, are preferred to supplements alone because the range of nutrients and the establishment of good dietary habits are enhanced by consuming food. In addition, nutrient interactions may be less and tolerance may be greater for minerals provided by food sources.[4-6]

Mineral supplements are readily available; however, their use does not compensate for poor food choices and an inadequate diet. Furthermore, the Food and Drug Administration (FDA) regulates dietary supplements under a different set of regulations than drug products (prescription and over-the-counter). As a result, the specific contents and contaminants of dietary supplements are not as rigorously monitored.[6]

Dietary Requirements

Mineral requirements depend on the needs for tissue synthesis in growing children and the balance among dietary supply, intestinal absorption, renal excretion, and bone exchange for these minerals. Several unique challenges exist in maintaining mineral homeostasis during infancy, childhood, and adolescence. To successfully adapt to extrauterine life, all neonates must adjust to the interruption of a continuous supply of minerals from the placenta at birth. This adaptation is usually achieved with appropriate nutrition support, even in critically ill and preterm neonates.[7] Nutrition requirements for Ca, P, and Mg remain high until skeletal growth is complete. Infants and adolescents have the greatest requirements because of their high growth rates.[8]

The average gain in skeletal growth over 1 year is > 25 cm for an infant, and it can be even greater for the preterm infant. The peak height gain is about 7–10 cm per year during adolescence. The recommended dietary reference intakes for Ca, P, and Mg are shown in Table 6-1.

Table 6-1. Dietary Reference Intake for Calcium, Phosphorus, and Magnesium[4,5]

| LIFE STAGE[a] | RDA (UL)[b,c] | | |
	CALCIUM, mg/d	PHOSPHORUS, mg/d	MAGNESIUM, mg/d
0–6 mo	200 (1000)	100	30
7–12 mo	260 (1000)	275	75
1–3 y	700 (2500)	460 (3000)	80 (65)
4–8 y	1000 (2500)	500 (3000)	130 (110)
Males			
9–13 y	1300 (3000)	1250 (4000)	240 (350)
14–18 y	1300 (3000)	1250 (4000)	410 (350)
Females			
9–13 y	1300 (3000)	1250 (4000)	240 (350)
14–18 y	1300 (3000)	1250 (4000)	360 (350)
Pregnancy			
14–18 y	1300 (3000)	1250 (3500)	400 (350)
Lactation			
14–18 y	1300 (3000)	1250 (4000)	360 (350)

Recommendation for calcium in Institute of Medicine[5] supersede those in Food and Nutrition Board, Institute of Medicine.[4] Recommendations for phosphorus and magnesium are based on reference 4.

[a] Adequate intake (AI) is an observed or experimentally determined estimate of nutrient intake by a group or groups of healthy people. AI is the only reference level provided for infants < 12 mo.

[b] Recommended dietary allowance (RDA) is the average daily dietary intake sufficient to meet the requirement of 97%–98% of healthy individuals at a specific life stage for each sex. For the RDA during pregnancy and lactation for other ages, check Institute of Medicine[5] and Food and Nutrition Board, Institute of Medicine.[4]

[c] Tolerable upper intake level (UL) for each life stage is indicated in parenthesis. For magnesium, the value applies to nonfood sources only. UL is the highest level of daily nutrient intake that is likely to pose no risk of adverse health effects to almost all individuals in the general population.

Absorption and Excretion

Intestinal absorption of Ca, P, and Mg involves a passive paracellular concentration-dependent process as well as a saturable active transcellular process. Vitamin D has some influence on active intestinal transport, but its role under normal circumstances appears to be much less than the passive diet-dependent process in the growing child. Renal reabsorption of these minerals also has passive and active transport components. It is highly efficient, but an excessive intake can overwhelm the renal excretory capacity, leading to elevated circulating levels for each of the minerals. Conversely, during deficient states, especially if abnormal loss from the gastrointestinal (GI) tract or the kidney occurs, renal conservation alone cannot prevent the development of abnormally low circulating concentrations. Normally, the growing child has net bone (and soft tissue) accretion of these minerals. Some exchange of these minerals typically occurs with bone modeling. The exchangeable portion may be increased during periods of stress and increased bone turnover. During extreme circumstances (eg, severe Ca or P deficiency in infants), it is not possible to protect the skeleton or to maintain mineral homeostasis.

Metabolism

Maintaining mineral homeostasis requires a complex interaction of hormonal and nonhormonal factors; adequate functioning of various body systems, particularly the renal, GI, skeletal, and endocrine systems; and adequate dietary intake. When assessing changes in serum concentrations of these minerals, understanding the interrelationships among them is vital. For example, hypomagnesemia may cause hypocalcemia due to the impaired secretion of parathyroid hormone (PTH) and impaired end organ responsiveness to PTH in maintaining Ca homeostasis. Serum Ca and P have a reciprocal relationship, and hypoalbuminemia can cause hypocalcemia secondary to decreased Ca binding, while the ionized Ca (unbound Ca) concentration remains normal.

Intake of minerals may interact with other nutrients including protein, sodium, potassium, iron, zinc, copper, and vitamin D at the intestine-kidney-bone axis. A significant positive or negative interaction may occur at the level of intestinal absorption, renal excretion, or metabolism. A positive effect is possible generally at low dietary intakes and a negative effect is possible at high intakes primarily as dietary supplements. Direct regulation on this axis by PTH, 1,25 dihydroxyvitamin D (1,25 $(OH)_2D$), and fibroblast growth factor-23 (FGF 23) and indirect regulation by growth-regulating hormones, including sex hormones, also significantly affect growth and mineralization of the skeleton and maintenance of normal circulating concentrations of the minerals. Thus, in the presence of abnormal circulating concentration of the minerals, it is vital to manage the underlying cause in addition to providing symptomatic treatment.

Deficiency States

In the United States, estimated Ca intakes from both food and dietary supplements are provided by the National Health and Nutrition Examination Survey. Mean dietary intake varies with life stage and by sex. Low dietary intake for Ca is common in older children. Groups with mean intakes below their respective estimated average requirement—and

Table 6-2. Dietary Sources of Calcium[10-12]

DIETARY CALCIUM (mg)[a]	CALCIUM-ENRICHED FOOD (mg)
Milk 240 mL (285–302)	Fortified orange and other fruit juices 180 mL (200–260)
Yogurt 8 oz (245–415)	Instant drink mix with 240 mL water (105–250)
Cheese single-wrapped 0.75 oz (120), others (150–200/oz)	Ready-to-eat cereals 1 cup (100–1000)
Chocolate pudding made with 120 mL 2% milk (153)	Breads/English muffins 30 g (30)
Sardines with bones 3 oz (325)	Tortilla corn one 6-inch diameter ~1.2 oz (46)
Salmon 3 oz (181)	Tortilla flour one 6-inch diameter ~1.75 oz (32)
Chinese cabbage 1 cup shredded and boiled (74)	Tofu 1/2 cup made with calcium sulfate (253)
Broccoli chopped 1 cup (70)	
Kale 1 cup (90)	

[a] Several servings of certain foods with less bioavailable calcium (eg, vegetables) are needed to achieve the same amount of calcium absorbed from 1 serving (240 mL or 8 oz) of milk.

thus with a prevalence of inadequacy in excess of 50% at the population level—include boys and girls aged 9–13 years and girls aged 14–18 years.[5,9] Preoccupation with being thin is common in adolescents, especially among girls, as is the misconception that all dairy foods are fattening. Many children and adults are unaware that low-fat milk contains at least as much Ca as does whole milk. A list of foods relatively high in Ca is shown in Table 6-2. Low Ca intake places children at risk for fractures, and both Ca and vitamin D deficiency are factors in the development of rickets in infants and young children.[13,14]

Risks for mineral deficiency escalate with increased requirement, decreased absorption or increased losses through the GI tract or the kidney, or disturbed metabolism. All rapidly growing infants, especially very low birth weight (<1.5 kg) preterm infants, are at risk for mineral deficiency because of increased requirement, intolerance to multiple nutrients during acute illness, and therapy-related interference with mineral retention or metabolism. Critically ill neonates or children who require parenteral nutrition (PN) often do not tolerate increased nutrient intake, especially the energy load. Thus, it is unrealistic to expect a critically ill child to achieve normal growth (ie, normal anabolic state). In critically ill preterm neonates, growth rarely reaches the in utero rate, thus the needs for minerals are correspondingly less compared to stable and growing patients. For preterm infants who are not receiving any medications that might interfere with mineral absorption, excretion, or metabolism, no convincing evidence exists for clinically significant mineral deficiency in the stable small preterm infant with adequate growth who is receiving adequate volumes (>150 mL/kg/d) of high-energy (≥24 kcal/oz) preterm infant formula or mother's milk fortified with commercial human milk fortifier containing protein, energy, and high mineral contents.

Malabsorption states, chronic therapy with loop diuretics, gastric acid inhibitors, or corticosteroids as well as heritable disorders of mineral metabolism are associated with abnormalities in mineral retention and/or metabolism.[1,2,4,5] In disease states, a deficiency involving multiple minerals and additional nutrients may be unmasked during therapy. This type of deficiency is best illustrated by the simultaneous development of hypophosphatemia, hypomagnesemia, and hypokalemia during refeeding of severely malnourished individuals.

Excess Intake and Adverse Effects

The most common risk factor for excessive intake of minerals is associated with increased parenteral intake of minerals arising from the unrealistic expectation of normal growth in the critically ill child. Minerals delivered via parenteral routes can exceed the excretory capacity, most commonly resulting in hyperphosphatemia and hypermagnesemia with associated hypocalcemia.[1,2,7] These findings may in part reflect "shifts" in minerals among various compartments, but they also suggest that delivery of minerals can exceed the body's needs.

Adverse effects from excess dietary intake of minerals occur rarely in pediatric ages. However, some healthy infants may possibly develop hyperphosphatemia and secondary hypocalcemia from feeding of standard infant formula. This situation results from a combination of higher intake of P from infant formulas relative to breast milk and the inability to eliminate the excess P because of immature kidney and parathyroid gland function.[1,2] Most of the adverse effects of excess mineral intake are due to excessive intake of supplements in pharmacologic doses and may result in serious morbidity and even mortality. The derivation of the current recommendation for the upper level of intake of Mg is based on the amount of supplement.[4]

Calcium
(1 mmol = 40 mg)

Biochemistry and Physiology

Ca is the most abundant mineral in the human body and accounts for about 1%–2% of adult human body weight. More than 99% of total body Ca is stored in the bones and teeth, where it functions to support their structure. Thus, Ca is critical for normal growth and development of the skeleton and teeth. The remaining 1% occurs throughout the body in blood, muscle, and other tissues and is critical to numerous physiological functions. In the circulation, ~50% of Ca is ionized and the rest is bound to albumin or complexed to small anions such as citrate, bicarbonate, and phosphate.

Optimal bodily function depends on maintaining the circulating total, and especially the ionized Ca concentration, within a narrow range. Ca exerts its effect either through a membrane-bound Ca-sensing receptor (a member of the G protein–coupled receptor family, expressed on numerous organs and tissues) or at the cellular level through the action of ionized Ca, which functions as both an extracellular and intracellular messenger. Its role as a secondary messenger is critical to numerous bodily functions including muscle contraction, blood vessel contraction and expansion, the secretion of hormones and enzymes, and message relay through the nervous system.[1,2]

The FDA authorized placement of a health claim on food labels that states, "The role of adequate Ca intake, or when appropriate, the role of adequate Ca and vitamin D intake, throughout life is linked to reduced risk of osteoporosis through the mechanism of optimizing peak bone mass during adolescence and early adulthood." However, further data are needed for other health claims.[5,15]

Sources

Ca is present in many dietary sources, with dairy products having the best bioavailability (Table 6-2) and accounting for >70% of dietary Ca intake in the United States.[4,5] Nonfat and reduced fat dairy products contain the same amount of Ca as regular dairy products. Some food sources (eg, fruit juices, fruit drinks, tofu, and cereals) are fortified with various Ca compounds that are well absorbed. Ca is present in human milk in relatively constant amounts between 200 and 250 mg/L. Various Ca salts are added to cow's milk formulas for term infants to provide at least 60 mg/100 kcal.[16] This Ca concentration is about 2-fold higher than that in human milk.[13] Ca-fortified formulas for small preterm infants may have Ca concentrations 4-fold to 6-fold higher than those in human milk.

Oral supplements such as Ca compounds containing carbonate and citrate are the most common although preparations containing other anions are available. Naturally occurring products (eg, oyster shell marketed as a Ca supplement) contain high levels of lead, mercury, and other potentially toxic contaminants.[17] Common parenteral supplements include calcium gluconate and calcium chloride, but other compounds are also available. The proportion of elemental Ca by weight varies with the Ca compound: 40% for carbonate, 38% for tribasic calcium phosphate, 21% for citrate, 13% for lactate, 9% for gluconate, and 6.4% for glubionate.[17,18]

Absorption, Excretion, and Metabolism

Gastric acid aids in the digestion of natural or Ca-fortified food or drink. Some Ca compounds such as calcium citrate are better absorbed than calcium carbonate in individuals with decreased gastric acid. About 90% of the Ca absorbed is through the small intestine and < 10% is absorbed through the large intestine. Paracellular absorption takes place throughout the small intestine and depends on the concentration gradient. Transcellular absorption takes place largely in the duodenum and is dependent on 1,25 $(OH)_2D$.

The efficiency of Ca absorption decreases with increased amounts of Ca consumed and with the presence of non-Ca components in the diet. These components include the type and amount of carbohydrate, phytic acid (whole grain bread, wheat bran, beans, seeds, nuts, grains, and soy isolates), and/or oxalic acid (spinach, collard greens, sweet potatoes, rhubarb, and beans) that may bind to Ca and prevent its optimal absorption. These plant substances do not appear to interfere with Ca absorption from other foods.

Ca is excreted through feces, urine, and sweat. Ca excretion can be increased by many factors including high dietary intake of sodium, protein, and caffeine. High potassium intake lowers urinary Ca, thereby affecting the net Ca absorption.[5,19] The effect of dietary P on Ca and bone metabolism is limited if Ca intake is adequate.[4] The detrimental effects of consuming foods high in phosphate, such as carbonated soft drinks, are probably due to milk being replaced with soda, not phosphate itself playing a role.[20] Chronic use of Mg antacids and potent loop diuretics such as furosemide can increase urinary Ca excretion. Aluminum antacids should not be used, especially for individuals with limited renal function, such as infants, because of potential aluminum toxicity.[21] Chronic therapy with a proton pump inhibitor results in multiple side effects including hypomagnesemia and raises risks for fractures.[22,23]

Retention of Ca generally reflects the body's need, which is usually higher in individuals undergoing rapid growth and may be > 60% of dietary intake. Adequate intakes of Ca that meet or exceed the amount needed to maintain a state of adequate nutrition in nearly all members of a specific age group of either sex are shown in Table 6-1. The pregnant and lactating adolescent theoretically could have an increased need for Ca because both bone mineralization of the mother and the fetus need support. A compensatory increase in Ca absorption may occur, however, and any decrease in bone mass during pregnancy and lactation is replenished upon return of ovarian function; therefore, no additional increase in dietary Ca intake is recommended.[5] However, adequate maternal diets except for very low Ca intake can lower the fetal bone mineral content. This situation can be prevented by an adequate Ca intake from diet or Ca supplementation.[24] At all ages,[25] particularly in young children, dietary Ca absorption is primarily regulated by Ca[26] rather than vitamin D[27] intake.

Ca and Mg homeostasis rely on dietary intake and 3 components:

- Absorption, excretion, and tissue accretion involving the primary target organs of GI tract, kidney, and bone;
- Direct modulation of transport and mobilization of these minerals, mainly PTH and the active vitamin D metabolite, 1,25 $(OH)_2D$, with additional modulation by other factors such as FGF 23;
- Sensors controlling the transport of Ca and Mg ions in tissues.[1,2]

Transient perturbation in Ca and P homeostasis occurs in some term infants fed regular infant formula. These formulas contain much greater P than human milk, and in some infants, formula ingestion coupled with immature renal function and PTH response to the high P load can result in hyperphosphatemia and hypocalcemia. These infants often present with seizures from hypocalcemia. Symptomatic support with Ca supplement for a few days and a switch to an infant formula with a P content comparable to that of human milk for several months are sufficient to return serum Ca and P concentrations to the normal range.[2] A feeding challenge with regular infant formula is warranted after a few months to ensure that the renal and PTH functions have matured sufficiently to handle the resumption of the increased dietary P load. If the infant does not quickly respond to this management approach, further endocrinology work-up is appropriate. A similar approach can be undertaken for preterm infants who develop hyperphosphatemia and hypocalcemia from excessive P load.

In pediatrics, the gut and kidney primarily act to retain Ca for the growth needs of the bone, hence a positive Ca balance always exists during growth. Dietary Ca, physical activity, and pubertal stage have independent effects on the rate of bone mineralization and therefore mineral retention.[28,29] Maintenance Ca intake should generally be in the form of foods because of the range of other nutrients present in various foods.[30] Foods fortified with Ca have increased the options for Ca-rich foods in the diet.[5,31]

Deficiency States

Risk factors for a deficient state include increased need, as in the rapidly growing infant, and the presence of disease states that affect Ca digestion, absorption, or metabolism. Physically active females, particularly those with secondary menstrual disorders, may have lower Ca absorption and decreased bone formation, and adequate Ca intake is important to their bone health.[32] Lactose-intolerant individuals may be at risk for Ca deficiency, not because they are unable absorb Ca, but rather because they avoid dairy products.[5] Drinking milk with a meal and other dietary options (eg, choosing aged cheeses such as Cheddar and Swiss, which contain little lactose; yogurt, which contains live active cultures that aid in lactose digestion; or lactose-reduced and lactose-free milk) may allow increased Ca intake.[33] Strict vegans[34] should include adequate amounts of nondairy sources of Ca in their daily diets; otherwise, they will likely need a Ca supplement to meet the recommended Ca intake.

Dietary Ca deficiency is a risk factor for fractures,[5] although it is usually not associated with clinical or biochemical manifestations unless the Ca intake is extremely low. In general, hypocalcemia does not occur solely because of low Ca intake; concomitant deficiency of vitamin D or Mg or associated medical problems are also present. Severe hypocalcemia may result in clinical signs and symptoms that may be subtle and vary with an individual's maturity. Preterm infants often manifest nonspecific symptomatology that may include irritability, jitteriness or lethargy, poor feeding with or without feeding intolerance, abdominal distention, apnea, cyanosis, and seizures. These features may be confused with manifestations of hypoglycemia, sepsis, meningitis, anoxia, intracranial bleeding, or narcotic withdrawal. The degree of irritability of the infant does not appear to correlate with serum Ca values. In more mature individuals, other symptoms and signs may include tetany from peripheral hyperexcitability of motor nerves. In chronic deficient states, Ca is mobilized from the skeleton to maintain Ca levels in the blood, which is a predisposing factor for suboptimal bone accretion. In young children, both Ca and vitamin D deficiency have key roles in the development of rickets.[13,14]

Resolution of hypocalcemia may not be possible until the underlying cause has been corrected. For example, hypocalcemia secondary to Mg deficit may not be correctable until Mg replacement therapy is initiated.

Excess Intake and Adverse Effects

Excess Ca intake can result in hypercalcemia (serum or plasma total Ca > 11 mg/dL or ionized Ca > 5.6 mg/dL, respectively) and its complications of polyuria and polydipsia, renal calculi, and metastatic calcification. High dietary Ca intakes and routine Ca supplementation generally do not cause hypercalcemia. However, high Ca intake has the potential to interfere with the absorption of other minerals such as iron, zinc, Mg, and P. Ca supplements can interact with several prescription and over-the-counter medications.[35,36] Ca decreases absorption of digoxin, fluroquinolones, levothyroxine, tetracycline, tiludronate disodium, phenytoin, and mineral oil or stimulant laxatives when taken simultaneously with these drugs. Thiazide diuretics can interact with calcium carbonate and vitamin D supplements, increasing the risk for hypercalcemia and hypercalciuria. Ca supplements from natural products such as oyster shell should be avoided because of possible toxic contaminants.

Hypercalcemia may be a manifestation of P deficiency (see Phosphorus section). Metastatic deposits of Ca precipitate in the infusion delivery system, in kidneys, and in other organs and increased mortality have been reported in neonates who received ceftriaxone simultaneously with parenteral solutions containing Ca.[37]

Phosphorus
(1 mmol = 31 mg)

Biochemistry and Physiology

P as phosphate is an essential constituent of all known protoplasm. P and phosphate are often used interchangeably, but the term phosphate actually means the inorganic freely available form. This measurable component is generally referred to as phosphorus (P).

Tissue P is ~0.5% of the body weight in the neonate and increases to ~1% in the adult because of greater bone and soft tissue mass. Structurally, P is incorporated in mineralized tissues of the skeleton and teeth, in biological membranes as phospholipids, and in cells as nucleotides and nucleic acids. About 85% of P is in the skeleton, primarily in the form of hydroxyapatite. Of the remainder, 14% is intracellular (primarily in the soft tissues) and 1% is extracellular in the circulation and interstitial fluid. Of the extracellular P, 70%

is organic and contained within phospholipids, and 30% is inorganic.[38] At pH 7.4, the mono-hydrogen and di-hydrogen form is in a ratio of about 4:1. For that reason, P is usually expressed in millimole rather than milli-equivalents per liter.

The serum or plasma P concentration is ~1–2 mmol/L (3.1–6.2 mg/dL) and is higher at younger ages. Plasma P concentrations of preterm infants is about 0.5 mmol higher, but it can be as high as 2.81 mmol/L (8.7 mg/dL) without affecting plasma Ca concentration.[1,2] This minute compartment of P is the major source of exchange of P associated with dietary uptake and absorption, renal excretion and reabsorption, and bone modeling and remodeling. This compartment is also the primary source of P for structural and high-energy phosphate in the cells of all tissues. When extracellular fluid P concentrations are low, cellular dysfunction follows.

A normal level of P in the extracellular fluid is necessary for cellular function and skeletal mineralization. The physiological functions include the maintenance of mineral and acid–base homeostasis, the temporary storage of the transfer of energy derived from metabolic fuels, and the activation of many catalytic proteins through phosphorylation.[38] Most of these processes involve the recycling of P. Thus, the role of dietary P is to support tissue growth and to replace excretory and cellular and dermal losses.[4]

Sources

P is ubiquitous in natural foods and is present in both organic and inorganic forms.[4,10,12] Various phosphate salts used in food processing for nonnutritive functions (eg, moisture retention, smoothness, and binding) provide significant contributions to dietary P intake. Cola soft drinks contain phosphoric acid as the acidulant and provide about 50 mg of P per 12 oz serving.[4] P intake from soft drinks can be substantial when multiple servings are consumed.

Dairy and meat products have high P density. Plants, nuts, and seeds are also significant sources of P. Animal or synthetic protein has more bioavailable P than soy or grain-based protein. P in plants (beans, peas, cereals, nuts) is present in the poorly digestible phytic acid. However, some phytate P is absorbed from the combined effect of food phytases, colonic bacteria enzymes, and yeast products.[4] Human milk has low P content, which decreases further with prolonged lactation, although the P bioavailability is higher than all other milks for infants. Compared to human milk, P content is higher in cow's milk by 5- to 6-fold, standard cow milk–based infant formula by about 2-fold, and soy-based infant formula by about 3-fold.[16] The Ca-P ratio varies widely in natural foods. However, both the Ca-P ratio and absolute quantities of these minerals are important to optimize mineral accretion in bone and soft tissue. P supplements are available as mono- and dibasic phosphates, in both oral and parenteral forms. They are usually used for medical indications such as PN and inherited metabolic defects.

Absorption, Excretion, and Metabolism

Net absorption of P ranges from 55% to 70% in adults and 65% to 90% in children and infants. The fractional P absorption is virtually constant across a broad range of intakes. The bulk of P absorption is passive (paracellular) and concentration dependent. A saturable, active transcellular sodium (Na^+)-dependent absorption involving the type IIb Na^+/phosphate cotransporter and facilitated by 1,25 $(OH)_2D$ also exists. P is not absorbed in the stomach but is absorbed throughout the small bowel. The fractional absorption of P and other minerals is lower from infant formulas compared to human milk, although the absolute amounts of each mineral absorbed from infant formulas are higher because of the much higher mineral content in infant formulas.

Medications or foods that bind P (antacids, phosphate binders, and Ca) can decrease the net amount of P absorbed by decreasing the free phosphate for absorption. Unabsorbed Ca complexes with phytic acid and can interfere with bacterial hydrolysis of phytate, decreasing P absorption.[4]

The kidney is a major regulator of P homeostasis. Renal P is reabsorbed primarily at proximal tubular cells (70%–80%). The remaining P is reabsorbed in the distal tubules. Renal P reabsorption is increased by the abundance of type IIa Na/phosphate cotransporter (Npt2a) protein at the basolateral basement membrane, and it requires the interaction of Npt2a with various scaffolding and regulatory proteins.[40] Renal P reabsorption is also increased by growth hormone, thyroid hormone, and 1,25 $(OH)_2D$. Renal P reabsorption is decreased by an increase in the circulating concentration of P or dietary P mediated by an increase in FGF 23. Although the effects are more minor, renal P reabsorption is decreased by volume expansion, metabolic acidosis, glucocorticoids, and calcitonin. FGF 23 and PTH are major phosphaturic hormones, and their secretion is increased by both dietary and circulating P.[39–41] Serum P increases as the total P intake and absorption exceeds the renal filtration and excretion for P.

The kidney can increase or decrease its P resorptive capacity to accommodate P needs. In infants and children, lower glomerular filtration rate is probably the main determinant of the higher serum P because P resorptive capacity is high even in the small preterm infant.[1] Healthy infants have lower serum P when breastfed compared to those fed infant formula.[1,42] The lowest level of renal excretory work to maintain normal P homeostasis during the first year is achieved with human milk as the major source of minerals. In deficient states, renal retention of filtered phosphate is almost complete even in the preterm infant.[1]

Deficiency States

Cellular storage of phosphate and the portion of P that can be mobilized from bone are limited. Thus, dietary P is required to maintain extracellular fluid P, which is the source of P for the tissue metabolic phosphate. Because P is ubiquitous in foods, dietary P deficiency rarely occurs unless the individual is subjected to near total starvation except in small preterm infants with selected milk feedings; for example, small preterm infants with prolonged exclusive feeding of mother's milk without multi-nutrient fortifier or those fed infant formula with low mineral content. In addition, P must be added to PN to prevent the development of P deficiency. Poorly managed PN with inadequate P content, inappropriate administration of fluid and electrolyte therapy that causes excessive renal P loss, or rapid refeeding in the setting of diabetic ketoacidosis or in severely malnourished patients, especially if accompanied by diarrhea, place an individual at risk for hypophosphatemia in addition to other electrolyte abnormalities.[1,2,43] Individuals with chronic aluminum antacid therapy and heritable defects of P metabolism can also manifest P deficiency. Chronic diuretic therapy that increases urine P can exacerbate the P deficit.

Clinical manifestations of P deficiency include anorexia, general debility, anemia, muscle weakness including respiratory compromise, bone pain, rickets and osteomalacia, increased susceptibility to infection, paresthesia, ataxia, confusion, and even death.[44] Cellular dysfunction and clinical manifestations can occur when the extracellular fluid P is < 0.65 mmol/L (2 mg/dL) and universally occurs when the extracellular fluid P is < 0.3 mmol/L (0.9 mg/dL). Plasma Ca may be elevated simultaneously to hypercalcemic levels, particularly in infants.[1,2]

Excess Intake and Adverse Effects

Essentially all the adverse effects of excess P intake from any source are the result of hyperphosphatemia. These effects include adjustments in the hormonal control system regulating Ca homeostasis and may be complicated by hypocalcemia and its adverse effects; ectopic (metastatic) cal-

cification, particularly of the kidney; and possible decreases in the intestinal absorption of Ca, iron, zinc, and copper. Hyperphosphatemia usually occurs in the setting of kidney disease and rarely occurs under normal circumstances. One exception is the development of hyperphosphatemia and secondary hypocalcemia in some healthy infants who consume standard infant formulas. This situation results from a combination of higher intake of P from infant formulas relative to breast milk and the inability to eliminate excess P because of immature renal and parathyroid functions. Clinically, this is exacerbated by the early introduction of solids or whole cow's milk to the infant.[1,2]

Magnesium
(1 mmol = 24 mg)

Biochemistry and Physiology

Mg is the fourth most abundant cation in the body and is the second most abundant intracellular cation. Total body Mg content is ~25 g (1000 mmol), of which ~60% resides in bone. About one-third of the skeletal Mg is exchangeable and serves as a reservoir for maintaining extracellular Mg concentration. The remaining Mg is in soft tissues such as muscle and organs, and ~1% is in extracellular fluid. Cellular Mg content is 6–9 mmol/kg net weight, and most of this Mg is localized in membrane structures (eg, microsome, mitochondria, plasma membrane).[45,46] The much smaller pool of free Mg in the cell is maintained at ~1 mmol/L and is in an exchanging equilibrium with membrane-bound Mg. This unbound intracellular Mg has a critical role in cellular physiology.[47] Intracellular Mg usually remains stable despite wide fluctuations in serum Mg. In Mg-deficient states, however, the intracellular content of Mg can be low despite normal serum concentrations. Serum Mg has a protein-bound (~30%) and an ultrafiltrable (~70%) portion. Of the latter, 70%–80% is in ionic form. The remainder is complexed to anions, particularly phosphate, citrate, and oxalate.

Mg is a required cofactor for >300 enzyme systems. It is critical for normal ATP function and glucose metabolism, and it is necessary for both aerobic and anaerobic metabolism. Mg is also important in cellular cytoskeleton contraction and at the myoneural junction; in this role, it can alter skeletal and cardiac muscle function. It catalyzes enzymatic processes pertaining to the transfer, storage, and use of energy; regulation of movement of potassium and Ca across cell membranes; and numerous other cell functions. Abnormalities in circulating Mg concentrations are associated with widespread cellular effects.

Sources

Mg is ubiquitous in foods, but the Mg content of foods varies substantially. Green leafy vegetables are rich in Mg because chlorophyll is the Mg chelate of porphyrin. Unpolished grains and nuts also have high Mg content, whereas meats and milk have intermediate levels. Refined foods generally have the lowest Mg content.[48,49] Water is a variable source of Mg, but "hard" water typically has higher concentrations of Mg salts.[4,49] Human milk contains adequate amounts of Mg, and infant formulas are mandated to contain at least 6 mg/100 kcal.[16] Supplements containing various Mg salts are readily available in oral forms. The proportion of elemental Mg by weight is 60.3% for oxide; 28% for carbonate; 16% for citrate; ~12% for chloride, acetate, and lactate; 9.7% for sulfate; 6.8% for phosphate; 6.4% for ascorbate; and 5.4% for gluconate.[18] Magnesium sulfate is available in parenteral form. Mg supplements may contribute a substantial portion of daily intake and are used as a basis for the derivation of tolerable upper intake levels.[4]

Absorption, Excretion, and Metabolism

The net absorption of Mg is about 40%–60%. Fractional intestinal absorption is inversely proportional to the amount of Mg ingested. Intestinal absorption occurs via a passive gradient-dependent paracellular and an active saturable vitamin D–dependent transcellular mechanism. Mg is absorbed throughout the entire intestinal tract, with maximal absorption at the distal jejunum and ileum.[4] Mg absorption is not significantly affected by other nutrients at usual dietary intake levels. It is lowered with high P intake, particularly in association with a high fiber and phytate intake, and at low protein intake.[4,50]

The kidney plays an important role in the homeostasis of divalent ions. Most of the ionized forms of Ca and Mg are reabsorbed at the proximal tubules and the thick ascending limb of Henle's loop via a passive paracellular pathway. Renal Ca and Mg reabsorption is dependent on salt and water reabsorption and rate of fluid flow. The distal convolute tubule and the connecting tubule are the sites where ionized Ca and ionized Mg are reabsorbed via an active transcellular transport, and this process determines the final plasma Mg concentrations.

Mg is often considered "a natural Ca antagonist," and Mg homeostasis is regulated similarly to but less tightly than Ca homeostasis. Renal Mg transport is also affected by both hormonal (PTH, calcitonin, glucagon, arginine vasopressin, 17β estradiol) and nonhormonal factors. High intake of glucose, sodium, Ca, and Mg and chronic excessive alcohol intake, as well as elevated serum Mg or Ca, depletion of potassium and phosphate, and metabolic acidosis inhibit Mg and Ca reabsorption, leading to increased urine excretion of both cations.[51] When hypocalcemia coexists with hypomagnesemia, the former may not respond to therapy until hypomagnesemia is corrected. Mg is increasingly being used as an adjunct therapy to treat asthma and cystic fibrosis in children and to halt preterm labor in mothers for neuroprotection of the fetus. The exact mechanisms of supplemental Mg therapy in these states remain to be elucidated.

Deficiency States

Mg deficiency is usually associated with malabsorption, increased losses from the gut or kidney, or upon refeeding of severe and chronically malnourished individuals. Loop diuretics, cisplatin, and tacrolimus are among the medications that result in increased renal Mg excretion and predisposition to Mg deficiency.[51] In addition, reports are increasing regarding patients with heritable defects of Mg transport that lead to Mg wasting and deficiency states.[52–54]

The typical deficit required to produce symptomatic hypomagnesemia is approximately 0.5–1 mmol (12–24 mg)/kg of body weight.[55] Hypomagnesemia is usually associated with a significant Mg deficit. These individuals often are at risk for concurrent hypocalcemia, hypokalemia, hypophosphatemia, and possible disturbance of acid–base status. The loss of other nutrients such as zinc through GI secretion may also be considerable. Hypomagnesemia often coexists with hypocalcemia.

Hypomagnesemia and hypocalcemia may have similar clinical manifestations. Prolonged dietary Mg deprivation in human adults leads to personality change, tremor, muscle fasciculation, spontaneous carpopedal spasm, and generalized spasticity as well as hypomagnesemia, hypocalcemia, and hypokalemia.[55] In infants, acute complications associated with clinical manifestations include seizure, apnea, cyanosis and hypoxia, electrocardiographic changes, bradycardia, and hypotension.

Excess Intake and Adverse Effects

Ingestion of Mg from natural foods has not been shown to exert any adverse effects. However, adverse effects of excess Mg intake have been reported for nonfood sources, such as various Mg salts for pharmacologic purposes, particularly in patients with renal dysfunction. The amount of Mg supplement is the basis from which the current upper limit of Mg intake is derived.[4] The primary initial manifestation of excessive Mg intake from nonfood sources is diarrhea (probably from its osmotic effect), which may be accompanied by nausea and abdominal cramping. Neuromuscular depression with floppiness and lethargy and respiratory depression are frequent clinical manifestations of severe neonatal hypermagnesemia in infants born to mothers who received Mg therapy prior to delivery.[1,2] Acute hypotonia, apnea, hypotension, and refractory bradycardia mimicking septic shock syndrome has been reported in premature infants accidentally overdosed with Mg in PN.[56] In adults with hypermagnesemia, hypotension and urinary retention occur at serum Mg concentrations of 1.67–2.5 mmol/L (4–6 mg/dL); central nervous system depression, hyporeflexia, and electrocardiographic abnormalities (ie, increased atrioventricular and ventricular conduction time) at 2.5–5 mmol/L (6–12 mg/dL); and respiratory depression, coma, and cardiac arrest above 5 mmol/L (12 mg/dL).[57]

Test Your Knowledge Questions

1. Which of the following statements on bioavailability of calcium is incorrect?
   A. Low-fat dairy products are a good source of bioavailable calcium.
   B. Presence of phytate in plants can decrease calcium bioavailability.
   C. Calcium supplement in food sources are bioavailable.
   D. Vitamin D is a major determinant of calcium bioavailability.

2. Which of the following statements on calcium absorption is incorrect?
   A. It is inversely related to dietary content of calcium.
   B. It is related to growth rate.
   C. It is decreased with lactose intolerance.
   D. Dietary zinc does not impair calcium absorption.

3. Which of the following statement about phosphorus is incorrect?
   A. It is ubiquitous in natural foods.
   B. Dietary intake of phosphorus is increased with increased consumption of processed foods.
   C. Soy or grain-based protein has more bioavailable phosphorus than animal protein.
   D. Phosphorus deficiency can result in hypercalcemia.

4. Low serum inorganic phosphate is associated with all of the following except:
   A. Increased PTH.
   B. Increased FGF 23.
   C. Vitamin D deficiency.
   D. Decreased renal function.

5. The following findings can be associated with magnesium deficit except:
   A. The deficit can result from chronic gastrointestinal losses.
   B. It can result in increased fecal fat loss.
   C. It can be associated with deficiency of other nutrients.
   D. It can result in hypocalcemia.

6. Which of the following statements about hypermagnesemia is incorrect?
   A. It can increase cardiac arrhythmia.
   B. It can increase respiratory failure.
   C. It can increase central nervous system depression.
   D. It can increase tendon reflex.

References

1. Koo WWK. Neonatal calcium, magnesium and phosphorus disorders. In: Lifshitz F, ed. *Pediatric Endocrinology: A Clinical Guide.* 5th ed. New York, NY: Marcel Dekker Inc; 2007:497–529.
2. Koo WWK, Tsang RC. Calcium and magnesium homeostasis. In: MacDonald MG, Seshia MMK, eds. *Avery's Neonatology—Pathophysiology and Management of the Newborn.* 7th ed. Philadelphia, PA: Lippincott-Williams and Wilkins. In press.
3. U.S. Food and Drug Administration. Guidance for industry: a food labeling guide. http://www.fda.gov/food/guidance-regulation/guidancedocumentsregulatoryinformation/labelingnutrition/ucm064916.htm. Updated November 22, 1013. Accessed July 10, 2014.
4. Food and Nutrition Board, Institute of Medicine. *Dietary Reference Intakes for Calcium, Phosphorus, Magnesium, Vitamin D and Fluoride.* Washington, DC: National Academy Press; 1997.
5. Institute of Medicine. 2011. *Dietary Reference Intakes for Calcium and Vitamin D.* Washington, DC: The National Academies Press.
6. U.S. Food and Drug Administration. Dietary supplements. http://www.fda.gov/AboutFDA/Transparency/Basics/ucm193949.htm. Updated June 3, 2010. Accessed October 14, 2014.
7. Koo WWK, McLaughlin K, Saba M. Nutrition support for the neonatal intensive care patients. In: Merritt R, ed. *The A.S.P.E.N. Nutrition Support Practice Manual.* 2nd ed. Silver Spring, MD: American Society for Parenteral and Enteral Nutrition; 2005:301–314.
8. Koo W, Walyat N. Vitamin D and skeletal growth and development. *Curr Osteoporos Rep.* 2013;11:188–193.
9. Bailey RL, Dodd KW, Goldman JA, et al. Estimation of total usual calcium and vitamin D intakes in the United States. *J Nutr.* 2010;140:817–822.
10. Pennington JAT, ed. *Bowes & Church's Food Values of Portions Commonly Used.* 19th ed. Philadelphia, PA: J. B. Lippincott; 2009.

11. Calcium content in foods. CalorieKing™ for Food Awareness Web site. http://www.calorieking.com. Accessed November 25, 2009.

12. USDA National Nutrient Database for Standard Reference. http://ndb.nal.usda.gov. Accessed July 10, 2014

13. Greer FR, Krebs NF; Committee on Nutrition. Optimizing bone health and calcium intakes of infants, children, and adolescents. *Pediatrics.* 2006;117:578–585.

14. Fischer PR, Thacher TD, Pettifor JM. Pediatric vitamin D and calcium nutrition in developing countries. *Rev Endocr Metab Disord.* 2008;9:181–192.

15. U.S. Food and Drug Administration. Guidance for industry: food labeling: health claims; calcium and osteoporosis, and calcium, vitamin D, and osteoporosis. http://www.fda.gov/food/guidanceregulation/guidancedocumentsregulatory-information/labelingnutrition/ucm152626.htm. Updated July 9, 2014. Accessed July 10, 2014.

16. U.S. Food and Drug Administration. Infant formula nutrient specifications. CFR 21.http://www.accessdata.fda.gov/scripts/cdrh/cfdocs/cfcfr/CFRSearch.cfm?CFR-Part=107&showFR=1&subpartNode=21:2.0.1.1.7.4. Updated September 1, 2014. Accessed October 14, 2014

17. Levenson D, Bockman R. A review of calcium preparations. *Nutr Rev.* 1994;52:221–232.

18. *Drug Facts and Comparisons* 2009. St. Louis, MO: Wolters Kluwer Health.

19. Standing Committee on the Scientific Evaluation of Dietary Reference Intakes, Food and Nutrition Board, Institute of Medicine. *Dietary Reference Intakes for Water, Potassium, Sodium, Chloride, and Sulfate.* Washington, DC: National Academy Press; 2004.

20. Heaney RP, Rafferty K. Carbonated beverages and urinary calcium excretion. *Am J Clin Nutr.* 2001;74:343–347.

21. Koo WWK, Kaplan LA. Aluminum and bone disorders: with specific reference to aluminum contamination of infant nutrients. *J Am Coll Nutr.* 1988;7:199–214.

22. Yang YX, Lewis JD, Epstein S, Metz DC. Long-term proton pump inhibitor therapy and risk of hip fracture. *JAMA.* 2006;296:2947–2953.

23. Proton pump inhibitors information. U.S. Food and Drug Administration Web site. http://www.fda.gov/drugs-safety/informationbydrugclass/ucm213259.htm. Updated February 9, 2012. Accessed July 10, 2014.

24. Koo WWK, Walters JC, Esterlitz J, Levine RJ, Bush AJ, Sibai B. Maternal calcium supplementation and fetal bone mineralization. *Obstet Gynecol.* 1999;94:577–582.

25. Bronner F. Recent developments in intestinal calcium absorption. *Nutr Rev.* 2009;67:109–113.

26. Oramasionwu GE, Thacher TD, Pam SD, Pettifor JM, Abrams SA. Adaptation of calcium absorption during treatment of nutritional rickets in Nigerian children. *Br J Nutr.* 2008;100:387–392.

27. Thacher TD, Obadofin MO, O'Brien KO, Abrams SA. The effect of vitamin D_2 and vitamin D_3 on intestinal calcium absorption in Nigerian children with rickets. *J Clin Endocrinol Metab.* 2009;94:3314–3321.

28. Slemenda CW, Reister TK, Hui SL, Miller JZ, Christian JC, Johnston CC Jr. Influences on skeletal mineralization in children and adolescents: evidence for varying effects of sexual maturation and physical activity. *J Pediatr.* 1994;125:201–207.

29. Specker BL. Evidence for an interaction between calcium intake and physical activity on changes in bone mineral density. *J Bone Miner Res.* 1996;11:1539–1544.

30. Fulgoni VL 3rd, Keast DR, Auestad N, Quann EE. Nutrients from dairy foods are difficult to replace in diets of Americans: food pattern modeling and an analyses of the National Health and Nutrition Examination Survey 2003-2006. *Nutr Res.* 2011;31:759–765.

31. Dietary supplement fact sheet: calcium. National Institutes of Health, Office of Dietary Supplements Web site. http://ods.od.nih.gov/factsheets/calcium.asp. Reviewed November 21, 2013. Accessed July 10, 2014.

32. Nattiv A. Stress fractures and bone health in track and field athletes. *J Sci Med Sport.* 2000;3:268–279.

33. U.S. Food and Drug Administration. Problems digesting dairy products? http://www.fda.gov/downloads/forconsumers/consumerupdates/ucm143705.pdf. Published October 2009. Accessed July 10, 2014.

34. Key TJ, Appleby PN, Rosell MS. Health effects of vegetarian and vegan diets. *Proc Nutr Soc.* 2006;65:35–41.

35. Shannon MT, Wilson BA, Stang CL. *Health Professionals Drug Guide.* Stamford, CT: Appleton & Lange; 2000.

36. Jellin JM, Gregory P, Batz F, Hitchens K. *Pharmacist's Letter/Prescriber's Letter Natural Medicines Comprehensive Database.* 3rd ed. Stockton, CA: Therapeutic Research Facility; 2000.

37. U.S. Food and Drug Administration. Information for Healthcare Professionals: Ceftriaxone (marketed as Rocephin and generics). http://www.fda.gov/Drugs/DrugSafety/PostmarketDrugSafetyInformationforPatientsandProviders/DrugSafetyInformationforHeathcareProfessionals/ucm084263.htm#main. Updated April 21, 2009. Accessed October 14, 2014.

38. Nordin BEC. Phosphorus. *J Food Nutr.* 1988;45:62–75.

39. Takeda E, Taketani Y, Sawada N, Sato T, Yamamoto H. The regulation and function of phosphate in the human body. *Biofactors.* 2004;21:345–355.

40. Tenenhouse HS. Regulation of phosphorus homeostasis by the type IIa Na/phosphate cotransporter. *Annu Rev Nutr.* 2005;25:197–214.

41. Lederer E. Regulation of serum phosphate. *J Physiol.* 2014;592(Pt 18):3985–3995.

42. Specker BL, Lichtenstein P, Mimouni F, Gormley C, Tsang RC. Calcium-regulating hormones and minerals from birth to 18 months of age: a cross-sectional study. II. Effects of sex, race, age, season, and diet on serum minerals, parathyroid hormone, and calcitonin. *Pediatrics.* 1986;77:891–896.

43. Freiman I, Pettifor JM, Moodley GM. Serum phosphorus in protein energy malnutrition. *J Pediatr Gastroenterol Nutr.* 1982;1:547–550.

44. Lotz M, Zisman E, Bartter FC. Evidence for a phosphorus-depletion syndrome in man. *N Engl J Med.* 1968;278:409–415.

45. Elin RJ. Assessment of magnesium status. *Clin Chem.* 1987;33:1965–1970.
46. Reinhart RA. Magnesium metabolism: a review with special reference to the relationship between intracellular content and serum levels. *Arch Intern Med.* 1988;148:2415–2420.
47. Saris NE, Mervaala E, Karppanen H, Khawaja JA, Lewenstam A. Magnesium. An update on physiological, clinical and analytical aspects. *Clin Chim Acta.* 2000;294:1–26.
48. Egan SK, Tao SS, Pennington JA, Bolger PM. U.S. Food and Drug Administration's Total Diet Study: intake of nutritional and toxic elements, 1991-96. *Food Addit Contam.* 2002;19:103–125.
49. National Institutes of Health. Office of Dietary Supplements. Magnesium. http://ods.od.nih.gov/factsheets/magnesium.asp. Reviewed November 4, 2013. Accessed July 10, 2014.
50. Schwartz R, Walker G, Linz MD, MacKellar I. Metabolic responses of adolescent boys to two levels of dietary magnesium and protein. I. Magnesium and nitrogen retention. *Am J Clin Nutr.* 1973;26:510–518.
51. Quamme GA. Renal magnesium handling: new insights in understanding old problems. *Kidney Int.* 1997;52:1180–1195.
52. OMIM - Online Mendelian Inheritance in Man. National Center for Biotechnology Information Web site. http://www.ncbi.nlm.nih.gov/omim. Accessed July 10, 2014.
53. Hoorn EJ, Zietse R. Disorders of calcium and magnesium balance: a physiology-based approach. *Pediatr Nephrol.* 2013; 28:1195–1206.
54. Lainez S, Schingmann KP, Van der Wijst J, et al. New TRPM6 missense mutations linked to hypomagnesemia with secondary hypocalcemia. *Eur J Hum Genet.* 2014;22:497–504.
55. Shils ME. Experimental human magnesium depletion. *Medicine.* 1969;48:61–85.
56. Ali A, Walentik C, Mantych GJ, Sadiq HF, Keenan WJ, Noguchi A. Iatrogenic acute hypermagnesemia after total parenteral nutrition infusion mimicking septic shock syndrome: two case reports. *Pediatrics.* 2003;112:e70–e72.
57. Mordes JP, Wacker WE. Excess magnesium. *Pharmacol Rev.* 1978;29:273–300.

Test Your Knowledge Answers

1. The correct answer is **D**. Rationale: Vitamin D affects the active component of calcium absorption, which is quantitatively much less than passive calcium absorption and does not directly influence calcium bioavailability. The preferred source of calcium is from the diet because diets with high bioavailable calcium are generally nutrient dense, with multiple other critical nutrients. Foods fortified with Ca have increased the options for Ca-rich foods in the diet. Naturally occurring products (eg, oyster shell) marketed as calcium supplements have disadvantages and may contain high levels of lead, mercury, and other potentially toxic contaminants.

2. The correct answer is **C**. Rationale: No evidence exists that lactose-intolerant individuals have intrinsically impaired Ca absorption. Lactose-intolerant individuals may be at risk for Ca deficiency, not because they are unable to absorb Ca, but rather because they avoid dairy products. Drinking milk with a meal and other dietary options (eg, choosing aged cheeses such as Cheddar and Swiss, which contain little lactose; yogurt, which contains live active cultures that aid in lactose digestion; or lactose-reduced and lactose-free milk) may allow increased Ca intake. Intestinal calcium absorption is generally higher with growth and with lower calcium intake. High Ca intake may decrease zinc absorption, but no convincing evidence exists that normal dietary zinc intake affects Ca absorption.

3. The correct answer is **C**. Rationale: Animal or synthetic protein has more bioavailable phosphorus than soy or grain-based protein. Phosphorus in plants (beans, peas, cereals, nuts) is present in poorly digestible phytic acid and is less bioavailable than P from animal protein. Various phosphate salts used in food processing for nonnutritive functions (eg, moisture retention, smoothness, and binding) provide significant contributions to dietary P intake. Phosphorus deficiency occurs in selected clinical situations and can have serious consequences, including hypercalcemia.

4. The correct answer is **D**. Rationale: The kidney is a major regulator of circulating P, and impaired renal function results in hyperphosphatemia. PTH and FGF are phosphaturic, and an increase in either can lower serum P. Vitamin D deficiency in infants results in rickets and can be associated with hypophosphatemia.

5. The correct answer is **B**. Rationale: Magnesium absorption is independent of fat absorption. Gastrointestinal secretions have high Mg content. Magnesium deficiency can occur with chronic losses from the gastrointestinal tract and concomitantly with deficiency of multiple other nutrients. Magnesium deficiency can have serious consequences including hypocalcemia. The latter may not resolve unless Mg deficiency has been corrected.

6. The correct answer is **D**. Rationale: Hypermagnesemia is associated with neuromuscular depression and therefore decreases tendon reflex. Other statements are correct.

7

Water-Soluble Essential Micronutrients

Winston Koo, MBBS, FACN, CNS; **Judith Christie**, RN, MSN; **May Saba**, PharmD, BCNSP;
Mirjana Lulic-Botica, BSc, BCPS; and **Letitia Warren**, RD, CSP

CONTENTS

Learning Objectives

1. Review the physiological basis for the function and requirement common to the group and unique to the individual water-soluble essential micronutrients.
2. Define the common risk factors and special considerations in the development of deficiency state for these micronutrients.
3. Define the common manifestations and diagnosis of deficiency state for these micronutrients.
4. Describe the potential risks with excessive intake of these micronutrients.

Overview

Water-soluble essential micronutrients include the 8 B-complex vitamins: thiamin (vitamin B$_1$), riboflavin (vitamin B$_2$), niacin (vitamin B$_3$), vitamin B$_6$ (pyridoxine), folate (vitamin B$_9$), vitamin B$_{12}$, vitamin C, pantothenic acid (vitamin B$_5$), biotin (vitamin B$_7$), and choline. These micronutrients affect the function of all cells, and many have interrelated transport mechanisms, metabolism, and functions.[1-3] In pediatric subjects, these cellular functions additionally affect growth and development.

Some of these essential nutrients can be synthesized de novo from other nutrients (eg, niacin from tryptophan, choline from methylation of phosphatidylethanolamine) or from intestinal bacteria (eg, riboflavin, pyridoxine, vitamin B$_{12}$, pantothenic acid, and biotin), although in amounts inadequate to meet physiological demands.

One or more of these micronutrients are used to fortify many food and drink products, some nutrients such as choline are added to foods as a component of an emulsifying agent, and all water-soluble micronutrients are available as individual supplements or as part of multivitamin +/- multinutrient supplements.[4–9] All are available as oral and parenteral preparations except for choline, which is available in oral form only. Vitamin B_{12} is also available in an intranasal form.[4,7,10] Multivitamin preparations used for parenteral nutrition (PN) are shown in Table 7-1.

For healthy near-term or term infants, milk from well-nourished mothers ingesting a varied diet should be sufficient to provide all water-soluble essential micronutri-

ents for their daily needs. Small preterm infants have greater needs for these and other nutrients because of minimal or absent reserves and for catch-up growth. Human milk fortifier added to mother's milk raises the concentration of these nutrients to multiple folds higher than what is naturally present in human milk and should be sufficient for preterm infants tolerating adequate volumes of enteral intake.[3] For formula-fed infants, the use of commercial milk-based formula designed for term and preterm infants is expected to

Table 7-1. Content per Unit Dose of Multivitamin Preparations for Use With Parenteral Nutrition

INGREDIENT/DOSE	M.V.I. PEDIATRIC	INFUVITE PEDIATRIC	M.V.I. ADULT FOR AGES ≥ 11 Y	M.V.I.-12	INFUVITE ADULT
Unit dose volume, mL	5[a]	5[b]	10[c]	10[c]	10[c]
Fat-soluble vitamins					
Vitamin A (retinol), mg	0.7	0.7	1	1	1
Vitamin D (erogocalciferol,[d] cholecalciferol[e]), mcg	10[d]	10[e]	5[d]	5[d]	5[e]
Vitamin E (DL-α-tocopheryl acetate), mg	7	7	10	10	10
Vitamin K (phytonadione), mcg	200	200	150	none	150
Water-soluble vitamins					
Vitamin B_1 (thiamin), mg	1.2	1.2	6	6	6
Vitamin B_2 (riboflavin), mg	1.4	1.4	3.6	3.6	3.6
Vitamin B_3 (niacinamide), mg	17	17	40	40	40
Vitamin B_6 (pyridoxine), mg	1	1	6	6	6
Folic acid (vitamin B_9), mcg	140	140	600	600	600
Vitamin B_{12} (cyanocobalamin), mcg	1	1	5	5	5
Vitamin C (ascorbic acid), mg	80	80	200	200	200
Dexpanthenol (D-pentothenyl alcohol), mg	5	5	15	15	15
Biotin, mcg	20	20	60	60	60
Other					
Aluminum, mcg/L	42	30	43–183	43–78	70
Polysorbate 80, mg	50	50	160	160	140
Polysorbate 20, mg	0.8	–	2.8	2.8	–
Propylene glycol, g	–	–	3	3	3

Data from manufacturer product insert: Hospira, Inc., Lake Forest, IL for M.V.I. Pediatric (August 2007), M.V.I. Adult (February 2009), and M.V.I.-12 (February 2009). Baxter Inc, Deerfield, IL for Infuvite Pediatric (September 2007) and Infuvite Adult (February 2012), and from Vanek et al.[6] Manufacturers, products, and product information can change frequently.

[a]Single dose vial reconstitute to 5 mL

[b]Two single dose vials: vial 2 (1 mL) contains folic acid, biotin, and vitamin B, and vial 1 (4 mL) contains all the other vitamins. For both pediatric preparations, 5 mL is the daily dose for infants and children weighing 3 kg or more up to age 11 years, 3.25 mL (65% of daily dose) for infants weighing 1–3 kg, and 1.5 mL (30% of daily dose) for infants weighing < 1 kg. Multiple product shortages are an ongoing issue. In the event of no pediatric intravenous multivitamin availability, an adult intravenous multivitamin at a daily dose of 1 mL/kg and up to a maximum of 2.5 mL/d may be used for infants < 2.5 kg or < 36 weeks gestation (Hospira Package insert 8/2007).

[c]Supplied in one or more forms depending on manufacturer. Unit vial is a 2-chambered single-dose vial that must be mixed just prior to use and will provide one 10-mL dose. Dual vial is 2 vials labeled vial 1 (5 mL) and vial 2 (5 mL), with both vials to be used for a single 10-mL dose. Pharmacy bulk package consists of 2 vials labeled vial 1 (50 mL) and vial 2 (50 mL), and 5 mL of each vial provides 10 mL of a single dose.

be adequate.[3] Beyond infancy, a culturally appropriate varied diet ensures the adequacy of intake at all life stages because these essential nutrients are present in a wide range of food products,[1-3,8,9] although most children have relatively low consumption of fruit and vegetables rich in many water-soluble vitamins (WSVs).[11]

Digestion, Absorption, and Metabolism

Water-soluble dietary micronutrients are released with the digestion of foods and then absorbed in free form or as small molecular complexes. Absorption is usually by active transport at low nutrient intake and by passive diffusion at high intake. Absorption occurs mainly at the jejunum, except for cobalamin, which is absorbed only at the ileum under physiological conditions. Some absorption occurs at the stomach (niacin) and proximal colon (riboflavin, biotin).[12]

Postabsorptive transport usually occurs as an enzyme complex or bound to proteins. Erythrocytes may serve both as transporter and storage source. Tissue uptake is usually specific to each nutrient. Some of these essential nutrients have interrelated metabolism and function. The bioavailability of WSV supplements is generally similar to or better than that from dietary sources when tested under the same conditions.[1-4]

Dietary Reference Intake

The current dietary reference intakes (DRIs) of water-soluble essential micronutrients for pediatric populations are provided in Table 7-2. The recommended intake of these nutrients for patients requiring PN are shown in Table 7-3. The current reference values are subject to change as understanding of the relationship among vari-

Table 7-2. Dietary Reference Intake of Water-Soluble Essential Micronutrients in Pediatric Populations[1,2]

LIFE STAGE	THIAMIN (B₁), mg	RIBOFLAVIN (B₂), mg	NIACIN (B₃), mg	B₆ (PYRIDOXINE), mg	FOLATE (B₉), mcg	B₁₂ (COBALAMIN), mcg	VITAMIN C, mg	PANTOTHENIC ACID (B₅), mgª	BIOTIN (B₇), mcgª	CHOLINE, mgª
0–6 mª	0.2	0.3	2	0.1	65	0.4	40	1.7	5	125
7–12 mª	0.3	0.4	4	0.3	80	0.5	50	1.8	6	150
1–3 yᵇ	0.5	0.5	6 (15)	0.5 (30)	150 (300)	0.9	15 (400)	2	8	200 (1000)
4–8 yᵇ	0.6	0.6	8 (20)	0.6 (40)	200 (400)	1.2	25 (650)	3	12	250 (1000)
Males										
9–13 yᵇ	0.9	0.9	12 (20)	1.0 (60)	300 (600)	1.8	45 (1200)	4	20	375 (2000)
14–18 yᵇ	1.2	1.3	16 (30)	1.3 (80)	400 (800)	2.4	75 (1800)	5	25	550 (3000)
Females										
9–13 yᵇ	0.9	0.9	12 (20)	1.0 (60)	300 (600)	1.8	45 (1200)	4	20	375 (2000)
14–18 yᵇ	1.0	1.0	14 (30)	1.2 (80)	400 (800)	2.4	65 (1800)	5	25	400 (3000)
Pregnancy										
14–18 yᵇ	1.4	1.4	18 (30)	1.9 (80)	600 (800)	2.6	80 (1800)	6	30	450 (3000)
Lactation										
14–18 yᵇ	1.4	1.6	17 (30)	2.0 (80)	500 (800)	2.8	115 (1800)	7	35	550 (3000)
Highest intakeᶜ	11 mg at >51 y	11 mg at >70 y	35 mg at 51–70 y	3.9 mg at 19–30 y	1000 mcg at 51–70 y	36.8 mcg at 14–55 y	656 mg at 51–70 y	NA	NA	NA
ULᵈ	NA	NA	ᵉ	ᵉ	ᵉ	NA	ᵉ	NA	NA	ᵉ

AI, adequate intake; NA, not available; RDA, recommended dietary allowance; UL, tolerable upper intake level.

ªAI is the observed or experimentally determined estimate of nutrient intake by a group or groups of healthy people. AI is the only reference level provided for infants < 12 months, and for pantothenic acid, biotin, and choline at all life stages and for both sexes.

ᵇRDA is calculated as + 2 standard deviations of the estimated average requirement, or in its absence, a coefficient of variation of 10% - 15% for each standard deviation is assumed for a life stage and by sex.

ᶜHighest intake is the highest reported daily mean intake from both food and supplements at 95th percentile for any life stage or sex.

ᵈUL is the highest level of daily nutrient intake that is likely to pose no risk of adverse health effects to almost all individuals in the general population.

ᵉUpper limit for each life stage is indicated in parenthesis.

Table 7-3. Daily Parenteral Water-Soluble Vitamin Recommendations for Pediatric Patients[6]

	NEONATES PRETERM	NEONATES TERM	INFANTS	CHILDREN
Thiamin (vitamin B$_1$)	200–350 mcg/kg/d	1.2 mg/d	0.35–0.5 mg/kg/d	1.2 mg/d
Riboflavin (vitamin B$_2$)	150–200 mcg/kg/d	1.4 mg/d	0.15–0.2 mg/kg/d	1.4 mg/d
Niacin (vitamin B$_3$)	4–6.8 mg/kg/d	17 mg/d	4.0–6.8 mg/kg/d	17 mg/d
Vitamin B$_6$	150–200 mcg/kg/d	1000 mcg/d	0.15–0.2 mg/kg/d	1 mg/d
Folate (vitamin B$_9$)	56 mcg/kg/d	140 mcg/d	56 mcg/kg/d	140 mcg/d
Vitamin B$_{12}$	0.3 mcg/kg/d	1 mcg/d	0.3 mcg/kg/d	1 mcg/d
Vitamin C	15–25 mg/kg/d	80 mg/d	15–25 mg/kg/d	80 mg/d
Pantothenic acid (vitamin B$_5$)	1–2 mg/kg/d	5 mg/d	1–2 mg/kg/d	5 mg/d
Biotin (vitamin B$_7$)	5–8 mcg/kg/d	20 mcg/d	5–8 mcg/kg/d	20 mcg/d

No parenteral choline preparation.

ous nutrients increases and more data are available on the type and bioavailability of specific nutrients from naturally occurring dietary sources, fortification of foods and drinks, and supplements.

For infants, the DRI of each essential micronutrient is based on adequate intake (AI): the average daily intake of a specific nutrient in healthy infants fed principally human milk during the first and second 6 months after birth. For ages beyond 1 year, several sets of reference values are used and include AI, estimated average requirement (EAR), and recommended dietary allowance (RDA). Establishing AI depends on the availability of the content of the specific essential micronutrient in food-composition data, large-scale epidemiologic studies to determine the dietary and any supplement intake of the nutrient in groups of healthy people of both sexes, and at the specific life stage. These data in turn allow the determination of EAR, which is a daily nutrient intake value estimated to meet the requirement of half the healthy individuals, and RDA, which is the average daily dietary intake level that is sufficient to meet the nutrient requirement of nearly all (97%–98%) healthy individuals. If sufficient data are available, dose-response risk assessment to high intakes and setting of upper tolerable levels of intake (UL) are made. The absence or limitation of data in children and adolescents has often necessitated the derivation of EAR, RDA, and UL by extrapolation from adult data. AI is used when RDA cannot be determined.[1,2]

Increased Demands and Predisposition to Deficiency States

Many potential predispositions exist for the development of deficiency states (Table 7-4). Requirements for many WSVs generally increase with growth, pregnancy, lactation, physical exertion, fever, and conditions associated with increased metabolic needs. Other predisposing conditions that may result in poorer WSV status include health and dietary fads, including diets with high fat and a preponderance of low-nutrient density foods, and strict vegetarianism; medical conditions involving malabsorption states such as celiac disease, Crohn's disease, cystic fibrosis, anorexia nervosa, human immunodeficiency virus (HIV) infection, or acquired immunodeficiency syndrome (AIDS); prolonged therapy with certain medications; and extensive bariatric surgery involving the stomach or small intestine. Interruptions to manufacturing of parenteral vitamins and micronutrients also contribute to the risk of deficiency state in patients requiring substantial amounts of PN support.[6,13]

Most deficiency states are associated with deficiencies in more than one water-soluble essential micronutrient, either from poor intake, digestion, or absorption or because of interrelated metabolism.

Tobacco and alcohol also affect the needs for these nutrients. More than 15% of in-school youths in the United States are reported to be current cigarette smokers,[14] and an association exists between cigarette smoking and dieting in adolescents even in non-overweight individuals.[15] Smokers may have an increased need for antioxidant vitamins because of the oxidative stress from smoking.[1] There may also be a concomitant decreased intake because of inappropriate dieting.[15] Alcohol is used by more young people than tobacco and illicit drugs.[16] Alcohol abuse is often associated with poor dietary intake of many essential nutrients. In addition, alcohol can directly or indirectly interfere with the digestion, absorption, and metabolism of multiple essential water-soluble micronutrients.[1,2,17,18]

Deficiency of multiple micronutrients is commonly associated with HIV infection or AIDS. A complex interplay is likely between primary dietary deficiency, deficiencies sec-

Table 7-4. Predispositions to Deficiency of Water-Soluble Essential Micronutrients[a]

- Limited body store, particularly in infants and young children
- Inadequate endogenous synthesis
- Decreased intake
  - Parenteral nutrition without water-soluble vitamins[b]
  - Food faddism or severe dietary restrictions
  - Food refusal
  - Anorexia nervosa
- Decreased bioavailability
  - Cooking and storage of foods at high temperatures and prolonged periods
  - Addition of baking soda to vegetables
- Decreased absorption and/or increased loss
  - Celiac disease, Crohn's disease, cystic fibrosis, gastrointestinal bypass surgery, and any malabsorption states
- Nutrient-nutrient and nutrient-drug interaction (see Table 7-6)
- Mixed predispositions including some or all of above
  - Hyperemesis gravidarum
  - Chronic renal dialysis
  - Alcohol abuse
  - Human immunodeficiency virus infection

[a]More than one predisposition to the development of deficiency state is usually present.
[b]Occurs during production shortage of parenteral multivitamin preparation.

ondary to antiretroviral-induced or concomitant diarrheal diseases, and inflammation-suppressed circulating nutrient biomarkers. Micronutrient supplementation probably provides some overall benefits with respect to growth in children and pregnancy outcomes.[19,20] However, not all children with HIV infection have micronutrient deficiencies,[21] particularly in developed countries, and it is at least theoretically possible that certain micronutrients might exacerbate HIV infection.[19,22]

Certain drugs, including chronic diuretic therapy, through their actions on excretion or metabolism of certain nutrients also predispose individuals to deficiency states. Thus, the management of deficiency states must take into account all potential predisposing factors.[1–7,10,22–25]

Deficiency and toxicity states have many biochemical and clinical manifestations (Table 7-5). Isolated WSV deficiency is rare and often associated with problems in the manufacturing of nutrition products, secondary to restrictive dietary practice or inborn errors of metabolism. Thiamin deficiency with cardiac failure and encephalopathy was reported during a shortage of multivitamin preparation for patients requiring PN.[13] Biochemical deficiency of vitamin B_{12} as indicated by increased urinary methylmalonic acid has been reported in 2-month-old to 14-month-old infants

predominantly fed human milk from vegan mothers.[26] Inborn errors of metabolism or certain gene polymorphism associated with various aspects of digestion, absorption, transport, and metabolism of specific essential micronutrients may also result in deficiency of the specific micronutrient. These heritable predispositions to deficiency or dependency states have been reported for thiamin, riboflavin, niacin, vitamin B_6, folate, vitamin B_{12}, biotin, and vitamin C, and the number of disorders is expected to increase with improvements in molecular diagnostic techniques. Molecular diagnosis and genetic counselling are appropriate for the heritable defects.

Biochemical indicators of deficiency may be affected by laboratory technique. Normal ranges of laboratory values may vary with life stages and possibly other physiologic factors such as sex. Clinical manifestations of deficiency states may overlap and commonly include skin disorders, anemia, diarrhea, and impaired neurologic function.[1–3,27] Thus, interpretation of nutrient status must take into account these variables.

Management of Deficiency State and Supplementation and Toxicity

Treatment of a deficiency state requires an understanding of the primary cause, the possibility of deficiency in other nutrients, and concomitant therapies that may interfere with effective replacement therapy. Since all vitamins are pharmacologically active substances, potential nutrient-nutrient and nutrient-drug interactions (Table 7-6) can increase the likelihood of deficiency and toxicity, sometimes with serious consequences.

The initial treatment may require an amount of micronutrient that is 10-fold to 100-fold or greater than the daily requirement and delivered via a route that will ensure delivery to the tissues; for example, parenteral or intranasal delivery rather than oral if a significant malabsorption state is present. Correction of the underlying cause (if possible), continued monitoring for clinical response, and normalization of laboratory parameters are warranted. Thus, management of a deficiency state should be individualized, taking into account the cause, concomitant diet, and non-nutrition therapy. Close monitoring of patients requiring total PN—particularly those patients with abnormal gastrointestinal losses, organ failure, or preexisting nutrient deficiency—is critical to the clinical management. Fortification of selected nutrients, such as folic acid in the diet, is effective in the improvement of folate status of the population.

Table 7-5. Characteristics of Water-Soluble Essential Micronutrients[a]

MICRONUTRIENT	ADULT TISSUE STORE	BIOLOGICAL HALF-LIFE	DEFICIENCY—MAJOR CLINICAL MANIFESTATIONS	DEFICIENCY—BIOCHEMICAL ERYTHROCYTE (RC), BLOOD (WB), PLASMA (P), URINE (U)	TOXICITY
Thiamin (B$_1$)	~30 mg, mostly in erythrocytes and liver	9–18 d	Beriberi: wet, dry. Wernicke encephalopathy	↓ RC or WB thiamin pyrophosphate (TPP); ↑ RC transketolase activity with TPP	Rapid injection: anaphylactoid-like reaction
Riboflavin (B$_2$)	Very low	Minutes	Ariboflavinosis: pharyngitis, cheilosis, angular stomatitis, glossitis, seborrheic dermatitis	↓ RC riboflavin; ↑ RC erythrocyte glutathione reductase activity coefficient with flavin adenine dinucleotide (FAD) stimulation; ↓ 24 h urine riboflavin	Photo-oxidation of some amino acids
Niacin (B$_3$)	Not available	45 min	Pellegra: diarrhea, dementia, dermatitis	↓ RC nicotinamide adenine dinucleotide: nicotinamide adenine dinucleotide phosphate ratio; ↓ 24 h U niacin and its metabolites	Vasodilatory, nausea and vomiting, hepatitis, neurovisual disturbance, glucose intolerance
B$_6$ (pyridoxine)	160 mg, assume muscle has 80%	25 d	Seizures	↓ P pyridoxal phosphate, ↓ RC aspartate and alanine transferase saturation	Peripheral sensory neuropathy
Folate	12–30 mg, liver has ~50%	Erythrocyte, ~8 wk	Seizures, neuromotor disorder, developmental delay, megaloblastic anemia	↓ RC folate, ↑ P homocysteine	Exacerbates B12 deficient neuropathy
B$_{12}$ (cobalamin)	2–3 mg, liver has ≥ 50%	6 d	Macrocystic megaloblastic anemia, nervous system involvement	↓ P B12, ↑ P and U methylmalonic acid, and ↑ P homocysteine	Cyanocobalamin worsens Leber's optic atrophy, use hydroxycobalamin
Vitamin C	2 g	8–40 d	Scurvy	↓ P ascorbate < 0.2 mg/dL, ↓ RC and leukocyte ascorbate	Nausea, abdominal cramps, and diarrhea
Pantothenic acid	Not available	Not available	Gastrointestinal and nervous system	No consistent changes in RC, WB, or P	Not available
Biotin	Not available	2 h (postingestion elimination)	Seizures, developmental delay, rash, alopecia	↓ U biotin, ↑ 3 hydroxyisovaleric acid	Not available
Choline	Not available	43 h	Nonspecific	↓ P, RC, and tissue choline and phosphatidylcholine	Hypotension, cholinergic, fishy odor

[a]Insufficient data to provide quantitative data in some cells. Selected references.[1-7,10,22-25]

No evidence exists for adverse effects from the consumption of naturally occurring water-soluble nutrients in foods, presumably in part because of lowered fractional absorption at high intakes. The increasing practice of ingesting multinutrient supplements to provide an intake similar to daily need has no documented long-term benefit but is unlikely to result in any long-term side effects. Children at risk for WSV deficiencies may benefit from supplemental multivitamin preparations providing 50%–100% of the RDA with minimal risks.[3] Supplement use does not compensate for poor food choices and inadequate diet.

Dietary supplements in the form of multivitamins and multiminerals are taken regularly by more than 30% of children in the United States, with the lowest use reported among infants ≤1 year (11.9%) and teenagers 14–18 years old (25.7%) and highest use among children 4–8 years (48.5%).[28] Furthermore the content of each vitamin other than the D vitamins in commercial multivitamin preparations, particularly those for children 1 to 3 years, is higher than the DRI by as much as 900%.[29,30] Dietary supplements likely contribute a substantial amount to micronutrient intake.[31] However, challenges exist for accurate documen-

Table 7-6. Potential Nutrient-Nutrient and Nutrient-Drug Interactions of Water-Soluble Essential Micronutrients[a]

MICRONUTRIENT	NUTRIENT-NUTRIENT INTERACTION	NUTRIENT-DRUG INTERACTION
Thiamin (B_1)	Not available	↓ Plasma B_1 with or without ↑ requirement from excess alcohol, caffeine, chronic diuretics, and phenytoin
Riboflavin (B_2)	Deficiency can impair metabolism of vitamin B_6, folate, niacin, and iron. Divalent cations may chelate B_2 from tryptophan	↑ B2 metabolism from tricyclic antidepressant, phenothiazines, phenytoin, quinacrine, adriamycin, chronic alcohol
Niacin (B_3)	Riboflavin, pyridoxine, and iron needed for B_3 endogenous synthesis	↓ Endogenous production from isoniazid, 5 fluorouracil, or 6-mercaptopurine
B_6 (pyridoxine)	B_6 metabolism interacts closely with metabolism of riboflavin, niacin, zinc, and folate	↓ Plasma B_6 from binding to isoniazid, hydralazine, oral contraceptives, penicillamine, cycloserine, theophylline, L-dopa. B_6 ↓ plasma phenobarbital, phenytoin, L-dopa
Folate	Interacts closely with choline and B_{12} metabolism in the transfer of methyl group	↓ Plasma folate from aspirin, ibuprofen, naproxene, methotrexate, 5-fluorouracil, phenobarbital, phenytoin, primidone, pyrimethamine.
B_{12} (cobalamin)	Interacts closely with folate and choline metabolism in the transfer of methyl group	↓ Plasma or altered B_{12} metabolism from zidovudine, bile acid sequestrants, H_2 receptor antagonist, proton pump inhibitors, metformin, nitrous oxide
Vitamin C	Participates in redox reactions with glutathione, tocopherol, flavanoid, iron, copper; ↑ iron absorption	↓ Vitamin C cellular transport from proton pump inhibitors. ↑ Vitamin C excretion from aspirin. Vitamin C ↑ excretion of aspirin and acetaminophen but ↓ activity of β blocker, protease inhibitors, warfarin, and chemotherapy drugs that generate free radicals (eg, cyclophosphamide, chlorambucil, carmustine, busulfan, thiotepa, and doxorubicin)
Pantothenic acid (vitamin B_5)	Potential to compete with B_7 for intestinal and cellular uptake due to their similar structures	Not available
Biotin (vitamin B_7)	Potential to compete with B_5 for intestinal and cellular uptake due to their similar structures. Avidin (a protein found in raw egg white) binds biotin.	Not available
Choline	Interacts closely with folate and B_{12} metabolism in the transfer of methyl group	Choline requirement may ↑ from methotrexate, limiting the availability of methyl groups donated from folate derivatives

[a]Insufficient data in some cells in the table. Clinically significant adverse effects from these interactions are poorly defined in many instances. However, clinically significant adverse effects are more likely from certain medications in the presence of marginal nutrition status or excess use of selected water-soluble essential micronutrients. Chronic alcohol or tobacco use would exacerbate any clinical adverse effect. Also see text and selected references.[1–7,10,22–25]

tation of the micronutrient intake from these dietary supplements since the manufacturing of dietary supplements is not well regulated and the amount of micronutrients could be higher or lower than the label claims.[30] Legislative efforts are needed on the manufacturing process[30] to allow accurate estimates of overall micronutrient intake.

Energy drinks and vitamin water products contain variable amounts of WSVs and may contain extremely high amounts. For example, the label of a 2-oz energy shot product reports an excess of the daily requirement by 2000% for vitamin B6 and > 8000% for vitamin B_{12}.[3,24] At high intakes of supplements or if the individual has an underlying metabolic disorder that enhances or interferes with the action of a specific nutrient or the drug, clinical adverse effects may result from nutrient-nutrient and drug-nutrient interactions (Table 7-6). Detailed descriptions of some of these interactions may be obtained from multiple sources.[1–7,10,22–25]

Understanding is limited regarding the biochemical and genetic mechanisms whereby impaired metabolism of these essential micronutrients increases the risk for developmental anomalies and disease. Similarly, understanding of the mechanisms whereby elevated intake of these nutrients protects against these pathologies is also limited. Current initiatives to increase intake of some essential nutrients such as folic acid in human populations to ameliorate developmental anomalies and prevent disease, while effective, lack predictive value with respect to unintended adverse outcomes. Systematic studies of excessive intake of some water-soluble essential micronutrients for prolonged periods are extremely limited.[1–3] The lack of reported adverse effects does not mean that the potential for adverse effects from prolonged periods of high intakes does not exist. Nevertheless sufficient data are available to set the upper limit of intake for niacin, vitamin B_6, folate, vitamin C, and choline (Table 7-2).

Specific Nutrients

Thiamin (Vitamin B_1)

Biochemistry and physiology
Chemically, thiamin consists of substituted pyrimidine and thiazole rings linked by a methylene bridge. Thiamin exists mainly in various interconvertible phosphorylated forms: thiamin monophosphate, thiamin triphosphate, and ~80% as thiamin pyrophosphate (TPP). TPP, the coenzyme form of thiamin, is involved in 2 main types of metabolic reactions: decarboxylation of α-keto acids (eg, pyruvate, α-ketoglutarate, and branch-chain keto acids) and transketolation (eg, among hexose and pentose phosphates). Thiamin requirement is a function of carbohydrate intake and is critical to the metabolism of carbohydrates and branched-chain amino acids and the synthesis of neurotransmitters glutamate and γ-amino butyric acid, nicotinamide adenine dinucleotide phosphate (NADPH), and the pentose sugars deoxyribose and ribose.[1] TPP is also present in nerve membranes and activates a chloride channel for nerve conduction.

Source
Thiamin in the diet includes free thiamin, phosphorylated thiamin, and protein-phosphate complexes. Dietary sources include enriched, fortified, or whole grain rice; pasta and cereals; pork; eggs; yeast; legumes; and nuts. Thiamin is lost during processing to white flour, from milling of brown rice, and during cooking. Dairy products and most fruits contain little thiamin.

Thiamin in fortified foods and pharmaceutical preparations are usually thiamin salts: thiamin hydrochloride and thiamin mononitrate. Thiamin supplements are available in oral and injectable forms as thiamin salts or as part of multivitamin preparations. Lipid-soluble thiamin derivatives called allithiamins are also available and may be better absorbed at higher intakes.[10]

Absorption, metabolism, and excretion
Thiamin uptake by the small intestine and by cells within various organs is mediated by a saturable, high-affinity transport system. At high intake, absorption can occur by passive diffusion. Following absorption mainly at the jejunum, thiamin is transported by blood in both erythrocytes (~90%) and plasma. Nonphosphorylated thiamin is weakly bound to plasma proteins. The liver appears to be the major organ for phosphorylation of thiamin, although it can occur in all tissues.[18] After an oral dose of thiamin, peak urine excretion occurs in about 2 hours and is nearly complete after 4–6 hours. However, the biological half-life of the vitamin is much longer and estimated to be between 9 and 18 days. Total thiamin content in the adult human is estimated to be ~30 mg.

Deficiency state
Thiamin deficiency can occur with inadequate intake particularly during PN without added WSV,[13] from inadequate absorption or defective transport of the vitamin,[32] and excessive loss from multiple causes.[1,3] A state of severe depletion may occur in <3 weeks from a strict thiamin-deficient diet, but the most common cause of thiamin deficiency in affluent countries is alcoholism.[17,18] Alcohol abuse is often associated with poor dietary intake of many essential nutrients and decreased intestinal absorption and transport, and phosphorylation of thiamin. Patients with end-stage organ failure (especially of the liver) are at risk for deficiency of thiamin and multiple nutrients.

The classic clinical syndromes associated with deficiency of thiamin include beriberi or Wernicke's encephalopathy. Beriberi is traditionally classified as "dry" or "wet" form. Dry beriberi is characterized by a symmetrical peripheral neuropathy with progressive weakness, muscle wasting, difficulty walking, and ataxia, and is accompanied by paresthesia and loss of deep tendon reflex. Wet beriberi is secondary to cardiomyopathic congestive cardiac failure and edema. Infantile beriberi is characterized by shock at 2–3 months in a breastfed child with or without a preceding history of weak cry and poor feeding. It generally occurs in the exclusively breastfed infant whose mother has a subclinical thiamin deficiency.[33] Wernicke's encephalopathy is characterized by altered consciousness as well as the triad of ophthalmoplegia, nystagmus, and ataxia. It is generally seen in adults with alcohol abuse and malnutrition, although it has been reported in infants and children.[33,34]

Thiamin deficiency from feeding of unfortified soy infant formula due to manufacturing error has been reported.[33,35] Clinical presentation occurred between 2 and 12 months. Initial manifestations were nonspecific and included vomiting, lethargy, irritability, abdominal distention, diarrhea, respiratory symptoms, developmental delay, and failure to thrive. Respiratory and gastrointestinal infections were noted in many of the reported cases. Classic manifestation of ophthalmoplegia or death also occurred in several infants.

Thiamin deficiency in children and adults with clinical manifestations of beriberi or Wernicke's encephalopathy and severe lactic acidosis leading to death in some cases have been reported.[6,13] The onset of clinical manifestation began within weeks after a nationwide shortage of multivitamins for PN and clinical recovery was noted within days after the provision of parenteral thiamin.

Laboratory investigations show abnormal magnetic resonance imaging at the frontal lobes, basal ganglia, periaqueductal region, thalami, and the mammillary bodies, while magnetic resonance spectroscopy demonstrates a characteristic lactate peak.[36] Biochemical diagnosis of thiamin deficiency is by low TPP in erythrocyte and whole blood[37] or by the transketolase activation test.[38] The latter measures the whole blood or erythrocyte transketolase activity at baseline, which is increased after TPP is added if the individual is deficient.

For simple deficiency states, acute symptomatic improvement occurs rapidly within 1 day of treatment.[35] However, neurodevelopmental delay, particularly in receptive and expressive language,[39] and recurrent seizures[40] have been noted at up to 6 years of follow-up.

A number of inborn errors of metabolism may have significant clinical improvements following administration of pharmacologic doses of thiamin. For example, an autosomal recessive defect in folate-thiamin transporter SLC family[32] with a clinical triad including diabetes mellitus, sensorineural deafness, and thiamin-responsive megaloblastic anemia with ringed sideroblasts. Another mutation in the *SLC19A3* gene results in biotin-thiamin responsive basal ganglia disease with a variable onset from neonatal period to adulthood of seizures, ataxia, dystonia, and dysphagia. Prompt administration of biotin and thiamin early in the disease course results in partial or complete improvement within days.[41]

Supplementation

Prophylactic use of thiamin supplements may be warranted in malabsorption disorders. High-dose supplementation can result in interactions with chemotherapy agents or other high-dose vitamins.[1,3,24] Anaphylactic reaction with parenteral administration of thiamin has occasionally been reported, but toxic effects of thiamin excess have not been studied systematically.[1] The use of thiamin in the treatment of neurological disorders such as Parkinson's disease, Freidrich's ataxia, and multiple sclerosis remains ill defined.

Riboflavin (Vitamin B$_2$)

Biochemistry and physiology

Riboflavin (7, 8-dimethyl-10-ribityl-isoalloxazine) is a water-soluble, yellow, fluorescent compound. The primary form of riboflavin is an integral component of the coenzymes flavin mononucleotide (FMN) and flavin adenine dinucleotide (FAD), the predominant flavoenzyme in body tissues. These coenzymes are involved in multiple oxidation-reduction reactions integral to carbohydrate, protein, and fat metabolism and are involved in the metabolism of folate, pyridoxine, and niacin. Riboflavin-binding proteins expressed in fetuses of different species are evidently essential to normal fetal development.[42]

Source

More than 90% of dietary riboflavin is consumed as a complex of food protein with FAD and FMN and lesser amounts as free vitamin and traces of glycosides and esters. Animal protein (meat, dairy, and eggs) as well as green vegetables and fortified cereals are abundant sources.[8] Riboflavin may be synthesized by colonic bacteria, but the extent of its contribution to human needs is not known.[42]

Absorption, metabolism, and excretion

FAD and FMN from dietary protein are released by gastric acid digestion. They are then hydrolyzed to riboflavin by nonspecific pyrophosphatases and phosphatases in the upper small intestine. Riboflavin absorption is relatively poor compared to other WSVs, but it is increased when riboflavin is ingested along with other foods and in the presence of bile salts. Some divalent cations, such as copper, zinc, iron, and manganese, form chelates with riboflavin and lower its absorption.

Most absorption occurs in the small intestine via an active or facilitated transport system at low intakes and via passive diffusion at high intakes. A small amount is absorbed in the large intestine.[43] A small component of enterohepatic circulation also exists.

Riboflavin is transported in the circulation bound to albumin and immunoglobulins. It is phosphorylated to FMN and FAD in most tissues, particularly in the small intestine, liver, kidney, and heart. Intracellular phosphorylation is regulated by thyroid hormone, and production of FAD is under negative feedback control. Very little riboflavin is stored in body tissues, and excess riboflavin is excreted in the urine secondary to glomerular filtration and active tubular secretion as riboflavin (~60%–70%) and as a variety of flavin-related products. Riboflavin is more heat stable than thiamin but is very photosensitive.[43] It also interacts with an extensive list of drugs[23] (Table 7-6).

Deficiency state

Riboflavin deficiency is often accompanied by deficiencies of one or more of the other B vitamins, in part because of its role in the metabolism of niacin, pyridoxine, and folate. Chronically limited dietary meat or dairy intake (including infants after weaning) is a specific risk factor for riboflavin deficiency. Riboflavin deficiency is also found in protein energy malnutrition states, such as kwashiorkor and anorexia nervosa, and in patients with other risk factors such as malabsorptive states that are common to all water-soluble micronutrients. Symptoms and signs of mild deficiency state can be nonspecific. The more characteristic features of severe deficiency state of ariboflavinosis include pharyngitis, cheilosis, angular stomatitis, glossitis (magenta tongue), and seborrheic dermatitis involving nasolabial folds, flexural area of extremities, and the genital areas.

Diagnosis of riboflavin deficiency is by low erythrocyte riboflavin quantified by high-performance liquid chromatography and low 24-hour urinary excretion of riboflavin. Erythrocyte glutathione reductase activity coefficient from in vitro stimulation by FAD increased in the ranges of >40%, 20%–40%, and <20% are considered to be deficient, low, and acceptable levels of riboflavin status, respectively. Biochemical deficiency has been reported in infants receiving short-term phototherapy.[44]

Supplementation

Excess riboflavin turns urine yellow although no functional or structural adverse effects have been demonstrated in vivo after excess riboflavin intake. This is in part because of the limited absorption of ingested riboflavin. Nevertheless, riboflavin could theoretically increase photosensitivity to ultraviolet irradiation, and excess riboflavin would then increase the photosensitized oxidation of amino acids and proteins in infants receiving phototherapy for hyperbilirubinemia.

Multiple acyl-coenzyme A dehydrogenase deficiency, one of the heritable lipid storage myopathy conditions, is reported to be responsive to riboflavin in pharmacological doses.[45]

Niacin (Vitamin B₃)

Biochemistry and physiology

Niacin refers to nicotinamide (nicotinic acid amide), nicotinic acid (pyridine-3-carboxylic acid), and derivatives that exhibit the biological activity of nicotinamide. None of the forms are related to the nicotine found in tobacco although their names are similar.[46] The 2 major forms of niacin are chemically modified in the mitochondria to form coenzymes nicotinamide adenine dinucleotide (NAD) and nicotinamide adenine dinucleotide phosphate (NADP). About 200 enzymes require NAD and NADP, mainly to accept or donate electrons in the energy-producing oxidation-reduction (redox) reactions. NAD functions most often in energy-producing reactions during degradation (catabolism) of carbohydrate, fat, protein, and alcohol. NADP functions more often in biosynthetic (anabolic) reactions, such as in the synthesis of macromolecules including fatty acids and cholesterol. Non-redox enzymatic reactions important to DNA repair and stress responses, cell signaling, transcription, regulation of apoptosis, chromatin structure, and cell differentiation require separation of the niacin moiety from NAD and integration of ADP-ribose in these functions.[1,3,46]

Source

Unlike most of the WSVs, nicotinamide can be synthesized in the liver and kidney from tryptophan. This process requires adequate amounts of riboflavin, pyridoxine, and iron and is highly variable depending on multiple other factors. For instance, tryptophan is used also for protein synthesis, which takes priority over NAD and NADP synthesis. An estimated average of 60 mg of tryptophan produces 1 mg of niacin or niacin equivalent. However, dietary intake of niacin is needed to meet the daily requirements.

Good sources of niacin include yeast, meats, poultry, red fish (eg, tuna and salmon), cereals (especially fortified cereals), legumes, and seeds. Lesser amounts are found in milk, green leafy vegetables, coffee, and tea. In corn and wheat, niacin may be bound to sugar molecules as glycosides, which significantly decrease niacin bioavailability.[47]

Absorption, metabolism, and excretion

Intestinal glycohydrolases catalyze the release of nicotinamide from NAD. Nicotinic acid and nicotinamide are rapidly absorbed from the stomach and the intestine. They enter cells by simple diffusion and also by sodium-dependent facilitated transport across gut mucosa and erythrocytes.

The coenzymes NAD and NADP are synthesized in all tissues. Extracellular nicotinamide appears to regulate the tissue NAD but is itself under hepatic control. Hepatic NAD is hydrolyzed to provide nicotinamide for tissues that lack the ability to synthesize nicotinamide from tryptophan. The tissue store of niacin is in the form of NAD that is not bound to enzymes or as nicotinamide adenine mononucleotide synthesized from tryptophan and nicotinic acid. Excess niacin is methylated in the liver to N^1-methyl-nicotinamide and excreted in the urine either unchanged or as its 2-pyridone derivative.

Deficiency state
Several conditions uniquely predispose to niacin deficiency. These include carcinoid syndrome in which tryptophan is preferentially oxidized to 5-hydroxytryptophan and serotonin; prolonged treatment with isoniazid, 5-fluorouracil, or 6-mercaptopurine, which competes with the pyridoxine-derived coenzyme required in the tryptophan-niacin pathway; and Hartnup's disease, an autosomal recessive disorder that interferes with the absorption of the neutral amino acid, tryptophan.

The classic manifestation of severe niacin deficiency is pellagra, an Italian term meaning "rough skin." It is characterized by the triad of diarrhea, dermatitis, and dementia.[48] Gastrointestinal manifestations include glossitis, angular stomatitis, chelitis, and diarrhea in about 50% of patients. Skin lesions begin as painful erythema in sun-exposed areas. Vesicle or bullae formation may occur upon re-exposure to sun and the skin eventually becomes rough, hard, and scaly. Hair and nails tend to be spared. Neuropsychiatric manifestations include insomnia, fatigue, nervousness, irritability, apathy, and memory impairment. Dementia and death may occur in untreated cases.

Niacin status is determined by "niacin number," a decreased concentration of NAD relative to NADP in erythrocytes, and low levels of niacin and its metabolite N^1-methyl-nicotinamide and its 2-pyridone derivative in a 24-hour urine sample.

Supplementation
Niacin as a supplement or pharmacologic agent used primarily in the treatment of hyperlipidemia can result in clinical side effects. Both forms of niacin may result in similar side effects although nicotinamide results in less vasodilatory ef-

fects. High-dose niacin, as seen in energy drinks and energy shots, also causes flushing. Nicotinic acid as low as 30 mg daily is associated with vasodilatory effects including flushing, burning, tingling, an itching sensation, and gastrointestinal effects of nausea and vomiting. Some improvement may occur with gradual increase in dosage, coingestion of food, or the slow-release form of the supplement. Liver dysfunction is more common with the slow-release form. At high intakes of niacin, fulminant hepatitis and encephalopathy, glucose intolerance, and ocular effects of blurred vision, toxic amblyopia, macular edema, and cystic maculopathy also may occur.[1,24]

Vitamin B$_6$

Biochemistry and physiology
Vitamin B$_6$ comprises a group of 6 related compounds: pyridoxal (PL), pyridoxine (Pn), pyridoxamine (PM), and their respective 5'-phosphates (PLP, PnP, and PMP). The major forms in animal tissues are PLP and PMP; plant-derived foods contain primarily Pn and PnP, sometimes in the form of a glucoside.

PLP is a coenzyme for a multitude of enzymes involved in amino acid metabolism including aminotransferases, decarboxylases, racemases, and dehydratases. It is required for the conversion of tryptophan to both niacin and the neurotransmitter serotonin, homocysteine to cysteine, dopa to dopamine, as well as the synthesis of the inhibitory neurotransmitter γ-aminobutyric acid. Pyridoxine is a coenzyme for δ-aminolevulinate synthase, the rate-limiting first step in heme synthesis.

Source
Foods rich in pyridoxine include fruits and nuts (bananas, cantaloupe, walnuts), plants (green leafy vegetables, broccoli, peas, carrots, rice husks, brown rice, maize, wheat germ, yeast), and animal products (eggs, chicken, fish, beef), as well as fortified cereals. Microbial synthesis of B$_6$ is possible, but the extent to which it contributes to the physiological need is not known.

Absorption, metabolism, and excretion
Bioavailability of vitamin B$_6$ in a mixed diet is ~75%, with nonphosphorylated B$_6$ as the major form absorbed. Phosphatase-mediated hydrolysis of PLP and PMP precedes absorption by a nonsaturable passive diffusion transport of the nonphosphorylated form primarily at the jejunum and ileum. Pyridoxine glucoside is absorbed after deconjugation

by a mucosal glucosidase, and some is absorbed intact and then hydrolyzed in various tissues. The unphosphorylated forms of B_6 are absorbed and then converted to 5'-phosphate forms by pyridoxal kinase primarily in the liver. PnP and PMP are oxidized to PLP by PnP oxidase. PMP is also generated from PLP via aminotransferase reactions. PLP is bound to various proteins in tissues, which protects it from the action of phosphatases. Muscle, plasma, and erythrocytes (hemoglobin) have high capacity for PLP-protein binding. Albumin is the major PLP-binding protein in the circulation.

When the capacity for protein binding is exceeded, free PLP is rapidly hydrolyzed and nonphosphorylated forms of B_6 are released. Free PLP in the circulation is also dephosphorylated then reabsorbed or carried in the erythrocyte. Vitamin B_6 is found in various subcellular compartments but primarily in the mitochondria and cytosol.

In humans, the major excretory form is 4-pyridoxic acid, which accounts for about half the B_6 compounds in the urine. At high doses of pyridoxine, much of the dose is excreted unchanged. The body's B_6 content is estimated to be about 167 mg based on muscle biopsy data and the assumption that muscle represents about 80% of the store. The overall half-life of vitamin B_6 is about 25 days, but the muscle turnover for B_6 is much slower.[49]

Deficiency state

Isolated deficiency of pyridoxine is rare because its metabolism is intimately involved with multiple other nutrients including riboflavin, niacin, zinc, and folate. Lower plasma PLP may result from its binding to certain drugs (isoniazid, hydralazine, oral contraceptives, penicillamine, cycloserine, theophylline, and L-dopa [react with carbonyl group of PLP]); acetaldehyde, but not ethanol, decreases net PLP formation and may compete with PLP for protein binding. However, the extent to which these situations increase B_6 requirements is not known. Vitamin B_6 status is inversely associated with markers of inflammation, oxidative stress, and chronic inflammatory conditions, but the cause and effect relationship remains ill defined. Multiple autosomal recessive mutations in several genes that increase degradation of Pn (deficiency of α-aminoadipic semialdolase dehydrogenase [antiquitin] encoded by *ALDH7A1* gene) or decrease the production of PLP (deficiency of pyridox(am)ine 5'-phosphate oxidase, *PNPO* gene) result in deficiency of the respective vitamin B_6.

Clinical manifestations of the B_6-deficient state include seizures in infants fed milk formulas without fortification

by pyridoxine from an error in the manufacturing[50,51] and abnormal electroencephalograms in adults from experimental B_6 deficiency.[52] Both are reversed with reintroduction of B_6. Intractable neonatal or infantile seizure unresponsive to standard therapy should raise the concern for the presence of inborn errors of metabolism in vitamin B_6. They can be categorized as pyridoxine-dependent, pyridoxine-responsive, and pyridoxal phosphate–responsive conditions depending on the type of mutation and whether partial or complete expression of the gene mutation occurs. Plasma and cerebrospinal fluid samples should be collected for diagnostic testing before and after empiric therapy using Pn followed by PLP if unresponsive to Pn.[53] Oral folinic acid may be needed to improve response to Pn. Other clinical manifestations of B_6 deficiency are nonspecific and may include microcytic anemia, glossitis, seborrheic dermatitis, and depression.

Plasma PLP is probably the best indicator of B_6 status because it appears to reflect tissue stores.[54] Erythrocyte aspartate and alanine aminotransferase saturation by PLP or tryptophan metabolites are also useful indicators of relative B_6 status. Other biochemical markers and genetic testing may be needed with inborn errors of metabolism for vitamin B_6.[53]

Supplementation

The tolerable upper intake level for vitamin B_6 is set at 80 mg daily,[1] and high-dose pyridoxine supplement of 2–6 g daily for 2–40 months[55] or chronic intake at doses < 500 mg/d[56] may result in peripheral sensory neuropathy. The latter may improve slowly upon withdrawal of the supplement. The combination of high doses of both vitamin B_6 with vitamin B_{12} may result in a severe rosacea fulminans.[24]

Folate (Vitamin B_9)

Biochemistry and physiology

Folate is a generic term for this water-soluble B-complex vitamin. Most naturally occurring food folates are pteroyl glutamates containing 1–6 glutamate molecules joined in a peptide linkage to the γ-carboxyl of glutamate. Folic acid (pteroylmonoglutamic acid) is the most oxidized and stable form of folate. It consists of a *p*-aminobenzoic acid molecule linked at one end to a pteridine ring and at the other end to a glutamic acid molecule. It occurs rarely in food but is the form used in vitamin supplements and in fortified food products.

Folate is critical to the metabolism of nucleic and amino acids. It promotes cellular growth in general and is necessary for erythrocyte maturation. Folate is a substrate (5-methyl-tetrahydrofolate) and vitamin B_{12} is a coenzyme in the formation of 5,10-methylenetetrahydrofolate (MTHF) and thymidylate synthesis. In either folate or vitamin B_{12} deficiency, the megaloblastic changes in bone marrow and other replicating cells result from lack of MTHF. Folate and vitamin B_{12} deficiency are independent risk factors for neural tube defects including anencephaly and spina bifida.[54] Folic acid is the only WSV mandated as part of prenatal supplements for the prevention of neural tube defects.

Source

Natural sources include fresh green vegetables, liver, yeast, and some fruits. About 60% of children consume fewer fruits than recommended, and 93% of children consume fewer vegetables than recommended.[11] Thus generally lower intake of vegetables and fruits contributes to the potentially inadequate intake of folate. Significantly improved folate status as indicated by population survey of red cell and serum folate has been reported since the Food and Drug Administration in 1998 required the addition of folic acid to all enriched breads, cereals, flours, corn meal, pasta products, rice, and other cereal grain products sold in the United States.[57]

Absorption, metabolism, and excretion

Dietary folate equivalent has ~50% lower bioavailability compared with folic acid supplement. Food folates (polyglutamate derivatives) are hydrolyzed by conjugase enzymes to monoglutamate forms and then enter various cells by membrane carrier or folate-binding protein-mediated system. The folate transporter derives from the *SLC19* gene family of solute carriers and shares structural homology with the thiamin transporter.[32] Monoglutamates, mainly 5-methyl-tetrahydrofolate, are metabolized in the liver and other tissues to polyglutamate derivatives by the enzyme folylpolyglutamate synthetase. Polyglutamates are the forms retained in various tissues or found in blood or bile and are the forms needed for function as a coenzyme in single-carbon transfer reactions.

Folate catabolism involves cleavage of intracellular and circulatory polyglutamates to the monoglutamate form. Approximately two-thirds of the folate in plasma is protein bound, and albumin accounts for ~50% of the bound folate. Folates freely filter through the glomeruli and are secreted and reabsorbed by the renal tubules. The bulk of the urine excretory products are folate cleavage products mainly in the monoglutamate form. Extensive enterohepatic circulation of folate occurs.[58] The estimated total body folate content is between 12 and 28 mg, of which ~50% is in the liver.

Deficiency state

Low intake of fruits and vegetables in normal populations is a risk factor for folate deficiency.[11] Patients with malabsorptive states and those receiving folate antagonists such as methotrexate and other drugs that have antifolate activity, including pyrimethamine, trimethoprim, triamterene, trimetrexate, and sulfasalazine, require monitoring for folate status to ensure adequate dietary intake or folate supplementation. Several inborn errors in folate metabolism (MTHF reductase deficiency associated with mutations of alleles on chromosome 1),[59] and those with folate transport defects to the central nervous system or presence of autoantibody to folate receptor (cerebral folate deficiency)[60,61] predispose the affected individual to folate deficiency. Serum and red cell folate concentration are low in the former and normal in the latter. In cerebral folate deficiency, the transfer of folate from plasma to cerebrospinal fluid is low and cerebrospinal fluid MTHF concentration is low.

Clinical features of folate deficiency may begin during infancy and include retarded psychomotor development, poor social interaction, decelerating head growth, hypotonia, ataxia, dyskinesia, irritability, visual and hearing deficiency, and seizures. Some neurological manifestations may be reversible with folinic acid supplement. Onset of anemia is usually gradual, and clinical manifestations typically appear only at an advanced stage of anemia but may be earlier in the elderly.[61,62]

Megaloblastic anemia is the primary sign of deficiency. Deficiency states are confirmed with low red cell folate, which reflects tissue folate stores. Plasma folate reflects concurrent folate balance. Plasma total homocysteine concentrations increase when folate status is inadequate to convert homocysteine to methionine.

Supplementation

Excessive folate intake may precipitate or exacerbate neuropathy in individuals with vitamin B_{12} deficiency, and it has been implicated in delaying the diagnosis of pernicious anemia until after irreversible neurological damage has occurred.[61,62]

Vitamin B_{12} (Cobalamin)

Biochemistry and physiology

The term vitamin B_{12} is usually restricted to cyanocobalamin but can be used to refer to all potentially biologically active cobalamins, a group of cobalt-containing compounds (corrinoids) that contain the sugar ribose, phosphate, and a base (5,6-dimethyl benzimidazole) attached to the corrin ring. The cobalamin coenzymes active in human metabolism exist as methylcobalamin and 5-deoxyadenosylcobalamin. Methylcobalamin and folate are necessary for the remethylation of homocysteine to methionine by methionine synthase. Adenosylcobalamin is required for isomerization of L-methylmalonyl-CoA to succinyl-CoA with the enzyme L-methylmalonyl-CoA mutase. An adequate supply of B_{12} is essential for bone marrow, particularly the production of normal erythrocytes, and for neurological function.

Source

Cobalamin is found in foods of animal origin only. Meat, fish, poultry, cheese, milk, and eggs are good sources. Cereal and soy milks are fortified with varied amounts of B_{12}. Vitamin B_{12} content in breast milk is dependent on maternal diet, and colostrum has higher content than mature milk. In the United States and Canada, both cyanocobalamin and hydroxocobalamin are available commercially, although cyanocobalamin is most commonly used in supplements and pharmaceuticals. Vitamin B_{12} can be synthesized by intestinal bacteria, but this contribution to the body pool is not known and is likely to be limited.

Absorption, metabolism, and excretion

Cobalamin absorption and cellular uptake require an intact stomach, adequate transport proteins, pancreatic sufficiency, and a normally functioning terminal ileum.[12,25] Haptocorrin (HC, also known as transcobalamin I), gastric intrinsic factor (IF), and transcobalamin (TC, also known as transcobalamin II) are critical to B_{12} transport from food to cell. IF and HC, but not TC, are glycosylated proteins. Increasing specificity exists for binding to cobalamin in the order HC, TC, and IF.[63] Cobalamin bound to protein in food is released by the activity of hydrochloric acid and gastric protease in the stomach. Free cobalamin then binds to IF to form a cobalamin-IF complex. When synthetic vitamin B12 is added to fortified foods and dietary supplements, it is already in free form and binds to salivary HC. After proteolysis of HC in the duodenum, free cobalamin then binds to gastric parietal cell–produced IF. The cobalamin-IF complex is absorbed only in distal ileum under physiological conditions via endocytosis mediated by a specific receptor. In the enterocyte, the cobalamin-IF complex is degraded, and cobalamin is transported to the cells bound to TCs and taken up via endocytosis by a specific receptor on most cell types.

Vitamin B_{12} appears in circulation several hours after ingestion. If the circulating B_{12} exceeds the B_{12}-binding capacity of the blood, the excess is excreted in the urine. About 80% of circulating B_{12} is bound to the protein transcobalamin I (TCI) and the remainder to TCII or III. TCII is the form that delivers B_{12} to the tissues (~50% taken up by the liver) through specific receptors for TCII. HC in the plasma cannot facilitate cellular uptake of cobalamin except in hepatocytes.

In the presence of IF, an active enterohepatic circulation reabsorbs almost all B_{12} secreted into the bile. Unlike other WSVs, a large store of B_{12} exists, primarily in the liver. The average B_{12} content of liver is ~1 mcg/g in healthy adults. The average total body pool of B_{12} is estimated to be 2–3 mg. Daily loss of B_{12} is ~0.1%–0.2% of the B_{12} pool regardless of the size of the store, with the 0.2% value generally applicable to those with pernicious anemia.[64]

Deficiency state

Breastfed infants of mothers following a strict vegan diet, children receiving macrobiotic diets, and the elderly are at risk for B_{12} deficiency as are individuals lacking an intact stomach, distal ileum, pancreatic exocrine function, or IF.[26,65] Chronic use of proton pump inhibitors increases the risk for B_{12} deficiency by inhibition of intragastric proteolysis, thereby inhibiting the release of B_{12} from food prior to binding to HC and also inhibiting B_{12} binding to gastric IF.[66] Autoantibodies against parietal cell H^+K^+-adenosine triphosphate causing loss of gastric parietal cells or blocking the B_{12} binding site for IF result in B_{12} deficiency. Extensive gastrointestinal surgery involving gastric bypass or resection of ileum predisposes the individual to B_{12} deficiency and may even affect the fetus.[67] Genetic defects that involve deletions or defects of methylmalonic acid-CoA mutase, IF, TCII, enzymes in the pathway of cobalamin adenosyllation, and the cubilin or amnionless genes involved in the intestinal handling of B_{12} are reported to be associated with B_{12} deficiency.[3,25,68]

Clinical manifestations of B_{12} deficiency include macrocytic megaloblastic anemia and neurological problems. The latter include ataxia, muscle weakness, spasticity, incontinence, vision problems, dementia, psychosis, and mood disturbance. Impaired cognitive function has been demonstrated in adolescents with marginal cobalamin status.[69]

Decreased plasma B_{12} and elevated plasma and urine methylmalonic acid and plasma homocysteine are biochemical indicators of a functional B_{12} deficiency state. Plasma B_{12}

is considered as a less sensitive indicator of B_{12} deficiency compared to other biochemical changes.

Supplementation

Short-term studies up to 4 months indicate that oral B_{12} supplementation has similar efficacy to intramuscular treatment for B_{12} deficiency.[70,71] B_{12} fortification of foods to improve the population's B_{12} status has been advocated.[65] Intranasal delivery of B_{12} is possible but the bioavailability is ~10% of the intramuscular preparation. Periodic parenteral administration of high-dose B_{12} (1–5 mg) to patients with pernicious anemia (lack of IF) or malabsorptive defects supports the lack of adverse effects at high doses.

Energy drinks and shots contain vitamin B_{12} with variable amounts but can contain > 8000% of the daily value. Toxic reactions include urticaria, anaphylaxis, and exacerbation of and precipitation of acneiform eruptions.[3,24] High-dose vitamin B_{12} in combination with pyridoxine may cause the severe skin lesion rosacea fulminans.[24]

The use of cyanocobalamin is contraindicated in individuals with B_{12} deficiency who are at risk for Leber's optic atrophy, a genetic disorder caused by chronic cyanide (present in tobacco smoke, alcohol, and some plants) intoxication, because the latter may increase the risk of irreversible optic atrophy. Hydroxocobalamin, a cyanide antagonist,[72] can be used instead of cyanocobalamin.[1]

Vitamin C

Biochemistry and physiology

Ascorbic acid is the enolic form of an α-ketolactone (2,3-didehydro-L-threo-hexano-1,4-lactone). The 2 enolic hydrogen atoms give the compound its acidic character and provide electrons for its function as a reductant and antioxidant. Vitamin C refers to both ascorbic acid and dehydroascorbic acid. Ascorbic acid is the functional and primary in vivo form of the vitamin. Ascorbate is the free reduced form of ascorbic acid. Ascorbyl radical and dehydroascorbic acid are 1- or 2-electron oxidation products that readily reduce back to ascorbic acid in vivo, thus a relatively small amount of the vitamin is lost through catabolism.

Vitamin C is known to be an electron donor for 8 human enzymes. Three enzymes participate in collagen hydroxylation (also requires iron) and contribute to the biosynthesis of other connective tissue components including elastin, fibronectin, proteoglycans, bone matrix, and elastin-associated fibrillin. Two enzymes along with iron are required in carnitine synthesis, and 3 enzymes, dopamine-β-hydroxy-lase, peptidyl-glycine monooxygenase, and 4-hydroxyphenylpyruvatedioxygenase, are required in hormone and amino acid biosynthesis.

Vitamin C is an effective antioxidant because of its ability to donate electrons and its antioxidant effect operates in the aqueous phase both intracellularly and extracellularly. It participates in redox reactions with many other dietary and physiological compounds including glutathione, tocopherol, flavonoids, and the trace metals iron and copper. Antioxidation activities at the tissue level include protection of the eye, neutrophils, and sperm DNA, among many others. In the circulation, it protects against oxidation of plasma low-density lipoprotein. Ascorbate also provides antioxidant protection indirectly by regenerating other biological antioxidants such as glutathione and α-tocopherol back to their active state. Ascorbic acid functions as a reducing agent for mixed function oxidases in the microsomal drug-metabolizing system that inactivates a wide variety of substrates, such as endogenous hormones or xenobiotics including drugs, pesticides, or carcinogens that are foreign to humans. The vitamin is involved in the biosynthesis of corticosteroids and aldosterone and in the microsomal hydroxylation of cholesterol to bile acids.[3,4,73] One form of hereditary methemoglobinemia is reported to be responsive to vitamin C.[74]

Source

Almost 90% of vitamin C in the typical diet comes from fruits and vegetables. Citrus fruits, tomatoes, tomato juice, and potatoes are major sources. Other sources include brussel sprouts, cauliflower, broccoli, strawberries, cabbage, and spinach. Vitamin C content of foods can vary with growing condition, season, stage of maturity, cooking practice, and storage time prior to consumption.[7,9]

Absorption, metabolism, and excretion

Some 70%–90% of usual dietary intake of ascorbic acid is absorbed via a sodium-dependent active transport at low gastrointestinal ascorbate concentrations, while passive diffusion occurs at high concentrations. With large intakes of vitamin C, unabsorbed ascorbate is degraded in the intestine, a process that may account for the diarrhea and intestinal discomfort. Dehydroascorbic acid is the form of vitamin that primarily crosses the membranes of blood and intestinal cells, after which it is reduced intracellularly to ascorbic acid and localized mostly in the cytosol. Cellular transport of ascorbic acid and dehydroascorbic acid is mediated by tissue-specific cellular transport systems that allow for wide variation of tissue ascorbate concentrations. High levels are maintained in the pituitary and adrenal glands, leukocytes, eyes, and the brain, while low levels are found in plasma and saliva.

Both intracellular and plasma vitamin C exist predominantly in the free reduced form as ascorbate monoanion. Both the 1-electron and 2-electron oxidation products of the vitamin are readily reduced back to ascorbic acid in vivo—chemically and enzymatically—by glutathione and NADH–dependent and NADPH–dependent reductases, and relatively small amounts of the vitamin are lost through catabolism.

Vitamin C is actively secreted in human gastric juice. Proton pump inhibitor therapy lowers the concentration of vitamin C in gastric juice and may reduce the bioavailability of ingested vitamin C.

The kidney is capable of reabsorption of ascorbate, but renal excretion of ascorbate is greater with increased intake. Aspirin may increase urinary ascorbate.[7] Due to homeostatic regulation, the biological half-life of ascorbate varies widely from 8 to 40 days and is inversely related to the ascorbate body pool. A body pool of <300 mg is associated with scurvy, while maximum body pools are estimated to be about 2 g.

Deficiency state

In developed countries, population surveys show serum vitamin C concentrations are significantly lower in smokers and low-income persons, presumably reflecting the increased oxidative stress of smokers and low dietary consumption of vitamin C foods.[75] Clinical manifestation of vitamin C deficiency is quite rare but has been reported in children with severely restricted diets related to food faddism, psychiatric or developmental problems,[76] or end-stage organ disease with severely compromised nutrition.[77] Deficiency also has been reported in young children who ingest only well-cooked foods and few fruits and vegetables and are supplemented with ultra–heat-processed milk.[78]

The primary clinical manifestation of vitamin C deficiency is scurvy and reflects deterioration of elastic tissues. Clinical features include follicular hyperkeratosis, petechiae, ecchymoses, brittle coiled hairs, inflamed and bleeding gums, perifollicular hemorrhages, and impaired wound healing. Refusal to walk, with or without joint effusions and arthralgia, dyspnea, edema, weakness, fatigue, depression, and Sjögren syndrome (dry eyes and mouth) also can occur. Other findings include impaired bone growth, disturbed ossification, and subperiosteal hemorrhage.[27,79] In experimental subjects, gingival inflammation and fatigue were

among the most sensitive markers of deficiency without being frankly scorbutic. Scurvy usually occurs at a plasma concentration of <0.2 mg/dL (11 μmol/L), although leukocyte ascorbate concentration is considered a better measure of tissue reserve than plasma ascorbate concentration and is the preferred indicator of vitamin C status.[80]

Supplementation

Gastrointestinal disturbances such as nausea, abdominal cramps, and diarrhea have been reported at vitamin C intake of >3 g/d probably as a result of the osmotic effect of unabsorbed vitamin C. In vivo data do not clearly show a causal relationship between excess vitamin C intake by apparently healthy individuals and other adverse effects,[2] although increased urine oxalate excretion and development of oxalate stones may be possible.[81] However, individuals with hemochromatosis, glucose-6-phosphate dehydrogenase deficiency, and renal disorders may be more susceptible to adverse effects of excess vitamin C intake, which include excess iron absorption, pro-oxidant effects, and kidney (oxalate) stone formation. Additional risks exist for reduced vitamin B_{12} and copper levels, increased oxygen demand, dental enamel erosion, allergic response, and inhibited action of warfarin.[2,7] Vitamin C intake of 250 mg/d or higher has been associated with false-negative result for stool and gastric occult blood.[82] High-dose vitamin C supplement should be stopped before these laboratory tests, while taking into consideration of the biological half-life of about 8 days in the presence of a well-replenished ascorbate body pool.

Pantothenic Acid (Vitamin B_5)

Biochemistry and physiology

Pantothenic acid is a component of coenzyme A (CoA), which is involved in more than 70 enzymatic pathways. CoA, in forms such as acetyl-CoA and succinyl-CoA, plays an important role in the tricarboxylic acid cycle and in the synthesis of fatty acids and membrane phospholipids, amino acids, steroid hormones, vitamins A and D, porphyrin and corrin rings, and neurotransmitters, and acetylation and acylation of proteins and the synthesis of α-tubulin.

Source

Pantothenic acid is widely distributed in foods and found in high concentrations in organ meats, yeast, egg yolk, fresh vegetables, whole grains, and legumes. Intestinal microflora can synthesize pantothenic acid, but this contribution has not been quantified in humans.

Absorption, metabolism, and excretion

CoA in the diet is hydrolyzed in the intestinal lumen to dephospho-CoA, phosphopantethine, and pantethine, with the latter subsequently hydrolyzed to pantothenic acid. Intestinal absorption of pantothenic acid occurs through a saturable sodium-dependent active transport at low intakes, while passive diffusion occurs at high intakes.

Tissue CoA synthesis is regulated primarily by pantothenate kinase, an enzyme inhibited by feedback from the pathway end products, CoA and acyl-CoA. CoA is hydrolyzed to pantothenic acid in a multiple-step reaction and is excreted intact in the urine in proportion to dietary intake.

Deficiency state

Deficiency has been reported only with feeding semisynthetic diets[83] or an antagonist to the vitamin Ω-methyl pantothenic acid.[84] Clinical manifestations may be nonspecific and include irritability, restlessness, fatigue, apathy, malaise, sleep disturbances, nausea, vomiting and abdominal cramps, numbness, paresthesia, staggering gait, and increased sensitivity to insulin. Historically, pantothenic acid was implicated in the "burning feet" syndrome that affected prisoners of war in Asia during World War II.[85]

No data support the use of whole blood, plasma, or red cell concentrations as a marker of deficiency state. Urinary excretion of pantothenic acid is strongly dependent on dietary pantothenic acid.[83]

Supplementation

No subgroups of the population are distinctly susceptible to adverse effects of excess pantothenic acid.

Biotin (Vitamin B₇)

Biochemistry and physiology

Biotin is a cofactor for 5 mammalian carboxylases. These carboxylases catalyze the carboxylation of pyruvate to oxaloacetate, which serves as an intermediate in the tricarboxylic acid cycle. They also catalyze the carboxylation of propionyl-CoA to form D-methylmalonyl-CoA, which then undergoes isomerization to succinyl-CoA and enters into the tricarboxylic acid cycle, and that of acetyl-CoA to malonyl-CoA, which serves as a substrate for fatty acid elongation. The carboxylases are also active in the degradation of leucine.

Source

Biotin is widely distributed in natural foodstuffs, but its concentration varies substantially. Liver has the highest content, while fruits and most meats contain small amounts. The contribution of biotin synthesized by intestinal microflora to the body's needs has not been defined.

Absorption, metabolism, and excretion

Most dietary biotin is protein bound, although it also exists in free form. Biotinidase releases the free vitamin from the protein for absorption primarily in the proximal small intestine, but some occurs at the proximal colon. Absorption is by active transport at low concentrations and passive diffusion at high concentrations. Avidin, a protein found in appreciable amounts in raw egg white, binds to biotin and prevents its absorption. Specific receptors are probably involved in tissue uptake of biotin.[86]

About half of biotin undergoes metabolism to bisnorbiotin and biotin sulfoxide before excretion. In human urine and plasma, they are present in molar proportions of ~3:2:1. Two additional minor metabolites, bisnorbiotin methyl ketone and biotin sulfone, are also present in urine. The urinary excretion and serum concentrations of biotin and its metabolites increase roughly in the same proportion in response to either intravenous or oral administration of large doses of biotin.[87]

During normal breakdown of cellular proteins, biotin-containing enzymes are degraded to biocytin (ε-N-biotinyl-L-lysine) or short oligopeptides containing biotin-linked lysyl residues. Biotin is released from these oligopeptides by biotinidase, and the biotin is reused.[88]

Deficiency state

Clinical deficiency of biotin is uncommon but has been reported in individuals who consumed raw egg whites over long periods[89] or received PN without biotin supplementation.[90] Infantile seizures either alone or with other neurological or cutaneous findings, particularly in the presence of ketolactic acidosis and organic aciduria, are typical of biotinidase deficiency.[91] Infants manifest rash around the mouth, nose, and eyes as "biotin deficiency facies" after several months of biotin-free PN. This rash may extend to ears and perineal orifices. Alopecia totalis, hypotonia, lethargy, developmental delay, and withdrawn behavior may also occur. Similar manifestations including ataxia and paresthesia may occur in older children and adults. The list of inborn errors of metabolism that result in biotin dependency and various degrees of neurological and dermatologic abnormalities now extends to holocarboxylase synthetase deficiency and a defect in biotin transport.[92]

Biochemically, lymphocyte biotinylated 3-methylcrotonyl-CoA carboxylase and propionyl-CoA carboxylase are the most reliable single markers of biotin status. Urine excretion of biotin is decreased and 3-hydroxyisovaleric acid is increased, and reduced lymphocyte expression of SLC19A3, a potential biotin transporter, also occur in subjects with deficiency.[93]

Biotinidase deficiency results in a relative biotin deficiency through lack of adequate digestion of protein-bound biotin. It is treated with free (unbound) biotin at the estimated typical dietary intake of 50–150 mcg/d.[94]

Supplementation

Intakes of biotin at >10 mg/d in a variety of subjects at different life stages was not associated with documented adverse effects.[86]

Choline

Biochemistry and physiology

Choline is the major source of methyl groups in the diet. It is a precursor for acetylcholine, phospholipids, and the methyl donor betaine. Functionally, it plays a critical role in the structural integrity of cell membranes, methyl metabolism, cholinergic neurotransmission, transmembrane signaling, and lipid and cholesterol transport and metabolism.

Source

Choline in the diet is available as free choline or is bound as water-soluble esters (phosphocholine, glycerophosphocholine) or lipid-soluble esters (sphingomyelin, phosphatidylcholine). It is widely distributed in foods, with most in the form of phosphatidylcholine in membranes. Foods especially rich in choline compounds are milk, liver, eggs, and peanuts. Lecithin, a phosphatidylcholine-rich fraction prepared during commercial purification of phospholipids, is often used interchangeably with phosphatidylcholine. It is frequently added to food as an emulsifying agent and may be a significant source of choline.

Endogenous synthesis of choline occurs via sequential methylation of phosphatidylethanolamine catalyzed by the enzyme phosphatidylethanolamine N-methyltransferase and with S-adenosylmethionine as the methyl donor. However, it is insufficient to compensate for the lack of dietary choline.

Absorption, metabolism, and excretion

Choline can be absorbed as lipid-soluble esters through the lymph or as free choline into portal circulation. Pancreatic enzymes can liberate choline from its ester forms. The absorption through the small intestinal mucosa is by transporter proteins, which are probably unique for choline. Some choline may be metabolized by intestinal bacteria to form betaine (which may be absorbed and used as a methyl donor) and methyl amines (which are not methyl donors). Choline, folate, and B_{12} metabolism interactions are required for methyl transfer from MTHF to homocysteine to form methionine and tetrahydrofolate with the enzyme methionine synthase. Thus, the need for choline is modified by methionine, folic acid, and vitamin B_{12} and may be influenced by polymorphisms in genes involved in the metabolism of these nutrients.

All tissues accumulate choline by diffusion and mediated transport. A specific carrier mechanism transports free choline across the blood-brain barrier at a rate proportional to the serum choline concentration. Choline is required to form the phosphatidylcholine portion of very low-density lipoprotein particles needed for the transport of fat from the liver to the tissues. The liver and kidney also readily take up choline where a large proportion is oxidized to betaine. The methyl groups of betaine can be scavenged and reused in single-carbon metabolism.

Deficiency state

Though many foods contain choline, dietary intake varies at least 2-fold in humans. When deprived of dietary choline, most men and postmenopausal women developed signs of organ dysfunction (fatty liver or muscle damage), while less than half of premenopausal women developed such signs. This outcome is probably because estrogen can induce the gene (phosphatidylethanolamine-N-methyltransferase) that catalyzes endogenous synthesis of phosphatidylcholine, which can subsequently yield choline.[95] Individuals receiving PN devoid of choline but adequate for methionine and folate developed hepatic steatosis and elevated alanine aminotransferase. These abnormalities resolved in some individuals when a source of dietary choline was provided.[96] In addition to the sex-based influence, genetic polymorphisms and epigenetics also appear to influence susceptibility to choline deficiency.[95] Fasting plasma, erythrocyte, and tissue content of choline and phosphatidylcholine can be used as markers of choline status.

Supplementation

The critical adverse effect from high intake of choline is hypotension, with corroborative evidence on cholinergic side effects (eg, sweating, diarrhea, and fishy body odor).[1]

Test Your Knowledge Questions

1. All of the following conditions affect bioavailability of water-soluble essential micronutrients except:
   A. Temperature and duration of cooking
   B. Storage
   C. Source from food or supplement
   D. Exposure to light

2. Normal function of all of the following is necessary to prevent deficiency of water-soluble essential micronutrients except for:
   A. Stomach
   B. Pancreas
   C. Small bowel
   D. Large bowel

3. All of the following are true except:
   A. Deficiency in WSVs can occur with a high-fat, low-nutrient-density diet and excess consumption of alcohol and tobacco use.
   B. For nutrition deficiency in WSVs, after initial treatment and correction of predisposing cause, its recurrence can be prevented with the intake of same vitamins at the level of RDA.
   C. After the initial treatment of inborn error of metabolism of a specific WSV, the clinical manifestation can be prevented with the intake of same vitamin at the level of RDA.
   D. Excessive intake of some WSVs can mask or delay the manifestation of other WSVs.

4. All of the following are true except:
   A. Folate can result in megaloblastic anemia from a lack of 5,10-methylenetetrahydrofolate.
   B. Fresh green vegetables are good source of folate and vitamin B_{12}.
   C. Vitamin B_{12} can result in megaloblastic anemia from a lack of 5,10-methylenetetrahydrofolate.
   D. Excess folate intake may exacerbate clinical manifestation of deficiency in vitamin B_{12}.

5. All of the following may be a manifestation of inherited metabolic defects in water-soluble essential micronutrients except:
   A. Nutritional deficiency rickets
   B. Intractable seizures
   C. Skin disorders
   D. Anemia

6. All of the following samples obtained before and after treatment of suspected inborn error of metabolism for a WSV are likely to be useful except:
   A. Nail
   B. Cerebrospinal fluid
   C. Plasma
   D. Urine

References

1. Institute of Medicine, Food and Nutrition Board. *Dietary Reference Intakes for Thiamin, Riboflavin, Niacin, Vitamin B_6, Folate, Vitamin B_{12}, Pantothenic Acid, Biotin, and Choline.* Washington, DC: National Academy Press; 1998.

2. Institute of Medicine, Food and Nutrition Board. *Dietary Reference Intakes for Vitamin C, Vitamin E, Selenium, and Carotenoids.* Washington, DC: National Academy Press; 2000.

3. American Academy of Pediatrics Committee on Nutrition. Water soluble vitamins. In: Kleinman RE, Greer FR, eds. *Pediatric Nutrition.* 7th ed. Elk Grove Village, IL: *American Academy of Pediatrics*; 2014:495–516.

4. Medline Plus, National Institutes of Health. Drugs, supplements, and herbal information. http://www.nlm.nih.gov/medlineplus/druginformation.html. Accessed August 15, 2014.

5. National Institutes of Health. Dietary supplement label database. http://www.dsld.nlm.nih.gov/dsld/. Accessed August 1, 2014.

6. Vanek VW, Borum P, Buchman A, et al; Novel Nutrient Task Force, Parenteral Multi-Vitamin and Multi–Trace Element Working Group; and the American Society for Parenteral and Enteral Nutrition (A.S.P.E.N.) Board of Directors. AS-PEN position paper: recommendations for changes in commercially available parenteral multivitamin and multi-trace element products. *Nutr Clin Pract* 2012;27(4):440–491. Accessed August 1, 2014.

7. Linus Pauling Institute, Oregon State University. Micronutrient Information Center. http://lpi.oregonstate.edu/infocenter/vitamins.html. Accessed August 1, 2014.

8. USDA Food and Nutrition Information Center. Food composition. Vitamins and minerals. http://www.nal.usda.gov/fnic/foodcomp/search/. Accessed August 1, 2014.

9. Ball GFM. *Vitamins in Foods: Analysis, Bioavailability, and Stability.* Boca Raton, FL: Taylor and Francis; 2006.

10. *Drug Facts and Comparisons 2009.* St Louis, MO: Wolters Kluwer Health; 2009.

11. Kim SA, Moore LV, Galuska D, et al; Division of Nutrition, Physical Activity, and Obesity, National Center for Chronic Disease Prevention and Health Promotion, CDC. Vital signs: fruit and vegetable intake among children—United States, 2003–2010. *MMWR Morb Mortal Wkly Rep.* 2014;63(31):671–676.

12. Basu TK, Donaldson D. Intestinal absorption in health and disease: micronutrients. *Best Pract Res Clin Gastroenterol.* 2003;17:957–979.

13. Centers for Disease Control and Prevention (CDC). Lactic acidosis traced to thiamin deficiency related to nationwide shortage of multivitamins for total parenteral nutrition—United States, 1997. *MMWR Morb Mortal Wkly Rep.* 1997;46(23):523–528.

14. Rudatsikira E, Muula AS, Siziya S. Current cigarette smoking among in-school American youth: results from the 2004 National Youth Tobacco Survey. *Int J Equity Health.* 2009;8:10.

15. Seo DC, Jiang N. Associations between smoking and extreme dieting among adolescents. *J Youth Adolesc.* 2009;38:1364–1373.

16. National Center for Chronic Disease Prevention and Health Promotion. Healthy youth! Alcohol and drug use. http://www.cdc.gov/HealthyYouth/alcoholdrug/index.htm. Accessed August 1, 2014.

17. Singleton CK, Martin PR. Molecular mechanisms of thiamine utilization. *Curr Mol Med.* 2001;1:197–207.

18. Manzetti S, Zhang J, van der Spoel D. Thiamin function, metabolism, uptake, and transport. *Biochemistry.* 2014;53:821–835.

19. Mehta S, Fawzi W. Effects of vitamins, including vitamin A, on HIV/AIDS patients. *Vitam Horm.* 2007;75:355–383.

20. Allen LH, Peerson JM, Olney DK. Provision of multiple rather than two or fewer micronutrients more effectively improves growth and other outcomes in micronutrient-deficient children and adults. *J Nutr.* 2009;139:1022–1030.

21. Malik ZA, Abadi J, Sansary J, Rosenberg M. Elevated levels of vitamin B_{12} and folate in vertically infected children with HIV-1. *AIDS.* 2009;23:403–407.

22. Nevado J, Tenbaum SP, Castillo AI, Sánchez-Pacheco A, Aranda A. Activation of the human immunodeficiency virus type I long terminal repeat by 1 alpha, 25-dihydroxyvitamin D3. *J Mol Endocrinol.* 2007;38:587–601.

23. Erlich SD. Possible interactions with vitamin B2 (riboflavin). http://www.umm.edu/altmed/articles/vitamin-b2-000989.htm. Updated May 31, 2013. Accessed August 1, 2014.

24. Rogovik AL, Vohra S, Goldman RD. Safety considerations and potential interactions of vitamins: should vitamins be considered drugs? *Ann Pharmacother.* 2010;44:311–324.

25. Kozyraki R, Cases O. Vitamin B12 absorption: mammalian physiology and acquired and inherited disorders. *Biochimie.* 2013;95:1002–1007.

26. Specker BL, Black A, Allen L, Morrow F. Vitamin B-12: low milk concentrations are related to low serum concentrations in vegetarian women and to methylmalonic aciduria in their infants. *Am J Clin Nutr.* 1990;52:1073–1076.

27. Jen M, Yan AC. Syndromes associated with nutritional deficiency and excess. *Clin Dermatol.* 2010;28:669–685.

28. Picciano MF, Dwyer JT, Radimer KL, et al. Dietary supplement use among infants, children and adolescents in the United States, 1999–2002. *Arch Pediatr Adol Med.* 2007;161:978–985.

29. Madden MM, DeBias D, Cook GE. Market analysis of vitamin supplementation in infants and children: evidence from the dietary supplement label database. *JAMA Pediatr.* 2014;168:291–292.

30. Madden MM, Cook GE. Dietary supplementation in children and adolescents: supplementing with the "correct" amount. *JAMA Pediatr.* 2013;167:991–992.

31. Wallace TC, McBurney M, Fulgoni VL 3rd. Multivitamin/mineral supplement contribution to micronutrient intakes in the United States, 2007–2010. *J Am Coll Nutr.* 2014;33:94–102.

32. Ganapathy V, Smith SB, Prasad PD. SLC19: the folate/thiamin transporter family. *Pflugers Arch.* 2004;447:641–646.

33. Luxemburger C, White NJ, ter Kuile F, et al. Beri-beri: the major cause of infant mortality in Karen refugees. *Trans R Soc Trop Med Hyg.* 2003;97:251–255.

34. Davis RA, Wolf A. Infantile beriberi associated with Wernicke's encephalopathy. *Pediatrics.* 1958;21:409–420.

35. Fattal-Valevski A, Kesler A, Sela BA, et al. Outbreak of life-threatening thiamin deficiency in infants in Israel caused by a defective soy-based formula. *Pediatrics.* 2005;115:e233–e238.

36. Kornreich L, Bron-Harlev E, Hoffmann C, et al. Thiamin deficiency in infants: MR findings in the brain. *Am J Neuroradiol.* 2005;26:1668–1674.

37. Talwar D, Davidson H, Cooney J, St JO'Reilly D. Vitamin B(1) status assessed by direct measurement of thiamin pyrophosphate in erythrocytes or whole blood by HPLC: comparison with erythrocyte transketolase activation assay. *Clin Chem.* 2000;46:704–710.

38. Bayoumi RA, Rosalki SB. Evaluation of methods of coenzyme activation of erythrocyte enzymes for detection of deficiency of vitamins B1, B2, and B6. *Clin Chem.* 1976;22:327–335.

39. Fattal-Valevski A, Azouri-Fattal I, Greenstein YJ, Guindy M, Blau A, Zelnik N. Delayed language development due to infantile thiamine deficiency. *Dev Med Child Neurol.* 2009;51:629–634.

40. Fattal-Valevski A, Bloch-Mimouni A, Kivity S, et al. Epilepsy in children with infantile thiamine deficiency. *Neurology.* 2009;73:828–833.

41. Tabarki B, Al-Hashem A, Alfadhel M. Biotin-thiamin-responsive basal ganglia disease. http://www.ncbi.nlm.nih.gov/books/NBK169615/. Published November 21, 2013. Accessed August 1, 2014.

42. Powers HJ. Riboflavin (vitamin B-2) and health. *Am J Clin Nutr.* 2003;77:1352–1360.

43. Jusko WJ, Levy G. Absorption, metabolism, and excretion of riboflavin-5'-phosphate in man. *J Pharm Sci.* 1967;56:58–62.

44. Amin HJ, Shukla AK, Snyder F, Fung E, Anderson NM, Parsons HG. Significance of phototherapy-induced riboflavin deficiency in the full-term neonate. *Biol Neonate.* 1992;61:76–81.

45. Liang WC, Nishino I. Lipid storage myopathy. *Curr Neurol Neurosci Rep.* 2011;11:97–103.

46. DeLage B. Niacin. Micronutrient Information Center, Linus Pauling Institute, Oregon State University. http://lpi.oregonstate.edu/infocenter/vitamins/niacin. Updated July 2013. Accessed August 1, 2014.

47. Gregory JF 3rd. Nutritional properties and significance of vitamin glycosides. *Annu Rev Nutr.* 1998;18:277–296.

48. Hegyi J, Schwartz RA, Hegyi V. Pellagra: dermatitis, dementia, and diarrhea. *Int J Dermatol.* 2004;43:1–5.

49. Coburn SP. Location and turnover of vitamin B6 pools and vitamin B6 requirements of humans. *Ann N Y Acad Sci.* 1990;585:76–85.

50. Coursin DB. Convulsive seizures in infants with pyridoxine-deficient diet. *J Am Med Assoc.* 1954;154:406–408.

51. Bessey OA, Adam DJ, Hansen AE. Intake of vitamin B6 and infantile convulsions: a first approximation of requirements of pyridoxine in infants. *Pediatrics.* 1957;20:33–44.

52. Kretsch MJ, Sauberlich HE, Newbrun E. Electroencephalographic changes and periodontal status during short-term vitamin B-6 depletion of young, nonpregnant women. *Am J Clin Nutr.* 1991;53:1266–1274.

53. Dakshinamurti K, Dakshinamurti S. Neonatal epileptic encephalopathy: role of vitamin B-6 vitamers in diagnosis and therapy. *Am J Clin Nutr.* 2014;100:505–506.

54. Lui A, Lumeng L, Aronoff GR, Li TK. Relationship between body store of vitamin B6 and plasma pyridoxal-P clearance: metabolic balance studies in humans. *J Lab Clin Med.* 1985;106:491–497.

55. Schaumburg H, Kaplan J, Windebank A, et al. Sensory neuropathy from pyridoxine abuse. A new megavitamin syndrome. *N Engl J Med.* 1983;309:445–448.

56. Parry GJ, Bredesen DE. Sensory neuropathy with low-dose pyridoxine. *Neurology.* 1985;35:1466–1468.

57. McDowell MA, Lacher DA, Pfeiffer CM, et al. Blood folate levels: the latest NHANES results. *NCHS Data Brief.* 2008;6:1–8.

58. Weir DG, McGing PG, Scott JM. Folate metabolism, the enterohepatic circulation and alcohol. *Biochem Pharmacol.* 1985;34:1–7.

59. Tonetti C, Burtscher A, Bories D, Tulliez M, Zittoun J. Methylenetetrahydrofolate reductase deficiency in four siblings: a clinical, biochemical, and molecular study of the family. *Am J Med Genet.* 2000;91:363–367.

60. Ramaekers VT, Rothenberg SP, Sequeira JM, et al. Autoantibodies to folate receptors in the cerebral folate deficiency syndrome. *N Engl J Med.* 2005;352:1985–1991.

61. Stover PJ. Physiology of folate and vitamin B12 in health and disease. *Nutr Rev.* 2004;62:S3–S12.

62. Chan YM, Bailey R, O'Connor DL. Folate. *Adv Nutr.* 2013;4:123–125.

63. Wuerges J, Geremia S, Fedosov SN, Randaccio L. Vitamin B12 transport proteins: crystallographic analysis of beta-axial ligand substitutions in cobalamin bound to transcobalamin. *IUBMB Life.* 2007; 59:722–729.

64. Amin S, Spinks T, Ranicar A, Short MD, Hoffbrand AV. Long-term clearance of [57Co]cyanocobalamin in vegans and pernicious anaemia. *Clin Sci (Lond).* 1980;58:101–103.

65. Allen LH. How common is vitamin B-12 deficiency? *Am J Clin Nutr.* 2009;89:693S–696S.

66. Termanini B, Gibril F, Sutliff VE, Yu F, Venzon DJ, Jensen RT. Effect of long-term gastric acid suppressive therapy on serum vitamin B12 levels in patients with Zollinger-Ellison syndrome. *Am J Med.* 1998;104:422–430.

67. Celiker MY, Chawla A. Congenital B12 deficiency following maternal gastric bypass. *J Perinatology.* 2009;29:640–642.

68. Kapadia CR. Vitamin B12 in health and disease: part I-inherited disorders of function, absorption, and transport. *Gastroenterologist.* 1995;3:329–344.

69. Briani C, Dalla Torre C, Citton V, et al. Cobalamin deficiency: clinical picture and radiological findings. *Nutrients.* 2013;5:4521–4539

70. Vidal-Alaball J, Butler CC, Cannings-John R, et al. Oral vitamin B12 versus intramuscular vitamin B12 for vitamin B12 deficiency. *Cochrane Database Syst Rev.* 2005;3:CD004655.

71. Andrès E, Dali-Youcef N, Vogel T, Serraj K, Zimmer J. Oral cobalamin (vitamin B$_{12}$) treatment. An update. *Int J Lab Hematol.* 2009;31:1–8.

72. Shepherd G, Velez LI. Role of hydroxocobalamin in acute cyanide poisoning. *Ann Pharmacother.* 2008;42:661–669.

73. Lykkesfeldt J, Michels AJ, Frei B. Vitamin C. *Adv Nutr* 2014;5:16–18.

74. Jamal A. Hereditary methemoglobinemia. *J Coll Physicians Surg Pak.* 2006;16:157–159.

75. Schleicher RL, Carroll MD, Ford ES, Lacher DA. Serum vitamin C and the prevalence of vitamin C deficiency in the United States: 2003-2004 National Health and Nutrition Examination Survey (NHANES). *Am J Clin Nutr.* 2009;90:1252–1263.

76. Willmott NS, Bryan RA. Case report: scurvy in an epileptic child on a ketogenic diet with oral complications. *Eur Arch Paediatr Dent.* 2008;9:148–152.

77. Samonte VA, Sherman PM, Taylor GP, et al. Scurvy diagnosed in a pediatric liver transplant patient awaiting combined kidney and liver retransplantation. *Pediatr Transplant.* 2008;12:363–367.

78. Ratanachu-Ek S, Sukswai P, Jeerathanyasakun Y, Wongtapradit L. Scurvy in pediatric patients: a review of 28 cases. *J Med Assoc Thai.* 2003;86:S734–S740.

79. Fain O. Musculoskeletal manifestations of scurvy. *Joint Bone Spine.* 2005;72:124–128.

80. Thurnham DI. Micronutrients and immune function: some recent developments. *J Clin Pathol.* 1997;50:887–891.

81. Wandzilak TR, D'Andre SD, Davis PA, Williams HE. Effect of high dose vitamin C on urinary oxalate levels. *J Urol.* 1994;151:834–837.

82. Gogel HK, Tandberg D, Strickland RG. Substances that interfere with guaiac card tests: implications for gastric aspirate testing. *Am J Emerg Med.* 1989;7:474–480.

83. Fry PC, Fox HM, Tao HG. Metabolic response to a pantothenic acid deficient diet in humans. *J Nutr Sci Vitaminol (Tokyo).* 1976;22:339–346.

84. Hodges RE, Bean WB, Ohlson MA, Bleiler R. Human pantothenic acid deficiency produced by omega-methyl pantothenic acid. *J Clin Invest.* 1959;38:1421–1425.

85. Glusman M. The syndrome of "burning feet" (nutritional melagia) as a manifestation of nutritional deficiency. *Am J Med.* 1947;3:211–223.

86. Zempleni J, Kuroishi T. Biotin. *Adv Nutr.* 2012;3:213–214.

87. Wolf B, Grier RE, Secor McVoy JR, Heard GS. Biotinidase deficiency: a novel vitamin recycling defect. *J Inherit Metab Dis.* 1985;8 (suppl 1):53–58.

88. Mock DM, Heird GM. Urinary biotin analogs increase in humans during chronic supplementation: the analogs are biotin metabolites. *Am J Physiol.* 1997;272:E83–E85.

89. Baugh CM, Malone JH, Butterworth CE Jr. Human biotin deficiency. A case history of biotin deficiency induced by raw egg consumption in a cirrhotic patient. *Am J Clin Nutr.* 1968;21:173–182.

90. Mock DM, Baswell DL, Baker H, Holman RT, Sweetman L. Biotin deficiency complicating parenteral alimentation: diagnosis, metabolic repercussions, and treatment. *J Pediatr.* 1985;106:762–769.

91. Wolf B, Heard GS, Weissbecker KA, McVoy JR, Grier RE, Leshner RT. Biotinidase deficiency: initial clinical features and rapid diagnosis. *Ann Neurol.* 1985;18:614–617.

92. Mardach R, Zempleni J, Wolf B, et al. Biotin dependency due to a defect in biotin transport. *J Clin Invest.* 2002;109:1617–1623.

93. Eng WK, Giraud D, Schlegel VL, Wang D, Lee BH, Zempleni J. Identification and assessment of markers of biotin status in healthy adults. *Br J Nutr.* 2013;110:321–329.

94. Wolf B, Heard GS, McVoy JR, Raetz HM. Biotinidase deficiency: the possible role of biotinidase in the processing of dietary protein-bound biotin. *J Inherit Metab Dis.* 1984;7 (suppl 2):121–122.

95. Zeisel SH. Nutritional genomics: defining the dietary requirement and effects of choline. *J Nutr.* 2011 March;141(3):531–534.

96. Buchman AL, Dubin MD, Moukarzel AA, et al. Choline deficiency: a cause of hepatic steatosis during parenteral nutrition that can be reversed with intravenous choline supplementation. *Hepatology.* 1995;22:1399–1403.

Test Your Knowledge Answers

1. The correct answer is **C**. Bioavailability of WSV supplements is generally similar to that from dietary sources when tested under the same conditions. However, the bioavailability of some WSVs is usually negatively affected by high heat, prolonged cooking or storage, and light exposure.

2. The correct answer is **D**. Intact functioning of one of more of the organ systems is needed for the digestion, absorption, and transport of ingested water-soluble micronutrients. The absorption of these nutrients is usually completed prior to reaching the large bowel. Thus, the absence of intact large bowel is least likely to be associated with deficiency of WSVs.

3. The correct answer is **C**. Diets with high fat and a preponderance of low-nutrient-density foods have low content of WSVs. Alcohol abuse is often associated with poor dietary intake of many essential nutrients.

In addition, alcohol can directly or indirectly interfere with the digestion, absorption, and metabolism of multiple essential water-soluble micronutrients. Smokers may have an increased need for antioxidant vitamins because of the oxidative stress from smoking. There may also be a concomitant decreased intake because of inappropriate dieting. Unlike nutrition-deficiency states, individuals with an inborn error of metabolism involving a WSV generally require an intake greater than the RDA to remain symptom free. Excessive folate intake may precipitate or exacerbate neuropathy in individuals with vitamin B_{12} deficiency and has been implicated in delaying the diagnosis of pernicious anemia until after irreversible neurological damage has occurred.

4. The correct answer is **B**. Fresh green vegetables are a good source of folate but not vitamin B_{12}. Folate is critical to the metabolism of nucleic and amino acids; it promotes cellular growth in general and is necessary for the maturation of red cells. Folate is a substrate (5-methyl-tetrahydrofolate) and vitamin B_{12} is a coenzyme in the formation of MTHF and thymidylate synthesis. In either a folate or vitamin B_{12} deficiency, the megaloblastic changes in bone marrow and other replicating cells result from lack of MTHF. Excessive folate intake may precipitate or exacerbate neuropathy in individuals with vitamin B_{12} deficiency and has been implicated in delaying the diagnosis of pernicious anemia until after irreversible neurological damage has occurred.

5. The correct answer is **A**. Nutrition-deficiency rickets are typically a result of mineral (calcium and/or phosphorus deficiency) and/or vitamin D deficiency. Clinical manifestations of deficiency in WSVs may overlap and commonly include skin disorders, anemia, diarrhea, and impaired neurologic function.

6. The correct answer is **A**. In patients with a suspected inborn error of metabolism, the collection of plasma, cerebrospinal fluid, and urine before and after empiric therapy with pharmacological doses of a specific vitamin is useful to monitor the concentration of the vitamin, its metabolites, and other biochemical markers to aid in the diagnosis and therapy. Additional genetic testing may be warranted. Nail samples are unlikely to have any use in this situation.

8

Fat-Soluble Vitamins

Winston Koo, MBBS, FACN, CNS; **May Saba,** PharmD, BCNSP; **Mirjana Lulic-Botica,** BSc, RPh, BCPS; and **Judith Christie,** RN, MSN

CONTENTS

Learning Objectives

1. Review the physiological basis for the function and requirement common to the group and unique to a specific fat-soluble vitamin.
2. Define the common risk factors and special considerations in the development of fat-soluble vitamin deficiency.
3. Define the common manifestations and diagnosis of deficiency states for fat-soluble vitamins.
4. Describe the potential risks of excessive intake of fat-soluble vitamins.

Introduction

Achievement of adequate status for fat-soluble vitamins (A, D, E, and K) depends on adequate intake, intestinal digestion and absorption, cellular uptake, and metabolism. Vitamins D and K are produced endogenously in substantial, but variable, amounts. Fortification of some vitamins (eg, vitamin D) is widely practiced because of their limited distribution in commonly consumed natural foods. However, a varied dietary intake generally meets the dietary reference intake (DRI) of fat-soluble vitamins in the normal population (Table 8-1).

Nutrient requirements and biological actions of fat-soluble vitamins must be considered as part of total nutrition support since these vitamins have metabolic interactions with other nutrients. For example, zinc, energy, and protein metabolism affect vitamin A status through their effect on production of retinol-binding protein (RBP) and transthyretin; novel ligands (eg, secondary bile acids and long-chain polyunsaturated fatty acids) can activate vitamin D receptors leading to additional potential biological function for vitamin D; and antioxidants such as vitamin C, glutathione,

Table 8-1. Dietary Reference Intake for Fat-Soluble Vitamins[1-3]

LIFE STAGE	VITAMIN A, mcg RAE (1 mcg = 3.3 IU)	VITAMIN D,[a] IU (1 mcg = 40 IU)	VITAMIN E, mg	VITAMIN K,[a] mcg
0–6 mo[a]	400 (600)	400 (1000)	4	2.0
7–12 mo[a]	500 (600)	400 (1500)	5	2.5
1–3 y[b]	300 (600)	600 (2500)	6 (200)	30
4–8 y[b]	400 (900)	600 (3000)	7 (300)	55
9–13 y[b]	600 (1700)	600 (4000)	11 (600)	60
MALES				
14–18 y[b]	900 (2800)	600 (4000)	15 (800)	75
FEMALES				
14–18 y[b]	700 (2800)	600 (4000)	15 (800)	75
PREGNANCY[c]				
14–18 y[b]	750 (2800)	600 (4000)	15 (800)	75
LACTATION[c]				
14–18 y[b]	1200 (2800)	600 (4000)	19 (800)	75
UL	[d]	[d]	[d]	NA

AI, adequate intake; EAR, estimated average requirement; NA, not available; RAE, retinol activity equivalent; RDA, recommended dietary allowance; UL, upper limit.

[a]AI is the observed or experimentally determined estimate of nutrient intake by a group or groups of healthy people. Applicable for all ages for vitamins D and K.

[b]RDA is the average daily dietary intake sufficient to meet the requirement of 97%–98% of healthy individuals in a life stage based on sex. RDA = EAR + 2SD$_{EAR}$ or 1.2 EAR or 1.3 EAR. EAR is the daily intake of a nutrient estimated to meet the nutrient requirement of half of the healthy individuals in a life stage based on sex.

[c]RDA during pregnancy and lactation for other ages; check references 1–3.

[d]Upper limit for each life stage is indicated in parenthesis.

and ubiquinols can affect the regeneration of α-tocopherol, itself an antioxidant, and the requirement for vitamin E.

Consideration of specific clinical disorders and consequences of surgical and medical therapy is also warranted in the assessment and management of fat-soluble vitamin status. Details on specific situations are presented in Parts III and IV on disease states and their specific nutrition support.

Fat-soluble vitamin deficiency occurs more frequently in individuals with any disease state that impairs biliary and pancreatic secretions, intestinal mucosal function, micelle formation, and uptake into enterocytes. In addition, impaired chylomicron secretion can lower the digestion and absorption of all fat-soluble vitamins. Thus, severe hepatobiliary disorders, cystic fibrosis, and Whipple's disease are some of the diseases that predispose an individual to fat-soluble vitamin deficiency. Increasingly, inherited defects in absorption or metabolism of various vitamins are documented to contribute to deficiency states in an individual.

Decreased intake and absorption of fat-soluble vitamins and other nutrients often occur with severe dietary restriction and bariatric surgery in the treatment of extreme obesity. Interference with absorption of fat-soluble vitamins can occur with the use of bile salt or fat sequestrants, such as cholestyramine and orlistat, as adjunct therapy for hypercholesterolemia, hepatobiliary disorders, or extreme obesity, as well as from the use of mineral oil and other nonabsorbable lipids. Vitamin D metabolism is adversely affected by chronic glucocorticoid and phenobarbital therapy. Vitamin K metabolism is adversely affected by coumarin anticoagulant therapy.

In the general population, deficiency states from limited intake are more common for vitamins A and D than for vitamins E and K. Absence or inadequate endogenous production, especially when coupled with poor exogenous intake, increases the risk for deficiency of fat-soluble vitamins. Thus, infants living at high latitudes and exclusively breastfed for prolonged period are predisposed to vitamin D deficiency because inadequate sunlight exposure lowers vitamin D synthesis and breast milk has low vitamin D content. Restrictions in the variety of foods due to limited financial resources or fad diets contribute to the deficiency of fat-soluble vitamins. Concomitant deficit in other nutrients is also common in these circumstances.

Pregnancy and lactation result in added demands to the body's nutritional requirements, although the recommended dietary allowance (RDA) for fat-soluble vitamins remains the same as that for any age range except for an increase of ~7% for vitamin A during pregnancy and an increase of ~70% for vitamin A and ~25% for vitamin E during lactation.[1-3]

Ingestion of fat-soluble vitamins, often in some combination of multiple vitamins, is a common practice among healthy adults and children.[1-4] With the exception of vitamin A during infancy, the upper limit of DRI for fat-soluble vitamins is 2 to >50 times the RDA,[1-3] thus supplementation

in amounts similar to the daily requirements is unlikely to result in any adverse effect, although there is also no consistent reported benefit.

Bioavailability of the enteral supplement may be improved with the water-miscible form or with alteration in the physical form, although parenteral supplementation may still be needed in some patients with diseases that impair the absorption of fat-soluble vitamins.[1-3,5-9]

Table 8-2 lists the fat-soluble multivitamin preparations for parenteral nutrition. However, complete delivery of some parenteral nutrients may not be ensured particularly if prolonged storage is needed. For example, binding of vitamin A to intravenous bags and tubing, and photo-oxidation and lipid peroxidation of other nutrients have been reported. Thus, any patient on chronic parenteral or specific

Table 8-2. Content per Unit Dose of Fat-Soluble Multivitamin Preparations for Use With Parenteral Nutrition

INGREDIENT	M.V.I. PEDIATRIC	INFUVITE PEDIATRIC	M.V.I. ADULT FOR AGES ≥ 11 Y	M.V.I-12	INFUVITE ADULT
Unit dose volume, mL	5[a]	5[b]	10[c]	10[c]	10[c]
FAT-SOLUBLE VITAMINS					
Vitamin A (retinol), mg	0.7	0.7	1	1	1
Vitamin D (erogocalciferol,[d] cholecalciferol[e]), mcg	10[d]	10[e]	5[d]	5[d]	5[e]
Vitamin E (DL-α-tocopheryl acetate), mg	7	7	10	10	10
Vitamin K (phytonadione), mcg	200	200	150	none	150
OTHER					
Aluminum, mcg/L	42	30	43–183	43–78	70
Polysorbate 80, mg	50	50	160	160	140
Polysorbate 20, mg	0.8	–	2.8	2.8	–
Propylene glycol, g	–	–	3	3	3

Data from manufacturer product insert: Hospira, Inc., Lake Forest, IL for M.V.I. Pediatric (August 2007), M.V.I. Adult (February 2009), and M.V.I.-12 (February 2009). Baxter Inc., Deerfield, IL for Infuvite Pediatric (September 2007) and Infuvite Adult (February 2012), and from Linus Pauling Institute, Oregon State University.[7] Manufacturers, products, and product information can change frequently.

[a]Single-dose vial reconstituted to 5 mL.

[b]Two single-dose vials: vial 2 (1 mL) contains folic acid, biotin, and vitamin B, and vial 1 (4 mL) contains all the other vitamins. For both pediatric preparations, the 5 mL is the daily dose for infants and children weighing ≥ 3 kg up to age 11 years, 3.25 mL (65% of daily dose) for infants weighing 1–3 kg, and 1.5 mL (30% of daily dose) for infants weighing < 1 kg. Multiple product shortages are an ongoing issue. In the event of no pediatric intravenous multivitamin availability, an adult intravenous multivitamin at a daily dose of 1 mL/kg and up to a maximum of 2.5 mL/day may be used for infants < 2.5 kg or < 36 weeks of gestation (Hospira Package insert 8/2007).

[c]Supplied in one or more forms depending on manufacturer. Unit vial is a 2-chambered single-dose vial that must be mixed just prior to use and will provide one 10-mL dose. Dual vial is 2 vials labeled vial 1 (5 mL) and vial 2 (5 mL), with both vials to be used for a single 10-mL dose. Pharmacy bulk package consists of 2 vials labeled vial 1 (50 mL) and vial 2 (50 mL), and 5 mL of each vial provides 10 mL of a single dose.

enteral nutrition support requires monitoring of fat-soluble vitamins and overall nutritional status (see Part IV on specific nutrition support).

Adverse effects from consumption of fat-soluble vitamins naturally occurring in foods has been reported for vitamin A.[10] Chronic exposure to excess intake of vitamins A and D is well known to have toxic effects affecting many organ systems. In some cases, a single exposure to a large dose of some fat-soluble vitamins may be toxic and occasionally may be lethal. Certain individuals (eg, those with chronic alcohol abuse and liver dysfunction) may be at greater risk for adverse effects of excess intake or deficiency in fat-soluble vitamins and other nutrients. Cigarette consumption increases the demand on antioxidants in addition to its other adverse effects.[1–3] Any patient on pharmacological doses of fat-soluble vitamins should be under medical supervision.

Vitamin A

Biochemistry and Physiology
Vitamin A, or retinoids, refers to retinol and its derivatives including synthetic analogs that have the same β-ionone ring and similar biological activities. They also include provitamin A carotenoids that are the dietary precursor of retinol. The principal vitamin A compounds—retinol, retinal (retinaldehyde), retinoic acid, and retinyl esters—differ in the terminal C-15 group at the end of the side chain. The all-trans-isomer is the most common and stable form although many cis-isomers also exist.

Retinoids are critical to the maintenance of proper vision in the signal transmission of images to the visual cortex. They are necessary for cell differentiation and integrity of epithelial cells throughout the body, including normal differentiation of the cornea and conjunctival membranes, as well as for the photoreceptor rod and cone cells of the retina. Other critical functions include maintenance of immune function; expression of various genes that encode for structural and extracellular matrix proteins, enzymes, RBPs, and receptors; and embryonic development of hindbrain, eyes, ears, heart, and limbs. Provitamin A carotenoids must be converted to retinoids to exert vitamin A function. In addition, carotenoids are excellent antioxidants and may have other biological properties unrelated to their vitamin A activity.

Sources
Vitamin A is present in the diet as retinyl esters derived almost exclusively from animal sources (liver and fish liver oils, dairy products, kidney, and eggs). Most of the vitamin A in breast milk is in the form of retinyl palmitate in milk fat and is in greatest concentration in colostrum and transition milk. The vitamin A content of breast milk is generally lower in populations deficient in vitamin A but is still sufficient to prevent subclinical deficiency in exclusively breastfed infants during the first 6 months.[11] Cow's milk has relatively lower vitamin A content than human milk and averages ~40 IU/g fat.[12] The U.S. Food and Drug Administration encourages dairy producers to fortify reduced fat milk to 2000 IU/L.[12] Infant formulas are fortified with vitamin A at 250–750 IU/100 kcal.[13] High-temperature sterilization of milk increases isomerization of trans-retinol to cis-retinol by as much as 34%, thus reducing the stability and possibly bioavailability of vitamin A.[1]

Provitamin A carotenoids (mainly β-carotene) are distributed widely in green and yellow vegetables, oils, and fruits. Ripe colored fruits and cooked yellow tuber vegetables are more efficiently converted to vitamin A compared with dark green leafy vegetables.[1] Current estimates of total vitamin A intake from vegetable sources is about 26%–34% based on retinol activity equivalent (RAE).[1]

Supplements are available as retinol, retinyl esters (palmitate, acetate, and N-formyl aspartamate), retinaldehyde, or β-carotene, either alone or in a multivitamin formulation and in oral and parenteral forms.[6,14,15]

Vitamin A activity is expressed as RAEs (1 mcg RAE = 1 mcg all-trans-retinol = 2 mcg supplemental all-trans-β-carotene = 12 mcg dietary all-trans-β-carotene = 24 mcg other dietary provitamin A carotenoids = 3.3 IU of vitamin A activity).[1] The bioconversion of dietary provitamin carotenoids to RAE is estimated to be 12:1 (micrograms) based on the relative absorption efficiency of β-carotene from food and the functional carotene to retinol equivalency ratio. One RAE for dietary provitamin A carotenoids other than β-carotene is lower and set at 24 mcg.[1] The use of micrograms of RAE is preferred to micrograms of retinol equivalent (RE) or International Units (IUs) when calculating and reporting the amount of total vitamin A in mixed foods or assessing the amount of dietary and supplemental vitamin A consumed. RE was based on the earlier erroneous 2 times higher estimate of bioconversion of dietary carotenoids.[1]

Absorption and Metabolism
The efficiency of absorption of preformed vitamin A is about 70%–90%. Vitamin A supplements, particularly β-carotene, are generally better absorbed than the dietary vitamin sources. A water-miscible preparation of vitamin A supple-

ment is available for use in patients with fat malabsorption. There may be a maturation lag in the ability to absorb vitamin A in the preterm infant,[16] and the only effective means to elevate plasma retinol concentrations in preterm infants is via the parenteral route.[17]

Dietary retinyl esters are freed by acidic digestion and emulsified by bile salts to form micelles. These micelles are transported to the intestinal cells, where the retinyl ester is moved across the mucosal membrane and hydrolyzed, re-esterified, and then incorporated into chylomicrons within the cell and secreted into lymph. At physiological concentrations, cellular uptake and efflux of unesterified retinol by enterocytes is mediated by lipid transporters and is a saturable process, whereas at high pharmacological doses, the absorption of retinol is nonsaturable.[18] Portal route of absorption is possible under some circumstances.

Carotenoids are solubilized into micelles, from which they are absorbed into duodenal mucosal cells. Absorption of carotenoids is by passive diffusion and by a facilitated process that requires, at least for lutein, the class B-type 1 scavenger receptor.[19] The intestine, liver, lung, adipose, and other tissues possess β,β-carotene 15,15′ monooxygenase activity that allows the central cleavage of the β-carotene to form 2 molecules of retinal. The latter can be converted to other retinoids. Eccentric cleavage of carotenoids by other enzymes is also possible. The absorption efficiency of β-carotene has wide interindividual variation and is usually < 20%.[1,19] It is higher in the presence of dietary fat, from homogenized, juiced, or cooked vegetables, which allow the release of carotenoids, and during poor vitamin A status. It is lower in the presence of intestinal infections or infestations and at high dietary carotenoid intake.[20] β-Carotene significantly reduces lutein absorption when given simultaneously.[1]

Retinyl esters and carotenoids are transported to the liver in chylomicron remnants. Apoprotein E and several specific hepatic membrane receptors are required for the uptake of chylomicron remnants by the liver. Retinyl esters are hydrolyzed to retinol and then bound to RBP for release into the circulation. In the blood, holo-RBP associates with transthyretin to form a trimolecular complex with retinol in a 1:1:1 molar ratio for delivery to peripheral tissues. Retinoic acid, nuclear retinoic acid receptor and retinoid X receptors, cellular retinol, and retinoic acid binding proteins I and II are critical to the function of retinoids. Carotenoids are incorporated into very low-density lipoproteins and exported from the liver into the blood. They enter peripheral tissues via receptor uptake of lipoproteins and undergo further metabolism.

Retinoids are stored in the liver and other tissues including adipose tissue, bone marrow, lung, eye, kidney, and other organs. When vitamin A intake is adequate, > 90% of total body vitamin A is present in the liver. Vitamin A concentration of at least 20 mcg/g of liver in adults is suggested as the minimal acceptable reserve.[21] Regeneration of retinyl esters to form local storage pools (eg, in the retinal pigment epithelium) also occurs.

Typically, the majority of vitamin A metabolites are excreted in the urine and almost all of the excreted metabolites are biologically inactive. Thus, elevated plasma concentrations of retinol, RBP, and transthyretin can occur in chronic renal disease. Some retinoid metabolites are conjugated with glucuronic acid or taurine in the liver for excretion in bile.

Deficiency

Vitamin A deficiency is an endemic nutrition problem throughout much of the developing world and affects the health and survival of infants, young children, and pregnant and lactating women.[22] These life-stage groups represent periods when both nutrition stress is high and the diet is likely to be chronically deficient in vitamin A. Numerous clinical effects of vitamin A deficiency have been reported (Table 8-3), but the most specific manifestation is xerophthalmia. The latter include impaired dark adaptation and detrimental effect on cornea that could lead to irreversible blindness.

In developed countries, risk factors for vitamin A deficiency include fat malabsorption conditions, strict vegan diets, fad diets, and severely restricted intake of preformed vitamin A or provitamin A. Ethanol decreases liver vitamin

Table 8-3. Clinical Effects of Vitamin A Deficiency[1,23]

- Xerophthalmia[a]
  - o XN: Impaired dark adaptation (from slowed regeneration of rhodopsin) to night blindness
  - o XCj: Conjunctival dryness (xerosis), XB: keratinization (Bitot's spot)
  - o XCo: Corneal xerosis; XU/K: Corneal ulceration and/or keratomalacia of any part; XSc: Corneal scar in central part; XSp: Corneal scar in peripheral part
  - o XF: Xerophthalmia fundus
- Generalized dysfunction of cellular and humoral immunity with increased morbidity and mortality especially from measles and diarrhea
- Impaired iron mobilization from stores
- Defective lung function
- Follicular hyperkeratosis

[a]Classification according to Singh.[23]

A stores by increasing release of hepatic retinol independent of dietary intake and decreasing conversion of β-carotene to retinol, thus promoting vitamin A deficiency.[1] For any patient being treated for vitamin A deficiency, determining the presence of deficiencies in other nutrients and appropriate treatment is prudent because they may also detrimentally affect vitamin A status. For example, zinc deficiency decreases the synthesis and secretion of RBP and transthyretin and the synthesis of rhodopsin.

The level of retinol in the blood is under homeostatic control over a broad range of body stores and reflects body stores only when these are very low or very high.[11] In addition, low plasma retinol concentration can result from an inadequate supply of dietary protein, energy, or zinc because of decreased rate of synthesis of RBP, or it can result from acute or chronic infection because of decreased concentrations of the negative acute phase proteins, RBP and transthyretin, even when liver retinol is adequate.[1] Changes over time in plasma retinol concentration distributions within a population can be helpful to determine vitamin A status.[11] Plasma retinol at <0.70 μmol/L (1 μmol/L = 28.6 mcg/dL) reflects vitamin A inadequacy and at <0.35 μmol/L indicates vitamin A deficiency.[22] Simultaneous measurement of plasma RBP is helpful to assess the vitamin A status.

Other measures of vitamin A status, such as the relative dose response and modified relative dose response, immune function tests, conjunctival impression cytology, dark adaptation test, pupillary response test, and total liver reserve by isotope dilution, are abnormal in clinical vitamin A deficiency. However, none of these measures have sufficient data relating to the usual dietary intakes of individuals or populations to allow adequate determination of the vitamin A status. Some of these tests (eg, relative dose response and modified relative dose response) are subjected to other factors such as RBP production that can influence the outcome.[1,11,24]

Vitamin A supplementation reduces the risk of mortality among infants, young children, and pregnant and postpartum women in developing countries.[1,5,22,25–28] Night blindness significantly improved in a majority of affected persons with vitamin A or β-carotene supplementation.[25] The benefits of vitamin A supplementation in infectious diseases other than measles is less clear.[5,25]

In developed countries, intramuscular vitamin A supplement has a modest effect on reduction in oxygen requirement at 36 weeks postmenstrual age in those with birth weights < 1 kg.[17] Poor nutritional status is well known to impair wound healing. However, numerous nutrients including proteins, vitamin A, vitamin C, vitamin B complex, arginine, glutamine, iron, zinc, and selenium can have significant beneficial effects on wound healing and optimization of the immune system,[29] and no definitive data are available on the use of a single nutrient supplement for this purpose.

No evidence exists for a certain percentage of provitamin A carotenoids to meet the vitamin A requirement. However, in view of the health benefits of consumption of fruits and vegetables, 5 servings of fruits and vegetables daily could provide 5.2–6 mg/d of provitamin A, which is ~50%–65% of the men's RDA for vitamin A.[1]

Adverse Effects

Substantial data exist on the adverse effects of high vitamin A intake.[21,30] Individuals with preexisting liver disease, hyperlipidemia, severe protein malnutrition, or high alcohol intake may be distinctly susceptible to the adverse effects of preformed vitamin A intake. Short-term large doses and even a single dose > 150,000 mcg in adults[31] and proportionately lower in children can result in acute toxicity characterized by nausea, vomiting, headache, vertigo, blurred vision, muscular incoordination, and increased intracranial pressure. In infants, bulging of fontanels is also present.[21,32] Animal studies demonstrated that a similarly large single dose of vitamin A can be lethal.[33]

Chronic toxicity is usually associated with ingestion of large doses > 30,000 mcg/d for months or years. Clinical manifestations of chronic toxicity are varied and nonspecific and may include irritability, anorexia, skin desquamation, and liver abnormalities including elevated liver enzymes, fibrosis, and cirrhosis. In infants, additional nonhepatic manifestations include bulging fontanel, craniotabes, and laboratory findings of cortical hyperostosis, hypercalcemia, and hyperphosphatemia, and metastatic calcifications may occur at an intake between 5500 and 6750 mcg/d for 1–3 months.[1,32] In adults, findings for bone mineral loss and fractures are inconsistent.[1] Ethanol, while promoting a deficiency of vitamin A, also enhances vitamin A hepatotoxicity.[34] Care is needed with vitamin A supplementation in patients with renal dysfunction to avoid vitamin A toxicity because the kidney is the main route of excretion of vitamin A and its metabolites. Both acute and chronic vitamin A toxicity are associated with increased plasma retinyl ester concentrations.[35]

In humans, teratogenic effects, particularly neural crest defects, from naturally occurring metabolites of vitamin A (*trans*-retinoic acid, 13-*cis*-retinoic acid, and their oxo-derivatives) are well documented in women exposed during the first trimester. Limited data link teratogenic effects to high-dose preformed vitamin A (retinol and retinyl esters), and data are insufficient to determine the presence of toxic nonteratogenic developmental effects.[1,36] Adolescents using vitamin A or derivatives for the treatment of acne must be informed of the potential teratogenic effects and counseled on the need to avoid pregnancy during this therapy.

High-dose vitamin A supplementation is often used for the treatment and prevention of deficiency states. However, the potential for vitamin A toxicity under these circumstances exist and practitioners should consult the current recommendations of vitamin A dosing for specific conditions. Plasma retinol and RBP concentrations are not always reliable in detecting vitamin A toxicity, and plasma retinyl esters, normally not present, should be monitored.

High β-carotene intake has not been shown to cause hypervitaminosis A, but carotenodermia (a yellowish discoloration of the skin from hypercarotenemia) has been reported[37,38] and is reversed by discontinuing intake. A clinical intervention trial of β-carotene supplement based on its antioxidant activity resulted in a significant increase in the rate of lung cancer in smokers. This would suggest that excessive intake of the provitamin A carotenoids may have unintended consequences on the complex and intricately balanced natural antioxidant defense system.[39] Also, the combination of excess β-carotene and ethanol may result in hepatotoxicity.[1,34]

Vitamin D

Biochemistry and Physiology

Vitamin D (calciferol) refers to 2 fat-soluble seco-sterols: cholecalciferol (vitamin D_3) photosynthesized by the action of ultraviolet light (the most effective wavelengths are in the range of 290–315 nm) on a cholesterol precursor in the skin of vertebrates, and ergocalciferol (vitamin D_2) from the yeast and plant sterol. The term vitamin D without the subscript is frequently used generically to describe vitamins D_2 and D_3 and, correspondingly, their metabolites. The parent vitamin D compounds are biologically inert and considered as prohormones, which require 2 obligatory hydroxylation steps primarily in the liver and kidney to 25 hydroxyvitamin D (25 OHD) and 1,25-dihydroxyvitamin D (1,25 $(OH)_2D$), respectively. Quantitatively, 25 OHD is the major circulating metabolite. It is a good marker of vitamin D status because it reflects the cumulative effects of exposure to sunlight and dietary intake of vitamin D.[40] At physiological concentrations, 1,25 $(OH)_2D$ is the metabolite responsible for most, if not all, biological functions of vitamin D.

The classic actions of vitamin D include the maintenance of calcium homeostasis and bone mineralization in the prevention of rickets in children and osteomalacia in adults. These effects are mediated primarily through 1,25 $(OH)_2D$ binding of nuclear vitamin D receptor (VDR) and from participation in various feedback loops involving parathyroid hormone (PTH), calcitonin, and fibroblast growth factor-23. There is also 1,25 $(OH)_2D_3$-mediated gene regulation for several bone anabolic and resorbing factors. VDR is widely distributed in numerous organ systems, and 1,25 $(OH)_2D_3$-VDR effects include immunomodulation, antimicrobial action, detoxification, cell proliferation, apoptosis regulation, insulin secretion, skin integrity, and β-oxidation.[41,42] Numerous physiological functions are mediated by VDR, and disturbances in vitamin D pathways are associated with major human diseases such as cancer, infections, autoimmune diseases, cardiovascular and metabolic diseases, and disorders in muscle function, reproduction, and neurocognition. However, the evidence for major dysfunction from vitamin D deficiency other than the classic actions of mineral homeostasis and bone mineralization is limited.

Actions other than the classic VDR pathway, including modulation of miRNA function and the epigenetic regulation of genes,[43] are becoming better defined. VDR stimulation independent of 1,25 $(OH)_2D_3$ controls hair cycling and brain development. Novel ligands other than 1,25 $(OH)_2D_3$ including lithocolic acid, curcumin, γ-tocotrienol, and essential fatty acid derivatives may play additional specific roles in physiological functions and therapeutic potential for various diseases.[42–44]

Biological activity of vitamin D is expressed in IUs based on bioassays using cholecalciferol. The biological activity of 1 mcg of vitamin D is 40 IU and 1 mcg of 25 OHD is 200 IU (ie, 5 times more potent than cholecalciferol).[2] Both forms of vitamin D undergo the same metabolic fate and function similarly at least for the classic actions in the clinical prevention and treatment of rickets and osteomalacia.[45–47] The role of vitamin D_2 in other actions is not well defined.

Sources

Endogenous synthesis of vitamin D_3 requires exposure to sunlight or irradiation in the ultraviolet B range. It is extremely effective, and a 10-minute to 15-minute whole-body exposure to peak summer sun will generate and release up to 20,000 IU of vitamin D_3 into the circulation.[48,49] However, prolonged sunlight exposure increases the conversion of previtamin D_3 to inactive metabolites. Cutaneous production of vitamin D_3 is substantially diminished by decreased exposure to sunlight from seasonal changes or time of day, clouds, aerosols, thick ozone, higher latitude, aging, clothing, sunscreen use, and melanin pigmentation.[49] In dark-skinned individuals, endogenous synthesis of vitamin D is possible, although the rate of production is lower than in less pigmented individuals. The concern over hazards of ultraviolet radiation exposure have resulted in revised recommendations for sunlight exposure as a means of maintaining adequate vitamin D stores.[50] Thus, ensuring adequate vitamin D status in the presence of multiple factors that affect its endogenous synthesis requires attention to the use of dietary supplementation of vitamin D.

Foods naturally rich in vitamin D are limited to the flesh of fatty fish and fish liver oil and the liver and fat from aquatic mammals (eg, seals and polar bears). Thus, dietary intake of vitamin D from foods comes primarily from fortified milk products and other fortified foods such as breakfast cereals.[51,52] In the United States and Canada, the average intake of vitamin D is about 200–400 IU per day, with children tending to have greater intake than adults.[51] Human milk and cow's milk have very low vitamin D content (< 50 IU/L). In the United States, a vast majority of natural milk and all infant formulas are fortified with vitamin D_3 at 400 IU (10 mcg)/L[12] and 40–100 IU/100 kcal,[13] respectively. The amounts of vitamin D added to milk products were erratic during the early 1990s, but more recent testing of samples indicates that vitamin D fortification is more uniform.[12]

Vitamin D supplements as vitamin D_2 or D_3 are available either alone or as multivitamins in oral preparations. The use of vitamin D_2 as a food or dietary supplement is increasingly being replaced by vitamin D_3. The parent vitamin D compound is available in parenteral form only as part of multivitamin. The more potent vitamin D analog or hydroxylated vitamin D metabolites are available in the oral and parenteral forms and are most often used as part of the management of specific medical conditions. For example, vitamin D analogs with minimal or no calcemic effects are used for their antiproliferative and prodifferentiation actions.[14,15]

Absorption and Metabolism

Intestinal absorption of vitamin D and its metabolites requires normal bile and pancreatic secretions. Once absorbed from the intestine, it is incorporated into chylomicrons and transported through the lymphatic system. Both the endogenously synthesized and absorbed dietary vitamin D and its metabolites are transported in the circulation primarily by a specific vitamin D binding protein and also by albumin to the various tissues. Structural differences in the parent vitamin D_3, and vitamin D_2, and their metabolites alter both the binding to the carrier protein, vitamin D binding protein, and their metabolism. Data on bioavailability of vitamin D_3 vs D_2 is controversial with respect to the maintenance of circulating 25 OHD concentrations.[53,54]

Circulating parent vitamin D is short-lived because it is either stored in the fat or metabolized in the liver.[55] In the hepatic mitochondria, vitamin D 25 hydroxylase is regulated by vitamin D and its metabolites. The half-life of circulating 25 OHD is 10 days to 3 weeks.[56] Subsequent hydroxylation at the 1-carbon position to 1,25 $(OH)_2D$ in the kidney is tightly regulated, principally through the action of PTH in response to calcium and phosphorus levels. The half-life of 1,25 $(OH)_2D$ is ~4–6 hours.[57] It is possible that activated macrophages, some lymphoma cells, and cultured skin and bone cells also make 1,25 $(OH)_2D$ and exert paracrine or autocrine actions. Excessive unregulated production of 1,25 $(OH)_2D$ by activated macrophages and lymphoma cells is responsible for hypercalciuria and hypercalcemia.

Enterohepatic circulation of vitamin D and its metabolites is present but probably has a limited role in their conservation.[58] Further hydroxylation at the 24-carbon of 25 OHD and 1,25 $(OH)_2D$ is the initial step in the metabolic degradation of these 2 vitamin D metabolites, with the major metabolite (calcitroic acid) excreted in the urine.[59]

Deficiency

Clinical deficient states can result from lack of cutaneous production of vitamin D_3 with inadequate intake, impaired absorption or metabolism of vitamin D to its active form 1,25 $(OH)_2D$, or impaired recognition of 1,25 $(OH)_2D$ by its receptor. Drugs such as glucocorticoids inhibit vitamin D–dependent calcium absorption. Phenobarbital and phenytoin can alter the metabolism and circulating half-life of vitamin D metabolites. Chronic therapy with these medications predisposes patients to the effects of vitamin D deficiency.

Vitamin D deficiency results in inadequate mineralization, or demineralization, of the skeleton with occurrence of rickets in the developing skeleton and osteomalacia in adults. Rickets is characterized by widening at the ends of long bones, rachitic rosary, deformations include bowed legs and knock-knees, and frontal bossing of the skull. In addition, secondary hyperparathyroidism occurs as a homeostatic response to prevent a decrease in circulating ionized calcium from vitamin D deficiency. PTH mobilizes calcium from the skeleton, resulting in porotic bones, and conserves renal calcium but increases phosphorus excretion as reflected by low or absent urine calcium and increased urine phosphorus. Thus, vitamin D deficiency is characterized by a low circulating concentration of 25 OHD, normal fasting circulating calcium with low or low normal phosphorus, and elevated PTH, although hypocalcemia can occur in chronic vitamin D deficiency. Increased bone turnover with vitamin D deficiency is reflected by elevated bone alkaline phosphatase; collagenous bone proteins including hydroxyproline, pyridinoline, deoxypyridinoline, and N-teleopeptides and C-teleopeptides (amino- and carboxyl-terminal collagen crosslinks); and noncollagenous bone protein such as osteocalcin, in the circulation and/or urine. Clinical outcomes unrelated to calcium and bone, including cancer risk and immune defects, from population-based studies on vitamin D status are not well defined.[2]

Based on the traditional Gaussian distribution, the lower limit of serum or plasma 25 OHD is considered to be in the range of 10–15 ng/mL (1 nmol/L = 0.4 ng/mL). In the development of the DRIs, the Institute of Medicine committee's[2] conceptualization of integrated bone health outcomes and vitamin D exposure recommended concentrations of plasma or serum 25 OHD at <30 nmol/L, 30–49 nmol/L, 50–125 nmol/L, and >125 nmol/L (1 nmol/L = 0.4 ng/mL) as indicative of at risk for deficiency, at risk for inadequacy, sufficient, and possibly harmful, respectively. The committee additionally noted that serum 25 OHD concentrations above 75 nmol/L are not associated with increased benefit.[2,60] However, multiple publications based on circulating 25 OHD concentrations often as the sole criterion and sometimes using a higher cut point for vitamin D deficiency have led to controversy in the prevalence of vitamin D deficiency and conflicting recommendations for vitamin D intake.[2,61–63] Widespread occurrence of low circulating 25 OHD concentrations exists in children[64] and adults,[52] and a target of ≥ 50 nmol/L (20 ng/mL) is generally accepted to represent an adequate vitamin D status. The occasional clinical manifestation of rickets in nonsupplemented infants and children has prompted the recommendation to raise the daily vitamin D intake to 400 IU in infants and 600 IU in children.[2,5]

Adverse Effects

Vitamin D toxicity from prolonged exposure to natural sunlight has not been reported. Increased sunlight exposure leads to a decrease in endogenous production of vitamin D_3 by conversion of previtamin D_3 to inactive metabolites, inhibition of 25-hydroxylase enzymes results in decreased production of 25 OHD_3, and stimulation of 24-hydroxylase enzyme results in increased metabolic degradation of vitamin D metabolites. These processes contribute to the prevention of hypervitaminosis D and vitamin D toxicity.

Excessive vitamin D intake from supplements can result in hypervitaminosis D and is characterized by a considerable increase in plasma 25 OHD in the range of 400–1250 μmol/L (160–500 ng/mL).[65,66] Other vitamin D metabolites are also elevated, although the increase in 1,25 $(OH)_2D$ is generally elevated to a much lower extent.[66] Clinical toxicity is manifested through hypercalcemia, and its multiple debilitating effects include polyuria, polydipsia, depression, and metastatic calcification of soft tissues including the kidney, blood vessels, heart, and lung. These effects generally are seen with chronic supplementation in excess of 20,000 IU daily,[67] although toxicity can occur at lower doses. Toxicity from chronic intake of ergocalciferol appears to require significantly higher doses.[68] It is possible that this lower toxicity may be a result of its relatively low bioactivity compared to cholecalciferol.

High doses of vitamin D or its metabolites or analogs are often used for the treatment and prevention of deficiency states. However, the potential for vitamin D toxicity under these circumstances exist, and practitioners should consult the current recommendations of vitamin D dosing for specific conditions.

Vitamin E

Biochemistry and Physiology

Vitamin E has 8 naturally occurring forms, 4 tocopherols (α, β, γ, and δ), all in the RRR form, and 4 tocotrienols (α, β, γ, and δ). The RRR form of α-tocopherol is maintained in human plasma and occurs naturally in foods. Eight different stereoisomers in equal amounts are found in synthetic vitamin E (all rac-α-tocopherol): RRR, RSR, RRS, RSS, SRR, SSR, SRS, and SSS forms with structural differences at the side chain and at the ring/tail junction.

The various forms of vitamin E are not interconvertible in the human. The plasma concentration and biological activity of different forms of vitamin E are dependent primarily on the affinity of α-tocopherol transfer protein (α-TTP) for them. RRR α-tocopherol has the highest affinity for α-TTP. Other forms of vitamin E stereoisomers have much lower binding affinity to α-TTP.[3] They may have some biological functions,[69,70] and their intakes are reported as α-tocopherol equivalents.[3]

Vitamin E functions primarily as a nonspecific chain-breaking antioxidant acting as a peroxyl radical scavenger that prevents the propagation of free radical reaction and lipid peroxidation.[71] In addition to protecting cell membrane polyunsaturated fatty acids, thiol-rich proteins, and nucleic acids, vitamin E may play important roles in cell proliferation and differentiation, cell adhesion and arachidonic acid cascade through inhibition of protein kinase C activity, down-regulating expression of intercellular cell adhesion molecule (ICAM-1) and vascular cell adhesion molecule (VCAM-1), and up-regulating expression of cytosolic phospholipase A_2 and cyclooxygenase-1.[3] Opposing regulatory effects of vitamin E isomers such as the anti-inflammatory effect of α-tocopherol and the proinflammatory effect of γ-tocopherol might be responsible for the seemingly conflicting clinical outcomes.[72]

Current recommendations for vitamin E intake include only the 2R-stereoisomeric forms of α-tocopherol (RRR, RSR, RRS, SRR) since they are maintained in human plasma or tissue. Data on intakes from current surveys and nutrient content of foods are presented as α-tocopherol equivalents (α-TEs) and include all 8 naturally occurring forms of vitamin E, after adjustment for bioavailability using previously determined equivalencies. For example, γ-tocopherol is estimated to have only 10% of the bioactivity of α-tocopherol.

About 80% of the α-TE from foods is contributed by foods containing α-tocopherol. Thus, the intake of α-TE is usually greater than the intake of α-tocopherol alone.[3] The milligrams of α-tocopherol in a meal including fortified food or multivitamin is based on the following conversion factors:

= mg α-TE in a meal × 0.8 and/or
= IUs of the RRR-α-tocopherol compound × 0.67
= IUs of all rac-α-tocopherol compound × 0.45

If diets vary considerably from what might be considered typical in the United States or Canada, a conversion factor other than 0.8 might be more appropriate.[3] All forms of supplemental α-tocopherol are used to establish the tolerable upper intake level for vitamin E because all forms of vitamin E are absorbed.[3]

Sources

The main dietary sources of vitamin E are edible vegetable oils. All of the α-tocopherol present in natural foods is in the RRR-α-tocopherol form. Oils from wheat germ, sunflower, safflower, canola, olive, and cottonseed contain > 50% of the tocopherol as α-tocopherol. Soybean and corn oils contain ~10 times as much γ-tocopherol as α-tocopherol. Palm and rice bran oils contain high proportions of α-tocopherol, as well as various tocotrienols. Meat, poultry, fish, dairy products, nuts, grains, and fruit, especially the oils or fatty portions, are other sources of α-tocopherol.[3] Colostrum and breast milk are rich sources of vitamin E.[73] Infant formulas are fortified with a minimum of 0.7 IU/100 kcal.[13] Infant formulas fortified with the natural form of α-tocopherol have better bioavailability compared with those using the synthetic forms.[74]

Estimation of dietary intake of vitamin E is difficult because the source of oil is not always known with certainty and most nutrient databases, as well as nutrition labels, do not distinguish among the different tocopherols in food. Food preparation, such as deep frying using vegetable oil, leads to chemical structure modification and may result in functional discrepancy.[70] Vitamin E esters usually as acetate of either natural RRR or the synthetic mixture (all-rac) of α-tocopherol are used in food fortification, supplements, and pharmacological agents. Vitamin E supplements are available alone or as multivitamins in oral preparation. Vitamin E is available in parenteral form only as part of a multivitamin.[6,14,15] A water-miscible formulation of vitamin E, tocopheryl polyethylene glycol succinate 1000, is available but close monitoring of fat-soluble vitamin status is warranted since deficiency state can persist in severe fat malabsorption conditions.[9]

Absorption and Metabolism

Reports of vitamin E absorption from the intestinal lumen vary widely from 21% to 86%. In healthy humans, the esters are hydrolyzed and absorbed as efficiently as α-tocopherol. The absorption of various forms of vitamin E is independent and shows similar apparent efficiency.[3] Efficiency of absorption depends upon biliary and pancreatic secretions, micelle formation, uptake into enterocytes, and chylomicron secretion.[3] Vitamin E absorption is facilitated by dietary fat and is lowered following vitamin E supplementation.[75] During chylomicron catabolism, some vitamin E is distributed to all of the circulating lipoproteins. Chylomicron remnants, containing newly absorbed vitamin E, are taken up by the liver. The high affinity of hepatic α-TTP to α-tocopherol over all other vitamin E isomers is responsible for the preferential secretion of α-tocopherol with very low-density lipoprotein from the liver,[76] which is the main determinant of plasma vitamin E concentrations. Adipose tissue and muscle are other major storage sites for vitamin E.

Vitamin E rapidly transfers among lipoproteins and between lipoproteins and cell membranes, which may enrich cell membranes with vitamin E. The human plasma phospholipid transfer protein accelerates this process.[77] The RRR stereoisomer has roughly twice the availability of the all-rac forms. Tissue α-tocopherol concentrations largely reflect changes in plasma concentrations of α-tocopherol.[78] The 4 tocopherols are ultimately degraded by ω-oxidation and subsequent β-oxidations, followed by the elimination of the metabolites in the bile and in the urine. Excess α-tocopherol as well as forms of vitamin E not preferentially used is excreted unchanged in the stool and in bile. The decreased intestinal absorption and increased excretion of urinary vitamin E metabolites may limit the rise in plasma α-tocopherol (~3-fold) and vitamin E supplements providing > 150–200 mg daily may not promote higher tissue concentrations.[79]

When vitamin E intercepts a radical, α-tocopherol is oxidized to the tocopheryl radical, a 1-electron oxidation product. A tocopherol radical can be reduced (ie, to regenerate α-tocopherol) by other antioxidants including vitamin C, glutathione, and ubiquinols. The tocopherol radical can undergo further metabolism and is excreted in urine. It also may act as a pro-oxidant in the absence of a water-soluble antioxidant and oxidize other lipids in vitro. Whether this occurs in vivo is inconclusive. Vitamin E compounds other than RRR-α-tocopherol are preferentially metabolized and excreted.[3]

Deficiency

Vitamin E requirements increase with increased intake of polyunsaturated fatty acids, high-level physical activity, and cigarette smoking. However, the extent of increased requirement and the compensatory effects of other antioxidants are not defined. Intake of plant phenolic compounds and flavonoids may add to the total antioxidant pool. Cellular redox cycling is coupled to the energy status of the organism. Thus dietary deficiencies of niacin or riboflavin might result in insufficient reducing equivalents for recycling oxidized products.[3]

Plasma α-tocopherol concentrations < 12 μmol/L (0.5 mg/dL; 1 μmol/L = 0.042 mg/dL) are associated with increased infection, anemia, stunting of growth, and poor pregnancy outcome for mother and infant,[80] although overt clinical deficiency from low dietary intake of vitamin E in normal individuals without undue oxidative stresses has not been reported.[3] Clinical vitamin E deficiency occurs with fat malabsorption syndromes or with genetic defect in α-TTP or abetalipoproteinemia in which the hepatic reserve and circulating vitamin E are decreased.

Vitamin E deficiency causes axonal degeneration of the large myelinated axons and results in posterior column and spinocerebellar symptoms. Peripheral neuropathy is initially characterized by areflexia, with progression to ataxic gait, and by decreased vibration and position sensations. Ophthalmoplegia, skeletal myopathy, and pigmented retinopathy also may occur.[3,4,8] Neurological symptoms can progress if untreated and may be reversed if treated early. Increased erythrocyte fragility in vitro and hemolytic anemia with vitamin E deficiency are reversible with adequate replacement of vitamin E.

Vitamin E adequacy cannot be assessed with plasma α-tocopherol since states of increased plasma lipid concentrations are associated with increased plasma carriers for α-tocopherol, leading to higher circulating α-tocopherol concentrations. Abnormal lipoprotein metabolism with elevated plasma lipids does not necessarily increase α-tocopherol delivery to the tissues; however, a plasma α-tocopherol level at <12 μmol/L (0.5 mg/dL) is consistent with vitamin E inadequacy.[80] In subjects with elevated serum lipids (eg, in cholestasis), a ratio of serum α-tocopherol to serum total lipids of <0.6 mg/g indicates vitamin E deficiency regardless of serum α-tocopherol concentrations. In subjects with normal serum lipid concentrations (328–573 mg/dL), corrections are not necessary to assess whether α-tocopherol concentrations are within the normal range.[9,81] Hydrogen peroxide–induced hemolysis and lipid peroxidation biomarkers in plasma, urine, or breath are elevated during vitamin E depletion and are normalized upon vitamin E repletion. However, these markers are nonspecific and may vary with intake of other antioxidants.

Routine supplementation of vitamin E is recommended for specific disorders such as hepatobiliary disorder. However, no conclusive data support a high intake of vitamin E in the management of chronic illnesses involving the cardiovascular system, diabetes mellitus, cancer, central nervous system, cataracts, or immune function.[3]

Adverse Effects

All forms of vitamin E are absorbed and could contribute to vitamin E toxicity, although not all forms are maintained in plasma. Normal adults appear to tolerate oral tocopherol intake of 100–800 mg/d,[82] but adverse effects from the consumption of vitamin E as a supplement, food fortifier, or pharmacological agent are possible. Reports on hemorrhagic complications from high vitamin E intake in humans are contradictory. Individuals deficient in vitamin K or those on anticoagulant therapy may possibly be at an increased risk for coagulation defects.[3] Preterm infants with birth weights < 1.5 kg with elevated plasma vitamin E at a mean of 5.1 mg/dL have an increased incidence of sepsis and necrotizing enterocolitis.[83] Plasma α-tocopherol concentrations are not informative for assessing adverse effects because they plateau at ~3–4 times the values for nonsupplemented individuals.[3]

Vitamin K

Biochemistry and Physiology

Vitamin K belongs to the family of 2-methyl-1,4-naphthoquinones. Two naturally occurring compounds have vitamin K activity: phylloquinone (vitamin K_1) from plants and long-chain menaquinones (vitamin K_2) synthesized from intestinal bacteria. Menadione (vitamin K_3) is chemically synthesized and has better water solubility than the 2 natural forms. Structural differences in the isoprenoid side chain govern many facets of the metabolism of K vitamins, including the way they are transported, taken up by target tissues, and subsequently excreted.[84]

Vitamin K in its reduced form is a cofactor for γ-glutamyl carboxylase enzymes responsible for the posttranslational carboxylation of the glutamic acid (Glu) residues to γ-carboxyglutamyl (Gla) residues in a subclass of proteins known as vitamin K–dependent proteins (also known as γ-carboxylated proteins or Gla-proteins). The major Gla-proteins include certain proteins of the blood coagulation system: prothrombin (coagulation factor II); factors VII, IX, and X; protein C, protein S, and protein Z; and proteins expressed in mineralized tissues, osteocalcin and matrix Gla-protein.[85,86] Other putative non-cofactor functions of vitamin K include suppressing inflammation, preventing brain oxidative damage, and playing a role in sphingolipid synthesis.[1,86]

Sources

Vitamin K content in most foods is very low (< 10 mcg/100 g), and the majority is obtained from a few leafy green vegetables and 4 vegetable oils (soybean, cottonseed, canola, and olive) that contain high amounts. Hydrogenation of plant oils to form solid shortenings results in some conversion of phylloquinone to 2′,3′-dihydrophylloquinone, but it is uncertain whether these forms are metabolically and functionally identical. These forms of vitamin K are most prevalent in margarines, infant formulas, and prepared foods. Long-chain menaquinones have about 60% of the activity of phylloquinone. Menaquinones are produced in substantial amounts endogenously but are probably insufficient to meet the daily requirement for vitamin K.[87] Vitamin K is present in low concentrations in breast milk (< 5 mcg/L).[85] Commercial infant formulas are fortified with vitamin K (50–100 mcg/L) based on a minimum of 4 mcg/100 kcal.[13] Intravenous fat emulsions are another source of vitamin K, although the content varies with composition of the fat emulsion and manufacturing process.[88] Vitamin K supplements are available alone or as part of many, but not all, multivitamin preparations in oral and parenteral forms.[6,14,15]

Absorption and Metabolism

Phylloquinone absorption in the jejunum depends on the presence of bile and pancreatic secretions and is enhanced by dietary fat. Free phylloquinone is almost completely absorbed, but absorption of vitamin K from food sources is much lower and is generally < 20%.[1] Absorbed phylloquinone is secreted into lymph and enters the circulation. In the postprandial state, phylloquinone is transported mainly by triglyceride-rich lipoproteins (TRLs) and long-chain menaquinones mainly by low-density lipoproteins. Liver uptake and turnover of phylloquinone is rapid. TRL-borne phylloquinone uptake by some extrahepatic tissues (eg, osteoblasts) is an apoE-mediated process with the LRP1 receptor playing a predominant role. With limited vitamin K storage capacity, the body recycles vitamin K in the vitamin K oxidation-reduction cycle in order to reuse it multiple times.[84]

Both phylloquinone and menaquinones activate the steroid and xenobiotic receptor that initiates their catabolism. Vitamin K is excreted primarily in bile and also in urine after oxidative degradation of the phytyl side chain followed by glucuronide conjugation. The liver has the highest concentration of phylloquinone, and significant amounts are also present in the heart and other tissues. Hepatic reserve is rapidly depleted from restricted dietary intake.

Deficiency

Individuals at risk for vitamin K deficiency include those with severe fat malabsorption conditions (eg, hepatobiliary disorders) or those who have had bariatric surgery, especially with severe diet restriction. Prolonged use of broad-spectrum antibiotics may decrease vitamin K synthesis by intestinal bacteria. Long-term differences in dietary vitamin K intake modulate the response to coumarin anticoagulants, which act by blocking the vitamin K recycling. Elevated intake of vitamin E antagonizes vitamin K action probably through its effect on vitamin K absorption and metabolism.[1,89]

The classic sign of vitamin K deficiency is an increase in prothrombin time, and in severe cases, a hemorrhagic event.

Both abnormalities are responsive to vitamin K. However, other than the exclusively breastfed infant without vitamin K prophylaxis therapy, it is almost impossible to achieve this level of deficiency by simple restriction of vitamin K intake in any nutritionally adequate, self-selected diet in healthy individuals. The role of vitamin K in matrix-Gla formation would support its physiological activity in the metabolism of multiple organ systems, but to date its role in chronic diseases such as osteoporosis and atherosclerosis remains to be defined.

Prothrombin time; vitamin K–dependent factors II, VII, IX, and X; plasma phylloquinone and menaquinone concentrations; and proteins induced in vitamin K deficiency such as under-γ-carboxylated prothrombin (PIV-KA-II) and osteocalcin (ucOC) respond to alterations in dietary vitamin K and are helpful to assess relative changes in vitamin K status. However, prothrombin time is the only indicator of vitamin K status associated with adverse clinical effects. Vitamin K prophylaxis is recommended in newborn infants[5,90] and in conditions that predispose the patient to fat-soluble vitamin deficiency states.

Adverse Effects

Vitamin K toxicity is rare. Parenteral administration of a large amount of water-soluble synthetic vitamin K (vitamin K_3) has been associated with hemolytic anemia, hyperbilirubinemia, kernicterus[5] and with liver damage and anaphylactic reaction.[1] No adverse effects associated with other vitamin K supplements or from food have been reported in healthy individuals, although high dietary intake or supplemental vitamin K can inhibit the anticoagulation effect of vitamin K antagonists.

Test Your Knowledge Questions

1. Human milk is a good source of which fat-soluble vitamins?
   A. A and E
   B. D and A
   C. E and D
   D. K and A
2. Which of the following statements about vitamin A is correct:
   A. Vitamin A is present in abundance in green vegetables.
   B. Absorption decreases with presence of dietary fat.
   C. Biological activity is mediated directly as carotenoids.
   D. Retinoids have higher bioactivity potency than carotenoids.
3. Which of the following statements on endogenous synthesis of vitamin D is correct:
   A. Dark-skinned individuals cannot produce vitamin D.
   B. Chronic exposure to sunlight results in vitamin D toxicity.
   C. A brief period of sunlight exposure can generate a large amount of vitamin D.
   D. Sunscreen, clothing, and winter do not decrease the endogenous synthesis of vitamin D.
4. Which of the following statements concerning vitamin E is correct?
   A. Natural RRR-α-tocopherol has similar biopotency to all other naturally occurring vitamin E stereoisomers.
   B. Vegetable oils are poor sources of vitamin E.
   C. Synthetic (all-rac-α-tocopherol) vitamin E has greater biopotency than the natural RRR-α-tocopherol.
   D. Soybean and corn oils have much higher content of γ-tocopherol vs α-tocopherol.
5. Which of the following does not interfere with vitamin K action?
   A. Cholestyramine
   B. Chloroquine
   C. Orilstat
   D. Coumarin-type anticoagulants

References

1. Food and Nutrition Board, Institute of Medicine. *Dietary Reference Intakes for Vitamin A, Vitamin K, Arsenic, Boron, Chromium, Copper, Iodine, Iron, Manganese, Molybdenum, Nickel, Silicon, Vanadium, and Zinc.* Washington, DC: National Academy Press; 2001.
2. Institute of Medicine (IOM). 2011. *Dietary Reference Intakes for Calcium and Vitamin D.* Washington, DC: The National Academies Press.
3. Food and Nutrition Board, Institute of Medicine. *Dietary Reference Intakes for Vitamin C, Vitamin E, Selenium, and Carotenoids.* Washington, DC: National Academy Press; 2000.
4. Picciano MF, Dwyer JT, Radimer KL, et al. Dietary supplement use among infants, children and adolescents in the United States, 1999–2002. *Arch Pediatr Adol Med.* 2007;161:978–985.
5. American Academy of Pediatrics, Committee on Nutrition, Kleinman RE, Greer FR, eds. *Pediatric Nutrition Handbook.* 7th ed. Elk Grove Village, IL: American Academy of Pediatrics; 2014.
6. National Institutes of Health. Dietary supplement label database. http://www.dsld.nlm.nih.gov/dsld/. Accessed August 1, 2014.

7. Linus Pauling Institute, Oregon State University. Micronutrient Information Center. http://lpi.oregonstate.edu/infocenter/vitamins.html. Accessed August 1, 2014.

8. Papas KA, Sontag MK, Pardee C, et al. A pilot study on the safety and efficacy of a novel antioxidant rich formulation in patients with cystic fibrosis. *J Cyst Fibros.* 2008;7:60–67.

9. Shneider BL, Magee JC, Bezerra JA, et al; Childhood Liver Disease Research Education Network (ChiLDREN). Efficacy of fat-soluble vitamin supplementation in infants with biliary atresia. *Pediatrics.* 2012;130:e607–614.

10. Mahoney CP, Margolis MT, Knauss TA, Labbe RF. Chronic vitamin A intoxication in infants fed chicken liver. *Pediatrics.* 1980;65:893–897.

11. World Health Organization. *Indicators for Assessing Vitamin A Deficiency and Their Application in Monitoring and Evaluating Intervention Programmes.* Brown E, Akre J, eds. Geneva: World Health Organization; 1998. http://www.who.int/nutrition/publications/micronutrients/vitamin_a_deficiency/WHO_NUT_96.10/en/. Accessed August 25, 2014.

12. Murphy SC, Whited LJ, Rosenberry LC, Hammond BH, Bandler DK, Boor KJ. Fluid milk vitamin fortification compliance in New York state. *J Dairy Sci.* 2001;84:2813–2820.

13. U.S. Food and Drug Administration. Infant formula nutrient specifications. 21 CFR 107.100. http://www.accessdata.fda.gov/scripts/cdrh/cfdocs/cfcfr/CFRSearch.cfm?fr=107.100&SearchTerm=infant%20formula. Revised April 1, 2014. Accessed August 25, 2014.

14. *Drug Facts and Comparisons.* St. Louis, MO: Wolters Kluwer Health; 2009.

15. Medline Plus, National Institutes of Health. Drugs, supplements, and herbal information. http://www.nlm.nih.gov/medlineplus/druginformation.html. Updated January 3, 2014. Accessed August 25, 2014.

16. Koo WWK, Krug-Wispe S, Succop P, Tsang RC, Neylan M. Effect of different vitamin A intakes in very low birth weight infants. *Am J Clin Nutr.* 1995;62:1216–1220.

17. Darlow BA, Graham PJ. Vitamin A supplementation to prevent mortality and short and long-term morbidity in very low birthweight infants. *Cochrane Database Syst Rev.* 2011;(10):CD000501.

18. Harrison EH. Mechanisms of digestion and absorption of dietary vitamin A. *Annu Rev Nutr.* 2005;25:87–103.

19. Borel P, Drai J, Faure H, et al. Recent knowledge about intestinal absorption and cleavage of carotenoids [in French]. *Ann Biol Clin (Paris).* 2005;63:165–177.

20. Tang G, Qin J, Dolnikowski GG, Russell RM. Vitamin A equivalence of beta-carotene in a woman as determined by a stable isotope reference method. *Eur J Nutr.* 2000;39:7–11.

21. Olsen JA. Adverse effects of large doses of vitamin A and retinoids. *Semin Oncol.* 1983;10:290–293.

22. World Health Organization. Micronutrient deficiencies. Vitamin A deficiency. http://www.who.int/nutrition/topics/vad/en/. Accessed August 25, 2014.

23. Singh K. Modified classification of xerophthalmia. *Indian J Ophthalmol.* 1991;39:105–107.

24. Wasantwisut E. Application of isotope dilution technique in vitamin A nutrition. *Food Nutr Bull.* 2002; 23(3 suppl):103–106.

25. World Health Organization, United Nations Children's Fund, VACG Task Force. *Vitamin A Supplements: A Guide to Their Use in the Treatment and Prevention of Vitamin A Deficiency and Xerophthalmia.* 2nd ed. Geneva: World Health Organization; 1997. http://apps.who.int/iris/handle/10665/41947. Accessed August 25, 2014.

26. Haider BA, Bhutta ZA. Neonatal vitamin A supplementation for the prevention of mortality and morbidity in term neonates in developing countries. *Cochrane Database Syst Rev.* 2011;(10):CD006980. doi:10.1002/14651858.CD006980.pub2.

27. Gogia S, Sachdev HS. Vitamin A supplementation for the prevention of morbidity and mortality in infants six months of age or less. *Cochrane Database Syst Rev.* 2011;(10):CD007480. doi:10.1002/14651858.CD007480.pub2.

28. Imdad A, Yakoob MY, Sudfeld C, Haider BA, Black RE, Bhutta ZA. Impact of vitamin A supplementation on infant and childhood mortality. *BMC Public Health.* 2011;11(suppl 3):S20. doi:10.1186/1471-2458-11-S3-S20.

29. Agha-Mohammadi S, Hurwitz DJ. Potential impacts of nutritional deficiency of postbariatric patients on body contouring surgery. *Plast Reconstr Surg.* 2008;122(6):1901–1914.

30. Penniston KL, Tanumihardjo SA. The acute and chronic toxic effects of vitamin A. *Am J Clin Nutr.* 2006;83:191–201.

31. Bendich A, Langseth L. Safety of vitamin A. *Am J Clin Nutr.* 1989;49:358–371.

32. Persson B, Tunell R, Ekengren K. Chronic vitamin A intoxication during the first half year of life; description of 5 cases. *Acta Paediatr Scand.* 1965;54:49–60.

33. Macapinlac MP, Olson JA. A lethal hypervitaminosis A syndrome in young monkeys (*Macacus fascicularis*) following a single intramuscular dose of a water-miscible preparation containing vitamins A, D_2 and E. *Int J Vitam Nutr Res.* 1981;51:331–341.

34. Leo MA, Lieber CS. Alcohol, vitamin A, and beta-carotene: adverse interactions, including hepatotoxicity and carcinogenicity. *Clin Nutr.* 1999;69:1071–1085.

35. Krasinski SD, Russell RM, Otradovec CL, et al. Relationship of vitamin A and vitamin E intake to fasting plasma retinol, retinol-binding protein, retinyl esters, carotene, alpha-tocopherol, and cholesterol among elderly people and young adults: increased plasma retinyl esters among vitamin A-supplement users. *Am J Clin Nutr.* 1989;49:112–120.

36. World Health Organization, The Micronutrient Initiative. *Safe Vitamin A Dosage During Pregnancy and Lactation.* Geneva: World Health Organization; 1998. http://apps.who.int/iris/handle/10665/63838. Accessed August 25, 2014.

37. Lascari AD. Carotenemia. A review. *Clin Pediatr.* 1981;20:25–29.

38. Bendich A. The safety of beta-carotene. *Nutr Cancer.* 1988;11:207–214.

39. Black HS. Reassessment of a free radical theory of cancer with emphasis on ultraviolet carcinogenesis. *Integr Cancer Ther.* 2004;3:279–293.

40. Haddad JG Jr, Hahn TJ. Natural and synthetic sources of circulating 25-hydroxyvitamin D in man. *Nature.* 1973;244:515–517.

41. Jurutka PW, Bartik L, Whitfield GK, et al. Vitamin D receptor: key roles in bone mineral pathophysiology, molecular mechanism of action, and novel nutritional ligands. *J Bone Miner Res.* 2007;22(suppl 2):v2–10.

42. Haussler MR, Haussler CA, Bartik L, et al. Vitamin D receptor: molecular signaling and actions of nutritional ligands in disease prevention. *Nutr Rev.* 2008;66(10 suppl 2):S98–S112.

43. Lisse TS, Adams JS, Hewison M. Vitamin D and microRNAs in bone. *Crit Rev Eukaryot Gene Expr.* 2013;23(3):195–214.

44. Bouillon R, Lieben L, Mathieu C, Verstuyf A, Carmeliet G. Vitamin D action: lessons from VDR and Cyp27b1 null mice. *Pediatr Endocrinol Rev.* 2013;10(suppl 2):354–366.

45. Gordon CM, Williams AL, Feldman HA, et al. Treatment of hypovitaminosis D in infants and toddlers. *J Clin Endocrinol Metab.* 2008;93:2716–2721.

46. Bischoff-Ferrari HA, Willett WC, Wong JB, et al. Prevention of nonvertebral fractures with oral vitamin D and dose dependency: a meta-analysis of randomized controlled trials. *Arch Intern Med.* 2009;169:551–561.

47. Hollis BW. Circulating 25-hydroxyvitamin D levels indicative of vitamin D sufficiency: implications for establishing a new effective dietary intake recommendation for vitamin D. *J Nutr.* 2005;135:317–322.

48. Lehmann B. The vitamin D3 pathway in human skin and its role for regulation of biological processes. *Photochem Photobiol.* 2005;81:1246–1251.

49. Engelsen O, Brustad M, Aksnes L, Lund E. Daily duration of vitamin D synthesis in human skin with relation to latitude, total ozone, altitude, ground cover, aerosols and cloud thickness. *Photochem Photobiol.* 2005;81:1287–1290.

50. Balk SJ. Ultraviolet radiation: a hazard to children and adolescents. *Pediatrics.* 2011;127(3):e791–e817.

51. Calvo MS, Whiting SJ, Barton CN. Vitamin D fortification in the United States and Canada: current status and data needs. *Am J Clin Nutr.* 2004;80:1710S–1716S.

52. Yetley EA. Assessing the vitamin D status of the US population. *Am J Clin Nutr.* 2008;88:558S–564S.

53. Holick MF, Biancuzzo RM, Chen TC, et al. Vitamin D2 is as effective as vitamin D3 in maintaining circulating concentrations of 25-hydroxyvitamin D. *J Clin Endocrinol Metab.* 2008;93:677–681.

54. Armas LA, Hollis BW, Heaney RP. Vitamin D_2 is much less effective than vitamin D_3 in humans. *J Clin Endocrinol Metab.* 2004;89:5387–5391.

55. Mawer EB, Backhouse J, Holman CA, Lumb GA, Stanbury SW. The distribution and storage of vitamin D and its metabolites in human tissues. *Clin Sci.* 1972;43:413–431.

56. Mawer EB, Schaefer K, Lumb GA, Stanbury SW. The metabolism of isotopically labeled vitamin D_3 in man: the influence of the state of vitamin D nutrition. *Clin Sci.* 1971;40:39–53.

57. Kumar R. The metabolism and mechanism of action of 1,25-dihydroxyvitamin D_3. *Kidney Int.* 1986;30:793–803.

58. Clements MR, Chalmers TM, Fraser DR. Enterohepatic circulation of vitamin D: a reappraisal of the hypothesis. *Lancet.* 1984;1:1376–1379.

59. DeLuca HF. Evolution of our understanding of vitamin D. *Nutr Rev.* 2008;66(10 suppl 2):S73–S87.

60. Koo W, Walyat N. Vitamin D and skeletal growth and development. *Curr Osteoporos Rep.* 2013;11(3):188–193.

61. Holick MF, Binkley NC, Bischoff-Ferrari HA, et al. Evaluation, treatment, and prevention of vitamin D deficiency: an Endocrine Society clinical practice guideline. *J Clin Endocrinol Metab.* 2011;96:1911–1930.

62. Rosen CJ, Abrams SA, Aloia JF, et al. IOM committee members respond to endocrine society vitamin D guideline. *J Clin Endocrinol Metab.* 2011;97:1146–1152.

63. Braegger C, Campoy C, Colomb V, et al. Vitamin D in the healthy European pediatric population. *J Pediatr Gastroenterol Nutr.* 2013;56:692–701.

64. Rovner AJ, O'Brien KO. Hypovitaminosis D among healthy children in the United States: a review of the current evidence. *Arch Pediatr Adolesc Med.* 2008;162:513–519.

65. Jacobus CH, Holick MF, Shao Q, et al. Hypervitaminosis D associated with drinking milk. *N Engl J Med.* 1992;326:1173–1177.

66. Jones G. Pharmacokinetics of vitamin D toxicity. *Am J Clin Nutr.* 2008;88:582S–586S.

67. Heaney RP. Vitamin D: criteria for safety and efficacy. *Nutr Rev.* 2008;66(10 suppl 2):S178–S181.

68. Stephenson DW, Peiris AN. The lack of vitamin D toxicity with megadose of daily ergocalciferol (D2) therapy: a case report and literature review. *South Med J.* 2009;102:765–768.

69. Sen CK, Khanna S, Roy S. Tocotrienols: vitamin E beyond tocopherols. *Life Sci.* 2006;78:2088–2098.

70. Cornwell DG, Ma J. Studies in vitamin E: biochemistry and molecular biology of tocopherol quinones. *Vitam Horm.* 2007;76:99–134.

71. Traber MG, Atkinson J. Vitamin E, antioxidant and nothing more. *Free Radic Biol Med.* 2007;43:4–15.

72. Cook-Mills JM, Abdala-Valencia H, Hartert T. Two faces of vitamin E in the lung. *Am J Respir Crit Care Med.* 2013;188(3):279–284. doi:10.1164/rccm.201303-0503ED.

73. Debier C. Vitamin E during pre- and postnatal periods. *Vitam Horm.* 2007;76:357–373.

74. Stone WL, LeClair I, Ponder T, Baggs G, Barrett Reis B. Infants discriminate between natural and synthetic vitamin E. *Am J Clin Nutr.* 2003;77:899–906.

75. Lodge JK, Hall WL, Jeanes YM, Proteggente AR. Physiological factors influencing vitamin E biokinetics. *Ann N Y Acad Sci.* 2004;1031:60–73.

76. Traber MG, Burton GW, Hamilton RL. Vitamin E trafficking. *Ann N Y Acad Sci.* 2004;1031:1–12.

77. Kostner GM, Oettl K, Jauhiainen M, Ehnholm C, Esterbauer H, Dieplinger H. Human plasma phospholipid transfer protein accelerates exchange/transfer of alpha-tocopherol between lipoproteins and cells. *Biochem J.* 1995;305:659–667.

78. Burton GW, Traber MG, Acuff RV, et al. Human plasma and tissue alpha-tocopherol concentrations in response to sup-

plementation with deuterated natural and synthetic vitamin E. *Am J Clin Nutr.* 1998; 67:669–684.

79. Schultz M, Leist M, Petrizika M, Gassmann B, Brigelius-Flohe R. A novel urinary metabolite of α-tocopherol, 2,5,7,8-tetramethyl-2(2′ carboxyethyl)-6-hydroxychroman, as an indicator of adequate vitamin E supply? *Am J Clin Nutr.* 1995;62:1527S–1534S.

80. Traber MG. Vitamin E inadequacy in humans: causes and consequences. *Adv Nutr.* 2014; 5:503–514. doi:10.3945/an.114.006254.

81. Sokol RJ, Heubi JE, Iannaccone ST, Bove KE, Balistreri WF. Vitamin E deficiency with normal serum vitamin E concentrations in children with chronic cholestasis. *N Engl J Med.* 1984;310:1209–1212.

82. Farrell PM, Bieri JG. Megavitamin E supplementation in man. *Am J Clin Nutr.* 1975;28:1381–1386.

83. Johnson L, Bowen FW Jr, Abbasi S, et al. Relationship of prolonged pharmacologic serum levels of vitamin E to incidence of sepsis and necrotizing enterocolitis in infants with birth weight 1,500 grams or less. *Pediatrics.* 1985;75:619–638.

84. Shearer MJ, Newman P. Metabolism and cell biology of vitamin K. *Thromb Haemost.* 2008;100(4):530–547.

85. Greer FR. Vitamin K the basics—what's new? *Early Hum Dev.* 2010;86(suppl 1):S43–S47.

86. Benzakour O. Vitamin K dependent proteins: functions in blood coagulation and beyond. *Thromb Haemost.* 2008;100:527–529.

87. Booth SL, Suttie JW. Dietary intake and adequacy of vitamin K. *J Nutr.* 1998;128:785–788.

88. Chambrier C, Bannier E, Lauverjat M, Drai J, Bryssine S, Boulétreau P. Replacement of long-chain triglyceride with medium-chain triglyceride/long-chain triglyceride lipid emulsion in patients receiving long-term parenteral nutrition: effects on essential fatty acid status and plasma vitamin K1 levels. *JPEN J Parenter Enteral Nutr.* 2004;28:7–12.

89. Traber MG. Vitamin E and K interactions—a 50-year-old problem. *Nutr Rev.* 2008;66:624–629.

90. American Academy of Pediatrics Policy Statement. Committee on Fetus and Newborn. Controversies concerning vitamin K and the newborn. *Pediatrics.* 2003;112:191–192. Reaffirmed May 2006.

Test Your Knowledge Answers

1. The correct answer is **A**. Rationale: In healthy exclusively breastfed babies, human milk provides adequate vitamins A and E during the first 6 months. Daily vitamin D supplementation is recommended for all breastfeeding babies. Human milk vitamin K content is low, and all babies are recommended to receive a single intramuscular dose immediately after birth to prevent hemorrhagic disease of the newborn although no supplementation is needed thereafter. All infant formulas in the United States are fortified with fat-soluble vitamins, and no supplements are needed except for the first dose of vitamin K.

2. The correct answer is **D**. Rationale: Vitamin A is present in the diet as retinyl esters derived almost exclusively from animal sources. Intestinal absorption of vitamin A and provitamin A is enhanced in the presence of dietary fat. Provitamin A carotenoids must be converted to retinoids to exert vitamin A function. The bioconversion of dietary provitamin carotenoids to retinol activity equivalent (RAE) is estimated to be 12:1 (mcg:mcg) based on the relative absorption efficiency of β-carotene from food and the functional carotene to retinol equivalency ratio. One RAE for dietary provitamin A carotenoids other than β-carotene is lower and set at 24 mcg.

3. The correct answer is **C**. Rationale: Endogenous synthesis of vitamin D_3 requires exposure to sunlight or irradiation in the ultraviolet B range. It is extremely effective and 10–15 minutes of whole-body exposure to peak summer sun will generate and release up to 20,000 IU vitamin D_3 into the circulation. However, prolonged sunlight exposure increases the conversion of previtamin D_3 to inactive metabolites and prevents the risk of vitamin D toxicity. Cutaneous production of vitamin D_3 is substantially diminished by decreased exposure to sunlight from seasonal changes, time of day, clouds, aerosols, thick ozone, higher latitude, aging, clothing, sunscreen use, and melanin pigmentation. In dark-skinned individuals, endogenous synthesis of vitamin D is possible, although the rate of production is lower than less pigmented individuals.

4. The correct answer is **D**. Rationale: The main dietary sources of vitamin E are edible vegetable oils. All of the α-tocopherol present in natural foods is in the RRR-α-tocopherol form. Oils from wheat germ, sunflower, safflower, canola, olive, and cottonseed contain > 50% of the tocopherol as α-tocopherol. Soybean and corn oils contain ~10 times as much γ-tocopherol as α-tocopherol. Palm and rice bran oils contain high proportions of α-tocopherol, as well as various tocotrienols. Meat, poultry, fish, dairy products, nuts, grains, and fruit, especially the oils or fatty portions, are other sources of α-tocopherol.

5. The correct answer is **B**. Rationale: Chronic antibiotic use may decrease bacteria synthesis of vitamin K, although the antimalarial chloroquine has not been reported to interfere with vitamin K action. Cholestyramine, orilstat, and coumarin-type anticoagulants can interfere with absorption or action of vitamin K.

9

Fluids and Electrolytes

Gerald L. Schmidt, PharmD, BCNSP

CONTENTS

Learning Objectives

1. Describe factors that influence movement of fluid and electrolytes between the intracellular and extracellular fluid compartments.
2. Recommend appropriate treatments for fluid and electrolyte abnormalities.
3. Describe the differences in the treatment of acute and chronic electrolyte abnormalities.

Background

Water is the most abundant and probably the most important substance in the body. It is essential for digestion, absorption, transport, and utilization of nutrients as well as the excretion of waste products. The regulation of fluids and electrolyte balance is maintained by an elaborate system of interrelated regulatory systems to ensure proper cell function. Unfortunately, fluid and electrolyte imbalances are common, and severe imbalances can have a detrimental effect on major organ systems. This chapter will focus on fluid and electrolyte homeostasis as well as commonly encountered fluid and electrolyte abnormalities and the treatment of these disorders.

Fluid Distribution

Water, being the most abundant component of the body, makes up a large portion of total body weight. Adipose tissue is the least hydrated body tissue; therefore, obese patients will have a lower percentage of total body water (TBW) content.[1-3] TBW volume varies depending on age, weight, sex, and body fat percentage. Water accounts for about 80% of total body weight in premature infants, and this proportion decreases to 55%–60% of total body weight by 18 years of age.[4,5] TBW is divided into separate compartments: intracellular fluid (ICF; 32%–52% of total body weight), transcellular fluid (1.5%–2.5% of total body weight), and extracellular fluid (ECF; 16%–26% of total body weight). The ECF is further divided into the interstitial space (12%–19% of total body weight) and the intravascular space (4%–6% of total body weight).[6] Relative percentages in each compartment at various ages are presented in Table 9-1.

The primary factor that determines water distribution between the ICF and ECF compartments is osmotic pressure. Sodium is the predominant extracellular osmotic agent, and potassium is the predominant intracellular osmotic agent. The sodium-potassium-adenosine triphosphatase (Na^+-K^+-ATPase) pump maintains the sodium and potassium gradient in normal conditions by pumping 3 sodium ions extracellularly for every 2 potassium ions it pumps intracellularly. A disruption in the function of the Na^+-K^+-ATPase pump can have a significant effect on fluid distribution between the compartments.[3,6–8]

Fluid composition also plays an important role in fluid dynamics between the ICF and ECF. For example, when 100 mL of 5% dextrose (a solute-free solution) is administered intravenously to a patient, the dextrose is metabolized and the resultant water is proportionally distributed to all compartments. Approximately 65% of the fluid volume (65 mL) would go into the ICF, 32% (32 mL) would remain in the ECF, and 3% (3 mL) would go into the transcellular fluid compartment. Of the 32 mL remaining in the ECF, 25% (8 mL) would stay in the intravascular space and 75% (24 mL) would be in the interstitial space (Figure 9-1). If 100 mL of 0.9% sodium chloride was given, all 100 mL would stay in the ECF: 25% (25 mL) in the intravascular space and 75% (75 mL) in the interstitial space (Figure 9-2.)[9,10] The administration of a hypertonic solution (eg, 3% sodium chloride) has a different effect on fluid distribution. The increased tonicity of the 3% sodium chloride would create an osmotic gradient, pulling fluid into the ECF from the ICF. Thus, the ECF volume would increase as would the ECF and ICF osmolality. However, the ICF volume would decrease due to the fluid shift caused by the hypertonic fluid. The volume of the ECF increase would be determined by the volume of the hypertonic solution given.[9]

The balance between the ECF and ICF is important in fluid homeostasis, but these are not the only compartments that must be maintained. The ECF components, the intravascular space, and the interstitial space are maintained by Starling forces, which consist of plasma oncotic pressure and hydrostatic pressure. When fluid moves from the plasma to the interstitial space, edema occurs.[11] As vascular permeability increases, albumin leaks from the plasma to the interstitial space. This capillary leak reduces plasma oncotic pressure, which in turn causes fluid to move from the plasma to the interstitial space. If this happens quickly, and the plasma volume is not replaced, intravascular volume depletion can occur resulting in hypotension and poor perfusion.

Fluid Regulation

Ingestion of fluids is the primary source of fluid, although some water is generated from the oxidation of carbohydrates, proteins, and fat.[3,12] The majority of fluid losses are through urinary output, but fluid losses also occur via the skin and the respiratory and gastrointestinal (GI) tracts.[8] Sodium and fluid balance are closely linked. Disturbances of water balance lead to changes in plasma osmolarity and sodium balance, and changes in sodium balance result in changes in plasma osmolarity and fluid volume. To maintain

Table 9-1. Distribution of Total Body Water as a Percentage of Total Body Weight

AGE/LIFE STAGE	TOTAL BODY WATER	INTRACELLULAR	EXTRACELLULAR		TRANSCELLULAR
Premature infant	80%	52%	26%	Intravascular 6% Interstitial 19%	2.5%
3-mo-old infant	70%	46%	22%	Intravascular 5.5% Interstitial 16.5%	2%
6-mo-old infant	60%	39%	19%	Intravascular 5% Interstitial 14%	1.8%
10- to 18-y-old child/adolescent	Male 59% Female 57%	38% 36%	18%	Intravascular 4.5% Interstitial 13.5%	1.7%
Elderly patient	50%	32%	16%	Intravascular 4% Interstitial 12%	1.5%

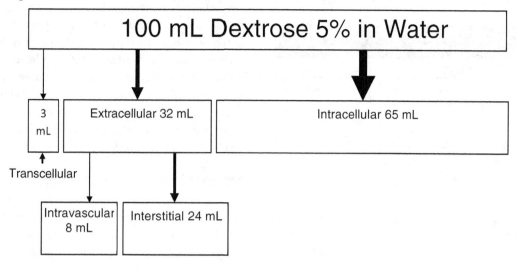

Figure 9-1. Fluid Distribution of 100 mL Dextrose 5% in Water

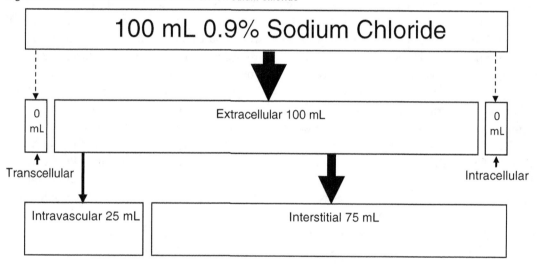

Figure 9-2. Fluid Distribution of 100 mL of 0.9% Sodium Chloride

a relatively normal serum osmolarity (290 ± 5 mOsm/L), the sodium to TBW ratio must be maintained in a relatively narrow range. When a fluid imbalance occurs, physiological feedback mechanisms are activated to either increase or decrease renal water excretion or to increase or decrease thirst, thereby influencing fluid intake.[13–17] An abnormality in either of these 2 mechanisms can have a significant effect on water and sodium balance. The treatment of a fluid imbalance requires identifying the condition that caused the abnormality and determining the time frame during which the abnormality occurred. Acute disturbances, changes occurring in 48 hours or less, are more frequently associated with significant signs and symptoms and should be cor-

rected acutely. Chronic disturbances developing over a longer period of time are typically asymptomatic and should be corrected less aggressively.[8,18]

Fluid Considerations and Requirements in Children

Normal daily fluid requirements can be estimated in a variety of ways. One of the most common ways, the Holliday-Segar formula, is a weight-based method (Table 9-2).[19,20] For example, by this method, a child weighing 27 kg would require a minimum of 1640 mL of fluid per day. This method is commonly used to estimate fluid requirements; however, it does not address fluid requirements in

Table 9-2. Calculating Estimated Fluid Requirements (Holliday-Segar Formula)

BODY WEIGHT	DAILY FLUID REQUIREMENT (HOLLIDAY-SEGAR)	FLUID REQUIREMENTS (4:2:1 SHORT CUT)
≤10 kg	100 mL/kg	4 mL/kg/h[a]
>10 kg to ≤20 kg	1000 mL + 50 mL/kg for wt > 10 kg	40 mL/h + 2 mL/kg/h > 10 kg
>20 kg	1500 mL + 20 mL/kg for wt > 20 kg	60 mL/h + 1 mL/kg > 20 kg

[a] This may underestimate fluid requirements by about 5% in young children; 5 mL/kg/h is often used to avoid this.

abnormal circumstances such as kidney failure or congestive heart failure.

Several conditions require adjustments in fluid intake for providing optimal care. After birth, a contraction of the ECF compartment takes place due to the loss of interstitial fluid, which results in a 5%–10% weight loss in healthy neonates, possibly more in premature infants.[21-26] Prematurity affects fluid balance. Premature infants may require as much as 200 mL/kg/d to maintain fluid balance due to their large insensible fluid losses. These losses are due partially to the large ratio of skin to body surface area and partially to the immaturity of the skin's barrier function, which leads to increased evaporative fluid loss.[27,28] Phototherapy and radiant warmers also increase water losses, often as much as 20–40 mL/kg/d.[29-32] Humidified incubators reduce fluid requirements by decreasing insensible losses. Daily insensible fluid losses are high during the first few weeks of life: often >100 mL/kg in neonates weighing < 750 g; 60 mL/kg in neonates weighing between 750 and 1000 g; and 35 mL/kg for neonates weighing 1001–1250 g.[33] This decrease in insensible fluid losses is due mainly to maturation and thickening of the skin shortly after birth. Antenatal corticosteroids that help progress lung maturation will also affect skin thickening, which reduces fluid losses via the skin. Therefore, premature infants whose mothers did not receive antenatal corticosteroids prior to birth may have excessive fluid losses for an extended period of time compared with those whose mothers received antenatal corticosteroids.[32] Other conditions that increase insensible water loss include omphalocele, gastroschisis, tachypnea, and administration of nonhumidified oxygen. Conditions that may require fluid restriction due to decreased fluid losses include, but are not limited to kidney and lung dysfunction and heart failure.

One relatively simple way to assess fluid balance in infants and neonates is by measuring their weight daily. For accurate measurements, it is important to use the same scale every day and to ensure that the patient has the same equipment attached (eg, armboards, diapers, and monitoring equipment). Rapid weight changes typically reflect changes in water balance. Another useful indicator for assessing fluid status is serum sodium concentrations. An increase in the serum sodium concentration with little weight gain or weight loss typically indicates dehydration, whereas a low serum sodium concentration along with weight gain typically indicates fluid overload.

Treatment of Fluid Imbalances

When assessing and/or treating fluid and electrolyte imbalances, the patient's volume status must be assessed to determine if he or she is euvolemic, hypervolemic, or hypovolemic. Patients who are euvolemic can usually self-regulate fluid status and require little more than maintenance fluids and electrolyte supplementation. Patients who are either hyper- or hypovolemic require additional assessment and may also require additional treatment. Conditions that affect fluid balance will also have an effect on the serum sodium concentration. When addressing fluid issues, assessing trends in the serum sodium concentration is essential for making the appropriate adjustment. Whenever possible, the underlying cause of the electrolyte disturbance should be treated, rather than just the serum sodium concentration. Dilutional hyponatremia (one form of hypervolemia) can occur from conditions in which fluid accumulates, such as in sepsis or in kidney or liver dysfunction, especially when ascites is present.[34] In general, chronic fluid disturbances take longer than 48 hours to develop, and patients typically do not exhibit signs and symptoms unless the fluid overload is severe, resulting in a very low serum sodium concentration (typically < 120 mEq/L). Overzealous diuresis or administration of hypertonic saline can result in an osmotic demyelination syndrome, brain injury caused by increasing (or decreasing) the serum sodium faster than 0.5 mEq/L/h or by more than 10 mEq/L in 24 hours.[18]

Hypovolemia

Hypovolemia is a condition in which TBW is decreased significantly enough to cause symptoms. The body can correct the problem by stimulating the thirst response, increasing antidiuretic hormone (ADH) release, or both. When the plasma osmolarity is increased or when the blood volume or pressure is reduced, the thirst response is stimulated.[35] In hypovolemia, the serum osmolarity increases and the blood volume decreases, which results in the release of ADH. The

ADH release increases the permeability of water in the collecting tubule, where water is then reabsorbed (ie, water retention). The resultant water retention will result in a more concentrated urine.[36,37] Signs and symptoms of hypovolemia include thirst, altered mental status, weakness, fatigue, neuromuscular irritability, agitation, seizures, and coma.[34] Other conditions that may lead to hypovolemia include GI hemorrhage, vomiting, diarrhea, excessive sweating, burns, diabetes insipidus, and excessive diuresis.[38] Various methods are used for correcting volume depletion, but 3 principles always apply: (1) the fluid deficit must be replaced with an appropriate fluid; (2) maintenance fluids must be provided on an ongoing basis; and (3) if continued ongoing losses are present (eg, gastric drainage, vomiting, diarrhea), the fluid must be replaced on an ongoing basis to prevent further deficits.

The fluid deficit can be calculated by using the following equation:

$$\text{Water deficit (L)} = {}^*\text{TBW} \times \text{wt (kg)} \times ([Na_{serum}\ (mEq/L)/140\ mEq/L] - 1);$$

*TBW = 0.8 in premature infants; 0.7 term to ≤ 6 months of age; and 0.6 > 6 months of age

Another method for calculating fluid deficits has been proposed by Roberts.[39] This method proposes calculating the fluid deficit based on estimated weight loss (Table 9-3).

In order to treat the patient appropriately, classifying dehydration as mild, moderate, or severe is necessary. Mild dehydration can be identified by the presence of dry mucous membranes with normal hemodynamic parameters.

Table 9-3. Clinical Assessment and Treatment of Dehydration in Infants and Adolescents

PATIENT GROUP	MILD DEHYDRATION	MODERATE DEHYDRATION	SEVERE DEHYDRATION
	Characterized by dry mucous membranes, oliguria	Characterized by dry mucous membranes, marked oliguria, tachycardia, poor skin turgor, and sunken fontanelles (infants only)	Characterized by dry mucous membranes, marked oliguria, tachycardia, poor skin turgor, and sunken fontanelles (infants only); hypotension and poor perfusion
EWL infants and children			
% dehydration	5	10	15
Fluid deficit, mL/kg	50	100	150
Fluid replacement	20 mL/kg bolus; then 15 mL/kg plus regular maintenance fluids over first 8 h; then 15 mL/kg plus regular maintenance fluids over next 16 h	20 mL/kg bolus; then 40 mL/kg plus regular maintenance fluids over first 8 h; then 40 mL/kg plus regular maintenance fluids over next 16 h	20 mL/kg bolus; then 65 mL/kg plus regular maintenance fluids over first 8 h; then 65 mL/kg plus regular maintenance fluids over next 16 h
			Patient may require > 1 bolus to resolve hypotension and tachycardia; for every additional bolus the fluid replacement would decrease by 10 mL/kg.
EWL adolescents			
% dehydration	3	5–6	7–9
Fluid deficit, mL/kg	30	50–60	70–90
Fluid replacement	10 mL/kg bolus; then 10 mL/kg plus regular maintenance fluids over first 8 h; then 10 mL/kg plus regular maintenance fluids over next 16 h	10 mL/kg bolus; then 20 mL/kg plus regular maintenance fluids over first 8 h; then 20 mL/kg plus regular maintenance fluids over next 16 h	10 mL/kg bolus; then 35 mL/kg plus regular maintenance fluids over first 8 h; then 35 mL/kg plus regular maintenance fluids over next 16 h
			Patient may require > 1 bolus to resolve hypotension and tachycardia; for every additional bolus the fluid replacement would decrease by 5 mL/kg

EWL, estimated weight loss.

Moderate dehydration can be defined as changes occurring in hemodynamic parameters that suggest intravascular depletion, like tachycardia, mild hypotension, and orthostasis. Severe volume depletion is defined by the presence of more profound hemodynamic compromise, such as moderate to severe hypotension, tachycardia, and poor perfusion. Clinical symptoms of mild, moderate, and severe hypovolemia generally correspond to a 5%, 10%, and 15% weight loss in infants, respectively, which can be detected if pre- and post-hypovolemia weights are available. In teenagers, mild, moderate, and severe hypovolemia corresponds to a 3%, 5%, and 7% loss in body weight, respectively. Fluid therapy must include replacement of the volume deficit as well as provision of maintenance fluids. Once the weight loss is estimated, the severity of dehydration is determined (mild, moderate, or severe). An appropriate amount of fluid to be administered in milliliters per kilograms is then determined based on severity of dehydration. An initial bolus of 20 mL/kg of an isotonic fluid (usually 0.9% sodium chloride) is given in infants and children and 10 mL/kg is given in adolescents; 50% of the remaining volume deficit is then given during the next 8–16 hours in addition to regular maintenance fluids. The remaining deficit is administered during the next 16–24 hours in addition to regular maintenance fluids.

For example, an infant weighing 5 kg has a 500-mL (10%) fluid deficit. Given the degree of fluid deficit (10% or more), an isotonic fluid bolus (20 mL/kg or 2% of the patient's body weight is 100 mL) would be indicated initially. After this bolus, the remaining deficit (8% or 400 mL) would be replaced as follows: 50% (200 mL) over the next 8 hours and 50% (200 mL) over the subsequent 16 hours. In addition to the deficit replacement, usual maintenance fluids (column 3 in Table 9-2) must be administered. If severely volume depleted, the patient will generally require more than one fluid bolus of 20 mL/kg to resolve the tachycardia, hypotension, and other symptoms. Once the tachycardia and hypotension have resolved, the fluid deficit and maintenance requirements can be calculated. In a teenager, the fluid deficit associated with mild, moderate, and severe dehydration is generally about 50% of that seen in an infant; therefore the initial bolus is generally 10 mL/kg rather than 20 mL/kg. Alternatively, as in adults, a fluid bolus of 500–1000 mL may be given initially and repeated based on hemodynamic response.

Hypertonic dehydration (hypernatremia) must be managed differently. In hypertonic dehydration, the fluid from the ICF compartment is drawn into the intravascular space. Rapid administration of fluid as already described may cause rapid fluid shifts that can result in cerebral edema and intracranial bleeding. In hypertonic dehydration, the fluid volume deficit is calculated and gradually replaced (usually over 48 hours).[40] However, the need for a fluid bolus is based on hemodynamic parameters. If the patient is hemodynamically compromised (hypotension, severe tachycardia), then a bolus of 10–20 mL/kg of an isotonic fluid is imperative to restore perfusion and normalize hemodynamic parameters. When severe symptomatic hypovolemic hypernatremia is being corrected, the underlying cause of the hypernatremia should be treated. In general, to prevent cerebral edema, the serum sodium should not be lowered at a rate that exceeds 0.5mEq/L/h or more than 10 mEq/L in 24 hours.

Hypervolemia

Hypervolemia, or increased TBW, causes a decreased serum osmolarity resulting in dilute urine by suppressing ADH secretion. The precise mechanism by which plasma osmolarity suppresses ADH release is unclear, but it probably is related to specialized cells that sense osmolarity changes and send messages to the neuroendocrine cells located in the hypothalamus or the organum vasculosum.[35] In most cases, the thirst response will be suppressed, ADH will be suppressed, and the excess water will be excreted by the kidneys. However, in conditions in which the low plasma osmolarity fails to inhibit ADH secretion (such as in severe low-output congestive heart failure), cell expansion, hypervolemia, and hyponatremia continue to progress.[41] Symptoms include headache, nausea, vomiting, muscle twitching, disorientation, depressed reflexes, and in severe cases, seizures and coma. Other conditions that may result in hypervolemia include kidney or liver failure with ascites, sepsis, cardiac failure, and syndrome of inappropriate antidiuretic hormone (SIADH).[42,43]

Electrolyte Assessment

Changes in the ECF compartment are responsible for the signs and symptoms associated with fluid and electrolyte imbalances. Therefore, the ECF compartment must be corrected to alleviate those signs and symptoms. Prior to any fluid or electrolyte treatment, the laboratory values must be validated. Treating electrolyte abnormalities based on inaccurate laboratory values can have serious consequences. Figure 9-3 presents an algorithm for assessing the validity of electrolyte laboratory values. The first step in assessing and treating fluid imbalances is determining the cause of the electrolyte imbalance. For example, is the hypokalemia a result of chronic diuretic therapy or is it due to an intra-

Figure 9-3. Laboratory Assessment

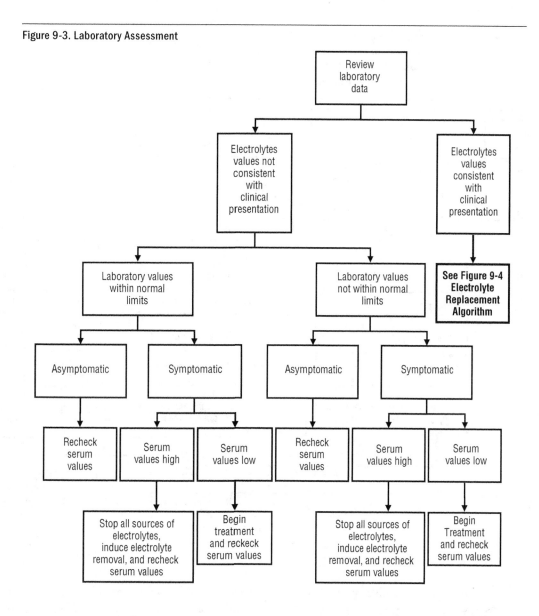

cellular shift secondary to a large dextrose infusion? Once the cause has been identified, the next step is to classify the event as either acute or chronic. The prescriber can then determine whether a supplemental infusion or a change in the maintenance solution is a more appropriate intervention to correct the abnormality. Acute problems should generally be treated with supplemental infusions, whereas chronic problems should usually be treated with maintenance solutions. The next step is to determine the relative safety range of the electrolyte to be corrected. For severe hypokalemia, it is typically safer to administer a relatively moderate potassium infusion and then recheck the serum potassium concentration before repeating the dose, rather than giving one large potassium supplemental infusion. If

the deficit was inappropriately assessed and the single supplementation was too high, the patient could develop hyperkalemia and its associated consequences. In a patient with severe hypomagnesemia, overestimating the magnesium supplementation will have little clinical impact on the patient. Therefore, the prescriber can be more aggressive with magnesium supplementation compared to potassium supplementation. The final step or criterion is to assess the acuity of the electrolyte imbalance. If the serum electrolyte concentration is critical or life threatening, then the problem should be treated acutely. After initial treatment, the maintenance solution can be adjusted, if necessary. Figure 9-4 presents an algorithm for the evaluation and treatment of electrolyte abnormalities.

Figure 9-4. Electrolyte Replacement Assessment Algorithm

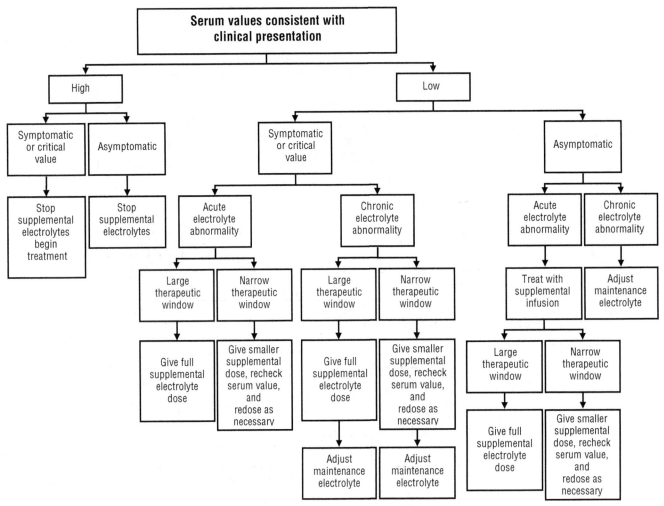

Reference values for normal serum electrolyte concentrations based on age appear at the beginning of each of the following electrolyte sections. These values are included to illustrate the differences in electrolyte concentrations for various age groups. Laboratory reference values will vary from institution to institution, and practitioners should use the reference values listed at their individual institutions for adjusting serum electrolyte values.

Sodium

Preterm Neonates:	130–140 mEq/L
Term Neonates/Infants:	133–146 mEq/L
Children/Adolescents:	135–145 mEq/L

Sodium is the most abundant extracellular cation in the body. It has 2 primary functions: fluid balance and mainte-

nance of membrane potential. The body maintains sodium homeostasis primarily by the renin-angiotensin-aldosterone system and ADH secretion. Other systems involved in sodium maintenance include the sympathetic nervous system, atrial natriuretic peptide, the kallikrein-kinin system, various intrarenal mechanisms, and other factors that regulate kidney and medullary blood flow.[44] The body maintains cell membrane potential by the Na^+-K^+-ATPase pump. Three sodium ions are pumped out of the cell for every 2 potassium ions that are pumped into the cell, which produces the negative charge in the cells that is necessary for normal functioning of nerves and muscle cells and the active transport of nutrients, such as glucose and amino acids.[45]

Normally the body's sodium losses match its sodium intake. The kidney can reabsorb up to 99% of the sodium presented to the renal tubules, so in times of a sodium intake deficit, serum sodium concentrations can be maintained. Daily sodium losses in these instances may be only a few milliequivalents. Medications can also affect sodium balance. Lactulose, 0.9% sodium chloride, and hypertonic saline can cause hypernatremia, and medications such as chlorpropamide, demeclocycline, and loop diuretics can cause hyponatremia. Diuretics can also cause sodium imbalances. Loop diuretics cause hypovolemic hypernatremia due to increased water loss relative to sodium loss, and overzealous use of thiazide diuretics causes hypovolemic hyponatremia. Sodium requirements vary depending on age group, and they also vary from patient to patient. In general, daily parenteral requirements for sodium are about 2–5 mEq/kg in term infants, children, and adolescents. In preterm infants, as little as 1 mEq/kg/d of sodium may maintain sodium concentrations, but in general 3–4 mEq/kg/d is recommended for the first week of life and then 3–6 mEq/kg/d in preterm infants < 28 weeks gestation.[46,47] Oral sodium requirements vary with age (Table 9-4). Figure 9-5 shows an algorithm for the adjustment of maintenance electrolytes in intravenous fluids.

Hyponatremia

Hyponatremia is defined as a serum sodium concentration < 135 mEq/L. It is one of the most common electrolyte disturbances found in the hospitalized patient. Signs and symptoms include headache, nausea, vomiting, muscle cramps, lethargy, restlessness, disorientation, and depressed reflexes, and they are more commonly seen with an acute decrease in the serum sodium concentration, typically below 125 mEq/L. Severe acute hyponatremia is life threatening; fortunately most cases of hyponatremia seen in hospitalized patients develop slowly and are less severe.

The assessment and treatment of hyponatremia begins with the assessment of serum osmolality or tonicity. An algorithm for this assessment can be found in Figure 9-6. **Hypertonic hyponatremia** is distinguished by a serum osmolality of >295 mOsm/L. It is typically caused by the excessive presence and/or administration of osmotically active agents such as mannitol and glucose. If the hyponatremia is a result of hyperglycemia, a closer approximation of the effective serum sodium concentration can be calculated. For every 100 g/dL increase in serum glucose concentration, a decrease of 1.6–2.4 mEq/L occurs in the serum sodium concentration.[48,49] For practical purposes and ease of calculations, 2 mEq/L can be added to the serum sodium level for every 100 g/dL of serum glucose concentration to approximate an effective serum sodium concentration.

Table 9-4. Oral Electrolyte Requirements by Age

AGE	SODIUM		POTASSIUM		MAGNESIUM		CALCIUM		PHOSPHORUS	
	mg	mEq	mg	mEq	mg	mEq	mg	mEq	mg	mmol
0 to <0.5 y	120	11	500	26	302	2.5	210	10.5	100	3
0.5 to <1 y	200	18	700	37	75	6	270	13.5	275	(9)
1 to <2 y	225	20	1000	53						
2 to <3 y					80	7	500	25	460	15
3 to <4 y										
4 to <5 y	300	27	1400	74						
5 to <6 y										
6 to <7 y					130	11	500	25	500	16
7 to <8 y	400	36	1600	89						
8 to <9 y										
9 to <10 y										
10 to <11 y					240	20				
11 to <12 y							1300	65	1250	40
12 to <13 y	500	45	2000	111						
≥13 y (M)					400	30				
≥13 y (F)					360	33				

Figure 9-5. Maintenance Electrolyte Replacement Flow Chart
Directions:
This flow chart is for the adjustment of maintenance electrolytes only.
The number in the box is the starting dose of electrolyte in mEq/kg or mmol/kg.
If the serum concentration is high, move up the arrow one step, if the serum concentration is low, move down the arrow one step.
For phosphorus, potassium, or magnesium, if the serum creatinine is > 1.5 mg/dL move up the arrow one step.

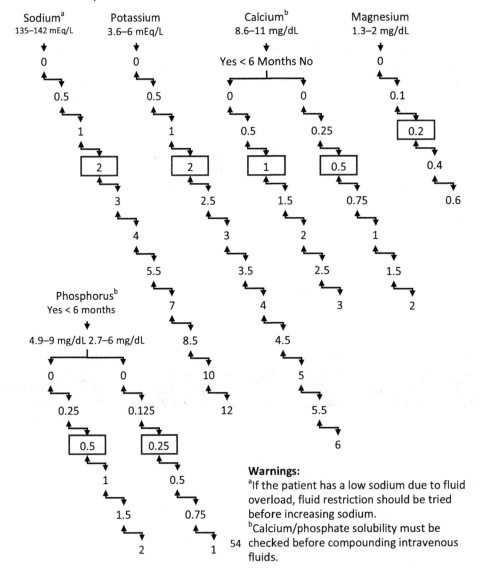

Warnings:
[a]If the patient has a low sodium due to fluid overload, fluid restriction should be tried before increasing sodium.
[b]Calcium/phosphate solubility must be checked before compounding intravenous fluids.

Isotonic hyponatremia is a less common condition in which the serum osmolality is within the normal range. It can be caused by an excess of plasma proteins or lipids. If the hyponatremia is a result of hypertriglyceridemia, a closer approximation of the effective serum sodium concentration can be calculated. One can add 1 mEq/L to the serum sodium level for every 450 mg/dL of serum triglyceride concentration to approximate an effective serum sodium concentration.

The assessment and treatment of **hypotonic hyponatremia** is more complex and always requires an assessment of the fluid status. Three types of hypotonic hyponatremia are possible: hypovolemic, euvolemic, and hypervolemic.

Figure 9-6. Evaluating Hyponatremia

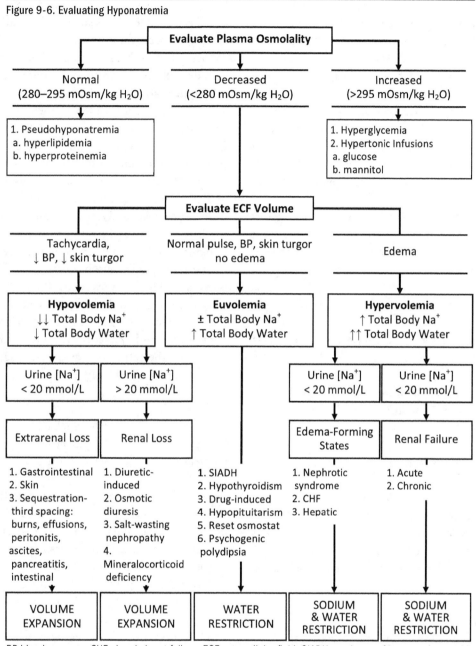

BP, blood pressure; CHF, chronic heart failure; ECF, extracellular fluid; SIADH, syndrome of inappropriate antidiuretic hormone. Adapted from Matarese LE, Gottschlich MM, eds. *Contemporary Nutrition Support Practice: A Clinical Guide.* Whitmire SJ. Fluids and electrolytes. p. 130. Copyright © 1998 with permission from Matarese Le, Gottschlich MM.

Hypovolemic hypotonic hyponatremia is characterized by a serum osmolality of <280 mOsm/L and signs of hypovolemia such as tachycardia, hypotension, or decreased skin turgor. Causes of hypovolemic hypotonic hyponatremia include diarrhea and other GI losses such as gastric suction, enterocutaneous fistulas, or necrotizing enterocolitis; thiazide diuretic-induced hyponatremia; and salt-wasting ne-

phropathy. In premature neonates, salt-wasting nephropathy can be severe, often requiring administration of 6 mEq/kg of sodium or more daily to maintain sodium and fluid balance.[22]

Euvolemic hypotonic hyponatremia is commonly associated with the SIADH. Common causes of SIADH include head trauma and brain malignancies. Other causes of euvolemic hypotonic hyponatremia include hypothyroidism and psychogenic polydipsia. Treatment usually consists of treating the underlying disorder. If conventional measures such as fluid restriction do not work with refractory SIADH, medications such as conivaptan or tolvaptan may be necessary, although little data exist to support their use in children.[36]

Hypervolemic hypotonic hyponatremia can be associated with kidney failure, liver failure with ascites, hyperaldosteronism, and heart failure. It may also occur during the first few days after birth due to fluid retention. The treatment for hypervolemic hypotonic hyponatremia is sodium and water restriction.

Treatment with hypertonic saline may be indicated if the serum sodium concentration is below 125 mEq/L or if the patient is symptomatic. The sodium deficit can be estimated by using the equation:

sodium deficit (mEq) = *TBW × wt (kg) × ($Na_{desired}$ − Na_{actual})

*TBW = 0.8 in premature infants; 0.7 in term infants to ≤ 6 months of age; and 0.6 in infants > 6 months of age

For example, a 7 kg neonate with a serum sodium of 127 and a desired serum sodium of 140 mEq/L would have a sodium deficit of 54.6 mEq.

(140 − 127) × 7 (kg) × 0.6 = 54.6 mEq

Typically no more than 30%–50% of the sodium deficit should be replaced over 6–12 hours. In general, the serum sodium should not be corrected at a rate that exceeds 0.5 mEq/L/h or more than 10 mEq/L in 24 hours in order to prevent the development of osmotic demyelination syndrome.[50]

Hypernatremia

Hypernatremia is defined as serum sodium concentration > 145 mEq/L. Hypernatremia usually develops under conditions of low or normal total body sodium, but it can also develop with an increase in total body sodium. Hypernatremia is typically a result of net water loss or hypotonic fluid loss. Causes of hypernatremia include lack of oral hydration, diarrhea, vomiting, overzealous diuresis, fever, and the inability to express a need for water (eg, infants, children, or patients who have altered mental status). The assessment of a patient with hypernatremia requires evaluation of fluid status. **Hypovolemic hypernatremia** is a condition in which excessive fluid losses occur due to either renal or nonrenal losses.

Renal losses may be due to diuretic use or increased solute diuresis from conditions such as glycosuria or azotemia. Excessive nonrenal fluid losses include diarrhea and excessive sweating (phototherapy or open bed warmers). Treatment includes volume expansion with hypotonic saline. **Euvolemic hypernatremia** is usually caused by high renal water losses versus sodium losses. Diabetes insipidus is the most common cause, and treatment involves water replacement. **Hypervolemic hypernatremia** can be caused by the excessive administration of isotonic or hypertonic saline or by mineralocorticoid excess, Cushing's syndrome, or adrenal malignancy. Management involves treating the underlying disorder, diuresis, and free water replacement. An algorithm for the evaluation and treatment of hypernatremia is shown in Figure 9-7. If the hypernatremia is due to sodium intake, then sodium intake must be decreased. If the hypernatremia is associated with hypovolemia, then rehydration should be started immediately. If the hypovolemia is mild and asymptomatic, then rehydration can be addressed by simply altering the oral fluid intake. If the hypovolemia is moderate to severe or if the patient is symptomatic, aggressive treatment should begin immediately.

Potassium

Newborns:	3.7–5.9 mEq/L
Infants:	4.1–5.3 mEq/L
Children/Adolescents:	3.4–4.7 mEq/L

Potassium is the primary ICF cation. Potassium is essential for cell metabolism and maintenance of resting membrane potential. Intracellular potassium concentration is approximately 140 mEq/L (ICF potassium concentration is equal to the ECF sodium concentration due to the action of the Na^+-K^+-ATPase pump).[51] Potassium distribution is also affected by factors that act on the Na^+-K^+-ATPase pump, such as insulin, catecholamines, and ECF pH; exercise; and cell breakdown.[3,52,53] Potassium is primarily excreted via the kidney. Potassium excretion varies based on serum potassium concentrations and the release of aldosterone and angiotensin II. A lack of aldosterone causes potassium retention, whereas an excess causes potassium depletion.[54] In times of a potassium deficit, urinary excretion drops significantly, but not entirely. If potassium intake significantly increases, urinary potassium excretion will increase as well as potassium excretion via nonrenal mechanisms (GI tract), a process known as potassium adaptation. In chronic kidney insufficiency, GI potassium losses may increase to 30%–50% of the ingested potassium.[55-57] Medications that

Figure 9-7. Evaluation of Hypernatremia

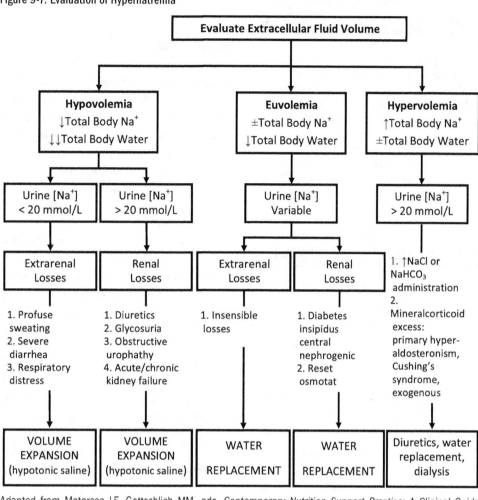

affect potassium concentrations are listed in Table 9-5. Supplementation in parenteral nutrition (PN) solutions or maintenance intravenous fluids should start at about 2–4 mEq/kg and may increase or decrease depending on kidney function, GI losses, and medication use.[39,46] Oral potassium requirements vary with age (Table 9-4). An algorithm for the adjustment of maintenance electrolytes in intravenous fluids is presented in Figure 9-5.

Hypokalemia

Hypokalemia is usually defined as a serum potassium concentration < 3.4 mEq/L. It is a common electrolyte abnormality seen in clinical practice, and typical causes are abnormal kidney or GI losses. Other causes of hypokalemia include medications, metabolic alkalosis, hyperaldosteronism, hypomagnesemia, catecholamines, and inadequate

intake. Signs and symptoms are nonspecific but include muscle weakness and cramping, dysrhythmias, paralysis, muscle necrosis, and possibly death. The treatment of hypokalemia depends on both the severity and the cause. Oral potassium supplements are available as a variety of salts, and the choice of agent depends on other concomitant electrolyte imbalances, cost, and patient preference. In an asymptomatic patient with mild to moderate hypokalemia, oral supplementation is preferred because of safety reasons (eg, no risk for potassium extravasation). Oral supplementation also reduces the risk of overcorrection causing hyperkalemia and too rapid correction causing dysrhythmias. Oral potassium liquid preparations often have an unpleasant taste, and all potassium supplements can be irritating to the GI tract, causing nausea, vomiting, and/or diarrhea. For mild to moderate potassium depletion, doses of 2–5

Table 9-5. Medications Affecting Potassium and Magnesium

HYPERKALEMIA	HYPOKALEMIA
Potassium-sparing diuretics	Loop diuretics
Nonsteroidal anti-inflammatory drugs	Thiazide diuretics
Angiotensin converting enzyme inhibitors	Fludrocortisones
Angiotensin-II receptor blockers	High-dose glucocorticoids
Trimethoprim	High-dose penicillins
Pentamidine	Phenolphthalein
Cyclosporine	Sodium polystyrene sulfonate
Tacrolimus	Sorbitol
Heparin	β_2-adrenergic agonists
Penicillin G potassium	Tocolytic agents
β-blockers	Theophylline
Succinylcholine	Caffeine
	Insulin/dextrose
HYPERMAGNESEMIA	**HYPOMAGNESEMIA**
Tocolytic agents	Cisplatinum
Magnesium-containing antacids	Foscarnet
Magnesium-containing enemas	Amphotericin B
	Aminoglycosides
	Thiazide diuretics

mEq/kg/d of potassium in divided doses, not to exceed 1–2 mEq/kg as a single dose, taken with plenty of fluid, are recommended.[58-60] Serum potassium should be rechecked approximately 2 hours after the initial dose is completed, and additional doses given, if needed.

The use of intravenous potassium supplementation should be reserved for patients who are symptomatic or have severe hypokalemia or when administration via the GI tract is contraindicated. Recommended doses range from 0.5 to 1 mEq/kg depending on the severity of the hypokalemia and kidney function. Generally, infusion rates should not exceed 0.5 mEq/kg/h, unless continuous cardiac monitoring is available. Potassium can be caustic to the vein, so to minimize irritation, the concentration for administration through a peripheral vein should not exceed 6 mEq/100 mL.[59-61] When intravenous potassium supplementation is administered, co-administration with dextrose may worsen the hypokalemia by stimulating insulin release, which promotes the intracellular shift of potassium. Concurrent hypomagnesemia may result in refractory hypokalemia due to increased renal potassium losses due to the kidney's attempt to conserve magnesium and impairment of the Na$^+$-K$^+$-ATPase pump.[62] As such, it is important to correct a low magnesium concentration while treating hypokalemia. Serum potassium should be rechecked approximately 1–2 hours after

the initial dose is completed, and additional doses given, if needed.

Hyperkalemia

Hyperkalemia is defined as a serum potassium concentration > 4.5 mEq/L. Higher serum concentrations may be clinically acceptable depending on the patient's age. Signs and symptoms of hyperkalemia include muscle twitching, cramping, weakness, ascending paralysis, electrocardiogram changes (eg, peaked T-waves, prolonged PR interval), and dysrhythmias (eg, bradyarrhythmias, ventricular fibrillation, and asystole). Hyperkalemia is one of the most dangerous electrolyte imbalances for premature infants. The immaturity of the kidneys results in a reduced glomerular filtration rate, urinary potassium excretion, acidosis, and an immature renal tubular response to aldosterone.[63] Hyperkalemia can occur from excessive potassium intake in the presence of altered kidney excretion or metabolic acidosis caused by conditions such as diabetic ketoacidosis and renal tubular acidosis. Metabolic acidosis causes hyperkalemia by causing a shift of potassium from the ECF to the ICF to balance the excess hydrogen ions that are moving into the ICF. Clinically significant hyperkalemia can also develop as a result of cell lysis (hemolysis) or tissue injury and death (eg, burns, rhabdomyolysis) in vivo due to the release of the ICF potassium into the serum.

Treatment of hyperkalemia depends on both the severity and the cause. All sources of potassium intake should be discontinued immediately and, if feasible, any medication that may contribute to hyperkalemia should be stopped or the dose reduced. If the potassium is significantly elevated or if the patient is symptomatic, intravenous calcium chloride should be administered immediately to reduce the excitability of the cardiac muscle. (It is important to note that calcium gluconate is generally not recommended in emergency situations.) Two basic mechanisms are used to treat hyperkalemia: shifting potassium into the ICF and removing potassium from the body. Insulin in combination with glucose, β_2-adrenergic agonists, and sodium bicarbonate will shift the potassium into the ICF. Loop and thiazide diuretics (loop to a greater extent than thiazide), cation exchange resins like sodium polystyrene, and dialysis all reduce potassium concentrations by directly removing potassium from the body (exchange resins and dialysis) or by increasing renal potassium excretion (diuretics). Serum potassium concentrations should be monitored frequently during treatment, especially in patients receiving dextrose and insulin, β_2-adrenergic agonists, and sodium bicarbonate because once these therapies are discontinued, potassium will shift back to the ECF compartment. Potassium concentrations should be monitored for at least 12 hours after the hyperkalemia has resolved to ensure that equilibration of potassium between the ICF and ECF is complete.[3]

Pseudohyperkalemia is common in infants and young children and can occur when red blood cells lyse during the blood-drawing process. In other words, the serum potassium detected in the sample is higher than the actual concentration due to hemolysis of the red blood cells during the blood-drawing process or while in the collection tube. This form of hyperkalemia is the most common form detected in pediatric patients with normal kidney function. If pseudohyperkalemia is suspected, and if the patient is asymptomatic and has normal kidney function, the serum potassium concentration should be repeated (rapid aspiration and the use of narrow gauge needles should be avoided when possible) before starting any treatment for hyperkalemia.

Magnesium

All Age Groups: 1.6–2.3 mg/dL

Magnesium is an essential cofactor in more than 300 enzymatic reactions, including those involved in glucose metabolism, fatty acid synthesis and breakdown, and DNA and protein metabolism. Magnesium plays a critical role in the functioning of the Na^+-K^+-ATPase pump, thus affecting neuromuscular transmission, cardiovascular excitability, vasomotor tone, and muscle contraction. Magnesium is also an integral component of bone and parathyroid hormone (PTH) secretion.[64,65] Magnesium is found primarily in the ICF, with only about 2% of total body stores found in the ECF. More than 50% of the magnesium in the body resides in bone. About 61% of serum magnesium is physiologically active in the ionized form, 33% protein bound, and 5% complexed to phosphate, citrate, and other compounds.

Magnesium homeostasis is maintained and regulated by the GI tract, kidney, and bone via PTH. Healthy individuals absorb between 30% and 40% of ingested magnesium. Magnesium is absorbed in the distal jejunum and ileum, and absorption is inversely proportional to the magnesium intake. Magnesium is primarily excreted via the kidneys with about 35% of ingested magnesium excreted in the urine. In the presence of high magnesium intake, renal excretion increases to maintain normal serum magnesium concentrations. Very little magnesium (1%–2%) is excreted via the feces. If a patient becomes magnesium depleted, the mineral is leached from the bones to maintain ECF magnesium concentrations. ECF magnesium is then sacrificed to the ICF to maintain normal metabolic functions.[66] Medications

that affect magnesium concentrations are listed in Table 9-5. Usual intravenous magnesium supplementation in PN solutions ranges from 0.25 to 0.5 mEq/kg daily but may be higher in patients with abnormal magnesium losses. Oral magnesium requirements vary with age (Table 9-4). Figure 9-5 shows an algorithm for the adjustment of maintenance electrolytes in intravenous fluids.

Hypomagnesemia

Hypomagnesemia is defined as a serum magnesium concentration < 1.6 mg/dL. It is a common condition seen in hospitalized patients. Signs and symptoms include apathy, depression, psychosis, muscle weakness, vertigo, ataxia, seizures, confusion, leg cramps, hyperactive tendon reflexes, anorexia, nausea, vomiting, paresthesia, Chvostek's and Trousseau's signs, spontaneous carpal-pedal spasm, and cardiac complications including dysrhythmias.[67] Hypomagnesemia can also contribute to the development of other electrolyte abnormalities. Hypomagnesemia may result in refractory hypokalemia because of increased renal potassium losses due to the kidney's attempt to conserve magnesium and impairment of the Na^+-K^+-ATPase pump.[62] Hypomagnesemia may also contribute to the development of hypocalcemia. Magnesium deficiency can impair parathyroid function, and hypomagnesemia accompanied by hypoparathyroidism is a common cause of neonatal hypocalcemia.[6,68]

Hypomagnesemia can be caused by decreased intake, increased excretion, or an intracellular shift of magnesium.[69] Excessive renal losses may occur in patients with acute tubular necrosis, renal tubular acidosis, Bartter's syndrome, or hyperaldosteronism, or they may be induced by medications such as amphotericin B, cisplatin, cyclosporine, aminoglycosides, and foscarnet.[70] Intracellular shifts can be caused by dextrose and/or insulin administration.

Because only about 1%–2% of total body magnesium is found in the ECF, serum concentrations are not a good reflection of total body magnesium stores. Treatment of hypomagnesemia is therefore empirical. The intravenous route is preferred in patients with moderate to severe hypomagnesemia because of the GI intolerance generally seen with large oral doses. Recommended doses are 0.2–0.4 mEq/kg (25–50 mg/kg), up to 16 mEq (2 g) every 8–12 hours for 2–3 doses.[71] A renal magnesium threshold exists for magnesium reabsorption; thus up to 50% of an individual magnesium dose will be eliminated via the kidneys if the magnesium is not distributed intracellularly.[72,73] In asymptomatic adults, a maximum infusion rate of 1 g (8 mEq)/h is recommended.[74,75] This infusion rate equates to about 0.1 mEq/kg/h in children. Supplemental magnesium doses may be reduced by 50% in patients with kidney dysfunction to lessen the risk of hypermagnesemia. However, reducing the dose by 50% may not be necessary in all cases; if only a one-time dose is given, the magnesium will not accumulate, and mild hypermagnesemia is well tolerated. Serum magnesium should be rechecked approximately 1–2 hours after the infusion is completed, and additional boluses given, if needed.

Hypermagnesemia

Hypermagnesemia is defined as a serum magnesium concentration > 2.4 mg/dL. Hypermagnesemia is usually well tolerated but can affect neurological, neuromuscular, and cardiac function when magnesium concentrations exceed 3 mg/dL.[76,77] Physical findings include nausea, vomiting, diaphoresis, flushing, depressed mental function, drowsiness, muscular weakness, hypotension, and bradycardia. Hypermagnesemia occurs primarily in the setting of kidney insufficiency in combination with continued magnesium intake. In the premature infant, the most common cause of hypermagnesemia is the placental transfer of magnesium during maternal treatment with magnesium sulfate for premature labor contractions. The effect that hypermagnesemia has on the ability to relax smooth muscle makes magnesium a viable treatment due to the low risk of harm to the neonate. The neonate with hypermagnesemia will have poor muscle tone, which will return to normal as the serum magnesium concentration decreases over approximately 2–5 days, depending on the severity of the initial hypermagnesemia and the neonate's kidney function.[78,79]

If patients with severe hypermagnesemia are symptomatic, intravenous calcium chloride should be administered immediately to reverse the cardiac and neuromuscular effects. Hemodialysis may be required to reduce the magnesium concentration to a safer value. Treatments for hypermagnesemia in an asymptomatic patient include dietary magnesium restriction, administration of a loop diuretic, and hemodialysis if severe kidney dysfunction is present and other methods are unsuccessful.[64,78]

Calcium

AGE GROUP	TOTAL CALCIUM	AGE GROUP	IONIZED (SI UNITS)
Preterm neonate	6.2–11 mg/dL	Preterm	1.75–2 mmol/L
Full-term neonate	7.6–10.4 mg/dL	Full-term <36 h Full-term 36–84 h	1.05–1.37 mmol/L 1.1–1.42 mmol/L
10 days–2 years 2 years–12 years >12 years	9–11 mg/dL 8.8–10.8 mg/dL 8.6–10 mg/dL	>84 h	1.2–1.38 mmol/L

Calcium is one of the most abundant ions in the body, accounting for 1%–2% of total body weight. Calcium is necessary for many physiological functions, including neuromuscular activity, preservation of cell membrane integrity, regulation of endocrine secretory activities, blood coagulation, activation of the complement system, and bone metabolism. Serum calcium concentrations are controlled by the parathyroid gland. When serum calcium is low, PTH secretion is stimulated, which increases bone resorption, augments renal calcium conservation, and activates vitamin D, which in turn increases calcium absorption from the GI tract. When serum calcium concentration is increased, the thyroid releases calcitonin, which acts to inhibit bone resorption and increase renal calcium excretion. Generally, serum calcium concentrations are maintained by either renal excretion of excess calcium or leaching of calcium from the bone.[80]

About 99% of the body's calcium is found in teeth and bone, with only 1% found in the serum. The body contains 3 forms of calcium: complexed, protein bound, and ionized. Complexed calcium is combined with nonprotein anions such as phosphate, carbonate, and citrate, and it is not available for physiological activity. Slightly less than half of the serum calcium is bound to protein, primarily albumin. A serum calcium measurement assesses total serum calcium, which includes the calcium bound to albumin and the free or ionized calcium. Therefore, if the serum albumin concentration is low, the serum total calcium concentration also will be low. Although not completely reliable in critically ill patients, serum calcium concentrations can be corrected for the degree of hypoalbuminemia, using the equation:

$$\text{Corrected calcium} = \text{measured total calcium (mg/dL)} + 0.8 \times [4 - \text{albumin (g/dL)}]$$

Alternatively, if the patient's albumin concentration is low, then the serum ionized calcium can be checked, which is the most accurate laboratory test for assessing the physiologically active calcium status. The serum pH and the phosphorus and albumin concentrations affect the amount of calcium that is ionized.[81–83] Supplementation of calcium in PN solutions ranges from 1 to 4 mEq/kg depending on the patient's age. Oral calcium requirements also vary with age (Table 9-4). An algorithm for the adjustment of maintenance electrolytes in intravenous fluids is presented in Figure 9-5.

Hypocalcemia

Measured hypocalcemia is commonly encountered in patients with hypoalbuminemia, but it does not require treatment unless the corrected calcium or ionized calcium is low. Signs and symptoms of hypocalcemia include hypotension, decreased myocardial contractility, prolonged QT interval, paresthesia, Chvostek's and Trousseau's signs, muscle cramps, tetany, and seizures. Causes of hypocalcemia include vitamin D deficiency or the inability to activate vitamin D, hyperphosphatemia, pseudohypoparathyroidism, decreased PTH activity, sepsis, rhabdomyolysis, and massive blood transfusions.[84] Medications can also cause hypocalcemia, and furosemide, phenobarbital, and phenytoin are particularly important in the premature infant.[85] Sulfur-containing amino acids (eg, cysteine) also increase renal calcium excretion. The increased renal calcium excretion seen with cysteine supplementation in PN solutions is counterbalanced by the increased solubility of calcium and phosphorus in PN solutions that contain cysteine hydrochloride due to the lower pH.[86,87]

Patients with severe hypocalcemia or acute symptomatic hypocalcemia require immediate treatment. Intravenous calcium is available commercially in 2 salt forms: chloride and gluconate. Calcium chloride contains 13.6 mEq of elemental calcium per gram; calcium gluconate contains 4.65 mEq of elemental calcium per gram. Because calcium chloride has 3 times the amount of elemental calcium as calcium gluconate, it is associated with a higher incidence of tissue necrosis if extravasation occurs.[88] For hypocalcemic tetany, 0.5–1 mEq/kg of calcium chloride infused over 5–10 minutes may be used; this dose may be repeated in 6 hours or followed with a continuous infusion with 2.5 mEq/kg/d of calcium chloride.[89,90] If hypomagnesemia is present, magnesium supplementation should be given to facilitate correction of hypocalcemia. In cases of hypocalcemia secondary to hyperphosphatemia, treating with an oral phosphate binder should be considered prior to giving intravenous calcium to prevent calcium/phosphate precipitation in soft tissues.

Hypercalcemia

Hypercalcemia is most often seen in patients with hyperparathyroidism or cancer with bone metastases. It can also occur with toxic serum concentrations of vitamin A or vitamin D, chronic ingestion of milk and/or calcium carbonate-containing antacids in the setting of kidney insufficiency, immobility, tuberculosis, and medications. Clinical signs and symptoms include fatigue, nausea, vomiting, constipation, anorexia, and confusion. In severe cases, cardiac dysrhythmias may be present. Mild hypercalcemia typically responds to fluid and ambulation. In severe hypercalcemia,

immediate treatment should be started to prevent acute kidney failure, obtundation, ventricular dysrhythmias, coma, and death. If a loop diuretic and intravenous fluid are used to treat hypercalcemia (eg, to increase calcium excretion), intravenous hydration with 0.9% sodium chloride should be started immediately to prevent dehydration. Hemodialysis may be necessary for patients with life-threatening hypercalcemia or those with kidney failure.[91] Bisphosphonates have been used to treat hypercalcemia of malignancy, but these are not effective in acute hypercalcemia due to their delayed onset of action.

Phosphorus

Newborn:	4.5–9 mg/dL
10 days–2 years:	4.5–6.7 mg/dL
2–12 years:	4.5–5.5 mg/dL
>12 years:	2.7–4.5 mg/dL

Phosphorus, mainly in the form of phosphate, is the primary intracellular anion in the body. It has many important functions including bone and cell membrane composition, maintenance of normal pH, and provision of energy-rich bonds (ATP), making it integral in all cellular functions that require energy. Phosphorus is required for glucose utilization, glycolysis, 2,3-diphosphoglycerate synthesis, neurological function, and muscle function.[92-94] Phosphorus homeostasis is maintained by GI absorption, renal excretion, PTH, and distribution between the ICF and ECF. Glucose and insulin, catecholamines, and alkalosis all cause an intracellular shift of phosphorus. Cell destruction and acidosis cause a shift to the ECF. Intravenous phosphorus requirements are 1–2.5 mmol/kg in premature infants and 0.5–1 mmol/kg/d in term infants and children up to 18 years of age. Oral phosphorus requirements vary with age (Table 9-4). An algorithm for the adjustment of maintenance electrolytes in intravenous fluids can be found in Figure 9-5.

Hypophosphatemia

Hypophosphatemia is defined as a serum phosphorus concentration below 2.7–4.5 mg/dL, depending on the patient's age.[95] Hypophosphatemia is common in critical illness, malnutrition, and alkalosis and in patients receiving phosphate binders (eg, aluminum-, magnesium-, and calcium-containing products, sevelamer, or sucralfate). Signs and symptoms of hypophosphatemia reflect neurologic, neuromuscular, cardiopulmonary, and hematologic dysfunction.[92-94] Primary causes of hypophosphatemia include inadequate intake of phosphate or the administration of large amounts of dextrose solutions in malnourished (refeeding syndrome) (Chapter 19).

Treatment of hypophosphatemia varies, depending on the serum phosphorus concentration and the presence of signs and symptoms. Mild asymptomatic hypophosphatemia can be treated with oral phosphate supplements, assuming that the GI tract is functional. However, oral supplements are not well absorbed and often cause diarrhea. Currently, no oral liquid phosphorus supplements are commercially available, but the saline enema containing monobasic and dibasic sodium phosphate (phosphate at 1.5 mmol/mL) can be used if a liquid preparation is needed. Patients with symptomatic or moderate to severe hypophosphatemia should be treated with intravenous phosphate. Three salt forms are available for replacing phosphate: sodium phosphate, potassium phosphate, and sodium glycerophosphate. Sodium phosphate provides 4 mEq sodium for every 3 mmol phosphate, potassium phosphate provides 4.4 mEq potassium for every 3 mmol phosphate, and sodium glycerophosphate provides 2 mEq of sodium for every 1 mmol of phosphate. In the order for phosphate, the dose should be in millimoles of phosphate rather than milliequivalents of the sodium or potassium component of the salt. A common recommendation for replacing phosphate is to provide up to 0.32 mmol/kg of phosphate for a serum phosphorus concentration < 1.5 mg/dL. However, this dose is often inadequate and multiple boluses may be required to restore normal phosphorus concentrations.[96,97] Higher doses have been recommended for phosphorus replacement in adults, and these higher supplemental doses have been used successfully in pediatric patients (Table 9-6). Serum phosphate concentrations should be checked 1–2 hours after the infusion is completed, and the patient should receive additional doses, as needed. Phosphate should be replaced no faster than 0.1–0.2 mmol/kg/h to allow the phosphate time to move intracellularly and to prevent possible hypocalcemia.[98] This rate usually necessitates a 4- to 6-hour infusion. If potassium phosphate is used to replace the phosphate, the infusion rate should be based on the potassium infusion rate. Electrocardiogram monitoring should accompany infusion of individual doses > 0.5

mEq/kg/h. Sodium phosphate is the preferred salt for phosphate supplementation.

Hyperphosphatemia

Hyperphosphatemia is defined as a serum phosphate concentration greater than 4.5–9 mg/dL, depending on the patient's age. Most patients are asymptomatic, but signs and symptoms may include anorexia, nausea, vomiting, dehydration, and neuromuscular irritability. The biggest concern with hyperphosphatemia is soft tissue and vascular calcification from elevated serum calcium and phosphorus concentrations.[99] Although various equations for predicting metastatic calcification are used, the equations are not accurate because of the variety of factors that determine in vivo calcium and phosphate solubility. Ionized calcium is much more reactive than phosphate, so hypercalcemia with a mild hyperphosphatemia has a higher probability of causing metastatic calcification than hyperphosphatemia with slightly increased serum calcium. With the newer phosphate-binding agents available, aluminum-containing antacids are no longer recommended for treating or preventing hyperphosphatemia in patients with kidney insufficiency because of the anemia, osteomalacia, and central nervous system toxicity experienced with the use of aluminum-containing agents in this patient population.[100,101]

Test Your Knowledge Questions

1. The intravenous administration of 100 mL of 0.9% sodium chloride to a patient will
   A. Increase the intracellular fluid (ICF) compartment by 67 mL and increase the extracellular fluid (ECF) compartment by 33 mL.
   B. Increase the ECF compartment by 100 mL, with a 25-mL increase in intravascular volume and a 75-mL increase in interstitial volume.
   C. Increase the ECF compartment by 100 mL, with a 75-mL increase in intravascular volume and a 25-mL increase in interstitial volume.
   D. Increase the ICF compartment by 100 mL.

2. A 1340-g neonate is placed on intravenous fluids/nutrition at 160 mL/kg/d. Over the next 5 days, the weight decreases to 1250 g due to extracellular fluid contraction seen after birth. On day 7, the patient's serum sodium concentration is 137 mEq/L. The patient continues to receive 160 mL/kg/d of intravenous fluids that contain 3 mEq/kg/d of sodium. Over the next 3 days, the patient's serum sodium concentration has decreased to 129 mEq/L. The patient does not appear to be fluid

Table 9-6. Phosphate Replacement in Adults

DEPLETION	REPLACEMENT, mmol/kg
Mild (2.3–3 mg/dL)	0.16
Moderate (1.6–2.2 mg/dL)	0.32
Severe (<1.5 mg/dL)	0.64

overloaded, septic, or suffering from necrotizing entero-colitis. The patient's weight has remained around 1250 g. What is the most appropriate way to correct the serum sodium concentration?

A. Increase the sodium concentration in the intravenous solution because the current sodium intake is inadequate to keep up with the renal and gastrointestinal sodium losses.

B. Decrease the maintenance intravenous fluid rate by 25% because the decrease in the serum sodium concentration is probably due to fluid overload.

C. Give 3% sodium chloride intravenously to replace the sodium deficit.

D. Decrease the maintenance intravenous fluid by 25% and give sodium chloride orally because the decrease in the serum sodium concentration is probably due to fluid overload, but the serum sodium concentration is a critical value; thus treatment must begin immediately.

3. An 8-year-old child who weighs 27 kg is admitted for nausea, vomiting, and failure-to-thrive. The patient is started on maintenance intravenous fluids containing $D_{10}W/0.2\%$ NaCl with KCl at 20 mEq/L. The following morning, the serum phosphorus concentration is 1.2 mg/dL, the potassium concentration is 3.2 mEq/L, and the magnesium concentration is 1.5 mg/dL. What is the most appropriate way to correct these serum electrolyte abnormalities?

A. Increase the amounts of magnesium, phosphorus/phosphate, and potassium in the maintenance intravenous fluid.

B. Keep the intravenous fluids the same and give oral or intravenous supplements of magnesium, phosphorus/phosphate, and potassium.

C. Keep the intravenous fluids the same, none of the serum levels are so critical that they would require acute treatment.

D. Increase the amounts of magnesium, phosphorus/phosphate, and potassium in the maintenance intravenous fluid and give oral or intravenous supplements of magnesium, phosphorus/phosphate, and potassium.

References

1. Steijaert M, Deurenberg P, Van Gaal L, De Leeuw I. The use of multi-frequency impedance to determine total body water and extracellular water in obese and lean female individuals. *Int J Obes Relat Metab Disord.* 1997;21(10):930–934.
2. Sartorio A, Malavolti M, Agosti F, et al. Body water distribution in severe obesity and its assessment from eight-polar bioelectrical impedance analysis. *Eur J Clin Nutr.* 2005;59(2):155–160.
3. Hellerstein S. Fluids and electrolytes: physiology. *Pediatr Rev.* 1993;14(2):70–79.
4. Bhatia J. Fluid and electrolyte management in the very low birth weight neonate. *J Perinatol.* 2006;26 Suppl 1:S19–S21.
5. Guignard JP, John EG. Renal function in the tiny, premature infant. *Clin Perinatol.* 1986;13(2):377–401.
6. Desai TK, Carlson RW, Geheb MA. Prevalence and clinical implications of hypocalcemia in acutely ill patients in a medical intensive care setting. *Am J Med.* 1988;84(2):209–214.
7. Galva C, Artigas P, Gatto C. Nuclear Na+/K+-ATPase plays an active role in nucleoplasmic Ca2+ homeostasis. *J Cell Sci.* 2012;125(Pt 24):6137–6147.
8. Lobo DN. Fluid, electrolytes and nutrition: physiological and clinical aspects. *Proc Nutr Soc.* 2004;63(3):453–466.
9. Bahrami S, Zimmermann K, Szelenyi Z, et al. Small-volume fluid resuscitation with hypertonic saline prevents inflammation but not mortality in a rat model of hemorrhagic shock. *Shock.* 2006;25(3):283–289.
10. Mange K, Matsuura D, Cizman B, et al. Language guiding therapy: the case of dehydration versus volume depletion. *Ann Intern Med.* 1997;127(9):848–853.
11. Jacob M, Chappell D. Reappraising starling: the physiology of the microcirculation. *Curr Opin Crit Care.* 2013;19(4):282–289.
12. Toney GM, Chen QH, Cato MJ, Stocker SD. Central osmotic regulation of sympathetic nerve activity. *Acta Physiol Scand.* 2003;177(1):43–55.
13. Sutsch G, Bertel O, Rickenbacher P, et al. Regulation of aldosterone secretion in patients with chronic congestive heart failure by endothelins. *Am J Cardiol.* 2000;85(8):973–976.
14. Quinn SJ, Williams GH. Regulation of aldosterone secretion. *Annu Rev Physiol.* 1988;50:409–426.
15. Weber KT. Aldosterone in congestive heart failure. *N Engl J Med.* 2001;345(23):1689–1697.
16. Thompson CJ, Bland J, Burd J, Baylis PH. The osmotic thresholds for thirst and vasopressin release are similar in healthy man. *Clin Sci (Lond).* 1986;71(6):651–656.
17. Robertson GL. Thirst and vasopressin function in normal and disordered states of water balance. *J Lab Clin Med.* 1983;101(3):351–371.
18. Harring TR, Deal NS, Kuo DC. Disorders of sodium and water balance. *Emerg Med Clin North Am.* 2014;32(2):379–401.
19. Holliday MA, Segar WE. The maintenance need for water in parenteral fluid therapy. *Pediatrics.* 1957;19(5):823–832.
20. Choong K, Bohn D. Maintenance parenteral fluids in the critically ill child. *J Pediatr (Rio J).* 2007;83(2 Suppl):S3–S10.
21. Lorenz JM, Kleinman LI, Ahmed G, Markarian K. Phases of fluid and electrolyte homeostasis in the extremely low birth weight infant. *Pediatrics.* 1995;96(3 Pt 1):484–489.
22. Modi N. Sodium intake and preterm babies. *Arch Dis Child.* 1993;69(1 Spec No):87–91.
23. Bauer K, Bovermann G, Roithmaier A, Gotz M, Proiss A, Versmold HT. Body composition, nutrition, and fluid bal-

ance during the first two weeks of life in preterm neonates weighing less than 1500 grams. *J Pediatr.* 1991;118(4 Pt 1):615–620.

24. Sankar MJ, Agarwal R, Mishra S, Deorari AK, Paul VK. Feeding of low birth weight infants. *Indian J Pediatr.* 2008;75(5):459–469.

25. Shaffer SG, Bradt SK, Hall RT. Postnatal changes in total body water and extracellular volume in the preterm infant with respiratory distress syndrome. *J Pediatr.* 1986;109(3):509–514.

26. Tang W, Ridout D, Modi N. Influence of respiratory distress syndrome on body composition after preterm birth. *Arch Dis Child Fetal Neonatal Ed.* 1997;77(1):F28–31.

27. Rutter N, Hull D. Water loss from the skin of term and preterm babies. *Arch Dis Child.* 1979;54(11):858–868.

28. Costarino A, Baumgart S. Modern fluid and electrolyte management of the critically ill premature infant. *Pediatr Clin North Am.* 1986;33(1):153–178.

29. Kjartansson S, Hammarlund K, Sedin G. Insensible water loss from the skin during phototherapy in term and preterm infants. *Acta Paediatr.* 1992;81(10):764–768.

30. Grunhagen DJ, de Boer MG, de Beaufort AJ, Walther FJ. Transepidermal water loss during halogen spotlight phototherapy in preterm infants. *Pediatr Res.* 2002;51(3):402–405.

31. Maayan-Metzger A, Yosipovitch G, Hadad E, Sirota L. Transepidermal water loss and skin hydration in preterm infants during phototherapy. *Am J Perinatol.* 2001;18(7):393–396.

32. Hartnoll G. Basic principles and practical steps in the management of fluid balance in the newborn. *Semin Neonatol.* 2003;8(4):307–313.

33. Chawla D, Agarwal R, Deorari AK, Paul VK. Fluid and electrolyte management in term and preterm neonates. *Indian J Pediatr.* 2008;75(3):255–259.

34. Keane M. Recognising and managing acute hyponatraemia. *Emerg Nurse.* 2014;21(9):32–36.

35. Zimmerman EA, Ma LY, Nilaver G. Anatomical basis of thirst and vasopressin secretion. *Kidney Int Suppl.* 1987;21:S14–19.

36. Ranadive SA, Rosenthal SM. Pediatric disorders of water balance. *Pediatr Clin North Am.* 2011;58(5):1271–1280.

37. Mange K, Matsuura D, Cizman B, et al. Language guiding therapy: the case of dehydration versus volume depletion. *Ann Intern Med.* 1997;127(9):848–853.

38. Mariscalco G, Musumeci F. Fluid management in the cardiothoracic intensive care unit: diuresis--diuretics and hemofiltration. *Curr Opin Anaesthesiol.* 2014;27(2):133–139.

39. Roberts KB. Fluid and electrolytes: parenteral fluid therapy. *Pediatr Rev.* 2001;22(11):380–387.

40. Finberg L. Hypernatremic (hypertonic) dehydration in infants. *N Engl J Med.* 1973;289(4):196–198.

41. Uretsky BF, Verbalis JG, Generalovich T, Valdes A, Reddy PS. Plasma vasopressin response to osmotic and hemodynamic stimuli in heart failure. *Am J Physiol.* 1985;248(3 Pt 2):H396–H402.

42. Ghali JK, Tam SW. The critical link of hypervolemia and hyponatremia in heart failure and the potential role of arginine vasopressin antagonists. *J Card Fail.* 2010;16(5):419–431.

43. Hori M. Tolvaptan for the treatment of hyponatremia and hypervolemia in patients with congestive heart failure. *Future Cardiol.* 2013;9(2):163–176.

44. Baram M, Kommuri A, Sellers SA, Cohn JR. ACE inhibitor-induced angioedema. *J Allergy Clin Immunol Pract.* 2013;1(5):442–445.

45. Hillmeister P, Persson PB. The kallikrein-kinin system. *Acta Physiol (Oxf).* 2012;206(4):215–219.

46. Wilkins BH. Renal function in sick very low birthweight infants: 3. Sodium, potassium, and water excretion. *Arch Dis Child.* 1992;67(10 Spec No):1154–1161.

47. Hartnoll G, Betremieux P, Modi N. Randomised controlled trial of postnatal sodium supplementation on body composition in 25 to 30 week gestational age infants. *Arch Dis Child Fetal Neonatal Ed.* 2000;82(1):F24–F28.

48. Katz MA. Hyperglycemia-induced hyponatremia—calculation of expected serum sodium depression. *N Engl J Med.* 1973;289(16):843–844.

49. Hillier TA, Abbott RD, Barrett EJ. Hyponatremia: evaluating the correction factor for hyperglycemia. *Am J Med.* 1999;106(4):399–403.

50. Holliday MA, Kalayci MN, Harrah J. Factors that limit brain volume changes in response to acute and sustained hyper- and hyponatremia. *J Clin Invest.* 1968;47(8):1916–1928.

51. Gomez-Sanchez CE, Oki K. Minireview: potassium channels and aldosterone dysregulation: is primary aldosteronism a potassium channelopathy? *Endocrinology.* 2014;155(1):47–55.

52. Horisberger JD, Lemas V, Kraehenbuhl JP, Rossier BC. Structure-function relationship of Na,K-ATPase. *Annu Rev Physiol.* 1991;53:565–584.

53. Rodriguez-Soriano J. Potassium homeostasis and its disturbances in children. *Pediatr Nephrol.* 1995;9(3):364–374.

54. Ganguly A. Primary aldosteronism. *N Engl J Med.* 1998;339(25):1828–1834.

55. Klevay LM, Bogden JD, Aladjem M, et al. Renal and gastrointestinal potassium excretion in humans: new insight based on new data and review and analysis of published studies. *J Am Coll Nutr.* 2007;26(2):103–110.

56. Mathialahan T, Sandle GI. Dietary potassium and laxatives as regulators of colonic potassium secretion in end-stage renal disease. *Nephrol Dial Transplant.* 2003;18(2):341–347.

57. Brown RS. Extrarenal potassium homeostasis. *Kidney Int.* 1986;30(1):116–127.

58. Strom BL, Carson JL, Schinnar R, et al. Upper gastrointestinal tract bleeding from oral potassium chloride. comparative risk from microencapsulated vs wax-matrix formulations. *Arch Intern Med.* 1987;147(5):954–957.

59. Taketomo C, Hodding J, Kraus D, eds. Potassium chloride. In: *Pediatric and Neonatal Dosage Handbook.* 20th ed. Hudson, OH: Lexicomp; 2013.

60. Phelps S, Hak E, Crill C, eds. Potassium chloride. In: *The Teddy Bear Book: Pediatric Injectable Drugs.* 9th ed. Bethesda, MD: American Society of Health-System Pharmacist Inc; 2010.

61. Unwin RJ, Luft FC, Shirley DG. Pathophysiology and management of hypokalemia: a clinical perspective. *Nat Rev Nephrol.* 2011;7(2):75–84.

62. Whang R, Whang DD, Ryan MP. Refractory potassium repletion. A consequence of magnesium deficiency. *Arch Intern Med.* 1992;152(1):40–45.

63. Subramanian S, Agarwal R, Deorari AK, Paul VK, Bagga A. Acute renal failure in neonates. *Indian J Pediatr.* 2008;75(4):385–391.

64. Reinhart RA. Magnesium metabolism. A review with special reference to the relationship between intracellular content and serum levels. *Arch Intern Med.* 1988;148(11):2415–2420.

65. Castiglioni S, Cazzaniga A, Albisetti W, Maier JA. Magnesium and osteoporosis: current state of knowledge and future research directions. *Nutrients.* 2013;5(8):3022–3033.

66. Quamme GA. Laboratory evaluation of magnesium status. renal function and free intracellular magnesium concentration. *Clin Lab Med.* 1993;13(1):209–223.

67. Weisinger JR, Bellorin-Font E. Magnesium and phosphorus. *Lancet.* 1998;352(9125):391–396.

68. Lee CT, Tsai WY, Tung YC, Tsau YK. Transient pseudohypoparathyroidism as a cause of late-onset hypocalcemia in neonates and infants. *J Formos Med Assoc.* 2008;107(10):806–810.

69. Ryzen E, Wagers PW, Singer FR, Rude RK. Magnesium deficiency in a medical ICU population. *Crit Care Med.* 1985;13(1):19–21.

70. Dacey MJ. Hypomagnesemic disorders. *Crit Care Clin.* 2001;17(1):155–173.

71. Taketomo C, Hodding J, Kraus D, eds. Magnesium sulfate. In: *Pediatric and Neonatal Dosage Handbook.* 20th ed. Hudson, OH: Lexicomp; 2013.

72. Topf JM, Murray PT. Hypomagnesemia and hypermagnesemia. *Rev Endocr Metab Disord.* 2003;4(2):195–206.

73. Oster JR, Epstein M. Management of magnesium depletion. *Am J Nephrol.* 1988;8(5):349–354.

74. Rose B, Post T. *Clinical Physiology of Acid-Base and Electrolyte Disorders.* 5th ed. New York, NY: McGraw-Hill; 2001.

75. Hebert P, Mehta N, Wang J, Hindmarsh T, Jones G, Cardinal P. Functional magnesium deficiency in critically ill patients identified using a magnesium-loading test. *Crit Care Med.* 1997;25(5):749–755.

76. Teng RJ, Wu TJ, Sharma R, Garrison RD, Hudak ML. Early neonatal hypotension in premature infants born to preeclamptic mothers. *J Perinatol.* 2006;26(8):471–475.

77. Whang R, Ryder KW. Frequency of hypomagnesemia and hypermagnesemia. Requested vs routine. *JAMA.* 1990;263(22):3063–3064.

78. Riaz M, Porat R, Hurt H. The effects of maternal magnesium sulfate treatment on newborns: a prospective controlled study. *J Perinatol.* 1998;18(6 pt 1):449–454.

79. Ramsey PS, Rouse DJ. Magnesium sulfate as a tocolytic agent. *Semin Perinatol.* 2001;25(4):236–247.

80. Chattopadhyay N, Mithal A, Brown EM. The calcium-sensing receptor: a window into the physiology and pathophysiology of mineral ion metabolism. *Endocr Rev.* 1996;17(4):289–307.

81. Chang WT, Radin B, McCurdy MT. Calcium, magnesium, and phosphate abnormalities in the emergency department. *Emerg Med Clin North Am.* 2014;32(2):349–366.

82. Jain A, Agarwal R, Sankar MJ, Deorari AK, Paul VK. Hypocalcemia in the newborn. *Indian J Pediatr.* 2008;75(2):165–169.

83. Bushinsky DA, Monk RD. Electrolyte quintet: calcium. *Lancet.* 1998;352(9124):306–311.

84. Moe SM. Disorders involving calcium, phosphorus and magnesium. *Prim Care Clin Office Pract.* 2008;35(2):215–237.

85. Schmidt GL, Baumgartner TG, Fischlschweiger W, Sitren HS, Thakker KM, Cerda JJ. Cost containment using cysteine HCl acidification to increase calcium/phosphate solubility in hyperalimentation solutions. *J Parenter Enteral Nutr.* 1986;10(2):203–207.

86. Wood RJ, Sitrin MD, Cusson GJ, Rosenberg IH. Reduction of total parenteral nutrition-induced urinary calcium loss by increasing the phosphorus in the total parenteral nutrition prescription. *J Parenter Enteral Nutr.* 1986;10(2):188–190.

87. Semple P, Booth C. Calcium chloride; a reminder. *Anaesthesia.* 1996;51(1):93.

88. Phelps S, Hak E, Crill C, eds. Calcium chloride. In: *The Teddy Bear Book: Pediatric Injectable Drugs.* 9th ed. Bethesda, MD: American Society of Health-System Pharmacists Inc; 2010.

89. Taketomo C, Hodding J, Kraus D, eds. Calcium chloride. In: *Pediatric and Neonatal Dosage Handbook.* 20th ed. Hudson, OH: Lexicomp; 2013.

90. Davis KD, Attie MF. Management of severe hypercalcemia. *Crit Care Clin.* 1991;7(1):175–190.

91. Zivin JR, Gooley T, Zager RA, Ryan MJ. Hypocalcemia: a pervasive metabolic abnormality in the critically ill. *Am J Kidney Dis.* 2001;37(4):689–698.

92. Peppers MP, Geheb M, Desai T. Endocrine crises. Hypophosphatemia and hyperphosphatemia. *Crit Care Clin.* 1991;7(1):201–214.

93. Knochel JP. The pathophysiology and clinical characteristics of severe hypophosphatemia. *Arch Intern Med.* 1977;137(2):203–220.

94. Worley G, Claerhout SJ, Combs SP. Hypophosphatemia in malnourished children during refeeding. *Clin Pediatr (Phila).* 1998;37(6):347–352.

95. Taketomo C, Hodding J, Kraus D, eds. Potassium phosphate. In: *Pediatric and Neonatal Dosage Handbook.* 20th ed. Hudson, OH: Lexicomp; 2013.

96. Goodman WG, Goldin J, Kuizon BD, et al. Coronary-artery calcification in young adults with end-stage renal disease who are undergoing dialysis. *N Engl J Med.* 2000;342(20):1478–1483.

97. Phelps S, Hak E, Crill C, eds. Potassium phosphate. In: *The Teddy Bear Book: Pediatric Injectable Drugs.* 9th ed. Bethesda, MD: American Society of Health-System Pharmacists Inc; 2010.

98. Ritz E. The clinical management of hyperphosphatemia. *J Nephrol.* 2005;18(3):221–228.

99. Clark CL, Sacks GS, Dickerson RN, Kudsk KA, Brown RO. Treatment of hypophosphatemia in patients receiving specialized nutrition support using a graduated dosing scheme: results from a prospective clinical trial. *Crit Care Med.* 1995;23(9):1504–1511.

100. Sperschneider H, Gunther K, Marzoll I, Kirchner E, Stein G. Calcium carbonate (CaCO3): an efficient and safe phos-

phate binder in haemodialysis patients? A 3-year study. *Nephrol Dial Transplant.* 1993;8(6):530–534.

101. Bhan I. Phosphate management in chronic kidney disease. *Curr Opin Nephrol Hypertens.* 2014;23(2):174–179.

Test Your Knowledge Answers

1. The correct answer is **B**. Fluid gains in the body compartments depend on the volume and osmolarity of the fluid administered. Administering 100 mL of 0.9% sodium chloride (154 mEq/L of sodium) will not alter the plasma osmolarity because it is iso-osmotic. The sodium will be held in the ECF by the Na^+-K^+-ATPase pump, and the water stays with the sodium. Therefore, all of the administered volume (100 mL) will stay in the ECF compartment. Because 25% of the ECF compartment is intravascular volume, the intravascular volume will increase by 25 mL, and because 75% of the ECF is interstitial volume, the interstitial volume will increase by 75 mL.

2. The correct answer is **A**. A low serum sodium concentration is the result of either an increase in TBW or a decrease in total body sodium with a subsequent decrease in TBW. The weight has not changed significantly over the past 3 days, and the sodium intake (3 mEq/kg/d)

may not be sufficient for a 1250-g neonate. Therefore, the renal and GI losses are probably exceeding the sodium intake, resulting in the decreased serum sodium concentration. The correct treatment would be to increase the sodium concentration in the maintenance intravenous fluids. The sodium chloride is not at a critical level, so acute replacement with 3% sodium chloride would not be necessary.

3. The correct answer is **B**. The low serum magnesium, phosphorus, and potassium concentrations are most likely a result of the intracellular shift seen in malnourished patients when dextrose is administered and should be treated acutely (oral or intravenous supplement). A supplemental intravenous infusion of sodium phosphate and magnesium sulfate would be more appropriate than adding sodium phosphate and magnesium sulfate to the maintenance intravenous solution. A serum potassium concentration of 3.2 mEq/L could be treated either orally or intravenously with a supplemental dose. Once the intracellular/extracellular electrolyte shifts have stabilized, (usually 2–3 days), decreases in serum concentrations would indicate an inadequate amount of electrolytes in the maintenance fluids and then maintenance fluids should be adjusted.

PART II

AGE-SPECIFIC NUTRITION FOR GROWTH AND DEVELOPMENT

10

Nutrition and Early Development

Ricardo Rueda, MD, PhD; Esther Castanys-Muñoz, PhD; Richard W. Gelling, PhD; José M. López-Pedrosa, PhD; Yen-Ling Low, PhD; Christina Sherry, PhD, RD; and Barbara Marriage, PhD, RD

CONTENTS

Learning Objectives

1. Achieve familiarity with the normal physiology and metabolism of the fetus and know nutrient deficiencies associated with adverse pregnancy outcomes.
2. Know common late adverse manifestations of early programming observed in epidemiologic and animal studies.
3. Be aware of potential mechanisms involved in late and transgenerational effects of early-life programming.

Introduction

Dietary inadequacy, imbalance, or excess can all impact fetal development. Some of these changes persist throughout life or leave the individual vulnerable to later environmental and dietary conditions that can adversely impact health and longevity. This chapter aims to provide an updated overview on the importance of nutrition during sensitive periods such as pregnancy and lactation, together with the crucial role it plays, not only on fetal development but also on the long-term health of the offspring.

We will first address how maternal dietary deficiencies during pregnancy and nutrition during lactation affect the fetus and the infant, respectively. In addition, the impact of nutrition and other stresses on fetal metabolism will be evaluated. We will then focus on how prenatal and postnatal programming effects are integrated, and a summary on the different animal models used in developmental programming studies will be presented. To conclude, the persistence of adverse effects across several generations and the implications for future health and current practice will be discussed.

Pregnancy

Physiology of Pregnancy

A healthy pregnancy is dependent on maternal nutrition status at conception and an adequate blood flow to deliver oxygen and nutrients to the placenta and fetus, as well as maintenance of the appropriate hormonal milieu (from maternal, fetal, and placental origins) to support placental and fetal development. Early in gestation, the placental to fetal weight ratio is high, and this ratio declines in later gestation. Initially, placental transport largely depends on increases in placental size, but later in pregnancy, both placental transport function and placental size must increase to meet the needs of the rapidly growing fetus.

The placenta acts as the main interface between mother and fetus and largely controls nutrient availability and consequently fetal growth. The primary barrier to placental nutrient transport is the syncytiotrophoblast, which features polarized microvillous maternal-facing membranes and fetal-facing baso-lateral membranes. This specialized multinucleated epithelial cell layer produces multiple hormones, expresses numerous nutrient transporters, and acts as the physical and immunological barrier between the maternal and fetal circulation. Highly permeable molecules, like respiratory gases, are transported bidirectionally across the syncytiotrophoblast, and their transport can be largely influenced by changes in blood flow. Less permeable nutrients and molecules are conveyed by both passive and active transport mechanisms intrinsic to the placenta. As such, alterations in placental transport can play a key role as mediator-integrator of maternal nutrition effects on fetal overgrowth and undergrowth and the later lifelong health outcomes associated with these conditions.[1]

The major energy source for the fetus is glucose, which is transported by facilitated diffusion and therefore largely driven by maternal-fetal concentration gradients.[2] It also uses lactate produced in the placenta and endogenously.[3] The fetal pancreas secretes insulin by mid-gestation and responds to variations in the glucose delivery rate. Normally the fetal liver is not active in gluconeogenesis. Fetal tissue glucose transporters and intracellular downstream metabolic regulators are modulated by glucose and insulin levels in the fetus. Insulin-responsive fetal tissues include the heart, liver, skeletal muscle, and adipose tissue. Fetal glucose oxidation is maintained even when fetal glucose supply is limited, which indicates that placental glucose uptake is not regulated by insulin: "…The fetus develops with mech-anisms that tend to keep its energy metabolism relatively constant, while growth is, at times of deficient energy supply, expendable."[4]

Amino acids are the second most important macronutrient in the fetus with at least 14 complex amino acid transporter systems on both of the syncytiotrophoblast membranes.[5] The transport of large neutral and branched-chain amino acids is the most directly proportional to their maternal concentration.[6] All amino acids except tryptophan are more highly concentrated in the placenta than in maternal blood. Leucine appears to have specific trophic effects on the placenta and the fetus, possibly because of its impact on the mammalian target of rapamycin (mTOR), which is a critical regulator of protein synthesis and is involved in placental nutrient sensing mechanisms.[7] Fetuses with intrauterine growth restriction (IUGR) have reduced fetal enrichment of leucine relative to the maternal circulation.[8] Other specific amino acids such as arginine also have not only nutrient effects but similar regulatory and developmental effects as well.[5]

When less oxygen, glucose, and amino acids are available to the fetus because of reduced umbilical vein blood flow (associated with placental transport insufficiency), fetal weight gain slows. Compensatory increases occur in fetal amino acid catabolism to minimize changes in fetal blood amino acid concentrations. This situation is associated with altered substrate distribution and changes in relative organ growth. When glucose (and other substrate) supply is limited and the fetus is relatively hypoglycemic, growth of the brain, kidney, and adrenals is protected to the detriment of other organs, such as spleen, liver, pancreas, and lung.[9] A redistribution of blood flow leads to slower growth, altered fetal liver metabolism, and reduced pancreatic β-cell mass or function, depending on the stage of pregnancy. The most common cause of IUGR is placental transport insufficiency (oxygen, glucose, amino acids), which may be related to local uterine factors, maternal malnutrition, advanced maternal diabetes, hypertension, or other maternal or placental pathology.[10,11]

Central metabolic mediators for regulatory hormone and metabolic changes in the fetus are fetal insulin, cortisol (increased levels of which are associated with reduced glucose uptake, increased gluconeogenesis, and slower fetal growth), and insulin-like growth factors (IGFs), which are critical for placental development and function and protein synthesis in fetal tissues.[12,13]

Common metabolic/hormonal derangements that influence organ growth and metabolic development of the fetus include hypoglycemia, hyperglycemia, maternal or gestational diabetes, and activation of the fetal hypothalamic-pituitary-adrenal (HPA) axis by a variety of intrauterine insults.[14,15] The fetus and its uteroplacental support system are highly adaptive to their vascular supply, oxygenation state, and metabolic substrate availability. In this formative stage of life, a multitude of responses at the fetal, organ, tissue, membrane, cytosolic, and nuclear levels determine the survival, health, and function of the fetus. Some of these adaptations are transient and others, particularly with prolonged exposure, appear to be permanent.[16] Epigenetic modifications of cells in specific organs help determine the final metabolic phenotype, which is a product of both genetic inheritance and developmental environmental influences on gene expression. Vulnerability to environmental and dietary influences appears to continue well past the time of birth. Fetal and early postnatal plasticity allows survival, but may also set the stage for later maladaptive metabolic responses, particularly to metabolic environments different from those experienced early in development (eg, food surfeits versus scarcity).[1,14]

Impact of Maternal Dietary Deficiencies on the Fetus

Maternal nutrition during pregnancy can exert long-lasting effects on the health of the offspring.[17] These effects may be due to undernutrition or deficit of specific nutrients or to an excess of energy or nutrients. Epidemiological and animal studies suggest that fetal adaptive responses to the intrauterine environment, including maternal malnutrition, overnutrition, or diabetes, may increase the risk of many chronic diseases in adulthood, including type 2 diabetes and coronary heart disease (CHD).[18] Animal studies also show that both maternal undernutrition and overnutrition reduce placental-fetal blood flow and slow fetal growth. Impaired placental synthesis of nitric oxide, a major vasodilator and angiogenesis factor, and polyamines, key regulators of DNA and protein synthesis, may provide an explanation for IUGR in response to the 2 extremes of nutrition problems with the same pregnancy outcome. Placental and fetal growth is the most vulnerable to maternal nutrition status during the peri-implantation period and the period of rapid placental development (the first trimester of gestation).

Extensive clinical research, using both observational and interventional study designs, has allowed some quantification of the effects of maternal anthropometric indices, dietary intake in pregnancy, and nutritional supplements with respect to measures of fetal size, maturity at birth, and developmental outcomes. Overall, these studies find a strong positive association between maternal prepregnancy nutrition status and the ability of a mother to nourish her growing fetus. Accumulating evidence also suggests that both periconceptional undernutrition and pregnancy undernutrition are important determinants of the length of gestation and fetal growth and development. Gestational weight gain and nutrition interventions during pregnancy appear able to modify this association by altering the rate of fetal growth, although the extent of the modification appears to be dependent on maternal baseline nutrition status and is modest.[19] Current estimates of nutrition needs are provided in Table 10-1.

Macronutrients

During pregnancy, extra energy (and therefore macronutrient intake) is required by the mother to support the growth of the fetus, placenta, and various maternal tissues, such as in the uterus and breast, and for the deposition of fat stores. In terms of maternal macronutrient status, deficiency of macronutrients, protein and carbohydrates, during pregnancy and gestation results in lower infant birth weight, a surrogate marker of fetal growth, and may predispose the offspring to insulin resistance, glucose intolerance, hypertension, and adiposity in adulthood.[20] Some studies have also demonstrated that a low-protein diet in utero has a deleterious effect on bone development in the offspring that persists into adulthood.[21] In these studies, the offspring displayed significant differences in bone structure and density at various sites. These differences are indicative of significantly altered bone turnover.[22]

Balanced protein-energy supplementation is designed to provide less than 25% of total energy content and is believed to be the most suitable supplement for malnourished pregnant women.[23] A Cochrane review published in 2012 found that balanced energy and protein supplementation in pregnant women is associated with clear increases in mean birth weight, with fewer stillbirths and fewer small-for-gestational-age (SGA) births. In contrast, high-protein supplementation or isocaloric protein supplementations (in which protein replaces an equal quantity of nonprotein energy) showed no benefit.[24] Hence, current evidence indicates that balanced protein-energy supplementation is an effective intervention to reduce the prevalence of low birth weight (LBW) and SGA births, especially in undernourished women.

Table 10-1. Recommended Daily Nutrient Intakes During Pregnancy

NUTRIENT	RECOMMENDED DAILY INTAKE
Water	3 L
Energy	Varies by age, pregnancy stage, body mass index, activity
Carbohydrate	175 g
Total fiber	28 g
Linoleic acid	13 g
Linolenic acid	1.4 g
Protein	71 g
Vitamin A	750–770 mcg[a]
Vitamin C	80–85 mg/d[a]
Vitamin D	15 mcg
Vitamin E	15 mg
Vitamin K	75–90 mcg[a]
Thiamin	1.4 mg
Riboflavin	1.4 mg
Niacin	18 mg
Vitamin B$_6$	1.9 mg
Folate	600 mcg
Vitamin B$_{12}$	2.6 mcg
Pantothenic acid	6 mg
Biotin	30 mcg
Choline	450 mg
Calcium	1000–1300 mg[a]
Chromium	29–30 mcg[a]
Copper	1000 mcg
Fluoride	3 mg
Iodine	220 mcg
Iron	27 mg
Magnesium	350–400 mg[a]
Manganese	2 mg
Molybdenum	50 mcg
Phosphorus	700–1250 mg[a]
Selenium	60 mcg
Zinc	11–12 mg[a]
Potassium	4.7 g
Sodium	1.5 g
Chloride	2.3 g

Data from Dietary Reference Intakes: Estimating Average Requirements and from Dietary Reference Intakes: Recommended Dietary Allowances and Adequate Intakes, Vitamins. Food and Nutrition Board, National Academies of Science Institute of Medicine. (http://fnic.nal.usda.gov/dietary-guidance/dietary-reference-intakes/dri-tables)

[a]Varies by age group.

Calcium

During pregnancy, the fetus exerts additional calcium demand on the mother as calcium is transferred across the placenta to support fetal skeletal mineralization. The additional demand can usually be achieved through calcium mobilization from the skeleton, increased intestinal calcium absorption efficiency, and enhanced renal calcium retention or greater dietary calcium intake of the mother.[25] Observational studies have generally found a positive relationship between maternal dietary calcium intake during pregnancy and bone outcomes of offspring, with positive bone outcomes seen in children at 9 years of age.[26] Calcium supplementation during pregnancy can be linked directly to increased bone density and bone length of neonates.

Apart from calcium's effect on bone health of fetus, 2 Cochrane systematic reviews have investigated whether calcium supplementation on a daily basis during pregnancy safely improved maternal and infant outcomes. Calcium supplementation during pregnancy was found to significantly reduce the risk of preeclampsia and high blood pressure (with or without proteinuria).[27,28]

Iron

A recent World Health Organization review found that iron supplementation during pregnancy was associated with reduced likelihood of having LBW babies compared with controls, and the mean birth weight was 30.81 g greater for infants whose mothers received iron during pregnancy (95% CI 5.94–55.68 g, 14 studies).[29] In addition, reduced iron availability for brain iron accretion is associated with persistent developmental and behavioral changes. Several conditions associated with fetal growth retardation or macrosomia, such as diabetes, placental insufficiency, and smoking, restrict iron availability during gestation and create a predisposition to later iron deficiency.[30]

Iodine

The importance of iodine for fetal growth and development is well established, and severe iodine deficiency during pregnancy results in cretinism. Strong evidence indicates that adequate iodine during pregnancy is important to support healthy neurodevelopment of the fetus.[31] Several intervention studies have shown that iodine supplementation during pregnancy in iodine-deficient mothers improved intelligence quotient (IQ) points in children several years later. Pregnancy seems to be a critical time period since children whose mothers were given iodine during pregnancy performed better on a psychomotor test than those who were supplemented from 2 years of age.[32] Ensuring adequate iodine intake in early life is an important way to promote healthy brain development in children.

Folic Acid and Vitamin B$_{12}$

Folic acid is very important both preconceptionally and periconceptionally in protecting the fetus from neural tube defects. In well-nourished populations, folic acid needs are usually met by dietary intake. However, in some countries (eg, the United States), pregnant women are advised to consume 600 mcg of folic acid per day to reduce the risk of neural tube defects (Table 10-1). Low maternal folate intake (< 240 mcg/d) has been associated with a greater than 3-fold increase in the risk of LBW and preterm delivery. A metabolic effect of folate deficiency is an elevation of homocysteine, and women with high homocysteine levels are more likely to have a reproductive history of preeclampsia, preterm delivery, LBW, or fetal growth restriction.[17] A study carried out in India has highlighted the major role that dietary methyl donors including B$_{12}$ and folate seem to play in fetal programming. Maternal low B$_{12}$ status along with normal to high folate status predicted later adiposity and insulin resistance in children. Thus, 1-C (methyl) metabolism seems to have a key role in fetal programming.[33]

Vitamin D

Vitamin D deficiency during pregnancy predisposes newborns to neonatal hypocalcemia and to later rickets. Maternal vitamin D status during pregnancy may have long-term effects on bone mineral accretion in childhood. Vitamin D insufficiency during pregnancy appears to be increasingly common in developed countries,[34] and the consequences may extend beyond the recognized influence of neonatal calcium deficiency and rickets. Several studies have also proposed low vitamin D concentrations during prenatal or early-life development as a cause of a greater risk of later development of multiple sclerosis, cancer, insulin-dependent diabetes mellitus, recurrent wheeze, and schizophrenia, though the evidence is still inconclusive.[35]

Vitamin E

The plasma concentration of α-tocopherol, the most common isomer of vitamin E, is positively related to fetal growth (birth weight for gestation), reduced SGA births, and increased risk of large-for-gestational-age births. Concentrations of α-tocopherol were positively related to the use of prenatal multivitamins before and during pregnancy and to vitamin E in the maternal diet. Emerging evidence suggests that the effect of vitamin E on fetal growth may occur via increased blood flow and nutrient supply to the fetus.[17]

Multiple Micronutrients

Few published studies have examined whether supplements of multiple micronutrients might be more beneficial than single micronutrients. Evidence exists for interactions of several micronutrients at the metabolic level. Little is yet known about the significance of these interactions for pregnancy outcomes, especially in developing countries where nutrient deficiencies rarely occur in isolation and multiple micronutrient deficiencies are common. A meta-analysis of global multinutrient supplementation studies found a small effect on birth weight between iron-folate supplementation and placebo.[36] A Cochrane review in 2012 found that supplementation with multiple micronutrients significantly affects SGA and LBW outcomes compared to supplementation with 2 or fewer micronutrients, no supplementation, or a placebo. Comparison of the multiple micronutrient supplementation with iron and folate showed similar beneficial effects on SGA and LBW outcomes.[37]

Lactation

Physiology of Lactation

Lactation is divided into 4 phases: (1) preparation of breasts (mammogenesis), (2) synthesis and secretion from the breast alveoli (lactogenesis), (3) ejection of milk (galactokinesis), and (4) maintenance of lactation (galactopoiesis). The first 2 phases constitute lactogenesis stage 1, which occurs in midpregnancy, and the last 2 phases are lactogenesis stage 2, which occurs 3–4 days postpartum.[38]

During pregnancy full alveolar development and maturation are induced by the hormones of pregnancy, including progesterone, prolactin, placental lactogen, glucocorticoid, and oxytocin. Each breast contains lobules with alveoli that are surrounded by myoepithelial cells and contain acinar cells, which produce milk. During early pregnancy, growth and development of the ductal trees occur along with further formation of lobules, which is followed by increased secretory activity and the alveoli starting to become engorged with milk.[39] Colostrum secretion, which is a sticky substance, can be squeezed from the breast by approximately the 12th week of pregnancy, and by about the 16th week, it will be thick and yellowish.

Major hormonal changes occur after delivery that allow for the onset of stage 2 of lactogenesis. The most important change is the withdrawal of progesterone and estrogen allowing prolactin to enable milk secretion. Progesterone levels decrease about 10-fold in the first few days after delivery. Upon infant suckling, nerves in the areola communicate to the hypothalamus and subsequently to the anterior and posterior pituitary gland, which secretes prolactin and oxytocin, respectively. Prolactin stimulates the production of milk in the alveolar cells, and oxytocin stimulates the myoepithelial cells to squeeze the alveoli and eject milk into the larger ducts for suckling by the infant. Prolactin is the most important hormone to lactation; although oxytocin controls the "let-down" of the milk, milk cannot be made without prolactin.[39]

Components of breast milk are secreted into the alveolar lumina in 5 distinct pathways, which operate in parallel to make the components of breast milk from precursors in the interstitial fluid and blood.

1) Exocytosis is the pathway used for the aqueous fraction of breast milk and is similar to that of other cells of the body.

2) Lipid synthesis and secretion are unique to the mammary gland. Through this pathway, triglycerides are synthesized from fatty acids and glycerol in the smooth endoplasmic reticulum of the alveolar cells. After the lipid droplet is enveloped in the apical plasma membrane, it is expelled as a milk-fat globule.

3) Transport across the apical membrane involves direct transport of monovalent ions, water, and glucose across the apical membrane. At this time, exact transport mechanisms are not well understood.

4) Transcytosis of interstitial molecules involves the transport of proteins from the interstitial space across the mammary epithelium. Immunoglobulin A is the most studied of these proteins. After being synthesized in the body, it binds to receptors on the basal surface of the alveolar cell, and the entire complex undergoes endocytosis and is transferred to the apical membrane. Many other proteins, hormones, and growth factors use a similar method, but are not as well studied.

5) The paracellular pathway involves the movement of substances between, rather than through the alveolar cells. During mature lactation, the tight junctions between cells do not allow substances to pass between them; however, it appears that immune cells can undergo diapedesis and be incorporated into the breast milk. The tight junctions can become more leaky during pregnancy, mastitis, and after involution.[38]

Impact of Maternal Nutrition During Lactation on the Infant

Lactation is one of the most nutritionally demanding times in a woman's life, with needs for almost all nutrients increased beyond those in pregnancy. The caloric expenditure of 6–9 months of lactation can exceed that of pregnancy by 42% and 98%, respectively.[40] To preserve the survival of the species, mammary glands are still able to produce a sufficient volume of breast milk for infant survival, even in times of poor maternal nutrition. However, the nutrition adequacy for optimal infant growth and development may still be at risk; therefore, the nutrition status of the lactating women is important to the nutrition received by the infant via breast milk.

Several nutrients are of greater importance than others in the maternal diet/body stores because their deficiency can more greatly impact their levels in breast milk. Such nutrients include B vitamins, choline, vitamins A and D, and iodine. However, many of the major minerals, including calcium, iron, and zinc, as well as calories and protein are not influenced by maternal intake/stores. Other breast milk nutrients, such as polyunsaturated fatty acids and carotenoids that are important for infant development, may also be influenced by maternal intake. Of the few studies that have looked at dietary intake of lactating women, many suggest that the nutrients in breast milk that are the most sensitive to maternal intake are the most likely to be deficient in the maternal diet.[41–43]

Since B vitamins are water soluble and not stored, these must come from the diet. Maternal deficiency of thiamin (B_1) and riboflavin (B_2) can rapidly impact breast milk concentration[44] of these vitamins, which are readily transported across the mammary gland into the milk. Supplementation may improve breast milk status for those who are undernourished.[45,46] A strong correlation exists between breast milk concentration and infant status and maternal intake.[47] Supplementation in well-nourished women does not seem to increase concentrations,[48] suggesting the presence of a feedback mechanism that ensures an adequate breast milk concentration with intake that is appropriate. Similar to the other B vitamins, infant status of vitamin B_6 is strongly related to maternal intake,[49,50] and B_6 supplementation in reasonably nourished women does demonstrate a significant increase in breast milk concentration.[51] Higher doses of 10 mg/d resulted in infants meeting the adequate intake for vitamin B_6.[50] Vitamin B_{12} may be of even greater concern for many, especially women who are following a strict

Table 10-2. Milk concentrations assumed for setting the adequate intake (AI) for the first 6 months of life compared to value in milk of deficient infants and percent of AI this represents.[1]

NUTRIENT	MILK CONCENTRATION/L ASSUMED FOR SETTING AI	MILK CONCENTRATION REPORTED FOR DEFICIENT INFANTS (REFERENCE)	AI CONSUMED BY DEFICIENT INFANTS %
Thiamin, mg	0.21	0.16 (16)[2]	60
Riboflavin, mg	0.35	0.21 (16)[3]	53
Vitamin B_6, mg	0.13	0.10 (16, 18, 59)[4]	80
Vitamin B_{12}, µg	0.42	<0.05[5]	16
Choline, mg	160	90 (48)[6]	56

[1]Milk intake was assumed to be 780 mL/d.

[2]Study selected because of larger sample size. Note that breast milk concentration was higher than in India (18) and Thailand (19).

[3]Selected based on largest sample size and clear evidence of deficiency in mothers and infants.

[4]Similar values from these studies in India, Gambia, and Egypt.

[5]Selected because of large sample size and evidence of deficiency in mothers and infants (44).

[6]Based on data from the only available low income country (Equador). Forty percent of samples were lower than this value. Infant choline status was not asessed.

Reprinted from Allen LH. B vitamins in breast milk: relative importance of maternal status and intake, and effects on infant status and function. *Adv Nutr.* 2012;3(3):362–369 with permission from the American Society for Nutrition.

vegetarian or vegan diet or for whom animal food sources are scarce because almost all B_{12} in the food chain is from animals. Little research has been done on B_{12} supplementation in lactating women; however, data do suggest that breast milk concentration may respond to B_{12} supplementation in undernourished women.[44,52] Finally, maternal choline intake is also correlated to breast milk and plasma concentrations, and choline supplementation can increase concentrations, which seem to be impacted by individual genotypes.[53] Given the impact of maternal nutrition on breast milk concentration of B vitamins, it is noteworthy that infants who are exclusively breastfed by mothers with a dietary deficiency are at significant risk of inadequate intake.[44]

The recommendation for vitamin A for lactating women is almost 70% greater than that during pregnancy, and it represents the largest increase for any single vitamin/mineral between pregnancy and lactation. On average, infants received approximately 400 mcg/d of vitamin A from breast milk during the first 6 months of lactation[54] and almost 60 times more vitamin A is transferred to the infant during this time than during gestation.[55] Vitamin A status of breast milk status is dependent on maternal stores. In parts of the world with low vitamin A intake and high rates of deficiency, the average vitamin A content of mature milk is about 1 µmol/L compared to about 7 µmol/L for well-nourished women, suggesting that infants may have subclinical vitamin A deficiency by 6 months of age.[55] Vitamin A supplementation in breast feeding women has been

shown to offer limited benefits to improving maternal and infant vitamin A deficiency.[56]

As described elsewhere (Chapter 11), vitamin D supplementation is recommended for all breastfed infants due to the low breast milk concentration, even in well-nourished women. Research has continued to determine whether larger doses of vitamin D to lactating women can result in adequate infant plasma vitamin D in breastfed infants. A few studies with supplement doses of at least 2000 IU vitamin D per day in lactating women have demonstrated that the level of circulating 25(OH)-D_2 in exclusively breastfed infants was similar to that in infants receiving the recommended 400 IU/d supplement.[57,58] These studies demonstrated that these higher doses appear to be safe, even though they are greater than the 600 IU/d recommended by the Institute of Medicine. Further research is needed in this area to determine the longer-term impact to the breastfeeding dyad regarding higher vitamin D supplementation.

Iodine deficiency is still a problem that is often overlooked because it is expected that this condition was mostly eliminated with iodized tabled salt, which was introduced in the United States in 1924. Deficiency during pregnancy can have a significant negative impact on cognitive outcomes in the infant that may not be reversible[31]; it is likely to also be of concern if breast milk is not adequate in iodine. Concern about the iodine intake of lactating women is ongoing because recent research has shown that lactating women are consuming only about 30% of the amount recommended by the Institute of Medicine.[43] Most salt intake is from packaged and processed foods, which do not used iodized salt. The other main dietary sources of iodine are seafood and dairy, the consumption of which are also well below recommendations.[43] It is not surprising that iodine intake is low and the risk for deficiency is high. The mammary gland is able to concentrate iodine, which is likely why infant iodine status may be maintained even if the mother has overt iodine deficiency.[59] Supplementation during pregnancy has been shown to improve maternal iodine status,[60] and breast milk concentration is related to maternal intake.[61] Therefore, given the important role iodine has in infant development and the concern of low dietary intakes, iodine is an important nutrient to monitor during lactation and supplement if needed.

Other nutrients in breast milk, such as polyunsaturated fatty acids, carotenoids, and docosahexaenoic acid (DHA) and lutein in particular, are predominant components in the infant brain[62] and eye[63] and have important roles in the development of these organs.[64,65] The consumption of dietary sources of these nutrients is well below recommendations of fatty fish (4-oz portion) 3 times per week and dark leafy greens 2 cups per week.[66] Given the strong correlation of breast milk DHA[67] and lutein[68] to maternal intake, these nutrients may be lacking for breastfed infants if maternal intake is low. Research has shown breast milk to be highly responsive to lutein[69] and DHA[70] supplementation, suggesting that women who are not consuming recommended amounts of fish and vegetables could benefit from supplementation.

Impact of Nutrition and Other Stresses on Fetal Metabolism, Organ Growth, and Development

Deprivation of nutrients and/or oxygen in utero alters fetal metabolism in a manner that changes body growth and the development of individual fetal tissues.[36] The effects of varying nutrient availability on fetal metabolism depend on the specific nature of the nutrition variation and on the duration, severity, and gestational age at the onset of the insult. Deprivation of oxidative substrates such as glucose produces a different metabolic response in the fetus from that seen from oxygen deprivation alone or in the presence of combined oxygen and substrate deficiency. These different nutrition challenges also have different effects on the uteroplacental tissues and on the fetal hormonal environment, both of which influence the availability and metabolic fate of specific nutrients in the fetus.[71]

Many of the nutritionally induced alterations in fetal metabolism and growth are likely to be mediated by hormonal changes in either the mother or the fetus. Dietary restriction is known to alter maternal concentrations of growth hormone, IGFs, insulin, glucocorticoids, leptin, thyroid hormones, and placental lactogen.[36] These hormones alter maternal metabolite concentrations, which in turn influence fetal substrate availability, particularly for metabolites crossing the placenta against a concentration gradient. In general, reducing fetal delivery of oxygen and nutrients lowers anabolic hormones (eg, insulin, IGFs, and thyroid hormones) and increases catabolic hormone concentrations (eg, cortisol, catecholamines, glucagons, and growth hormone). The anabolic hormones tend to increase the uptake and utilization of glucose and reduce the oxidation of amino acids. They also enhance protein accretion by stimulating protein synthesis, reducing proteolysis, or both. The catabolic hormones tend to increase fetal glucose production by activating hepatic gluconeogenesis. They also reduce protein accretion and fetal uptake of amino acids.

Work in animals convincingly demonstrates that prenatal stress can have a long-term effect on the function of the HPA axis in the offspring, also showing the variability and complexity of the possible effects. These effects vary depending on the nature of the stress, its timing in gestation, the genetic strain of the animal, the sex and age of the offspring, and whether basal or stimulated HPA axis responses are studied. Equivalent work in humans is only just starting, but experimental evidence suggests that there might be similar effects. These data are also very variable, but mostly suggest that prenatal stress or anxiety is associated with increased basal cortisol or increased cortisol reactivity in the offspring.[72]

Programming of the fetal HPA axis appears to play a central role in the link between fetal growth and long-term disease in adulthood (Figure 10-1). Molecular mechanisms underlying the developmental programming effects of excess glucocorticoids/prenatal stress include epigenetic changes in target gene promoters. Crucially, changes in gene expression persist long after the initial challenge, predisposing the individual to disease in later life. Intriguingly, the effects of a challenged pregnancy appear to be possibly transmitted to one or two subsequent generations, suggesting that these epigenetic effects persist.[73]

A wide variety of prenatal stress insults can have long-term effects on the behavioral and cognitive outcomes for the child.[72] Exposure of the fetus to elevated glucocorticoids appears to be the central link between prenatal stress and modification of HPA axis development and function. Evidence exists that antenatal stress/anxiety has a program-

Figure 10-1. Scheme of the role that programming of the fetal hypothalamic-pituitary-adrenal (HPA) axis during development plays in the link between fetal growth and long-term disease in adulthood. 11β-HSD, 11β-hydroxysteroid dehydrogenase; CNS, central nervous system; Dex, dexamethasone; GC, glucocorticoids.

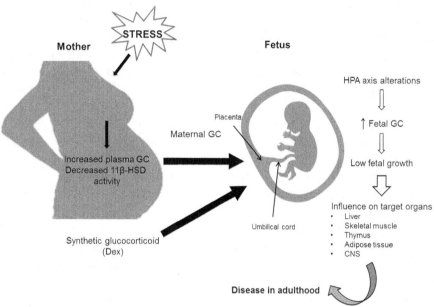

ming effect on the fetus that lasts at least until mid-childhood and results in higher rates of behavioral and emotional problems.[74] Cognitive and behavioral modifications have also been linked to alterations in HPA axis activity and prenatal glucocorticoid exposure. Prenatal stress has been associated with changes in memory and behavior and with depression, anxiety, chronic fatigue syndrome, and schizophrenia.[75] These alterations in HPA axis function, behavior, and cognition as a result of prenatal stress have been related to changes in brain corticosteroid receptor populations and alterations in hippocampal and hypothalamic neuronal development.[76]

Prenatal stress has also been linked to fetal programming of metabolic syndrome. In utero stress causes a predisposition to disease that is manifested only if additional stress, such as obesity or a high-fat diet (HFD), occurs later in postnatal life. This is exemplified by the increasing incidence of diabetes in low-income and middle-income countries, where the combination of poor nutrition in utero and overnutrition in later life is common.[77] Effects of in utero stress differ according to the particular timing of its occurrence during pregnancy, and the differences can be explained by the cellular events that occur during those particular periods of pregnancy. However, glucose intolerance is independent of the time of stress occurrence. Stress in early gestation leads to a greater risk of an abnormal atherogenic lipid profile, obesity in women, and coronary artery disease.

Stress in the second trimester of pregnancy, during which the numbers of nephrons increases rapidly, is associated with an increase in the risk for microalbuminuria. Finally, stress during the third trimester of pregnancy, when fat deposition occurs, has a relatively higher effect in reducing birth weight. Additional windows of sensitivity include the preconception and early postnatal periods.[77]

The influence of maternal prenatal stress on offspring immune system development has also been described. The hypothesis is that the impact of maternal prenatal stress and anxiety on the fetal immune system alters the maternal HPA axis, ultimately altering the function of the child's HPA axis, with a higher set point or greater reactivity of the infant HPA axis predicting a suppressed immune response. Another hypothesis is that immunological changes in the mother associated with maternal prenatal stress and anxiety, such as proinflammatory cytokines, could cross the placenta and/or alter placental function, consequently exposing the fetus to an elevated immune response early in development.[78]

Numerous studies in animals and humans have demonstrated that synthetic glucocorticoid administration can also promote HPA hyperactivity. Synthetic glucocorticoids are poorly catabolized by placental 11β-hydroxysteroid dehydrogenase type 2 (11β-HSD2) and readily pass to the fetus.[79] Fetal glucocorticoid exposure alters the expression of glucocorticoid receptors and impacts every level of the HPA axis. Synthetic glucocorticoids are often administered to women threatened with preterm delivery to enhance fetal lung maturation and reduce morbidity and mortality at a time point in gestation when endogenous fetal cortisol levels would normally be quite low. Due to recent clinical observations and animal studies of this practice, concerns have been voiced by international expert groups. In spite of these concerns, administration of repeated doses of antenatal corticosteroids to pregnant patients continues to be common clinical practice.[73]

Because regulation of energy and food intake under stress is important for survival, it is not surprising that the HPA axis not only drives appropriate stress responses but also is tightly intertwined with the regulation of appetite.[80] The early-life environment has a critical role in programming the circuitry that later integrates stress and feeding behavior. A hyperactive HPA axis, programmed as a result of a stressful early-life environment, can lead to excess glucocorticoids and an exacerbation of glucocorticoids typical appetite-stimulatory effects. Glucocorticoid interactions with feeding-related hormones such as leptin and insulin are also affected. In addition, the early-life environment also has specific influences on brain development, such as ensuring appropriate connectivity between the various parts of the hypothalamus necessary for regulating feeding. Stress and the early-life nutrition environment can acutely affect this brain development leading to abnormal feeding behavior long term.[81]

History and Epidemiology of Fetal Origins of Disease

Hypothesis

Early nutrition programming is the concept that nutrition experiences in early life can program an individual's metabolism and development and influence later health outcomes. In a landmark study in 1962, McCance[82] observed that the size of a weanling rat could be altered to vary inversely with the number of littermates suckled by the dam. Further experimental work in both rats and pigs illustrated that the earlier in life the animal was exposed to undernutrition, the more permanent the effects on adult size, despite attempts to obtain catch-up growth.[83] Competition among fetuses for intrauterine food supply or littermates for milk may lead to periods of undernutrition during critical periods of development. The fetus or neonate adapts by slowing the rate of cell division in certain organs in such a way as to permanently change or program metabolism and growth potential. The influence of nutrition during

pregnancy and early postnatal life has an impact on later health outcomes.

Barker and colleagues proposed the "developmental or fetal origins of adult disease" in humans in 1986. The hypothesis was based on observations that the highest rates of CHD in a geographical region of England were associated with increased infant mortality in the same population decades earlier.[84] Further epidemiological evidence was provided by 2 large studies of males from Hertfordshire and Sheffield, England, that demonstrated a strong correlation between the variables LBW, low weight for length at 1 year, and small head circumference and death from CHD.[85,86] It is of interest to note that the relationship between LBW and CHD was related to slow fetal/infant growth rather than prematurity. The association between reduced size at birth and risk factors for CHD, including obesity, hypertension, hyperlipidemia, and non-insulin dependent diabetes (NIDDM), has been confirmed from cohort studies in various countries.[87-92] A systematic review of 80 studies found that there was a 2-mm Hg decrease in systolic blood pressure per kilogram increase in birth weight.[91] A review of 48 papers examining the relationship of birth weight and later glucose and insulin metabolism demonstrated that LBW was correlated with adverse glucose and insulin metabolism, possibly related to insulin resistance.[92] Fetal overnutrition in infants of diabetic mothers may also cause an increased risk of glucose intolerance and NIDDM in later life.[93] A study in Pima Indians demonstrated a U-shaped relationship between birth weight and prevalence of NIDDM with high birth weight explained by the presence of gestational diabetes.[94] The epidemiological evidence is substantial that events occurring during intrauterine life may have profound implications for future health.

Expansion to Postnatal Growth Period

Although nutrition effects during fetal life have been shown to be important determinants of susceptibility to later health effects, postnatal events modify the influence of prenatal growth. In evaluations of the fetal origins of disease hypothesis, it has been recognized that adjusting for early weight gain and current body size is important. Numerous epidemiological studies show that the highest risk for cardiovascular disease and associated disorders occurs in adults who were small at birth and became overweight or obese during childhood or adulthood.[87,95-98] The "thrifty phenotype" hypothesis proposed by Hales and Barker[99] postulates that the fetus selectively distributes nutrients to certain organs during periods of undernutrition, leading to permanent metabolic changes that bolster the chances of survival during periods of limited postnatal nutrition. If adequate food becomes available postnatally, the prenatal metabolic adaptations to undernutrition could then be detrimental, and obesity and related metabolic disorders may develop.[100]

Lucas[101] proposed the term "programming" to explain the mechanism whereby an early stimulus or insult occurring at a critical or sensitive period results in a permanent or long-term change. Recent evidence suggests that rapid weight gain during infancy may be associated with an increased incidence of childhood or adult obesity and cardiovascular risk factors. The majority of the studies show consistent associations between LBW and rapid weight gain in infancy with increased risk of CHD. Conversely, an observational study from Helsinki demonstrated that slow weight gain during infancy followed by a rapid weight gain after 1 year of age increased the risk of CHD, irrespective of birth size.[96] A systematic review of 15 studies examining the role of rapid growth in infancy and childhood on later obesity found 13 publications that demonstrated a significant association of early rapid growth with obesity prevalence in later life.[102] Another systematic review that evaluated both size at birth and rate of growth in infancy concluded that infants who are at the highest end of the distribution for weight or who grew rapidly during infancy are at increased risk of subsequent obesity.[103] Although controversy exists as to the specific periods of infancy and childhood that predict later adiposity, several observational studies have indicated that weight gain in the first half of infancy may be a critical period.[104–106] In formula-fed infants for whom repeated measures of infant weight gain were available, Stettler and colleagues showed that rapid weight gain in the first week of life was associated with risk of overweight in adulthood.[107]

Several reviews have demonstrated that breastfeeding may reduce the risk of later obesity, but the current literature is controversial. The benefits of breastfeeding have been suggested to be due to slower growth in the breastfed compared to the formula-fed infant. The differences in growth rate between breastfed and formula-fed infants are greatest in the first few weeks of life, a critical period for programming of obesity.[107] In a recent meta-analysis, formula-fed infants were found to consume a substantially higher volume of milk of greater energy density and protein content in early life, which, as shown previously, could potentially program a greater risk of long-term obesity.[108]

Observational studies support the hypothesis that early postnatal nutrition plays an important role in the development of obesity and related cardiovascular risk factors, but

limited experimental evidence exists on the effects of early nutrition programming in term infants. In a recent study, SGA term infants randomly assigned to a nutrient-enriched formula at birth had higher diastolic blood pressure at 6–8 years, and the diastolic blood pressure was greater in children who had more rapid weight gain from birth to 9 months.[109] Support for the "growth acceleration hypothesis" in term infants was demonstrated in a study that utilized multiple measurements of growth from birth to 5 years in relation to blood pressure.[110] Rapid increases in weight in the first 6 months of life predicted elevated diastolic blood pressure in adults, independent of fetal growth.[110] LBW and rapid postnatal growth are associated with later elevated blood pressure indicating the importance of both prenatal and postnatal factors in the programming of later health effects. Improved maternal nutrition and prevention of rapid percentile-crossing weight gain in infants could have a substantial impact on the development of adult chronic diseases.

Integration of Prenatal and Postnatal Programming Effects

Epidemiological and prospective data support the concept that events occurring in early life are associated with later risk of obesity, cardiovascular disease, diabetes, and metabolic syndrome. Gluckman and colleagues[1] use the term "developmental plasticity" (defined as the ability of an organism to develop in various ways, depending on the particular environment or setting) to help provide a framework for the observations on the impact of early growth on later health.

The first models to explain the developmental origins of health and disease (DOHaD) idea were the thrifty phenotype hypothesis and the "fetal salvage" hypothesis, which proposes that a fetus adapts to survive a deprived intrauterine environment.[99,111] These hypotheses were later expanded to include the postnatal environment and termed a "predictive adaptive response."[112] The risk of disease is increased when the postnatal environment does not match what is predicted prenatally. In these programming or integrated responses, environmental events at critical time periods can produce different phenotypes from a given genotype (plasticity). These processes may be mediated in part by epigenetic modulation of regulatory or developmental genes.[1] Epigenetics is the chemical modification of gene expression without changes in the inherited DNA code sequence. Epigenetic changes include DNA methylation, histone modifications, and alternation to noncoding RNAs. The mechanisms underlying epigenetic programming and developmental plasticity are still unclear, but the link between nutrition imbalances, epigenetic modifications, and later health outcomes is well accepted.[18,113]

Early Programming in the Premature Infant
The greatest body of evidence of early programming in humans comes from longitudinal studies in preterm infants. Prospective interventional studies performed by Singhal et al[114] in preterm infants demonstrated the importance of early nutrition for long-term health outcomes. Over 900 preterm infants were randomly assigned in 2 parallel trials to receive (a) banked breast milk or preterm formula or (b) standard term formula or preterm formula. The preterm infants fed breast milk for a period of 4 weeks had improved lipid profiles,[115] lower blood pressure,[116] lower leptin concentrations, and decreased insulin resistance[117,118] at 13–16 years compared to the infants fed preterm (nutrient-enriched) formula. The lipoprotein profile, C-reactive protein (a marker for the low-grade inflammatory response associated with the atherosclerotic process), and blood pressure did not differ significantly between infants randomized to standard infant formula and those fed preterm formula.[115,116] The ratio of leptin to fat mass (a marker of obesity) was significantly higher in children fed the preterm formula compared with the children who received breast milk or standard term formula.[117] Fasting 32-33 split proinsulin concentration (a marker of insulin resistance) was significantly higher in children who received preterm formula, and further analysis demonstrated that differences in weight gain (or loss) in the first 2 weeks of life was the only factor related to later proinsulin concentrations, irrespective of size at birth.[118] These landmark studies provide the first experimental clinical evidence that faster postnatal growth and a nutrient-dense diet may be a risk factor for later cardiovascular disease.

Although slower growth in preterm infants may have benefits for later health outcomes, the risks of adverse consequences on cognition and bone health must be considered. Numerous studies have demonstrated that growth restriction in preterm infants is associated with long-term short stature and cognitive deficits. Preterm infants fed standard formula compared to nutrient-enriched formula demonstrated a significant reduction in IQ and neurocognitive impairment at 7–8 years of age.[119] Higher bone mineralization and improved linear growth in childhood has been reported in preterm infants fed a preterm formula versus unfortified breast milk or standard formula.[120,121] Clear benefits exist for the use of specialized formulas in preterm infants relative to term formulas to support brain development and bone growth, and these benefits outweigh the later risks of cardiovascular disorders. Short-term advantages of dietary supplementation of at risk infants have also been demonstrated in developing countries where more rapid weight gain up to 2 years of age was associated with decreased hospital admissions and reduced mortality.[122] Further research is needed to determine optimal growth to achieve cognitive and bone benefits (in preterm infants) and short-term health benefits in at risk populations while minimizing the longer-term risk of chronic disease. Additional research to assess the impact of early nutrition in term infants is needed, but it is difficult from an ethical point of view to perform clinical intervention studies.

Animal Models
Apart from the obvious ethical constraints, many factors limit the clinical investigation in humans, including small sample size, methodological difficulties, and genetic heterogeneity, as well as differences in disease and (intensive care) treatment. Therefore, animal models are an invaluable tool to study physiological, metabolic, and cellular events related to early nutrition in both neonatal and later life under highly controlled circumstances; moreover, they are essential to the search of the mechanisms involved in developmental programming. The use of animal models enables a strong level of control over confounding factors, the measurement of invasive endpoints, and the characterization of downstream events not only in the mother but also in the offspring across the whole life span. By far the most common models used are rodents (eg, mouse, rat, and guinea pig); however, a variety of large animals (eg, sheep, pig, and nonhuman primates) have also been widely used.

Sex-specific differences in offspring outcomes from developmental programming are demonstrated in both rodents and large animals.[123] Therefore, male and female development could be treated by researchers as separate models in which sexual dimorphism should be considered when applying the results of developmental programming studies to designing diagnostic, preventive, and therapeutic approaches.[124]

Animal Models of Dietary Manipulation
Most animal models for investigating early nutrition programming have focused on inducing poor fetal growth as a consequence of maternal caloric restriction, prenatal low-protein intake, and maternal iron deficiency during pregnancy. However, during recent years there has been an

increasing need for models that mimic the impact of maternal overnutrition upon fetal development and long-term health. Several obesogenic animal models, mainly rodents, have shown a relatively common phenotype of metabolic disorders in offspring, but the magnitude of effects differed with the timing of the nutrition challenge and diet composition.[125] Collectively, these studies demonstrate that dietary manipulation during pregnancy in rodent models can lead to permanent alterations in postnatal physiological function and disease risk.

Maternal Protein Restriction Model

One of the most widely studied rodent models is the maternal protein restriction model. In this model, striking parallels exist with the development of type 2 diabetes and/or the metabolic syndrome. Rats are fed a low-protein (5%–8%) diet during pregnancy that restricts the growth of the offspring.[126] If such offspring are cross-fostered to mothers fed a control diet (20% protein) during lactation, they gain weight rapidly and have similar body weights to controls by weaning (21 days of age). However, this catch-up growth has a detrimental effect on longevity. Maternal protein restriction, even during lactation, has been shown to have long-term effects on the structure and function of individual organs such as the endocrine pancreas.[127]

Moreover, nutrition restriction is one of the most common experimental methods of fetal insult used to investigate the mechanisms of programmed hypertension. Offspring of nutrient-restricted sheep showed lower blood pressure than those of normally fed animals, but began to develop relative hypertension as they aged. A reduction of nephron number was observed when the nutrition insult coincided with the nephrogenic period.[128]

Severe food restriction during pregnancy has also been shown to induce acute IUGR in rats. In addition to suffering hypertension in adulthood, these offspring have increased fasting plasma insulin compared to controls.[129]

Studies in rodent models indicate that fetal undernutrition determines adult adiposity.[130] It is unclear whether the increase in central adiposity is related to increased food intake or reduced energy expenditure, although evidence suggests that both may be involved. Rats subjected to intrauterine protein restriction exhibited increased preference for high-fat foods. Feeding energy-dense foods to rats that were undernourished in utero promoted a greater degree of obesity than noted in animals with adequate nutrition in fetal life. Programming of appetite may stem from remodeling of hypothalamic structures that control feeding and pro-

gramming of the expression of genes involved in responses to orexigenic hormones.

Maternal Obesogenic Model

Early studies of dietary manipulation to induce overnutrition involved feeding dams with a HFD and/or high-sugar purified diet or a "cafeteria diet." These obesogenic models were designed to mimic the dietary habits in Western society. The phenotypic outcome of the offspring exposed to a maternal obesogenic diet during development varies based on the species, diet composition, timing, and length consumption.[131]

Several studies in rodents have demonstrated that a HFD alters maternal food intake, substrate utilization, body composition, glucose and lipid metabolism, leptin levels, and placental nutrient transport.[132,133] In addition, chronic HFD feeding leads to maternal obesity, which is itself a major risk factor for adverse effects on the offspring.

Maternal HFD in utero has been shown to enhance the susceptibility of the offspring to develop obesity, insulin and leptin resistance, hypertension, fatty pancreas disease, hepatic steatosis, and nonalcoholic fatty liver disease.[133] It has also been reported that maternal adiposity, and not dietary fat per se, induces hyperleptinemia and insulin resistance in offspring, as well as an increased body weight that persists into adulthood.[134] Even mild maternal overnutrition has been shown to induce increased adiposity, glucose intolerance, and altered brain appetite regulators in offspring.[135]

High-fat exposure in utero results in remodeling of the bone structure of the offspring in a sexually dimorphic manner, and a HFD has been shown to affect bone structure and length.[136] These data provide insight into the effect of a maternal HFD on the skeletal structure of the offspring, and how these alterations may lead to the development of future diseases such as osteoporosis.

Although, little is known about the effect of maternal HFD exposure on offspring behavior, it is suggested that it may increase anxiety behaviors in the offspring via alterations in the GABAergic and neurotrophin systems in early life.[137]

Sheep and nonhuman primate models are studied less than rodent models, but some evidence from them strongly suggests that exposure to a maternal HFD predisposes offspring to altered growth and metabolic sequelae, data that closely parallel those from rodent models. Interestingly, in the nonhuman primate models many of the negative effects induced by the maternal HFD were reversible when the diet was switched postnatally or prior to pregnancy. In contrast, switching the diets in rodents did not completely reverse the effects.[133]

Maternal Iron Deficiency

Iron deficiency and anemia are common during pregnancy, particularly in the developing world. Maternal anemia is associated with LBW and increased rates of perinatal mortality and morbidity. In the rat, maternal iron restriction causes fetal growth retardation and has been shown to affect blood pressure, glucose tolerance, and serum triglyceride in the adult offspring.[138] Many studies have shown that iron deficiency during pregnancy results in long-term adverse consequences in neurodevelopment for the offspring.[139] These animal studies have demonstrated that early iron deficiency affects neuronal and glial energy metabolism, monoamine metabolism, and myelination.

Animal Models Induced by Endocrine or Paracrine Mechanisms

Studies in a variety of animal models (sheep, rats, mice, guinea pigs, and nonhuman primates) have shown that early-life exposure to glucocorticoids may lead to adverse metabolic effects.[73] Prenatal glucocorticoid excess, either from endogenous overproduction due to maternal stress or through exogenous administration to the mother or fetus, reduces birth weight, causes hypertension and hyperglycemia, and alters behavior in the offspring.[140] These effects may also be transmitted across generations without further exposure to glucocorticoids, an observation that supports an epigenetic mechanism.[141]

Studies on rat offspring exposed to an excess of prenatal glucocorticoids have shown that they undergo catch-up growth postnatally and normalize body weight by the time they wean.[142] Accumulating data in rodents suggest that prenatal glucocorticoid overexposure programs an adverse adult cardiovascular, metabolic, skeletal muscle, neuroendocrine, and behavioral phenotype.[143] The phenotypic outcome is similar to that of the low-protein model.[144] Fetal glucocorticoid overexposure may be a common mechanism for mediating fetal growth retardation and metabolic programming. This suggestion is based on the observation that dietary protein restriction during rat pregnancy reduces the activity of 11β-HSD2, which serves as a placental barrier to maternal glucocorticoids.[142]

Circulating glucocorticoid concentrations are tightly controlled by activation of the HPA axis, whose regulation can be programmed by nutrient restriction. In fetal rats, nutrient restriction results in blunted diurnal patterns of adrenocorticotropic hormone at 4 weeks postnatal age, alterations in basal plasma corticosterone in adulthood, and altered basal HPA axis activity.[145]

Animal Models Induced by Surgical Manipulation

Reduction in placental blood flow and consequent restriction of oxygen, nutrient transport, and fetal growth can be produced in the rat by uterine artery ligation in late gestation, uterine and umbilical artery embolism, or carunclectomy.[142,146] In this model of IUGR, at 2 weeks of age, offspring have reduced numbers of nephrons. This nephron deficit is associated with impaired renal function at 2 weeks despite compensatory hypertrophy of remaining nephrons. In female offspring, after uterine artery ligation, growth restriction is associated with increased fasting blood glucose levels and with impaired glucose tolerance and lower insulin secretion during a glucose tolerance test.[142] Thompson et al[147] showed that epigenetic dysregulation occurred in fetuses with IUGR near genes regulating processes abnormal in IUGR islet, such as vascularization, β-cell proliferation, insulin secretion, and cell death.

Third and Future Generation Effects

Adverse events during pregnancy can affect not only the offspring but also subsequent generations, regardless of whether they are exposed (multigenerational exposure) or unexposed (intergenerational or transgenerational inheritance) to the adverse effects, thus perpetuating the problem.[148] In a UK study examining the relationship of adult blood pressure to the mother's fetal growth and size at birth, reduced fetal growth was associated with increased blood pressure in the next generation.[149] The researchers concluded that if the growth of a female fetus is restricted, changes in her physiology and metabolism occur that lead to elevated blood pressure in the next generation. This suggests that malnourishment of the mothers during development affects her progeny's health.

The Dutch famine, which occurred toward the end of World War II (winter 1944–1945), constitutes a unique opportunity to study the effects of severe undernutrition during pregnancy on the health of future generations. Studies have shown that adults who were born during the Dutch famine and whose mothers had inadequate nutrition during the first 2 trimesters of pregnancy were more likely to be obese and have abnormal lipid profiles than adults whose mothers had poor nutrition during the third trimester.[150] Infants born to mothers who were malnourished during the third trimester were leaner but had impaired glucose tolerance. In addition, individuals who were of normal birth weight born to severely malnourished mothers went on to deliver smaller babies in the next generation.[150] One explanation for the intergenerational effects on birth weight is that the hormonal environment of the uterus of the undernourished mother may affect the developing germ cells that will form the next generation.[151] Another study has reported that grandchildren of the women who were pregnant during the famine had increased neonatal adiposity and poor health later in life.[152] These data indicate that maternal undernutrition during gestation may have effects on the offspring's later health that are transmitted to subsequent generations. A possibly similar transgenerational transmission of longevity propensity has been identified for males in epidemiologic studies of food supply during early spermatogenesis.[153] A recent study has shown that fluctuations in food availability during grandparents' development had an impact on their granddaughter's cardiovascular mortality, supporting transmission through the paternal line.[154]

Although the mechanisms behind these relationships are poorly understood, epigenetic dysregulation of the *IGF-2* gene has been proposed. IGF-2 is a key factor in human development and growth and is maternally imprinted. Individuals who were prenatally exposed to malnutrition during the Dutch famine had less DNA methylation of the *IGF-2* gene compared with their unexposed same-sex siblings 6 decades later.[155] Interestingly, a recent epidemiological study observed a similar degree of *IGF-2* hypomethylation in newborns from obese fathers. This suggests that, besides in utero exposures to nutrition or environmental factors, paternal malnutrition has a heritable influence on *IGF-2* and may therefore impact subsequent generations.[156] These data support the hypothesis that early-life environmental conditions cause epigenetic changes in humans that persist throughout life.

Implications for Future Health

The influence of dietary inadequacy or imbalance and other stressors on morphological and functional changes during pregnancy and early infancy, and their adult consequences, has become a rapidly growing research area during the last years. We are now beginning to understand the molecular determinants of these changes and the dietary and environmental factors controlling them. Both overnutrition and undernutrition in utero and in early life can increase risks for adverse metabolic outcomes including type 2 diabetes, cardiovascular disease, and obesity. The seriousness of these events is amplified by evidence that certain potentially ad-

verse epigenetic effects induced in the female fetus may persist through at least an additional generation.

Current agricultural production and food distribution and changes in diet and activity patterns are associated with a historically high prevalence of obesity, diabetes, and their complications. As many as a third of today's children in some states are destined to become diabetic, given obesity rates and genetic predisposition. In developed countries, many of these individuals may represent the second or third generation of families expressing this phenotype. Many come from environments with a history of food and micronutrient scarcity. In many parts of the world, these contrasting nutrition states coexist contemporaneously. In India we now have the phenomenon of the "thin, fat Indian," which has given India the distinction of having the world's highest rate of diabetes, despite a lower ranking for obesity. Based on what is emerging from the DOHaD literature and the investigation of epigenetics, we can expect the consequences of dietary scarcity and surfeit and their coexistence to exert adverse effects in future generations in the absence of fresh insights on how to intervene to break this cycle. An inability to meet potential major population increases in health care costs related to morbidity patterns associated with DOHaD-associated conditions could itself become a driver of morbidity and mortality, as well as a potential source of economic and political instability. Already, it is estimated that today's children in the United States will, for the first time in generations, not live longer than their parents.

Recent evidence also suggests that severe stress experienced during pregnancy may impact the developing fetus to produce increased susceptibility for childhood and adult obesity and alterations in metabolic function. Reduced glucocorticoid output in response to stress in pregnancy may have important consequences for conserving energy supply to the fetus or fetuses, modulating immune system adaptations, and protecting against adverse fetal programming by glucocorticoids. Understanding the mechanisms underpinning this adaptation in pregnancy may provide insights for manipulating HPA axis responsiveness in later life, particularly in the context of resetting HPA axis hyperactivity associated with prenatal stress exposure, which may underlie several major pathologies, including metabolic, cognitive, and mood disorders.[157] Therefore, to prevent complex common health disorders, more emphasis should be placed on the well-being of women of reproductive age prior to conception and across gestation to more effectively address health-related and disease risk–related issues in their offspring.[158]

Implications for Current Practice

What implications can be drawn from current knowledge in this area for nutrition advice in the practice of obstetrics, pediatrics, neonatology, and public health? Given that preconceptual nutrition status is at least as important as nutrition status during pregnancy, planned pregnancies in mature women with good nutrition status is a highly desirable starting point. This requires approaches to maximizing nutrition status of fertile women of childbearing age beyond an exclusive focus on pregnancy and lactation, especially if pregnancies are likely to be unplanned. During pregnancy, adequate energy, protein, and micronutrients, including methyl donors, can be expected to have a salutary effect on developmental outcomes related to fetal nutrition status. Some evidence indicates excesses of fat and protein during pregnancy are to be avoided, and long-chain n-3 fatty acids, especially docosahexaneoic acid, may have beneficial impacts on mental, visual, and behavioral development. Monitoring fetal growth, maternal weight gain, and maternal blood sugar can detect deviations from expected developmental patterns.

Lactation is also one of the most nutritionally demanding times in a woman's life, with increased need for almost all nutrients. The nutrition status of the lactating women is important to the nutrition received by the infant via breast milk. Consequently, maintaining and optimizing the nutrition status of lactating women may have a considerable impact on promoting optimal infant growth and development.

For term infants, it appears to be desirable to continue on a relative growth trajectory (percentile) similar to that experienced in utero. Traditionally, "normalizing" the growth of infants with in utero growth retardation has been accepted as the de facto goal of good nutrition. Based on more recent findings, these children may be metabolically more suited to a slower rate of growth. Percentile crossing in infancy and later appears to increase risk of the DOHaD-associated conditions. In the first 2 weeks of life and after about 4 months of age, breastfeeding may lead to less weight gain than formula feeding and can be viewed as particularly beneficial in this population. An important medical concern in such infants is to support brain development, but most of the data on the importance of early nutrition for brain development come from studies of premature infants. It remains largely unknown if nutritional supplementation and growth acceleration are beneficial in this regard for term infants with retarded growth. For infants in underdeveloped countries who develop extrauterine growth retardation later in infancy and early childhood, short-term nutritional supplementation has been found to reduce acute morbidity and mortality (as well as progression of their malnutrition).

Premature infants, especially extremely low birth weight (ELBW) infants, are at high risk of extrauterine growth restriction. Given their immature development and body composition, these infants' nutrition requirements exceed those of term infants. In infants with ELBW, developmental achievement and reduced neurological complications are associated with higher growth rates. Premature infants, both in-hospital and following hospital discharge, are very responsive to nutrition supplementation. Data from Singhal and Lucas[114] have demonstrated that rapid growth should not be encouraged for this population, based on higher blood pressure, leptin, blood lipids, and split proinsulin values in premature infants when fed premature formula compared to term formula or human milk. However, in their studies, these markers of cardiovascular risk were not elevated above those for typical term infants. These same investigators demonstrated developmental disadvantages in these infants at least through childhood from receiving standard term formulas versus more nutrient-rich premature formula. Interestingly, while premature infants fed premature formula grew faster than breastfed infants, their neurodevelopmental status was not better. Bone mineralization is improved in premature infants given mineral-rich premature and postdischarge formulas compared to standard term formulas. However, this may not persist into adulthood.[159]

Human milk with human milk fortifier is the currently recommended approach for small premature infants because it can preserve the beneficial nutrition and immunological effects of human milk, while providing additional energy, protein, minerals, and other micronutrients. For formula-fed premature infants, premature, not term, formula is recommended. However, no evidence exists that postdischarge formulas have improved developmental outcomes more than standard term formulas after hospital discharge. Nevertheless, in the smallest infants, they have been observed to enhance head growth. U.S. data from Ehrenkranz et al[160] on the positive developmental outcome of encouraging early growth in premature infants dictate against any go-slow approach for these infants to possibly reduce markers of future cardiovascular risk (to values below those observed in healthy term infants).

Future Research Needs

Nutrition and early development present a rich area for potential investigation at all levels of biological research. At the molecular level, we need specific descriptions of the molecular changes underlying the DOHaD phenomenon in various organs and the mechanisms controlling these molecular changes, including nutrition influences. In physiology, opportunities remain to explore the developmental impact of organ-specific effects of general and nutrient-specific undernutrition and overnutrition at various stages of fetal and infant development.[161] The epidemiologists, who did much to initiate this field of research, can tell us more about the similarities and differences of effects of various stressors (eg, gestational malnutrition versus diabetes) on the expression of DOHaD-related morbidity. More remains to be done to elucidate the relation of intrauterine and postnatal effects (and their interaction). Clinical investigators can prospectively study the developmental impact of growth acceleration in various populations and age groups of infants and young children, looking at infection and immune outcomes, cardiovascular and metabolic risk factors, bone health, and neurodevelopment. There may be better versus worse times or target populations for catch-up growth. Great potential appears to exist in exploring very early or later drug or hormonal interventions to reverse the underlying molecular basis of some DOHaD-associated conditions.

More research is needed on the effects of intrauterine stress exposure on child metabolic function and obesity risk, using a multilevel approach, to develop specific diagnostic and primary or secondary intervention strategies.[158] Novel biomarkers of in utero stress need to be identified, and advanced high-throughput technology is required to discern the cellular mechanisms that are altered by in utero stress.[77] Future work needs to consider more potentially relevant variables including timing and the nature of prenatal exposure, method of delivery, birth weight, genetic vulnerabilities in mother and offspring, sex of offspring, age at testing, and nature of the postnatal care; in addition, the underlying mechanisms, such as the epigenetic changes in relevant genes, need to be considered.[72] Preliminary human evidence shows that methylation levels of genes involved in glucocorticoid action are altered by the early-life environment. Further detailed longitudinal studies are needed to confirm whether such changes are identifiable at birth and hence may represent useful biomarkers of risk.[140] The preimplantation period is particularly sensitive to stress, and artificial reproductive technology constitutes a potential new form of preimplantation stress. Additional studies are needed to follow up children conceived by artificial reproductive technology. Finally, strategies, such as specific nutrients or hormones, to counteract the effect of in utero stress are needed. Such research could be particularly important for populations in developing countries.[77]

Test Your Knowledge Questions

1. The dominant fuel source for the healthy fetus is
   A. Fatty acids because they are the richest source of energy
   B. Amino acids because they promote rapid growth
   C. Galactose, because the fetus cannot utilize glucose
   D. Glucose transported from the maternal circulation
2. Nutrition programming is a process that
   A. Is specific to the fetus
   B. Occurs only in animals
   C. Occurs early in life and may extend beyond a single generation
   D. Is a transient response to nutrient availability
3. Upward growth-percentile crossing in infancy and early childhood
   A. Reduces short-term infectious mortality and leads to lower adult blood pressure
   B. Has been associated with increased risk for development of features of the metabolic syndrome
   C. Helps prevent subsequent rebound obesity
   D. Improves glucose control later in life

Acknowledgments

The authors of this chapter for the second edition of this text wish to thank Russell J. Merritt, MD, PhD, FAAP, for his contributions to the first edition of this text.

References

1. Gluckman PD, Hanson MA, Cooper C, Thornburg KL. Effect of in utero and early-life conditions on adult health and disease. *N Engl J Med.* 2008;359(1):61-73.
2. Hay WW Jr. Placental-fetal glucose exchange and fetal glucose metabolism. *Trans Am Clin Climatol Assoc.* 2006;117:321–339; discussion 339–340.
3. Sparks JW, Hay WW Jr, Bonds D, Meschia G, Battaglia FC. Simultaneous measurements of lactate turnover rate and umbilical lactate uptake in the fetal lamb. *J Clin Invest.* 1982;70(1):179–192.
4. Hay WW Jr. Recent observations on the regulation of fetal metabolism by glucose. *J Physiol.* 2006;572(Pt 1):17–24.
5. Grillo MA, Lanza A, Colombatto S. Transport of amino acids through the placenta and their role. *Amino Acids.* 2008;34(4):517–523.
6. Battaglia FC. In vivo characteristics of placental amino acid transport and metabolism in ovine pregnancy—a review. *Placenta.* 2002;23(Suppl A):S3–S8.
7. Jansson N, Rosario FJ, Gaccioli F, et al. Activation of placental mTOR signaling and amino acid transporters in obese women giving birth to large babies. *J Clin Endocrinol Metab.* 2013;98(1):105–113.
8. Battaglia FC. Clinical studies linking fetal velocimetry, blood flow and placental transport in pregnancies compli-

cated by intrauterine growth retardation (IUGR). *Trans Am Clin Climatol Assoc.* 2003;114:305–313.

9. Myers RE, Hill DE, Holt AB, Scott RE, Mellits ED, Cheek DB. Fetal growth retardation produced by experimental placental insufficiency in the rhesus monkey. I. Body weight, organ size. *Biol Neonate.* 1971;18(5):379–394.

10. Bloomfield FH, Spiroski AM, Harding JE. Fetal growth factors and fetal nutrition. *Semin Fetal Neonatal Med.* 2013;pii:S1744-165X(13)00022-X.

11. Wu G, Imhoff-Kunsch B, Girard AW. Biological mechanisms for nutritional regulation of maternal health and fetal development. *Paediatr Perinat Epidemiol.* 2012;26(Suppl 1):14–26.

12. de Onis M, Villar J, Gulmezoglu M. Nutritional interventions to prevent intrauterine growth retardation: evidence from randomized controlled trials. *Eur J Clin Nutr.* 1998;52(Suppl 1):–S.

13. Shiell AW, Campbell DM, Hall MH, Barker DJ. Diet in late pregnancy and glucose-insulin metabolism of the offspring 40 years later. *BJOG.* 2000;107(7):890–895.

14. Burdge GC, Lillycrop KA. Nutrition, epigenetics, and developmental plasticity: implications for understanding human disease. *Annu Rev Nutr.* 2010;30(1):315–339.

15. McMillen IC, MacLaughlin SM, Muhlhausler BS, Gentili S, Duffield JL, Morrison JL. Developmental origins of adult health and disease: the role of periconceptional and foetal nutrition. *Basic Clin Pharmacol Toxicol.* 2008;102(2):82–89.

16. Georgieff MK. The role of iron in neurodevelopment: fetal iron deficiency and the developing hippocampus. *Biochem Soc Trans.* 2008;36(Pt 6):1267–1271.

17. Scholl TO. Maternal nutrition before and during pregnancy. *Nestle Nutr Workshop Ser Pediatr Program.* 2008;6179-89.

18. Martin-Gronert MS, Ozanne SE. Maternal nutrition during pregnancy and health of the offspring. *Biochem Soc Trans.* 2006;34(Pt 5):779–782.

19. Morton SMB. Maternal nutrition and fetal growth and development. In: Gluckman PD, Hanson MA, eds. *Developmental Origins of Health and Disease.* Cambridge, United Kingdom: Cambridge University Press; 2006:98–129.

20. Lakshmy R. Metabolic syndrome: role of maternal undernutrition and fetal programming. *Rev Endocr Metab Disord.* 2013;14(3):229–240.

21. Lanham SA, Roberts C, Cooper C, Oreffo RO. Intrauterine programming of bone. Part 1: alteration of the osteogenic environment. *Osteoporos Int.* 2008;19(2):147–156.

22. Lanham SA, Roberts C, Perry MJ, Cooper C, Oreffo RO. Intrauterine programming of bone. Part 2: alteration of skeletal structure. *Osteoporos Int.* 2008;19(2):157–167.

23. Imdad A, Bhutta ZA. Maternal nutrition and birth outcomes: effect of balanced protein-energy supplementation. *Paediatr Perinat Epidemiol.* 2012;26(Suppl 1):178–190.

24. Ota E, Tobe-Gai R, Mori R, Farrar D. Antenatal dietary advice and supplementation to increase energy and protein intake. *Cochrane Database Syst Rev.* 2012;9CD000032.

25. Olausson H, Goldberg GR, Laskey MA, Schoenmakers I, Jarjou LM, Prentice A. Calcium economy in human pregnancy and lactation. *Nutr Res Rev.* 2012;25(1):40–67.

26. Hacker AN, Fung EB, King JC. Role of calcium during pregnancy: maternal and fetal needs. *Nutr Rev.* 2012;70(7):397–409.

27. Buppasiri P, Lumbiganon P, Thinkhamrop J, Ngamjarus C, Laopaiboon M. Calcium supplementation (other than for preventing or treating hypertension) for improving pregnancy and infant outcomes. *Cochrane Database Syst Rev.* 2011(10):CD007079.

28. Hofmeyr GJ, Lawrie TA, Atallah AN, Duley L. Calcium supplementation during pregnancy for preventing hypertensive disorders and related problems. *Cochrane Database Syst Rev.* 2010(8):CD001059.

29. World Health Organization Guideline: daily iron and folic acid supplementation in pregnant women. Geneva: World Health Organization; 2012.

30. Rao R, Georgieff MK. Iron in fetal and neonatal nutrition. *Semin Fetal Neonatal Med.* 2007;12(1):54-63.

31. Bath SC, Steer CD, Golding J, Emmett P, Rayman MP. Effect of inadequate iodine status in UK pregnant women on cognitive outcomes in their children: results from the Avon Longitudinal Study of Parents and Children (ALSPAC). *Lancet.* 2013;382(9889):331–337.

32. O'Donnell KJ, Rakeman MA, Zhi-Hong D, et al. Effects of iodine supplementation during pregnancy on child growth and development at school age. *Dev Med Child Neurol.* 2002;44(2):76–81.

33. Yajnik CS, Deshmukh US. Maternal nutrition, intrauterine programming and consequential risks in the offspring. *Rev Endocr Metab Disord.* 2008;9(3):203–211.

34. Vandevijvere S, Amsalkhir S, Van Oyen H, Moreno-Reyes R. High prevalence of vitamin D deficiency in pregnant women: a national cross-sectional survey. *PLoS One.* 2012;7(8):e43868.

35. Berti C, Biesalski HK, Gartner R, et al. Micronutrients in pregnancy: current knowledge and unresolved questions. *Clin Nutr.* 2011;30(6):689–701.

36. Fowden AL, Ward JW, Forhead A. Control of fetal metabolism: relevance to developmental origins of health and disease. In: Gluckman PD, Hanson MA, ed. Developmental Origins of Health and Disease. Cambridge, United Kingdom: Cambridge University Press; 2006:143–158.

37. Haider BA, Bhutta ZA. Multiple-micronutrient supplementation for women during pregnancy. *Cochrane Database Syst Rev.* 2012;11CD004905.

38. Neville MC. Anatomy and physiology of lactation. *Pediatr Clin North Am.* 2001;48(1):13–34.

39. Riordan J, Wambach K. *Breastfeeding and Human Lactation.* 4th ed. Sudbury, MA: Jones and Bartlett Publishers; 2010.

40. Picciano MF. Nutrient composition of human milk. *Pediatr Clin North Am.* 2001;48(1):53-67.

41. Durham HA, Lovelady CA, Brouwer RJ, Krause KM, Ostbye T. Comparison of dietary intake of overweight postpartum mothers practicing breastfeeding or formula feeding. *J Am Diet Assoc.* 2011;111(1):67–74.

42. Lovelady CA, Stephenson KG, Kuppler KM, Williams JP. The effects of dieting on food and nutrient intake of lactating women. *J Am Diet Assoc.* 2006;106(6):908–912.

43. Pratt NS, Sherry CL. Lactating women consume less than the recommendations for many nutrients. *FASEB J.* 2014;28(1):Suppl 810.1.

44. Allen LH. B vitamins in breast milk: relative importance of maternal status and intake, and effects on infant status and function. *Adv Nutr.* 2012;3(3):362–369.

45. Prentice AM, Roberts SB, Prentice A, et al. Dietary supplementation of lactating Gambian women. I. Effect on breast-milk volume and quality. *Hum Nutr Clin Nutr.* 1983;37(1):53–64.

46. Deodhar AD, Rajalakshmi R, Ramakrishnan CV. Studies on human lactation. IV. Lactic and malic dehydrogenases and xanthine oxidase in breast milk and their variation with the progress of lactation and dietary vitamin supplementation. *Acta Paediatr.* 1964;53:101–104.

47. Kodentsova VM, Vrzhesinskaya OA. Evaluation of the vitamin status in nursing women by vitamin content in breast milk. *Bull Exp Biol Med.* 2006;141(3):323–327.

48. Thomas MR, Sneed SM, Wei C, Nail PA, Wilson M, Sprinkle EE 3rd. The effects of vitamin C, vitamin B6, vitamin B12, folic acid, riboflavin, and thiamin on the breast milk and maternal status of well-nourished women at 6 months postpartum. *Am J Clin Nutr.* 1980;33(10):2151–2156.

49. Kang-Yoon SA, Kirksey A, Giacoia G, West K. Vitamin B-6 status of breast-fed neonates: influence of pyridoxine supplementation on mothers and neonates. *Am J Clin Nutr.* 1992;56(3):548–558.

50. Chang SJ, Kirksey A. Pyridoxine supplementation of lactating mothers: relation to maternal nutrition status and vitamin B-6 concentrations in milk. *Am J Clin Nutr.* 1990;51(5):826–831.

51. Hamaker BR, Kirksey A, Borschel MW. Distribution of B-6 vitamers in human milk during a 24-h period after oral supplementation with different amounts of pyridoxine. *Am J Clin Nutr.* 1990;51(6):1062–1066.

52. Duggan C, Srinivasan K, Thomas T, et al. Vitamin B-12 supplementation during pregnancy and early lactation increases maternal, breast milk, and infant measures of vitamin B-12 status. *J Nutr.* 2014;144(5):758–764.

53. Fischer LM, da Costa KA, Galanko J, et al. Choline intake and genetic polymorphisms influence choline metabolite concentrations in human breast milk and plasma. *Am J Clin Nutr.* 2010;92(2):336–346.

54. Institute of Medicine. *Dietary Reference Intakes for Vitamin A, Vitamin K, Arsenic, Boron, Chromium, Copper, Iodine, Iron, Manganese, Molybdenum, Nickel, Silicon, Vanadium and Zinc.* Washington, DC: National Academy of Sciences, Institute of Medicine, Food and Nutrition Board; 2001.

55. Stoltzfus RJ, Underwood BA. Breast-milk vitamin A as an indicator of the vitamin A status of women and infants. *Bull World Health Organ.* 1995;73(5):703–711.

56. Oliveira-Menegozzo JM, Bergamaschi DP, Middleton P, East CE. Vitamin A supplementation for postpartum women. *Cochrane Database Syst Rev.* 2010;(10):CD005944.

57. Hollis BW, Wagner CL. Vitamin D requirements during lactation: high-dose maternal supplementation as therapy to prevent hypovitaminosis D for both the mother and the nursing infant. *Am J Clin Nutr.* 2004;80(6 Suppl):1752S–1758S.

58. Wagner CL, Hulsey TC, Fanning D, Ebeling M, Hollis BW. High-dose vitamin D3 supplementation in a cohort of breast-feeding mothers and their infants: a 6-month follow-up pilot study. *Breastfeed Med.* 2006;1(2):59–70.

59. Zimmermann MB. The impact of iodised salt or iodine supplements on iodine status during pregnancy, lactation and infancy. *Public Health Nutr.* 2007;10(12A):1584–1595.

60. Charlton KE, Yeatman H, Brock E, et al. Improvement in iodine status of pregnant Australian women 3years after introduction of a mandatory iodine fortification programme. *Prev Med.* 2013;57(1):26–30.

61. Kurtoglu S, Akcakus M, Kocaoglu C, et al. Iodine status remains critical in mother and infant in Central Anatolia (Kayseri) of Turkey. *Eur J Nutr.* 2004;43(5):297–303.

62. Innis SM. Dietary (n-3) fatty acids and brain development. *J Nutr.* 2007;137(4):855–859.

63. Vishwanathan R, Kuchan MJ, Sen S, Johnson EJ. Lutein is the predominant carotenoid in infant brain: preterm infants have decreased concentrations of brain carotenoids. *J Pediatr Gastroenterol Nutr.* 2014;59(5):659–665.

64. Zimmer JP, Hammond BR Jr. Possible influences of lutein and zeaxanthin on the developing retina. *Clin Ophthalmol.* 2007;1(1):25–35.

65. Innis SM. Impact of maternal diet on human milk composition and neurological development of infants. *Am J Clin Nutr.* 2014;99(3):734S–741S.

66. U.S. Department of Agriculture, Department of Health and Human Services. *Dietary Guidelines for Americans.* Washington, DC: Government Printing Office; 2010.

67. Fidler N, Sauerwald T, Pohl A, Demmelmair H, Koletzko B. Docosahexaenoic acid transfer into human milk after dietary supplementation: a randomized clinical trial. *J Lipid Res.* 2000;41(9):1376–1383.

68. Cena H, Castellazzi AM, Pietri A, Roggi C, Turconi G. Lutein concentration in human milk during early lactation and its relationship with dietary lutein intake. *Public Health Nutr.* 2009;12(10):1878–1884.

69. Sherry CL, Oliver JS, Renzi LM, Marriage BJ. Lutein supplementation increases breast milk and plasma lutein concentrations in lactating women and in infant plasma concentrations but does not affect other carotenoids. *J Nutr.* 2014;144(8):1256–1263.

70. Meldrum SJ, D'Vaz N, Casadio Y, et al. Determinants of DHA levels in early infancy: differential effects of breast milk and direct fish oil supplementation. *Prostaglandins Leukot Essent Fatty Acids.* 2012;86(6):233–239.

71. Fowden AL, Forhead A. The role of hormones in intrauterine development. In: Barker DJ, ed. *Fetal Origins of Cardiovascular and Lung Disease.* New York, NY: Marcel Dekker Inc; 2000:199–228.

72. Glover V, O'Connor TG, O'Donnell K. Prenatal stress and the programming of the HPA axis. *Neurosci Biobehav Rev.* 2010;35(1):17–22.

73. Braun T, Challis JR, Newnham JP, Sloboda DM. Early-life glucocorticoid exposure: the hypothalamic-pituitary-adrenal axis, placental function, and long-term disease risk. *Endocr Rev.* 2013;34(6):885–916.

74. O'Connor TG, Heron J, Golding J, Glover V. Maternal antenatal anxiety and behavioural/emotional problems in chil-

dren: a test of a programming hypothesis. *J Child Psychol Psychiatry*. 2003;44(7):1025–1036.

75. Sloboda D, Newnham J, Moss T, Challis J. The fetal hypothalamic-pituitary-adrenal axis: relevance to developmental origins of health and disease. In: Gluckman PD, Hanson MA, ed. *Developmental Origins of Health and Disease*. Cambridge, United Kingdom: Cambridge University Press; 2006:191–205.

76. Welberg LA, Seckl JR. Prenatal stress, glucocorticoids and the programming of the brain. *J Neuroendocrinol*. 2001;13(2):113–128.

77. Rinaudo P, Wang E. Fetal programming and metabolic syndrome. *Annu Rev Physiol*. 2012;74(1):107–130.

78. Marques AH, O'Connor TG, Roth C, Susser E, Bjorke-Monsen AL. The influence of maternal prenatal and early childhood nutrition and maternal prenatal stress on offspring immune system development and neurodevelopmental disorders. *Front Neurosci*. 2013;7:120.

79. Seckl JR, Holmes MC. Mechanisms of disease: glucocorticoids, their placental metabolism and fetal 'programming' of adult pathophysiology. *Nat Clin Pract Endocrinol Metab*. 2007;3(6):479–488.

80. Adam TC, Epel ES. Stress, eating and the reward system. *Physiol Behav*. 2007;91(4):449–458.

81. Spencer SJ. Perinatal programming of neuroendocrine mechanisms connecting feeding behavior and stress. *Front Neurosci*. 2013;7:109.

82. McCance RA. Food, growth, and time. *Lancet*. 1962;2(7258):671–676.

83. Widdowson EM, McCance RA. A review: new thoughts on growth. *Pediatr Res*. 1975;9(3):154–156.

84. Barker DJ, Osmond C. Infant mortality, childhood nutrition, and ischaemic heart disease in England and Wales. *Lancet*. 1986;1(8489):1077–1081.

85. Barker DJ, Osmond C, Simmonds SJ, Wield GA. The relation of small head circumference and thinness at birth to death from cardiovascular disease in adult life. *BMJ*. 1993;306(6875):422–426.

86. Barker DJ, Winter PD, Osmond C, Margetts B, Simmonds SJ. Weight in infancy and death from ischaemic heart disease. *Lancet*. 1989;2(8663):577–580.

87. Frankel S, Elwood P, Sweetnam P, Yarnell J, Smith GD. Birthweight, body-mass index in middle age, and incident coronary heart disease. *Lancet*. 1996;348(9040):1478–1480.

88. Stein CE, Fall CH, Kumaran K, Osmond C, Cox V, Barker DJ. Fetal growth and coronary heart disease in south India. *Lancet*. 1996;348(9037):1269–1273.

89. Leon DA, Lithell HO, Vagero D, et al. Reduced fetal growth rate and increased risk of death from ischaemic heart disease: cohort study of 15 000 Swedish men and women born 1915-29. *BMJ*. 1998;317(7153):241–245.

90. Forsen T, Osmond C, Eriksson JG, Barker DJ. Growth of girls who later develop coronary heart disease. *Heart*. 2004;90(1):20–24.

91. Huxley RR, Shiell AW, Law CM. The role of size at birth and postnatal catch-up growth in determining systolic blood pressure: a systematic review of the literature. *J Hypertens*. 2000;18(7):815–831.

92. Newsome CA, Shiell AW, Fall CH, Phillips DI, Shier R, Law CM. Is birth weight related to later glucose and insulin metabolism?—A systematic review. *Diabet Med*. 2003;20(5):339–348.

93. Dabelea D, Pettitt DJ. Intrauterine diabetic environment confers risks for type 2 diabetes mellitus and obesity in the offspring, in addition to genetic susceptibility. *J Pediatr Endocrinol Metab*. 2001;14(8):1085–1091.

94. McCance DR, Pettitt DJ, Hanson RL, Jacobsson LT, Knowler WC, Bennett PH. Birth weight and non-insulin dependent diabetes: thrifty genotype, thrifty phenotype, or surviving small baby genotype? *BMJ*. 1994;308(6934):942–945.

95. Fall CH, Osmond C, Barker DJ, et al. Fetal and infant growth and cardiovascular risk factors in women. *BMJ*. 1995;310(6977):428–432.

96. Eriksson JG, Forsen T, Tuomilehto J, Osmond C, Barker DJ. Early growth and coronary heart disease in later life: longitudinal study. *BMJ*. 2001;322(7292):949–953.

97. Eriksson JG, Forsen T, Tuomilehto J, Winter PD, Osmond C, Barker DJ. Catch-up growth in childhood and death from coronary heart disease: longitudinal study. *BMJ*. 1999;318(7181):427–431.

98. Rich-Edwards JW, Kleinman K, Michels KB, et al. Longitudinal study of birth weight and adult body mass index in predicting risk of coronary heart disease and stroke in women. *BMJ*. 2005;330(7500):1115.

99. Hales CN, Barker DJ. Type 2 (non-insulin-dependent) diabetes mellitus: the thrifty phenotype hypothesis. *Diabetologia*. 1992;35(7):595–601.

100. Ozanne SE, Hales CN. Early programming of glucose-insulin metabolism. *Trends Endocrinol Metab*. 2002;13(9):368–373.

101. Lucas A. Programming by early nutrition in man. *Ciba Found Symp*. 1991;156:38–50; discussion 50–55.

102. Monteiro PO, Victora CG. Rapid growth in infancy and childhood and obesity in later life—a systematic review. *Obes Rev*. 2005;6(2):143–154.

103. Baird J, Fisher D, Lucas P, Kleijnen J, Roberts H, Law C. Being big or growing fast: systematic review of size and growth in infancy and later obesity. *BMJ*. 2005;331(7522):929.

104. Stettler N, Zemel BS, Kumanyika S, Stallings VA. Infant weight gain and childhood overweight status in a multicenter, cohort study. *Pediatrics*. 2002;109(2):194–199.

105. Stettler N, Kumanyika SK, Katz SH, Zemel BS, Stallings VA. Rapid weight gain during infancy and obesity in young adulthood in a cohort of African Americans. *Am J Clin Nutr*. 2003;77(6):1374–1378.

106. Dennison BA, Edmunds LS, Stratton HH, Pruzek RM. Rapid infant weight gain predicts childhood overweight. *Obesity (Silver Spring)*. 2006;14(3):491–499.

107. Stettler N, Stallings VA, Troxel AB, et al. Weight gain in the first week of life and overweight in adulthood: a cohort study of European American subjects fed infant formula. *Circulation*. 2005;111(15):1897–1903.

108. Hester SN, Hustead DS, Mackey AD, Singhal A, Marriage BJ. Is the macronutrient intake of formula-fed infants greater than breast-fed infants in early infancy? *J Nutr Metab*. 2012;2012:891201.

109. Singhal A, Cole TJ, Fewtrell M, et al. Promotion of faster weight gain in infants born small for gestational age: is there an adverse effect on later blood pressure? *Circulation.* 2007;115(2):213–220.

110. Ben-Shlomo Y, McCarthy A, Hughes R, Tilling K, Davies D, Smith GD. Immediate postnatal growth is associated with blood pressure in young adulthood: the Barry Caerphilly Growth Study. *Hypertension.* 2008;52(4):638–644.

111. Cianfarani S, Germani D, Branca F. Low birthweight and adult insulin resistance: the "catch-up growth" hypothesis. *Arch Dis Child Fetal Neonatal Ed.* 1999;81(1):F71–F73.

112. Gluckman PD, Hanson MA. The consequences of being born small—an adaptive perspective. *Horm Res.* 2006;65(Suppl 3):5–14.

113. Jimenez-Chillaron JC, Diaz R, Martinez D, et al. The role of nutrition on epigenetic modifications and their implications on health. *Biochimie.* 2012;94(11):2242–2263.

114. Singhal A, Lucas A. Early origins of cardiovascular disease: is there a unifying hypothesis? *Lancet.* 2004;363(9421):1642–1645.

115. Singhal A, Cole TJ, Fewtrell M, Lucas A. Breastmilk feeding and lipoprotein profile in adolescents born preterm: follow-up of a prospective randomised study. *Lancet.* 2004;363(9421):1571–1578.

116. Singhal A, Cole TJ, Lucas A. Early nutrition in preterm infants and later blood pressure: two cohorts after randomised trials. *Lancet.* 2001;357(9254):413–419.

117. Singhal A, Farooqi IS, O'Rahilly S, Cole TJ, Fewtrell M, Lucas A. Early nutrition and leptin concentrations in later life. *Am J Clin Nutr.* 2002;75(6):993–999.

118. Singhal A, Fewtrell M, Cole TJ, Lucas A. Low nutrient intake and early growth for later insulin resistance in adolescents born preterm. *Lancet.* 2003;361(9363):1089–1097.

119. Lucas A, Fewtrell MS, Morley R, et al. Randomized trial of nutrient-enriched formula versus standard formula for post-discharge preterm infants. *Pediatrics.* 2001;108(3):703–711.

120. Chan GM. Growth and bone mineral status of discharged very low birth weight infants fed different formulas or human milk. *J Pediatr.* 1993;123(3):439–443.

121. Fewtrell MS, Prentice A, Jones SC, et al. Bone mineralization and turnover in preterm infants at 8-12 years of age: the effect of early diet. *J Bone Miner Res.* 1999;14(5):810–820.

122. Victora CG, Barros FC, Horta BL, Martorell R. Short-term benefits of catch-up growth for small-for-gestational-age infants. *Int J Epidemiol.* 2001;30(6):1325–1330.

123. Maloney CA, Hay SM, Young LE, Sinclair KD, Rees WD. A methyl-deficient diet fed to rat dams during the peri-conception period programs glucose homeostasis in adult male but not female offspring. *J Nutr.* 2011;141(1):95–100.

124. Aiken CE, Ozanne SE. Sex differences in developmental programming models. *Reproduction.* 2013;145(1): R1–R13.

125. Li M, Sloboda DM, Vickers MH. Maternal obesity and developmental programming of metabolic disorders in offspring: evidence from animal models. *Exp Diabetes Res.* 2011;2011:592408.

126. Martin-Gronert MS, Ozanne SE. Experimental IUGR and later diabetes. *J Intern Med.* 2007;261(5):437–452.

127. Dahri S, Snoeck A, Reusens-Billen B, Remacle C, Hoet JJ. Islet function in offspring of mothers on low-protein diet during gestation. *Diabetes.* 1991;40(Suppl 2) :115–120.

128. Gopalakrishnan GS, Gardner DS, Dandrea J, et al. Influence of maternal pre-pregnancy body composition and diet during early-mid pregnancy on cardiovascular function and nephron number in juvenile sheep. *Br J Nutr.* 2005;94(6):938–947.

129. Vickers MH, Breier BH, Cutfield WS, Hofman PL, Gluckman PD. Fetal origins of hyperphagia, obesity, and hypertension and postnatal amplification by hypercaloric nutrition. *Am J Physiol Endocrinol Metab.* 2000;279(1):E83–E87.

130. Sarr O, Yang K, Regnault TR. In utero programming of later adiposity: the role of fetal growth restriction. *J Pregnancy.* 2012;2012:134758.

131. Armitage JA, Lakasing L, Taylor PD, et al. Developmental programming of aortic and renal structure in offspring of rats fed fat-rich diets in pregnancy. *J Physiol.* 2005;565(Pt 1):171–184.

132. Ainge H, Thompson C, Ozanne SE, Rooney KB. A systematic review on animal models of maternal high fat feeding and offspring glycaemic control. *Int J Obes (Lond).* 2010;35(3):325–335.

133. Williams L, Seki Y, Vuguin PM, Charron MJ. Animal models of in utero exposure to a high fat diet: a review. *Biochim Biophys Acta.* 2014;1842(3):507–519.

134. White CL, Purpera MN, Morrison CD. Maternal obesity is necessary for programming effect of high-fat diet on offspring. *Am J Physiol Regul Integr Comp Physiol.* 2009;296(5):R1464–R1472.

135. Hartil K, Vuguin PM, Kruse M, et al. Maternal substrate utilization programs the development of the metabolic syndrome in male mice exposed to high fat in utero. *Pediatr Res.* 2009;66(4):368–373.

136. Lanham SA, Roberts C, Hollingworth T, et al. Maternal high-fat diet: effects on offspring bone structure. *Osteoporos Int.* 2010;21(10):1703–1714.

137. Peleg-Raibstein D, Luca E, Wolfrum C. Maternal high-fat diet in mice programs emotional behavior in adulthood. *Behav Brain Res.* 2012;233(2):398–404.

138. Lewis RM, Petry CJ, Ozanne SE, Hales CN. Effects of maternal iron restriction in the rat on blood pressure, glucose tolerance, and serum lipids in the 3-month-old offspring. *Metabolism.* 2001;50(5):562–567.

139. Harvey L, Boksa P. Do prenatal immune activation and maternal iron deficiency interact to affect neurodevelopment and early behavior in rat offspring? *Brain Behav Immun.* 2013;pii:S0889-1591(13)00463-7.

140. Reynolds RM. Glucocorticoid excess and the developmental origins of disease: two decades of testing the hypothesis—2012 Curt Richter Award Winner. *Psychoneuroendocrinology.* 2013;38(1):1–11.

141. Matthews SG, Phillips DI. Transgenerational inheritance of stress pathology. *Exp Neurol.* 2012;233(1):95–101.

142. Ozanne SE. Metabolic programming in animals. *Br Med Bull.* 2001;60:143–152.

143. Maniam J, Antoniadis C, Morris MJ. Early-life stress, HPA axis adaptation, and mechanisms contributing to later health outcomes. *Front Endocrinol (Lausanne).* 2014;5:73.

144. Zambrano E, Nathanielsz PW. Mechanisms by which maternal obesity programs offspring for obesity: evidence from animal studies. *Nutr Rev.* 2013;71(Suppl 1):S42–S54.

145. Langley-Evans SC. Fetal programming of CVD and renal disease: animal models and mechanistic considerations. *Proc Nutr Soc.* 2013;72(3):317–325.

146. Armitage JA, Khan IY, Taylor PD, Nathanielsz PW, Poston L. Developmental programming of the metabolic syndrome by maternal nutritional imbalance: how strong is the evidence from experimental models in mammals? *J Physiol.* 2004;561(Pt 2):355–377.

147. Thompson RF, Fazzari MJ, Niu H, Barzilai N, Simmons RA, Greally JM. Experimental intrauterine growth restriction induces alterations in DNA methylation and gene expression in pancreatic islets of rats. *J Biol Chem.* 2010;285(20):15111–15118.

148. Drake AJ, Liu L. Intergenerational transmission of programmed effects: public health consequences. *Trends Endocrinol Metab.* 2010;21(4):206–213.

149. Barker DJ, Shiell AW, Barker ME, Law CM. Growth in utero and blood pressure levels in the next generation. *J Hypertens.* 2000;18(7):843–846.

150. Stein AD, Lumey LH. The relationship between maternal and offspring birth weights after maternal prenatal famine exposure: the Dutch Famine Birth Cohort Study. *Hum Biol.* 2000;72(4):641–654.

151. Benyshek DC. The "early life" origins of obesity-related health disorders: new discoveries regarding the intergenerational transmission of developmentally programmed traits in the global cardiometabolic health crisis. *Am J Phys Anthropol.* 2013;152(Suppl 5):779–793.

152. Painter RC, Osmond C, Gluckman P, Hanson M, Phillips DI, Roseboom TJ. Transgenerational effects of prenatal exposure to the Dutch famine on neonatal adiposity and health in later life. *BJOG.* 2008;115(10):1243–1249.

153. Pembrey ME, Bygren LO, Kaati G, et al. Sex-specific, male-line transgenerational responses in humans. *Eur J Hum Genet.* 2006;14(2):159–166.

154. Bygren LO, Tinghög P, Carstensen J, et al. Change in paternal grandmothers' early food supply influenced cardiovascular mortality of the female grandchildren. *BMC Genet.* 2014;15:12.

155. Heijmans BT, Tobi EW, Stein AD, et al. Persistent epigenetic differences associated with prenatal exposure to famine in humans. *Proc Natl Acad Sci U S A.* 2008;105(44):17046–17049.

156. Soubry A, Schildkraut JM, Murtha A, et al. Paternal obesity is associated with IGF2 hypomethylation in newborns: results from a Newborn Epigenetics Study (NEST) cohort. *BMC Med.* 2013;11:29.

157. Brunton PJ. Resetting the dynamic range of hypothalamic-pituitary-adrenal axis stress responses through pregnancy. *J Neuroendocrinol.* 2010;22(11):1198–1213.

158. Entringer S. Impact of stress and stress physiology during pregnancy on child metabolic function and obesity risk. *Curr Opin Clin Nutr Metab Care.* 2013;16(3):320–327.

159. Fewtrell MS, Williams JE, Singhal A, Murgatroyd PR, Fuller N, Lucas A. Early diet and peak bone mass: 20 year follow-up of a randomized trial of early diet in infants born preterm. *Bone.* 2009;45(1):142–149.

160. Ehrenkranz RA, Dusick AM, Vohr BR, Wright LL, Wrage LA, Poole WK. Growth in the neonatal intensive care unit influences neurodevelopmental and growth outcomes of extremely low birth weight infants. *Pediatrics.* 2006;117(4):1253–1261.

161. Beardsall K, Diderholm BM, Dunger DB. Insulin and carbohydrate metabolism. *Best Pract Res Clin Endocrinol Metab.* 2008;22(1):41–55.

Test Your Knowledge Question Answers

1. The correct answer is **D**.
2. The correct answer is **C**.
3. The correct answer is **B**.

11

Human Milk

Jacqueline J. Wessel, MEd, RDN, CNSC, CSP, CLE

 Podcast

CONTENTS

Learning Objectives

1. List 3 benefits of the use of human milk for the infant.
2. Describe the rationale for human milk fortification for the premature infant.
3. State the American Academy of Pediatrics recommendation for the use of vitamin D with an exclusively human milk–fed infant.

Introduction

Breastfeeding is advocated throughout the world. The American Academy of Pediatrics (AAP), the Canadian Pediatric Society, the International Pediatric Association, the World Health Organization (WHO), and others all have policies that recommend breastfeeding as the preferred method of feeding for infants.[1-4] The Healthy People 2010 goals proposed by the U.S. Surgeon General include breastfeeding initiation rates of 75% and continued breastfeeding rates of 50% at 6 months and 25% at 12 months.[5] Currently, the initiation goal is being met; however, the goals for duration and for exclusivity of breastfeeding are not being met. In the 2011 Surgeon General Call to Action to Support Breastfeeding report,[6] the breastfeeding rates for black infants were about 50% lower than those for white infants at birth, 6 months, and 12 months, even when controlling for the family's income or educational level.

The advantages of breastfeeding are numerous and include nutritional, immunologic, bonding, and societal benefits (Table 11-1). Human milk is considered the gold standard for protective nutrients for the infant.[7] Some of the immunological protection seen with the use of human milk may be attributed to the establishment of beneficial bacteria in the gastrointestinal tract of the infant. Human milk contains

Table 11-1. Benefits of Breastfeeding

ROLE	BENEFIT
Mother	Improved mother-infant bonding
	More rapid uterine involution
	Postpartum weight loss
	Decreased incidence of premenopausal breast cancer
	Decreased incidence of ovarian cancer
	May protect against development of osteoporosis
Infant	Antibacterial factors: secretory IgA, IgM, IgG, IgD, *Bifidobacterium* growth factor, lactoferrin, complement C1-9, factor binding proteins, lysozyme, lactoperoxidase, macrophages, neutrophils, B and T lymphocytes, lipid, growth factors, nucleotides, and vitamins A, E, C[1,14,15]
	Decreased incidence of gastrointestinal illness, respiratory illness, otitis media, urinary tract infections, sudden infant death syndrome[16-22]
	Lower incidence of allergies, even with a family history of atopy[23-27]
	May have lower incidence of later chronic diseases such as celiac disease, Crohn's disease, lymphoma, specific genotypes of diabetes mellitus type I[28-33]
Society	Reduced time off work for mothers of breastfed infants for infant illnesses
	Reduced healthcare costs[1]

probiotics, including *Bifidobacterium bifidum* and *Lactobacillus,*[7] and other factors, such as prebiotic oligosaccharides, that promote the growth of these bacteria.[8] The bifidus flora of the breastfed infant is thought to activate the immune system and defend against pathogens.[7,9] Breastfed infants have been found to have more diarrhea-free days in the first 6 months of life than nonbreastfed infants.[9] A large study from the Philippines showed that nonbreastfed infants had a 10-fold increase in diarrhea compared to breastfed infants.[10] In the case of a common cause of diarrhea, *Campylobacter jejuni,* breastfed infants were protected during the time that they were breastfeeding, even though the specific antibody concentration is highest in colostrum, decreases over the next few weeks, but then remains constant throughout lactation.[9] The bacterial colonization pattern of the human milk–fed infant differs from that of formula-fed infants. Some term infant formulas have now added prebiotics and some have added probiotics.[11]

The infant's intestinal host defense is immature at birth, and breast milk helps the infant ward off antigens and microbes during this vulnerable time.[7] Secretory IgA levels are low in term newborns at birth and for the first 30 days[12]; in hu-

man milk, secretory IgA is at its highest level as a percentage of the total protein during this time. The activation of secretory IgA-producing cells in the intestine is dependent on the initial colonization of the gut by *Bifidobacteria* and *Lactobacilli* contained in human milk and stimulated for growth by the nondigestible oligosaccharides also contained in human milk.[7, 13]

Lactation Science

The major limitation to the provision of human milk is inadequate supply for the premature or hospitalized infant. Mothers of infants who cannot yet breastfeed either due to illness or prematurity are dependent upon a breast pump for initiation and maintenance of their milk supply. The science of lactation has made great strides in providing mothers with more efficient breast pumps with newly designed breast pump suction patterns to mimic the sucking patterns of healthy term infants.[34] These patterns make the maintenance of lactation more efficient and comfortable. Research has also shown that hand expression and hands on pumping in combination with traditional pumping increase the fat content and therefore caloric content of human expressed milk.[35] More information is available elsewhere.[36]

Breast Milk and Maternal Medications

Health professionals are often asked questions about the use of medications in mothers who are lactating. Riordan and Auerbach state that 3 "knowns" exist about medications and breast milk: (1) most drugs pass into breast milk; (2) almost all medications appear in only small amounts, usually < 1% of the maternal dosage; and (3) very few drugs are contraindicated for breastfeeding women.[37-39] That does not mean, however, that caution should not be taken when prescribing medications to lactating women. Hale's *Medications and Mother's Milk* is a useful reference that is updated regularly and compiles the known data about medications, assigning a risk code.[39] The evaluation of the safety of medications for premature infants depends on 3 factors according to Hale: (1) the amount of medication in the milk, (2) the oral bioavailability of the medication, and (3) the ability of the infant to clear the medication.[40] Some of the drugs of concern in general are the chemotherapeutic agents, radioactive isotopes, drugs of abuse, lithium, ergotamine, and drugs that suppress lactation. Antihistamines may reduce milk supply. The Academy of Breastfeeding Medicine has a clinical protocol on the use of galactogogues for use for initiation, maintenance, or augmentation of milk supply.[41]

LactMed is a database on medications and other chemicals to which breastfeeding mothers may be exposed, including information on alternatives, and possible adverse effects on the infant. LactMed is part of the National Library of Medicine's Toxicology Data Network. It is available at the Web site http://toxnet.nlm.nih.gov/cgi-bin/sis/htmlgen?-LACT or as a free application for iPhone/iPod Touch and Android devices. The information is based on scientific references and is updated monthly.[42]

A grave concern is what to do about the mother who wants to breastfeed or pump but also admits to using drugs of abuse. Marijuana is now legal to use in some states in the United States, further complicating the identification of what substances are considered drugs of abuse. The Academy of Breastfeeding Medicine has useful, practical guidelines,[43] and the AAP has an older guideline[44] as well as recommendations regarding breastfeeding and drug use in its 2012 guidelines.[45] In general, adequately nourished mothers who are narcotic dependent but enrolled and participating in a drug treatment program and who have had consistent prenatal care with no other contraindications (such as infection with human immunodeficiency virus [HIV]), are supported in their decision to breastfeed their infants. Breastfeeding is sometimes used as part of a methadone weaning program.[46] A bigger question may be what are the short-term and long-term implications for the prenatally exposed fetus; whether the positive effects of human milk can alter any deleterious effects is not yet known.[43]

Tobacco is also considered a drug, and smoking is strongly discouraged.[45] If a mother cannot quit, breastfeeding is superior to formula feeding and can protect the infants against some of the hazards of smoking[47,48]; however, the protective effect of exclusive breastfeeding for 6 months against developing allergic respiratory symptoms may be lost when the mother is a smoker.[49] Breastfeeding mothers who smoke have been noted to have a shorter duration of breastfeeding.[50,51] Sleep/awake cycles of breastfed infants appear to be disrupted in association with maternal smoking, with shorter periods of sleep after an acute episode of smoking.[52]

Contrary to popular thought, alcohol is not a galactogogue, and drinking alcoholic beverages is not recommended.[45] At higher doses alcohol can block the release of oxytocin, which stimulates milk ejection.[53] More information regarding minimizing alcohol exposure to the breastfeeding infant is available elsewhere.[54]

Contraindications to the Use of Human Milk

Very few absolute contraindications exist regarding the use of breast milk. They include inborn errors of metabolism, although some of these conditions may allow for a small amount of human milk to be used under the guidance of a metabolic dietitian in combination with a metabolic diet. In the industrialized world, HIV-positive mothers have been discouraged from breastfeeding; however, in the developing world, the benefits of breastfeeding appear to outweigh the risk of acquiring HIV infection from human milk.[45]

Breastfeeding

In 1991 the WHO and United Nations International Children's Fund (UNICEF) established an international program to promote breastfeeding, the Baby Friendly Hospital Initiative (BFHI).[4] This incorporated a 10-step program to promote and support breastfeeding (Table 11-2).

The management of the breastfeeding dyad requires skill and knowledge to achieve a successful outcome for both the mother and infant. Unfortunately, reports continue to occur about hypernatremic dehydration among exclusively breastfed neonates due to inadequate intake with potentially devastating consequences. The recommendation from analyses of these reports is for close and regular follow-up of breastfed infants by a healthcare provider.[55–57]

Evidence-based guidelines from the Academy of Breastfeeding Medicine are available that provide recommendations

Table 11-2. Ten Steps to Successful Breastfeeding[3]

EVERY FACILITY PROVIDING MATERNITY SERVICES AND CARE FOR NEWBORN INFANTS SHOULD:
1. Have a written breastfeeding policy that is routinely communicated to all healthcare staff.
2. Train all health care staff in skills necessary to implement this policy.
3. Inform all pregnant women about the benefits and management of breastfeeding.
4. Help mothers initiate breastfeeding within 30 minutes after birth.
5. Show mothers how to breastfeed and how to maintain lactation even if they should be separated from their infants.
6. Give newborn infants no food or drink other than breast milk, unless medically indicated.
7. Practice rooming in—allow mothers and infants to remain together—24 hours a day.
8. Encourage breastfeeding on demand.
9. Give no artificial teats or pacifiers (also called dummies or soothers) to breastfeeding infants.
10. Foster the establishment of breastfeeding support groups and refer mothers to them on discharge from the hospital or clinic.

Reprinted with permission from Baby-Friendly USA Web site http://www.babyfriendlyusa.org. Accessed December 31, 2009.

for best practice in the management of term, late preterm, and premature infants.[58,59] Late preterm infants with gestational ages between 34 and 36 6/7 weeks are at particular risk for lactation problems because these infants may appear to be competent early in breastfeeding when they are not and may fool even experienced mothers. These infants may have difficulty extracting milk and stimulating the mother to produce an adequate milk supply.[60,61] Late preterm infants are more likely to require rehospitalization in the first 2 weeks after birth and have poor lactation outcomes such as early cessation of breastfeeding, jaundice, dehydration, and poor growth.[62,63] Their mothers are also at risk for delayed lactogenesis.[64] Wight et al[65] and Meier et al[64,66,67] describe strategies to work with the mother-infant dyad in establishing and maintaining maternal milk supply and adequate intake for the infant.

The mothers of premature or sick term infants have the challenge of pumping their milk. Strategies to facilitate pumping are available.[64–67] A discussion of these is beyond the scope of this chapter, and interested readers are referred to the book by Wight et al[65] and to several works by Paula Meier PhD, RN.[33,63,66–68] Meier has written extensively on the promotion of lactation in an inner-city newborn intensive care unit (NICU) setting,[66] evaluation of the efficiency of different breast pumps,[33,67] and the role of nipple shields in facilitating milk transfer for preterm infants.[68]

Human Milk and the Premature Infant: The Relationship Between Human Milk and Necrotizing Enterocolitis

For the premature infant the use of breast milk offers a particular advantage in decreasing the incidence of necrotizing enterocolitis (NEC).[69,70] Research by Meinzen-Derr et al[71] suggested a dose-related association of breast milk feeding, with a reduction in risk of NEC or death in extremely low birth weight infants. In a trial by Cristofalo et al[72] comparing outcomes between the use of premature infant formula and the use of donor human milk and human milk–derived fortifier, the incidence of both medical and surgical NEC was higher in the formula-fed group. Other studies using human milk and donor human milk with human milk–derived fortifier have shown a decreased incidence of NEC as compared to human milk with bovine fortification.[73–75] One often-quoted study uses premature formula instead of donor milk in the bovine protein group.[73] Only the latest study by Herrmann and Carroll[75] had a low baseline level of NEC, and the study again showed an advantage for the exclusively human milk diet including human milk–derived fortification.

Walker,[7] Schanler et al,[76] Schanler,[77] and Kleinman and Walker[78] have suggested a protective effect against infection in premature infants who are fed their own mother's milk, sometimes termed the enteromammary immune system. Although pasteurization alters some nutritional and immunological properties of donor human milk, a meta-analysis has shown that it still conveys protection against NEC.[79] The 2012 AAP recommendation is that pasteurized donor human milk, appropriately fortified, should be used if the mother's own milk is unavailable or its use is contraindicated.[45] The current thoughts are that a combination of genetic predisposition, intestinal immaturities, and microbial dysbiosis combine to induce NEC.[80] New information about the fecal microflora of premature infants before and during NEC suggest that a difference in flora exists between these infants and those who do not get NEC, characterized by unusual intestinal microbial species and a lower diversity of flora.[81–83] Prolonged empirical antibiotic use is associated with these unusual microbial patterns as well.[84,85]

Preterm Breast Milk

No agreement exists on the macronutrient content of human milk from mothers of preterm infants. Some researchers have described increased amounts of protein, sodium, chloride, and iron for 3 weeks[86] to approximately 1 month after delivery.[87–89] Others have reported no difference between preterm and term milk in protein content at different stages[90,91] and a lower protein value.[90–93] For optimal growth, preterm infants need augmentation of breast milk because of their increased needs for protein, phosphorus, calcium, and zinc.[94,95] Previously it was thought that, at least in terms of bone mineralization, the bone density of infants born prematurely would normalize as they grew into childhood.[96] Chan et al[97] demonstrated that premature infants < 1.5 kg at birth continue to show lower bone mineral content and density and tend to be significantly smaller for age than their term counterparts when studied at 5–9 years of age. Fortification is an acceptable method of augmenting breast milk for a premature infant.[44,97]

Breast Milk Fortification

Fortification is added to human milk for premature infants to meet their high nutrient needs. The optimal population, method, time, and product for fortification remains to be determined; however, a general consensus exists that all infants with a birth weight < 1500 g should be fortified.[98–104]

Many different methods of fortification now exist (Table 11-3), including powdered human milk fortifier with

Table 11-3. Nutrient Composition of Human Milk and Fortified Human Milk Based on Intake of 120 kcal/kg

TYPE OF MILK OR FORTIFIED MILK	CALORIES	PROTEIN	CALCIUM	PHOSPHORUS
Preterm milk[105]	120 cal/kg	2.5 g/kg	44.6 mg/kg	23.2 mg/kg
Term milk[106]	120 kcal/kg	1.6 g/kg	50 mg/kg	25 mg/kg
Preterm milk with Enfamil Human Milk Fortifier Acidified Liquid[107]	120 cal/kg	4.8 g/kg	174 mg/kg	96 mg/kg
Preterm milk with Similac Human Milk Fortifier (powder)[108]	120 cal/kg	3.6 g/kg	207 mg/kg	117 mg/kg
Preterm milk with Similac Human Milk Fortifier Concentrated Liquid[108]	120 kcal/kg	3.6 g/kg	210 mg/kg	118 mg/kg
Preterm milk with Similac Human Milk Fortifier Extensively Hydrolyzed Protein Concentrated Liquid[108]	120 kcal/kg	4.3 g/kg	158.4 mg/kg	102 mg/kg
Preterm/term milk 1:1 with Similac Special Care 30 cal/oz[108]	125 cal/kg	4.35 g/kg preterm milk 3.75 g/kg term milk	174 mg/kg	95.6 mg/kg
Prolact+4 H2MF[109]	120 cal/kg	Fortifies up to 3.45 g/kg	Added minerals, variable	Added minerals, variable
ESPGHAN recommended intake for preterm infants[94]	110-135 cal/kg	4-4.5 g/kg/d (infants < 1000 g) 3.5-4 g/kg/d (infants 1000-1800 g)	120-140 mg/kg	60-90 mg/kg
Koletzko et al[110]	110-130 cal/kg	3.5-4.5 g/kg	120-200 mg/kg	60-140 mg/kg

ESPGHAN, European Society of Pediatric Gastroenterology, Hepatolology, and Nutrition.

bovine protein, liquid human milk fortifier with bovine protein, liquid acidified human milk fortifier with bovine protein, a new liquid human milk fortifier with hydrolyzed protein, and liquid human milk–derived fortifier. In addition, higher calorie (30 calorie) premature formula can be mixed in a 1:1 mixture or other ratios with breast milk. The final nutrient content can vary significantly depending on the fortifier selected. Most clinicians prefer a human milk fortifier in order to use the maximal amount of human milk. Higher protein intake from human milk fortifier has been associated with better linear growth.[111]

Osmolality increases when fortifier is added to breast milk,[112,113] but there do not appear be differences in the incidence of side effects[114] or NEC[114] or alterations in gastric emptying.[115] Two recent papers, however, describe problems as a result of using powdered fortifier in infants < 1000 g. One center described an association with bowel obstruction,[116] and another center reported a calcium stone ileus.[117] A comparison between the use of the acidified liquid human milk fortifier with a powdered bovine protein containing fortifier noted that the use of the acidified product was associated with poorer growth and clinically significant acidosis.[118] Concern has been expressed about how the addition of an acidified product affects human milk. A study of 100 samples of human milk found a 76% reduction in white cells,

56% decrease in lipase activity, and 14% decrease in total protein; however, the crematocrit increased 36%.[119]

Controversy has existed concerning the effect of iron, one of the ingredients in human milk fortifiers, on the antimicrobial properties of human milk. A comparison of 2 powdered fortifiers, one with iron and one without, showed decreased bacteriostatic properties of human milk with the iron-containing fortifier added.[120] In an in vitro study, human milk with an iron-containing fortifier was found to have a reduced antimicrobial effect against *Escherichia coli*, *Staphylococcus*, *Enterobacter sakazakii*, and Group B streptococcus,[120] and against *E. coli*, *Staphylococcus aureus*, *Pseudomonas aeruginosa*, and *Candida albicans* in a second study[121] when these organisms were added to human milk. Iron is proposed to undermine the antibacterial effects of lactoferrin, which are known to be lessened when it is saturated with iron.[120] Other research using the same methodology showed that the human milk–derived fortifier did not affect the bacteriostatic effects of human milk.[122] In another study, no effect was seen in the counts of resident flora and *E. sakazakii* when the iron-containing fortifier was added to fresh milk within a time span of 6 hours.[123]

The human milk–derived liquid fortifier, Prolact H2MF comes as +4, +6, +8, and +10 with increasing amounts of calories and protein.[109] A cream supplement is now available to augment calories from human milk fat.[109] As discussed previously, studies have shown decreased incidence of NEC with the use of this fortifier.[73–75] This product is much more expensive at $6.75/mL (2014 pricing; Cincinnati Childrens Hospital, oral communication, May 2014) than traditional human milk fortifiers. However, a cost analysis on the use of this fortification showed a cost savings $8167 per infant compared to the cost of medical or surgical treatment for NEC.[124] Many centers have seen a need to increase the density of these products to 26 or 28 kcal/oz. This increases the volume of fortification and uses less of the mother's own milk, but so far studies have not shown any problem with this fortification. Increased density does increase the cost, however. This product is frozen and is available in volumes that would be added to human milk to make a final volume of 100 mL.[109]

Adjustable and Targeted Fortification of Human Milk

Adjustable and targeted fortification are strategies that individualize the fortification of human milk. The adjustable fortification work was initially studied by Moro et al.[125] Adjustable fortification studies by Arslangolu et al[126] have looked at using serum blood urea nitrogen (BUN) tests, specifically looking at a lower BUN at a steady fluid intake, to give additional protein through increasing the fortification at first, then giving protein at different levels above the fortification. They were aiming for a BUN level of 9–14 mg/dL,[126] and infants in their study were given more fortification so that protein content increased. Growth was improved vs historical controls, with weight and head circumference (HC) showing statistical significance and length just missing significance.[126] An updated version of their protocol is now available.[127] Miller et al[128] also used this method with BUN with infants < 31 weeks. They saw less growth failure but did not see improvements in length or HC. Another study by Alan et al,[129] using a similar premise but adding twice as much protein as in the 2 previous studies without adding additional fortifier, revealed significant improvements in weight, length, and HC growth.

Targeted fortification of human milk uses analysis of the milk to guide individualized fortification. This approach was first described by Pohlberger et al[130] in a research method type analysis, and other authors have now taken this process to the bedside.[131–134] Some have used this technique to fortify protein,[126–130] while others have used it to fortify all nutrients including both carbohydrate and fat.[134] Because the literature has described protein as a limiting nutrient for

growth, especially linear growth,[111] clinicians are typically not accustomed to fortifying the other macronutrients. In this algorithm, the dietary prescription is determined after the analysis of human milk in the NICU laboratory. This targeted method of fortifying milk resulted in better growth, and future plans are to include body composition to look at lean body mass.[134]

In some cases, a term infant cannot tolerate full-volume feedings because of a disease process. A higher calorie human milk can be made for these infants, but it does not use the same products as for the preterm infant because the levels of calcium and phosphorus may be too high. An individualized approach is necessary based on the prescribed volume and the calorie, protein, and mineral needs for that infant. Term infant formula may be used to augment breast milk to keep a good protein, carbohydrate, and lipid ratio.

A concept sometimes called lacto-engineering may also be used to increase calories, using the higher calorie hindmilk to augment the caloric content of feedings. This will not alter the need for fortification for a preterm infant, but it can help supply additional calories. A creamatocrit is a measurement for estimating the fat content and therefore the caloric content of a human milk sample.[135,136] The Creamatocrit Plus (Medela Inc, McHenry, IL) instrument is available and computes calories and fat grams from that measurement.[137] Some units have incorporated this measurement into their clinical program.[138,139] Mothers have been taught to perform this test in the clinical setting.[140]

The traditional method is to use microhematocrit tube, which is filled with milk and spun in a centrifuge. The layer of fat is measured as with a blood hematocrit.[134,136] Regression equations are as follows[136]:

- Fresh breast milk: Energy (kcal/dL) = 5.99 × creamatocrit (%) + 32.5.
- Frozen breast milk: Energy (kcal/dL) = 6.20 × creamatocrit (%) + 35.1.

A recent paper compared the results of creamatocrit testing with mid-infrared spectroscopy and laboratory analysis.[141] The laboratory analysis and the spectroscopy methods showed no statistical difference in fat and energy.[141] The creamatocrit method overestimated the fat and therefore the energy content of human milk, with mean values of these samples 21.8 ± 3.4 kcal/oz as compared to 17.1 ± 2.9 kcal/oz.[141]

Research is being conducted on the content of hindmilk.[142] There do not appear to be any significant differences in creamatocrit values in the milk of mothers of preterm, small for gestational age, and term infants.[143] The creamatocrit values appear to increase until 16 weeks post partum and then decline.[143] The circadian variation of fat content in human milk has been evaluated, and although spot values may be misleading, consistent sampling does show a trend in 2 studies for samples expressed at night to have greater fat content.[144,145] The vitamin A and E levels also appear to be 1.6 times higher in hindmilk than foremilk, something to consider when planning fortification.[146]

Banked Human Milk

The use of donor milk has increased substantially in the last few years; in 2011 the 13 North American milk banks distributed more than 2 million ounces of donor human milk.[147] The Human Milk Banking Association of North America has guidelines for screening, collection, processing, storage, and distribution of donor milk[148] as well as guidelines for establishing a donor milk bank.[149] Seventeen milk banks are currently active in North America, with 4 more in development.[147] The milk is pasteurized to avoid any viral or bacterial contamination.[147] Pasteurization reduces the immunomodulatory proteins in human milk. A study by Akinbi et al[150] showed that the concentrations of lysozyme, lactoferrin, lactoperoxidase, and secretory immunoglobulin A were reduced 50%–82% in pasteurized donor milk. The activities of lysozyme and lactoperoxidase were 74%–88% lower in donor milk than in freshly expressed human milk.[150] Proliferation of bacterial pathogens in pasteurized donor milk was enhanced 1.8-fold to 4.6-fold compared with fresh or frozen human milk, highlighting the need for stringent procedures for handling of this milk.[150]

Banked donor pasteurized human milk is used in many nurseries for premature infants, either as a bridge to feed early if the mother's own milk is not yet in, or as a substitute for the mother who cannot supply sufficient milk or who has chosen not to pump. Some nurseries use donor milk for the first month after delivery for very low birth weight infants. An advantage of using the mother's own milk is the enteromammary system, which provides targeted antibodies for the infant from the antigens that are present in the mother's (and baby's) environment.[80] Donor milk may be collected from preterm or term mothers; obviously, a much greater pool is available from mothers of term infants. If donor-banked term milk is used for a preterm infant, supplemental protein, calcium, phosphorus, and zinc will be needed because the levels of these nutrients are lower in donor term milk than in preterm milk.[151]

Growth issues are prevalent when donor milk is used. Others have noted the lower protein content of donor human milk, which is often from a mother who is in a different stage of lactation. The lowered protein milk is very suitable for the mother's own infant (who may at this time of lactation be eating foods), but not for a premature infant. Many centers use additional fortification for this milk, especially in protein content, and some also add zinc because the zinc content of this "older infant" milk may be lower. Some centers use additional sodium supplementation, either guided by a low urine sodium or added as part of their protocol.

Vitamin D

The latest statement regarding vitamin D from the AAP is to supplement with 400 IU/d beginning soon after birth.[152] This replaces the 2003 statement that recommended 200 IU beginning in the first 2 months after birth.[153] Rickets, an example of extreme vitamin D deficiency, continues to be reported in the United States and other Western countries, predominantly in the breastfed population and in infants with darker skin pigmentation.[152,154,155] Historically we relied upon the effect of sunlight on our skin to stimulate synthesis of vitamin D from cholesterol as our main source. Breast milk normally has very little vitamin D. In a lactating mother supplemented with 400 IU of vitamin D, the vitamin content of her own milk ranges from < 25 to 78 IU/L.[152] Some research on providing women with very large doses of vitamin D shows an increased content of the vitamin in their milk.[156] At this time, research is needed concerning the safety and efficacy of this method prior to recommendation to a larger population.[156] A concern now also exists about the age at which direct sunlight exposure may be initiated.[157] Following these guidelines, vitamin D supplementation is necessary. More vitamin D-only products are now available.

Iron

The iron content in human milk is very low, although the iron is in a form that is more bioavailable compared with that in fortified infant formula.[158] Iron needs in the first 6 months of life for a breastfed infant rely on the infant's stores at birth.[159] In healthy breastfed term infants iron deficiency before 6 months of age is sometimes observed, but it is uncommon.[159] Typically at 4–6 months, iron-rich complementary foods are added to the infant's diet, although the newer guidelines are for exclusive breastfeeding for 6 months.[45] (However, according to the 2011 Infant study, 40% of infants received foods in the first 4 months of life.[6]) The WHO recommends meats for the first food for breastfed infants.[6] Meats have the advantage of being a rich source of iron and zinc.

Premature infants do not have the same iron stores as term infants, and both term and preterm infants who are hospitalized may have blood sampled for testing, further depleting their iron stores. Premature infants typically receive iron supplementation due to their low stores at birth, and the beneficial effect has been documented in the literature[159,160] Iron deficiency in infants is concerning because it appears to lead to developmental delay, which is irreversible.[161] Premature infants who are breastfed exclusively for 6 months may be at increased risk of iron deficiency. Ziegler et al[160] studied the effect of early (at 1 month) iron administration on breastfed term infants and found that it was feasible and well tolerated by most infants.

Growth of Breastfed Infants

Growth of breastfed infants differs from that of formula-fed infants. The WHO has published a growth curve based on infant growth data from one site in the United States as well as sites in Brazil, Ghana, India, Norway, and Oman.[162] The intention was to choose sites where breastfeeding was commonly practiced and provide lactation support to mothers to help them comply with the feeding standards required to construct this growth curve. The factors were exclusive or predominate breastfeeding for the first 4 months, introduction of complementary food between 4 and 6 months, and partial breastfeeding to be continued until at least 12 months.[163] Comparing the 2000 Centers for Disease Control and Prevention (CDC) growth curve to the WHO curve, the growth trajectory of breastfed infants is notably different, with breastfed infants growing more rapidly in the first 2 months and less rapidly from 3 to 12 months in relation to the CDC curve. Linear growth is higher until 4 months. The growth trajectories show that infants in the CDC curve are heavier and shorter than the WHO reference population.[164]

Breast Milk Safety and Administration

In 2001, a powdered infant formula, Portagen (which was not a standard formula for preterm infants), was used and prepared in a NICU for preterm infants. A 33-week infant became ill and died; the cerebral spinal culture grew *E. sakazakii*. Because this is a rare cause of neonatal meningitis, the state health board and the CDC became involved. In the investigation, it was found that not only opened cans of the formula contained the bacteria but also the unopened cans as well. This finding launched an investigation into the bacterial counts of powdered formula; unlike liquid concentrate or ready to feed, powdered formula is not sterile.[165,166] In 2002, the CDC stated that formula products should be based on nutritional needs

with alternatives to powder forms used whenever possible; in addition, hang times were limited to 4 hours.[165] The European Society of Pediatric Gastroenterology, Hepatolology, and Nutrition had similar recommendations in 2004.[167] The Food and Drug Administration issued a letter to professionals with similar recommendations.[168] These statements have implications for the use of powdered human milk fortifiers as well as the use of expressed breast milk. Safety remains a paramount concern in the provision of any nutrition to the preterm or term infant. Detailed guidelines published by the Academy of Nutrition and Dietetics Association (AND) have been established for the collection, labeling, transport, storage, and administration of expressed breast milk (Tables 11-4 and 11-5).[169] The Human Milk Banking Association of North America also published guidelines for the handling of breast milk in hospitals, daycare settings, and the home.[171] The following are some of the AND key points:

- Mothers are encouraged to express milk, ideally as soon as possible after birth (or breastfeed if the infant is able).[172]
- Mothers are encouraged to pump every 2–3 hours or at least 8 times in 24 hours, using a hospital grade pump; using a double kit not only saves time but also increases hormone levels, leading to increased milk production.[172]
- Breast milk should be stored in sterile or aseptic food grade plastic or glass containers that are built to withstand long-term freezing. They need to have close-fitting caps that provide an airtight closure; a nipple is not an acceptable cap.[169]
- Labels should indicate the contents: expressed breast milk, infant's name, medical record or identification number, date and time of milk expressed, medications or supplements taken by the mother, date and time of

Table 11-4. Academy of Nutrition and Dietetics Recommendations for Human Milk Storage for Hospitalized Infants[169]

STORAGE METHOD	TEMPERATURE	LENGTH OF TIME RECOMMENDED
Room temperature	25°C, 75°F	≤ 4 h
Cooler with ice packs	15°C, 59°F; fresh milk	24 h
Refrigerator, thawed milk	4°C, 39°F	24 h feeding when possible
Refrigerator, fortified milk	4°C, 39°F	24 h
Refrigerator, fresh milk	4°C, 39°F	48 h
Freezer, home unit		3 mo
Freezer	−20°C, −4°F	6-12 mo
Freezer	−70°C, −94°F	≥ 12 mo

Table. 11-5. Academy of Breastfeeding Medicine: Storage Duration of Fresh Human Milk for Use With Healthy Full-Term Infants[170]

LOCATION	TEMPERATURE	DURATION	COMMENTS
Countertop, table	Room temperature (up to 77°F or 25°C)	6–8 h	Containers should be covered and kept as cool as possible; covering the container with a cool towel may keep milk cooler.
Insulated cooler bag	5°F–39°F or −15°C to 4°C	24 h	Keep ice packs in contact with milk containers at all times, limit opening cooler bag.
Refrigerator	39°F or 4°C	5 d	Store milk in the back of the main body of the refrigerator.
Freezer			
Freezer compartment of a refrigerator	5°F or −15°C	2 wk	Store milk toward the back of the freezer, where temperature is most constant. Milk stored for longer durations in the ranges listed is safe, but some of the lipids in the milk undergo degradation, resulting in lower quality.
Freezer compartment of refrigerator with separate doors	0°F or −18°C	3–6 mo	
Chest or upright deep freezer	−4°F or −20°C	6–12 mo	

milk expiration, whether pasteurized donor milk or not, fortifiers added, and caloric density. The expiration will depend on whether the milk is fresh or frozen. Labels should be double-checked prior to feeding to avoid the risk of feeding the wrong milk to an infant. Guidelines exist for the management of misadministration of human milk as well.[169]

- Frozen milk should not be transported in ice because it is warmer than frozen milk and could thaw the milk. Blue ice containers freeze at a colder temperature and are acceptable for use.[169]
- Length of time milk may be stored varies with different storage temperatures.[169]

Continuous Infusion of Human Milk

Because breast milk is not homogenized, separation of fat may occur when breast milk is used in tube feedings, with resultant loss of fat and calories.[173-178] Research has shown a 17% fat loss in intermittent feeding, but a 34% loss in a continuous tube feeding.[177] The decrease in fat content of fresh human milk is significantly lower than that in thawed human milk.[178,179] While some nurseries never use human milk in a continuous feeding setup due to the losses, others take the approach that despite not being ideal, it may be the best therapy for an infant. They will accept and try to minimize the losses via the tube. Techniques include using a shortened tubing length and tilting the feeding pump syringe upward between 25° and 40°,[174] as well as transitioning to bolus feedings when possible. A study by Brennan-Behm et al[178] found that there was a mean calorie loss of 2.77–2.32 kcal/oz using standard and microbore tubing when feeding in a continuous fashion. The wand ultrasound homogenization method may prove helpful in these situations as well.[180] The hang time for breast milk should be 4 hours, and the syringe and tubing should be changed every 4 hours.[181]

Only the human milk to be given per feed should be warmed. Excessive heat could harm the infant and destroy factors such as IgA and enzymes. Several newer warming systems are now available. Any milk left in a bottle should be discarded if it is not to be fed immediately for enteral supplementation.[169]

Hospitals should have policies to cover the misadministration of breast milk. Unfortunately this continues to be a problem in nurseries, and strategies have been employed to decrease the incidence of misadministration.[182-184] A thorough schematic is presented in the Infant Feedings Academy of Nutrition and Dietetics Manual.[169]

Cytomegalovirus (CMV) transfer in human milk continues to be a concern. Human milk has been implicated in the acquisition of CMV and CMV sepsis-like syndrome in infants.[185-189] Freezing at −20°C has been discussed as a method of decreasing the viral load of CMV in breast milk. Freezing at this temperature does not appear to decrease secretory IgA, lysozyme, lactoferrin, C3 complement, or the function of cells in breast milk.[185,189] While freezing at −20°C for various time periods does appear to decrease viability of CMV, it is not certain what freezing time period is safe for high viral loads and what would be necessary to achieve 100% inactivity. A recent meta-analysis estimated that 0.3%–4.5% of very low birth weight and premature infants in the United States may develop CMV sepsis-like syndrome from breast milk–acquired CMV infection.[189] A full review of this issue is beyond the scope of this article and a comprehensive review is available.[189]

Human Milk Use in the Infant With Chylothorax

Infants may acquire chylothorax from a chest surgery, or it may occur spontaneously. Chyle accumulates in the pleural space and respiratory compromise can result. Typically the enteral nutrition administered is either devoid or low in long-chain fat and higher in medium-chain triglycerides; however, one previously used infant formula is no longer recommended on the label to be used for infants < 1 year of age.[190,191] Adding medium-chain triglyceride oil can add calories but does not give essential fatty acids, which are only contained in long-chain fats. If the plan is to have no long-chain fat, intravenous lipids would need to be used to supply essential fatty acids. Clinicians have used innovative methods to "defat" human milk so it can be fed to these infants.[191-193] A comparison of the methods is available.[193] Case reports using defatted human milk and full fat human milk are also available.[192,194,195]

Summary

More information is appearing every day to document the beneficial effects of human milk on the infant and mother. New information—from citing the benefits of human milk to improve gut maturation as compared with formula[196] to new information on the impact of the immune cells in human milk[197]—is exciting. The job of the healthcare provider is to translate this information to mothers to give them the information that human milk is very important to their infant. We also must advocate for policies that offer mothers lactation support not only in the beginning but throughout lactation.

Test Your Knowledge Questions

1. Why is the late preterm infant at particular risk for lactation problems?
   A. The infant may be mislabeled as a term infant and treated as such.
   B. The infant may have difficulty extracting milk sufficiently.
   C. The infant appears competent at breastfeeding when he or she is not.
   D. The mothers of these infants are at risk for delayed lactogenesis.
   E. All of the above.
2. Can the use of higher calorie hindmilk from the use of lacto-engineering replace fortification in a preterm infant?
   A. Yes
   B. No
3. Could there be nutrition problems affecting growth with the use of donor banked human milk for preterm infants?
   A. Yes
   B. No

References

1. Kleinman RE, ed. *Pediatric Nutrition Handbook.* 6th ed. Elk Grove Village, IL: American Academy of Pediatrics; 2009:55.
2. Canadian Paediatric Society Nutrition Committee, American Association of Pediatrics Committee on Nutrition. Breast-feeding; a commentary in celebration of the international year of the child. 1979. *Pediatrics.* 1978;65:591–601.
3. International Pediatric Association: Recommendations for action programmes to encourage breastfeeding. *Acta Paediatr Scand.* 1976;65:275–277.
4. WHO/UNICEF. Protecting, promoting, and supporting breastfeeding; the special role of maternity services, a joint WHO/UNICEF statement. Geneva, Switzerland: World Health Organization; 1989.
5. U.S. Department of Health and Human Services. *Healthy People 2010: Understanding and Improving Health and Objectives for Improving Health.* Vols. 1, 2. 2nd ed. Washington, DC: U.S. Department of Health and Human Services; 2000.
6. Surgeon General Call to Action Support of Breastfeeding http://www.surgeongeneral.gov/library/calls/breastfeeding/. Accessed May 22, 2014.
7. Walker A. Breast milk as the gold standard for protective nutrients. *J Pediatr.* 2010; 156; S3–S7.
8. Lawrence RA, Lawrence RM. *Breastfeeding: A Guide for the Medical Profession.* 6th ed. St. Louis, MO: Mosby; 2005:187.
9. Ruiz-Palacios GM, Calva JJ, Pickerington LK. Protection of breast-fed infants against *Campylobacter* diarrhea by antibodies in human milk. *J Pediatr.* 1990;116:707–713.
10. Clavino NR. Mode of feeding and its effect on infant mortality and morbidity. *J Trop Pediatr.* 1982;28:287–294.
11. Fanaro S, Vigi V. Infant formulas supplemented with prebiotics: intestinal microbiota and immune responses. *Minerva Pediatr.* 2008;60:327–335.
12. Xanthou M, Bines J, Walker WA. Human milk and intestinal host defense in the newborn: an update. *Adv Pediatr.* 1995;42:171–208.
13. Hanson LA, Korolkova M. The role of breastfeeding in prevention of neonatal infection. *Semin Neonatol.* 2002;7:275–281.
14. Newburg DS, Walker WA. Protection of the neonate by the immune system of developing gut and of human milk. *Pediatr Res.* 2007;61:2–8.
15. Hatakka K, Savilahti E, Pönkä A, et al. Effect of long-term consumption of probiotic milk on infections in children attending day care centres: double blind, randomised trial. *BMJ.* 2001;322:1327.
16. May JT. Microbial contaminants and antimicrobial properties of human milk. *Microbiol Sci.* 1988;5:42–46.

17. Goldman AS, Garza C, Nichols BL, Goldblum RM. Immunologic factors in human milk during the first year of lactation. *J Pediatr.* 1982;100:563–567.

18. Howie PW, Forsyth JS, Ogston SA, Clark A, Florey CD. Protective effect of breast feeding against infection. *BMJ.* 1990;300(6716):11–16.

19. Duncan B, Ey J, Holberg CJ, Wright AJ, Martinez FD, Taussig LM. Exclusive breastfeeding for at least 4 months protects against otitis media. *Pediatrics.* 1993;91:867–872.

20. Aniansson G, Alm B, Andersson B, et al. A prospective cohort study on breastfeeding and otitis media in Swedish infants. *Pediatr Infect Dis J.* 1994;12:183–188.

21. Paradise JL, Elster BA, Tan L. Evidence in infants with cleft palate that breast milk protects against otitis media. *Pediatrics.* 1994;94:853–860.

22. Pisacane A, Graziano L, Mazzarella G, Scarpellino B, Zona G. Breastfeeding and urinary tract infections. *J Pediatr.* 1992;120:87–89.

23. Vennemann MM, Bajanowski T, Brinkmann B, et al; GeSID Study Group. Does breastfeeding reduce the risk of sudden infant death syndrome? *Pediatrics.* 2009;123:e406–e410.

24. Saarinen UM, Kajosaari M, Backman A, Siimes MA. Prolonged breastfeeding as prophylaxis for atopic disease. *Lancet.* 1979;2:163–166.

25. Kramer MS. Does breastfeeding help protect against atopic disease? Biology, methodology and a golden jubilee of controversy. *J Pediatr.* 1988;112:181–190.

26. Thygarajan A, Burks AW. American Academy of Pediatrics recommendations on the effects of early nutritional interventions on the development of atopic disease. *Curr Opin Pediatr.* 2008;20:698–702.

27. Greer FR, Sicherer SH, Burks W; ; American Academy of Pediatrics Committee on Nutrition; American Academy of Pediatrics Section on Allergy and Immunology. Effects of nutritional interventions on the development of atopic disease in infants and children; the role of maternal diet restriction, timing of introduction of complementary foods, and hydrolyzed formulas. *Pediatrics.* 2008;121:183–190.

28. Hanson LA, Adlerberth I, Carlsson B, et al. Host defense of the neonate and the intestinal flora. *Acta Paediatric Scand Suppl.* 1989;351:122–125.

29. Ivarsson A, Hernell O, Stenlund H, Persson LA. Breastfeeding protects against celiac disease. *Am J Clin Nutr.* 2002;75:914–921.

30. Koletzko S, Sherman P, Corey M, et al. Role of infant feeding practices in development of Crohn's disease in childhood. *BMJ.* 1989;298:1617–1618.

31. Gerstein HC. Cow's milk exposure and type I diabetes mellitus. A critical overview of the clinical literature. *Diabetes Care.* 1994;17:13–19.

32. Savilahti E, Saarinen KM. Early infant feeding and type I diabetes. *Eur J Nutr.* 2009;48(4):243–249.

33. Davis MK, Savitz DA, Graubard BI. Infant feeding and childhood cancer. *Lancet.* 1988;2:365–368.

34. Meier PP, Engstrom JL, Janes JE, Jegier BJ, Loera F. Breast pump suction patterns that mimic the human infant during breastfeeding: greater milk output with less time spent pumping for breast pump-dependent mothers with premature infants [erratum in *J Perinatol.* 2012;32(2):160]. *J Perinatol.* 2012;32:103–110.

35. Morton J, Wong RJ, Hall JY, et al. Combining hand techniques with electric pumping increases the caloric content of milk in mothers of preterm infants. *J Perinatol.* 2012;32:791–796.

36. Riordan J, Wambach K. *Breastfeeding and Human Lactation.* 4th ed. Sudbury, MA: Jones and Bartlett; 2010.

37. Riordan J. Drugs and breastfeeding. In: Riordan J, Auerbach K, eds. *Breastfeeding and Human Lactation.* 2nd ed. Sudbury, MA: Jones and Bartlett; 1998:163–219.

38. Kleinman RE, ed. *Pediatric Nutrition Handbook.* 6th ed. Elk Grove Village, IL: American Academy of Pediatrics; 2009:71.

39. Hale T. *Medications and Mothers Milk.* 15th ed. Amarillo, TX: Hale Publishing, LP; 2012.

40. Hale T. Medications in breastfeeding mothers of preterm infants. *Pediatr Ann.* 2003;337–347.

41. Academy of Breastfeeding Medicine Protocol Committee. ABM clinical protocol #9: use of galactogogues in initiating or augmenting the rate of maternal milk secretion. *Breastfeed Med.* 2011;6:41–46.

42. U.S. National Library of Medicine. LactMed: a ToxNet database. http://toxnet.nlm.nih.gov/cgi-bin/sis/htmlgen?-LACT. Accessed December 2014.

43. Jansson LM. ABM clinical protocol #21: guidelines for breastfeeding and the drug-dependent woman. *Breastfeed Med.* 2009;4:225–228.

44. American Academy of Pediatrics Committee on Drugs. Transfer of drugs and other chemicals into human milk. *Pediatrics.* 2001;108:776–789.

45. Section on Breastfeeding. Breastfeeding and the use of human milk. *Pediatrics.* 2012;129:e827–841.

46. Jansson LM, Choo R, Velez ML, Lowe R, Huestis MA. Methadone maintenance and long-term lactation. *Breastfeed Med.* 2007;3:34–37.

47. Dorea JG. Maternal smoking and infant feeding: breastfeeding is better and safer. *Matern Child Health J.* 2007;11:287–291.

48. Yilmaz G, Hizli S, Karacan K, Yurdakök K, Coşkun T, Dilmen U. Effect of passive smoking on growth and infection rates of breast-fed and non-breast-fed infants. *Pediatr Int.* 2009;51:352–358.

49. Guedes HT, Souza LS. Exposure to maternal smoking in the first year of life interferes in breast-feeding protective effect against the onset of respiratory allergy from birth to 5 years. *Pediatr Allergy Immunol.* 2009;20:30–34.

50. Amir LH. Maternal smoking and reduced duration of breastfeeding: a review of possible mechanisms. *Early Hum Dev.* 2001;64:45–67.

51. Amir LH, Donath SM. Does maternal smoking have a negative physiological effect on breastfeeding? The epidemiological evidence. *Breastfeed Rev.* 2003;11:19–29.

52. Mennella JA, Yourshaw LM, Morgan LK. Breastfeeding and smoking: short-term effects on infant feeding and sleep. *Pediatrics.* 2007;120:497–502.

53. Anderson PO. Alcohol and breastfeeding. *J Hum Lact.* 1995;11:321–323.

54. Schulte P. Minimizing alcohol exposure of the breastfeeding infant. *J Hum Lact.* 1995;11:317–319.

55. Wang AC, Chen SJ, Yuh YS. Breastfeeding associated neonatal hypernatremic dehydration in a medical center: a clinical investigation. *Acta Paediat Taiwan.* 2007;48:186–190.

56. Unal S, Arhan E, Kara N, Uncu N, Aliefendioğlu D. Breastfeeding associated hypernatremia: retrospective analysis of 169 term newborns. *Pediatr Int.* 2008;50:29–34.

57. Yaseen H, Salem M, Darwich M. Clinical presentation of hypernatremic dehydration in exclusively breast-fed neonates. *Indian J Pediatr.* 2004;71:1059–1062

58. Evans A, Marinelli KA, Taylor JS, et al. ABM clinical protocol #2: guidelines for hospital discharge of the breastfeeding term newborn and mother: "the going home protocol," revised 2014. *Breastfeed Med.* 2014;9:3–8.

59. Academy of Breastfeeding Medicine. ABM clinical protocol #10: breastfeeding the late preterm infant (34(0/7) to 36(6/7) weeks gestation) (first revision June 2011). *Breastfeed Med.* 2011;6:151–156.

60. Nagulesapillai T, McDonald SW, Fenton TR, Mercader HF, Tough SC. Breastfeeding difficulties and exclusivity among late preterm and term infants: results from the all our babies study. *Can J Public Health.* 2013;104:e351–e356.

61. McDonald SW, Benzies KM, Gallant JE, McNeil DA, Dolan SM, Tough SC. A comparison between late preterm and term infants on breastfeeding and maternal mental health. *Matern Child Health J.* 2013;17:1468–1477.

62. Wight N. Breastfeeding the borderline (near-term) infant. *Pediatr Ann.* 2003;32:329–336.

63. Meier PP, Furman LM, Degenhardt M. Increased lactation risk for late preterm infants and mother: evidence and management strategies to protect breastfeeding. *J Midwifery Womens Health.* 2007;52:579–587.

64. Meier PP, Enstrom JL, Patel AL. Improving the use of human milk during and after the NICU stay *Clin Pediatr.* 2010; 37:217–245.

65. Wight NE, Morton JA, Kim JH. *Best Medicine: Human Milk in the NICU.* Amarillo, TX: Hale Publishing, LP; 2008.

66. Meier PP, Engstrom JL, Mingolelli SS, Miracle DJ, Kiesling S. The Rush Mothers' Milk Club: breastfeeding interventions for mothers with very-low-birthweight infants. *J Obstet Gynecol Neonatal Nurs.* 2004;33:164–172.

67. Meier PP, Engstrom JL, Hurst NM, et al. A comparison of the efficiency, comfort and convenience of two hospital-grade electric breast pumps for mothers of very low birth weight infants. *Breastfeed Med.* 2008;3:141–120.

68. Meier PP, Brown LP, Hurst NN, et al. Nipple shields for preterm infants: effect on milk transfer and duration of breastfeeding. *J Hum Lact.* 2000;16:106–114.

69. Schanler RJ. The use of human milk for premature infants. *Pediatr Clin North Am.* 2001;48:207–219.

70. Sisk PM, Lovelady CA, Dillard RG, Gruber KJ, O'Shea TM. Early human milk feeding is associated with a lower risk of necrotizing enterocolitis in very low birth weight infants. *J Perinatol.* 2007;27:428–433.

71. Meinzen-Derr J, Poindexter B, Wrage L, Morrow AL, Stoll B, Donovan EF. Role of human milk in extremely low birth weight infants' risk of necrotizing enterocolitis or death. *J Perinatol.* 2009;29:57–62.

72. Cristofalo EA, Schanler RJ, Bianco CL, et al. Randomized trial of exclusive human milk versus preterm formula diets in extremely premature infants. *J Pediatr.* 2013;163:1592–1595.

73. Sullivan S, Schanler RJ, Kim JH, et al. An exclusively human milk-based diet is associated with a lower rate of necrotizing enterocolitis than a diet of human milk and bovine-milk-based products. *J Pediatr.* 2010;156:562–567.

74. Abrams SA, Schanler RJ, Lee ML, Rechtman DJ. Greater mortality and morbidity in extremely preterm infants fed a diet containing cow milk protein products. *Breastfeed Med.* 2014;9:382–395.

75. Herrmann K, Carroll K. An exclusively human milk diet reduces necrotizing enterocolitis. *Breastfeed Med.* 2014; 4:184–190.

76. Schanler RJ, Lau C, Hurst NM, et al. Randomized trial of donor human milk versus preterm formula as substitutes for mothers' own milk in the feeding of extremely low birth-weight infants. *Pediatrics.* 2005;116:400–406.

77. Schanler RJ. Mother's own milk, donor human milk, and preterm formulas in the feeding of extremely premature infants. *J Pediatr Gastroenterol Nutr.* 2007;48:S175–S177.

78. Kleinman RE, Walker WA. The enteromammary immune system. *Dig Dis Sci.* 1979;24:876–882.

79. Quigley MA, McGuire W. Formula milk versus donor breast milk for feeding preterm or low birth weight infants. *Cochrane Database Syst Rev.* 2007; 4:CD002971.

80. Neu J. Necrotizing enterocolitis. In: Koletzko B, Poindexter B, Uauy R, eds. *World Review of Nutrition and Dietetics. Vol. 110: Nutritional Care of Preterm Infants.* Basel, Switzerland: Karger; 2014:253–263.

81. Wang Y, Hoenig JD, Malin KJ, et al. 16S rRNA gene-based analysis of fecal microbiota from preterm infants with and without necrotizing enterocolitis. *ISME J.* 2009; 3:944–954.

82. Mai V, Young CM, Ukhanova M, et al. Fecal microbiota in premature infants prior to necrotizing enterocolitis. *PLoS One.* 2011;6:e20647.

83. Morrow AL, Lagomarcino AJ, Schibler KR, et al. Early microbial and metabolomic signatures predict later onset of necrotizing enterocolitis in preterm infants. *Microbiome.* 2013;1:13.

84. Kuppala VS, Meinzen-Derr J, Morrow AL, Schibler KR. Prolonged empirical antibiotic treatment is associated with adverse outcomes in premature infants. *J Pediatr.* 2011;159:720–725.

85. Greenwood C, Morrow AL, Lagomarcino AJ, et al. Early empiric antibiotic use in preterm infants is associated with lower bacterial diversity and higher relative abundance of Enterobacter. *J Pediatr.* 2014;pii:S0022-3476(14)00011-0. doi: 10.1016/j.jpeds.2014.01.010.

86. Chazpak N, Ruiz JG, KMC Team. Breast milk composition in a cohort of preterm infants' mothers followed in a ambulatory program in Colombia. *Acta Paediatr.* 2007;96:1735–1739.

87. Lawrence RA, Lawrence RM. *Breastfeeding: A Guide for the Medical Profession.* 6th ed. St. Louis, MO: Mosby; 2005:445.
88. Bauer J, Gens J. Longitudinal analysis of macronutrients and mineral in human milk produced by mothers of preterm infants. *Clin Nutr.* 2011;30:215–220.
89. Hibberd CM, Brooke OG, Carter ND, Haug M, Harzer G. Variations in the composition of breast milk during the first 5 weeks of lactation: Implications for the feeding of preterm infants. *Arch Dis Child.* 1982;657:658–662.
90. Ballard O, Morrow AL. Human milk composition: nutrients and bioactive factors. *Pediatr Clin North Am.* 2013;60:49–74.
91. Hsu YC, Chen CH, Lin MC, Tsai CR, Liang JT, Wang TM. Changes in preterm breast milk nutrient content in the first month. *Pediatr Neonatol.* 2014;320:1–6.
92. Arslanoglu S, Moro GE, Ziegler EE. Preterm infants fed fortified human milk receive less protein than they need. *J Perinatol.* 2009;29:489–492.
93. Paul VK, Singh M, Srivastata LM, Arora NK, Deorari AK. Macronutrient and energy content of breast milk of mothers delivering prematurely. *Indian J Pediatr.* 1997;64:379–382.
94. Morales Y, Schanler RJ. Human milk and clinical outcomes in VLBW infants: how compelling is the evidence of benefit? *Semin Perinatol.* 2007;31:83–88.
95. Mukhopadhyay K, Narang A, Mahajan R. Effect of human milk fortification in appropriate for gestation and small for gestation preterm babies: a randomized trial. *Indian Pediatrics.* 2007;44:286–290.
96. Carey DE, Rowe JC, Goetz CA, Horak E, Clark RM, Goldberg B. Growth and phosphorus metabolism in premature infants fed human milk, fortified human milk, or special premature formula. *Am J Dis Child.* 1987;141:511–515.
97. Chan GM, Armstrong C, Moyer-Mileur L, et al. Growth and bone mineralization in children born prematurely. *J Perinatol.* 2008; 28:619–623.
98. Embleton ND. Optimal nutrition for preterm infants: putting the ESPGHAN guidelines into practice. *J Neonatal Nurs.* 2013;19:130–133.
99. Kim JH, Chan CS, Vaucher YE, Stellwagen LM. Challenges in the practice of human milk nutrition in the neonatal intensive care unit. *Early Hum Dev.* 2013;89:S35–S38.
100. Maggio L, Costa S, Gallini F. Human milk fortifiers in very-low-birth weight infants. *Early Hum Dev.* 2009;85:S59–S61.
101. Embleton ND. Optimal protein and energy intakes in preterm infants. *Early Hum Dev.* 2007;83:831–837.
102. Ziegler EE. Breast milk fortifiers. *Acta Paediatr.* 2011;90:720–723.
103. Agostoni C, Buonocore G, Carnielli VP, et al; ESPGHAN Committee on Nutrition. Enteral nutrient supply for preterm infants: commentary from the European Society of Pediatric Gastroenterology, Hepatolology, and Nutrition Committee on Nutrition. *J Pediatr Gastroenterol Nutr.* 2010;50:85–91.
104. Groh-Wargo S, Sapsford A. Enteral nutrition support of the preterm infant in the neonatal intensive care unit. *Nutr Clin Pract.* 2009;24:363–376.
105. Sapsford A. Composition of human milk and selected enteral products. In: Groh Wargo S, Thompson M, Cox JH, eds. *Nutrition for the High Risk Neonate.* 3rd ed. Chicago: Precept Press; 2000:684.
106. Valentine CJ, Morrow AL. Human milk feeding of the high risk neonate. In: Neu J, ed. *Gastroenterology and Nutrition.* 2nd ed. Neonatology Questions and Controversies. Philadelphia, PA: Saunders, Elsevier Imprints; 2012:206.
107. MeadJohnson Nutrition. Web site. http://www.mjn.com. Accessed June 2014.
108. Abbott Nutrition. Web site. http://www.abbottnutrition.com. Accessed June 2014.
109. Prolacta. Web site. http://www.prolacta.com. Accessed June 2014.
110. Koletzko B, Poindexter B, Uuay R. Recommended nutrient intake levels for stable, fully enteral fed very low birthweight infants. In: Koletzko B, Poindexter B, Uuay R, eds. *Nutritional Care of Preterm Infants: Scientific Basis and Practical Guidelines.* Basel, Switzerland: Karger; 2014:297–299.
111. Olsen IE, Harris CL, Lawson ML, et al. Higher protein intake improves length, not weight, z scores in preterm infants. *J Pediatr Gastroenterol Nutr.* 2014;58:409–416.
112. Janjindamai W, Chotsampancharoen T. Effect of fortification on the osmolality of human milk. *J Med Assoc Thai.* 2006; 99:1400–1403.
113. Fenton TR, Belik J. Routine handling of milk fed to preterm infants can significantly increase osmolaloty. *J Pediatr Gastroenterol Nutr.* 2002;35(3):298–302.
114. Bhat BA, Gupta B. Effects of human milk fortification on mortality factors in very low birthweight infants. *Ann Saudi Med.* 2003;23:28–31.
115. Yigit S, Akgoz A, Memisoglu A, Akata D, Ziegler EE. Breast milk fortification: effect on gastric emptying. *J Matern Fetal Neonatal Med.* 2008;21:843–846.
116. Stanger J, Zwicker K, Albersheim S, Murphy JJ 3rd. Human milk fortifier: an occult cause of bowel obstruction in extremely premature neonates. *J Pediatr Surg.* 2014;49:724–726.
117. Murase M, Miyazawa T, Taki M, et al. Development of fatty acid calcium stone ileus after initiation of human milk fortifier. *J Pediatr Gastroenterol Nutr.* 2013;55:114–116.
118. Thoene M, Hanson C, Lyden E, Dugick L, Ruybal L, Anderson-Berry A. Comparison of the effect of two human milk fortifiers on clinical outcomes in premature infants. *Nutrients.* 2014;6:261–275.
119. Erickson T, Gill G, Chan GM. The effects of acidification on human milk's cellular and nutritional content. *J Perinatol.* 2013;33:371–373.
120. Chan GM. Effect of powdered human milk fortifier on the antibacterial actions of human milk. *J Perinatol.* 2003;23:620–623.
121. Ovali F, Ciftci I, Cetinkaya Z, et al. Effects of human milk fortifier on the antimicrobial properties of human milk. *J Perinatol.* 2006;26:761–763.
122. Chan GM, Lee MI, Rechman DJ. Effects of a human milk-derived human milk fortifier on the antibacterial actions of human milk. *Breastfeed Med.* 2007;2:205–208.
123. Telang S, Berseth CL, Ferguson PW, et al. Fortifying fresh human milk with commercial human milk fortifiers does

not affect the bacterial growth during 6 hours at room temperature. *J Am Diet Assoc.* 2005;105:567–572.

124. Ganapathy V, Hay JL, Kim JH. Costs of necrotizing enterocolitis and cost-effectiveness of exclusively human milk-based products in feeding extremely premature infants. *Breastfeed Med.* 2012;7:29–37.

125. Moro GE, Minoli I, Ostrom M, et al. Fortification of human milk: evaluation of a novel fortification scheme and of a new fortifier. *J Pediatr Gastroenterol Nutr.* 1995;20:162–172.

126. Arslanoglu S, Moro GE, Ziegler EE. Adjustable fortification of human milk fed to preterm infants: does it make a difference? *J Perinatol.* 2006;26:614–621.

127. Arslanoglu S, Bertino E, Coscia A, Tonetto P, Giuliani F, Moro GE. Update of adjustable fortification regimen in preterm infants: a new protocol. *J Biol Regul Homeost Agents.* 2012;26:65–67.

128. Miller J, Makrides M, Gibson RA, et al. Effect of increasing protein content of human milk fortifier on growth in preterm infants born < 31 wk gestation: a randomized controlled trial. *Am J Clin Nutr.* 2012;95:648–655.

129. Alan S, Atasay B, Cakir U, et al. An intention to achieve better postnatal growth postnatal in-hospital-growth for preterm infants: adjustable protein fortification of human milk. *Early Hum Develop.* 2013;89:1017–1023.

130. Polberger S, Räihä NC, Juvonen P, Moro GE, Minoli I, Warm A. Individualized protein fortification of human milk for preterm infants: comparison of ultrafiltrated human milk protein and a bovine whey protein fortifier. *J Pediatr Gastroenterol Nutr.* 1999;29:332–338.

131. Corvaglia L, Aceti A, Paoletti V, et al. Standard fortification of preterm human milk fails to meet recommended protein intake: bedside evaluation by near-infrared reflectance analysis. *Early Hum Develop.* 2010;86:237–240.

132. Corvaglia L, Battistini B, Paoletti V, Aceti A, Capretti MG, Faldella G. Near infrared reflectance analysis to reflect human milk's nitrogen and fat content in neonatal intensive care unit. *Arch Dis Child Fetal Neo Ed.* 2008;993:372–375.

133. de Halleux B, Close A, Stalport S, Studzinski F, Habibi F, Rigo J. Advantages of individualized fortification of human milk for preterm infants [in French]. *Arch Pediatr.* 2007;14:S5–S10.

134. Rochow N, Fusch G, Choi A, et al. Target fortification of breast milk with fat, protein, and carbohydrates for preterm infants. *J Pediatr.* 2013;163:1001–1007.

135. Lawrence RA, Lawrence RM. *Breastfeeding: A Guide for the Medical Profession.* 6th ed. St. Louis, MO: Mosby; 2005:693.

136. Lucas A, Gibbs JAH, Lyster RLI, Baum JD. Creamatocrit: simple clinical technique for estimating fat concentration and energy value of human milk. *Br Med J.* 1978;1:1018–1020.

137. Medela Web site. http://www.medelabreastfeedingus.com/for-professionals/lc-information. Accessed February 2009.

138. Meier PP, Engstrom JL, Zuleger JL, et al. Accuracy of a user-friendly centrifuge for measuring creamatocrit on mothers' milk in a clinical setting. *Breastfeed Med.* 2006;1:79–87.

139. Meier PP, Engstrom JL, Murtaugh MA, et al. Mothers' milk feedings in the neonatal intensive care nursery: accuracy of the creamatocrit technique. *J Perinatol.* 2002;22:646–649.

140. Griffith TL, Meier PP, Bradford LP, Bigger HR, Engstrom JL. Mothers' performing creamatocrit measures in the NICU: accuracy, reactions, and cost. *J Obstet Gynecol Neonatal Nurs.* 2000;29:249–257.

141. O'Neill EF, Radmacher PG, Sparks B, Adamkin DH. Creamatocrit analysis of human milk overestimates fat and energy content when compared to a human milk analyzer using mid-infrared spectroscopy. *J Pediatr Gastroenterol.* 2013;56:569–572.

142. Wang CD, Chu PS, Mellen BG, Shenai JP. Creamatocrit and the nutrient composition of human milk. *J Perinatol.* 1999;19:343–346.

143. Chatterjee R, Chatterjee S, Datta T, Roy B, Marimuthu P. Longitudinal study of human milk creamatocrit and weight gain in exclusively breastfed infants. *Indian Pediatr.* 1997;34:901–904.

144. Lubetzky R, Mimouni FB, Dollberg S, Salomon M, Mandel D. Consistent circadian variations in creamatocrit over the first 7 weeks of lactation: a longitudinal study. *Breastfeed Med.* 2007;2:15–18.

145. Weber A, Loui A, Jochum F, Bührer C, Obladen M. Breast milk from mothers of very low birthweight infants: variability in fat and protein content. *Acta Paediatr.* 2001;90:772–775.

146. Bishara R, Dunn MS, Merko SE, et al. Nutrient composition of hindmilk is produced by mothers of very low birth weight infants born at less than 28 weeks gestation. *J Hum Lact.* 2008;24:159–167.

147. Human Milk Banking Association of North America. Web site. http://www.HMBANA.org. Accessed May 21, 2014.

148. Human Milk Banking Association of North America. 2011 Best Practice for Expressing, Storing and Handling Human Milk in Hospitals, Homes, and Child Care Settings. 3rd ed. Fort Worth, TX: HMBANA. 2011.

149. Human Milk Banking Association of North America. *Guidelines for the Establishment and Operation of a Donor Human Milk Bank.* 2013. Fort Worth, TX: HMBANA.

150. Akinbi H, Meinzen-Derr J, Auer C, et al. Alterations in the host defense properties of human milk following prolonged storage or pasteurization. *J Pediatr Gastroenterol Nutr.* 2010;51:347-52.

151. Wojcik KY, Rechtman DJ, Lee, ML, et al. Macronutrient analysis of a nationwide sample of breast milk. *J Am Diet Assoc.* 2009; 109:137–140.

152. Wagner CL, Greer FR; American Academy of Pediatrics Section on Breastfeeding; American Academy of Pediatrics Committee on Nutrition. Prevention of rickets and vitamin D deficiency in infants, children, and adolescents. *Pediatrics.* 2008:122:1142–1152.

153. Gartner LM, Greer FR; American Academy of Pediatrics Section on Breastfeeding; American Academy of Pediatrics Committee on Nutrition. Prevention of rickets and vitamin D deficiency: new guidelines for vitamin D intake. *Pediatrics.* 2003;111:908–910.

154. Kreiter SR, Schwartz RP, Kirkman HN, et al. Nutritional rickets in African American breastfed infants. *J Pediatr.* 2000;137:153–157.

155. Ward LM. Vitamin D deficiency in the 21st century: a persistent problem among Canadian infants and mothers. *CMAJ.* 2005;172:769–770.

156. Wagner CL, Hulsey TC, Fanning D, et al. High dose vitamin D supplementation in a cohort of breastfeeding mothers and their infants; a six month follow-up pilot study. *Breastfeed Med.* 2006;1:59–70.

157. American Academy of Pediatrics, Committee on Environmental Health. Ultraviolet light: a hazard to children. *Pediatrics.* 1999;104:328–333.

158. Chantry CJ, Howard CR, Auinger P. Full breastfeeding duration and risk for iron deficiency in U.S. infants. *Breastfeeding Med.* 2007;2:63–73.

159. Steinmacher J, Pohlandt F, Bode H, et al. Randomized trial of early versus late enteral iron supplementation in infants with a birth weight of less than 1301 grams: neurocognitive development at 5.3 years' corrected age. *Pediatrics.* 2007;120:538–546.

160. Ziegler EE, Nelson SE, Jeter JM. Iron supplementation of breastfed infants from an early age. *Am J Clin Nutr.* 2009;89(2):525–532.

161. Lozoff B, Jimenez E, Hagen J, et al. Poorer behavioral and developmental outcome more than 10 years after treatment for iron deficiency. *Pediatrics.* 2000;105:E51.

162. World Health Organization. The WHO Child Growth Standards. www.who.int/childgrowth/standards/en. Accessed January 30, 2009.

163. WHO Multicentre Growth Reference Study Group. Breastfeeding in the WHO Multicentre Growth Reference Study. *Acta Paediatr Suppl.* 2006;450:16–26.

164. de Onis M, Onyango AW. The Centers for Disease Control and Prevention 2000 growth charts and the growth of breastfed infants. *Acta Paediatr.* 2003;92:413–419.

165. Centers for Disease Control and Prevention (CDC). *Enterobacter sakazakii* infections associated with the use of powdered infant formula—Tennessee 2001. *MMWR Morb Mortal Wkly Rep.* 2002;51:297–300.

166. Bowen AB, Braden CR. Invasive *Enterobacter sakazakii* disease in infants. *Emerg Infect Dis.* 2006;12:1185–1189.

167. EPGHAN Committee on Nutrition, et al. Preparation and handling of powdered infant formula: A commentary by the ESPGHAN Committee on Nutrition. *J Pediatr Gastroenterol Nutr.* 2004;39:320-322.

168. Food and Drug Administration. Health professionals letter on *Enterobacter sakazakii* infections associated with use of powdered (dry) infant formulas in neonatal intensive care units. http://www.fda.gov/Food/RecallsOutbreaksEmergencies/SafetyAlertsAdvisories/ucm111299.htm. Published April 11, 2002. Revised October 10, 2002.

169. Sapsford A, Lessen R. Expressed human milk. In: Robbins ST, Meyers M, eds. *Infant Feedings: Guidelines for Preparation of Formula and Breastmilk in Health Care Facilities.* 2nd ed. Chicago: American Dietetic Association; 2011:40–70.

170. Centers for Disease Control and Prevention. Proper handling and storage of human milk. http://www.cdc.gov/breastfeeding/recommendations/handling_breastmilk.htm. Updated March 4, 2010. Accessed December 2014.

171. Human Milk Banking Association of North America. *2006 Best Practice for Expressing, Storing and Handling of Mother's Own Milk in Hospital and at Home.* Raleigh, NC: Human Milk Banking Association of North America; 2006.

172. Spatz DL. State of the science: use of human milk and breastfeeding for vulnerable infants. *J Perinatol Neonatal Nurs.* 2006;20:51–55.

173. Greer FR, McCormic A, Loker J. Changes in fat concentration of human milk during delivery by intermittent bolus and continuous mechanical pump infusion. *J Pediatr.* 1984;105;745–749.

174. Narayan I, Singh B, Harvey D. Fat loss during feeding of human milk. *Arch Dis Child.* 1984;59:475–477.

175. Stocks RJ, Davies DP, Allen F, Sewell D. Loss of breastmilk nutrients during tube feeding. *Arch Dis Child.* 1985;60:164–166.

176. Rogers SP, Hicks PD, Hamzo M, Veit LE, Abrams SA. Continuous feeding of fortified human milk lead to nutrient losses of fat, calcium, and phosphorus. *Nutrients.* 2010;2:230–240.

177. Brooks C, Vickers AM, Aryal S. Comparison of lipid and calorie loss from donor milk among 3 methods of simulated gavage feeding: one hour, 2 hour, and intermittent gavage feedings. *Adv Neonatal Care.* 2013;13:131–138.

178. Brennan-Behm M, Carlson GE, Meier P, Engstrom J. Caloric loss from expressed mother's milk during continuous gavage infusion. *Neonatal Netw.* 1994;13:27–32.

179. Igawa M, Murase M, Mizuno K, Itabashi K. Is fat content of human milk decreased by infusion? *Pediatr Int.* 2014;56:230–233.

180. Martinez FE, Desai ID, Davidson AGF, Nakai S, Radcliffe A. Ultrasonic homogenization of expressed human milk to prevent fat loss during tube feeding. *J Pediatr Gastroenterol Nutr.* 1987;6:593–597.

181. Bankhead R, Boullata J, Brantley S, et al. Enteral nutrition practice recommendations. *JPEN J Parenter Enteral Nutr.* 2009;33:122–167.

182. Zeilhofer UB, Frey B, Zandes J, Bernet V. The role of critical incident monitoring in detection and prevention of breast milk confusions. *Eur J Pediatr.* 2009;168(10):1277–1279.

183. Dougherty D, Giles V. From breast to bottle: quality assurance for breast milk management. *Neonatal Netw.* 2000;19:21–25.

184. Drenckpohl D, Bowers L, Cooper B. Use of the six signs methodology to reduce incidence of breast milk administration errors in the NICU. *Neonatal Netw.* 2007;26:161–166.

185. Schleiss MR. Role of breast milk in the acquisition of cytomegalovirus infection: recent advances. *Curr Opin Pediatr.* 2006;18:48–52.

186. Omarsdottir S, Caspar C, Zweyberg Wirgart B, Grillner L, Vanpée M. Transmission of cytomegalovirus in extremely preterm infants through breast milk. *Acta Paediatr.* 2007;96:492–494.

187. Lawrence RA. Storage of human milk and the influence of procedures on immunological components of human milk. *Acta Paediatr Suppl.* 1999;88:14–18.

188. Lawrence RM. Cytomegalovirus in human breast milk: risk to the premature infant. *Breastfeeding Med.* 2006;1:99–107.

189. Lanzieri TM, Dollard SC, Josephson CD, Schmid DS, Bialek SR. Breast milk-acquired cytomegalovirus infection and disease in VLBW and premature infants. *Pediatrics.* 2013;131:e1937–e1945.

190. Peitersen B, Jacobsen B. Medium chain triglycerides for treatment of spontaneous, neonatal chylothorax. Lipid analysis of the chyle. *Acta Paediatr Scand.* 1977;66(1):121–125.

191. Chan GM, Lechtenberg E. The use of fat-free human milk in infants with chylous pleural effusion. *J Perinatol.* 2007;27:434–436.

192. Lessen R. Use of skim breast milk for an infant with chylothorax. *Infant Child Adolesc Nutr.* 2009;1:303–310.

193. Drewniak MA, Lyon AW, Fenton TR. Evaluation of fat separation and removal methods to prepare low-fat breast milk for fat-intolerant neonates with chylothorax. *Nutr Clin Pract.* 2013;28:599–602.

194. Hamdan MA, Gaeta ML. Octreotide and low-fat breast milk in postoperative chylothorax. *Ann Thorac Surg.* 2004;77(6):2215–2217.

195. Roehr CC, Jung A, Curcin OA, Proquitte H, Hammer H, Wauer RR. Loculated neonatal chylothorax treated with octreotide: complete recovery while on unrestricted full fat breast milk. *Ann Thorac Surg.* 2005;80:1981–1982.

196. Reisinger KW, de Vaan L, Kramer BW. Breast-feeding improves gut maturation compared with formula feeding in preterm babies. *J Pediatric Gastroenterol Nutr.* 2014;59:720–724.

197. Bode L, McGuire M, Rodriguez JM, et al. It's alive: microbes and cells in human milk and their potential benefits to mother and infant. *Adv Nutr.* 2014;5:571–573.

Test Your Knowledge Answers

1. The correct answer is **E**. Some of these infants have been shown to have an insufficient suck and negative pressure needed for good milk extraction. They may fool mothers, and if this problem persists, the mother's milk supply may dwindle. This may cause dehydration as well as poor growth and create a cycle that can lead to lactation failure. Encouraging mothers to pump to stimulate milk supply is helpful; also, the use of teat weights to determine whether sufficient milk is transferred can also be helpful. Further information is included in references 39 and 40.

2. The correct answer is **B**. Although calories are important, which will be supplied in greater amounts with the higher fat content of hindmilk, the premature infant needs fortification for protein, calcium, phosphorus, magnesium, and zinc.

3. The correct answer is **A**. Donor banked human milk may often be from donations of mothers of term infants. This milk would have lower protein content than the milk from a mother of a preterm infant. The pasteurization process alters some of the properties of human milk as well. There will be increased needs for supplemental protein, calcium, and phosphorus.

12

Infant Formulas and Complementary Feeding

Kelly Green Corkins, MS, RD, LDN, CNSC; and **Allison Beck,** MS, RD, LDN, CSP, CNSC

 Podcast

CONTENTS

Learning Objectives

1. Explain the basic composition of infant formulas and their regulation.
2. Discuss reasons for functional ingredients in infant formulas.
3. Differentiate types of infant formulas and appropriate use.
4. Describe how to increase calorie concentrations.
5. Summarize reasoning behind current guidelines for introducing complementary foods to an infant's diet.

Introduction

The World Health Organization recommends human milk as the sole source of nutrition for healthy full-term infants from birth to 6 months of age.[1] The American Academy of Pediatrics (AAP) supports this recommendation. Breastfeeding provides benefits to the infant that infant formula cannot. Breastfeeding promotes gastrointestinal development and function, provides immune support, and bolsters neurodevelopment.[2] A mother might not always be able to breastfeed, or she may choose not to breastfeed due to cultural, social, or health reasons. Iron-fortified infant formulas are appropriate substitutes for human milk. A mother should be encouraged to breastfeed or to provide as much expressed human milk as possible, even if she chooses to supplement breastfeeding with formula or needs to supplement for medical reasons.[3]

Because human milk is the optimal source of nutrition for an infant, the first infant formulas were developed to be similar to human milk in composition.[4] Even with the latest functional ingredients added (docosahexaenoic acid [DHA] and arachidonic acid [ARA], nucleotides, probiotics, prebiotics), infant formulas still cannot provide the hormones, immunoglobulins, enzymes, and live cells that are in human milk.[3] Standard term infant formulas and term infant formulas modified for symptoms of intolerance are formulated using cow's milk or soy as a base. Because infant formula manufacturers may never be able to completely replicate the composition of human milk, modifications and research continue with more emphasis on promoting growth and development similar to the breastfed infant.[5]

Regulation

An infant formula is defined by the Federal Food, Drug, and Cosmetic Act (FDCA) as "a food which purports to be or is represented for special dietary use solely as a food for infants by reason of its simulation of human milk or its suitability as a complete or partial substitute for human milk."[6] Infant formulas designed to meet a specific medical need (ie, premature infant formulas) are considered "exempt" because the nutrition requirements of infants with certain medical conditions differ from those of healthy infants. Exempt formulas are not exempt from monitoring or regulation, however, and they need to meet certain criteria developed for those products. All infant formula manufacturers must begin with safe ingredients that are approved for use in infant formulas, or are generally recognized as safe (GRAS).[6]

The Infant Formula Act of 1980 (revised 1986), an amendment to the FDCA, was developed due to an incident involving inadequate chloride in a soy-based formula that resulted in metabolic acidosis in several infants.[7] The Food and Drug Administration (FDA) is responsible for monitoring the manufacturers that make infant formulas. Federal regulations exist on quality control, labeling, nutrient levels, formula recall, new product notification, and exempt products. Levels for 29 nutrients and maximum levels for 9 nutrients have been established. Manufacturers are required to declare on the label the minimum levels of each nutrient provided, and the manufacturer must analyze each batch of formula to ensure the declared levels of all essential nutrients are being provided. The FDA reviews the analysis records and will perform tests on the formula to monitor the manufacturers.[5] The concentration of nutrients in infant formula is higher than in human milk because of the decreased bioavailability in infant formula.[3,8]

Types of Infant Formulas

Information included in this section and the accompanying tables is up-to-date as of the time of publication. For the most current information, please visit the manufacturers' Web sites (Table 12-1).

Table 12-1. Infant Formula Manufacturer Web Sites

MANUFACTURER	PRODUCT LINE	WEB SITE
Abbott Nutritionals	Similac	www.abbottnutrition.com
Mead Johnson	Enfamil	www.meadjohnson.com
Nestle Gerber	Good Start	www.medical.gerber.com
Nutricia	Neocate and other products	www.nutricia-na.com
Perrigo Nutritionals	Bright Beginnings Parent's Choice	www.perrigonutritionals.com
Vitaflo	Some modulars	www.vitaflousa.com

Standard Milk-Based Term Infant Formulas

Standard milk-based infant formulas (Table 12-2) are designed to meet the needs of healthy, term infants from birth to 1 year of age. These formulas are cow's milk–based and iron fortified. Standard infant formula contains more protein compared to breast milk and usually has a lower whey-to-casein ratio. Formula composition, both micronutrient and macronutrient components, varies between manufacturers, though most provide 20 cal/oz based on standard mixing instructions. Most formula-fed infants will consume one of these products. Subgroups of standard milk-based term infant formulas are organic, lower calorie/lower protein (19 kcal/oz), and breast milk supplementation.

Organic

Organic formulas are milk based and meet all the same guidelines of infant formula. In order to be labeled organic, the formula ingredients must be certified organic and meet U.S. Department of Agriculture regulations under the Organic Foods Production Act. Ingredients must be produced without added growth hormones, or antibiotics. Pesticides used to grow ingredients or in the plants used to feed animals that product the products must meet specific guidelines.[9]

Lower Calorie/Lower Protein

Reduced energy infant formula is now available from some manufacturers. This change is meant to reflect the variable caloric density of breast milk and to address the obesity problem in the United States as it relates to infant feeding choices. Limited research exists to support this change, and no studies have looked at the risks and benefits of this decreased calorie density in U.S. infants.[10]

Breast Milk Supplementation

Formula manufacturers have developed formulas intended to be used when supplementing the breastfed infant with

Table 12-2. Standard Milk-Based Infant Formulas (per 100 Calories)—Standard Dilution Is 0.67 kcal/mL (20 kcal/oz) or 0.63 kcal/mL (19 kcal/oz)

PRODUCT (MANUFACTURER)	PROTEIN gm (% kcal) SOURCE	CHO gm (%kcal) SOURCE	FAT gm (%kcal) SOURCE	Na mg	K mg	Ca mg	Phos mg	Vit D IU	Fe mg	OSMOLALITY mOsm	COMMENTS
Enfamil Premium (Mead Johnson)	2 (8.5%) whey, nonfat milk	11.3 (43.5%) lactose, GOS, polydextrose	5.3 (48%) palm olein, soy oil, coconut oil, high oleic sunflower oils	27	108	78	43	60	1.8	300	added nucleotides DHA 17 mg, ARA 34 mg PRSL 19.1/100 cal added prebiotics—GOS, polydextrose
Enfamil Newborn (Mead Johnson)	2.1 (8.5%) nonfat milk, whey protein concentrate	11.2 (43.5%) lactose, GOS, polydextrose	5.3 (48%) palm olein, soy oil, coconut oil, high oleic sunflower oil	27	108	78	43	75	1.8	300	added nucleotides DHA 17 mg, ARA 34 mg PSRL 19.1/100 cal added prebiotics—GOS, polydextrose
Enfamil for Supplementing (Mead Johnson)	2.3 (9%) partially hydrolyzed nonfat milk and whey protein concentrated solids (soy)	10.8 (43%) corn syrup solids	5.3 (48%) palm olein, oil, soy oil, coconut oil, high oleic sunflower oil	36	108	82	46	75	1.8	230	added nucleotides DHA 17 mg, ARA 34 mg PRSL 21/100 cal
Good Start Gentle (Gerber)	2.2 (9%) whey protein concentrate (from cow's milk, enzymatically hydrolyzed, reduced in minerals)	11.6 (46%) corn maltodextrin, lactose, GOS	5.1 (46%) palm olein, soy oil, coconut oil, high oleic safflower or sunflower oil	27	108	67	38	60	1.5	250	4.6 mg/100 cal added nucleotides DHA 0.32%, ARA 0.64% PRSL 19.6/100 cal added prebiotic—GOS
Good Start Gentle for Supplementing (Gerber)	2.2 (9%) whey protein concentrate (enzymatically hydrolyzed, reduced in minerals)	11.2 (46%) lactose, corn maltodextrin	5.1 (46%) palm olein, soy oil, coconut oil, high oleic safflower or sunflower oil	27	108	67	38	75	1.5	250	4.6 mg/100 cal added nucleotides DHA 0.32%, ARA 0.64% PRSL 19.6/100 cal added probiotic—Bifidobacterium lactis
Similac Advance Stage 1 20 kcal/oz (Abbott Nutrition)	2.07 (8%) nonfat milk, whey protein concentrate	11.2 (43%) lactose, GOS	5.4 (49%) high high oleic safflower oil, soy oil, coconut oil	24	105	78	42	75	1.8	310	added nucleotides DHA 0.15%, ARA 0.40% PRSL 18.7/100 cal added prebiotic—GOS
Similac Advance Stage 1 19 kcal/oz (Abbott Nutrition)	2.07 (8%) nonfat milk and whey protein concentrate	11.2 (43%) lactose, GOS	5.4 (49%) high high oleic safflower oil, soy oil, coconut oil	25	110	82	44	75	1.9	310	added nucleotides DHA 0.15%, ARA 0.40% PRSL 19.1/100 cal added prebiotic—GOS
Similac Advance Stage 2 19 kcal/oz (Abbott Nutrition)	2.2 (8%) nonfat milk and whey protein concentrate	10.6 (43%) lactose, GOS	5.6 (49%) high oleic safflower oil, soy and coconut oils	25	110	118	64	75	1.9	310	added nucleotides DHA 0.15%, ARA 0.40% PRSL 20.5/100 cal added prebiotic—GOS
Similac Advance Organic (Abbott Nutrition)	2.07 (8%) organic nonfat dry milk	10.9 (43%) organic maltodextrin, organic lactose, organic sugar, FOS	5.4 (49%) organic high oleic sunflower oil, organic soy oil, organic coconut oil	24	105	78	42	60	1.8	225	DHA 0.15%, ARA 0.40% PRSL 18.7/100 cal unmodified whey:casein 18:82 added prebiotic—FOS
Similac for Supplementation (Abbott Nutrition)	2.07 (8%) nonfat milk, whey protein concentrate	11.3 (43%) lactose, GOS	5.4 (49%) high oleic safflower oil, soy oil, coconut oil	25	110	82	44	75	1.9	290	added nucleotides DHA 0.15%, ARA 0.40% PRSL 19.1/100cal added prebiotic—GOS
Store Brands* Advantage (Perrigo Nutritionals)	2.07 (8%) nonfat milk, whey protein concentrate	10.7 (42%) lactose, maltodextrin, GOS	5.6 (50%) palm olein, soy oil, coconut oil, high oleic safflower or sunflower	24	105	78	42	60	1.8	280	added nucleotides DHA, ARA
Store Brands* Organic (Perrigo Nutritionals)	2.2 (9%) organic nonfat milk	10.6 (42%) organic glucose syrup solids, organic maltodextrin	5.3 (48%) organic vegetable oils (palm or palm olein, high oleic safflower or sunflower, coconut, soy)	23	84	78	42	60	1.8	225	added nucleotides DHA, ARA 60:40 whey-to-casein ratio
Store Brands* Premium (Perrigo Nutritionals)	2.1 (8%) nonfat milk, whey protein concentrate	11 (44%) lactose	5.3 (48%) palm olein, soy oil, coconut oil, high oleic safflower or sunflower oil	27	108	78	43	60	1.8	294	added nucleotides DHA, ARA added prebiotic—GOS

*Perrigo Nutritionals makes Store Brands for Walmart, Sam's Club, Walgreens, CVS, Target, and Babies R Us as well as Bright Beginnings. Check product labels for the most accurate and up-to-date information.

GOS, galacto-oligosacchides; FOS, fructo-oligosaccharides.

formula. Each manufacturer has developed a formula with a slight modification from other formulas in their line of standard term infant formulas. Evidence is limited that these breast milk supplementation formulas make any significant difference in comparison with other standard term formulas.

Term Formulas Designed for Symptoms of Intolerance

Formulas designed for symptoms of intolerance (Table 12-3) are milk based or soy based and are appropriate for the full-term infant. Modifications include partial hydrolysis of the protein, reduced lactose, probiotics, and added rice starch.

Partially Hydrolyzed Protein

Formulas containing partially hydrolyzed protein are not considered hypoallergenic and are not intended to be used for treatment of any allergic condition or disease. Partially hydrolyzed protein formulas contain reduced or no lactose, and each product differs by the type of protein hydrolyzed and degree of hydrolysis; therefore, all partially hydrolyzed protein formulas cannot be assumed to offer identical benefits.[11] Even if the products contain the same type of partially hydrolyzed protein, techniques used to hydrolyze the protein may be different and therefore result in different end products.

The benefits of one specific partially hydrolyzed 100% whey protein has been studied, and research demonstrates that it may decrease the risk of atopic dermatitis in infants with a family history of allergic disease.[11,12] A product with partially hydrolyzed whey and casein has been shown to decrease fussiness, gas, and crying.[13]

Reduced Lactose/Lactose-free

Lactose is only present in mammalian milk. Reduced lactose formulas have similar calorie, protein, fat, and micronutrient content as standard milk-based formulas. In some products the lactose is reduced to compensate for the increased osmolality due to the hydrolyzed protein. Polysaccharides are used instead of the disaccharide lactose. There is also one low lactose product that adds a probiotic.

Parents with lactose intolerance may assume their infants are also lactose intolerant. However, most babies make adequate amounts of lactase, and congenital lactase deficiency is extremely rare. Milk-based lactose-free formulas are not indicated in galactosemia because they may contain small amounts of lactose or galactose.

Added Rice Starch

Added rice starch formulas are standard milk-based infant formulas designed to thicken in the acidic environment of the stomach to decrease spitting-up episodes.[9] These formulas have not been shown to decrease episodes of gastroesophageal reflux (GER) and so are not indicated as a medical treatment of GER. Rice starch is added as part of the carbohydrate content; therefore, the macronutrient distribution remains consistent with standard milk-based infant formulas. Rice cereal may be added to standard infant formula to achieve a similar effect; however, it increases the caloric density, increases the carbohydrate concentration (altering macronutrient distribution) and may result in clogged bottle nipples. Added rice starch formulas are not substitutes for thickened formula indicated for risk of aspiration.

Currently, 2 added rice starch products are on the market; one of the products is lactose-free, while the other has reduced lactose. Each product has studies to support that the added rice starch decreases episodes of spitting up and supports normal growth in healthy term infants.[14,15]

Soy-Based Formulas

Soy-based formulas (Table 12-4) are designed to meet the needs of healthy infants from birth to 1 year of age. The protein source is soy, supplemented with methionine to make it a complete protein source.

These formulas are fortified with iron and are lactose-free. It is estimated that about 25% of infants consuming formula will consume a soy-based formula. Soy-based infant formulas have higher calcium and phosphorus than standard cow's milk–based formulas because of reduced bioavailability secondary to phytates.[16] Soy-based formulas offer no advantage over cow's milk–based formulas except for a few indications. Indications for soy-based formula are infants with galactosemia or hereditary lactase deficiency (rare), or if a vegetarian human milk substitute is requested.[17]

Soy-based formulas are not recommended for premature infants because they are not designed to meet the premature infant's specific needs.[17] Soy milk protein is no less allergenic than cow's milk protein.[3] Infants with documented cow's milk allergy should not be given a soy formula because 10%–14% of these babies will also have a sensitivity to soy protein.[18,19] Infants with acute gastroenteritis who were previously well can be managed with rehydration and continued use of human milk or their usual cow's milk–based formula at the standard dilution.[17]

Premature or Low Birth Weight Formulas

Premature or low birth weight formulas (Table 12-5) come in ready-to-feed nurser bottles that are available for hospital use only. These formulas are milk based and designed to meet the

Table 12-3. Infant Formulas for Symptoms of Intolerance (per 100 Calories)—Standard Dilution Is 0.67 kcal/mL (20 kcal/oz) or 0.63 kcal/mL (19 kcal/oz)

PRODUCT (MANUFACTURER)	PROTEIN gm (% kcal) SOURCE	CHO gm (% kcal) SOURCE	FAT gm (% kcal) SOURCE	Na mg	K mg	Ca mg	Phos mg	Vit D IU	Fe mg	OSMOLAL-ITY mOsm	COMMENTS
Enfamil A.R. (Mead Johnson)	2.5 (10%) nonfat milk	11.3 (44%) lactose, rice starch, malto-dextrin, GOS	5.1 (46%) palm olein, soy oil, coconut oil, high oleic sunflower oil	40	108	78	53	60	1.8	240 liquid 230 powder	DHA 17 mg, ARA 34 mg PRSL 23/100 cal
Enfamil Gentlease (Mead Johnson)	2.3 (9%) partially hydrolyzed nonfat milk and whey protein concentrate solids (soy)	10.8 (43%) corn syrup solids	5.3 (48%) palm olein, soy oil, coconut oil, high oleic sunflower oil	36	108	82	46	60	1.8	220 liquid 230 powder	DHA 17 mg, ARA 34 mg PRSL 21/100 cal 60:40 whey-to-casein ratio ~80% less lactose
Enfamil Reguline (Mead Johnson)	2.3 (9%) partially hydrolyzed nonfat milk and whey protein concentrate	11.1 (43%) lactose, corn syrup solids, GOS, polydextrose (liquid also contains rice starch)	5.3 (48%) palm olein, soy oil, coconut oil, high oleic sunflower oil	36	108	82	46	60	1.5	260 liquid 250 powder	DHA 17 mg, ARA 34 mg PRSL 21/100 cal added prebiotics
Similac Expert Care for Diarrhea (Abbott Nutrition)	2.66 (11%) soy protein isolate, L-methionine	10.1 (40%) corn syrup solids, sucrose	5.46 (49%) soy oil, coconut oil	44	108	105	75	60	1.8	240	no DHA or ARA soy protein lactose-free added soy fiber (6 gm/L)
Similac Sensitive - 19 kcal/oz (Abbott Nutrition)	2.14 (9%) milk protein isolate	11.1 (43%) malto-dextrin, sugar, GOS	5.4 (49%) high oleic safflower oil, soy oil, coconut oil	32	110	88	59	60	1.9	200	DHA 0.15%, ARA 0.40% PRSL 20.3/100 cal very low lactose
Similac Sensitive for Spit-up (Abbott Nutrition)	2.14 (9%) milk protein isolate	10.96 (43%) corn syrup, rice starch, sugar, GOS	5.4 (49%) high oleic safflower oil, soy oil, coconut oil	30	107	84	56	60	1.8	180	DHA 0.15%, ARA 0.40% PRSL 19.9/100 cal very low lactose
Similac Total Comfort - 19 kcal/oz (Abbott Nutrition)	2.32 (9%) whey protein hydrolysate	11 (42%) corn syrup solids, sugar, GOS	5.4 (49%) high oleic safflower oil, soy oil, coconut oil	46	121	105	70	60	1.9	140	DHA 0.15%, ARA 0.40% added nucleotides PRSL 22.5/100 cal reduced lactose
Good Start Soothe (Gerber)	2.2 (9%) 100% whey partially hydrolyzed	11.2 (46%) malto-dextrin, lactose	5.1 (46%) palm olein, soy oil, coconut oil, high oleic safflower or sunflower, single cell oil	27	108	190	106	60	2	195	0.32% DHA, 0.64% ARA 4.6 mg/100 cal added nucleotides 70% less lactose probiotic added—L. reuteri PRSL 19.5/100 cal
Store Brands* Added Rice Starch (Perrigo Nutritionals)	2.5 (10%) nonfat milk	11 (44%) rice starch, maltodextrin, lactose	5.1 (46%) palm olein, soy oil, coconut oil, high oleic safflower or sunflower	40	108	78	53	60	1.8	206	DHA, ARA
Store Brands* Gentle (Perrigo Nutritionals)	2.3 (9%) nonfat milk, whey protein hydrolysate	10.8 (43%) corn syrup solids	5.3 (48%) palm olein, coconut oil, soy oil, high oleic safflower or sunflower oil	36	108	82	46	60	1.8	190	DHA, ARA 60:40 whey-to-casein ratio 75% less lactose than standard
Store Brands* Sensitivity (Perrigo Nutritionals)	2.14 (9%) whey protein concentrate, milk protein isolate	10.9 (43%) corn syrup solids	5.4 (48%) palm olein, coconut oil, soy oil, high oleic safflower or sunflower oil	30	107	84	56	60	1.8	198	DHA, ARA added nucleotides reduced lactose

*Perrigo Nutritionals makes Store Brands for Walmart, Sam's Club, Walgreens, CVS, Target, and Babies R Us as well as Bright Beginnings. Check product labels for the most accurate and up-to-date information.
GOS, galacto-oligosacchrides.

special nutrition needs of preterm infants (born < 37 weeks gestation) and/or infants born < 1500 g (which is considered very low birth weight) while in the hospital, if human milk is not available. The unique characteristics of this group of formulas include increased protein, carbohydrate blends of lactose and glucose polymers, fat blends containing a portion of fat as medium-chain triglycerides to promote fat absorption, and increased calcium and phosphate to promote net mineral retention and bone mineralization.[20,21] Premature infant formulas are available with low iron or with iron fortification. They are

Table 12-4. Soy-Based Infant Formulas (per 100 Calories)—Standard Dilution for Soy-Based Formulas Is 0.67 kcal/mL (20 kcal/oz)

PRODUCT (MANUFACTURER)	PROTEIN gm (% kcal) SOURCE	CHO gm (%kcal) SOURCE	FAT gm (%kcal) SOURCE	Na mg	K mg	Ca mg	Phos mg	Vit D IU	Fe mg	OSMOLAL-ITY mOsm	COMMENTS
Enfamil Prosobee (Mead Johnson)	2.5 (10%) soy protein isolate, L-methionine	10.6 (42%) corn syrup solid	5.3 (48%) palm olein, soy oil, coconut oil, high oleic sunflower oil	36	120	105	69	60	1.8	170 liquid 180 powder	DHA 17 mg, ARA 34 mg PRSL 23/100 cal
Good Start Soy (Gerber)	2.5 (10%) enzymatically hydrolyzed soy protein isolate, L-methionine	11 (44%) corn maltodextrin, sucrose	5.1 (46%) palm olein, soy oil, coconut oil, high oleic safflower or sunflower oil	40	116	105	63	60	1.8	180	DHA 0.32%, ARA 0.64% PRSL 23.1100 cal
Similac Soy Isomil—20 kcal/oz (Abbott Nutrition)	2.45 (10%) soy protein isolate, L-methionine	10.4 (41%) corn syrup, sugar, FOS	5.46 (49%) high oleic safflower oil, soy oil, coconut oil	44	108	105	75	60	1.8	200	DHA 0.15%, ARA 0.40% PRSL 22.8/100 cal
Similac Soy Isomil—19 kcal/oz (Abbott Nutrition)	2.45 (10%) soy protein isolate, L-methionine	10.4 (41%) corn syrup, sugar, FOS	5.46 (49%) high oleic safflower oil, soy oil, coconut oil	46	110	110	79	60	1.9	200	
Store Brands* Soy (Perrigo Nutritionals)	2.5 (10%) soy protein isolate	10.6 (42%) corn syrup	5.3 (48%) palm olein, coconut oil, soy oil, high oleic safflower or sunflower oil	36	120	105	69	60	1.8	164	DHA, ARA

*Perrigo Nutritionals makes Store Brands for Walmart, Sam's Club, Walgreens, CVS, Target, and Babies R Us as well as Bright Beginnings. Check product labels for the most accurate and up-to-date information.
FOS, fructo-oligosaccharides.

also available in ready-to-feed nursers in a variety of calorie concentrations and a higher protein option. One of the 3 formulas available has partially hydrolyzed 100% whey protein. The other 2 formulas contain intact whey and casein proteins.

Premature Discharge Formulas

Premature discharge formulas (Table 12-6) are designed to meet the nutrition needs of the infant born prematurely or the infant with low birth weight who is transitioning home. These formulas are milk based with higher levels of calcium and phosphorus than standard term infant formulas. They provide a nutrient intake that is between a preterm and term formula, and the calorie concentration at standard dilution is higher than standard term infant formulas. A Cochrane Review from 2012 concluded that there is insufficient evidence for current recommendations for the use of premature discharge formulas.[22] Premature discharge formulas are still commonly recommended, however, and manufacturers have studies that these formulas support appropriate growth for the premature or low birth weight infant upon discharge from the hospital.

Specialized Infant Formulas

Extensively Hydrolyzed Protein

Formulas containing extensively hydrolyzed protein (Table 12-7) are considered hypoallergenic according to AAP and FDA standards, meaning that most children with cow's

milk protein sensitivity will not have an allergic reaction to these formulas. The protein in these formulas is extensively hydrolyzed by heat or enzymes, resulting in free amino acids and small peptides. The fat content is made up of long-chain triglycerides from polyunsaturated vegetable oil to supply essential fatty acids (EFAs) and varying amounts of medium-chain triglycerides. These formulas are lactose-free and because of the hydrolyzed protein have a higher osmolarity. Protein hydrolysates are recommended for infants intolerant of cow's milk and soy proteins and those with significant malabsorption due to gastrointestinal or hepatobiliary disease.[3,23] These products are safe for the general population, but they cost significantly more than standard term infant formulas and should only be used with medical advice.

Amino Acid-Based

Amino acid–based infant formulas (Table 12-8) are considered nonallergenic and are indicated in extreme protein hypersensitivity or when intolerance symptoms persist on an extensively hydrolyzed formula.[24] Approximately 2%–10% of infants with cow's milk protein allergy develop persistent symptoms despite therapy with extensively hydrolyzed protein formula and thus require an amino acid–based formula.[25] Using an amino acid–based formula has no additional benefit if an extensively hydrolyzed protein formula is effective. Other indications for the amino acid–based formulas include eosinophilic gastrointestinal disorders,

Table 12-5. Premature Infant Formulas (per 100 Calories)—Standard Dilution Is 0.67 kcal/mL (20 kcal/oz), 0.8 kcal/mL (24 kcal/oz), or 1 kcal/mL (30 kcal/oz)

PRODUCT (MANUFACTURER)	PROTEIN gm (% kcal) SOURCE	CHO gm (%kcal) SOURCE	FAT gm (%kcal) SOURCE	Na mg	K mg	Ca mg	Phos mg	Vit D IU	Fe mg	OSMOLAL-ITY mOsm	COMMENTS
Enfamil Premature 20 cal/oz (low iron or iron fortified) (Mead Johnson)	3 (12%) nonfat milk, whey protein concentrate	11 (44%) corn syrup solids, lactose	5.1 (44%) MCT, soy oil, high oleic vegetable oil	58	98	165	83	240	0.5 1.8	240	28 mg/L added nucleotides DHA 17 mg, ARA 34 mg PRSL 27/100 cal Ca:Phos ratio—2:1
Enfamil Premature 24 cal/oz (low iron or iron fortified) (Mead Johnson)	3 (12%) non-fat milk, whey protein concentrate	11 (44%) corn syrup solids, lactose	5.1 (44%) MCT, soy oil, high oleic vegetable oil	58	98	165	83	240	0.5 1.8	300	34 mg/L added nucleotides DHA 17 mg, ARA 34 mg PRSL 27/100 cal Ca:Phos ratio—2:1
Enfamil Premature 24 cal/oz High Protein (Mead Johnson)	3.5 (14%) nonfat milk, whey protein concentrate	10.5 (42%) corn syrup solids, lactose	5.1 (44%) MCT, soy oil, high oleic sunflower and/or safflower oil	58	98	165	83	240	1.8	300	added nucleotides DHA 17 mg, ARA 34 mg PRSL 30/100 cal Ca:Phos ratio—2:1
Enfamil Premature 30 cal/oz (Mead Johnson)	3 (12%) nonfat milk, whey protein concentrate	11 (43%) malto-dextrin	5.1 (45%) MCT, soy oil, high oleic sunflower oil	58	102	165	83	240	1.8	320	added nucleotides DHA 17 mg, ARA 34 mg PRSL 27/100 cal Ca:Phos ratio—2:1
Good Start Premature 20 cal/oz (Gerber)	3 (12%) enzymat-ically hydrolyzed whey protein isolate	10.5 (42%) lactose, maltodextrin	5.2 (47%) MCT, high oleic safflower or sunflower oil, soy oil, single cell oil	55	120	164	85	180	1.8	229	added nucleotides DHA 0.32%, ARA 0.64% Ca:Phos ratio—1.9 PRSL 27.7/100 cal
Good Start Premature 24 cal/oz (Gerber)	3 (12%) enzymat-ically hydrolyzed whey protein isolate (from cow's milk)	10.5 (42%) malto-dextrin, lactose	5.2 (46%) MCT, soy oil, high oleic safflower or sun-flower oil	55	120	164	85	180	1.8	275	added nucleotides DHA 0.32%, ARA 0.64% Ca:Phos ratio—1.9:1 PRSL 27.7/100 cal
Good Start Premature 24 cal/oz High Protein (Gerber)	3.6 (14%) enzymat-ically hydrolyzed whey protein isolate (from cow's milk)	9.7 (39%) malto-dextrin, lactose	5.2 (47%) MCT, high oleic safflower or sunflower oil, soy oil, single cell oil	55	120	164	85	180	1.8	299	added nucleotides DHA 0.32%, ARA 0.64% Ca:Phos ratio—1.9:1 PRSL 31.3/100 cal
Good Start Premature 30 cal/oz (Gerber)	3 (12%) enzymat-ically hydrolyzed whey protein isolate (from cow's milk)	10.5 (42%) malto-dextrin, lactose	5.2 (46%) MCT, soy oil, high oleic safflower or sun-flower oil	55	120	164	85	180	1.8	341	added nucleotides DHA 0.32%, ARA 0.64% Ca:Phos ratio—1.9:1 PRSL 27.7/100 cal
Similac Special Care 20 cal/oz (Abbott Nutrition)	3 (12%) nonfat milk, whey protein concentrate	10.3 (41%) corn syrup solids, lactose	5.43 (47%) MCT, soy oil, coconut oil	43	129	180	100	150	1.8	235	DHA 0.25%, ARA 0.40% PRSL 27.8/100 cal Ca:Phos ratio—1.8:1
Similac Special Care 24 cal/oz (Abbott Nutrition)	3 (12%) nonfat milk, whey protein concentrate	10.3 (41%) corn syrup solids, lactose	5.43 (47%) MCT, soy oil, coconut oil	43	129	180	100	150	1.8	280	DHA 0.25%, ARA 0.40% PRSL 27.8/100 cal Ca:Phos ratio—1.8:1
Similac Special Care 24 cal/oz High Protein (Abbott Nutrition)	3.3 (13%) nonfat milk, whey protein concentrate	10 (40%) corn syrup solids, lactose	5.43 (47%) MCT, soy oil, coconut oil	43	129	180	100	150	1.8	280	DHA 0.25%, ARA 0.40% PRSL 29.5/100 cal Ca:Phos ratio—1.8:1
Similac Special Care 30 cal/oz (Abbott Nutrition)	3 (12%) nonfat milk, whey protein concentrate	7.73 (31%) corn syrup solids, lactose	6.61 (57%) MCT, soy oil, coconut oil	43	129	180	100	150	1.8	325	DHA 0.21%, ARA 0.33% PRSL 27.8/100 cal Ca:Phos ratio—1.8:1

transitioning from parenteral to enteral feedings, and short bowel syndrome.[25] These formulas should only be used with medical advice and under medical supervision.

Carbohydrate-Free

Carbohydrate-free formulas (Table 12-9) are designed for the management of carbohydrate metabolism disorders and carbohydrate malabsorption issues (eg, glucose-galactose malabsorption).[26] These formulas require a carbohydrate source. The physician or healthcare professional prescribes

a carbohydrate to be added to the formula, and it is usually titrated up to make the formula 20 kcal/oz.[27]

Reduced Fat/Modified Fat

Reduced or modified fat formulas (Table 12-10) can be used in conditions of decreased bile salts, fat malabsorption, defective lymphatic transport of fat, chylothorax, or long-chain 3-hydroxyacyl-CoA dehydrogenase deficiency. Due to the risk of essential fatty acid deficiency (EFAD), these formulas should only be used under the supervision of a physician. Pa-

Table 12-6. Premature Discharge Infant Formulas (per 100 Calories)—Standard Dilution for These Formulas Is 0.73 kcal/mL (22 kcal/oz)

PRODUCT (MANUFACTURER)	PROTEIN gm (% kcal) SOURCE	CHO gm (%kcal) SOURCE	FAT gm (%kcal) SOURCE	Na mg	K mg	Ca mg	Phos mg	Vit D IU	Fe mg	OSMOLAL-ITY mOsm	COMMENTS
Enfamil Enfacare (Mead Johnson)	2.8 (11%) whey protein concentrate, nonfat milk	10.4 (42%) powder: lactose, corn syrup solids RTU: malto-dextrin, lactose	5.3 (47%) high oleic sunflower or safflower oil, soy oil, MCT, coconut oil	35	105	120	66	70	1.8	310 powder 250 liquid	42 mg added nucleotides DHA 17 mg, ARA 34 mg PRSL 25/100 cal
Similac Neosure (Abbott Nutrition)	2.8 (11%) nonfat milk, whey protein concentrate	10.1 (40%) corn syrup solids, lactose	5.5 (49%) soy oil, coconut oil, MCT	33	142	105	62	70	1.8	250	DHA 0.15%, ARA 0.40% PRSL 25.2/100 cal

*Check product labels for the most accurate and up-to-date information.

Table 12-7. Extensively Hydrolyzed Protein Infant Formulas (per 100 Calories)—Standard Dilution Is 0.67 kcal/mL (20 kcal/oz)

PRODUCT (MANUFACTURER)	PROTEIN gm (% kcal) SOURCE	CHO gm (%kcal) SOURCE	FAT gm (%kcal) SOURCE	Na mg	K mg	Ca mg	Phos mg	Vit D IU	Fe mg	OSMOLAL-ITY mOsm	COMMENTS
Nutramigen (Mead Johnson)	2.8 (11%) casein hydrolysate, L-cystine, L-tyrosine, L-tryptophan	10.3 (41%) corn syrup solids, modi-fied corn starch	5.3 (48%) palm olein, soy oil, coco-nut oil, high oleic sunflower oil	47	110	94	52	50	1.8	260 concentrate 270 RTU 8,32 oz 320 RTU 2 oz	DHA 17 mg, ARA 34 mg PRSL 25/100 cal lactose- and sucrose-free *only available in liquid forms
Nutramigen with Enflora LGG (Mead Johnson)	2.8 (11%) casein hydrolysate, L-cystine, L-tyrosine, L-tryptophan	10.3 (41%) corn syrup solids, modi-fied corn starch	5.3 (48%) palm olein, soy oil, coco-nut oil, high oleic sunflower oil	47	110	94	52	50	1.8	300	DHA 17 mg, ARA 34 mg PRSL 25 100 cal added probiot-ic—Lactobacillus GG *only available in powder
Pregestimil (Mead Johnson)	2.8 (11%) casein hydrolysate	10.2 (41%) corn syrup solids, modi-fied corn starch	5.6 (48%) MCT, soy oil, corn oil, high oleic safflower or sunflower oil RTU-no corn oil	47	110	94	52	50	1.8	290 liquid 320 powder	DHA 17 mg, ARA 34 mg PRSL 25/100 cal 55% MCT
Similac Expert Care Alimentum (Abbott Nutrition)	2.75 (11%) casein hydrolysate, L-cys-tine, L-tyrosine, L-tryptophan	10.2 (41%) sugar, modified tapioca starch	5.54 (48%) high oleic safflower oil, MCT, soy oil	44	118	105	75	45	1.8	370	DHA 0.15%, ARA 0.40% PSRL 25.3/100 cal

*Check product labels for the most accurate and up-to-date information.

Table 12-8. Free Amino Acid Infant Formulas (per 100 Calories)—Standard Dilution Is 0.67 kcal/mL (20 kcal/oz)

PRODUCT (MANUFACTURER)	PROTEIN gm (% kcal) SOURCE	CHO gm (%kcal) SOURCE	FAT gm (%kcal) SOURCE	Na mg	K mg	Ca mg	Phos mg	Vit D IU	Fe mg	OSMOLAL-ITY mOsm	COMMENTS
Elecare for Infants (Abbott Nutrition)	3.1 (15%) free L-amino acids	10.7 (42%) corn syrup solids	4.8 (43%) high oleic safflower oil, MCT, soy oil	45	150	116	84.2	60	1.8	350 (at 20 cal/oz)	DHA 0.15%, ARA 0.40% PRSL 28/100 cal 33% MCT
Neocate Infant DHA & ARA (Nutricia)	2.8 (11.2%) free amino acids	10.8 (43.1%) corn syrup solids	5.1 (45.7%) refined vegetable oil (MCT, high oleic sunflower oil, sunflower oil, canola oil)	39.1	109	116	82.2	72.9	1.5	340 (at 20 cal/oz)	DHA 0.35%, ARA 0.35% 4.8 mg/100 kcal added nucleotides PSRL 25/100 cal
Puramino (Mead Johnson)	2.8 (11%) free amino acids	10.3 (41%) corn syrup solids, modi-fied tapioca starch	5.3 (48%) palm olein, soy oil, coco-nut oil, high oleic sunflower oil	47	110	94	52	50	1.8	350	DHA 17 mg, ARA 34 mg PRSL 25/100 cal

*Check product labels for the most accurate and up-to-date information.

Table 12-9. Carbohydrate-Free Formulas (per 100 Calories)

PRODUCT (MANUFACTURER)	PROTEIN gm (% kcal) SOURCE	CHO gm (%kcal) SOURCE	FAT gm (%kcal) SOURCE	Na mg	K mg	Ca mg	Phos mg	Vit D IU	Fe mg	OSMOLAL-ITY mOsm	COMMENTS
RCF* (Abbott Nutrition)	3.0 (12%) soy protein isolate, L-methionine	10.1 (40%) selected by physician or healthcare professional	5.3 (48%) high oleic safflower oil, coconut oil, soy oil	44	108	105	75	60	1.8	168 (will vary based on type of CHO)	*based on preparation with 54 gm CHO and 12 oz water added to 13 oz of concentrate no DHA/ARA PRSL 25.8/100 cal
3232A** (Mead Johnson)	2.8 (11%) extensively hydrolyzed casein, L-cystine, L-tyrosine, L-tryptophan	13.4 (54%) choice by physician, modified tapioca starch as stabilizer	4.2 (35%) MCT, corn oil	43	109	94	63		1.88	360 (corn syrup solids) 430 (sucrose) 640 (glucose)	**based on preparation with 59 gm CHO at 20 kcal/oz PRSL 25/100 cal

*Check product labels for the most accurate and up-to-date information.

Table 12-10. Modified Fat Formulas (per 100 Calories)

PRODUCT (MANUFACTURER)	PROTEIN gm (% kcal) SOURCE	CHO gm (%kcal) SOURCE	FAT gm (%kcal) SOURCE	Na mg	K mg	Ca mg	Phos mg	Vit D IU	Fe mg	OSMOLAL-ITY mOsm	COMMENTS
Enfamil Enfaport (Mead Johnson)	3.5 (14%) calcium caseinate, sodium caseinate	10.2 (41%) corn syrup solids	5.5 (45%) MCT (84%), soy oil	30	115	94	52	50	1.8	280-30 cal/oz	17 mg DHA, 34 mg ARA 84% MCT PRSL 28/100 cal *comes in RTU, 30 cal/oz Water can be added to dilute to lower concentrations
Monogen (Nutricia)	2.97 (12%) whey protein concentrate, L-amino acids	16.1 (64%) corn syrup solids	2.62 (24%) MCT (as fractionated coconut oil), walnut oil	48	86	61	48	63	1	250-22 cal/oz 370-30 cal/oz	essential fatty acid ratio n6:n3 of 6.2:1 80% MCT *for > 1 y old
Lipistart (Vitaflo)	3.09 (12%) whey protein isolate (from milk), sodium caseinate (from milk)	12.2 (47%) dried glucose syrup	4.56 (41%) fractionated coconut oil, soy oil	57	111	108	79	81	1.1	180-20 cal/oz	*for > 1 y old

*Check product labels for the most accurate and up-to-date information.

tients on these formulas for an extended period of time need to be evaluated for signs and symptoms of EFAD. Addition of EFAs at a volume of 3%–5% of total kilocalories may be indicated with some of the formulas with lower levels of the long-chain fatty acids to meet EFA needs and prevent deficiency.

Reduced Mineral

The mineral content of reduced mineral formula (Table 12-11) is close to that of human milk and is designed to treat calcium disorders.[27] This formula may also be used for infants with impaired renal function. An additional source of iron may need to be considered. Infants consuming this formula should be monitored by a medical professional.

Functional Ingredients in Infant Formulas

DHA/ARA

Long-chain polyunsaturated fatty acids (LCPUFAs) have been shown to play an important role in the neurodevelopment of infants. DHA and ARA are the most abundant LCP-

UFAs in the brain; DHA is also found in retinal cells.[28–30] DHA and ARA can be obtained from dietary sources or by endogenous conversion of their precursors, α-linolenic acid (18:3 ω3) and linoleic acid (18:2 ω6).[29,30] DHA and ARA occur naturally in breast milk with levels varying based on maternal diet.

During pregnancy, DHA and ARA are transported across the placenta to the fetus. Fetuses can synthesize DHA and ARA after 26 weeks gestation, though the amount produced is highly variable.[30] After birth, DHA and ARA are provided via breast milk or infant formula supplemented with DHA/ARA. Infants fed formula without supplementation have been shown to have lower levels of DHA in the brain.[30]

Nucleotides

Dietary nucleotides are nonprotein, nitrogenous compounds found in high concentrations in breast milk.[31] They play key roles in many biological processes and are sometimes described as being "conditionally essential" in infancy.

Table 12-11. Reduced Mineral Infant Formula (per 100 Calories)

PRODUCT (MANUFACTURER)	PROTEIN gm (% kcal) SOURCE	CHO gm (%kcal) SOURCE	FAT gm (%kcal) SOURCE	Na mg	K mg	Ca mg	Phos mg	Vit D IU	Fe mg	OSMOLAL-ITY mOsm	COMMENTS
Similac PM 60/40 (Abbott Nutrition)	2.2 (9%) whey protein concentrate, sodium caseinate	10.2 (41%) lactose	5.6 (50%) high oleic safflower oil, soy oil, coconut oil	24	80	56	28	0.7	280	no DHA & ARA PRSL 18.3/100 cal	42 mg added nucleotides DHA 17 mg, ARA 34 mg PRSL 25/100 cal

Nucleotides serve as nucleic acid precursors and coenzyme constituents as well as physiologic mediators.[31-33]

Some research suggests that nucleotide supplementation enhances growth and maturation of the gut and enhances mucosal recovery after intestinal injury. Nucleotides also play an important role in immune function by stimulating lymphocyte differentiation and proliferation.[31-33] Nucleotide-supplemented formula has been shown to support normal growth in infants.[31,32]

Prebiotics and Probiotics

Prebiotics are fermentable carbohydrates that are not fully digested in the small intestine. Prebiotics promote growth of normal gut flora, thus preventing the proliferation of pathogenic bacteria.[34,35] Fermentation of prebiotics produces short-chain fatty acids that can be used by colonocytes for energy. Fructo-oligosaccharides and galacto-oligosacchrides are the main prebiotics found in breast milk and infant formula.[34]

Probiotics are nonpathogenic bacteria that alter the microflora of the host. They can help interfere with the adherence of pathogenic bacteria, increase immunological barrier function of the intestine, and modulate the inflammatory response.[34-36]

Bifidobacteria are the predominant species of bacteria found in the intestines of breastfed infants. Some studies have shown *Bifidobacterium lactis* to be protective against necrotizing enterocolitis due to its effect on gut barrier function.[34-36] *Lactobacillus rhamnosus* GG is also found in the intestine of infants. It has been shown in numerous studies to reduce duration of diarrhea in infants and may also be protective against necrotizing enterocolitis.[36] Infant formula with prebiotics and/or probiotics may be beneficial for infants experiencing gastrointestinal distress during and after illness or use of antibiotics.

Forms of Infant Formula and Mixing Guidelines

Infant formula is available in 3 forms: ready-to-feed, liquid concentrate, and powder, though not all formulas are available in all 3 forms. All forms are nutritionally complete and are regulated, but small differences exist between them due to differences in processing.[8,37] Liquid concentrate and powder forms require the addition of potable water to reconstitute and can be mixed to various caloric dilutions according to the special need of the infant.

Ready-to-feed formula is the most commonly used form in hospitals because it is considered commercially sterile. It is convenient and limits opportunity for contamination. Manufacturers provide many different formulas in standard caloric dilution and some formulas at higher caloric concentrations in convenient ready-to-feed nurser bottles. Consumers can purchase ready-to-feed formula at standard dilution in quart-sized bottles or single-serving nurser bottles. Ready-to-feed formula is the most expensive form because the consumer is paying for the convenience.

Liquid concentrate is also considered commercially sterile, but because it needs to be mixed with water to make a standard dilution, it offers more opportunity for potential contamination than ready-to-feed. Liquid concentrate is the second choice in hospitals and can be used to make higher-caloric concentrations. It is easy to mix for consumers and offers some financial savings over ready-to-feed.

Powder is not sterile and must be mixed with water. Because it is not sterile, it may contain pathogenic bacteria.[38] Powder formula has been associated with *Enterobacter sakazakii* contamination and infection in immunocompromised neonates in healthcare facilities.[39] Because of the population that they serve, hospitals should only use powder if no other option is available.[40,41] Reconstituted powder formulas have been safely consumed by millions of infants worldwide over the past half century, so parents of healthy newborns should continue to feel comfortable using powder infant formulas. Consumers choose it because it is the least expensive form and can be quickly mixed at any location when needed. The European Society for Pediatric Gastroenterology, Hepatology, and Nutrition Committee on Nutrition recommends that in the home, powder infant formulas should be freshly prepared for each feeding and any remaining formula be discarded to minimize potential risk of contamination.[41,42] If larger quantities are mixed, no more than a 24-hour supply should be mixed and refrigerated.[41]

Water

When it is from a municipal supply, water from the tap is adequate to use for preparing formula for infants at home with a normal immune system and who are fed orally.[43] Water used for formula preparation does not have to be boiled. Municipal tap water is more regulated than bottled water. Municipal water and bottled water are considered sterile.[41] Municipal tap water is fluoridated, whereas most bottled water is not. Bottled water or infant fluoridated bottled water may be a good choice when tap water is from a well because well water may contain high levels of certain minerals. In hospitals only chilled, sterile water is recommended in formula preparation.[41]

Infants consuming either human milk or infant formula exclusively do not need additional water in their diets. Human milk or infant formula mixed to standard dilution provides adequate free water for hydration in hot or dry climates and if the infant is febrile.

Standard Dilution

Standard dilution of most term infant formulas is 20 kcal/oz. Careful attention must be given to the calorie concentration on the label because lower calorie formulas are now on the market. The standard dilution for these formulas is 19 kcal/oz. This small difference may not make a significant difference for the healthy term infant, but may be significant for the infant with special healthcare needs. Standard dilution for the premature discharge formulas is 22 kcal/oz. When mixing formulas, healthcare professionals should suggest that parents read the manufacturer instructions on the can because instructions may vary by manufacturer and by product. When mixing powdered formulas, only use the scoop that comes with that particular formula because scoop sizes are different for each formula.

Increasing Caloric Concentration

For special feeding situations in which fluid volume may be limited, many of which are discussed in detail in this book, both powdered infant formula or infant formula concentrate can be reconstituted (Tables 12-12–12-14) to provide formula with more concentrated calories than standard dilution.[27] Concentrated liquids from all manufacturers contain 40 kcal/oz, but not all manufacturers have the same size container for the concentrated formula (13 or 12.1 oz). The powdered formulas are each different with regard to amount of calories per gram and grams per household measures. Also some formula powders may need to be a packed measure. All of these differences make it important to make recipes for concentrating formula specifically for each product.[41]

Table 12-12. Increasing Calorie Concentration With Formula Concentrate

CALORIE CONCENTRATION	FORMULA BRAND	AMOUNT CONCENTRATE (oz)	WATER TO ADD (oz)	APPROX. YIELD (oz)
20 kcal/oz (0.67 kcal/mL)	Enfamil/Similac	13	13	26
	Good Start	12.1	12	24
22 kcal/oz (0.73 kcal/mL)	Enfamil/Similac	13	11	24
	Good Start	12.1	10	22
24 kcal/oz (0.8 kcal/mL)	Enfamil/Similac	13	9	22
	Good Start	12.1	8	20
27 kcal/oz (0.9 kcal/mL)	Enfamil/Similac	13	6	19
	Good Start	12.1	6	18

*All concentrates are standard 40 kcal/oz or 1.33 kcal/mL.

Table 12-13. Increasing Calorie Concentration With Powder Infant Formula—Standard Dilution 19 kcal/oz

CALORIE CONCENTRATION	AMOUNT OF POWDER TO ADD*	WATER TO ADD (oz)	APPROX. YIELD (oz)
19 kcal/oz (0.63 kcal/mL)	4 scoops	8	8.8
21 kcal/oz (0.7 kcal/mL)	4 scoops	7	7.8
23 kcal/oz (0.76 kcal/mL)	5 scoops	8	9
26 kcal/oz (0.86 kcal/mL)	5 scoops	7	8

*Only use the scoop provided for the specific formula. Scoop sizes vary from product to product even within the same manufacturer.

Table 12-14. Increasing Calorie Concentration With Powder Infant Formula—Standard Dilution 20 kcal/oz

CALORIE CONCENTRATION	AMOUNT OF POWDER TO ADD*	WATER TO ADD (oz)	APPROX. YIELD (oz)
20 kcal/oz (0.67 kcal/mL)	4 scoops	8	9
22 kcal/oz (0.73 kcal/mL)	4 scoops	7	8
24 kcal/oz (0.8 kcal/mL)	5 scoops	8	9
27 kcal/oz (0.9 kcal/mL)	5 scoops	7	8

*Only use the scoop provided for the specific formula. Scoop sizes vary from product to product even within the same manufacturer.

When calories are being concentrated to >24 kcal/oz using only infant formula concentrate or powdered infant formula and less water, potential renal solute load (PRSL) must be considered. Protein, sodium, chloride, potassium, and phosphorus all contribute to PRSL, and a higher PRSL can contribute to more rapid dehydration.[44] In certain medical conditions the increase calorie concentration may be indicated, but should only be done under close monitoring by medical professionals. Increasing the concentration of formula also increases that osmolarity of the formula, so tolerance and fluid status should be monitored by a medical professional when formula is mixed to provide increased calorie concentration.

Modular Macronutrients

Modular macronutrients can be used to increase caloric concentration. Modulars are available as protein, carbohydrate, fat, and combinations of macronutrients. The fat and/or carbohydrate modulars may not add as significantly to the PRSL and osmolality as concentrating the formula with less water, and fat and/or carbohydrate modulars should be considered for concentrating calories > 24 cal/oz. Modular macronutrients will not increase the concentration of micronutrients like concentrating just the formula powder or concentrate. This may be desirable in some situations (renal insufficiency) and not desirable in other situations (increased calcium and phosphorus needs in prematurity). Another consideration is that the modular products will alter the macronutrient distribution. Modulars can be used to customize the formula to meet a specific need of the patient.

Modulars can be added to the formula when mixing, or they can be mixed with water and delivered as a bolus through the tube separate from formula. To boost caloric intake of formula, some common food products or ingredients may also be used (eg, vegetable oil or corn starch). These ingredients may not be ideal, but they are much less expensive and easier to purchase than the manufactured modulars.

Increasing Concentration of Breast Milk

Infants born prematurely often have caloric and nutrient deficits, even at discharge, and although breast milk is the best choice for feeding these infants, it may not meet all of the caloric and nutrient needs of the infant with significant comorbidities.[45] Expert opinion and studies show that preterm infants discharged from the hospital at suboptimal weight being fed breast milk should continue to be supplemented to ensure adequate nutrient intake.[46,47] Some healthcare professionals suggest adding premature infant formula or term infant formula concentrate or powder to expressed breast milk to increase the caloric and nutrient density.[3,41,48] When using powder, remember that powder is not commercially sterile.[41] Evidence for or against this practice is lacking, and a potential exists for error. Close medical monitoring is suggested.[47]

Introducing Complementary Foods to the Infant's Diet

The AAP recommends exclusive breastfeeding for up to 6 months of age.[2] No nutrition indication exists for starting complementary foods any earlier than 4–6 months of age, and starting solids as early as 4 months of age has not shown any adverse effects on growth.[3] There may be a link to earlier introduction of solids (within the 4–6 month range) and overweight in adulthood.[49]

Each infant develops at his or her individual rate. An infant is usually ready for solid foods when birth weight has doubled, truncal stability permits sitting with support, and neuromuscular maturation has been achieved.[3] Other signs may include frequently putting things in the mouth or leaning forward and opening the mouth to indicate a desire for food.[3]

Introducing foods in any certain order does not have supporting evidence, but the first food is usually iron-fortified cereal. Consideration should be given to introducing meats early in the process since they are good sources of iron. The general rule is to add 1 "single-ingredient" food at a time and wait 3–5 days before introducing a new food, watching for possible intolerances or allergic reactions.[3] Some parents want to make their own baby foods. Parents should cook the food until soft and put it in a baby food grinder or blender until the desired consistency is reached. For infants just starting on solid foods, the consistency should be a smooth puree. Older infants can tolerate small consistent-sized bits in their food. Parents should avoid adding salt or sugar.[3]

A good time to advance textures to minced or diced foods and other finger foods is when the infant starts teething. Parents should be aware that "rub on" teething medications can interfere with chewing and swallowing because muscles in the throat can become numb. Careful observation is advised.

Juice

After 6 months of age fruit juice can be introduced in a cup and should be limited to 4–6 oz daily.[50] Only 100% fruit juice should be offered. Juice is not a nutritionally necessary addition to the diet of an infant. Fruit juice displaces the more nutrient-dense human milk or infant formula; therefore, if juice is introduced, it should be used in limited amounts. Infants should not be offered juice in a bottle or in a cup that can be carried around, and they should not consume juice just before bed because of the increased risk for dental caries. Overconsumption of juice can lead to osmotic diarrhea due to the high fructose and sorbitol content.[3]

Milk

Cow's milk (whole, 2%, 1%, skim), goat or any other animal milk, or any plant-based beverage (soy, almond, coconut, rice) other than infant formula should be avoided during the first year of life. These milks and plant-based beverages are not fortified with vitamins and minerals at the levels recommended for infants and have been associated with protein calorie malnutrition.[3]

Foods to Avoid the First Year

Foods that are difficult to chew or can easily choke a child or be aspirated should be avoided up to about 4 years of age. Foods to avoid include, but are not limited to, hot dogs, nuts, grapes, raisins, raw carrots, popcorn, and rounded candies.[3]

Honey is another food to avoid during the first year of life. Honey can contain a bacteria that produces the toxin that results in botulism. Botulism is potentially very serious and can result in death if not diagnosed and treated properly in the infected infant.[3]

With the increasing prevalence of obesity and research to support that healthy eating habits are established early in life, high-fat or high-sugar foods are not needed in an infant's diet. These foods are high in calories and offer limited nutritional value and should be avoided during the first year of life.[51]

Toddler Formulas

Toddlers consuming adequate amounts of nutrients, especially iron, from solid foods do not need a toddler formula. Whole cow's milk is adequate and appropriate after 1 year of age. Toddler formulas (Table 12-15) are an option if nutrient intake is a concern because they contain higher amounts of iron, vitamin C, and vitamin E than cow's milk and contain nutrients such as zinc that cow's milk does not contain, but that a toddler usually gets in a varied, healthy diet. The calcium and phosphorus levels of the toddler formulas are higher than infant formulas to match the needs of the growing toddler. Toddler formulas contain DHA and ARA.

The standard dilution for these products is 0.67 kcal/mL (20 kcal/oz).

Test Your Knowledge Questions

1. Which formula(s) is indicated for cow's milk protein allergy in an infant?
   A. Similac Sensitive
   B. Enfamil Nutramigen
   C. Good Start Gentle
   D. Goat's milk with added vitamins and minerals

2. What is the standard dilution of premature discharge formulas?
   A. 19 kcal/oz
   B. 20 kcal/oz
   C. 22 kcal/oz
   D. 24 kcal/oz

3. According to the Federal Food, Drug, and Cosmetic Act, infant formulas that meet a specific medical need are considered
   A. Exempt
   B. GRAS (generally recognized as safe)
   C. Specialized
   D. Medical foods

4. Prebiotics are
   A. Oligosaccharides
   B. Complex dietary carbohydrates that are not digestible by humans
   C. The fuel for beneficial bacteria in the gut
   D. All of the above

Acknowledgments

The authors of this chapter for the second edition of this text wish to thank Timothy Sentongo, MD, for his contributions to the first edition of this text.

Table 12-15. Toddler Formulas (per 100 Calories)

PRODUCT (MANUFACTURER)	PROTEIN gm (% kcal) SOURCE	CHO gm (%kcal) SOURCE	FAT gm (%kcal) SOURCE	Na mg	K mg	Ca mg	Phos mg	Vit D IU	Fe mg	OSMOLALITY mOsm	COMMENTS
Gerber Graduate Gentle (Gerber)	2.2 (9%) whey protein concentrate (from cow's milk, enzymatically hydrolyzed, reduced in minerals)	11.6 (45%) lactose, corn maltodextrin, GOS	5.1 (46%) palm olein, soy oil, coconut oil, high oleic safflower or sunflower oil	27	108	190	106	60	2	180	added nucleotides DHA 0.32%, ARA 0.64% PRSL 21.9/100 cal
Gerber Graduate Protect (Gerber)	2.2 (9%) whey protein concentrate (from cow's milk, enzymatically hydrolyzed, reduced in minerals)	11.2 (45%) lactose, corn maltodextrin	5.1 (46%) palm olein, soy oil, coconut oil, high oleic safflower or sunflower oil	27	108	190	106	60	2	180	added nucleotides DHA 0.32%, ARA 0.64% PRSL 21.9/100 cal added probiotic—Bifidobacterium lactis
Enfagrow Toddler Transitions Gentlease (Mead Johnson)	2.6 (10%) partially hydrolyzed nonfat milk, whey protein concentrate	10.5 (42%) corn syrup solids	5.3 (48%) palm olein, coconut oil, soy oil, high oleic sunflower oil	40	130	195	130	60	2	230	DHA 17 mg, ARA 34 mg PRSL 26/100 cal reduced lactose
Enfagrow Toddler Transitions (Mead Johnson)	2.6 (10%) nonfat milk	10.8 (42%) lactose, corn syrup solids, GOS, polydextrose	5.3 (48%) palm olein, soy oil, coconut oil, high oleic sunflower oils	36	130	200	130	60	2	270	DHA 17 mg, ARA 34 mg PRSL 26/100 cal
Similac Go & Grow Stage 3 Milk Based (Abbott Nutrition)	3 (12%) nonfat milk	10.2 (39%) lactose, GOS	5.4 (49%) high oleic safflower oil, soy and coconut oils	30	150	195	130	60	2	300	DHA 0.15%, ARA 0.40% PRSL 27.5/100 cal
Store Brands* Stage 2 Formula (Perrigo Nutritionals)	2.6 (10%) nonfat milk	10.5 (42%) corn syrup solids, lactose	5.3 (48%) palm olein, soy oil, coconut oil, high oleic safflower oil	36	130	195	130	60	2	282	DHA, ARA
Gerber Graduate Soy (Gerber)	2.8 (11%) enzymatically hydrolyzed soy protein isolate	10.9 (44%) corn maltodextrin, sucrose	5.0 (45%) palm olein, soy oil, coconut oil, high oleic safflower or sunflower oil	40	116	190	106	60	2	180	DHA 0.32%, ARA 0.64%
Similac Go & Grow Soy Based (Abbott Nutrition)	2.8 (11%) soy protein isolate, L-methionine	10.3 (41%) corn syrup solids, sugar, fructo-oligosaccharides (FOS)	5.4 (48%) high oleic safflower oil, soy oil, coconut oil	44	120	195	130	60	2	200	DHA 0.15%, ARA 0.40% PRSL 23.7/100 cal
Enfagrow Toddler Transitions Soy (Mead Johnson)	3.3 (13%) soy protein isolate, L-methionine	11.8 (47%) corn syrup solids	4.4 (40%) palm olein, soy oil, coconut oil, high oleic sunflower oils	36	120	195	130	60	2	230	DHA 17 mg, ARA 34 mg PRSL 30/100 cal
Nutramigen with Enflora LGG Toddler (Mead Johnson)	2.5 (10%) casein hydrolysate	12.8 (51%) corn syrup solids, fructose, modified corn starch	4.3 (39%) palm olein oil, soy oil, coconut oil and high oleic sunflower oil	37	122	130	72	60	1.6	300	DHA 17 mg, ARA 34 mg lactose-free PRSL 24/100 cal added probiotic—Lactobacillus GG

*Perrigo Nutritionals makes Store Brands for Walmart, Sam's Club, Walgreens, CVS, Target, and Babies R Us.
Check product labels for the most accurate and up-to-date information.
GOS, galacto-oligosaccharides.

References

1. World Health Organization. The World Health Organization's infant feeding recommendation. http://www.who.int/nutrition/topics/infantfeeding_recommendation/en/. Accessed May 29, 2014.

2. American Academy of Pediatrics, Section on Breastfeeding. Breastfeeding and the use of human milk. *Pediatrics.* 2012;129(3):e827–e841.

3. Kleinman RE, Greer FR eds. *Pediatric Nutrition.* 7th ed. Elk Grove Village, IL: American Academy of Pediatrics; 2014.

4. Schulman AJ. A concise history of infant formula (twists and turns included). *Contemp Ped.* 2003;20(2):91–103.

5. Aggett PJ, Agostini C, Goulet O, et al; European Society of Pediatric Gastroenterology, Hepatology and Nutrition (ESPGHAN) Committee on Nutrition. The nutritional and safety assessment of breast milk substitutes and other dietary products for infants: a commentary by the ESPGHAN Committee on Nutrition. *J Pediatr Gastroenterol Nutr.* 2001;32:256–258.

6. Federal Food, Drug, and Cosmetic Act, § 412, Title 21 Code of Federal Regulations 106, 107.

7. Infant metabolic acidosis and soy-based formula—United States. *MMWR Morb Mortal Wkly Rep.* 1996;45(45):985–988. http://www.cdc.gov/mmwr/preview/mmwrhtml/00044475.htm. Accessed December 1, 2008.

8. Klish WJ. Special infant formulas. *Pediatr Rev.* 1990;12:55–62.

9. Gold MV. Organic production/organic food: information access tools. http://www.nal.usda.gov/afsic/pubs/ofp/ofp.shtml. Updated March 27, 2013. Accessed June 13, 2014.

10. Greer FR, Abrams SA. What pediatricians need to know about low calorie/low protein formulas. *AAP News.* 2014;35:13.

11. von Berg A, Koletzko S, Filipiak B, et al; German Infant Nutritional Intervention Study Group. Certain hydrolyzed formulas reduce the incidence of atopic dermatitis but not that of asthma; three year results of the German Infant Nutrition Intervention Study. *J Allergy Clin Immunol.* 2007;119(3):7118–7125.

12. Vandenplas Y, De Greef E, Devreker T. Treatment of cow's milk protein allergy. *Pediatr Gastroenterol Hepatol Nutr.* 2014;17 (1):1–5.

13. Berseth CL, Johnston WH, Stolz SI, Harris CL, Mitmesser SH. Clinical response to 2 commonly used switch formulas occurs in 1 day. *Clin Pediatr.* 2009;48(1):58–65.

14. Vanderhoof JA, Moran JR, Harris CL, Merkel KL, Orenstein SR. Efficacy of a pre-thickened infant formula: a multicenter, double-blind, randomized, placebo-controlled parallel group trial in 104 infants with symptomatic gastroesophageal reflux. *Clin Pediatr.* 2003;41:483–495.

15. Lasekan JB, Linke HK, Oliver JS, et al. Milk-based infant formula containing rice starch and low lactose reduced common regurgitation in healthy term infants: a randomized, blinded and prospective trial. *J Am Coll Nutr.* 2014;33(2):136–146.

16. Mimouni F, Campaigne B, Naylan M, Tsang RC. Bone mineralization in the first year of life in infants fed human milk, cow-milk formula or soy-based formula. *J Pediatr.* 1993;122(3):348–354.

17. Bhatia J, Greer F; American Academy of Pediatrics Committee on Nutrition. Use of soy protein-based formulas in infant feeding. *Pediatrics.* 2008;121;1062–1068.

18. Zeigler RS, Sampson HA, Bock SA, et al. Soy allergy in infant and children with IgE-associated cow's milk allergy. *J Pediatr.* 1999;134(5):614–622.

19. Klemola T, Vanto T, Juntunen-Blackman K, Kalimo K, Korpela R, Verjonen E. Allergy to soy formula and to extensively hydrolyzed whey formula in infants with cow's milk allergy: a prospective, randomized study with a follow-up to the age of 2 years. *J Pediatr.* 2002;140(2):219–224.

20. Picaud JC, Decullier E, Plan O, et al. Growth and bone mineralization in preterm infants fed preterm formula or standard term formula after discharge. *J Pediatr.* 2008;153:616–621.

21. Klein CJ. Nutrient requirements for preterm infant formulas. *J Nutr.* 2002;132(suppl 16-I):1395S–1577S.

22. Young L, Embleton ND, McCormick FM, McGuire W. Multinutrient fortification of human breast milk for premature infants following hospital discharge. *Cochran Database Syst Rev.* 2013;2:CD004866.

23. American Academy of Pediatrics Committee on Nutrition. Hypoallergenic infant formulas. *Pediatrics.* 2000;106:346–349.

24. Sicherer SH, Noone SA, Koerner CB, Christie L, Burks AW, Sampson HA. Hypoallergenicity and efficacy of an amino acid-based formula in children with cow's milk and multiple food hypersensitivities. *J Pediatrics.* 2001;138:688–693.

25. Hill DJ, Murch SH, Rafferty K, Wallis P, Green CJ. The efficacy of amino acid-based formulas in relieving symptoms of cow's milk allergy: a systematic review. *Clin Exp Allergy.* 2007;37:808–822.

26. Wright EM. Glucose galactose malabsorption. *Am J Physiol.* 1998;275(5):G879–G882.

27. Joeckel RJ, Phillips SK. Overview of infant and pediatric formulas. *Nutr Clin Prac.* 2009;24:356–362.

28. Agostoni C, Riva E. Role and function of long-chain polyunsaturated fatty acids in infant nutrition. In: Raiha NC, Rubaltelli FF, eds. *Infant Formula: Closer to the Reference.* Nestle Nutrition Workshop Series. Pediatric Program. Vol 47 Suppl. Philadelphia, PA: Lippincott Williams & Wilkins; 2002.

29. Hadders-Algra M. Effect of long-chain polyunsaturated fatty acid supplementation on neurodevelopmental outcome in full-term infants. *Nutrients.* 2010;2:790–804.

30. Qawasmi A, Landeros-Weisenberger A, Leckman JF, Bloch MH. Meta-analysis of long-chain polyunsaturated fatty acid supplementation of formula and infant cognition. *Pediatrics* 2012;129:1141–1149.

31. Singhal A, Kennedy K, Lanigan J, et al. Dietary nucleotides and early growth in formula-fed infants: a randomized controlled trial. *Pediatrics.* 2010;126:e946–e953.

32. Carver JD. Advances in nutritional modifications of infant formulas. *Am J Clin Nutr.* 2003;77:1550S–1554S.

33. Hess JR, Greenberg NA. The role of nucleotides in the immune and gastrointestinal systems: Potential clinical applications. *Nutr Clin Pract.* 2012;27:281–294.

34. Patel RM, Denning PW. Therapeutic use of prebiotics, probiotics and postbiotics to prevent necrotizing enterocolitis: what is the current evidence? *Clin Perinatol.* 2013;40(1):11–25.

35. Murguia-Peniche T, Mihatsch WA, Zegarra J, Supapannachart S, Ding ZY, Neu J. Intestinal mucosal defense system, part 2: Probiotics and prebiotics. *J Pediatr.* 2013;162:S64–S71.

36. Wall, R, Ross, RP, Ryan CA, et al. Role of gut microbiota in early infant development. *Clin Med Pediatr.* 2009;3:45–54.

37. Borschel MW, Baggs GE, Barrett-Reis B. Growth of healthy term infants fed ready-to-feed ad powdered forms of an extensively hydrolyzed casein-based infant formula: a randomized, blinded, control trial. *Clin Pediatr.* 2014;53(6):585–592.

38. Drudy D, Mullane NR, Quinn T, Wall PG, Fanning F. *Enterobacter sakazakii:* an emerging pathogen in powdered infant formula. *Clin Infect Dis.* 2006;42:996–1002.

39. *Enterobacter sakazakii* infections associated with the use of a powdered infant formula—Tennessee 2001. *MMWR Morb Mortal Wkly Rep.* 2002;51(14):298–300. http://www.cdc.gov/mmwr/preview/mmwrhtml/mm5114a1.htm. Accessed March 20, 2009.

40. Whaley T, Robbins S. Strategies for Implementing the Guidelines for Handling of Infant Feeding. *Building Block for Life.* 2004:27(3).

41. Robbins ST, Meyers R (eds). *Infant Feedings: Guidelines for Preparation of Human Milk and Formula in Health Care Facilities.* Chicago, IL: Academy of Nutrition and Dietetics; 2011.

42. Agostoni C, Axelsson I, Goulet O, et al; ESPGHAN Committee on Nutrition. Preparation and handling of powdered infant formula: a commentary by the ESPGHAN Committee on Nutrition. *J Pediatr Gastroenterol Nutr.* 2004;39(4):320–322.

43. Mueller C, Nestle M. Regulation of medical foods: toward a rational policy. *Nutr Clin Pract.* 1995;10:8–15.

44. Ziegler EE, Fomon SJ. Potential renal solute load of infant formulas. *J Nutr.* 1989;119:1785–1788.

45. Groh-Wargo S, Sapsford A. Enteral nutrition support of the preterm infant in the neonatal intensive care unit. *Nutr Clin Pract.* 2009;24(3):363–376.

46. ESPGHAN Committee on Nutrition; Aggett PJ, Agostoni C, Axelsson I, et al. Feeding preterm infants after hospital discharge: a commentary by the ESPGHAN Committee on Nutrition. *J Pediatr Gastroenterol Nutr.* 2006;42(5):596–603.

47. O'Connor DL, Khan S, Weishuhn K, et al. Growth and nutrient intakes of human milk fed preterm infants provided with extra energy and nutrients after hospital discharge. *Pediatrics.* 2008;121:766–776.

48. Academy of Breastfeeding Medicine. Clinical Protocol #12, Transitioning the breastfeeding/breastmilk-fed premature infant from the neonatal intensive care unit to home. http://www.bfmed.org. September 17, 2004. Accessed October 8, 2009.

49. Schack-Nielsen L, Sorensen TI, Mortensen EL, Michealsen KF. Late introduction of complementary feeding, rather than duration of breastfeeding, may protect against adult overweight. *Am J Clin Nutr.* 2010;91:619–627.

50. Committee on Nutrition. American Academy of Pediatrics: the use and misuse of fruit juice in pediatrics. *Pediatrics.* 2001;107:1210–1213.

51. Grummer-Strawn LM, Scanlon KS, Fern SB. Infant feeding and feeding transitions during the first year of life. *Pediatrics.* 2008;122:S36–S42.

Test Your Knowledge Answers

1. The correct answer is **B**.
2. The correct answer is **C**.
3. The correct answer is **A**.
4. The correct answer is **D**.

13

Enteral Formulas

Kelly Green Corkins, MS, RD, LDN, CNSC; and **Wednesday Marie A. Sevilla**, MD, MPH

 Podcast

CONTENTS

Learning Objectives

1. Explain the regulation of pediatric and adult formulas.
2. Differentiate pediatric formulas from adult products and describe the target populations.
3. Describe the benefits and contraindications to the blenderized diet administered through a gastrostomy tube.
4. Understand the clinical basis for the use of functional ingredients in enteral formulas.
5. Describe the advantages and disadvantages of both open and closed systems for enteral formula administration.

Introduction

Enteral nutrition (EN) is nourishment administered into the gastrointestinal tract, either orally or through a feeding tube. Enteral feeding is preferred to parenteral nutrition when the gastrointestinal tract is functioning and accessible. Some medical situations or conditions may make enteral feedings less safe, such as an open chest or when high doses of vasodilators are being administered. In situations when oral feeding is not possible, tube feedings should be considered.[1,2] The choice of enteral formula to be used should be based on a complete nutrition assessment that includes individualized estimation of protein and energy needs. The patient's specific diagnoses and comorbidities should also be considered; for example, calcium and phosphorous needs in renal disease or remnant intestinal length in patients with short bowel syndrome.[3]

Regulation of Enteral Products

Enteral formulas for both adult and pediatric patients fall under the category of medical foods defined in the Orphan Drug Amendments of 1988 as "a food which is formulated to be consumed or administered enterally under the supervision of a physician and which is intended for the specific dietary management of a disease or condition for which distinctive nutritional requirements, based on recognized scientific principles, are established by medical evaluation."[4] The definition of medical foods was incorporated into the Federal Food, Drug and Cosmetic Act, and 5 criteria are listed to qualify the characteristics of medical foods[5]: 1) it is a specially formulated and processed product for the partial or exclusive feeding of a patient by means of oral intake or enteral feeding tube; 2) it is intended for dietary management of a patient with a limited or impaired capacity to digest or absorb ordinary foodstuffs or certain nutrients, or who has other special medically determined nutrient requirements that cannot be achieved by the modification of the normal diet alone; 3) it provides nutrition support specifically modified for the management of the unique needs that result from the specific disease or condition, as determined by appropriate medical evaluation; 4) it is intended to be used under medical supervision; and 5) it is intended only for a patient receiving active and ongoing medical supervision, with the patient requiring medical care including instruction on the use of medical food.

Although infant formulas are regulated by the U.S. Food and Drug Administration, medical foods are not. Congress passed the Infant Formula Act of 1980, making infant formulas distinct from other formulations for special dietary use. While infant formulas are subject to regulation applying to quality control, labeling, nutrient requirements, formula recall, notification for new products, and exempt products, medical foods are regulated minimally with only the application of Good Manufacturing Practices for conventional foods. This makes the veracity of enteral formula labeling and product claims dependent on the specific vendor. Thus, the American Society for Parenteral and Enteral Nutrition recommends that medical professionals interpret the content and health claims of enteral formulas with caution until more specific regulations are in place.[6]

Types of Enteral Formulas

Some lines of enteral products are designed to meet the specific needs of pediatric patients (Table 13-1),[2] but disease-specific pediatric formulas are limited. These pediatric products usually meet the micronutrient needs of children 1–10 years of age in 1000–1100 mL/d. Adult formulas can be considered when disease-specific pediatric formulas are not available.

Information included in this section and tables is current as of the time of publication. For the most current information, please visit the manufacturers' Web sites (Table 13-2) or refer to the product labels.

Oral Supplements

Oral supplements are usually polymeric (intact) and have additional sucrose for enhanced taste. They are available in

Table 13-1. Enteral Formulas

CATEGORY OF FORMULA	USES	POTENTIAL POPULATIONS
Oral supplements	Limited diet variety, limited diet volume, unable to take solid foods, increased calorie needs that are difficult to meet with food alone	Autism, gastrointestinal disorders, or cystic fibrosis; overly picky eater
Polymeric enteral formulas	Normal functioning gastrointestinal tract, unable to consume adequate calories orally	Dysphagia, neurologic disorders, cerebral palsy
Semielemental formulas	Malabsorption issues, malfunctioning gastrointestinal tract, unable to take adequate calories from foods	Crohn's flare, cystic fibrosis, dysmotility, short bowel syndrome
Elemental formulas	Allergic responses, malfunctioning gastrointestinal tract, malabsorption issues	Allergies, dysmotility, short bowel syndrome
Specialized formulas	See product labels/handbooks for each product	
Adult formulas	Consider when higher percent protein is needed	Cerebral palsy, neuromuscular disorders
Modulars	Modify macronutrient content of foods or formulas to meet special needs of a patient	
	Protein: Meet protein needs with low calorie expenditure	Cerebral palsy, neuromuscular disorders
	Carbohydrate/fat: Meet high calorie needs without giving excessive protein	Congenital heart disease, renal disease

Table 13-2. Enteral Formula Manufacturer Web Sites

MANUFACTURER	PRODUCT/PRODUCT LINES	WEBSITE
Abbott Nutrition	Elecare Pediasure Vital	www.abbottnutrition.com
Nestle	Boost Compleat Nutren Peptamen Vivonex	www.nestle-nutrition.com
Nutricia	Neocate Ketocal Pepdite Jr.	www.nutricia-na.com
Perrigo Nutritionals	Bright Beginnings	www.perrigonutritionals.com
Vitaflo	Lipistart Renastart	www.vitaflousa.com

a variety of flavors. As the name implies, these formulas are intended to be used to supplement a limited oral diet and may not be indicated for sole-source nutrition, while others are also indicated for tube feeding and sole-source nutrition.

Not all of the oral supplements included in Table 13-3 are designed specifically for pediatric patients, but they may be used in the pediatric population. Adult products may be chosen for taste, cost, or availability. When using an adult product for a child, special attention should be given to assure appropriate macronutrient and micronutrient intakes are achieved. The oral supplements in Table 13-3 are polymeric. Information on oral supplements or products designed for both oral consumption and tube feeding that are intended to meet more disease-specific or condition-specific needs are in other tables in this chapter.

Pediatric Polymeric Enteral Formulas

The polymeric enteral formulas are designed for long-term sole-source nutrition.[2] As shown in Table 13-4, these products are available with and without fiber and come in different caloric densities (1 kcal/mL and 1.5 kcal/mL). The polymeric products are usually milk based and lactose-free. Only one product is soy protein based. These products are indicated for the tube-fed pediatric patients with normal gastrointestinal function whose nutrition needs cannot be met orally.[3]

Pediatric Semielemental Enteral Formulas

Semielemental products, or peptide-based formulas, are designed to meet the needs of the pediatric patient with gastrointestinal conditions that result from malabsorption or maldigestion (Table 13-5). They are given as supplemental or sole-source nutrition, and some are flavored for oral consumption. The protein content is peptides made from heat or enzymatically hydrolyzed whey, soy, or pork protein, and these products usually contain a percentage of the fat as medium-chain triglycerides for better absorption. The proportion of macronutrients in semielemental formulas is similar to that of polymeric formulas. Semielemental products are lactose-free and gluten-free with a kosher option, but contain milk and soy ingredients. Caloric formulations are available in 1.0 and 1.5 kcal/mL.

Pediatric Elemental Enteral Formulas

Elemental products, or amino acid–based formulas, are also used in pediatric patients with malabsorption due to a compromised gastrointestinal tract or with multiple food protein allergies. The protein source of elemental formulas are 100% free amino acids, with the caloric distribution from protein ranging from 10% to 15%. Carbohydrates provide 42%–63% of calories and fats give 25%–45%. This wide range allows for individual tailoring for different conditions. Most elemental formulas have a higher osmolarity than semielemental formulas because of the smaller particles (amino acids vs peptides). Many of these products are only available in powder form and must be reconstituted with water (Table 13-6).

Pediatric Specialized Enteral Formulas

A limited number of products (Table 13-7) are designed to meet disease-specific needs of the pediatric patient. In some cases an adult product may be the best choice. If an adult product is chosen, special attention must be given to the micronutrient intake to assure that the needs of the growing child are met.[3]

Adult Enteral Formulas Commonly Used in Pediatrics

Adult enteral formulas (Table 13-8) are commonly used in pediatric patients because of the higher protein content (25% of calories from protein). Due to the higher protein concentration, protein needs can be met without the use of modular protein and without exceeding calorie needs. Since these products are not made specifically for pediatric patients, special attention needs to be given to micronutrient intake.[3]

Table 13-3. Oral Supplements (Per Serving)

PRODUCT (MANUFAC-TURER)	SVG SIZE kcal/ SVG	kcal/ mL	PROTEIN, g (%kcal) SOURCE	CHO, g (%kcal) SOURCE	FAT, g (%kcal) SOURCE	Na mg	K mg	Ca mg	Phos mg	Fe mg	OSMOLALITY mOsm	FIBER g	COMMENTS
Boost Kid Essentials (Nestle)	8 oz 237 kcal	1	7.1 g (12%) sodium and calcium casienates, whey protein concentrate	32 g (54%) sugar, malto-dextrin	9 g (34%) high oleic sunflower oil, soybean oil, MCT	130	270	280	210	3.3	600 (Ch) 550 (Va) 570 (Str)	0	Flavors: Va, Ch, Str, lactose-free, gluten-free, low-residue, kosher
Boost Kid Essentials 1.5 (Nestle)	8 oz 355 kcal	1.5	10 g (11%) sodium and calcium casienates, whey protein concentrate	39 g (44%) maltodextrin, sugar	17.8 g (45%) soybean oil, high oleic sunflower oil, MCT	164	309	309	235	3.3	390 (Va)	0	Flavors: Va, Ch, Str, lactose-free, gluten-free, low-residue, kosher
Boost Kid Essentials 1.5 w/fiber (Nestle)	8 oz 355 kcal	1.5	10 g (11%) sodium and calcium casienates, whey protein concentrate	39 g (44%) maltodextrin, sugar, partial-ly hydrolyzed guar gum	17.8 g (45%) soybean oil, high oleic sunflower oil, MCT	164	309	309	235	3.3	405	6.8 (sol) 2.2 (insol)	Flavors: Va only, lactose-free, gluten-free, kosher
Bright Beginnings Soy Pediatric Drink (PBM Nutritionals)	8 oz 240 kcal	1	7 g (12%) soy protein isolate	26 g (43%) sucrose, corn maltodextrin, scFOS, inulin, oligofructose	12 g (45%) high oleic safflower or sunflower oil, soy oil, MCT	90	370	230	214	3.3	n/a	3	Va only, contains DHA, no milk protein
CIB Essentials Powder w/ skim milk (Nestle)	9 oz 220 kcal	0.8	13 g (25%) nonfat milk	39 g (73%) lactose, maltodextrin, sugar	0.5 g (2%) milk fat	220	640	500	500	4.5	n/a	0	Flavors: Ch, Va, DkCh, Ch Malt, Str
CIB Essentials Powder w/ whole milk (Nestle)	9 oz 280 kcal	1	13 g (18%) whole milk	39 g (55%) lactose, maltodextrin, sugar	8.2 g (26%) milk fat	214	554	489	481	4.5	n/a	0	Flavors: Ch, Va, DkCh, Ch Malt, Str
CIB Essentials RTD (Nestle)	325 mL 250 kcal	0.8	14 g (22%) nonfat milk, complete milk protein	34 g (58%) sugar, lactose, maltodextrin	5 g (20%) corn oil, milk fat	180	330	500	500	4.5		0	Flavors: Va, Ch, low residue, kosher, low-cholesterol shelf stable
CIB Essentials Powder No Sugar Added w/skim milk (Nestle)	9 oz 150 kcal	0.6	13 g (33%) nonfat milk	24 g (63%) lactose, inulin, malto-dextrin	0.5 g (4%) milk fat	168	595	500	500	4.5	n/a	0	Flavors: Ch, Va, Str, (Str only in variety package)

Table 13-3. (Continued) Oral Supplements (Per Serving)

PRODUCT (MANUFAC-TURER)	SVG SIZE kcal/ SVG	kcal/ mL	PROTEIN, g (%kcal) SOURCE	CHO, g (%kcal) SOURCE	FAT, g (%kcal) SOURCE	Na mg	K mg	Ca mg	Phos mg	Fe mg	OSMOLALITY mOsm	FIBER g	COMMENTS
CIB Essentials No Sugar Added RTD (Nestle)	325 mL 150 kcal	0.5	13 g (32%) nonfat milk, complete milk protein	16 g (40%) lactose, maltodextrin	5 g (28%) corn oil, milk fat	240	540	500	500	4.5		0	Flavors: Ch only, low residue, kosher, low cholesterol, shelf stable
CIB Lactose-Free (Nestle)	8 oz 250 kcal	1	8.75 g (14%) calcium casienate	33.1 g (51%) corn syrup solids, sugar	9.2 g (35%) canola oil, corn oil	220	312	125	125	2.25	480 (Va) 490 (Ch)	0	Flavors: Va, Ch, lactose-free, gluten-free, low-residue, kosher
CIB Lactose-Free Plus (Nestle)	8 oz 375 kcal	1.5	13 g (14%) calcium casienate	44 g (47%) corn syrup solids, sugar	17 g (39%) canola oil, corn oil	292	467	187	187	3.4	620	0	Flavors: Va, Ch, lactose-free, gluten-free, low-residue, kosher
CIB Lactose-Free VHC (Nestle)	8 oz 560 kcal	2.25	22.5 g (16%) calcium casienate, potassium casienate, isolated soy protein	49.2 g (34%) corn syrup solids, sugar	30.6 g (50%) canola oil, corn oil	290	440	308	308	5.6	950	0	Flavors: Va only, lactose-free, gluten-free, low-residue, kosher, use with fluid restrictions
Pediasure (Abbott)	8 oz 237 kcal	1	7 g (12%) milk protein concentrate, whey proetin concentrate, soy protein concentrate	31 g (53%) sucrose, corn maltodextrin, scFOS	9 g (35%) high oleic safflower oil, soy oil, MCT	90	310	230	200	3.3	480	1.7 (insol) 1 (sol)	Flavors: Va, Ch, Str, Ban, Ber, kosher, gluten-free, lactose-free
Pedisure w/fiber (Abbott)	8 oz 237 kcal	1	7 g (12%) milk protein concentrate, whey proetin concentrate, soy protein concentrate	32 g (53%) sucrose, corn maltodextrin, scFOS, soy fiber	9 g (35%) high oleic safflower oil, soy oil, MCT	90	310	230	200	3.3	480	3.2 (insol) 1 (sol)	Flavors: Va, kosher, gluten-free, lactose-free
Pediasure 1.5 (Abbott)	8 oz 350 kcal	1.5	14 g (16%) milk protein concentrate	38 g (43%) corn malto-dextrin	16 g (41%) high oleic safflower oil, soy oil, MCT	90	390	350	250	2.7	370	0	Va only
Pedisure 1.5 w/fiber (Abbott)	8 oz 350 kcal	1.5	14 g (16%) milk protein concentrate	39 g (43%) corn maltodextrin, scFOS	16 g (41%) high oleic safflower oil, soy oil, MCT	90	390	350	250	2.7	370	3	Va only

Ban, banana; Ber, berry; CIB, Carnation Instant Breakfast; CHO, carbohydrate; Ch, chocolate; DkCh, dark chocolate; insol, insoluble; MCT, medium-chain triglycerides; RTD, ready to drink; scFOS, short-chain fructooligosaccharides; sol, soluble; Str, strawberry; Svg, serving; Unfl, unflavored; Va, vanilla.

Table 13-4. Pediatric Polymeric Enteral Products (Per 1000 mL)

PRODUCT (MANUFAC-TURER)	kcal/mL	% H₂O	PROTEIN, g (%kcal) SOURCE	CHO, g (%kcal) SOURCE	FAT, g (%kcal) SOURCE	Na mg	K mg	Ca mg	Phos mg	Fe mg	OSMOLALITY mOsm	FIBER g	COMMENTS
Boost Kid Essentials (Nestle)	1	84	30 g (12%) sodium and calcium casienates, whey protein concentrate	135 g (54%) sugar, malto-dextrin	38 g (34%) high oleic sunflower oil, soybean oil, MCT	550	1140	1181	886	14	Van 550 Ch 600 Str 570	0	Flavors: Va, Ch, Str, lactose-free, gluten-free, low-residue, kosher
Boost Kid Essentials 1.5 (Nestle)	1.5	72	42 g (11%) sodium and calcium casienates, whey protein concentrate	165 g (44%) maltodextrin, sugar	75 g (45%) soybean oil, high oleic sunflower oil, MCT	690	1300	1300	990	14	Va 390	0	Flavors: Va, Ch, Str, lactose-free, gluten-free, low-residue, kosher
Boost Kid Essentials 1.5 w/fiber (Nestle)	1.5	71	10 g (11%) sodium and calcium casienates, whey protein concentrate	39 g (44%) maltodextrin, sugar, partially hydrolyzed guar gum	17.8 g (45%) soybean oil, high oleic sunflower oil, MCT	690	1300	1300	990	14	405	9	Flavors: Va only, lactose-free, gluten-free, kosher
Bright Beginnings Soy Pediatric Drink (Perigo Nutritionals)	1	n/a	29 g (12%) soy protein isolate	26 g (43%) sucrose, corn maltodextrin, scFOS, inulin, oligofructose	50 g (45%) high oleic safflower or sunflower oil, soy oil, MCT	374	1539	956	890	13.75	n/a	12.5	Va only, contains DHA, no milk protein
Compleat Pediatric (Nestle)	1	82	38 g (15%) chicken, sodium casienate (from milk), pea puree	130 g (50%) cranberry juice concentrate, corn syrup solids, green bean puree, partially hydrolyzed guar gum, peach puree	39 g (35%) canola oil, MCT	770	1600	1440	1000	13	380	6	lactose-free, gluten-free

Blenderized or Pureed Diets Through Feeding Tubes

Blenderized (or pureed) tube feedings are simply a variety of foods pureed in a blender to be fed through a gastrostomy tube. This concept is not new; the first attempt at tube feedings in the 1800s were mixtures of foods.[7] This chapter describes some of the many manufactured tube-feeding products available, including one product made with blenderized food. Even with the wide variety of products available for many different diseases and conditions, interest in blenderized tube feedings has been renewed.

This renewed interest may be due to the changing healthcare environment. An increasing number of insurance companies are not paying for tube-feeding formulas because they are considered "food." The manufactured tube-feeding products are more expensive than preparing meals for a child. The blenderized diet requires the initial investment in a high-quality blender to meet the daily demands of pureeing large volumes of food. Another reason caregivers may desire using a blenderized diet may be that food is nurturing and parents want to be involved with their child's care.[8] Whatever the reason, careful consideration must be given before initiating blenderized tube feeding. Benefits of blenderized tube feeding may be improved regulation of bowel movements and decreased gagging, retching, and vomiting[9]; however, limited research exists on the risks and benefits.

Table 13-4. (Continued) Pediatric Polymeric Enteral Products (Per 1000 mL)

PRODUCT (MANUFAC-TURER)	kcal/mL	% H$_2$0	PROTEIN, g (%kcal) SOURCE	CHO, g (%kcal) SOURCE	FAT, g (%kcal) SOURCE	Na mg	K mg	Ca mg	Phos mg	Fe mg	OSMOLALITY mOsm	FIBER g	COMMENTS
Nutren Jr. (Nestle)	1	85	30 g (12%) milk protein concentrate, whey protein concentrate	110 g (44%) maltodextrin, sucrose	49.6 g (44%) soybean oil, canola oil, MCT	460	1320	1000	800	14	350	0	Va only, closed system, lactose-free, gluten-free, low residue, kosher
Nutren Jr. Fiber (Nestle)	1	85	30 g (12%) milk protein concentrate, whey protein concentrate	110 g (44%) maltodextrin, sucrose	49.6 g (44%) soybean oil, canola oil, MCT	460	1320	1000	800	14	350	6	Va only, closed system, lactose-free, gluten-free, kosher
Pediasure Enteral Formula (Abbott)	1	85	30 g (12%) milk protein concentrate	133 g (53%) corn maltodextrin, sucrose	40 g (35%) high oleic safflower oil, soy oil, MCT	380	1310	972	845	14	335	0	Va only, kosher, gluten-free, lactose-free
Pediasure Enteral Formula w/fiber and ScFOS (Abbott)	1	85	30 g (12%) milk protein concentrate	138 g (53%) corn maltodextrin, sucrose, fructooligosaccharides, oat fiber, soy fiber	40 g (35%) high oleic safflower oil, soy oil, MCT	380	1310	972	845	14	335	8 (insol) 3 (sol)	Va only, kosher, gluten-free, lactose-free
Pediasure 1.5 (Abbott)	1.5	78	59 g (16%) milk protein concentrate	160 g (43%) corn maltodextrin	67.5 g (41%) high oleic safflower oil, soy oil, MCT	380	1645	1477	1055	11.4	370	0	Va only
Pediasure 1.5 w/fiber (Abbott)	1.5	78	59 g (16%) milk protein concentrate	164 g (43%) corn maltodextrin, scFOS	67.5 g (41%) high oleic safflower oil, soy oil, MCT	380	1645	1477	1055	11.4	370	3	Va only

Ban, banana; Ber, berry; CHO, carbohydrate; Ch, chocolate; insol, insoluble; MCT, medium-chain triglycerides; scFOS, short-chain fructooligosaccharides; sol, soluble; Str, strawberry; Svg, serving; Va, vanilla.

Blenderized tube feeding is not appropriate for all patients, even if the parent or caregiver is motivated and desires to use this type of feeding. Contraindications include gastrostomy tube < 10 French, jejunostomy tube or feeding into the jejunum, continuous feedings, immunocompromised patient, volume limit of <30 oz/d, multiple food allergies or intolerances, lack of electricity or refrigeration.[10-12] Some additional concerns related to blenderized tube feeding include food-borne illness due to improper preparation or handling of the food items, inconsistent or uncertain nutrient content, and increased risk for clogging the tube.[9,11,13,14] Potential complications include nutrient deficiencies, electrolyte disturbances, and increased wear on the gastrostomy tube.

Open communication between the caregiver and healthcare professionals, especially a registered dietitian, must be established before considering the diet for a patient. This communication is key to preventing many of the potential complications of the diet.[8]

Modular Macronutrients

Modular macronutrients can be used to increase the calorie concentration of liquid ready-to-use enteral formulas. Modular products (Table 13-9) are available as protein (intact or extensively hydrolyzed), carbohydrate (modified starch), fat (medium-chain or long-chain triglycerides), or combinations of macronutrients. Modular macronutrients will not increase the concentration of micronutrients but will alter

Table 13-5. Peptide-Based Pediatric Formulas (Per 1000 mL)

PRODUCT (MANUFAC-TURER)	kcal/mL	% H₂O	PROTEIN, g (%kcal) SOURCE	CHO, g (%kcal) SOURCE	FAT, g (%kcal) SOURCE	Na mg	K mg	Ca mg	Phos mg	Fe mg	OSMOLALITY mOsm	FIBER g	COMMENTS
Pepdite Jr. (Nutricia)	1	n/a	31 g (12%) hydrolyzed protein (pork and soy)	106 g (42%) corn syrup solids, (banana flavor also has sucrose)	50 g (46%) fractionated coconut oil, canola oil, high oleic safflower oil	410	1360	1130	940	14	430 (Unfl) 440 (Ban)	0	Flavors: Unfl, Ban, dairy-free, 1–51 g pkt = 240 kcal 1 pkt + 7 oz water = 8 oz @ 1 kcal/mL
Peptamen Jr. (Nestle)	1	85	30 g (12%) enzymatically hydrolyzed whey protein	138 g (55%) maltodextrin, corn starch	38.4 g (33%) MCT, soy bean oil, canola oil	460	1320	1000	800	14	260 (Unfl) 380 (Va/Ch) 400 (Str)	0	Flavors: Unfl, Va, Ch, Str, lactose-free, gluten-free, low residue, closed system
Peptamen Jr. Fiber (Nestle)	1	84	30 g (12%) enzymatically hydrolyzed whey protein	137 g (55%) maltodextrin, corn starch, pea fiber, oligofructose, inulin	38.4 g (33%) MCT, soy bean oil, canola oil	460	1320	1000	800	14	390	3.8 (insol) 3.5 (sol)	Va only, lactose-free, gluten-free
Peptamen Jr. 1.5 (Nestle)	1.5	77	45 g (12%) enzymatically hydrolyzed whey protein	180 g (53%) maltodextrin, corn starch, oligofructose, inulin	68 g (33%) MCT, soy bean oil, canola oil	692	1980	1652	1352	20.8	450	5.4 (sol)	Unfl only, closed system
Peptamen Jr. with PREBIO (Nestle)	1	85	30 g (12%) enzymatically hydrolyzed whey protein	137 g (55%) maltodextrin, corn starch, oligofructose, inulin	38.4 g (33%) MCT, soy bean oil, canola oil	460	1320	1000	800	14	365	3.6	Va only, lactose-free, gluten-free
Vital Jr. (Abbott)	1	84	30 g (12%) whey protein hydrolysate	133.8 g (53%) corn maltodextrin, sucrose, fructooligosaccharide	40.5 g (35%) structured lipids, MCT, canola oil	717	1350	1055	844	13.9	390	3 (insol) 3 (sol)	Flavors: Va, Str, gluten-free, lactose-free, low residue, kosher
PER SERVING													
Pepdite Jr. (Nutricia) 240 kcal/8 oz svg	1	n/a	7.4 g (12%) hydrolyzed protein (pork and soy)	25.5 g (42%) corn syrup solids (banana flavor also has sucrose)	12 g (46%) fractionated coconut oil, canola oil, high oleic safflower oil	98	327	271	225	3.3	430 (Unfl) 440 (Ban)	0	Flavors: Unfl, Ban, dairy-free, 1–51 g pkt = 240 kcal 1 pkt + 7 oz water = 8 oz @ 1 kcal/mL
Peptamen Jr. (Nestle) 250 kcal/8 oz svg	1	85	7.5 g (12%) enzymatically hydrolyzed whey protein	34.4 g (55%) maltodextrin, corn starch	9.6 g (33%) MCT, soy bean oil, canola oil	115	330	250	200	3.5	260 (Unfl) 380 (Va/Ch) 400 (Str)	0	Flavors: Unfl, Va, Ch, Str, lactose-free, gluten-free, low residue, closed system
Vital Jr. (Abbott) 237 kcal/8 oz svg	1	84	7.1 g (12%) whey protein hydrolysate	31.7 g (53%) corn maltodextrin, sucrose, fructooligosaccharide	9.5 g (35%) structured lipids, MCT, canola oil	170	320	250	200	3.3	390	1.4	Flavors: Va, Str, gluten-free, lactose-free, low residue, kosher

Ban, banana; CHO, carbohydrate; Ch, chocolate; insol, insoluble; MCT, medium-chain triglycerides; pkt, packet; sol, soluble; Str, strawberry; svg, serving; Unfl, unflavored; Va, vanilla.

Table 13-6. Pediatric Elemental Formulas (Per 1000 mL)

PRODUCT (MANUFAC-TURER)	kcal/ mL	% H₂O	PROTEIN, g (%kcal) SOURCE	CHO, g (%kcal) SOURCE	FAT, g (%kcal) SOURCE	Na mg	K mg	Ca mg	Phos mg	Fe mg	OSMOLALITY mOsm	FIBER g	COMMENTS
Elecare Jr. (Abbott)	1	84	31 g (15%) free amino acids	106.7 g (42%) corn syrup solids	49 g (43%) high oleic safflower oil, MCT, soy oil	459	1526	1174	854	18	590	0	Flavors: Unfl, Va, Unfl with DHA and ARA; gluten-free, lactose-free
Neocate Splash (Nutricia)	1	84	30 g (12%) free amino acids	105 g (42%) maltodextrin, sugar	51 g (46%) high oleic sunflower oil, MCT (modified palm kernel and/ or corn oil), canola oil	500	1370	1180	800	15	670 (Unfl) 740 (Gra) 790 (O-P)	0	Flavors: Unfl, Gra, O-P, gluten-free, flavored versions have artificial flavors and sucralose
Neocate Jr. Unfl (Nutricia)	1	85	33 g (13%) free amino acids	104 g (42%) corn syrup solids	50 g (45%) fractionated coconut oil, canola oil, high oleic safflower oil	410	1370	1130	697	15	590	0	
Neocate Jr. flavored (Nutricia)	1	84	35 g (14%) free amino acids	110 g (44%) corn syrup solids, (Ch - sucrose)	47 g (42%) fractionated coconut oil, canola oil, high oleic safflower oil	435	1450	1200	738	16	680 (Trop) 700 (Ch)	0	Flavors: Trop, Ch
Neocate Jr. w/prebiotics (Nutricia)	1	84	33 g (13%) free amino acids	104 g (42%) corn syrup solids, fructool-igosaccharides, inulin	50 g (45%) fractionated co-conut oil, canola oil, high oleic safflower oil	410	1370	1130	697	15	570	4 g	
Vivonex Pediatric (Nestle)	0.8	89	24 g (12%) free amino acids	130 g (63%) maltodextrin, corn starch modified	24 g (25%) MCT, soybean oil	400	1200	970	800	10	360	0	lactose-free, gluten-free, low residue
PER SERVING													
Neocate Splash (Nutricia) 237 kcal/8 oz svg	1	84	7.1 g (12%) free amino acids	24.9 g (42%) maltodextrin, sugar	12.1 g (46%) high oleic sunflower oil, MCT (modified palm kernel and/ or corn oil), canola oil	47.4	220	147	147	1.8	670 (Unfl) 740 (Gra) 790 (O-P)	0	Flavors: Unfl, Gra, O-P, gluten-free, flavored versions have artificial flavors and sucralose
Neocate Jr.- flavored (Nutricia) 240 kcal/8 oz svg	1	84	8.64 g (14%) free amino acids	26.7 g (44%) corn syrup solids, (Ch - sucrose)	11.3 g (42%) fractionated co-conut oil, canola oil, high oleic safflower oil	105	352	291	180	4	680 (Trop) 700 (Ch)	0	Flavors: Trop, Ch
Neocate Nutra (Nutricia) 175 kcal/37 g svg	n/a	n/a	3 g (7%) free amino acids	24.9 g (57%) corn syrup sol-ids, cornstarch, sugar	7 g (36%) non-hydroge-nated coconut oil, high oleic sunflower oil, canola oil, sunflower oil	14.1	0.14	247	126	2.2	n/a	0	Unfl, semisolid food for oral use only

ARA, arachidonic acid; CHO, carbohydrate; Ch, chocolate; DHA, docosahexaenoic acid; Gra, grape; MCT, medium-chain triglycerides; O-P, orange pineapple; svg, serving; Trop, tropical; Unfl, unflavored; Va, vanilla.

Table 13-7. Pediatric Specialized Enteral Formulas (Per 1000 mL)

PRODUCT (MANUFAC-TURER)	kcal/mL	% H₂O	PROTEIN, g (%kcal) SOURCE	CHO, g (%kcal) SOURCE	FAT, g (%kcal) SOURCE	Na mg	K mg	Ca mg	Phos mg	Fe mg	OSMOLALITY mOsm	FIBER g	COMMENTS
KetoCal 3:1 (Nutricia)	1	n/a	22 g (8.8%) milk protein	10 g (4.1%) lactose	97 g (87.1%) refined vegetable oil (palm and soy)	411	1360	1140	801	16	180	0	Unflavored enteral or oral feedings
KetoCal 4:1 (Nutricia)	1.44	n/a	30 g (8.4%) dry whole milk	6 g (1.6%) corn syrup solids	144 g (90%) hydrogenated soybean oil, refined soybean oil	600	2160	1600	1300	22	197	0	Vanilla only enteral or oral feedings
Monogen (Nutricia)	1	n/a	27 g (11%) whey protein concentrate	160 g (64%) corn syrup solids	27.8 g (25%) fractionated coconut oil, walnut oil	472	850	606	472	10	370	0	
Portagen (Mead Johnson)	1	n/a	35.4 g (14%) sodium casienate	114.6 g (46%) corn syrup solids, sucrose	48 g (40%) MCT, corn oil	552	1250	938	708	18.75	350	0	NOT NUTRITIONALLY COMPLETE. If used long term, supplementation of essential fatty acids and ultra trace minerals should be considered

MCT, medium chain triglycerides.

Table 13-8. Adult Enteral Products Commonly Used in Pediatrics (Per 1000 mL)

PRODUCT (MANUFAC-TURER)	kcal/mL	% H₂O	PROTEIN, g (%kcal) SOURCE	CHO, g (%kcal) SOURCE	FAT, g (%kcal) SOURCE	Na mg	K mg	Ca mg	Phos mg	Fe mg	OSMOLALITY mOsm	FIBER g	COMMENTS
Nutren Replete (Nestle)	1	85	62.4 g (25%) calcium and potasium caseinate	113 g (45%) maltodextrin	34 g (30%) canola oil, MCT, soy lecithin	876	1500	1000	1000	18	300 (Unfl) 350 (Va)	0	Flavors: Unfl, Va, lactose-free, gluten-free, low residue, kosher
Nutren Replete Fiber (Nestle)	1	84	62.4 g (25%) calcium and potasium caseinate	113 g (45%) maltodextrin, soy polysaccharides	34 g (30%) canola oil, MCT, soy lecithin	876	1500	1000	1000	18	310 (Unfl) 390 (Va)	14	Flavors: Unfl, Va, lactose-free, gluten-free, kosher
Promote (Abbott)	1	84	62.5 g (25%) sodium caseinate, soy protein isolate	130 g (52%) corn maltodextrin, sucrose	26 g (23%) soy oil, MCT, safflower oil	1000	1980	1200	1200	18	340	0	Va only, kosher, gluten-free, lactose-free, low residue
Promote w/fiber (Abbott)	1	83	62.5 g (25%) sodium caseinate, soy protein isolate	138.3 g (50%) corn maltodextrin, sucrose, oat fiber	28.2 g (25%) MCT, safflower oil, soy lecithin	1300	2100	1200	1200	18	380	14.4	Va only, kosher, gluten-free, lactose-free

CHO, carbohydrate; MCT, medium-chain triglycerides; Unfl, unflavored; Va, vanilla.

Table 13-9. Modular Macronutrients

PRODUCT (MANUFAC-TURER)	kcal	PROTEIN, g (%kcal) SOURCE	CHO, g (%kcal) SOURCE	FAT, g (%kcal) SOURCE	Na mg	K mg	Ca mg	Phos mg	Fe mg	OSMOLALITY mOsm	FIBER g	COMMENTS
Super Soluble Duocal (Nutricia) Per 100 g	492	None	72.7 g (59%) hydrolyzed cornstarch	22.3 g (41%) vegetable oils (corn, coconut), medium chain triglycerides (coconut oil, pal kernel oil), mono and diglycerides, diacetyl tartaric acid esters of monoglycerides	<20	<5	<5	<5	none	310	0	gluten-free, lactose-free, sucrose-free and fructose-free; completely soluble in water, liquids, and moist foods without altering tases
Benecalorie (Nestlé) Per 107 mL	800	17 g calcium ca-seinate (milk)	None	80 g high oleic sun-flower oil, mono and diglycerides							0	lactose-free, gluten-free, low residue, kosher, cholesterol-free
Beneprotein (Nestlé) Per 100 mL	357	86 g (100%) whey protein isolate (milk)	None	None			285				0	lactose-free, gluten-free, low residue, kosher
MCT Oil (Nestle) Per 100 mL	770	None	None	93 coconut oil							0	lactose-free, gluten-free, kosher
Microlipid (Nestle) Per 100 mL	450	None	None	50 safflower oil						62	0	lactose-free, kosher
Nutrisource Fiber (Nestle) Per 100 g	375	None	100 g partially hy-drolyzed guar gum	None							75	lactose-free, gluten-free, kosher
MCT Procal (Vitaflo) Per 100 mL	657	12.5 g	20.6 g	63.1 g	245	625	450	435			0	contains milk, gluten-free
ProMod Liquid Protein (Abbott) Per 100 mL	330	33 g hydrolyzed collagen	47g glycerin; no simple sugars	None	183	66		316			0	lactose-free, gluten-free, low residue

CHO, carbohydrates.

macronutrient distribution of the product. Modular protein and carbohydrate may significantly alter osmolarity of the formula and may result in intolerance. Specific macronutrients may be used to modify a formula to meet disease-specific needs.

Functional Ingredients in Enteral Formulas

Fiber/Prebiotics
Fibers are structural and storage plant-derived carbohydrate compounds that are not broken down by intestinal digestive enzymes.[15,16] Traditionally grouped into soluble and insolu-ble forms, dietary fiber exerts many benefits. These include, but are not limited to, normalization of colonic motility and regularity of bowel movements, promotion of normal colonic cell proliferation, and maintenance of the colonic microbiome balance with overall effects on immune function, digestion, and absorption.[17] Historically, enteral formulas did not contain additional fiber due to concerns about its viscous nature and the possibility of clogging feeding tubes.[16] With known current recommendations for daily fiber intake in adults and children (14 g of dietary fiber per 1000 kcal ingested for adults), the importance of supplementation in patients receiving enteral formulas has been emphasized.

Currently, the European Society for Parenteral and Enteral Nutrition, as reported through the Fiber Consensus Panel, recommends that fiber (specifically partially hydrolyzed guar gum) can be utilized to prevent EN–induced diarrhea in postsurgical and critically ill patients.[18] However, limitations exist for its use. A fiber-free enteral formula should be considered in patients at risk for bowel obstruction or ischemia.[16]

A prebiotic is a nondigestible component in food that exerts beneficial effects by stimulating growth and activity of select bacteria in the colon.[18] With the end effect of better health, much research has been done on these food components, which include oligosaccharides and polysaccharides. Roberfroid[19] further detailed specific criteria for an ingredient to be named a prebiotic:

1. Resistance to digestion and modification by gastric acid, hydrolysis of intestinal enzymes, and gastrointestinal digestion;
2. Fermentation by microflora in the intestines;
3. Selective stimulation of the growth and/or activity of intestinal bacteria that contribute to health and well-being.

Among the most extensively studied prebiotics are inulin, oligofructose, trans-galactooligosaccharides, and lactulose. Since the discovery of prebiotics a little over a decade ago, they have been included in commercially available infant and pediatric formulas. The addition of prebiotics to infant formulas arose from previous studies characterizing the substantial prebiotic content of human milk.[20] A limited amount of robust data examine the effects of prebiotics in the pediatric population, but it has been suggested that prebiotics can prevent the development of atopic eczema and infections.

EN formulas usually contain a mixture of fibers from various sources. Examples of fiber sources are soy polysaccharides, partially hydrolyzed guar gum, acacia gum, resistance starch, cellulose, and outer pea fiber. A group of fibers—inulin, oligofructose and fructo-oligosaccharides—are categorized as inulin-type fructans and are the most studied prebiotic fibers.[17] The Fiber Consensus Panel recommends that patients receiving EN be provided with a mixture of bulking and fermentable fibers in order to conceptually promote a balanced intake of fiber similar to a regular diet.[17,18] The consumption of a fiber blend provides advantages such as maintained production of short-chain fatty acids for colon health and increasing tolerance to different fibers and the enteral formula itself by minimizing gastrointestinal symptoms such as bloating, flatulence, and abdominal pain.[17]

Some of the developed fiber blends and their effects are listed in Table 13-10.

Table 13-10. Fiber Blends

PRODUCT/COMPANY	FIBERS	STUDY RESULTS
Prebio (Nestle)	Soluble	Increase in lactobacilli population, Improved IgG response to vaccination[21-23]
Nutricia Multifibre (Nutricia)	Soluble Insoluble	Decreased laxative use[24,25]
Jevity Fructo-oligosaccharide (Abbott)	Soluble Insoluble	Improvement in gastrointestinal symptoms, More formed stools[26]

Structured Lipids

Initially developed in the 1980s, structured lipids or structured triglycerides consist of triglycerides with medium-chain fatty acids and a long-chain fatty acid. Structured lipids are produced through chemical interesterification, enzyme-catalyzed interesterification with lipases, or by genetic engineering.[27] Chemical interesterification is an inexpensive method but is less specific, while lipase inter-esterification is more expensive and more specific. The medium-chain fatty acid at the sn-1 and sn-3 position of the glycerol backbone and the long-chain fatty acid at the sn-2 position have the advantage of enhanced lipid absorption, provision of polyunsaturated fatty acids, improved lymphatic absorption of fat-soluble vitamins, and correction of essential fatty acid deficiency.

Docosahexaenoic Acid/Arachidonic Acid

Some of the specialized formulas for younger children contain the long-chain polyunsaturated fatty acids (LCPUFAs), docosahexaenoic acid (DHA), and arachidonic acid (ARA). DHA and ARA are synthesized from the dietary EFAs α-linolenic acid (ω-3) and linoleic acid (ω-6), respectively. Endogenous synthesis of LCPUFAs begins in the first days of life.[28] DHA and ARA are the major fatty acids in neural tissues, and DHA is a major component of photoreceptor cells.[29] Refer to Chapter 12 for more information.

Forms and Administration of Enteral Formulas

Pediatric formulas are available in 2 forms: ready-to-use liquid and powder. Ready-to-use liquid is the most commonly used form in hospitals because it is considered commercially sterile, but some of the specialty formulas only come in powder. Powder is not sterile and must be mixed with water. Because it is not sterile, it may contain pathogenic bacteria.[30] Powder infant formula has been associated with *Enterobacter sakazakii* contamination in immunocompromised neonates in healthcare facilities.[31] Because of the population that they serve, hospitals should only use powder when no other option is available.[32] For more information on mixing powder formulas see Chapter 12.

Open vs Closed Systems

Ready-to-use liquid is available in "single serving" containers, which can be decanted into a bag for tube feeding (open system), or larger "daily amounts," which can be spiked and infused through the tube (closed system). A closed system for delivery of enteral formulas offers some advantages over an open system. With a closed system, less manipulation is needed, and labor and labor costs are decreased.[33–35] The cost savings of the closed system is primarily in the labor. Cost comparisons of the products, including waste, indicates the closed system is more expensive.[33] Another advantage of decreased manipulations is increased time the product is infused, resulting in increased volume of tube feeding received by the patient.[34–36]

Older research studies indicated that the closed system was safer because less manipulation meant less risk for contamination and infection in the patient.[35] A recent study in a pediatric hospital showed that when recommended enteral feeding practices are followed, decanted formula has a lower-than-expected rate of bacterial growth.[37] Also, aseptic technique must be used when spiking the closed system because this is a manipulation that can cause bacterial contamination.[34]

One significant limitation of the closed system is limited product selection, particularly in the pediatric specialty products. The product in the closed system cannot be manipulated to meet specific needs or disease states.[38] Since the main advantage to the open system is that the product can be modified for individual needs, many hospitals have both open and closed systems available.

Test Your Knowledge Questions

1. Enteral formulas are regulated on what parameters?
   A. Nutrient requirements
   B. Health claims
   C. Good Manufacturing Practices
   D. All of the above

2. Which is a contraindication to using a blenderized tube feeding?
   A. Continuous tube feeding
   B. Gastrostomy tube > 10 French
   C. Daily volume > 30 oz
   D. Cost of the food

3. What is the most significant advantage of an open system for tube feeding?
   A. Decreased manipulation of product
   B. Increased cost of labor
   C. Ability to modify the formula
   D. Easier to spike without contaminating the product

4. Prebiotics are:
   A. Oligosaccharides
   B. Complex dietary carbohydrates that are not digestible by humans
   C. The fuel for beneficial bacteria in the gut
   D. All of the above

References

1. Kleinman RE, Greer FR, eds. *Pediatric Nutrition.* 7th ed. Elk Grove Village, IL: American Academy of Pediatrics; 2014.
2. Axelrod D, Kazmerski K, Iyer K. Pediatric enteral nutrition. *JPEN J Parenter Enteral Nutr.* 2006;30(1):S21–S26.
3. Joeckel RJ, Phillips SK. Overview of infant and pediatric formulas. *Nutr Clin Prac.* 2009;24:356–362.
4. Grants and contracts for development of drugs for rare diseases and conditions. 21 USC §360ee(b)(3).
5. Nutrition labeling of food. 21 CFR 101.9(j)(8).
6. Bankhead R, Boullata J, Brantley S, et al; A.S.P.E.N. Board of Directors. Enteral nutrition practice recommendations. *JPEN J Parenter Enteral Nutr.* 2009;33:122–167.
7. Harkness L. The history of enteral nutrition therapy: from raw eggs and nasal tubes to purified amino acids and early postoperative jejunal delivery. *J Am Diet Assoc.* 2002;102(3):399–404.
8. Bobo E, Stone K. Blenderized formula for tube feeding. *Dietetics Practice Section Newsletter* 2013;Fall: 4–8.
9. Pentiuk S, O'Flaherty T, Santoro K, Willging P, Kaul A. Pureed by gastrostomy tube diet improves gagging and retching in children with fundoplication. *JPEN J Parenter Enteral Nutr.* 2011;35(3):375–379.
10. Novak P, Wilson KE, Ausderau K, Cullinane D. The use of blenderized tube feedings. *Infant, Child, & Adolescent Nutrition.* 2009;1(1):21–23.
11. Mortensen MJ. Blenderized tube feeding clinical perspectives on homemade tube feeding. *PNPG Post.* 2006;17(1):1–4.
12. Klein MD, Morris SE. *Homemade Blended Formula Handbook.* Tucson, AZ: Mealtime Notions LLC; 2007.
13. Campbell SM. An anthology of advances in enteral tube feeding formulations. *Nutr Clin Prac.* 2006;21(4):411–415.

14. Moe G. Invited review: Enteral feeding and infection in the immunocompromised patient. *Nutr Clin Prac.* 1991;6(2):55–64.

15. Khoshoo V, Sun S, Storm H. Tolerance of an enteral formula with insoluble and prebiotic fiber in children with compromised gastrointestinal function. *J Am Diet Assoc.* 2010;110:1728–1733.

16. Malone A. Enteral formula selection: a review of selected product categories. *Prac Gastroenterol.* 2005; June:44–74.

17. Klosterbuer A, Roughead ZF, Slavin J. Benefits of dietary fiber in clinical nutrition. *Nutr Clin Pract.* 2011;26:625–635.

18. Meier R, Gassull MA. Consensus recommendations on the effects and benefits of fibre in clinical practice. *Clin Nut Suppl.* 2004;1:73–80.

19. Roberfroid M. Prebiotics: the concept revisited. *J Nutr.* 2007;137:830S–837S.

20. Thomas DW, Greer FR; Committee on Nutrition, Section of Gastroenterology, Hepatology and Nutrition of the American Academy of Pediatric. Clinical report probiotics and prebiotics in pediatrics. *Pediatrics.* 2010;126:1217–1231.

21. Zheng S, Steenhout P, Kuiran D, et al. Nutritional support of pediatric cancer patients consuming an enteral formula with fructo-oligosaccharides. *Nutr Res.* 2006;26:154–162.

22. Zheng S. Enteral formula with fructo-oligosaccharides in nutritional support of pediatric cancer patients. *Am J Clin Nutr.* 2002:430S.

23. Van de Wiele T, Boon N, Possemiers S, Jacos H, Vestrate W. Inulin-type fructans of longer degree of polymerization exert more pronounced in vitro prebiotic effects. *J Appl Microbiol.* 2007;102:452–460.

24. Hoekstra JH, Szajweska H, Zikri Ma, et al. Oral rehydration solution containing a mixture of non-digestible carbohydrates in the treatment of acute diarrhea: a multicenter randomized placebo controlled study on behalf of the ESPGHAN working group on intestinal infections. *J Pediatr Gastroenterol Nutr.* 2004;39:239–245.

25. Evans S, Daly A, Davies P, MacDonald A. Fiber content of enteral feeds for the older child. *J Hum Nutr Diet.* 2009;22:414–421.

26. Van Aerde J, Alarco P, Lam W, et al. Tolerance and safety of energy-dense enteral formulae for young children. *Int Pediatr.* 2003;18:95–99.

27. Roy CC, Bouthillier L, Seidman E, Levy E. New lipids in enteral feeding. *Curr Opin Clin Nutr Metab Care.* 2004;7:117–122.

28. Agostoni C, Riva E. Role and function of long-chain polyunsaturated fatty acids in infant nutrition. In: Raiha NC, Rubaltelli FF, eds. *Infant Formula: Closer to the Reference.* Philadelphia, PA: Lippincott Williams & Wilkins; 2002. Nestlé Nutrition Workshop Series. Pediatric Program. Vol. 47 Suppl.

29. Martinez M. Tissue levels of polyunsaturated fatty acids during early human development. *J Pediatr.* 1992;120:S129–S138.

30. Drudy D, Mullane NR, Quinn T, Wall PG, Fanning F. *Enterobacter sakazakii*: an emerging pathogen in powdered infant formula. *Clin Infect Dis.* 2006;42:996–1002.

31. Centers for Disease Control and Prevention. *Enterobacter sakazakii* infections associated with the use of a powdered infant formula—Tennessee 2001. *MMWR Morb Mortal Wkly Rep.* 2002;51(14):298–300. http://www.cdc.gov/mmwr/preview/mmwrhtml/mm5114a1.htm. Accessed March 20, 2009.

32. Whaley T, Robbins S. Strategies for implementing the guidelines for handling of infant feeding. *Building Block for Life.* 2004:27(3).

33. Phillips W, Roman B, Glassman K. Economic impact of switching from an open to closed enteral nutrition feeding system in an acute setting. *Nutr Clin Prac.* 2013;28(4):510–514.

34. Storm H. Closed systems: point in: closed-system enteral feedings: point-counterpoint. *Nutr Clin Prac.* 2000;15:193–197.

35. Wagner DR, Elmore MF, Knoll DM. Evaluation of "closed" vs "open" systems for the delivery of peptide-based enteral diets. *JPEN J Parenter Enteral Nutr.* 1994;18(5):453–457.

36. Vanek VW. Closed versus open eternal delivery system: a quality improvement study. *Nutr Clin Prac.* 2000;15(5):234–243.

37. Lyman B, Gebhards S, Hensley C, Roberts C, San Pablo W. Safety of decanted enteral formula hung for 12 hours in a pediatric setting. *Nutr Clin Prac.* 2011;26(4):451–456.

38. Skipper A. Closed systems: point in: closed-system enteral feedings: point-counterpoint. *Nutr Clin Prac.* 2000;15:197–200.

Test Your Knowledge Answers

1. The correct answer is **C**.
2. The correct answer is **A**.
3. The correct answer is **C**.
4. The correct answer is **D**.

14

Obesity and Metabolic Syndrome

Kalyan Ray Parashette, MD, MPH; and **Sandeep K. Gupta,** MD

CONTENTS

Learning Objectives

1. Identify the components of metabolic syndrome in adults and children.
2. Describe the most common reasons why the metabolic syndrome, as a diagnosable entity, has not been accepted in the pediatric population.
3. Learn about the Expert Committee and Expert Panel Recommendations in pediatric practice.

Introduction

Since the early 1900s evidence has suggested the coexistence of chronic disorders associated with diabetes mellitus and coronary heart disease (CHD).[1] It wasn't until the years between 1980 and 1990 that scientists developed an understanding of the mechanisms underlying the connection between obesity, hypertension, hyperlipidemia, and type 2 diabetes mellitus (DM) and its relationship to increased cardiovascular disease (CVD) risk. Metabolic syndrome was a term first used to describe how environmental and genetic factors work together to produce this constellation of chronic metabolic disorders.[1] However, it was the earlier work of Reaven[2] that set the precedent for how the metabolic syndrome is understood within the clinical world today. In 1988, Reaven's Banting Lecture described the relationship between hyperinsulinemia, glucose intolerance, hypertension, and free-fatty acid metabolism and their association with CVD. Reaven hypothesized that the state of insulin resistance was the driver for metabolic change and represented the common pathophysiological link between these otherwise unrelated metabolic events.[2]

Through the 1990s, distinct perspectives on the etiology of metabolic syndrome began to emerge, coupled with the inclusion of additional biomarkers such as measures of insulin resistance and markers of pro-inflammation to augment the original components. This newfound knowledge resulted in several monikers being applied: "syndrome X," "the deadly quartet," and "the insulin resistance syndrome." However, in 1999 the term metabolic syndrome reappeared, now evolved from a hypothesis to a clinical entity. It is an emerging diagnosis applied to the adult population and, to a lesser extent, pediatrics. The diagnosis of metabolic syndrome has been subject to criticism because much remains unknown about the cumulative risk of its components and the utility of making this diagnosis.[3,4] Despite these criticisms, identification of metabolic syndrome and its component disorders among adults or children offers useful information about the patient's metabolic risk, particularly that associated with future cardiovascular morbidity and mortality.[5]

What Is the Metabolic Syndrome in Adults?

The early work of Hanefeld and Leonhardt[6] and Reaven[2] described the metabolic syndrome as a constellation of metabolic risk factors including obesity, hypertension, dyslipidemia, and glucose intolerance, all of which are associated with increased cardiovascular mortality. However, today, the metabolic syndrome is no longer viewed as a novel concept, but has surfaced as a diagnosable entity. The controversy begins with the criteria used. Currently, there are 6 sets of diagnostic criteria widely accepted for metabolic syndrome. These include definitions from the World Health Organization (WHO),[7] the National Cholesterol Education Program, Adult Treatment Panel III (NCEP-ATP III),[8] the American College of Endocrinology (ACE),[9] the International Diabetes Federation (IDF),[10] American Heart Association (AHA)/National Heart, Lung, and Blood Institute (NHLBI),[11] and a joint statement from the IDF, NHLBI, AHA, World Heart Federation (WHF), International Atherosclerosis Society (IAS), and International Association for the Study of Obesity (IASO).[12] Their components, key features, and intervention strategies are summarized in Table 14-1.

The ATP III is widely used criteria in the United States as it is a simple tool to use in the clinical setup. The AHA and NHLB metabolic syndrome criteria are similar to ATP III criteria with slight changes. In 2009, IDF, NHLBI, AHA, WHF, IAS, and IASO proposed a unified criterion for metabolic syndrome. Presence of 3 out of 5 risk factors was needed to classify an individual as having metabolic syndrome. Each of the 5 risk factors, except waist circum-

ference, was assigned a single set of cutoff points. The committee recommended use of population-specific and country-specific definitions to measure waist circumference until new data emerge.

Fundamentally, the components of each of the metabolic syndrome definitions are similar and feature a measure of body fatness, hypertension, triglycerides, high-density lipoprotein (HDL) cholesterol, and some measure of glucose intolerance. Yet, it is important to note the distinctive arrangement of diagnostic criteria and the management focus of the 6 definitions. In addition, the lack of a single set of criteria for metabolic syndrome in adults has created confusion among practitioners and hampered determinations of the specificity and sensitivity of the metabolic syndrome diagnosis, as well as its prevalence.[13] Experts offer several reasons why a consensus definition for metabolic syndrome has not been reached.

Evidence has failed to identify appropriate cut point values for any given metabolic component. Worldwide adoption of Westernized eating and physical activity behaviors has resulted in an increased prevalence of obesity, diabetes, stroke, and heart disease in what were once healthy populations. Researchers have learned that the degree of metabolic risk associated with developing CVD is distinct among people with diverse ethnic backgrounds. One good example is the differences of dyslipidemias among various ethnic groups. In African American population, the standard cutoff values for triglycerides and HDL cholesterol predicted insulin resistance is only 17%.[14] Furthermore, insulin resistance and triglycerides were found to be inversely correlated (ie, as insulin levels rose with insulin resistance, triglycerides fell). In this way, markers for dyslipidemia within the range of normal may prove insensitive and fail to identify individuals, particularly African Americans, who are insulin resistant and at risk for cardiovascular damage.[15] Furthermore, ethnic differences in metabolic risk have been reported for measures of waist circumference and hypertension among African Americans, Hispanics, whites, Iranians, and Asians.[13,16–19] These findings justify the need to assess the obese patient with a tailored approach to capture global metabolic risks.

Etiology

Controversy around the metabolic syndrome has surrounded the criteria used to make the diagnosis. Because the etiological underpinnings of the metabolic syndrome are substantially altered by ethnic variability it is difficult to build a single, all-inclusive definition.[1,4,13] Since Reaven,

Table 14-1. Etiology and Diagnostic Criteria of the Metabolic Syndrome in Adults

	DIAGNOSTIC CRITERIA	KEY FEATURES	RECOMMENDATIONS
A joint statement from IDF, NHLBI, AHA, WHF, IAS, and IASO (2009)[12]	Three or more of the following: 1) Abdominal obesity (population and country specific) 2) Elevated triglycerides 3) Low HDL cholesterol 4) Hypertension 5) Raised fasting plasma glucose	The organization attempted to unify the definitions of metabolic syndrome. A single set of cut points except waist circumference should be used. Presently, national or regional cut points for waist circumference can be used. Further work on waist circumference is needed.	At the national level, modification of lifestyle of the general population to reduce obesity and to increase physical activity is needed. On an individual level, we need to identify patients with metabolic syndrome and reduce multiple risk factors including lifestyle risk factors.
IDF (2006)[10]	A measure of body fatness characterized by 1) Abdominal obesity Plus 2 or more of the following: 2) Elevated triglycerides 3) Low HDL cholesterol 4) Hypertension 5) Raised fasting plasma glucose	The etiological perspective focuses on the need to establish a universally accepted definition for metabolic syndrome in research and clinical practice.	IDF recommends lifestyle changes including reducing calorie intake, increasing physical activity, and altering dietary habits to mitigate risk.
AHA/NHLBI (2005)[11]	Three or more of the following: 1) Abdominal obesity 2) Elevated triglycerides 3) Low HDL cholesterol 4) Hypertension 5) Elevated fasting plasma glucose	The features are similar to ATP III criteria except for a decrease in the threshold for elevated fasting glucose from 110 to 100 mg/dL.	AHA/NHLBI recommends weight loss, regular moderate intensity physical activity, limitation of an atherogenic diet, and treatment of metabolic risk factors as appropriate.
ACE (2003)[9]	1) An individual with risk factors for metabolic syndrome Plus 2 or more of the following: 2) Insulin resistance characterized by impaired glucose tolerance or high fasting glucose 3) Elevated triglycerides 4) Low HDL cholesterol 5) Hypertension	The society proposed to identify an individual with proposed risk factor including ethnicity, use of BMI (instead of waist circumference) as an index of obesity and differentiate metabolic syndrome (insulin resistance syndrome) from type 2 diabetes mellitus.	ACE recommends improving insulin sensitivity with lifestyle changes (lose 5%–10% of bodyweight) and using insulin sensitizing agents.
NCEP-ATP III (2001)[8]	Three or more of the following: 1) Abdominal obesity 2) Elevated triglycerides 3) Low HDL cholesterol 4) Hypertension 5) Raised fasting plasma glucose	The etiological perspective focuses on risk for cardiovascular disease that is attributed to environmental and genetic causes.	To control risk, NCEP-ATP III recommends weight control and physical activity as target therapeutic interventions.
WHO (1998)[7]	A measure of glucose intolerance characterized by 1) Impaired glucose tolerance 2) Impaired fasting glucose 3) Diabetes 4) Insulin resistance Plus 2 or more of the following: 4) Abdominal obesity 5) Elevated triglycerides 6) Low HDL cholesterol 7) Hypertension 8) Microalbuminuria	The etiological perspective focuses on ameliorating risk for type 2 diabetes mellitus which is attributed to the state of insulin resistance.	To control risk, WHO recommends weight control, physical activity, and the use of insulin sensitizing agents as target therapeutic interventions.

ACE, American College of Endocrinology; AHA, American Heart Association; BMI, body mass index; HDL, high-density lipoprotein; IAS, International Atherosclerosis Society; IASO, International Association for the Study of Obesity; IDF, International Diabetes Federation; NCEP-ATP III, National Cholesterol Education Program, Adult Treatment Panel III; NHLBI, National Heart, Lung, and Blood Institute; WHF, World Heart Federation; WHO, World Health Organization.

the basic connecting point uniting the various components has been insulin resistance. Yet even in this there is controversy. Some believe that the primary pathway leading to the metabolic syndrome is the result of glucose intolerance and diabetes,[13] whereas others suggest that glucose has no direct role in the metabolic syndrome or insulin resistance.[20,21] These individuals promote the surprising hypothesis that disordered fat metabolism, not glucose metabolism, is the etiologic prime mover for development of insulin resistance and, as a result, metabolic syndrome. Although the current research has not yet detailed the sequence of events leading to the insulin-resistant state that precedes the metabolic syndrome, mounting evidence supports the role of abnormal fat metabolism.[20,21]

Synergistic Risk and Treatment

Is the risk of metabolic syndrome greater than the sum of its parts? In other words, is it truly a syndrome? Even Reaven[4] challenged the idea that the diagnosis of the metabolic syndrome was itself a clinical entity of greater value than its individual components. From a clinical standpoint, the influence of the metabolic syndrome suggests to the practitioner the presence of CVD risk and therefore should be fully evaluated and aggressively treated.[4] Evidence implies that after adjusting for each of its individual components, the metabolic syndrome is no longer associated with early CVD mortality.[22] In an analysis of subjects with and without diabetes in the presence or absence of the metabolic syndrome, those with diabetes and metabolic syndrome had the highest prevalence (19.2%) of CHD mortality, followed by individuals with metabolic syndrome only (13.9%). Despite this significant association of metabolic syndrome and CVD mortality, multivariate analysis confirmed the presence of elevated blood pressure, diabetes, and low HDL cholesterol, not metabolic syndrome, were significant predictors for CHD.[23] Similarly, the evaluation of metabolic syndrome and the 11-year risk of incident CVD confirmed that when all 5 metabolic syndrome parameters are considered, metabolic syndrome as a whole does not incur greater CVD risk when compared with the sum of the individual components.[24]

Even though data suggest that metabolic syndrome does not incur risk greater than the sum of its parts, individuals with diagnoses for the cluster of disorders that compose metabolic syndrome suffer greater cardiovascular morbidity and mortality compared with individuals without the syndrome. According to the NCEP-ATP III Framingham Risk Score, approximately one-third of individuals with

the metabolic syndrome are classified as "high risk."[25] As demonstrated in the Framingham Offspring and San Antonio Heart Study, the predicted risk of CHD in individuals with the metabolic syndrome was significant (11.8% and 9.8%, respectively) in comparison with individuals without the metabolic syndrome (7% and 6.8%, respectively). Studies looking at incident CVD mortality indicate a 2-fold increase among individuals having metabolic syndrome compared to those without the syndrome.[23,24,26]

What Is the Metabolic Syndrome in Children?

Metabolic syndrome in children is also a constellation of factors including central obesity, hypertension, dyslipidemia, and insulin resistance as described in adults. No consensus definition in the pediatric population exists, despite the syndrome being widely studied among adolescents. Defining metabolic syndrome in pediatrics with a set value for a potential risk factor is even more challenging than in an adult population. Eight commonly used sets of diagnostic criteria for pediatric metabolic syndrome are described in Table 14-2.

Depending on the criteria used to classify the syndrome, prevalence among obese children and adolescents ranges from 26% to 49.7%.[27-34] However, there are a few fundamental problems with metabolic syndrome in children and adolescents.[35] Lack of consensus on etiology, age, and developmentally appropriate cut point measures for components of metabolic syndrome in children; and the effects of growth stage, puberty, and ethnicity as well as emerging evidence on the role of nontraditional risk factors all need to be considered. This discussion will focus briefly on issues such as cut-points, puberty, and nontraditional risk factors including the proinflammatory state and anatomical changes to the vasculature. Brambilla et al[35] offer a more complete review of the major and minor concerns with metabolic syndrome in children and adolescents. Furthermore, a scientific statement from the AHA was released in 2009. In this update to the 2003 report, the AHA provides a more comprehensive synopsis of the current advancements, challenges, and limitations to applying the metabolic syndrome to the child and adolescent populations.[36]

Metabolic Syndrome Controversies in Children

Pediatric-specific cut points that are sensitive to age, gender, and ethnicity have not been adapted for the majority of the metabolic syndrome components,[27,35,37] thus making it difficult to classify the syndrome as a diagnosable entity in the pediatric population. The pediatric population goes through

Table 14-2. Diagnostic Criteria of the Metabolic Syndrome in Pediatrics

GROUP/STUDY	CRITERIA	OBESITY	TRIGLYCERIDE	HDL-C	BLOOD PRESSURE (mm Hg)	GLUCOSE
IDF (2007)[27] 10–16 y	Abdominal obesity and any 2 risk factors	WC ≥ 90%ile	≥150 mg/dL	<40 mg/dL	Systolic ≥ 130 Diastolic ≥ 85	Fasting ≥ 100 mg/dL, or known type 2 DM
Modified NCEP ATP III (2007)[28]	3 or more of the following	WC ≥ 90%ile	>95%ile	<5%ile	>95%ile of either SBP/DBP	Impaired glucose tolerance
Goodman (2005)[29]	Insulin resistance or DM and 2 additional risk factors	BMI ≥ 95%ile	≥150 mg/dL	≤35 mg/dL (male) or ≤39 mg/dL (female)	≥130/85	Fasting ≥ 110 mg/dL or DM
Ford (2005)[30]	3 or more of the following	WC ≥ 90%ile	≥110 mg/dL	≤40 mg/dL	≥90%ile	Fasting ≥ 110 mg/dL
de Ferranti (2004)[31]	3 or more of the following	WC > 75%ile	≥1.1 mmol/L (100 mg/dL)	<1.3 mmol/L (50 mg/dL)	>90%ile	Fasting ≥ 6.1 mmol/L (110 mg/dL)
Weiss (2004)[32]	3 or more of the following	BMI > 97 or BMI Z score > –2	>95%ile	<5%ile	>95%ile	Impaired glucose tolerance (2 h, >140 mg/dL)
Cruz (2004)[33]	3 or more of the following	WC ≥ 90%ile	≥90%ile	≤10%ile	>90%ile	Impaired glucose tolerance
Cook (2003)[34]	3 or more of the following	WC ≥ 90%ile	≥110 mg/dL	≤40 mg/dL	≥ 90%ile	Fasting ≥ 110 mg/dL

BMI, body mass index; DBP, diastolic blood pressure; DM, diabetes mellitus; HDL-C, high-density lipoprotein cholesterol; IDF, International Diabetes Federation; NCEP ATP III, National Cholesterol Education Program, Adult Treatment Panel III; SBP, systolic blood pressure; WC, waist circumference.

various physiological changes, especially during the adolescent period. Various studies[38–41] reported changes in insulin resistance, lipid profile, body fat, and blood pressure as subject grew from late childhood to adolescence. With the constant changes in these factors, more than set values is needed to define metabolic syndrome in the pediatric population. Also, wide variations in pediatric-specific cut-points have been found across studies,[42] with many assigning arbitrary threshold values with no proven basis to predict future health risk.[28] One example that is subject to much debate is the value of waist circumference to substantiate metabolic syndrome risk in children. Some argue that measurements of visceral fat are the single most predictive anthropometric value of the metabolic syndrome compared with other measures of body fatness.[43] However, in children, percentile values for waist circumference are poorly established across age groups. Furthermore, the currently established cut-point references for waist circumference in children are not suitable for all ethnic populations because most guidelines result from studies conducted in white, European descendents.[44] Even if the appropriate, age-specific cut points are established for children, the value of waist circumference is arbitrary because no standardized protocol has been accepted for obtaining its measurement in clinical practice.[45]

The other limitation of metabolic syndrome in pediatrics is instability related to its diagnosis. The instability in diagnosis is noted even in obese patients. Up to 40%–55% of adolescents lost the diagnosis of metabolic syndrome over a 3-year to 9-year follow-up.[46–48] This outcome is related to changes in the body's metabolic milieu that occur during the years of puberty. The combined metabolic effects of growth hormone and insulin-like growth factor 1 (IGF-1) are associated with a normal state of mild insulin resistance, which follows the onset of puberty.[49] Furthermore, this phenomenon appears to be independent of body fat.[50] Thus, from the standpoint of the metabolic syndrome, puberty-induced insulin resistance complicates the task of attributing insulin resistance to the normal pubertal changes versus the metabolic consequences of overweight and obesity.

Epidemiology of Metabolic Syndrome in Children

The prevalence of metabolic syndrome in pediatrics is not uniform due to use of different criteria. The prevalence among the general population ranges from 2% to 9% and among school aged children from 4% to 8%. In a National Health and Nutrition Examination Survey (NHANES) survey, 9% of U.S. adolescents met the criteria for metabolic syndrome using modified ATP III diagnostic criteria. Depending on the criteria used to classify the syndrome, prevalence among obese children and adolescents ranges from 26% to 49.7% in the severely obese.[31-34] Epidemiological studies suggest that increase in severity of obesity increases the prevalence of metabolic syndrome. Racial/ethnic distribution of metabolic syndrome in pediatrics is comparable to adults.

The diagnosis of metabolic syndrome in childhood increases the odds of developing the metabolic syndrome and type 2 DM in adulthood by 9-fold and 11-fold, respectively.[51] The metabolic predictors track quite well across childhood, through young adulthood and into adulthood.[51,52] If overweight status continues past the first decade of life, excess body weight tracks into adulthood for 80% of subjects.

Pathophysiology of Metabolic Syndrome in Children

Metabolic syndrome in children is a potential risk factor for premature development of type 2 DM and atherosclerotic CVD. While the exact pathophysiology of metabolic syndrome in children is unknown, insulin resistance and obesity are thought to play key roles.

Insults to the cardiovascular system are associated with obesity and insulin resistance in childhood and adolescence, and formation of plaques and fatty streaks, deposited in the blood vessel walls, are associated with abnormal lipids and high blood pressure. All of these abnormalities have been found among obese children and adolescents. For example, excess body weight drives metabolic change resulting in insulin resistance and vascular dysfunction, and over time, anatomical changes to the arterial wall begin to develop which are thought to be the earliest indicators of risk for CVD.[53,54] Further damage to the blood vessel wall compromises arterial distensibility, resulting in vascular resistance and high blood pressure ensues. Disruption of the anatomical and physiological integrity of the vascular system appears to develop silently during childhood, even as young as age 5. The persistence of these anatomical vascular changes signifies a new wave of "nontraditional" cardiovascular risk factors that, like hypertension and dyslipidemia, need to be evaluated and treated aggressively. These changes may possibly be reversed through interventions such as physical activity and proper nutrition.[55-57]

Since Reaven's lecture in 1988, another major finding has occurred that has expanded our perspective on the metabolic syndrome. Chronic inflammation has been found not only to be closely associated with obesity in adults, children, and adolescents but also with each element of the metabolic syndrome.[58-61] This interconnectedness shapes the development of CVD. Among a number of actions, chronic inflammation, as identified by the biomarker high-sensitivity C-reactive protein (CRP), promotes platelet adhesion, a critical step in the expansion of atherosclerotic plaques. Further, in CVD the atherosclerotic lesion is expanded and made unstable by the influx of inflammatory cells, resulting in heart disease and stroke.[62] This link between the immune-inflammatory system and the body's metabolism is a consequence of cytokines secreted from excess adipose tissue.

Far from being a passive storage site for triglycerides, the adipocyte produces a vast array of chemokines with paracrine and endocrine functions,[63,64] including several proinflammatory cytokines. Not all adipocytes are the same. Visceral fat is far more inflammatory than peripheral fat, explaining why waist circumference, as a proxy for visceral fat, is such a key sign when assessing risk in obese patients.[65,66] Such adipokines released from metabolically active adipose tissue include tumor necrosis factor-α (TNF-α), CRP, and interleukin (IL)-6, all of which have been implicated in accelerating the atherosclerotic process.[63,64] Obesity and the subsequent proinflammatory state are suspected as the underlying mechanisms responsible for the progression of insulin resistance. Consequently, the triad of obesity, inflammation, and insulin resistance is associated with the metabolic syndrome in children. Children and adolescents who are morbidly obese are more insulin resistant and present with higher levels of inflammatory biomarkers including IL-6, intracellular adhesion molecule-1, and E-selectin, compared to lean counterparts.[61,65] In obese children and adolescents, the presence of traditional metabolic syndrome components is associated with nontraditional risk factors such as CRP and IL-6.[66-69] Furthermore, early functional and morphological changes to cardiovascular function, measured by intima-media thickness and flow-mediated dilation, are present with markers of inflammation and the metabolic syndrome.[58,62,70]

Risk Factors for Metabolic Syndrome in Children

There are several risk factors for metabolic syndrome in children. These risk factors can be evident at a young age. The pediatrician should use these risk factors to identify children at risk for metabolic syndrome. Family history, race, socioeconomic status, eating, and physical activity behaviors all can contribute to the future health risk of a child for development of metabolic syndrome.

Increased Weight/Adiposity

The pediatric population has higher rate of increase in adiposity compared to the adult population.[41] In a longitudinal study, a child's increased weight gain was associated with increased hyperinsulinemia/insulin resistance and concurrent changes in triglycerides.[41] In other pediatric studies, prevalence of metabolic syndrome increased with increased weight.[32,34] In the NHANES cross-sectional survey, 30% of overweight adolescents met the criteria for metabolic syndrome compared to 4% across the survey.[34] Increased truncal obesity correlates with abnormal blood pressure and increased low-density lipoprotein (LDL), triglyceride, lipoprotein, and insulin as well as decreased HDL.[71–74] Similarly, increased waist-to-height ratio is associated with increased metabolic and cardiovascular risk.[74,75]

Dietary Habits

Sugar-sweetened beverage intake is associated with insulin resistance, obesity (including truncal obesity), dyslipidemia, and increased inflammatory markers.[76–79] Sugar-sweetened beverages contribute to obesity due to high sugar content, low satiety, high glycemic load, abundance of excess energy storage, and incomplete compensation for total energy.[80,81] Several studies have shown that consumption of low sugar-sweetened beverage with increased physical activity decreases insulin resistance and triglycerides and increases HDL cholesterol.[76–79] Another study showed that consumption of a low-energy and low glycemic index diet improved children's lipid profile (triglycerides, LDL, cholesterol-normalized).[82] Epidemiological evidence suggests that fruit and vegetable consumption may be protective against the development of childhood obesity.[83]

Physical Inactivity

Sedentary lifestyle behaviors have been implicated as a potential cause of pediatric overweight and obesity. A recent study showed that 35% of boys and 25% of girls watch 4 or more hours of television each day.[84] Irrespective of socioeconomic status and race, children who watch more television are less physically active and are more overweight.[85] Furthermore, television watching also influences appetite, particularly if the child is already overweight or obese. In one study looking at Saturday morning television broadcasts, more than 50% of the commercials featured promoted food items and over 90% of these food-oriented commercials featured high-sugar/salt and high-fat foods.[86] As Halford et al[87,88] found, overweight and obese children respond to such advertisements by consuming more calories and choosing more snack foods after viewing such broadcasts. Schmitz et al[89] showed that physical inactivity is associated with traits of metabolic syndrome in pediatrics. This is further strengthened by observation in clinical trials that exercise improved insulin sensitivity in adults.[90,91] Studies in children showed improvement in all facets of metabolic syndrome including improved insulin sensitivity, dyslipidemia, obesity, cardiorespiratory fitness and blood pressure with regular physical activity.[76,79,89,92] Balducci et al[93] and Rubin et al[94] showed a reduction in inflammatory markers in patients with metabolic syndrome who were engaged in exercise. The reduction was independent of weight loss.

Genetic Factors

Several studies found that genetics play an important role in metabolic syndrome.[95–97] The genetic factors were found to influence metabolic syndrome–related traits such as central obesity, insulin resistance, dyslipidemia, hypertension, and endothelial dysfunction.[98–101] Having a first-degree relative with type 2 DM doubled a child's risk for developing the disease.[102] The components of the metabolic syndrome are documented to track across generations. A study in the pediatric population showed that presence of metabolic syndrome in parents was a risk factor for adolescent obesity and insulin resistance.[103] In the Northern Manhattan Family Study, the heritability of metabolic syndrome components was strikingly significant.[104] Among overweight and obese Hispanic youth, genetic determinants appear to predict the components of metabolic syndrome, with 68% and 60% of children, respectively, reporting a family history of diabetes and cardiovascular disease.[105] Familial clustering of metabolic syndrome from family studies and twin studies are also suggestive of the role of shared environment.

Tobacco Exposure

Twenty-one percent of U.S. adolescents are actively engaged in smoking. Additionally, 67% of adolescents are exposed to environmental tobacco smoke.[106] Growing evidence suggests that smoking is a potential risk factor for pediatric metabolic syndrome. The smoke exposure could be active and/ or passive. Maternal smoking during pregnancy and early childhood increase the risk of overweight and obesity.[107] Also, children exposed to parental smoking have elevated blood pressure, obesity, dyslipidemia, and increased inflammatory markers.[108–111] In a NHANES survey study nearly 20% of adolescents exposed to cigarette smoke met the criteria for metabolic syndrome compared to 5.6% of non-exposed adolescents.[106] The study also showed a dose-response relationship between tobacco smoke and metabolic syndrome. Smoke exposure alters vascular structure and function, resulting in early development of atherosclerosis and hypertension.[106,112–117]

Race/Ethnicity

The highest prevalence of metabolic syndrome is seen in Mexican-Americans (13%) followed by non-Hispanic whites (11%) and non-Hispanic blacks (2.5%).[31,34,118] This difference is less in girls compared with boys.[119] However, the rate of increase in adiposity is higher in blacks compared to whites, but only among females, and is independent of baseline adiposity.[41] Mexican-American adolescent males have less hypertension compared with non-Hispanic adolescent males.[119] Non-Hispanic black girls have less hypertriglyceridemia compared with others. The prevalence of metabolic syndrome is lower in blacks (blacks have lower triglycerides at baseline) as compared to Mexican-Americans and non-Hispanic whites, using same serum lipid criteria.[120,121] However, when an ethnicity-specific lipid threshold is used, the prevalence of metabolic syndrome is similar among all 3 ethnicity groups.[32] Hence, ethnicity-specific criteria are needed for diagnosis of metabolic syndrome.[32,122]

Socioeconomic Status

Low socioeconomic status is highly associated with the development of overweight and obesity among American children.[123–125] Lower cumulative family income is significantly associated with the onset of health conditions that limit childhood activities and require treatment by a pediatrician. However, in other countries lower socioeconomic class does not necessarily indicate higher prevalence of health risk. In fact, Chinese and Russian children from upper-level income groups are reported to have a higher incidence of overweight and obesity compared with middle and lower socioeconomic groups, an indication of access to a more Western lifestyle. Furthermore, when socioeconomic status is a factor along with race/ethnicity, the risk for obesity is even greater.

For example, Hispanic and black children from lower socioeconomic groups are significantly at greater risk for obesity than their white counterparts.[85]

Clinical Features of Metabolic Syndrome in Children

Obesity

About 17% of U.S. children and adolescents are obese.[126] The prevalence of obesity is highest in non-Hispanic black and Hispanic populations followed by whites and also increases with the age of a child and the presence of paternal obesity. Childhood obesity is associated with insulin resistance, inflammation, abnormal blood pressure, and compromised vascular function.[127] It is also associated with dyslipidemia including increased LDL, triglycerides, apolipoproteins, and triacylglycerol as well as decreased HDL.[71–74] Obesity, specifically central obesity, is the key component of pediatric metabolic syndrome. Depending on the metabolic syndrome definition used, obesity is measured by either body mass index (BMI) or waist circumference. While BMI is a standard tool to assess obesity, it measures subcutaneous adiposity and not visceral adiposity.[128] Thus, BMI is a less sensitive indicator of central adiposity in children.[129] Growing evidence suggests that waist circumference and waist to hip ratio are ideal parameters to measure central adiposity as well as a better predictor of cardiovascular risk factors.[71–75] Though both waist circumference and waist to hip ratio are components of childhood metabolic syndrome, waist to height ratio (>0.5) is preferred over waist circumference because it does not need age-specific and sex-specific cutoff points.

Hypertension

Hypertension is an essential component of pediatric metabolic syndrome,[130] and its development is likely multifactorial. Insulin resistance and subsequent development of hyperinsulinemia are critical for the development of hypertension through a variety of mechanisms that include 1) renal sodium retention; 2) vascular smooth muscle growth; 3) endothelial dysfunction; 4) increased sympathetic tone; and 5) impaired vasodilation resulting in hypertension.[96,131–133] Other mechanisms include reduced bioavailability of nitric oxide due to increased oxidative stress, excess glucocorticoid, increased free fatty acids, and increased leptin levels.[134–138] Sinaiko et al[139] showed that level of blood pressure was associated with cluster features of metabolic syndrome but not with individual components (insulin level, triglycerides, HDL, BMI) of metabolic syndrome.

Acanthosis Nigricans

Insulin resistance and subsequent hyperinsulinemia initiate a series of cascading metabolic events signaling total body changes in metabolism. Ultimately the clustering of metabolic parameters, as seen in the metabolic syndrome, brings attention to the serious health risks that are associated with insulin resistance and obesity. Furthermore, such metabolic changes identify individuals with the most urgent need for lifestyle intervention. Essentially, identifying certain physical signs may alert clinicians early in the clinical course.

Risk associated with family history, socioeconomic status, nutrition, and physical activity behaviors may be effective screening tools for prevention activities. However, as evidence suggests, a substantial number of children and teens already have acquired the first signs of metabolic changes, which will with time place a serious health burden on their cardiovascular system. Unlike family history, ethnicity, lifestyle, behavior, and BMI that predict future health burdens, the skin sign of acanthosis nigricans represents a physical manifestation of existing metabolic change.

Acanthosis nigricans is characterized by hyperpigmented velvety plaques on body folds, seen mainly on the neck. Several studies indicate that acanthosis nigricans is relatively common among children and adolescents, particularly those who are obese. In a broad population the prevalence of acanthosis nigricans among African American, Hispanic, and white youth is 19.4%, 23.1%, and 4.9%, respectively.[140] However, when overweight and obese subpopulations are examined specifically, rates of acanthosis nigricans are much higher. Among an ethnically diverse sample of obese children, acanthosis nigricans was seen in 46%. With rates of obesity beyond the 99th percentile, children present with acanthosis nigricans 70% of the time.[140]

National directives have recognized acanthosis nigricans screening as a noninvasive tool to identify burgeoning changes in metabolism that are associated with numerous risk factors for CVD, including abnormal lipid and glucose metabolism.[141–144] Pediatricians are urged to obtain laboratory tests on overweight and obese children who present with acanthosis nigricans including a complete fasting lipid profile, fasting glucose, and markers of liver function.[145]

Dyslipidemia

Dyslipidemia, specifically hypertriglyceridemia and low HDL cholesterol, are strongly associated with insulin resistance.[73,75,146] Hyperinsulinemia causes increased hepatic lipogenesis due to increased flux of free fatty acid into the liver.[147,148] This causes increased production of triglycerides as very low-density lipoprotein (VLDL) leading to hyperlipidemia. An inverse relationship exists between the plasma insulin level and the HDL level.[149] Also, hyperinsulinemia causes increased clearance of HDL, resulting in a low HDL level.[150,151]

Dyslipidemia is an integral feature of metabolic syndrome. Dyslipidemia is associated with visceral fat and abdominal obesity. The abnormal lipid profile has the potential to cause premature atherosclerotic changes. One of the limitations of using cutoff values for triglycerides is its variability with ethnicity. Blacks have less frequent hypertriglyceridemia.[120,121] Thus, there is need to integrate this variability when diagnosing an individual with metabolic syndrome using current diagnostic criteria.

Insulin Resistance

Insulin resistance leads to compensatory hyperinsulinemia, impaired fasting glucose level, impaired glucose tolerance, and subsequent type 2 DM.[152,153] The exact etiology for development of insulin resistance is unclear, and the following hypotheses are proposed: 1) increased free fatty acid influx from abdominal fat in obese patients and induces hepatic insulin resistance; 2) intracellular fatty acyl interferes with insulin signaling pathway; 3) release of proinflammatory cytokines in obese patients (TNF-α and IL-6) promotes insulin resistance; 4) reduced adiponectin level in obese patients; and 5) excess glucocorticoid levels.[154–158]

Children undergo a transient physiological insulin resistance state during pubertal growth. This is secondary to physiological increases in growth hormone, IGF-1, and sex hormones during puberty.[159,160] However, long-term insulin resistance is associated with elevated blood pressure, increased weight gain, and development of cardiovascular risk factors.[161–163] Twenty-four percent of obese adolescents with impaired glucose tolerance developed type 2 DM over a 12-month follow-up.[164,165]

Nonalcoholic Fatty Liver Disease

Nonalcoholic fatty liver disease (NAFLD) has also been implicated as an adverse consequence of carrying excess weight in childhood. In general it is estimated that 38% of obese children have NAFLD.[166] The relationship between NAFLD and the presence or development of the metabolic syndrome is less understood, particularly in the pediatric population. However, evidence shows a positive correlation between increased levels of aminotransferases and the number of metabolic syndrome risk factors present

Table 14-3. Laboratory Testing Guidelines Based on Age, BMI Percentile, and Risk Factors Present

LABORATORY TESTING PARAMETERS[a]	FASTING LIPID PROFILE (CHOLESTEROL, HDL, LDL, AND TRIGLYCERIDES)	FASTING GLUCOSE (EVERY 2 Y)	HEPATIC FUNCTION (ALT AND AST; EVERY 2 Y)
AGE 2-9 Y			
BMI % 85th-95th (with no additional risk factors)	X		
BMI % ≥85th-95th (with additional risk factors)	X		
BMI % ≥95th-99th (with or without additional risk factors)	X		
BMI % ≥99th (with or without additional risk factors)	X		
AGE 10-18 Y			
BMI % 85th-95th (with no additional risk factors)	X		
BMI % ≥85th-95th (with additional risk factors)	X	X	X
BMI % ≥95th-99th (with or without additional risk factors)	X	X	X
BMI % ≥99th (with or without additional risk factors)	X	X	X

ALT, alanine aminotransferase; AST, aspartate aminotransferase; BMI, body mass index; HDL, high-density lipoprotein; LDL, low-density lipoprotein.
[a]Risk factors refer to those risks found during the assessment of family history and physical examination. The laboratory guidelines recommended by the Expert Committee[145] are merely baseline recommendations. Any concerns found during the assessment of the family history and/or physical examination should be evaluated and monitored.

among children diagnosed with NAFLD.[167] Schwimmer et al[168] demonstrated that children with NAFLD have significantly more CVD risk factors associated with the metabolic syndrome than children without NAFLD. Although more studies are needed to determine the pathophysiology, natural history, and treatment of NAFLD,[169] an Expert Committee recognized that biomarkers for liver function, alanine aminotransferase and aspartate aminotransferase, are reasonable markers for NAFLD and are an important part of the laboratory assessment of the obese child.[145] The Expert Committee recommendations appear later in this chapter (Table 14-3).

Polycystic Ovarian Syndrome

Polycystic ovarian syndrome (PCOS) is a clinical disorder characterized by menstrual dysfunction, hyperandrogenism, and polycystic ovaries.[170] Females with PCOS have increased risk of metabolic syndrome, type 2 DM, and CVD.[171,172] Adolescents with PCOS were 4.5 times as likely to have metabolic syndrome compared to age-matched controls despite adjusting for BMI. Childhood PCOS pre-

dicts adulthood metabolic syndrome.[173] In females, excess visceral adiposity increases androgen precursor synthesis resulting in hyperandrogenism. Also, excess visceral adiposity causes defective insulin receptor signal transduction resulting in insulin resistance. Rossi et al[174] in a cross-sectional study found that adolescents girls with PCOS had higher glucose intolerance and increased plasminogen activator inhibitor compared to BMI matched controls. Stuckey et al[175] reported clustering of cardiovascular and metabolic risk factors in women with PCOS.

Inflammation

Obesity is considered to be a low-grade proinflammatory condition, with the liver and visceral adipose tissue playing a role in induction of inflammation.[32,176] The adipose tissue releases proinflammatory cytokines (IL-6, IL-8, monocyte chemoattractant protein-1, TNF-α),[177,178] which induce lipolysis and hepatic synthesis of free fatty acid.[179] These cytokines also decrease insulin receptor signaling resulting in insulin resistance. The hepatic insulin resistance initiates an innate immune response resulting in production of CRP, fibrinogen, and clotting factors,[178] which if unchecked can induce thrombogenesis. Various inflammatory markers including CRP, TNF-α, IL-18, IL-6, and adipocytokines are associated with metabolic syndrome.[177,180,181] Elevated CRP is associated with obesity, insulin resistance, dyslipidemia, and elevated blood pressure in children.[182,183] CRP is localized to atherosclerotic plaques and associated with poor cardiovascular outcomes.[184-190] Adiponectin is an anti-inflammatory agent, and its production is attenuated in obese patients,[191] leading to an inverse correlation between adiponectin and metabolic syndrome.[192,193] Despite the strong evidence of ongoing inflammation in metabolic syndrome, inflammatory markers are currently not part of metabolic syndrome diagnostic criteria.

Diagnostic Evaluation for Metabolic Syndrome in Children

Laboratory analysis is required for overweight and obese children to identify health risks that may be otherwise hidden. It is important to note that Expert Committee[145] guidelines on further laboratory testing mirror most of the components of the metabolic syndrome. Table 14-3 lists the tests that should be drawn at what degree of obesity and at what age. The physician should also explore concerns raised during the history and physical exam, which should be investigated fully along with the testing recommended for all overweight children.

Early Identification of Children at Risk for Metabolic Syndrome

The imperative raised in the original concept of the metabolic syndrome remains, which was to identify insulin-resistant individuals at greatest risk for CVD and in most urgent need for lifestyle intervention.[4] The overweight pediatric patient represents the leading edge of cardiovascular risk. A comprehensive approach to the assessment of metabolic syndrome and its components allows the pediatrician to observe the development of metabolic risk at its earliest stages and intervene to arrest the prospect of lifelong CVD risk. The following steps, as per evidence-based guidelines,[145,194] should be considered when assessing a child's health risk in a practice-based setting.

BMI percentile: At least annually, but ideally at each well child visit, the child's height and weight should be measured and the BMI percentile value should be calculated and plotted on the growth chart. The pediatrician should be looking for BMI percentile trends that show an increasing

weight-for-height trajectory and classify the child as underweight, normal weight, overweight, or obese.[145,195]

Blood pressure: A crucial part of the child's physical exam should be the blood pressure, but it must be obtained using the correct cuff size at rest. The results are then assessed using tables comparing systolic and diastolic readings against normal values for the child's height percentile to ascertain "at risk" values over the 90th percentile and "hypertensive" values above the 95th percentile.[196]

Blood pressure should be measured annually starting at 3 years of age. The result should be reviewed with parents and managed as appropriate. Blood pressure should be measured in children younger than 3 years of age in the presence of a history of renal/cardiac/urologic disorders or a history of admission to the neonatal intensive care unit.[194]

Family health history: Family health history is a strong indicator of future health risk for a child, particularly if the risk is identified in a first-degree relative. However, unlike other health risks, family health history is not modifiable. It does, however, represent an important context for a discussion about a child's risk for chronic diseases that are fueled by excess body weight.

Tobacco exposure: Tobacco exposure should be explored at every visit. The goal is to identify parents and caregivers who smoke and recommend a smoke-free environment, antismoking counseling, and referral as needed.

Behaviors (nutrition and physical activity): A targeted history should capture information about nutrition and physical activity habits of the overweight or obese child and the family. This information should serve as the baseline and basis for prevention and intervention counseling directed both at the child and the family.

A focused review of systems and targeted physical examination: The focused review of systems and targeted physical examination of the child should be comprehensive in nature and include, but not be limited to, the presence of anxiety, polyuria/dipsia, headaches, sleep problems, and abdominal pain (a focused review of systems); acanthosis nigricans; the presence of dysmorphic features, hirsutism, and extreme acne; tonsillar hypertrophy; abdominal tenderness; unexpected rates of linear growth; and undescended testicles.

These recommendations emphasize the need for risk identification to occur sooner in the child's life, rather than later, because identification of these health risks ultimately leads to the establishment of an intervention program targeted at reducing obesity-related comorbidities and controlling body weight.

Management of Metabolic Syndrome in Children

Due to the lack of a standard definition to diagnose the metabolic syndrome in the adult and pediatric populations, the best course of treatment for individuals with the syndrome remains to be determined. Experts disagree on whether the metabolic syndrome should be treated differently from the treatment prescribed for the individual components of the syndrome. Some counsel a more comprehensive approach to treatment for patients with the metabolic syndrome. Yet what we do know is the chronic disease components that derive the metabolic syndrome are a direct result of excess adiposity and subsequent insulin resistance. Therefore, national directives established by an expert committee may be used as a guideline to assess overweight and obese children and adolescents for health risks and mediate with the appropriate lifestyle and treatment interventions.

Irrespective of the ability to make a formal diagnosis of the metabolic syndrome in the pediatric population, evidence of the clustering of the metabolic syndrome components in children and adolescents suggests that 1) the body's metabolic milieu adapts to the presence of excess body fat, 2) the clustering of metabolic risk factors imply greater risk for CVD mortality for affected individuals compared with peers who do not present with the metabolic syndrome phenotype, and 3) the collective and individual metabolic risks represent a high-risk finding among children and adolescents. Developing metabolic risk at a young age implies that the health burden of cardiovascular damage will be greatly amplified by time the child ages into adulthood. CVD morbidity and mortality are the ultimate outcomes for individuals who carry metabolic risk. The younger the child is when metabolic risk is acquired, the higher the likelihood of tracking these components into adulthood.[197-199] The fundamental goal in the initial treatment is optimal nutrition, increased physical activity/physical fitness, and weight maintenance.

Nutrition and Physical Activity Behaviors

A recent review by the members of the Academy of Nutrition and Dietetics examined the relationship between eating and sedentary behaviors on the development of overweight and obesity in childhood.[82] Consuming large amounts of sugar-sweetened beverages and fruit juices was found to increase caloric intake and displace more nutritious foods from the diet. Although at this time evidence is lacking to support the relationship between sugar-sweetened beverages, fruit juices, and increased adiposity, epidemiological evidence has suggested that fruit and vegetable consump-

tion may be protective against the development of childhood obesity.[82]

Physical activity: In light of the sedentary behaviors that children and adolescents are displaying today, recent national recommendations emphasize that children participate in at least 1 hour of moderate to vigorous physical activity each day.[145] These recommendations are based on evidence from a systematic review that highlights the effects of physical activity on health and behavioral outcomes.[200] Children who participate in higher levels of physical activity are leaner. For those children who are overweight and obese, physical activity has been shown to reduce total body fat provided these children are physically active for 30–60 minutes 3–7 days per week. When examining variables of cardiovascular health, a consistent level of physical activity improves HDL cholesterol and triglycerides in high-risk children. Changes to the cardiovascular risk profile have been found to occur irrespective of any significant changes in weight reduction.[200]

For obese children and adolescents already presenting with early CVD risk, the use of exercise training has been supported as one management strategy. Irrespective of significant reductions in weight, exercise training demonstrates marked improvement in endothelial dysfunction. Worsening endothelial dysfunction, measured by flow-mediated dilation, is a predictor of future adverse cardiovascular events and correlates with measures of body fatness. Children who perform exercise training, particularly high-intensity exercise training, show marked improvement in vascular function.[55,56,201]

The physiological and functional changes to the vasculature develop silently during childhood and are fueled by obesity. As mentioned, the damage is amenable to repair if detected early and intervention is administered.

Weight loss: The underlying driver of metabolic dysfunction is excess adipose tissue. Evidence shows that for the obese patient a modest reduction in excess body weight of as little as 5%–7% induces significant health benefits, including a decrease in triglycerides, LDL, and VLDL cholesterols; raised HDL cholesterol; lowered blood pressure; and improvements in insulin action with improved glucose status.[57,202]

Physical activity alone is documented to alter CVD risk. In the prevention of coronary artery disease, individuals who are more physically active cut their risk in half, compared with sedentary individuals. In adults, comprehensive lifestyle interventions that include physical activity result in modest reductions in body fat (5%–7%) and demonstrate significant health benefits, starting with a lowered insulin resistance.[57,202] Irrespective of weight loss, exercise alone still demonstrates improvement of CVD outcomes. Among individuals with established CVD, exercise-only interventions significantly reduce cardiac mortality and total mortality by 31% and 27%, respectively.[203]

Nutrition: Optimal nutrition, particularly a diet rich in fruits, vegetables, and low-fat dairy (as described in the Dietary Approaches to Stop Hypertension [DASH] diet), has been shown to prevent increases in blood pressure during early childhood.[204] The DASH diet significantly improved measures of systolic and diastolic blood pressure among adolescents with documented hypertension.[205]

Mounting evidence in support of optimal nutrition, physical activity, and weight maintenance to ameliorate obesity and therefore lessen CVD risk has prompted the Expert Committee[145] to establish 9 core messages for pediatricians to reinforce as preventive and treatment strategies, applicable for both low-risk and high-risk children. Evidence-informed prevention and treatment goals should focus on

1) Limiting sugar-sweetened beverages
2) Encouraging a healthful diet with at least 9 servings of fruits and vegetables daily
3) Limiting television and screen time to 2 hours a day or less
4) Eating breakfast daily
5) Limiting eating out away from home
6) Encouraging family meals
7) Limiting portion sizes
8) Engaging in 1 hour or more of moderate to vigorous physical activity each day
9) Breastfeeding exclusively until 6 months of age

For some *high-risk* children, optimal nutrition, physical activity, and weight maintenance efforts are ineffective at controlling weight and reducing the burden of comorbidities and a more aggressive intervention is required. Lipid-lowering drug therapies, particularly statins, have been approved for use in children, as young as 8 years of age at the highest risk.[206] It is important to emphasize that pharmacological treatments have demonstrated safety and effectiveness among *high-risk children and adolescents only*[194,207] and are not recommended for children presenting with moderate laboratory values or risk. Similarly, bariatric weight-loss surgery has been used in the United States as a treatment option for morbidly obese adolescents as a means to mitigate the comorbidities of excess body weight.[208] An expert panel of pediatricians and surgeons has recommended that candidates demonstrate certain physical and psychological readi-

ness before receiving bariatric surgery.[209] Therefore, whether the treatment for the obese child includes pharmacological or surgical intervention, it is crucial for the practitioner to assess the risk status of the child. Utilizing practice-ready tools and guidelines provided by the Expert Committee/Panel[145,194] can assist the practitioner in evaluating risk and making decisions on the appropriate treatment course for the obese child or adolescent.

While the management of individual component of metabolic syndrome is beyond the scope of this book, information on management of most components including hypertension and dyslipidemia can be found in the Expert Panel on Integrated Guidelines for Cardiovascular Health and Risk Reduction in Children and Adolescents: Summary Report.[194]

Summary

In the decade following Reaven's Banting Lecture in 1988, the metabolic syndrome evolved from a concept to a diagnosis. Despite providing useful information on metabolic risk and the susceptibility for developing CVD, the clinical utility of the metabolic syndrome diagnosis remains controversial among researchers in adult and pediatric medicine. Among children and adolescents, the lack of consensus on the definition of the metabolic syndrome is compounded by 1) the inability to define metabolic thresholds using pediatric-specific cut points, 2) the role of natural metabolic changes during puberty, and 3) the application of emerging, nontraditional CVD risk factors in the metabolic syndrome definition. But the very presence of the metabolic syndrome in the pediatric population suggests that a shift in metabolism fueled by excess body weight is underway. Further, the presence of risk factors in early childhood means that damage to the cardiovascular system has begun. When metabolic risk factors present in a cluster, the clinical course and health outcomes for that child are compromised, unless interventions are undertaken. The Expert Committee on the Assessment, Prevention, and Treatment of Child and Adolescent Overweight and Obesity underscored the role of the clinician in identifying metabolic risk factors at the earliest stage possible, instituting treatment, and following up closely. Identification of metabolic risk in a child may prove beneficial for several reasons: 1) the threat of evolving cardiovascular damage throughout the lifespan can be reversed, if identified early and coupled with aggressive lifestyle changes, and 2) weight management is easier due to growth, along with the potential to influence home and school environments. Practice-ready guidelines emphasize a

6-step approach to assessing health risk in practice. For children at any risk level, the Expert Committee recommends evidence-based counseling supported by the 9 core messages for prevention and treatment. For children presenting with substantial health risks associated with the metabolic syndrome, pediatricians should focus on a comprehensive intervention strategy, including optimal nutrition, physical activity, weight maintenance, and, when appropriate, pharmacological and/or surgical intervention.

Test Your Knowledge Questions

1. A teenage Hispanic girl presents to your clinic with excessive weight gain and dark pigmentation over the neck for the last several years. Her blood work done through her primary care provider's office shows elevated alanine aminotransferase of 80 U/L. You are concerned about metabolic syndrome. What constitutes metabolic syndrome?
   A. Abdominal obesity, hypertension, fasting hyperglycemia, and hypertriglyceridemia
   B. Abdominal obesity, acanthosis nigricans, hypertension, and polycystic ovaries
   C. Abdominal obesity, nonalcoholic fatty liver, high HDL level, and history of smoking
   D. Glucose intolerance, high HDL, low triglyceride, and obesity
   E. Family history of heart disease, obesity, acanthosis nigricans, and low HDL level

2. You are seeing an adolescent African American girl in your multidisciplinary obesity clinic with a fourth year medical student. A medical student asks about risk factors for metabolic syndrome. Which one of the following is not a risk factor for metabolic syndrome?
   A. Visceral adiposity
   B. Poor dietary habits
   C. Sedentary lifestyle
   D. Tobacco exposure
   E. Higher education
   F. Genetic factors

3. After identifying a 5-year-old child with a body mass index > 95th percentile, what would be the most *inappropriate* next step in the child's care?
   A. Obtain a detailed family history
   B. Discuss lifestyle behaviors
   C. Perform a targeted physical exam and review of stems
   D. Obtain a laboratory analysis
   E. Simply monitor the child's weight over the next 12 months

Acknowledgments

The authors of this chapter for the second edition of this text wish to thank Michelle Battista, PhD, and Robert Murray, MD, for their contributions to the first edition of this text. We have edited and updated relevant clinical information.

References

1. Leslie BR. Metabolic syndrome: historical perspectives. *Am J Med Sci.* 2005;330:264–268.

2. Reaven GM. Role of insulin resistance in human disease. *Diabetes.* 1988;37:1595–1606.

3. Kahn R, Buse J, Ferrannini E, Stern M. The metabolic syndrome: time for a critical appraisal. *Diabetologia.* 2005;48:1684–1699.

4. Reaven GM. The metabolic syndrome: is this diagnosis necessary? *Am J Clin Nutr.* 2006;83:1237–1247.

5. Blaha MJ, Bansal S, Rouf R, Golden SH, Blumenthal RS, DePilippis AP. A practical "ABCDE" approach to the metabolic syndrome. *Mayo Clin Proc.* 2008;83:932–943.

6. Hanefeld M, Leonhardt W. Das metabolische Syndrom. Deutsche Gesundheit Wesen 1981;36:545–552.

7. Alberti KG, Zimmet PZ. Definition, diagnosis and classification of diabetes mellitus and its complications. Part 1: diagnosis and classification of diabetes mellitus provisional report of a WHO consultation. *Diabet Med.* 1998;15:539–553.

8. Expert Panel on Detection, Evaluation, and Treatment of High Blood Cholesterol in Adults. Executive Summary of the Third Report of the National Cholesterol Education Program (NCEP) Expert Panel on Detection, Evaluation, and Treatment of High Blood Cholesterol in Adults (Adult Treatment Panel III). *JAMA.* 2001;285:2486–2497.

9. Einhorn D, Reaven GM, Cobin RH, et al. American College of Endocrinology position statement on the insulin resistance syndrome. *Endocr Pract.* 2003;9(3):237–252.

10. International Diabetes Federation. The IDF consensus worldwide definition of the metabolic syndrome. http://www.idf.org/webdata/docs/IDF_Meta_def_final.pdf. Published 2006. Accessed December 14, 2014.

11. Grundy SM, Cleeman JI, Daniels SR, et al. Diagnosis and management of the metabolic syndrome: an American Heart Association/National Heart, Lung, and Blood Institute Scientific Statement. *Circulation.* 2005;112(17):2735–2752.

12. Alberti KG, Eckel RH, Grundy SM, et al. Harmonizing the metabolic syndrome: a joint interim statement of the International Diabetes Federation Task Force on Epidemiology and Prevention; National Heart, Lung, and Blood Institute; American Heart Association; World Heart Federation; International Atherosclerosis Society; and International Association for the Study of Obesity. *Circulation.* 2009;120(16):1640–1645.

13. Kahn JM, Beevers DG. Management of hypertension in ethnic minorities. *Heart.* 2005;91:1105–1109.

14. Sumner AE, Finley KB, Genovese DJ, Criqui MH, Boston RC. Fasting triglyceride and triglyceride-HDL cholesterol ratio are not markers of insulin resistance in African Americans. *Arch Intern Med.* 2005:165:1395–1400.

15. Sumner AE, Cowie CC. Ethnic differences in the ability of triglyceride levels to identify insulin resistance. *Atherosclerosis.* 2008;196:696–703.

16. Zhu S, Heymsfield SB, Toyoshima H, Wang Z, Piertrobelli A, Heshka S. Race-ethnicity-specific waist circumference cutoffs for identifying cardiovascular disease risk factors. *Am J Clin Nutr.* 2005;81:409–415.

17. Esteghamati A, Ashraf H, Rashidi A, Meysamie A. Waist circumference cut-off points for the diagnosis of metabolic syndrome in Iranian adults. *Diabetes Res Clin Prac.* 2008;82:104–107.

18. Oka R, Kobayashi J, Yagi K, et al. Reassessment of the cutoff values of waist circumference and visceral fat area for identifying Japanese subjects at risk for the metabolic syndrome. *Diabetes Res Clin Pract.* 2008;79:474–481.

19. Ferdinand KC, Saunders E. Hypertension related morbidity and mortality in African Americans—why we need to do better. *J Clin Hypertens.* 2006;8:21–31.

20. Unger J. Reinventing Type 2 diabetes: pathogenesis, treatment, and prevention. *JAMA.* 2008;299:1185–1187.

21. Lewis GF, Carpentier A, Adeli K, Giacca A. Disordered fat storage and mobilization in the pathogenesis of insulin resistance and type 2 diabetes. *Endocr Rev.* 2002; 23:201–229.

22. Iribarren C, Go AS, Husson G, et al. Metabolic syndrome and early-onset coronary artery disease: is the whole greater than its parts? *J Am Coll Cardiol.* 2006;48:1800–1807.

23. Alexander CM, Landsman PB, Teutsch SM, Haffner SM. NCEP-defined metabolic syndrome, diabetes, and prevalence of coronary heart disease among NHANES III participants age 50 years and older. *Diabetes.* 2003;52:1210–1214.

24. McNeill AM, Rosamond WD, Girman CJ, et al. The metabolic syndrome and 11 year risk of incident cardiovascular disease in the atherosclerosis risk in communities. *Diabetes Care.* 2005;28:385–390.

25. Hoang KC, Ghanderhari H, Lopez VA, Barboza MG, Wong ND. Global coronary heart disease assessment of individuals with the metabolic syndrome in the U.S. *Diabetes Care.* 2008;31:1405–1409.

26. Tong W, Lai H, Yang C, Ren S, Dai S, Lai S. Age, gender, and metabolic syndrome related coronary heart disease in U.S. adults. *Int J Cardiol.* 2005;104:288–291.

27. Zimmet P, Alberti KG, Kaufman F, et al; IDF Consensus Group. The metabolic syndrome in children and adolescents: an IDF consensus report. *Pediatr Diabetes.* 2007;8:299–306.

28. Jolliffe CJ, Janssen I. Development of age-specific adolescent metabolic syndrome criteria that are linked to the Adult Treatment Panel III and International Diabetes Federation criteria. *J Am Coll Cardiol.* 2007;49(8):891–898.

29. Goodman E, Daniels SR, Morrison JA, Huang B, Dolan LM. Contrasting prevalence of and demographic disparities in the World Health Organization and National Cholesterol Education Program Adult Treatment Panel III definitions of metabolic syndrome among adolescents. *J Pediatr.* 2004;145(4):445–451.

30. Ford ES, Ajani UA, Mokdad AH; National Health and Nutrition Examination. The metabolic syndrome and concentrations of C-reactive protein among U.S. youth. *Diabetes Care.* 2005;28(4):878–881.

31. de Ferranti SD, Gauvreau K, Ludwig DS, Neufeld EJ, Newburger JW, Rifai N. Prevalence of the metabolic syndrome in American adolescents: findings from the third national health and nutrition examination survey. *Circulation.* 2004;110:2494–2497.

32. Weiss R, Dziura J, Burgert TS, et al. Obesity and the metabolic syndrome in children and adolescents. *N Engl J Med.* 2004;89:108–113.

33. Cruz ML, Weigensberg MJ, Huang TT, Ball G, Shaibi GQ, Goran MI. The metabolic syndrome in overweight Hispanic youth and the role of insulin sensitivity. *J Clin Endocrinol Metab.* 2004;89(1):108–113.

34. Cook S, Weitzman M, Auinger P, Nguyen M, Dietz WH. Prevalence of metabolic syndrome phenotypes in adolescents: findings from the third national health and nutrition examination survey, 1998-1994. *Pediatr Adolesc Med.* 2003;157:821–827.

35. Brambilla P, Lissau I, Flodmark CE, et al. Metabolic risk factor clustering estimation in children: to draw a line across pediatric metabolic syndrome. *Int J Obes.* 2007;31:591–600.

36. Steinberger J, Daniels SR, Eckel RH, et al. Progress and challenges in metabolic syndrome in children and adolescents: a scientific statement from the American Heart Association Atherosclerosis, Hypertension, and Obesity in the Young Committee of the Council on Cardiovascular Disease in the Young; Council on Nursing; and Council on Nutrition, Physical Activity, and Metabolism. *Circulation.* 2009;119:628–647.

37. Huang TT. Finding thresholds of risk for components of the pediatric metabolic syndrome. *J Pediatr.* 2008;152:158–159.

38. Moran A, Jacobs DR, Jr., Steinberger J, et al. Changes in insulin resistance and cardiovascular risk during adolescence: establishment of differential risk in males and females. *Circulation.* 2008;117(18):2361–2368.

39. Dai S, Fulton JE, Harrist RB, Grunbaum JA, Steffen LM, Labarthe DR. Blood lipids in children: age-related patterns and association with body-fat indices: Project HeartBeat! *Am J Prev Med.* 2009;37(1 suppl):S56–S64.

40. Labarthe DR, Dai S, Fulton JE, Harrist RB, Shah SM, Eissa MA. Systolic and fourth- and fifth-phase diastolic blood pressure from ages 8 to 18 years: Project HeartBeat! *Am J Prev Med.* 2009;37(1 suppl):S86–S96.

41. Srinivasan SR, Myers L, Berenson GS. Rate of change in adiposity and its relationship to concomitant changes in cardiovascular risk variables among biracial (black-white) children and young adults: The Bogalusa Heart Study. *Metabolism.* 2001;50(3):299–305.

42. Ford ES, Li C. Defining the metabolic syndrome in children and adolescents: will the real definition please stand up? *J Pediatr.* 2008;152:160–164.

43. Moreno LA, Pineda I, Rodriguez G, Fleta J, Sarria A, Bueno M. Waist circumference for the screening of metabolic syndrome in children. *Acta Pediatr.* 2002;91:1307–1312.

44. Seidell JC, Perusse L, Despres JP, Bouchard C. Waist and hip circumference have independent and opposite effects on

cardiovascular disease risk factors: the Quebec family study. *Am J Clin Nutr.* 2001;74:315–321.

45. Moreno LA, Joyanes M, Mesana MI, et al; AVENA Study Group. Harmonization of anthropometric measurements for a multicenter nutrition survey in Spanish adolescents. *Nutrition.* 2003;19:481–486.

46. Goodman E, Daniels SR, Meigs JB, Dolan LM. Instability in the diagnosis of metabolic syndrome in adolescents. *Circulation.* 2007;115(17):2316–2322.

47. Stanley TL, Chen ML, Goodman E. The typology of metabolic syndrome in the transition to adulthood. *J Clin Endocrinol Metab.* 2014;99(3):1044–1052.

48. Gustafson JK, Yanoff LB, Easter BD, et al. The stability of metabolic syndrome in children and adolescents. *J Clin Endocrinol Metab.* 2009;94(12):4828–4834.

49. Moran A, Jacobs DR Jr, Steinberger J, et al. Association between the insulin resistance of puberty and the insulin-like growth factor/growth hormone axis. *J Clin Endocrinol Metab.* 2002;87:4817–4820.

50. Hannon TS, Janosky J, Arslanian SA. Longitudinal study of physiological insulin resistance and metabolic changes of puberty. *Pediatr Res.* 2006;60:759–763.

51. Morrison JA, Fredman LA, Wang P, Glueck CJ. Metabolic syndrome in childhood predicts adult metabolic syndrome and type 2 diabetes mellitus 25-30 years later. *J Pediatr.* 2008;152:201–206.

52. Katzmarzyk PT, Pérusse L, Malina RM, Bergeron J, Després JP, Bouchard C. Stability indicators of the metabolic syndrome from childhood and adolescence to young adulthood: the Quebec family study. *J Clin Epidemiol.* 2001;54:190–195.

53. Groner JA, Joshi M, Bauer JA. Pediatric precursors of adult cardiovascular disease: noninvasive assessment of early vascular changes in children and adolescents. *Pediatrics.* 2006;118(4):1683–1691.

54. Woo KS, Chook P, Yu CW, et al. Overweight in children is associated with arterial endothelial dysfunction and intima-media thickness. *Int J Obes Relat Metab Disord.* 2004;28:852–857.

55. Meyer AA, Kundt G, Lenschow U, Schuff-Werner P, Kienast W. Improvement of early vascular changes and cardiovascular risk factors in obese children after a six-month exercise program. *J Am Coll Cardiol.* 2006;7:1865–1870.

56. Watts K, Beye P, Siafarikas A, et al. Exercise training normalizes vascular dysfunction and improves central adiposity in obese adolescents. *J Am Coll Cardiol.* 2004;19:1823–1827.

57. McBride PE, Einerson JA, Grant H, et al. Putting the diabetes prevention program into practice: a program for weight loss and cardiovascular disease reduction with metabolic syndrome or type 2 diabetes mellitus. *J Nutr Health Aging.* 2008;12:745s–749s.

58. Ferri C, Croce G, Confini V, et al. C-reactive protein: interaction with the vascular endothelium and possible role in human atherosclerosis. *Curr Pharm Des.* 2007;13:1631–1645.

59. Valle M, Maros R, Gascon F, Canete R, Zafra MA, Morales R. Low-grade systemic inflammation, hypoadiponectinemia and a high concentration of leptin are present in very young obese children, and correlate with metabolic syndrome. *Diabetes Metab.* 2005;3:55–62.

60. Soriano-Guillen L, Hernandez-Garcia B, Pita J, Dominguez-Garrido N, Del Rio-Camacho G, Rovira A. High-sensitivity C-reactive protein is a good marker of cardiovascular risk in obese children and adolescents. *Eur J Endocrinol.* 2008;159:R1–R4.

61. Poirier P, Giles TD, Bray GA, et al. Obesity and cardiovascular disease: pathophysiology, evaluation and effect of weight loss. *Arterioscler Thromb Vasc Biol.* 2006;26:968–976.

62. Pai JK, Pischon T, Ma J, et al. Inflammatory markers and the risk of coronary heart disease in men and women. *N Engl J Med.* 2004;351:2599–2610.

63. Wozniak SE, Gee LL, Wachtel MS, Frezza EE. Adipose tissue: the new endocrine organ? A review article. *Dig Dis Sci.* 2009;54(9):1847–1856.

64. Antuna-Puente B, Feve B, Fellahi S, Bastard JP. Adipokines: the missing link between insulin resistance and obesity. *Diabetes Metab.* 2008;34:2–11.

65. Fox CS, Massaro JM, Hoffmann U, et al. Abdominal visceral and subcutaneous adipose tissue compartments: association with metabolic risk factors in the Framingham Heart Study. *Circulation.* 2007;116:39–48.

66. Pou KM, Massaro JM, Hoffmann U, et al. Visceral and subcutaneous adipose tissue volumes are cross-sectionally related to markers of inflammation and oxidative stress: the Framingham Heart Study. *Circulation.* 2007;116:1234–1241.

67. Lee S, Bacha F, Gungor N, Arslanian S. Comparison of different definitions of pediatric metabolic syndrome: relation to abdominal adiposity, insulin resistance, adiponectin, and inflammatory biomarkers. *J Pediatr.* 2008;152:177–184.

68. Retnakaran R, Zinman B, Connelly PW, Harris SB, Hanley AJG. Nontraditional risk factors in pediatric metabolic syndrome. *J Pediatr.* 2006;148:176–182.

69. Langenberg C, Bergstrom J, Scheidt-Nave C, Pfeilschifter J, Barrett-Connor E. Cardiovascular death and the metabolic syndrome: role of adiposity signaling hormones and inflammatory markers. *Diabetes Care.* 2006;29:1363–1369.

70. Kapiotis S, Holzer G, Schaller G, et al. A pro-inflammatory state is detectable in obese children and is accompanied by functional and morphological vascular changes. *Arterioscler Thromb Vasc Biol.* 2006;26:2541–2546.

71. Maffeis C, Pietrobelli A, Grezzani A, Provera S, Tato L. Waist circumference and cardiovascular risk factors in prepubertal children. *Obes Res.* 2001;9(3):179–187.

72. Freedman DS, Serdula MK, Srinivasan SR, Berenson GS. Relation of circumferences and skinfold thicknesses to lipid and insulin concentrations in children and adolescents: the Bogalusa Heart Study. *Am J Clin Nutr.* 1999;69(2):308–317.

73. Freedman DS, Dietz WH, Srinivasan SR, Berenson GS. The relation of overweight to cardiovascular risk factors among children and adolescents: the Bogalusa Heart Study. *Pediatrics.* 1999;103(6 pt 1):1175–1182.

74. Savva SC, Tornaritis M, Savva ME, et al. Waist circumference and waist-to-height ratio are better predictors of cardiovascular disease risk factors in children

than body mass index. *Int J Obes Relat Metab Disord.* 2000;24(11):1453–1458.

75. Maffeis C, Banzato C, Talamini G; Obesity Study Group of the Italian Society of Pediatric Endocrinology and Diabetology. Waist-to-height ratio, a useful index to identify high metabolic risk in overweight children. *J Pediatr.* 2008;152(2):207–213.

76. Bremer AA, Auinger P, Byrd RS. Relationship between insulin resistance-associated metabolic parameters and anthropometric measurements with sugar-sweetened beverage intake and physical activity levels in US adolescents: findings from the 1999-2004 National Health and Nutrition Examination Survey. *Arch Pediatr Adolesc Med.* 2009;163(4):328–335.

77. Kosova EC, Auinger P, Bremer AA. The relationships between sugar-sweetened beverage intake and cardiometabolic markers in young children. *J Acad Nutr Diet.* 2013;113(2):219–227.

78. Ambrosini GL, Oddy WH, Huang RC, Mori TA, Beilin LJ, Jebb SA. Prospective associations between sugar-sweetened beverage intakes and cardiometabolic risk factors in adolescents. *Am J Clin Nutr.* 2013;98(2):327–334.

79. Bremer AA, Byrd RS, Auinger P. Differences in male and female adolescents from various racial groups in the relationship between insulin resistance-associated parameters with sugar-sweetened beverage intake and physical activity levels. *Clin Pediatr.* 2010;49(12):1134–1142.

80. Dubois L, Farmer A, Girard M, Peterson K. Regular sugar-sweetened beverage consumption between meals increases risk of overweight among preschool-aged children. *J Am Diet Assoc.* 2007;107(6):924–934; discussion 934–935.

81. Harrington S. The role of sugar-sweetened beverage consumption in adolescent obesity: a review of the literature. *J Sch Nurs.* 2008;24(1):3–12.

82. Weker H. Simple obesity in children. A study on the role of nutritional factors [in Polish]. *Med Wieku Rozwoj.* 2006;10(1):3–191.

83. Academy of Nutrition and Dietetics. Factors associated with childhood overweight. http://andeal.org/topic.cfm?menu=5296. Accessed on October 27, 2014.

84. Marshall SJ, Gorely T, Biddle SJH. A descriptive epidemiology of screen-based media use in youth: a review and critique. *J Adolesc.* 2006;29:333–349.

85. Singh SG, Kogan MD, Van Dyck PC, Siahpush M. Racial/ethnic, socioeconomic, and behavioral determinants of childhood and adolescent obesity in the United States: analyzing independent and joint associations. *Ann Epidemiol.* 2008;18:682–695.

86. Kotz K, Story M. Food advertisements during children's Saturday morning television programming: are they consistent with dietary recommendations? *J Am Diet Assoc.* 1994;29:1296–1300.

87. Halford JC, Gillespie J, Brown V, Pontin EE, Dovey TM. Effect of television advertisements of foods on food consumption in children. *Appetite.* 2004;42:221–225.

88. Halford JC, Boyland EJ, Hughes GM, Stacey L, McKean S, Dovey TM. Beyond brand-effect of television food advertisements on food choice in children: the effects of weight status. *Public Health Nutr.* 2008;11:897–904.

89. Schmitz KH, Jacobs DR Jr, Hong CP, Steinberger J, Moran A, Sinaiko AR. Association of physical activity with insulin sensitivity in children. *Int J Obes Relat Metab Disord.* 2002;26(10):1310–1316.

90. Holloszy JO, Schultz J, Kusnierkiewicz J, Hagberg JM, Ehsani AA. Effects of exercise on glucose tolerance and insulin resistance. Brief review and some preliminary results. *Acta Med Scand Suppl.* 1986;711:55–65.

91. Eriksson KF, Lindgarde F. Prevention of type 2 (non-insulin-dependent) diabetes mellitus by diet and physical exercise. The 6-year Malmo feasibility study. *Diabetologia.* 1991;34(12):891–898.

92. Farpour-Lambert NJ, Aggoun Y, Marchand LM, Martin XE, Herrmann FR, Beghetti M. Physical activity reduces systemic blood pressure and improves early markers of atherosclerosis in pre-pubertal obese children. *J Am Coll Cardiol.* 2009;54(25):2396–2406.

93. Balducci S, Zanuso S, Nicolucci A, et al. Anti-inflammatory effect of exercise training in subjects with type 2 diabetes and the metabolic syndrome is dependent on exercise modalities and independent of weight loss. *Nutr Metab Cardiovasc Dis.* 2010;20(8):608–617.

94. Rubin DA, Hackney AC. Inflammatory cytokines and metabolic risk factors during growth and maturation: influence of physical activity. *Med Sport Sci.* 2010;55:43–55.

95. Bosy-Westphal A, Onur S, Geisler C, et al. Common familial influences on clustering of metabolic syndrome traits with central obesity and insulin resistance: the Kiel obesity prevention study. *Int J Obes (Lond).* 2007;31(5):784–790.

96. Balletshofer BM, Rittig K, Enderle MD, et al. Endothelial dysfunction is detectable in young normotensive first-degree relatives of subjects with type 2 diabetes in association with insulin resistance. *Circulation.* 2000;101(15):1780–1784.

97. Tang W, Hong Y, Province MA, et al. Familial clustering for features of the metabolic syndrome: the National Heart, Lung, and Blood Institute (NHLBI) Family Heart Study. *Diabetes Care.* 2006;29(3):631–636.

98. Mitchell BD, Kammerer CM, Mahaney MC, et al. Genetic analysis of the IRS. Pleiotropic effects of genes influencing insulin levels on lipoprotein and obesity measures. *Arterioscler Thromb Vasc Biol.* 1996;16(2):281–288.

99. Hong Y, Pedersen NL, Brismar K, de Faire U. Genetic and environmental architecture of the features of the insulin-resistance syndrome. *Am J Hum Genet.* 1997;60(1):143–152.

100. Rainwater DL, Mitchell BD, Mahaney MC, Haffner SM. Genetic relationship between measures of HDL phenotypes and insulin concentrations. *Arterioscler Thromb Vasc Biol.* 1997;17(12):3414–3419.

101. Xiang AH, Azen SP, Raffel LJ, et al. Evidence for joint genetic control of insulin sensitivity and systolic blood pressure in hispanic families with a hypertensive proband. *Circulation.* 2001;103(1):78–83.

102. Dallo FJ, Weller SC. Effectiveness of diabetes mellitus screening recommendations. *Proc Natl Acad Sci U S A.* 2003;100:10574–10579.

103. Pankow JS, Jacobs DR Jr, Steinberger J, Moran A, Sinaiko AR. Insulin resistance and cardiovascular disease risk factors in children of parents with the insulin resistance (metabolic) syndrome. *Diabetes Care.* 2004;27(3):775–780.

104. Lin HF, Boden-Albala B, Juo SH, Park N, Rundek T, Sacco RL. Heritabilities of the metabolic syndrome and its components in the Northern Manhattan study. *Diabetologia.* 2005;48:2006–2012.

105. Butte NF, Comuzzie AG, Cole SA, et al. Quantitative genetic analysis of the metabolic syndrome in Hispanic children. *Pediatr Res.* 2005;58:1243–1248.

106. Weitzman M, Cook S, Auinger P, et al. Tobacco smoke exposure is associated with the metabolic syndrome in adolescents. *Circulation.* 2005;112(6):862–869.

107. Raum E, Kupper-Nybelen J, Lamerz A, Hebebrand J, Herpertz-Dahlmann B, Brenner H. Tobacco smoke exposure before, during, and after pregnancy and risk of overweight at age 6. *Obesity.* 2011;19(12):2411–2417.

108. Simonetti GD, Schwertz R, Klett M, Hoffmann GF, Schaefer F, Wuhl E. Determinants of blood pressure in preschool children: the role of parental smoking. *Circulation.* 2011;123(3):292–298.

109. Khanolkar AR, Byberg L, Koupil I. Parental influences on cardiovascular risk factors in Swedish children aged 5-14 years. *Eur J Public Health.* 2012;22(6):840–847.

110. Feldman J, Shenker IR, Etzel RA, et al. Passive smoking alters lipid profiles in adolescents. *Pediatrics.* 1991;88(2):259–264.

111. Neufeld EJ, Mietus-Snyder M, Beiser AS, Baker AL, Newburger JW. Passive cigarette smoking and reduced HDL cholesterol levels in children with high-risk lipid profiles. *Circulation.* 1997;96(5):1403–1407.

112. Celermajer DS, Adams MR, Clarkson P, et al. Passive smoking and impaired endothelium-dependent arterial dilatation in healthy young adults. *N Engl J Med.* 1996;334(3):150–154.

113. Juonala M, Magnussen CG, Raitakari OT. Parental smoking produces long-term damage to vascular function in their children. *Curr Opin Cardiol.* 2013;28(5):569–574.

114. Juonala M, Magnussen CG, Venn A, et al. Parental smoking in childhood and brachial artery flow-mediated dilatation in young adults: the Cardiovascular Risk in Young Finns study and the Childhood Determinants of Adult Health study. *Arterioscler Thromb Vasc Biol.* 2012;32(4):1024–1031.

115. Kallio K, Jokinen E, Saarinen M, et al. Arterial intima-media thickness, endothelial function, and apolipoproteins in adolescents frequently exposed to tobacco smoke. *Circ Cardiovasc Qual Outcomes.* 2010;3(2):196–203.

116. Kallio K, Jokinen E, Hamalainen M, et al. Decreased aortic elasticity in healthy 11-year-old children exposed to tobacco smoke. *Pediatrics.* 2009;123(2):e267–e273.

117. Magnussen CG, Smith KJ, Juonala M. When to prevent cardiovascular disease? As early as possible: lessons from prospective cohorts beginning in childhood. *Curr Opin Cardiol.* 2013;28(5):561–568.

118. Batey LS, Goff DC Jr, Tortolero SR, et al. Summary measures of the insulin resistance syndrome are adverse among Mexican-American versus non-Hispanic white children: the Corpus Christi Child Heart Study. *Circulation.* 1997;96(12):4319–4325.

119. Walker SE, Gurka MJ, Oliver MN, Johns DW, DeBoer MD. Racial/ethnic discrepancies in the metabolic syndrome begin in childhood and persist after adjustment for environmental factors. *Nutr Metab Cardiovasc Dis.* 2012;22(2):141–148.

120. Becker DM, Yook RM, Moy TF, Blumenthal RS, Becker LC. Markedly high prevalence of coronary risk factors in apparently healthy African-American and white siblings of persons with premature coronary heart disease. *Am J Cardiol.* 1998;82(9):1046–1051.

121. Morrison JA, Friedman LA, Harlan WR, et al. Development of the metabolic syndrome in black and white adolescent girls: a longitudinal assessment. *Pediatrics.* 2005;116(5):1178–1182.

122. Deboer MD. Underdiagnosis of metabolic syndrome in non-Hispanic black adolescents: a call for ethnic-specific criteria. *Curr Cardiovasc Risk Rep.* 2010;4(4):302–310.

123. Goodman E. The role of socioeconomic status gradients in explaining differences in US adolescents health. *Am J Public Health.* 1999;89:1522–1528.

124. Chen E, Martin AD, Matthews KA. Trajectories of socioeconomic status across children's lifetime predict health. *Pediatrics.* 2007;120:e297–e303. doi:10.1542/peds.2006-3098.

125. Wang Y. Cross national comparison of childhood obesity: the epidemic and the relationship between obesity and socioeconomic status. *Int J Epidemiol.* 2001;30:1129–1136.

126. Skinner AC, Skelton JA. Prevalence and trends in obesity and severe obesity among children in the United States, 1999-2012. *JAMA Pediatr.* 2014;168(6):561–566.

127. Tounian P, Aggoun Y, Dubern B, et al. Presence of increased stiffness of the common carotid artery and endothelial dysfunction in severely obese children: a prospective study. *Lancet.* 2001;358(9291):1400–1404.

128. Brambilla P, Bedogni G, Moreno LA, et al. Crossvalidation of anthropometry against magnetic resonance imaging for the assessment of visceral and subcutaneous adipose tissue in children. *Int J Obes.* 2006;30(1):23–30.

129. Reilly JJ, Dorosty AR, Emmett PM, et al; Avon Longitudinal Study of Pregnancy and Childhood Study Team. Identification of the obese child: adequacy of the body mass index for clinical practice and epidemiology. *Int J Obes Relat Metab Disord.* 2000;24(12):1623–1627.

130. Ferrannini E, Buzzigoli G, Bonadonna R, et al. Insulin resistance in essential hypertension. *N Engl J Med.* 1987;317(6):350–357.

131. Haynes WG, Morgan DA, Walsh SA, Mark AL, Sivitz WI. Receptor-mediated regional sympathetic nerve activation by leptin. *J Clin Invest.* 1997;100(2):270–278.

132. DeFronzo RA, Cooke CR, Andres R, Faloona GR, Davis PJ. The effect of insulin on renal handling of sodium, potassium, calcium, and phosphate in man. *J Clin Invest.* 1975;55(4):845–855.

133. Egan BM. Insulin resistance and the sympathetic nervous system. *Curr Hypertens Rep.* 2003;5(3):247–254.

134. Tripathy D, Mohanty P, Dhindsa S, et al. Elevation of free fatty acids induces inflammation and impairs vascular reactivity in healthy subjects. *Diabetes.* 2003;52(12):2882–2887.

135. Wang M. The role of glucocorticoid action in the pathophysiology of the Metabolic Syndrome. *Nutr Metab.* 2005; 2(1):3.

136. Limberg JK, Harrell JW, Johansson RE, et al. Microvascular function in younger adults with obesity and metabolic syndrome: role of oxidative stress. *Am J Physiol Heart Circ Physiol.* 2013;305(8):H1230–H1237.

137. Virdis A, Neves MF, Duranti E, Bernini G, Taddei S. Microvascular endothelial dysfunction in obesity and hypertension. *Curr Pharm Des.* 2013;19(13):2382–2389.

138. Correia ML, Rahmouni K. Role of leptin in the cardiovascular and endocrine complications of metabolic syndrome. *Diabetes Obes Metab.* 2006;8(6):603–610.

139. Sinaiko AR, Steinberger J, Moran A, Prineas RJ, Jacobs DR Jr. Relation of insulin resistance to blood pressure in childhood. *J Hypertens.* 2002;20(3):509–517.

140. Nguyen TT, Keil MF, Russell DL, et al. Relation of acanthosis nigricans to hyperinsulinemia and insulin sensitivity in overweight African American and white children. *J Pediatr.* 2001;138(4):474–480.

141. Mukhtar Q, Cleverley G, Voorhees RE, McGrath JW. Prevalence of acanthosis nigricans and its association with hyperinsulinemia in New Mexico adolescents. *J Adoles Health.* 2001;28:372–376.

142. Sinha S, Schwartz RA. Juvenile acanthosis nigricans. *J Am Acad of Dermatol.* 2007;57:502–508.

143. Ice CL, Murphy E, Minor VE, Neal WA. Metabolic syndrome in fifth grade children with acanthosis nigricans: results from the CARDIAC project. *World J Pediatr.* 2009;5:23–30.

144. Guran T, Turan S, Akcay T, Bereket A. Significance of acanthosis nigricans in childhood obesity. *J Paediatr Child Health.* 2008;44:338–341.

145. Barlow S; Expert Committee. Expert committee recommendations regarding the prevention, assessment, and treatment of child and adolescent overweight and obesity: summary report. *Pediatrics.* 2007;120:S164–S192.

146. Bao W, Srinivasan SR, Wattigney WA, Berenson GS. Persistence of multiple cardiovascular risk clustering related to syndrome X from childhood to young adulthood. The Bogalusa Heart Study. *Arch Intern Med.* 1994;154(16):1842–1847.

147. Adiels M, Olofsson SO, Taskinen MR, Borén J. Overproduction of very low-density lipoproteins is the hallmark of the dyslipidemia in the metabolic syndrome. *Arterioscler Thromb Vasc Biol.* 2008;28(7):1225–1236.

148. Kwiterovich PO Jr. Clinical relevance of the biochemical, metabolic, and genetic factors that influence low-density lipoprotein heterogeneity. *Am J Cardiol.* 2002;90(8A):30i–47i.

149. Cominacini L, Zocca I, Garbin U, et al. High-density lipoprotein composition in obesity: interrelationships with plasma insulin levels and body weight. *Int J Obes.* 1988;12(4):343–352.

150. Pascot A, Lemieux I, Prud'homme D, et al. Reduced HDL particle size as an additional feature of the atherogenic dyslipidemia of abdominal obesity. *J Lipid Res.* 2001;42(12):2007–2014.

151. Goff DC Jr, D'Agostino RB Jr, Haffner SM, Otvos JD. Insulin resistance and adiposity influence lipoprotein size and subclass concentrations. Results from the Insulin Resistance Atherosclerosis Study. *Metabolism.* 2005;54(2): 264–270.

152. Dolan LM, Bean J, D'Alessio D, et al. Frequency of abnormal carbohydrate metabolism and diabetes in a population-based screening of adolescents. *J Pediatr.* 2005;146(6):751–758.

153. Weiss R, Dufour S, Taksali SE, et al. Prediabetes in obese youth: a syndrome of impaired glucose tolerance, severe insulin resistance, and altered myocellular and abdominal fat partitioning. *Lancet.* 2003;362(9388):951–957.

154. Roden M, Price TB, Perseghin G, et al. Mechanism of free fatty acid-induced insulin resistance in humans. *J Clin Invest.* 1996;97(12):2859–2865.

155. Santomauro AT, Boden G, Silva ME, et al. Overnight lowering of free fatty acids with Acipimox improves insulin resistance and glucose tolerance in obese diabetic and nondiabetic subjects. *Diabetes.* 1999;48(9):1836–1841.

156. Shulman GI. Cellular mechanisms of insulin resistance. *J Clin Invest.* 2000;106(2):171–176.

157. Bergman RN, Kim SP, Catalano KJ, et al. Why visceral fat is bad: mechanisms of the metabolic syndrome. *Obesity.* 2006;14(suppl 1):16S–19S.

158. Kadowaki T, Yamauchi T, Kubota N, Hara K, Ueki K, Tobe K. Adiponectin and adiponectin receptors in insulin resistance, diabetes, and the metabolic syndrome. *J Clin Invest.* 2006;116(7):1784–1792.

159. Amiel SA, Sherwin RS, Simonson DC, Lauritano AA, Tamborlane WV. Impaired insulin action in puberty. A contributing factor to poor glycemic control in adolescents with diabetes. *N Engl J Med.* 1986;315(4):215–219.

160. Moran A, Jacobs DR Jr, Steinberger J, et al. Insulin resistance during puberty: results from clamp studies in 357 children. *Diabetes.* 1999;48(10):2039–2044.

161. Taittonen L, Uhari M, Nuutinen M, Turtinen J, Pokka T, Akerblom HK. Insulin and blood pressure among healthy children. Cardiovascular risk in young Finns. *Am J Hypertens.* 1996;9(3):194–199.

162. Odeleye OE, de Courten M, Pettitt DJ, Ravussin E. Fasting hyperinsulinemia is a predictor of increased body weight gain and obesity in Pima Indian children. *Diabetes.* 1997;46(8):1341–1345.

163. Bao W, Srinivasan SR, Berenson GS. Persistent elevation of plasma insulin levels is associated with increased cardiovascular risk in children and young adults. The Bogalusa Heart Study. *Circulation.* 1996;93(1):54–59.

164. Weiss R, Taksali SE, Tamborlane WV, Burgert TS, Savoye M, Caprio S. Predictors of changes in glucose tolerance status in obese youth. *Diabetes Care.* 2005;28(4):902–909.

165. Weiss R. Impaired glucose tolerance and risk factors for progression to type 2 diabetes in youth. *Pediatr Diabetes.* 2007;8(suppl 9):70–75.

166. Schwimmer JB, Deutsch R, Kahen T, Lavine JE, Stanley C, Behling C. Prevalence of fatty liver in children and adolescents. *Pediatrics.* 2006;118:1388–1393.

167. Manco M, Marcellini M, Devito R, Comparcola D, Sartorelli MR, Nobili V. Metabolic syndrome and liver histology in paediatric non-alcoholic steatohepatitis. *Int J Obes.* 2008;32:381–387.

168. Schwimmer JB, Pardee PE, Lavine JE, Blumkin AK, Cook S. Cardiovascular risk factors and the metabolic syndrome in pediatric non-alcoholic fatty liver disease. *Circulation.* 2008;15:277–283.

169. Barshop NJ, Sirlin CB, Schwimmer JB, Lavine JE. Review article: epidemiology, pathogenesis and potential treatment of paediatric non-alcoholic fatty liver disease. *Aliment Pharmacol Ther.* 2008;28:13–24.

170. Setji TL, Brown AJ. Polycystic ovary syndrome: update on diagnosis and treatment. *Am J Med.* 2014;127(10):912–919.

171. Cussons AJ, Watts GF, Burke V, Shaw JE, Zimmet PZ, Stuckey BG. Cardiometabolic risk in polycystic ovary syndrome: a comparison of different approaches to defining the metabolic syndrome. *Hum Reprod.* 2008;23(10): 2352–2358.

172. Coviello AD, Legro RS, Dunaif A. Adolescent girls with polycystic ovary syndrome have an increased risk of the metabolic syndrome associated with increasing androgen levels independent of obesity and insulin resistance. *J Clin Endocrinol Metab.* 2006;91(2):492–497.

173. Glueck CJ, Morrison JA, Daniels S, Wang P, Stroop D. Sex hormone-binding globulin, oligomenorrhea, polycystic ovary syndrome, and childhood insulin at age 14 years predict metabolic syndrome and class III obesity at age 24 years. *J Pediatr.* 2011;159(2):308–313.e302.

174. Rossi B, Sukalich S, Droz J, et al. Prevalence of metabolic syndrome and related characteristics in obese adolescents with and without polycystic ovary syndrome. *J Clin Endocrinol Metab.* 2008;93(12):4780–4786.

175. Stuckey BG, Opie N, Cussons AJ, Watts GF, Burke V. Clustering of metabolic and cardiovascular risk factors in the polycystic ovary syndrome: a principal component analysis. *Metabolism.* 2014;63(8):1071–1077.

176. Ode KL, Frohnert BI, Nathan BM. Identification and treatment of metabolic complications in pediatric obesity. *Rev Endocr Metab Disord.* 2009;10(3):167–188.

177. Greenberg AS, McDaniel ML. Identifying the links between obesity, insulin resistance and beta-cell function: potential role of adipocyte-derived cytokines in the pathogenesis of type 2 diabetes. *Eur J Clin Invest.* 2002;32(suppl 3):24–34.

178. Gustafson B, Hammarstedt A, Andersson CX, Smith U. Inflamed adipose tissue: a culprit underlying the metabolic syndrome and atherosclerosis. *Arterioscler Thromb Vasc Biol.* 2007;27(11):2276–2283.

179. Marette A. Mediators of cytokine-induced insulin resistance in obesity and other inflammatory settings. *Curr Opin Clin Nutr Metab Care.* 2002;5(4):377–383.

180. Warnberg J, Marcos A. Low-grade inflammation and the metabolic syndrome in children and adolescents. *Curr Opin Lipidol.* 2008;19(1):11–15.

181. Nemet D, Wang P, Funahashi T, et al. Adipocytokines, body composition, and fitness in children. *Pediatr Res.* 2003;53(1):148–152.

182. Sutherland JP, McKinley B, Eckel RH. The metabolic syndrome and inflammation. *Metab Syndr Relat Disord.* 2004;2(2):82–104.

183. Cook DG, Mendall MA, Whincup PH, et al. C-reactive protein concentration in children: relationship to adiposity and other cardiovascular risk factors. *Atherosclerosis.* 2000;149(1):139–150.

184. Ridker PM. C-reactive protein and the prediction of cardiovascular events among those at intermediate risk: moving an inflammatory hypothesis toward consensus. *J Am Coll Cardiol.* 2007;49(21):2129–2138.

185. Hatanaka K, Li XA, Masuda K, Yutani C, Yamamoto A. Immunohistochemical localization of C-reactive protein-binding sites in human atherosclerotic aortic lesions by a modified streptavidin-biotin-staining method. *Pathol Int.* 1995;45(9):635–641.

186. Ridker PM, Buring JE, Cook NR, Rifai N. C-reactive protein, the metabolic syndrome, and risk of incident cardiovascular events: an 8-year follow-up of 14 719 initially healthy American women. *Circulation.* 2003;107(3):391–397.

187. Mendall MA, Patel P, Ballam L, Strachan D, Northfield TC. C reactive protein and its relation to cardiovascular risk factors: a population based cross sectional study. *BMJ.* 1996;312(7038):1061–1065.

188. Visser M, Bouter LM, McQuillan GM, Wener MH, Harris TB. Elevated C-reactive protein levels in overweight and obese adults. *JAMA.* 1999;282(22):2131–2135.

189. Moran A, Steffen LM, Jacobs DR Jr, et al. Relation of C-reactive protein to insulin resistance and cardiovascular risk factors in youth. *Diabetes Care.* 2005;28(7):1763–1768.

190. Abd TT, Eapen DJ, Bajpai A, Goyal A, Dollar A, Sperling L. The role of C-reactive protein as a risk predictor of coronary atherosclerosis: implications from the JUPITER trial. *Curr Atheroscler Rep.* 2011;13(2):154–161.

191. Lee S, Kwak HB. Role of adiponectin in metabolic and cardiovascular disease. *J Exerc Rehabil.* 2014;10(2):54–59.

192. Nascimento H, Costa E, Rocha S, et al. Adiponectin and markers of metabolic syndrome in obese children and adolescents: impact of 8-mo regular physical exercise program. *Pediatr Res.* 2014;76(2):159–165.

193. Lim S, Quon MJ, Koh KK. Modulation of adiponectin as a potential therapeutic strategy. *Atherosclerosis.* 2014;233(2):721–728.

194. Expert Panel on Integrated Guidelines for Cardiovascular Health and Risk Reduction in Children and Adolescents; National Heart, Lung, and Blood Institute. Expert panel on integrated guidelines for cardiovascular health and risk reduction in children and adolescents: summary report. *Pediatrics.* 2011;128(suppl 5):S213–S256.

195. Murray R, Battista M. Managing the risk of childhood overweight and obesity in primary care practice. *Curr Probl Pediatr Adoles Health Care.* 2009;39:145–166.

196. National High Blood Pressure Education Program Working Group on High Blood Pressure in Children and Adoles-

cents. The fourth report on the diagnosis, evaluation, and treatment of high blood pressure in children and adolescents. *Pediatrics.* 2004;114(2 suppl 4th report):555–576.

197. Freedman DS, Khan LK, Serdula MK, Dietz WH, Srinivasan SR, Berenson GS. Racial differences in the tracking of childhood BMI to adulthood. *Obes Res.* 2005;13:928–935.

198. Katzmarzyk PT, Pérusse L, Malina RM, Bergeron J, Després JP, Bouchard C. Stability indicators of the metabolic syndrome from childhood and adolescence to young adulthood: the Quebec family study. *J Clin Epidemiol.* 2001;54:190–195.

199. Morrison JA, Fredman LA, Wang P, Glueck CJ. Metabolic syndrome in childhood predicts adult metabolic syndrome and type 2 diabetes mellitus 25-30 years later. *J Pediatr.* 2008;152:201–206.

200. Strong WB et al. Evidence based physical activity for school-age youth. *J Pediatr.* 2005;146:732–737.

201. Hopkins ND, Stratton G, Tinken TM, et al. Relationships between measures of physical fitness, physical activity, body composition, and vascular function in children. *Atherosclerosis.* 2009;204:244–249.

202. Racette SB, Weiss EP, Hickner RC, Holloszy JO. Modest weight loss improves insulin action in African Americans. *Metabolism.* 2005;54:960–965.

203. Thompson PD, Buchner D, Pina IL, et al; American Heart Association Council on Clinical Cardiology Subcommittee on Exercise, Rehabilitation, and Prevention; American Heart Association Council on Nutrition, Physical Activity, and Metabolism Subcommittee on Physical Activity. Exercise and physical activity in the prevention and treatment of atherosclerotic cardiovascular disease: a statement from the Council of Clinical Cardiology and the Counsel on Nutrition, Physical Activity and Metabolism. *Circulation.* 2003;24:3109–3116.

204. Moore LL, Singer MR, Bradlee ML, et al. Intake of fruits, vegetables and dairy products in early childhood and subsequent blood pressure changes. *Epidemiology.* 2005;16:4–11.

205. Couch SC, Saelens BE, Levin L, Dart K, Falciglia G, Daniels S. The efficacy of a clinic based behavioral nutrition intervention emphasizing a DASH-type diet for adolescents with elevated blood pressure. *J Pediatr.* 2008;152:494–502.

206. Daniels SR, Greer FR, and the Committee on Nutrition. Lipid screening and cardiovascular health in childhood. *Pediatrics.* 2008;122:198–208.

207. McCrindle BW, Urbina EM, Dennison BA, et al; American Heart Association Atherosclerosis, Hypertension, and Obesity in Youth Committee; American Heart Association Council of Cardiovascular Disease in the Young; American Heart Association Council on Cardiovascular Nursing. Drug therapy of high-risk lipid abnormalities in children and adolescents: a scientific statement from the American Heart Association Atherosclerosis, Hypertension, and Obesity in Youth Committee, Council of Cardiovascular Disease in the Young, with the Council on Cardiovascular Nursing. *Circulation.* 2007;115:1948–1967.

208. Spear BA, Barlow SE, Ervin C, et al. Recommendations for treatment in children and adolescents with overweight or obesity. *Pediatrics.* 2007;120:S254–S288.

209. Inge TH, Krebs NF, Garcia VF, et al. Bariatric surgery for severely overweight adolescents: concerns and recommendations. *Pediatrics.* 2004;114(1):217–223.

Test Your Knowledge Answers

1. The correct answer is **A.**
2. The correct answer is **E.**
3. The correct answer is **E.**

15

Lipid Disorders

Elizabeth L. Wright, MS, RD, CSP, LDN; **Megan Dougherty,** RD, CSP, LDN, CNSC; and **Kristi Drabouski,** RD, CSP, LDN, CNSC

CONTENTS

Learning Objectives

1. Understand cardiovascular disease risk and the etiologies of lipid disorders.
2. Describe how to screen for lipid disorders and interpret laboratory results.
3. Discuss the role of dietary factors and physical activity in treating lipid disorders.

Background

Cardiovascular disease (CVD) is the leading cause of death both globally and in the United States, and it is more prevalent for those with low to middle income levels.[1-3] Although death occurs in adulthood, the risk factors and risk behaviors leading to CVD begin in early childhood and adolescence.[4] Risk factors include family history, age, sex, nutrition/diet, physical inactivity, tobacco exposure, high blood pressure, abnormal blood lipid levels, overweight/obesity, diabetes mellitus, predisposing conditions, metabolic syndrome, inflammatory markers, perinatal factors, and certain medications. Blood lipid levels can be easily monitored throughout the lifespan. The specific abnormal serum cholesterol levels include a high concentration of total cholesterol (TC), high low-density lipoprotein (LDL) cholesterol, high non–high-density lipoprotein (non-HDL), a low concentration of high-density lipoprotein (HDL) cholesterol, and high triglycerides (TGs). Nutrition intervention during childhood plays a critical role in CVD prevention and dyslipidemia treatment to reduce the risk of CVD.

Types of Lipid Disorders

Dyslipidemias can be defined as abnormalities, including both deficiency and overproduction, in lipid and lipoprotein metabolism.[4] Dyslipidemias are determined by age, sex, and racial cutoffs. Primary lipid disorders are caused by genetic or environmental factors. Dyslipidemia can also be due to secondary causes.

Primary Lipid Disorders

Types of primary lipid disorders include familial hypercholesterolemia (FH), familial defective apolipoprotein B, familial combined hyperlipidemia (FCH), polygenic hypercholesterolemia, familial hypertriglyceridemia, severe hypertriglyceridemia, familial hypoalphalipoproteinemia, and dysbetalipoproteinemia.[4] Of these, the most common types found in children and adolescents are FH and FCH. Polygenic hypercholesterolemia is also common but may not occur until after adolescence.

Familial Hypercholesterolemia

FH is typically caused by mutations in genes that affect LDL receptors, and 2 types of the disorder exist, heterozygous FH (FH) and homozygous FH (HoFH).[5] People with FH have inherited a mutated gene from one parent and have LDL cholesterol levels > 160 mg/dL with either normal or low HDL cholesterol levels and TC levels exceeding 230 mg/dL.[4] This form is more common, affecting approximately 1 in 500 people.[5] Symptoms are not present in childhood, but an acceleration of atherosclerosis and premature CVD is present, which then causes a coronary event in 50% of men and 25% of women with FH by the age of 50 years.[4] People with HoFH have inherited 2 mutated genes and have LDL cholesterol levels > 500 mg/dL with low HDL cholesterol levels, thus leading to TC levels of 600–1000 mg/dL.[4,5] This form is rare, affecting approximately 1 in 1 million people.[5] In HoFH, physical manifestations begin in infancy and childhood with the presence of xanthomata and tendonous xanthomata, with CVD developing by the second decade. People with HoFH may respond to medications, but many will need LDL apheresis with a goal of palliation of the disease until genetic therapy or pharmacotherapy becomes available.[4]

Familial Combined Hyperlipidemia

FCH is characterized by elevated TC levels, TG levels, or both in affected people and their first-degree relatives, with variable lipid and lipoprotein patterns.[6] The exact genetic defect or mechanism is not known, and several defects or

mechanisms may possibly be involved.[7] However, hepatic very low-density lipoprotein (VLDL) overproduction appears to be the underlying cause.[8] Presently, FCH has an estimated prevalence of 1%–2% in the general population worldwide and 10%–20% in survivors of myocardial infarction.

Polygenic Hypercholesterolemia

Polygenic hypercholesterolemia is caused by a combination of genetic susceptibility and environmental factors such as diet, weight, and physical inactivity.[6] LDL cholesterol levels are elevated but generally milder than in FH. If obesity is present, some children may have high TG levels and low HDL cholesterol levels. Prevalence is approximately 1 in 10–20 adults depending on age. No symptoms are noted but an increased risk exists for coronary heart disease. Children with polygenic hypercholesterolemia often respond well to nutrition and lifestyle behavior modifications.

Secondary Causes

Secondary causes of dyslipidemia include endocrine, metabolic, renal, hepatic, and storage disease; inflammatory and infectious conditions within the body; and certain medications.[4] Specific conditions seen in pediatrics include but are not limited to diabetes, chronic kidney disease, nephrotic syndrome, obstructive liver disease, alagille syndrome, systemic lupus erythematosis, post solid organ transplantation, anorexia nervosa, obesity, and childhood cancer survival. Certain medications include progestins, anabolic steroids, glucocorticoids, psychotherapeutic drugs, and retinoic acid acne treatment. Treatment of secondary causes usually normalizes lipid levels unless compounding factors are present.

Screening and Laboratory Interpretation

Tables 15-1 and 15-2 indicate who should be screened for lipid disorders and the screening procedure. Interpretation of the resultant fasting lipid profile is delineated in Figure 15-1.

Nutrition Management

The emphasis on a healthy diet and lifestyle is key in the prevention of CVD and treatment of abnormal blood lipid levels.[9] To prevent CVD in all children ≥ 2 years old, recommendations include a daily diet with total fat < 30% of total calories, saturated fat < 10% of total calories, avoidance of trans fat, monounsaturated and polyunsaturated fats up to 20% of total calories, and dietary cholesterol < 300 mg/d.[4] Furthermore, CVD prevention also includes increasing

Table 15-1. Screening Guidelines[4]

Whom to screen?

1. Universal screening once between ages 9 and 11 years and once between ages 17 and 21 years[a]
2. Any patient ≥ 2–8 or 12–16 years of age with any of the following CVD risk factors:
   - A parent, grandparent, aunt, or uncle with CVD before age ≤ 55 years (male) or ≤ 65 years (female). CVD includes myocardial infarction, sudden cardiac death, coronary bypass surgery, balloon angioplasty, angina pectoralis, coronary atherosclerosis, peripheral vascular disease, or stroke
   - A parent with a total cholesterol ≥ 240 mg/dL
   - A family history that is not available (adopted child)
   - Other cardiovascular risk factors: obesity (BMI ≥ 95th percentile), smoking, diagnosed hypertension, type 1 or type 2 diabetes, chronic renal disease, nephrotic syndrome, end-stage renal disease, post renal transplant, chronic inflammatory disease, Kawasaki disease with current or regressed coronary aneurysms, HIV infection, post-orthotopic heart transplant
   - Treatment with retinoid acid, anticonvulsants, or oral contraceptives

BMI, body mass index; CVD, cardiovascular disease.
[a]No universal screening needed between ages 12 and 16 years because total cholesterol and low-density lipoprotein levels decrease significantly by 10%–20% during puberty, then elevate again to prepuberty levels.[4]

Table 15-2. Laboratory Testing[4]

How to screen?

- For universal screening, obtain non-fasting lipid profile (non-FLP) that includes
  - Total cholesterol (TC)
  - High-density lipoprotein cholesterol (HDL)
  - Non-HDL cholesterol (calculate using TC minus HDL)[a]
- If non-HDL >145 mg/dL or HDL <40 mg/dL, then obtain FLP twice, then average and including
  - Triglycerides (TGs)
  - Low-density lipoprotein cholesterol (LDL)
- If cardiovascular disease risk factors are present, obtain FLP twice, then average. FLPs may be obtained 2 weeks to 3 months apart.

[a]Non-HDL has been found to be a more predictive indicator of atherosclerosis.[4]

Figure 15-1. Interpretation of Lipid Profile[4]

TC < 170 mg/dL LDL < 110 mg/dL Non-HDL < 120 mg/dL TGs (0–9 years old) < 75 mg/dL, (10–19 years old) < 90 mg/dL HDL ≥ 45 mg/dL	• Acceptable lipid profile • Recheck lipid profile if any of the CVD risk factors develop with patient or patient's family

TC ≥ 200 mg/dL
LDL ≥ 130 mg/dL
Non-HDL ≥ 145 mg/dL
TGs (0–9 years old) ≥ 100 mg/dL,
(10–19 years old) ≥ 130 mg/dL
HDL < 45 mg/dL
	• Confirm with FLP twice, then average
	• Consider referral to lipid specialist, especially if LDL ≥ 250 mg/dL or TGs ≥ 500 mg/dL
	• Initiate appropriate nutrition management
	• Recheck levels in 3–6 months
	• Consider pharmacological intervention for high-risk patients
	• Consider further assessment
	  ○ Evaluate for secondary causes
	  ○ Evaluate for familial disorders
	  ○ Screen family members

CVD, cardiovascular disease; FLP, fasting lipid profile; HDL, high-density lipoprotein; LDL, low-density lipoprotein; TC, total cholesterol; TGs, triglycerides.

CVD, unflavored reduced fat cow's milk is considered safe and appropriate, but its use should be discussed with child's primary care provider.[4] Additional dietary management for high-risk patients should always be tailored based on individual lipid profile and involve counseling with a lipid specialist and registered dietitian or other skilled clinician to ensure effective nutrition intervention while maintaining appropriate growth and development.

Dietary Cholesterol

Dietary cholesterol is found in animal-based foods and can be reduced by limiting foods such as butter, egg yolk, high-fat meat, beef, poultry with skin, and whole milk dairy products. Although limiting dietary cholesterol has less of a serum lipid lowering effect and has a more variable response among individuals than limiting saturated and trans fats, it is still important because cholesterol and saturated fat are found together in most foods.[11] In general, LDL may be decreased by 3%–5% if dietary cholesterol is restricted to < 200 mg/d. In addition, an increase of 100 mg/d of dietary cholesterol increases total serum cholesterol by 2–3 mg/dL.

Dietary Fats

Saturated Fats

Limiting saturated fats can help to lower LDL levels.[11] Saturated fat is found more in animal-based than plant-based

consumption of fruits, vegetables, fish, whole grains, and reduced-fat dairy products, while reducing the intake of fruit juice, sugar-sweetened beverages and foods, and salt.[10] For children ≥ 2 years old at risk for CVD, the daily diet should be further restricted to saturated fat < 7% of total calories and dietary cholesterol to < 200 mg/d. For children between 12 months and 2 years of age who are overweight, obese, or have a family history of obesity, dyslipidemia, or foods. A major source of saturated fat is red meat (fatty beef and lamb), but dairy products (cream, butter, cheese, and other dairy products made with whole milk) are also commonly overlooked as a source of saturated fat in children's diets. Plant-based sources of saturated fat are mainly found in tropical oils (coconut, palm, and palm kernel), which are often used in commercially baked goods. To reduce saturated fat intake, whole milk dairy products may be replaced with low-fat or nonfat ("skim") dairy products, and leaner cuts of meat may be recommended. Low-fat, reduced fat, and baked cookies, crackers, and other baked goods should be consumed instead of full-fat versions. Using additional saturated fat in the cooking process should be limited. Low-fat cooking methods such as broiling, grilling, steaming, microwaving, poaching, or baking are preferable to frying.[12] Saturated fats should be limited to < 7% total calories in children with high cholesterol.[4] This can be achieved by reading food labels and choosing products with <2 g of saturated fat per serving.

Trans Fats

Trans fats, or hydrogenated fats, are produced when fat is hydrogenated to make it solid at room temperature. In the process of hydrogenation, bonds in the *cis* position are switched to the *trans* position, which has been shown to increase LDL and decrease HDL cholesterol in people who consume the trans fats. Trans fats are found mostly in stick margarine, high-fat baked goods, shortening, commercial frying oils, and fried snack foods. Examples of these foods are doughnuts, pastries, biscuits, crackers, cookies, potato and tortilla chips, french fries, and other bakery and snack foods. Trans fats should be avoided in the diet for all children ≥ 2 years old.[4] Nutrition labels are allowed to list 0 g of fat per serving if the product contains < 0.5 g of trans fat per serving. Therefore, to ensure a food is completely free of trans fat, it is important to check the ingredients for hydrogenated and/or partially hydrogenated oils.[13]

Monounsaturated and Polyunsaturated Fats

Children with dyslipidemia are encouraged to replace saturated and trans fats with the healthier monounsaturated and polyunsaturated fats, which decrease LDL cholesterol levels.[4] Monounsaturated fats are found in avocados, peanuts, and many other nuts and seeds and in vegetable oils such as olive, canola, peanut, sunflower, and sesame oil.[14] Polyunsaturated fats are found in walnuts and sunflower seeds, fatty fish (salmon, tuna, mackerel, herring, and trout), and vegetable oils such as soybean, corn, and safflower oils.[15] It is important to note that while these fats are healthy, they are still calorically dense and should be limited as recommended by the Dietary Guidelines for Americans, especially for weight maintenance or loss.[10]

Simple Carbohydrates

Simple sugars and carbohydrates, found in foods such as sweetened beverages, desserts, snacks, and white breads and other refined starches, raise triglycerides more than saturated and trans fats. Patients with hypertriglyceridemia primarily need to limit their intake of simple carbohydrates and replace them with complex carbohydrates.[4,16] Sugar-sweetened beverage consumption in young children, aged 3–11 years, has been reported to have a positive association with decreased HDL cholesterol levels as well.[17] Intake of 100% fruit juice is recommended to be no more than 4–6 oz per day.[18] For children who are overweight or obese and have high triglycerides, limiting dietary fat, especially saturated and trans fats, and increasing physical activity should also be recommended in addition to limiting simple carbohydrates because obesity will have a direct effect on triglyceride levels.[10] Instructing patients to limit their intake of sugar-sweetened beverages and choosing food products with no more than 12 g of sugar per serving can help decrease the overall amount of sugar in their diet.

Fiber

Fiber combined with a low-fat diet may help to improve cholesterol levels further. Soluble fiber such as oat bran, psyllium, pectin, and guar gum primarily decreases LDL cholesterol levels and has some effect on increasing HDL cholesterol levels.[19] An increase in soluble fiber of 5–10 g/d may reduce LDL by 3%–5%.[6] One study found that children who consumed psyllium fiber along with a diet low in dietary fats and cholesterol, lowered LDL cholesterol by an additional 5%–10%.[20] Fiber binds to bile acids and decreases cholesterol absorption. Specific guidelines for the suggested amount of fiber intake for children with dyslipidemia currently do not exist and remain controversial. However, general guidelines for estimating adequate fiber intake in children are found in the Dietary Reference Intake and are generally much higher than most children and adolescents consume, which is 14 g of fiber per 1000 estimated calories needed per day for older children and adolescents.[4,21] Another commonly used method is adding 5 to the child's age to obtain the recommended daily intake of fiber in grams.[22] Meeting dietary fiber requirements can be achieved by increasing intake of whole fruit and vegetables by consuming them at each meal and snack time, aiming for at least 5 servings per day. Children are also recommended to have half of their grains intake as whole grains by consuming whole grain/high-fiber foods in place of refined grain products.[18,23] This can be achieved by reading food labels and choosing products with at least 3 g fiber per serving.

Plant Sterols/Stanols

Plant sterols and stanols are essential components of cell membranes in plants, and they are structurally similar to cholesterol. Plant stanols are saturated sterols and have no double bonds. They inhibit absorption of dietary cholesterol and decrease re-absorption of cholesterol from bile. Plant sterols are found naturally in foods but not in large quantities. They have been incorporated into products such as margarine/butter spreads, oatmeal, and some snacks and are also available as chews and capsules. Several studies have shown improved LDL cholesterol levels in adults consuming plant sterols, but fewer studies have been done in children and adolescents.[24,25] A randomized control study in children using 2 g of plant sterol in margarine per day decreased LDL cholesterol levels by 8%.[26] More recently, a small prospective study fortified a yogurt-based drink with 2 g of plant sterols, and children consumed the drink daily for 6–12 months.[27] LDL cholesterol and small dense LDL cholesterol levels decreased significantly in the children, but the levels remained higher than in the control group. The Expert Panel recommends 2 g/d of plant sterols and stanols for children and adolescents > 2 years old.[4] However, plant sterols may theoretically have the potential to decrease levels of fat-soluble vitamins such as vitamin A (β-carotene) or vitamin E (α-tocopherol).[26] One study showed lower levels of β-carotene with normal vitamin A levels after adults consumed 2–3 g of plant stanol esters daily.[28] However, fortification of vitamin A in phytosterol-enriched milk resulted in significantly improved levels of LDL cholesterol levels with no change in concentration of β-carotene.[29] Vitamin deficiencies can typically be prevented by increasing intake of food sources of both vitamin A and vitamin E. A multivitamin may be considered if additional risk factors for vitamin deficiency are present.[26]

Omega-3 Fatty Acids

The ω-3 fatty acids docosahexaenoic acid (DHA) and eicosapentaenoic acid (EPA) are found in fish oils and ocean fish (herring, mackerel, salmon, and sardines) and lower TG levels by inhibiting VLDL and *apolipoprotein B* synthesis. While fish intake alone has been shown to be cardioprotec-

tive, it has no effect on TC, LDL, or HDL cholesterol levels and has only been shown to lower TG levels. Still, the Expert Panel recommends increasing fish consumption for CVD prevention; no specific guidelines exist for pediatrics, but the recommendation for adults is 2–3 servings per week.[30] Intake of fish and seafood alone may not meet the ω-3 fatty acid amount needed to decrease TG levels significantly, therefore DHA and EPA supplementation maybe needed. DHA and EPA may be synthesized from α-linolenic acid, which is found in flaxseed oil, canola oil, soy oil, and walnuts. DHA/EPA supplementation of 2–4 g/d in adults, showed a decrease in TG levels by 10%–20%. However, prescription forms of this supplementation are not currently approved by the U.S. Food and Drug Administration (FDA) for use in children. Supplementation of 1–2 g/d of DHA/EPA may be recommended for children with triglycerides > 500 mg/dL.[4,16] It should be noted that over-the-counter fish oil supplements are often dosed with the total grams of fish oil, but one should pay attention to total grams of combined DHA and EPA and not total grams of fish oil in dosing supplements for the treatment of high triglycerides.

Soy Protein

The effect of soy on lowering cholesterol remains controversial. While some studies show soy isoflavones can decrease LDL cholesterol levels and TG levels and increase HDL cholesterol levels, others show little or no effect. Although a daily intake of 25 g of soy in adults may decrease TC and LDL cholesterol levels from 1.5% to 4.5%, this may be related more to the use of soy as a substitute for foods high in saturated fat.[31,32] No recommendations have been made for children. While the cholesterol-lowering benefits of soy remain controversial, soy can provide polyunsaturated fatty acids, fiber, vitamins, and minerals beneficial for cardiovascular and overall health.[19]

Enteral Nutrition Management

No studies have specifically focused on patients with dyslipidemia receiving specialized enteral nutrition supplementation. However, the same principles for oral intake can be used for enterally fed patients > 2 years old. For those with elevated LDL cholesterol levels, a diet low in fat and high in soluble fiber is recommended. Many standard pediatric formulas designed for tube feeding (milk protein based, 1 cal/mL) provide approximately 35%–45% of calories from fat. Many standard adult formulas designed for tube feeding (milk protein based, 1 cal/mL) provide approximately 30%–35% of calories from fat.[33,34] Lower fat and fat-free formulas are available and typically contain an increased amount of carbohydrate. Note that higher calorie formulas (>1.0 cal/mL) have a higher amount of fat to increase calories. Most standard pediatric and adult formulas do not contain fiber. Choose a formula that has added fiber or add a fiber supplement to provide the recommended amount of fiber. For patients with elevated TG levels, recommendations are to monitor carbohydrate intake. Choose a formula with lower carbohydrate content. Note many formulas designed for oral intake have a higher amount of carbohydrates for palatability because they come in a variety of flavors such as vanilla, chocolate, and strawberry.

Parenteral Nutrition Management

Elevated TG levels may occur in >30% of patients receiving parenteral nutrition (PN). These levels can occur due to multiple issues including prematurity, infection, inflammation, hypothyroidism, renal and liver failure, insulin resistance, medications, and prolonged PN use. They can also occur with an excessive amount of macronutrients such as carbohydrates or fat and possibly phytosterols. If left untreated, elevated TG levels may cause complications such as pancreatitis, lipid pneumonitis, an impaired immune system, and neurologic changes. Treatment for patients on PN with elevated TG levels include withholding the intravenous fat emulsion (IVFE) or adding carnitine or heparin to the PN solution. Changing to an alternative IVFE, such as one that is fish oil based, has been shown to lower TG levels significantly.[35]

Fats and Carbohydrates

An excessive amount of fat or carbohydrates can cause elevated TG levels in the patient receiving PN. High lipid infusion rates (>0.15 g/kg/h) may exceed the rate of metabolism and can lead to an accumulation of lipids in the liver cells, causing an increase in serum TG levels and impairing liver function. In this situation, IVFE is held for 4–6 hours to allow for clearance of fat from the blood. It may need to be held for several days but must be restarted to avoid essential fatty acid deficiency (EFAD). EFAD can develop with an intake of fat < 1%–2% of total calories in children and < 4%–5% of total calories in infants. Signs and symptoms of deficiency can appear in as little as 1–2 weeks.[35] Preterm infants need at least 0.25 g/kg/d IVFE to meet essential fatty acid requirements. Some hospitals limit the amount to 3 g/kg/d. Neonates < 32 weeks gestation, small for gestational age, or extremely low birth weight, may not be able to tolerate IVFE doses higher than 2 g/kg/d. The rate of lipid clear-

ance is decreased in preterm infants, causing elevated TG levels mainly due to immature enzyme systems, limited adipose tissue mass, and hepatic immaturity. The infants may also not be able to tolerate high glucose infusion rates if the IVFE is limited to <1 g/kg/d to prevent development intestinal failure-associated liver disease.[36,37]

Oil Source of IVFE

Soybean oil–based IVFE is the main product available for use in the United States. This type of oil is high in phytosterols, mainly sitosterol, campesterol, and stigmasterol, which are absorbed in small amounts in the small intestine and slowly metabolized by the liver. Long-term use of soybean oil–based IVFE may lead to a progressive increase and accumulation of phytosterols in cell membranes and plasma lipoproteins, which has been associated with the development of cholestasis in children on PN.[36,38] Along with prolonged PN, an accumulation of parenteral phytosterols may contribute to the development of intestinal failure-associated liver disease in neonates.[39] Soybean oil–based IVFE can predispose patients to high TG levels. The amount of phospholipid content varies with different concentrations of IVFE, its volume, and the rate of administration. The use of 10% is discouraged in children because of the high phospholipid content per gram of fat. Therefore, the use of 20% IVFE is encouraged.[35]

Soybean oil–based IVFE can also predispose patients to elevated TG levels because it is rich in ω-6 fatty acids. Fish oil–based IVFE, used mainly in Europe and not approved for use in the United States, contains more ω-3 fatty acids and very little ω-6 fatty acids. Omega-3 fatty acids have hypolipidemic activity, thus reducing TG concentration by reducing VLDL. Patients who have been able to receive fish oil–based IVFE have had a significant decrease in TG levels and blood glucose levels.[35]

Carnitine and Heparin

Carnitine is responsible for transporting long-chain fatty acids into the mitochondria for fatty acid oxidation to produce energy. The compound is biosynthesized from the amino acids lysine and methionine. Most neonates, especially those who are premature and weigh < 5 kg, have been found to be carnitine deficient.[40] Preterm infants usually have reduced stores because carnitine accretion happens in the last trimester of gestation. Carnitine can be supplemented in the PN solution at a dose of 2–5 mg/kg/d.[41] Supplementation as high as 10–20 mg/kg/d has been used in patients with elevated TG levels and those on PN longer than 7 days.[42] Carnitine has also been shown to lower TC levels and increase HDL levels.[35]

Heparin stimulates lipoprotein lipase activity by degrading TGs into fatty acid and glycerol. This activity is depressed in preterm infants. Infants receiving 1 U/mL heparin had lower TG levels than those receiving 0.5 U/mL or no heparin in PN solution.[37]

Physical Activity

Physical activity is beneficial for children and adolescents with dyslipidemia due to its effects on raising HDL cholesterol levels and decreasing TG and TC levels. Improvement of LDL cholesterol levels and insulin resistance have also been documented.[4] In addition, physical activity plays a critical role in maintaining an appropriate weight, which also affects blood lipid levels. Physical activity should be encouraged in all patients with dyslipidemia unless another medical condition contraindicates this. Current physical activity guidelines recommend that children have at least 60 minutes of moderate to vigorous physical activity daily, including vigorous physical activity at least 3 days per week.[4,43] Table 15-3 provides a summary of dietary interventions and physical activity recommendations for specific lipid abnormalities.

Pharmacologic Intervention

Statins, Bile Acid–Binding Resins, and Cholesterol-Absorption Inhibitors

Medications may be considered in conjunction with nutrition and physical activity interventions for patients 8 years and older with an LDL ≥ 190 mg/dL, especially in children with family members with CVD and in the presence of CVD risk factors. Statin therapy may be considered for children ages 10 years and older with LDL ≥ 160–189 mg/dL and a family

history of CVD and multiple CVD risk factors.[4] HMG-CoA reductase inhibitors, or statins, are the recommended class of medications to lower LDL cholesterol levels in pediatric patients. Statins have been shown to be safe and effective in lowering cholesterol in a number of clinical trials, though they have generally been short term.[44–47] Patients, however, need to be monitored closely for liver and muscle side effects. Bile acid–binding resins form another class of cholesterol-lowering medications, but they are not routinely recommended in pediatrics due to limited effectiveness and poor compliance, mainly due to gastrointestinal side effects such as gas, bloating, constipation, and cramps. Cholesterol-absorption inhibitors are the newest class and are often combined with other medications such as statins, but they have not yet been extensively studied in children; therefore, usage is not approved.[4]

Antioxidants

Antioxidants have been suggested as a possible treatment for dyslipidemia because oxidized LDL is implicated in plaque development. Although daily supplementation of vitamins C and E may improve endothelial function, large-scale clinical trials have not shown any benefit related to the primary or secondary prevention of CVD.[31,48] Studies in children are limited, and antioxidant vitamin supplementation is not currently recommended to manage dyslipidemia.[48]

Red Yeast Rice Extract

Red yeast rice extract supplements contain mevinic acids, or monacolins, with monacolin K having the highest concentration. Monacolin K is chemically identical to lovastatin, a statin therapy used to treat dyslipidemia.[49] Only one study has shown that the use of red yeast rice supplements in children ages 8–16 years lowers TC and LDL cholesterol levels.[50] One popular red yeast rice supplement called Cholestatin was removed from the market by the FDA for

Table 15-3. Summary of Nutrition and Physical Activity Recommendations for Specific Lipid Abnormalities[4,10,16,43]

LIPID ABNORMALITY	FIBER	SIMPLE CARBOHYDRATES	DIETARY CHOLESTEROL	TRANS FATS	SATURATED FATS	ω-3 FATS	PHYSICAL ACTIVITY
High LDL	Increase	DGA	<200 mg	Avoid	<7% total calories	DGA	Increase
High TGs	DGA	Decrease	<200 mg	Avoid	<7% total calories	Increase	Increase
Low HDL	DGA	DGA	<200 mg	Avoid	<7% total calories	DGA	Increase

DGA, Dietary Guidelines for Americans, 2010; HDL, high-density lipoprotein; LDL, low-density lipoprotein; TGs, triglycerides.

containing the prescription drug lovastatin. Many red yeast rice supplements are on the market, but their effectiveness is questionable without monacolin K as the active ingredient. Most of these supplements may also contain citrinin, a nephrotoxin. The amount of active ingredient in the supplements is not standardized, and they are largely unregulated.[49,51] Therefore, their use in children may be detrimental and is not recommended at this time.

Niacin

Niacin may help with the decrease of both LDL cholesterol and TG levels and raise HDL cholesterol levels. It may be used in conjunction with statin therapy in children with elevated TG levels ≥ 200–499 mg/dL and elevated non-HDL cholesterol levels ≥ 145 mg/dL, if the LDL cholesterol target level has been achieved. Adverse reactions include flushing and hepatic toxicity, and niacin can cause an increase in fasting blood glucose levels. Use of niacin supplementation is not recommended for children under the age of 2 years old.[4] There has been very few studies published and minimal research done on the use of niacin supplements in children.[52] Safety and efficacy of the supplement has not been evaluated; therefore, its use should be cautionary.[53]

Test Your Knowledge Questions

1. What is the acceptable level for LDL cholesterol in a fasting lipid profile in children and adolescents?
   A. <120 mg/dL
   B. <110 mg/dL
   C. <150 mg/dL

2. What percentage of saturated fats is recommended by the National Heart, Lung, and Blood Institute and American Academy of Pediatrics in children with high cholesterol?
   A. ≤20% total calories per day
   B. <10% total calories per day
   C. ≤30% total calories per day
   D. ≤7% total calories per day

3. In which lipid profile would ω-3 fatty acid supplementation be beneficial for a pediatric patient?
   A. LDL 200 mg/dL, triglycerides 80 mg/dL, HDL 50 mg/dL
   B. LDL 110 mg/dL, triglycerides 550 mg/dL, HDL 25 mg/dL
   C. LDL 120 mg/dL, triglycerides 150 mg/dL, HDL 25 mg/dL
   D LDL 180 mg/dL, triglycerides 100 mg/dL, HDL 30 mg/dL

Acknowledgments

The authors of this chapter for the second edition of this text wish to thank Shirley Huang, MD, and Melanie Katrinak, RD, CSP, LDN, for their contributions to the first edition of this text.

References

1. World Health Organization. Global status report on non-communicable diseases 2010. http://www.who.int/nmh/publications/ncd_report2010/en. Published April 2011. Accessed May 30, 2014.
2. Kochanek KD, Xu J, Murphy SL, Minino AM, Kung HC. Deaths: final data for 2009. *Natl Vital Stat Rep.* 2011;60(3): 1–117.
3. Fryar CD, Chen TC, Li X. Prevalence of uncontrolled risk factors for cardiovascular disease: United States, 1999–2010. *NCHS Data Brief.* 2012;(103):1–8.
4. Expert Panel on Integrated Guidelines for Cardiovascular Health and Risk Reduction in Children and Adolescents. Expert panel on integrated guidelines for cardiovascular health and risk reduction in children and adolescents: summary report. *Pediatrics.* 2011;5(128)(suppl):S213–S256.
5. Ziajka PE. Management of patients with homozygous familial hypercholesterolemia. *Am J Manag Care.* 2013;19(13) (suppl):S1–S5.
6. Expert Panel on Detection, Evaluation, and Treatment of High Blood Cholesterol in Adults. Executive Summary of the Third Report of the National Cholesterol Education Program (NCEP) Expert Panel on Detection, Evaluation, and Treatment of High Blood Cholesterol in Adults (Adult Treatment Panel III). *JAMA.* 2001;285(19):2486–2497.
7. Goldberg AC. Dyslipidemia. The Merck Manual for Health Care Professionals. http://www.merckmanuals.com/professional/endocrine_and_metabolic_disorders/lipid_disorders/dyslipidemia.html. Updated October 2013. Accessed May 28, 2014.
8. Veerkamp MJ, de Graaf J, Bredie JH, Hendriks JCM, Demacker PNM, Stalenhoef AFH. Diagnosis of familial combined hyperlipidemia based on lipid phenotype expression in 32 families: results of a 5-year follow-up study. *Arterioscler Thromb Vasc Biol.* 2002;22:274–282.
9. Rose G. Sick individuals and sick populations. *Int J Epidemiol.* 1985;14(1):32–38.
10. U.S. Department of Health and Human Services. 2010 dietary guidelines for Americans. http://www.health.gov/dietaryguidelines/2010.asp. Accessed June 5, 2014.
11. Howell WH, McNamara DJ, Tosca MA, Smith BT, Gaines JA. Plasma lipid and lipoprotein responses to dietary fat and cholesterol; a meta-analysis. *Am J Clin Nutr.* 1997;65:1747–1764.
12. American Heart Association. Saturated fats. http://www.heart.org/HEARTORG/GettingHealthy/NutritionCenter/HealthyEating//Saturated-Fats_UCM_301110_Article.jsp. Updated September 25, 2014. Accessed December 3, 2014.
13. American Heart Association. Trans fats. http://www.heart.org/HEARTORG/GettingHealthy/NutritionCenter/Healthy

Eating/Trans-Fats_UCM_301120_Article.jsp. Updated August 5, 2014. Accessed December 3, 2014.

14. American Heart Association. Monounsaturated fats. http://www.heart.org/HEARTORG/GettingHealthy/NutritionCenter/HealthyEating/Monounsaturated-Fats_UCM_301460_Article.jsp. Updated August 5, 2014. Accessed December 3, 2014.

15. American Heart Association. Polyunsaturated fats. http://www.heart.org/HEARTORG/GettingHealthy/NutritionCenter/HealthyEating/Polyunsaturated-Fats_UCM_301461_Article.jsp. Updated October 20, 2014. Accessed December 3, 2014.

16. Bamba V. Update on screening, etiology, and treatment of dyslipidemia in children. *J Clin Endocrinol Metab.* http://press.endocrine.org/doi/pdf/10.1210/jc.2013-3860. Published May 21, 2014. Accessed June 4, 2014.

17. Kosova E, Auinger P, Bremer AA. The relationships between sugar-sweetened beverage intake and cardiometabolic markers in young children. *J Acad Nutr Diet.* 2013;113(2):219–227.

18. American Heart Association. Dietary recommendations for healthy children. http://www.heart.org/HEARTORG/GettingHealthy/HealthierKids/HowtoMakeaHealthyHome/Dietary-Recommendations-for-Healthy-Children_UCM_303886_Article.jsp. Updated September 10, 2014. Accessed December 3, 2014.

19. Dalidowitz C. Nutrition management of dyslipoproteinemia. In: Nevin-Folino NL, ed. *Pediatric Manual of Clinical Dietetics.* 2nd ed. Chicago, IL: American Dietetic Association; 2003:319–340.

20. Kwiterovich PO Jr. Recognition and management of dyslipidemia in children and adolescents. *J Clin Endocrinol Metab.* 2008;93(11):4200–4209.

21. Food and Nutrition Board, Institute of Medicine. *Dietary Reference Intakes for Energy, Carbohydrate, Fiber, Fat, Fatty Acids, Cholesterol, Protein, and Amino Acids (Macronutrients).* Washington DC: National Academy Press; 2005.

22. Marcason W. What is the "age+5" rule for fiber? *J Am Diet Assoc.* 2005;105(2):301–302.

23. United States Department of Agriculture. MyPlate: grains. What foods are in the grains group? http://www.choosemyplate.gov/food-groups/grains.html. Accessed May 20, 2014.

24. McKenney JM, Jenks BH, Shneyvas E, et al. A soft gel dietary supplement containing esterified plant sterols and stannous improves the blood lipid profile of adults with primary hypercholesterolemia: a randomized, double-blind, placebo-controlled replication study. *J Acad Nutr Diet.* 2014;114(2):244–249.

25. Eussen ST, de Jong N, Rompelberg CJ, Garssen J, Verschuren WM, Klugel OH. Dose-dependent cholesterol-lowering effects of phytosterols/phytostanol-enriched margarine in statin users and statin non-users under free-living conditions. *Public Health Nutr.* 2011;14(10):1823–1832.

26. Tammi A, Ronnemaa T, Miettinen TA, et al. Effects of gender, apolipoproteína E phenotype and cholesterol-lowering by plant stanol esters in children: the STRIP study. Special Turku Coronary Risk Factor Intervention Project. *Acta Paediatr.* 2002;91(11):1155–1162.

27. Garoufi A, Vorre S, Soldatou A, et al. Plant sterols-enriched diet decreases small dense LDL cholesterol levels in children with hypercholesterolemia; a prospective study. *Ital J Pediatr.* 2014; 40:42.

28. Gylling H, Hallikainen M, Nissinen MJ, Miettinen TA. The effect of a very high daily plant stanol ester intake on serum lipids, carotenoids, and fat-soluble vitamins. *Clin Nutr.* 2010; 29(1):112–118.

29. Petroglanni M, Kanellakis S, Moschonis G, Manios Y. Fortification of vitamin A in a phytosterol enriched milk maintains plasma beta-carotene levels. *J Food Sci Technol.* 2014;51(1):196–199.

30. Dalidowitz C. Disorders of lipid metabolism. In: Leonberg B, ed. *Pediatric Nutrition Care Manual.* Chicago, IL: American Academy of Nutrition and Dietetics; 2014.

31. Fletcher B, Berra K, Ades P, et al. Managing abnormal blood lipids: a collaborative approach. *Circulation.* 2005;112:3184–3209.

32. Erdman JW Jr. AHA Science Advisory. Soy protein and cardiovascular disease: a statement for healthcare professionals from the Nutrition Committee of the AHA. *Circulation.* 2000;106:2555–2559.

33. Nestle Health Science. Nestle Nutrition. Products and applications. http://www.nestle-nutrition.com/Public/Default.aspx. Accessed October 1, 2014.

34. Abbott. Abbott Nutrition for Healthcare Professionals. All products by brand. http://abbottnutrition.com/brands/products/nutritional-products. Accessed October 1, 2014.

35. Gura K, Strijbosch R, Arnold S, McPherson C, Puder M. The role of an intravenous fat emulsion composed of fish oil in a parenteral nutrition-dependent patient with hypertriglyceridemia. *Nutr Clin Pract.* 2007;22:664–672.

36. Vanek VW, Seider DL, Allen P, et al; Novel Nutrient Task Force, Intravenous Fat Emulsions Workgroup; American Society for Parenteral and Enteral Nutrition Board of Directors. A.S.P.E.N. position paper: clinical role for alternative intravenous fat emulsions. *Nutr Clin Pract.* 2012;27(2):150–192.

37. Lim MS, Choi CW, Kim B, Yang HR. Clinical factors affecting lipid metabolism and optimal dose of heparin in preterm infants on parenteral nutrition. *Ped Gastro Hep Nutr.* 2013;16(2):116–122.

38. Forchielli ML, Bersani G, Tala S, Grossi G, Puggioli C, Masi M. The spectrum of plant and animal sterols in different oil-derived intravenous emulsions. *Lipids.* 2010;45(1):63–71.

39. Kurvinen A, Nissinen MJ, Andersson S, et al. Parenteral plant sterols and intestinal failure-associated liver disease in neonates. *J Pediatr Gastroenterol Nutr.* 2012;54(6):803–811.

40. Winther B, Jackson D, Mulroy C, MacKay M. Evaluation of serum carnitine levels for pediatric patients receiving carnitine-free and carnitine supplemented parenteral nutrition. *Hosp Pharm.* 2014;49(6):549–553.

41. Borum PR. Carnitine in parenteral nutrition. *Gastroenterology.* 2009;137(5 suppl):S129–S134.

42. Crill CM, Helms RA. The use of carnitine in pediatric nutrition. *Nutr Clin Pract.* 2007;22(2):204–213.

43. U.S. Department of Health and Human Services. 2008 physical activity guidelines for Americans. http://www.health.gov/paguidelines. Accessed May 21, 2014.

44. Lambert M, Lupien PJ, Gagne C, et al. Treatment of familial hypercholesterolemia in children and adolescents: effect of lovastatin. Canadian Lovastatin in Children Study Group. *Pediatrics.* 1996;97(5):619–628.

45. Wiegman A, Hutten BA, de Groot E, et al. Efficacy and safety of statin therapy in children with familial hypercholesterolemia: a randomized controlled trial. *JAMA.* 2004;292(3):331–337.

46. Avis HJ, Vissers MN, Stein EA, et al. A systemic review and meta-analysis of statin therapy in children with familial hypercholesterolemia. *Arterioscler Thromb Vasc Biol.* 2007;27:1803–1810

47. Eiland LS, Luttrell PK. Use of statins for dyslipidemia in the pediatric population. *J Pediatr Pharmacol Ther.* 2010;15:160–172.

48. Engler MM, Engler MB, Malloy MJ, et al. Antioxidants vitamins C and E improve endothelial function in children with hyperlipidemia: Endothelial Assessment of Risk From Lipids in Youth (EARLY) Trial. *Circulation.* 2003;108:1059–1063.

49. Cunningham E. Is red yeast rice safe and effective for lowering serum cholesterol? *J Am Diet Assoc.* 2011;111(2):324.

50. Guardamagna O, Abello F, Baracco V, Stasiowska B, Martino F. The treatment of hypercholesterolemic children: efficacy and safety of a combination of red yeast rice extract and policosanols. *Nutr Metab Cardiovasc Dis.* 2011;21(6):424–429.

51. Childress L, Gay A, Zargar A, Ito MK. Review of red yeast rice content and current Food and Drug Administration oversight. *J Clin Lipidol.* 2013;7(2):117–122.

52. McCrindle BW, Urbina EM, Dennison BA, et al. Drug therapy of high-risk lipid abnormalities in children and adolescents: a scientific statement from the American Heart Association Atherosclerosis, Hypertension, and Obesity in Youth Committee, Council of Cardiovascular Disease in the Young, with the Council on Cardiovascular Nursing. *Circulation.* 2007;115:1948–1967.

53. Pasquali SK, Li JS. Prevention of future cardiovascular disease in high-risk pediatric patients: a role for lipid lowering therapy? *Circ Cardiovasc Qual Outcomes.* 2008;1:131–133.

Test Your Knowledge Answers

1. The correct answer is **B**. The Expert Panel on Integrated Guidelines for Cardiovascular Health and Risk Reduction in Children and Adolescents has set <110 mg/dL LDL cholesterol level as the acceptable level. Less than 120 mg/dL is the acceptable level for young adults, 20–24 years old. An LDL cholesterol level ≥ 130 mg/dL is considered high.

2. The correct answer is **D**. Children with elevated LDL cholesterol, non-HDL cholesterol, and TG levels should further restrict their diet from no more than 10% saturated fats of total calories to ≤7% saturated fats of total calories.

3. The correct answer is **B**. Children with elevated TG levels ≥ 200–499 mg/dL may be considered for ω-3 fatty acid supplementation along with increased fish intake, 25%–30% calories from fat, ≤7% of total calories from saturated fat, <200 mg/d of cholesterol, avoidance of trans fats, decreased sugar intake along with no sweetened drinks, and increased intake of complex carbohydrates.

16

Childhood Overweight and Obesity: Efficacy and Safety of Popular Diets and Weight Control Programs

Catherine Christie, PhD, RDN, LDN, FAND; **Claudia Sealey-Potts**, PhD, RDN FAND; **Corinne Labyak**, PhD, RDN; and **Judith C. Rodriguez**, PhD, RDN, FAND

CONTENTS

Learning Objectives

1. Describe the importance of weight maintenance vs weight loss recommendations for children and adolescents.
2. Critique one of the discussed popular diets for use with children.
3. Describe 3 positive characteristics of a weight-loss plan discussed for use with adolescents.
4. Assess the efficacy of a balanced macronutrient low-kilocalorie diet for use with children.

Background

The incidence and prevalence of childhood overweight and obesity has increased worldwide. In 2010, the number of overweight children under the age of 5 years was estimated to be over 42 million, with 35 million living in developing countries.[1] In the United States, obesity has more than doubled in children and quadrupled in adolescents in the past 30 years.[2,3] However, among 2–5 year old children, obesity has declined based on the Centers for Disease Control and Prevention's National Health and Nutrition Examination Survey data.[2] The percentage of children aged 6–11 years in the United States who were obese increased from 7% in 1980 to nearly 18% in 2012. Similarly, the percentage of adolescents aged 12–19 years who were obese increased from 5% to nearly 21% over the same period.[2,3] In 2012, more than one-third of children and adolescents were overweight or obese.[2] Childhood and adolescent obesity are associated with multiple health risks and adverse effects during childhood as well as later in life, such as sleep problems, bone and joint problems, endocrine disorders, respiratory problems, gastrointestinal problems, skin conditions, diabetes, nonalcoholic fatty liver disease, and other cardiovascular risk factors as well as social and psychological problems related to poor self-esteem.[4]

Children and adolescents who are obese are also likely to be obese as adults[5-9] and are therefore more at risk for adult health problems such as heart disease, type 2 diabetes, stroke, and osteoarthritis.[8] Increased risks for certain types of cancers have been linked to conditions of overweight and obesity, including cancer of the breast, colon, endometrium, esophagus, kidney, pancreas, gall bladder, thyroid, ovary, cervix, and prostate, as well as multiple myeloma and Hodgkin's lymphoma.[9] One study reported that children who became obese as early as age 2 were also more likely to be obese as adults.[7]

Healthy lifestyle habits, including appropriate food choices and regular physical activity, can lower the risk of becoming obese and the concomitant risk for chronic diseases.[6] The dietary and physical activity behaviors of children and adolescents are influenced by many sectors of society, including families, communities, schools, child care settings, medical care providers, faith-based institutions, government agencies, the media, and the food and beverage and entertainment industries. Schools play a particularly critical role by establishing a safe and supportive environment with policies and practices that support healthy behaviors. Schools also provide opportunities for students to learn about and practice healthy eating and physical activity behaviors.

Dietary intake data are also of concern. The Total Healthy Eating Index-2010 score is a measure of overall diet quality.[10] For children ages 2–17 years in 2003–2004, 2005–2006, and 2007–2008, total scores ranged from 47% to 50% of the maximum score, and the differences were not statistically significant. The average scores for all the components of the Healthy Eating Index-2010 survey were below the standards, indicating that the diet quality of children and adolescents fell short of dietary recommendations.[10] In addition, during the 7 days before the survey, 4.8% of students had not eaten fruit or consumed 100% fruit juices; 5.7% of students had not eaten vegetables (green salad, potatoes [excluding French fries, fried potatoes, or potato chips], carrots, or other vegetables); 17.3% of students had not consumed milk; 11.3% of students had consumed a can, bottle, or glass of soda or pop (not counting diet soda or diet pop) 3 or more times per day; and 13.1% of students had not eaten breakfast.[10] The diet quality scores of children and adolescents would be improved by increasing the intake of vegetables, especially dark greens and beans; replacing refined grains with whole grains; substituting seafood for some meat and poultry; and decreasing the intake of sodium (salt) and empty calories from solid fats and added sugars.[10]

Successful, scientifically sound weight-loss measures with dietary, physical activity, and social support components are needed to assist youth. According to the Youth Risk Behavior Survey, which is part of the Youth Risk Behavior Surveillance System, a large number of adolescents use unhealthy methods to lose or maintain weight, evidenced by the finding that during the 30 days preceding the survey, 12.2% of students went without eating for 24 hours or more, 4.3% had vomited or taken laxatives, and 5.1% had taken diet pills, powders, or liquids without a doctor's advice.[10]

Systematic reviews of childhood obesity and expert committee recommendations have emerged over the last several years,[11-14] and all agree that child and adolescent obesity treatment should

- be directed at motivated families in which the child and/or parents perceive obesity to be a problem and are willing to make lifestyle changes
- be directed at the entire family rather than just the overweight/obese child
- aim for weight maintenance in children unless body mass index (BMI) is > 99th percentile
- be more intensive and comprehensive than has been the norm
- combine changes in diet plus changes in physical activity and/or reduction in sedentary behavior

The current definitions state that if BMI is greater than or equal to the 95th percentile based on sex-specific and age-specific reference data from the Centers for Disease Control and Prevention growth charts, the child is "obese," and if BMI is between the 85th and 94th percentiles for sex and age, the child is "overweight" (Table 16-1).

Clinical Approach to the Overweight/Obese Child or Adolescent

The Academy of Nutrition and Dietetics evidence-based analysis of pediatric overweight literature on intervention programs reports strong evidence for multicomponent, family-based programs for children between the ages of 5 and 12 and limited evidence for multicomponent, family-based programs for adolescents. Formats may vary with adolescents and parents together or separated. The components included diet, physical activity, nutrition counseling, and parent or caregiver participation.[15,16]

Interventions should be based on the family's readiness to change.[14] Parents and family members should be counseled that the following behaviors have been associated with an increased risk of childhood and adolescent obesity:

Table 16-1. Weight Recommendations According to Age and BMI Percentile[14]

AGE	TARGET
2-5 y	
BMI of 85th-94th percentile	Weight maintenance until BMI of <85th percentile or slowing of weight gain, as indicated by downward deflection of BMI curve.
BMI of ≥95th percentile	Weight maintenance until BMI of <85th percentile; however, if weight loss occurs with healthy, adequate-energy diet, then it should not exceed 1 lb/mo. If greater loss is noted, then patient should be monitored for causes of excessive weight loss.
6-11 y	
BMI of 85th-94th percentile	Weight maintenance until BMI of <85th percentile or slowing of weight gain, as indicated by downward deflection of BMI curve.
BMI of 95th-98th percentile	Weight maintenance until BMI of <85th percentile or gradual weight loss of ~1 lb/mo. If greater loss is noted, then patient should be monitored for causes of excessive weight loss.
BMI of ≥99th percentile	Weight loss not to exceed average of 2 lb/wk. If greater loss is noted, then patient should be monitored for causes of excessive weight loss.
12-18 y	
BMI of 85th-94th percentile	Weight maintenance until BMI of <85th percentile or slowing of weight gain, as indicated by downward deflection of BMI curve.
BMI of 95th-98th percentile	Weight loss until BMI of <85th percentile, no more than average of 2 lb/wk. If greater loss is noted, then patient should be monitored for causes of excessive weight loss.
BMI of ≥99th percentile	Weight loss not to exceed average of 2 lb/wk. If greater loss is noted, then patient should be monitored for causes of excessive weight loss.

BMI, body mass index.

Reproduced with permission from *Pediatrics*, Vol. 120, p. 254. Copyright © 2007 by the American Academy of Pediatrics.

- Restriction of highly palatable foods
- Consumption of high-calorie foods at meals and snacks consumed both at and away from home
- Increased portion size of meals
- Skipping breakfast

The following health behaviors were included in recommendations by the American Academy of Pediatrics[12,17]:

- Consumption of ≥5 servings of fruits and vegetables per day
- Limits of ≤2 hours of screen time per day; no television, computers, or video games in the room where the child sleeps; no television during dinner; and no television or other entertainment media if the child is < 2 years of age
- ≥ 1 hour of physical activity per day

Use of Popular Diets

Parents of overweight or obese children may be overweight themselves and often look to popular diets as a means of losing weight. Because these diets are often adopted by the family and modified for children or adolescents, a discussion of the use of popular diets for pediatric patients is warranted.

Family-friendly popular diets include elements of healthy eating that are applicable or can be easily modified to safely include children. Popular diets can be categorized into 7 major types: behavioral, food-focused, reduced macronutrient content, food group guides or exchange systems, food timing or specific combinations of meals and snacks, commercial meal or snack replacements, and an "other" category for plans that do not fit in any previous category.[18] Within each category of weight-loss diets, many are effective in reducing weight because regardless of the plan or claim, the principal goal is to lower caloric intake by prescribing limits on food intake. However, the scientific evidence consistently concludes that successful weight loss should be coupled with a plan that enables the dieter to manage weight over a lifetime.[18] The more extreme the plan, the more difficult it is to follow over the long term. The key for lifelong weight management is following a plan individualized to each person's needs. Kilocalorie-controlled and portion-controlled diets seem to be more conducive to long-term compliance than fat-restricted and carbohydrate-restricted diets.[18]

According to the Weight Control Registry,[19] adults who are successful at losing weight and keeping it off individualize their changes in lifestyle to include eating and exercise behaviors that they can sustain for a lifetime. Therefore, when considering any change in eating behavior, individuals should consider nutrition, food variety, moderate portions, ease of including these into their lifestyle, ways to continue them for an extended time, and how to add physical activity and reduce sitting time. For many, the term "diet" evokes thoughts of something temporary. The resultant "on-off" mindset produces short-term change only and does not address the underlying behaviors that created the need to change eating behaviors in the first place.

Successful weight-reduction programs reduce body weight and body fat gradually by decreasing caloric intake and increasing caloric expenditure. Individual plans may also include healthful foods such as fruits and vegetables in the diet. An increase in physical activity builds or maintains muscle mass and, together with aerobic activity, determines the utilization of body fat reserves and thus the metabolic rate or the rate of kilocalories being burned. Diets that promise immediate or fast weight loss are not recommended because they defy the scientific basis for metabolism, particularly in children because their normal growth and development may be inhibited. Such claims are at best misleading and at worst, potentially harmful. The mathematics of energy balance estimates that fat loss occurs at the rate of 1–2 pounds per week, even when a person severely restricts caloric intake. Weight loss greater than the recommended 1–2 pounds per week can only occur by losing muscle mass and water in addition to fat.[20]

Before undertaking a diet, families should set reasonable and reachable goals for weight loss with their healthcare provider and a registered dietitian. A plan for changing the diet for the family should first be evaluated to ensure that it is compatible with lifestyle and health needs. The family should be able to foresee continuing the plan indefinitely. A lifestyle change is required to prevent periods of on-and-off dieting and regression to the previous habits that initially caused weight gain. On-and-off dieting contributes to weight regain and could negatively impact health and affect chronic disease progression.

Meta-analysis of Intervention Programs for Children and Adolescents

A meta-analysis was recently published evaluating 52 studies published between 2000 and 2011.[21] The overall effect size was .068 ($P < .001$) with no significant differences between programs offered during school or after school. Programs working with children aged 15–19 were most effective ($r = .133$), and programs working with boys and girls were more effective ($r = .110$) than those working with girls alone ($r = .073$). Program effectiveness was higher with older children, in programs including physical activity and nutrition education combined with parental involvement, and lasting at least 1 year.

Lifelong Weight Management

Overweight and obese individuals can lose weight by following lower calorie diets that vary widely in macronutrient composition. Although caloric composition has been used to promote many varied diets over the years, caloric restriction rather than macronutrient composition is the key determinant of weight loss. Further research is needed to determine the optimal dietary macronutrient composition for improving specific comorbid conditions, such as impaired glycemic control, hypertension, and/or cardiovascular disease risk.

Wadden et al[22] reported that:

The choice of a diet also should address patient preferences, particularly those related to ease of dietary adherence.[23] A successful reducing diet is one that an individual can adhere to for several months to lose 5%–10% of initial weight. Greater weight loss is desirable because it is associated, in a linear manner, with greater improvements in cardiovascular disease risk factors, including hemoglobin A_{1c} (HbA$_{1c}$), blood pressure, triglycerides, and high-density lipoprotein cholesterol.[24] Although dietary interventions for hypertension and other comorbid conditions have shifted to the prescription of dietary patterns, such as the Dietary Approaches to Stop Hypertension (DASH) diet,[25,26] such approaches must be combined with calorie restriction to induce clinically meaningful weight loss (as they have in some recent trials).[27,28] To achieve long-term weight loss, most obese individuals must consciously restrict their energy intake, whether by reducing portion sizes, decreasing the energy density of the diet, counting calories (or specific macronutrients), or some combination of these approaches.[29]

Behavioral modification is also an important component of weight management programs.

Types of Popular Diets

Although a myriad of popular diets exist, most share common claims or principles that enable them to be grouped into a few categories.

Behavioral Weight-Management Plans

Behavioral weight management focuses on changing behaviors related to food intake rather than focusing solely on the foods themselves:

- Plan what to eat in advance
- Make physical activity an integral part of the day
- Eat 3 daily meals that include carbohydrates, proteins, and fats
- Enjoy fresh foods and flavorful fruits and vegetables in season
- Focus on smaller portions of high-quality foods
- Do not skip meals or induce feelings of deprivation
- Avoid obsessing about eating and dieting
- Eat without stuffing oneself or feeling guilty
- Change one's environment to avoid overeating or eating foods one does not really want
- Simply get back on track following a relapse

Behavioral plans emphasize the importance of assessing and creating an environment that increases cues for healthy eating and activity behaviors and minimizes the cues for unhealthy eating and activity behaviors. Helping participants create personal food environments that minimize unhealthy food-related decisions and/or unhealthy food exposure and maximize healthy food-related decisions and/or exposure may be very helpful for long-term weight loss and maintenance.

While not exclusive to this diet, behavioral approaches to weight loss that include portion control, regular physical activity, self-efficacy and self-regulation, and the monitoring of eating and weight have been shown to be effective for successful long-term weight management in adults.[16] These principles are also recommended for children and adolescents.[14] Behavioral strategies to help overweight children and their families include establishing a regular meal and snack pattern; eating smaller portions at meals and snacks; limiting second helpings to fresh fruit and nonstarchy vegetables; selecting lower calorie dairy products; eating more foods that are baked, broiled, grilled, or boiled instead of fried to reduce calories; selecting healthful snacks that include leaner protein along with fresh fruit, vegetables, or whole grain bread and cereals; and when eating out, selecting more healthful options or splitting larger servings to share with other family members or peers.[13]

The focus of behavioral change programs may also influence outcomes. A 2008 study by Epstein et al[30] looked at increasing healthy eating vs reducing high energy–dense foods to treat pediatric obesity. After a 24-month family-based behavioral treatment that focused on increasing fruits and vegetables and low-fat dairy vs reducing intake of high energy–dense foods, children in the increased health foods group showed greater reduction in BMI compared to children in the reduced high energy dense food group at 12 and 24 months. Parent change followed the same pattern as child change and were significantly correlated ($P < .001$).[30]

Food-Focused Weight-Loss Plans

One of the oldest and most well-known examples of a food-focused weight-loss plan is the grapefruit diet. Although grapefruit is credited with containing a special fat-burning enzyme, no scientific evidence exists to substantiate that claim. Another popular food-focused diet is the cabbage soup diet. Weight loss achieved through the grapefruit, cabbage soup, or any other "one food" diet is the result of limited food selection, reduced caloric intake, and loss of fluid. Complex carbohydrates and snacks between meals are forbidden, while most vegetables and all meat and fish are allowed. Meals comprise eggs, meat or fish, salads, vegetables, skim milk, tomato juice, and unlimited amounts of black coffee or tea. Each meal is accompanied by half a grapefruit or half a cup of unsweetened grapefruit juice. If no behavioral or lifestyle changes are instituted, it is likely that weight lost will be regained over time.[18] This type of plan would not be recommended for children or adolescents due to the potential for nutrient deficiencies, severely restricted caloric intake, and excessive weight loss.

A variation of this type of food focused diet is the Raw Food Diet. This diet includes only foods that have not been cooked, processed, microwaved, irradiated, genetically engineered, or exposed to pesticides and herbicides. It includes fresh vegetables, fruits, nuts, berries, seeds, and herbs in their unprocessed state. Weight loss achieved through the use of this diet is the result of very limited food selection and significant calorie reduction. The claim that cooking food significantly reduces vitamins in food as well as other plant phytochemicals is not supported by scientific evidence. This plan would not be recommended for children or adolescents due to the potential for severely restricted caloric intake and excessive weight loss.

Reduced Macronutrient Content Plans

The best known of the low-carbohydrate plans may be the Atkins Diet[31] followed by the South Beach Diet.[32] The most recent Atkins diet promotes 5 nutrition rules: a high consumption of protein, high consumption of fiber, substantial vitamin and mineral intake, low amounts of sugar, and the elimination of trans fats. Although physical activity is encouraged with the diet plan, the main focus is on high-protein, low-carbohydrate eating. Short-term research studies tracking the progress of adults on the diet have reported high levels of satiety, a temporary improvement in blood lipids and glucose levels, some loss of body fat, and the sparing of muscle protein.[33,34] Despite the up-and-down popularity of the Atkins or Atkins-type diets, plans that focus on healthier fats may produce better health outcomes. For example, in a 2-year trial, researchers concluded Mediterranean-style diets that are not necessarily lower in fat but focus on healthier fats and lower carbohydrate diets may be more effective alternatives to low-fat diets. The more positive effects on lipids with the low-carbohydrate diet and on glycemic control with the Mediterranean-style diet indicate that diets should be tailored to individual preferences and health risks.[35] Whereas reducing intake of simple sugars may be appropriate for children and adolescents, low-carbohydrate plans should not be universally recommended due to the potential low intake of fiber, nutrients, and kilocalories to support growth and development.

The South Beach Diet,[32] a variation on the carbohydrate-restricted diet is divided into 3 phases. Phase I allows lean meats, chicken, egg or egg substitutes, fish, olive oil, vegetables, salads, nuts, and some low-fat milk. Phase II introduces lower glycemic-index carbohydrates in limited amounts. Fruits are recommended for lunch or dinner, but not breakfast. Whole grain bread, sweet potatoes, and brown or wild rice in modest portions replace white bread, white potatoes, and white rice. Mashed, steamed cauliflower replaces mashed potatoes. Sandwiches are replaced by fillings in lettuce wraps. This phase lasts for 2 weeks or until the desired weight is lost. If overindulgence occurs during this phase, the recommendation is to return to Phase I for 1 week. Phase III is the lifelong maintenance phase where the emphasis is on the "good" carbohydrates and fats with restriction of the "bad" carbohydrates and fats. This low-kilocalorie, high-protein, lower-carbohydrate plan allows healthy fats, high-fiber foods, and selected carbohydrates in moderate amounts. The evidence suggests that moderate intake of carbohydrates, proteins, and healthy fats facilitates weight management in adults.[15] This plan is adaptable for use with children particularly in Phase III. However, the entire family should be committed to focusing on the consumption of more than 5 fruits and vegetables per day, min-

imizing sweetened beverages, increasing physical activity and reducing sedentary behaviors such as screen time, eating breakfast daily, limiting high-calorie meals and snacks outside the home including at fast-food venues and other restaurants, eating family meals at home at least 5 or 6 times per week, allowing children to self-regulate their meals, and avoiding overly restrictive behaviors.[14]

The Pritikin Diet[36] and the Dean Ornish Diet[37] are the most well-known of the low-fat diets that are still being used. Both diets were originally developed for the prevention and treatment of heart disease and also became popular as weight-loss diets. The Pritikin plan comprises a total caloric breakdown of 10% fat, 10%–15% protein, and 75%–80% carbohydrates with 35 g of fiber, less than 100 mg of cholesterol, and 600 mg of sodium. Exercise and stress management are integral to the plan. Encouraged as a life-long commitment, this restrictive, very low-fat, high-fiber plan requires extensive menu planning and may be difficult to implement because it entails careful label reading and product comparison.[18] In addition, no studies have evaluated the use of this diet in children or adolescents.

Like the Pritikin plan, the Dean Ornish Diet[37] allows only 10% of kilocalories from fat. It also limits sugar and honey. The restriction on fat and simple sugars prevents individuals from consuming excess kilocalories, and the high-fiber content contributes to a feeling of fullness. In addition, the diet promotes whole foods and a high intake of phytochemicals from plant-based foods and forbids meat, nuts, seeds, avocados, white flour, white rice, and fried foods. The diet also advocates a comprehensive lifestyle change including stress management training, smoking cessation, meditation, and moderate exercise. Strong scientific evidence supports the plan's claim to reverse the risk of heart disease in adults and the resulting weight loss is due to the caloric restriction.[37] However, no studies have evaluated the use of this diet in children or adolescents.

The newest diet in this category is the Paleo Diet[38] written by Loren Cordain, PhD. It is a high-protein, high-fiber eating plan that allows fresh lean meats, eggs and fish, fruits and vegetables, nuts and seeds, and "healthier" fats such as olive oil and coconut oil. The diet claims that by changing eating to resemble cavemen or Stone Age humans, weight can be lost and chronic diseases such as diabetes, heart disease, and cancer can be avoided. Foods that are not allowed on the diet included processed foods, wheat and other grains and legumes, dairy, potatoes, salt, refined sugar, and refined vegetable oils such as canola. No large randomized clinical trials have been conducted, but short-term studies with very small sample sizes comparing the Paleo diet to other eating plans have reported decreases in calorie intake, weight, and HbA_{1c} after 12 weeks.[39–43] These studies were all done in adults and this plan would not be recommended for children or adolescents due to the potential for nutrient deficiencies due to the restriction of dairy, grains, and legumes.

Food Group Guides/Exchange Systems

One example of a food group or exchange plan is the Volumetrics Weight-Control Plan.[44] Food choices are based on kilocalorie density. Fat, fiber, protein, and water content of foods all affect energy or kilocalorie density. By eating predominantly filling, low kilocalorie–dense foods, smaller portions of a few high kilocalorie–dense foods can be included, and the person will still lose weight due to the overall kilocalorie restriction. Low energy–dense foods include fruits and vegetables, skim milk, broth-based soups, fat-free salad dressings, pasta, cooked high-fiber grains, potatoes, legumes, low-fat meats, salads, low-fat soups, low-fat cheeses, cottage cheese, frozen yogurt, and kilocalorie-free beverages. This diet is complemented by regular exercise and behavior management, which includes keeping a food and exercise log, not skipping meals, identifying and managing cues to overeating, managing stress, and making a plan to handle setbacks. No foods are forbidden, and treats are allowed as long as the predominant eating style has a low-kilocalorie density.

Strong scientific evidence shows that reducing caloric intake combined with exercise and behavior management produces weight loss in adults.[16] No studies have evaluated the use of this diet in children or adolescents; however, it does contain many of the elements recommended (eg, focusing on > 5 fruits and vegetables per day, minimizing sweetened beverages, increasing physical activity and reducing sedentary behaviors as well as eating breakfast daily, limiting meals outside the home including at fast-food venues and other restaurants, allowing the child to self-regulate his or her meals, and avoiding overly restrictive behaviors).[14]

Food Timing/Meals and Snacks Combinations

A popular example of this category is the Suzanne Somer's diet and eating plan.[45] According to the diet in her many popular books, eating fat does not cause weight gain, sugar is more fattening than fat, and carbohydrates are not essential in the diet. According to Ms. Somers, weight gain is caused by hormonal imbalances and successful weight loss depends on keeping insulin stable following digestion. This stability is achieved by eating certain foods in specific combinations, cutting carbohydrate intake, and eliminating sugars and refined carbohydrates, starchy foods, white flour, caffeine, and "funky" foods. Meals should not be skipped and after eating fruit, the dieter should wait 20 minutes before consuming other foods. This diet has 2 levels. Level 1 is the most restrictive and is designed to initiate weight loss. Level 2 is the maintenance phase and introduces some protein, fat, and carbohydrate combinations. The rationale for the diet's effectiveness is not substantiated by scientific data; however, weight loss may be achieved due to the many food restrictions and the total caloric intake of the structured meals.[18] This type of plan would not be recommended for children or adolescents due to the lack of scientific validity in the premise, the potential for nutrient deficiencies, and severely restricted caloric intake.

Commercial Meal/Snack Replacements

One of the largest commercial weight-loss programs is Weight Watchers.[46] Weight Watchers International, Inc. has more than 1.5 million members attending 50,000 weekly meetings around the world. Weight Watchers was one of the first programs to incorporate a walking program and to emphasize physical activity as a necessary part of dieting. The POINTS Weight-Loss System assigns a point value to activities and food that is determined by the number of kilocalories, total fat, and dietary fiber in a defined serving. Each person is given a daily POINTS target that will lead to a caloric deficit that translates into 1–2 pounds per week weight loss. A second plan called the Core Plan focuses on choosing foods with low energy density. By routinely monitoring hunger cues and with an allowance for periodic "indulgences," the Core Plan has been shown to produce weight losses equal to the POINTS system. Strong evidence supports a lifestyle plan that includes regular monitoring and support systems using commonly available foods. The emphasis on portion control and low energy–density foods can be translated to many food settings, and the recipes help teach dieters to prepare dishes lower in kilocalories. Members do pay a fee for the weight-loss services including those on the Internet and for Weight Watchers–branded food items.[18] Weight Watchers does not recommend its plan for children and instead discusses children's needs in terms of 2 goals: ensuring the child grows and develops normally and helping the child reach a healthy weight. Weight maintenance strategies are recommended for children as young as 3 years of age[47] and weight gain in overweight young children should be limited to 2 pounds for every inch of growth.[48] Over age 4, it is recommended that the child maintain weight until the BMI drops down into the normal range, below the 85th percentile.[48]

Jenny Craig is a commercial diet plan that focuses on pre-packaged meals restricting calories and portion size. Instruction is provided for using knowledge gained regarding meal composition and portion size for after an individual finishes the plan. Participants meet weekly for one-on-one counseling with a Jenny Craig consultant. Consultants are not registered dietitian nutritionists but do have access to ones affiliated with the company. Diets are designed around current goals, fitness habits, motivation, and stress eating. They also encourage the concept of choosing low energy–dense foods to fill up, such as soups, salads, and raw vegetables. Special programs are available for people with type 2 diabetes. Vitamin/mineral supplements are recommended, and participants eat 3 meals and 2 snacks a day. Dessert is included in the dinner meal. Incentives are given with potential return of half the registration fee if participants keep the weight off after losing it. The Jenny Craig system is designed for adults and is not recommended for children or adolescents.[49]

Other Plans

Eat Right for Your Type was on the *New York Times* bestseller list and remains a popular diet plan today. The book provides 4 diets based on the blood types O, A, B, and AB. People with type O blood are described as hunters, who need a diet with lean high-protein, chemical-free meat, poultry, and fish with limited grains, beans, and legumes. Those with type A blood, the cultivators, need to eat predominantly vegetarian with fish and an emphasis on vegetables, tofu, grains, beans, legumes, and fruit. Type B, the nomads, should eat meat (no chicken), dairy, grains, beans, legumes, vegetables, and fruit. Type AB, the enigma, can eat a mixed diet in moderation including meat, seafood, dairy, tofu, beans, legumes, grains, vegetables, and fruit. Each blood type has a long list of forbidden foods including specific meats and poultry, seafood, dairy, eggs, oils and fats, nuts and seeds, beans, legumes, cereals, breads, muffins, grains, pasta, vegetables, fruit, juices, fluids, spices, condiments, herbal teas, and other beverages.

Each of the blood-type diets consists of whole, unprocessed foods, and all recommend the consumption of vegetables, which provide fiber, health-promoting nutrients, and phytochemicals. Physical activity, stress management, and reduction of health risks in the environment are integrated into each plan. However, no scientific evidence validates the claim that a diet should be defined by blood type. By limiting specific foods and sometimes food groups, those who follow the diet can lose weight, but the elimination of spe-

cific foods and groups is based on a premise without adequate scientific evidence.[18] A recent systematic review of evidence concluded "no evidence currently exists to validate the purported health benefits of blood type diets."[50] This diet plan is not recommended for children or adolescents.

Diets Designed for Use With Children and Adolescents

Balanced Macronutrient Low-Kilocalorie Diets

Evidence does suggest that short-term and long-term reduced energy (900–1200 kcal) may be an effective part of a multicomponent weight-management program in children 6–12 years of age.[16] In the adolescent population, the use of reduced energy (not less than 1200 kcal) is generally effective for short-term weight loss, but without a continued dietary intervention, weight is regained.[16]

Traffic Light Diet

The Traffic Light Diet was designed to promote weight loss, provide adequate kilocalories and nutrients for growth and development, and be easy to follow.[51] The diet divides foods into 5 categories, with the foods in each category separated into 3 color groups: green, yellow, and red. These colors correspond to the colors of a traffic light and signify GO (green), eat as much as you like of these foods; approach with CAUTION (yellow), eat in moderate amounts; and STOP (red), rarely or occasionally eat. Green foods are those foods that contain < 20 kcal per average serving and are found only in the vegetable and "free foods" categories. Yellow foods are staple foods that provide most of the nutrition from the protein, grain, fruit and vegetable, and milk and dairy food groups; a child should eat these foods in recommended amounts to obtain adequate nutrition. Red foods are foods that are high in calories from sugar or fat and exceed the caloric value of a yellow food, thereby providing low nutrient density. Initially, participants were limited to 4 red foods per week and 900–1200 calories, with some later studies using 1200–1500 calories.[51,52]

Results from a study by Epstein et al[52] showed that the parent and child intervention with diet and self-monitoring by both parent and child (group I) was clearly superior to diet and self-monitoring by the child alone (group II) and no diet or self-monitoring (group III, the control group). After 8 months and 21 months of treatment, the results for children in the 3 treatment groups were similar. Children's weight decreased by 16.6%, 18.6%, and 16.1% in groups I, II, and III, respectively. However, after 5 years, the children in group I maintained their relative weight change (–13.6%), while children in group II were at baseline (+3.3%) and the children in group III were heavier (+7%).[52]

MyPlate

MyPlate was designed by the US Department of Agriculture to replace the Food Guide Pyramid and is a general online guide for diet and exercise primarily for adults; however, it also includes a plan for preschool children.[53] MyPlate is also part of a larger initiative based on the *2010 Dietary Guidelines for Americans* to help consumers and their families make healthier food choices.[54] MyPlate illustrates the 5 food groups using a plate, which is familiar to most, and shows relational portions of various food groups.

The following nutrition messages are emphasized in the online material.

Balancing Calories
- Enjoy your food, but eat less
- Avoid oversized portions

Foods to Increase
- Make half your plate fruits and vegetables
- Make at least half your grains whole grains
- Switch to fat-free or low-fat (1%) milk

Foods to Reduce
- Compare sodium in foods like soup, bread, and frozen meals—and choose foods with lower numbers
- Drink water instead of sugary drinks

Formative research was done to ascertain what consumers knew about healthy eating and nutrition and what gaps in knowledge currently existed. The following is an excerpt from the final report[54]: "Overall, the qualitative research revealed that consumers know the basics about healthy eating. However, notable deficiencies still remain, particularly when it comes to weight management, a key recommendation from the 2010 *Dietary Guidelines for Americans*. Specifically, a lack of knowledge regarding portion sizes and total daily calorie limit may hinder consumer efforts to achieve and maintain a healthy weight, indicating a need for supportive resources and tools on calorie management and portion sizes." No studies evaluating the use of the MyPlate materials have been published.

Multidisciplinary Behavior Change Programs

Two examples of multidisciplinary behavior change programs for overweight children and their families are SHAPEDOWN and KidShape. Both were developed in academic medical centers and are offered in community settings such as hospitals or clinics with interdisciplinary teams of health professionals. They often include the disciplines of nutrition, exercise physiology, endocrinology, psychology, family therapy, adolescent medicine, family medicine, and/or behavioral and developmental pediatrics.

SHAPEDOWN incorporates behavioral techniques to address underlying issues of a child's or adolescent's weight. Included are problem solving, communication, and parenting skills (eg, limit setting and nurturing). In addition, cognitive therapy, stress management techniques, and body image therapies are used.[55] SHAPEDOWN was shown to produce significant long-term outcomes in a controlled study of 66 adolescents followed for 15 months who were randomly assigned to experimental or control groups. No significant differences were apparent between groups in any of the variables studied at the beginning of the study. The SHAPEDOWN group at the end of the treatment (3 months) and at 1-year follow-up (15 months) significantly decreased relative weight and significantly improved weight-related behavior, self-esteem, depression, and knowledge. The control group made no significant improvement in any of these variables except self-esteem.[56]

KidShape is a 9-week comprehensive family-based pediatric weight management program for overweight children and their families. Classes are divided into 3 major parts including a registered dietitian teaching adults and kids together about healthy eating for weight loss, separate meetings for adults and children with a mental health professional to learn to change habits and behaviors and receive group support, and meetings for adults to discuss their specific questions, while kids participate in 30 minutes of aerobic exercise; during 2 weeks adults and kids exercise together.[57] Program effectiveness was evaluated in a study of 1022 families from 24 community-based and hospital-based sites in Pennsylvania and California from 2004 through 2006.[58] Food records, activity logs, program questionnaires, and participant BMIs were obtained at the beginning and the end of the program. Statistically significant improvements in BMI, eating, physical activity, and self-esteem were reported.[36] A follow-up study looked at a convenience sample of 86 children at 3 months, 88 children at 6 months, 30 children at 12 months, and 15 children at 18–24 months after completion of the KidShape program. Graduates of the program maintained a significant change in BMI up to 24 months after the program and reported continued improvement in eating and physical activity.[59]

Conclusion

Many diets will result in weight loss or weight maintenance in adults and children because they lower and control caloric intake. The scientific evidence is strong that a successful weight-loss or weight-maintenance plan for children and adolescents should include reduced kilocalorie intake though consumption of ≥5 servings of fruits and vegetables per day and minimization or elimination of sugar-sweetened beverages (which are both present in a balanced macronutrient reduced kilocalorie diet and the Traffic Light Diet) as well as the behavioral components (eg, eating breakfast daily, limiting meals outside the home including at fast-food venues and other restaurants, eating family meals at least 5 or 6 times per week, allowing the child to self-regulate his or her meals, and avoiding overly restrictive behaviors). Long-term weight management happens when a plan is individualized to a family's needs and preferences. Kilocalorie-controlled and portion-controlled diets such as the balanced macronutrient low-calorie diets and the Traffic Light Diet have been studied over time and may be more conducive to long-term compliance in families than low-fat and carbohydrate-restricted diets.

Reviewing the various categories of popular and fad diets indicates that all have strengths and weaknesses and have the potential to result in weight loss in adults. However, for children and adolescents, these diets have not been studied due to potential risks for growing children and adolescents due to elimination of key food groups, greater-than-recommended caloric restriction, adverse behavioral patterns of eating, and/or lack of scientific evidence for the basis of the diet's recommendations. The key requirement for dietary treatment of overweight children and adolescents is to initiate and maintain lifelong healthy eating habits that focus on unhealthy weight in the short term and foster improved health outcomes in the long term. Family involvement, and particularly parental or caregiver involvement, in weight control, weight maintenance, and weight-loss interventions is associated with weight loss in children, and the use of behavior change techniques as an integral part of the program improves weight outcomes for both children and parents.[60]

Test Your Knowledge Questions

1. According to the Academy of Nutrition and Dietetics Evidence Analysis Library, which of the following clinical approaches had positive effects when working with overweight/obese children ages 5–12?
   A. Multicomponent, school-based
   B. Behavioral, family-based
   C. Multicomponent, family-based
   D. Diet, family-based

2. The parents of an 8-year-old child have decided to implement changes that will promote healthier lifestyle habits among all the family members. Which one of the following changes is recommended when there is readiness to change?
   A. Adding a salad or vegetable to lunch and dinner meals
   B. Substituting the dinner soda with a caffeine-free beverage
   C. Limiting family television viewing time to 3 hours a day
   D. Taking the family for a 30-minute walk after dinner

3. Diets that have been studied for use with children or adolescents include
   A. MyPlate and The (Children's) Atkins Plan
   B. The Traffic Light Diet and Behavior Change
   C. The Traffic Light Diet and the Pritikin Plan
   D. The Volumetrics and the Exchange Plans

4. Many of the popular/fad diets commonly used by adults are generally not recommended for children for all of the following reasons except:
   A. Their potential negative risks to a growing child related to the elimination or decrease of a key food group
   B. Greater than recommended caloric restriction
   C. Promotion of an adverse eating pattern
   D. Adequate scientific data for use in children for the diet/plan

Acknowledgments

The authors of this chapter for the second edition of this text wish to thank Julia A. Watkins, PhD, MPH, for her contributions to the first edition of this text.

References

1. World Health Organization. Global Strategy on Diet, Physical Activity and Health. http://www.who.int/dietphysicalactivity/childhood/en/. Accessed May 22, 2014.
2. Ogden CL, Carroll MD, Kit BK, Flegal KM. Prevalence of childhood and adult obesity in the United States, 2011-2012. *JAMA*. 2014;311(8):806–814.
3. National Center for Health Statistics. *Health, United States, 2011: With Special Features on Socioeconomic Status and Health*. Hyattsville, MD: U.S. Department of Health and Human Services; 2012.
4. National Institutes of Health, National Heart, Lung, and Blood Institute. *Disease and Conditions Index: What Are Overweight and Obesity?* Bethesda, MD: National Institutes of Health; 2010.

5. Guo SS, Chumlea WC. Tracking of body mass index in children in relation to overweight in adulthood. *Am J Clin Nutr.* 1999;70:S145–148.

6. Freedman DS, Khan LK, Serdula MK, Dietz WH, Srinivasan SR, Berenson GS. The relation of childhood BMI to adult adiposity: the Bogalusa Heart Study. *Pediatrics.* 2005;115:22–27.

7. Freedman D, Wang J, Thornton JC, et al. Classification of body fatness by body mass index-for-age categories among children. *Arch Pediatr Adolesc Med.* 2009;163:801–811.

8. Freedman DS, Khan LK, Dietz WH, Srinivasan SR, Berenson GS. Relationship of childhood obesity to coronary heart disease risk factors in adulthood: the Bogalusa Heart Study. *Pediatrics.* 2001;108:712–718.

9. Kushi LH, Byers T, Doyle C, et al; American Cancer Society 2006 Nutrition and Physical Activity Guidelines Advisory Committee. American Cancer Society guidelines on nutrition and physical activity for cancer prevention: reducing the risk of cancer with healthy food choices and physical activity. *CA Cancer J Clin.* 2006;56:254–281.

10. Centers for Disease Control and Prevention. youth risk behavior surveillance system—2011 national overview. http://www.cdc.gov/healthyyouth/yrbs/pdf/us_overview_yrbs.pdf. Accessed May 22, 2014.

11. Washington R. Overview of the expert recommendations for the assessment, prevention, and treatment of child and adolescent overweight and obesity. *Obes Manage.* 2008;2:20–23.

12. Barlow SE; Expert Committee. Expert committee recommendations on the assessment, prevention, and treatment of child and adolescent overweight and obesity. *Pediatrics.* 2007;120(suppl 4):S163–S288.

13. Kirk S, Scott BJ, Daniels SR. Pediatric obesity epidemic: treatment options. *J Am Diet Assoc.* 2005;105:S44–S51.

14. Spear BA, Barlow SE, Ervin C, et al. Recommendations for treatment of child and adolescent overweight and obesity. *Pediatrics.* 2007;120;S254–288.

15. American Dietetic Association. Position of the American Dietetic Association: individual-, family-, school-, and community-based interventions for pediatric overweight. *J Am Diet Assoc.* 2006;106:925–945.

16. Academy of Nutrition and Dietetics. Evidence analysis library. http://andevidencelibrary.com. Accessed May 21, 2014.

17. American Academy of Pediatrics. Media and children. http://www.aap.org/en-us/advocacy-and-policy/aap-health-initiatives/Pages/Media-and-Children.aspx. Accessed May 21, 2014.

18. Rodriguez J. *The Diet Selector.* Philadelphia, PA: Running Press; 2007.

19. National Weight Control Registry. Research findings. http://www.nwcr.ws/Research/published%20research.htm. Accessed May 27, 2014.

20. Evans SA, Parsons AD, Overton JM. Homeostatic responses to caloric restriction: influence of background metabolic rate. *J Appl Physiol.* 2005;99(4):1336–1342.

21. Vasques C, Magalhaes P, Cortinhas A, Mota P, Leitao J, Lopes VP. Effects of intervention programs on child and adolescent BMI: a meta-analysis study. *J Phys Act Health.* 2014;11:426–444.

22. Wadden TA, Webb VL, Moran CH, Bailer BA. Lifestyle modification for obesity: new developments in diet, physical activity, and behavior therapy. *Circulation.* 2012;125;1157–1170.

23. Dansinger ML, Gleason JA, Griffith JL, Selker HP, Schaefer EJ. Comparison of the Atkins, Ornish, Weight Watchers, and Zone diets for weight loss and heart disease risk reduction: a randomized trial. *JAMA.* 2005; 293:43–53.

24. Wing RR, Jeffery RW, Burton LR, Thorson C, Nissinoff KS, Baxter JE. Food provision vs structured meal plans in the behavioral treatment of obesity. *Int J Obes Relat Metab Disord.* 1996;20:56–62.

25. Wing RR, Lang W, Wadden TA, et al; Look AHEAD Research Group. Benefits of modest weight loss in improving cardiovascular risk factors in overweight and obese individuals with type 2 diabetes. *Diabetes Care.* 2011; 34:1481–1486.

26. Appel LJ, Champagne CM, Harsha DW, et al; Writing Group of the PREMIER Collaborative Research Group. Effects of comprehensive lifestyle modification on blood pressure control: main results of the PREMIER clinical trial. *JAMA.* 2003; 289:2083–2093.

27. Sacks FM, Svetkey LP, Vollmer WM, et al; DASH-Sodium Collaborative Research Group. Effects on blood pressure of reduced dietary sodium and the Dietary Approaches to Stop Hypertension (DASH) diet. *N Engl J Med.* 2001; 344:3–10.

28. Hollis JF, Guillon CM, Stevens VJ, et al; Weight Loss Maintenance Trial Research Group. Weight loss during the intensive intervention phase of the weight-loss maintenance trial. *Am J Prev Med.* 2008; 35:118–126.

29. Appel LJ, Clark JM, Yeh HC, et al. Comparative effectiveness of weight-loss interventions in clinical practice. *N Engl J Med.* 2011; 365:1959–1968.

30. Epstein LH, Paluch RA, Beecher MD, Roemmich JN. Increasing healthy eating vs. reducing high energy-dense foods to treat pediatric obesity. *Obesity.* 2008;16;318-326.

31. Atkins RC. *Atkins New Diet Revolution.* New York, NY: M. Evans & Co; 2002.

32. Agatson A. *The South Beach Diet.* New York, NY: Random House; 2003.

33. Sharman MJ, Gomez AL, Kraemer WJ, Volek JS. Very low-carbohydrate and low-fat diets affect fasting lipids and postprandial lipemia differently in overweight men. *J Nutr.* 2004;134:880–885.

34. Brehm BJ, Seeley RJ, Daniels SR, et al. A randomized trial comparing a very low carbohydrate diet and a kilocalorie-restricted low fat diet on body weight and cardiovascular risk factors in healthy women. *J Clin Endocrin Metab.* 2003;88(4):1617–1623.

35. Shai I, Schwarzfuchs D, Henkin Y, et al. Weight loss with a low-carbohydrate, Mediterranean, or low-fat diet. *N Engl J Med.* 2008;359:229–241.

36. Pritikin R. *The New Pritikin Program.* New York, NY: Simon & Schuster; 2000.

37. Ornish D. *Eat More Weight Less.* New York, NY: Harper Collins; 1993.

38. Cordain L. *The Paleo Diet.* Hoboken, NJ: John Wiley & Sons, Inc; 2011.

39. Jönsson T, Granfeldt Y, Ahrén B, et al. Beneficial effects of a Paleolithic diet on cardiovascular risk factors in type 2 diabetes: a randomized cross-over pilot study. *Cardiovasc Diabetol.* 2009;8:35.

40. Lindeberg S, Jönsson T, Granfeldt Y, et al. A Paleolithic diet improves glucose tolerance more than a Mediterranean-like diet in individuals with ischaemic heart disease. *Diabetologia.* 2007;50(9):1795–1807.

41. Jönsson T, Granfeldt Y, Erlanson-Albertsson C, et al. A paleolithic diet is more satiating per calorie than a Mediterranean-like diet in individuals with ischemic heart disease. *Nutr Metab (Lond).* 2010;7:85.

42. Frassetto LA, Schloetter M, Mietus-Synder M, et al. Metabolic and physiologic improvements from consuming a paleolithic, hunter-gatherer type diet. *Eur J Clin Nutr.* 2009;63(8):947–955.

43. Osterdahl M, Kocturk T, Koochek A, Wändell PE. Effects of a short-term intervention with a paleolithic diet in healthy volunteers. *Eur J Clin Nutr.* 2008;62(5):682–685.

44. Rolls B, Barnett RA. *The Volumetrics Eating Plan.* New York, NY: Harper Collins; 2005.

45. Somers S. *Eat Great, Lose Weight.* New York, NY: Random House; 1999.

46. WeightWatchers. Home page. http://www.weightwatchers.com. Accessed December 10, 2008.

47. Barlow S, Dietz W. Obesity evaluation and treatment: expert committee recommendations. *Pediatrics.* 1998;102(3):E29.

48. Daniels SR, Arnett DK, Eckel RH, et al. Overweight in children and adolescents: pathophysiology, consequences, prevention and treatment. *Circulation.* 2005;111:1999–2012.

49. U.S. News and World Report. Best weight loss diets. http://health.usnews.com/best-diet/best-weight-loss-diets. Accessed October 20, 2014.

50. Cusack L, De Buck E, Compernolle V, Vandekerckhove P. Blood type diets lack supporting evidence: a systematic review. *Am J Clin Nutr.* 2013;98:99-104.

51. Epstein LH, Valoski A, Wing RR, McCurley J. Ten-year follow-up of behavioral, family based treatment for obese children. *JAMA.* 1990;264:2519–2523.

52. Epstein LH, Valoski A, Wing RR, McCurley J. Ten-year outcomes of behavioral family-based treatment for childhood obesity. *Health Psychol.* 1994;13:373–383.

53. U.S. Department of Agriculture. MyPlate eating guide. http://www.ChooseMyPlate.gov. Accessed May 21, 2014.

54. U.S. Department of Agriculture, Center for Nutrition Policy and Promotion. Development of *2010 Dietary Guidelines for Americans*: Consumer Messages and New Food Icon—Executive Summary of Formative Research. http://www.choosemyplate.gov/food-groups/downloads/MyPlate/ExecutiveSummaryOfFormativeResearch.pdf. Published June 2011. Accessed May 27, 2014.

55. SHAPEDOWN. About SHAPEDOWN. http://www.shapedown.com/SD_About.html. Accessed May 21, 2014.

56. Mellin LM, Slinkard LA, Irwin CE Jr. Adolescent obesity intervention: validation of the SHAPEDOWN program. *J Am Diet Assoc.* 1987;87:333–338.

57. KidShape2.0. Information and description. http://www.kidshape.net/. Accessed May 21, 2014.

58. Rivard CW, Neufeld N. A comprehensive outcome analysis of a multi-site, multi state family-based pediatric weight management program. *J Am Diet Assoc.* 2007;107(8):A-11.

59. Rivard CW, Neufeld N. A long-term comprehensive evaluation of a family based pediatric weight management program implemented in multiple community based and hospital based sites. *J Am Diet Assoc.* 2008;109(9):A-94.

60. McLean N, Griffin L, Toney K, Hardeman W. Family involvement in weight control, weight maintenance and weight-loss interventions: a systematic review of randomized trials. *Int J Obes Relat Metab Disord.* 2003;27:987–1005.

Test Your Knowledge Answers

1. The correct answer is **C**. The Academy of Nutrition and Dietetics evidence-based analysis of pediatric overweight literature on intervention programs reported positive effects from one specific kind of intervention: multicomponent, family-based programs for children between the ages of 5 and 12. The components included were behavioral counseling, promotion of physical activity, parent training/modeling, dietary counseling, and nutrition education.

2. The correct answer is **A**. Interventions should be based on the family's readiness to change and include the following recommendations: consumption of ≥5 servings of fruits and vegetables per day; minimization or elimination of sugar-sweetened beverages; limits of ≤2 hours of screen time per day, no television in the room where the child sleeps, and no television if the child is < 2 years of age; and ≥ 1 hour of physical activity per day.

3. The correct answer is **B**. The Traffic Light Diet was designed to promote weight loss, provide adequate kilocalories and nutrients for growth and development, and be easy to follow. Behavior change was designed as a general guide for diet and exercise in adults; however, it has been used as a dietary component in childhood weight management programs.

4. The correct answer is **D**. For children and adolescents, these diets have not been studied due to potential risks for growing children and adolescents from elimination of key food groups, greater than recommended caloric restriction, adverse behavioral patterns of eating, and/or lack of scientific evidence for the basis of the diet's recommendations. The key requirement for dietary treatment of overweight children and adolescents is to initiate and maintain lifelong healthy eating habits that focus on unhealthy weight in the short term and foster improved health outcomes in the long term.

17

Pediatric Sports Nutrition

Jackie Buell, PhD, RD, ATC, CSSD; Diane L. Habash, PhD, MS, RD, LD; and Jessica Buschmann, MS, RD, LD

CONTENTS

Learning Objectives

1. Provide practitioners with the primary fueling concerns for young athletes.
2. Provide practitioners with the current evidence-based trends in sports nutrition.
3. Provide practitioners with potential interview advice and resources when counseling parents and children about fueling for sport.

Introduction

Evidence-based sports nutrition recommendations are not well established for child and adolescent athletes due to the sparse studies on this protected population. It is common to extrapolate studies from adult athletes to younger athletes while prioritizing the extra energy and nutrients to support growth and development. The few studies on child and adolescent sports nutrition topics will be presented within appropriate sections.

The young athlete differs from his or her nonathletic peers in the energy and nutrients needed to support training activities. The current dietary reference intakes for energy (Table 17-1) provide age-based and sex-based estimations for a spectrum of activity levels including active and very active adjustments.[1] The "active" activity factor is likely most appropriate for recreational activities in which participation is an average of an hour or so per day. Activities with a more intense time commitment would demand the "very active" adjustment for calorie intake. It may be important to realize that recent reviews suggest that heavy acute exercise or chronic exercise has an uncoupling effect on appetite and energy balance,[2] so some athletes may need specific guidance on how much food they need to reach body mass goals for

Table 17-1. Institutes of Medicine, Food and Nutrition Board, National Academy of Sciences Dietary Reference Intakes for Energy for Children and Adolescents[a]

BOYS	
3–8 y	EER = 88.5 – (61.9 × age [y]) + PA × (26.7 × weight [kg] + 903 x height [m]) + 20 kcal
9–18 y	EER = 88.5 – (61.9 × age [y]) + PA × (26.7 × weight [kg] + 903 x height [m]) + 25 kcal
	PA = 1.00, sedentary 1.13, low active 1.26, active 1.42, very active
GIRLS	
3–8 y	EER = 135.3 – (30.8 × age [y]) + PA × (10.0 × weight [kg] + 934 × height [m]) + 20 kcal
9–18 y	EER = 135.3 – (30.8 × age [y]) + PA × (10.0 × weight [kg] + 934 × height [m]) + 25 kcal
	PA = 1.00, sedentary 1.16, low active 1.31, active 1.56, very active

EER, estimated energy requirement; PA, physical activity.

[a]Data from *Dietary Reference Intakes for Energy, Carbohydrate, Fiber, Fat, Fatty Acids, Cholesterol, Protein, and Amino Acids (Macronutrients)*. Washington, DC: The National Academies Press; 2005.[1]

growth and sport. Nutrition should be personalized to the metabolism and goals of the athlete, so monitoring body changes and performance are important.

The tech-savvy practitioner might benefit from the interactive tool found on the Food and Nutrition Center's Web site at http://fnic.nal.usda.gov/fnic/interactiveDRI/. The tool allows the user to simply enter a patient's demographic information and check the selection boxes for the nutrients to be calculated; the generic answers will be provided for a mixed diet aligned with the current public guidelines. While the adjustment for energy is likely adequate for young athletes, the adjustments for other nutrients, such as carbohydrate and protein, may not support current fueling strategies. Ensuring adequate protein to support activity and muscle growth in lieu of some of the tool-suggested carbohydrate would better align with current sports nutrition guidelines. Similarly, the public nutrition education tool, ChooseMyPlate,[3] is not designed to meet the needs of the competitive athlete. Sports Nutrition has become a common focus of specialty study among registered dietitians (RDs), and the nutrition recommendations would be more personalized for the goals and body of each athlete with the help of a seasoned Sports RD (Certified Specialist in Sports Dietetics [CSSD] credential).

Low energy availability has been identified as a significantly detrimental issue in athletes of all ages. Energy availability is the amount of energy leftover (per kilogram lean mass) after daily consumption is adjusted for the amount of exercise.[4]

Energy Availability = (Calories in – Calories in Exercise)/kg Lean Body Mass

The International Olympic Committee has recently released a position statement on the relative energy deficiency in sport (RED-S) to supplement the prior literature on the female athlete triad.[5] Males are included in the RED-S paradigm, and the increased number of physiological detriments covers much more than menstrual dysfunction and bone health. The position statement includes an algorithm for return to normal physiological function as well as participation and return to play guidance for the medical staff. Less is known about the energy availability needs and influences for younger athletes, but after an athlete has finished puberty the current literature promotes 45 kcal/kg lean mass for optimal fueling and considers anything less than 30 kcal/kg lean mass as inadequate.[6] *Energy balance should be intentional according to the goals of the athlete.*

Macronutrient Needs

Distribution in Diet

Carbohydrates

Carbohydrates (CHOs) are considered the primary fuel for intense sporting activity,[7] and current sports nutrition position statements provide guidance relative to body weight for adults.[8,9] While some literature has suggested that children may need even more CHOs than adults,[10] Montfort-Steiger and Williams[11] challenge whether pre-pubertal athletes have developed similar glycolytic pathways to benefit from chronic high CHO ingestion. Substrate utilization is commonly and noninvasively determined by treadmill testing or cycling for aerobic capacity (indirect calorimetry), and many studies demonstrate lower respiratory quotients in children before puberty, demonstrating a greater reliance on fats at a given workload compared with older children or adults.[11,12] Data from lactate production studies in children would also suggest less reliance on CHOs, but it is unclear how diet manipulation may influence these studies. Similar to adult females, postmenarcheal adolescent females with normal reproductive hormones are likely better fat burners than male counterparts. Thus, CHO-feeding techniques used in adults may not be presumed as critical in pre-pubertal athletes or females. However, studies on children consuming CHOs during exercise show that children may be able to better utilize exogenous CHOs during intense exercise, and there is a clear benefit to time to exhaustion (Riddell).[13] Statements about substrate utilization are limited because prior studies on children and adolescents rarely control for long-term CHO intake, last longer than 1 hour, or include measures of muscle glycogen stores. *Care should be taken not to overfeed CHOs to young athletes at the expense of fat in the diet. The focus should be on a balanced diet with adequate CHOs to support training. Young athletes do seem to use exogenous CHOs well during exercise.*

The type of CHOs consumed may provide additional health or performance benefits. The Dietary Guidelines for Americans[14] encourage whole grains over processed grains or sugar-sweetened beverages for the health benefits of the whole grains. Traditional CHO wisdom would encourage more simple forms of CHO immediately before or during exercise to facilitate rapid absorption and delivery to the working muscle. The performance trials completed with young athletes typically use sports drink types of preparations. Limited data demonstrate the potential influence of low glycemic foods on children or adolescent performance. Intui-

tively, if the fueling strategy includes CHOs, a longer-lasting CHO (ie, one with slower gastrointestinal absorption) that is well-tolerated by the athlete's gut would provide a more sustained support of CHO-driven (high-intensity) exercise. While complex CHOs from foods are certainly more health promoting over the course of time, simple CHO sources taken during exercise from multiple sugars may benefit prolonged high-intensity exercise (eg, well-formulated sports drinks).[15]

Sports drinks, energy drinks, and sugar-sweetened beverages are commonly sought sources of exercise CHOs in youth populations. The American Academy of Pediatrics has issued a clinical report to discourage the use of these products due to the additional empty calories, artificial ingredients, and potential stimulants, although the academy qualifies that the statement does not apply to use for athletes.[16] Research demonstrates that 30%–50% of young athletes may be using energy drinks, and this is not an age-appropriate strategy for fueling or performance.[17] It has been reported in children that exogenous CHO consumption during activity will extend the time to high-intensity sprint exhaustion after extended endurance exercise,[17,18] thus justifying the appropriate use of formulated sports drinks in activities that last longer than about 45 minutes. The frequency, intensity, and length of sporting events as well as level of maturity will likely drive the needed CHOs in the young athlete's diet.

Finally, the central nervous system is responsive to blood glucose levels, with the young brain requiring more glucose than adult brains. As muscle glycogen decreases in adults with high-intensity exercise, fatigue ensues and some of the fatigue may be due to low blood glucose to the central nervous system.[19] Coordination and response time could possibly be mediated by CHO availability to the central nervous system as well. In adults, recent studies on mouth-rinsing with CHO indicate a clear role for the influence of CHOs on central mechanisms.[20] Studies on young athletes are sparse in these areas of research.

Protein

Protein is most respected as the nutrient that provides building blocks for new growth and tissue repair. Protein can be used as an energy source, but relative contributions are likely small as long as energy content of the diet is adequate. Current sports nutrition guidelines support that athletes need more protein than nonathletes.[8,9,21] The likely optimal range for adult athletes is supported between 1.2 and 1.7 g/kg of body weight. While the literature suggests that young people may be more efficient in how they handle body protein, child and adolescent athletes may need up 1.8–2.0 g/kg depending on goals (weight loss, weight gain, endurance, or strength). Boisseau et al[21] have documented nitrogen balance work that justifies male adolescent athletes (14-year-old soccer players) at a recommended dietary allowance of about 1.4 g/kg, but 2 of the 11 subjects were still in negative nitrogen balance. Aerenhouts et al[22] studied Flemish sprint athletes of both sexes and calculated a mean protein need of about 1.5 g/kg. While it is often a concern that too much protein may harm the liver and kidneys, no evidence supports high protein intakes being harmful in athletes with healthy liver and kidneys.[23]

Protein quality should also be assessed to support growth and muscle recovery. While the current dietary guidelines encourage the consumption of a plant-based diet, vegan athletes would need to include a wide variety of plant proteins in the diet to achieve protein quality. Athletes who consume animal products, such as dairy, meat, and eggs, are easily able to meet good-quality protein needs. Anecdotally, it is common for youth to have protein at 1 or 2 meals daily, instead of supporting the muscle throughout the day. Including multiple protein snacks and protein-centric meals throughout the day is currently recommended for the best lean mass response.[24,25]

Fats

Fats are critical for athletes to consume and are the preferred fuel for lower intensity activities.[7] The intramuscular triglyceride stores are an important fuel contributor to endurance exercise. Even though the current fueling paradigm suggests that athletes consume a high-CHO diet, eating enough fat to support the intramuscular fat stores is also important to proper fueling, especially for thin athletes who struggle to maintain body weight. Neutral advice is to consume fats within the current recommendation of 20%–35% of calories[1] with a balanced ratio of 1:1:1 for saturated, polyunsaturated, and monounsaturated fatty acids, respectively. This simply means consuming plant fats within the opportunities in which the athlete is choosing condiments or toppings such as olives, salad dressings, avocadoes, or nuts to achieve better balance. Low-fat diets are not in the young athlete's best fueling interest.

Fat is an important precursor to hormonal health, which illustrates the fundamental contributions that nutrients play in growth and development across the lifespan and in our immune systems. Dietary fat is important to balance for the overall health of the body, and no compelling evidence exists that young athletes would benefit from a low-fat diet. Young athletes should not be consuming low-fat (< 20% calories) diets. In the face of an obesity epidemic, it is important to evaluate overweight athletes for too much energy and fat in the training diet.

Many adult endurance athletes practice a keto-adapted diet in which the consumption of CHO is quite low to encourage the body to up-regulate the fat-metabolism enzymes during aerobic activity to tap the unlimited fat stores of the body during the very long distances.[26] Children are likely better at fat-burning (aerobic) pathways over glycolytic pathways.[11,12] Keto-adapting diets have been used in children to treat specific medical conditions, such as epilepsy or autism,[27] but have not been explored for fueling endurance sport. Even though young athletes may demonstrate lower respiratory quotients during exercise, CHOs still contribute to exercise, and exogenous CHOs may improve performance during intense exercise. For variety, nutrient balance, and growth, it is likely best to leave CHOs in the child and adolescent athlete's diet.

As the nutrition literature for the child and adolescent athlete grows, practitioners will be less reliant on adapting adult recommendations. Table 17-2 summarizes the current macronutrient suggestions of the adult athlete's diet, and provides rationale of child differences.

Table 17-2. Current Adult Sports Nutrition Macronutrient Guidelines[a]

MACRONUTRIENT	ADULT RECOMMENDATION	YOUTH DIFFERENCE
Carbohydrate	≥ 6 g/kg relative to workload	May be slightly less in children and female adolescents, similar for male adolescents
Protein	1.2–1.7 g/kg	Well supported around 1.5 g/kg in adolescents
Fat	20%–35% of calories in isocaloric diet	Similar in children but toward the high end of the range, fat phobia is poorly founded in child and adolescent athletes

[a]Data from Rodriguez et al,[8] Maughan and Shirreffs,[9] and Desbrow et al.[28]

Hydration

Ensuring adequate hydration is a safety concern as well as a performance advantage.[29-31] The goal of the sports nutrition program for an athlete is to maintain hydration throughout the day as well as throughout participation. Current guidelines suggest limiting loss of fluids to <2% of total body compared to precompetition weights.[30] These same guidelines suggest volumes and frequency for the adult athlete with the goal of maintaining light straw-colored urine and a consistent body weight according to the scale. It is sometimes useful to have a urine color chart to engage athletes in this hydration conversation.

A child athlete should consume 6 mL/lb of body weight during participation to be followed with 2 mL/lb/h after exercise to rehydrate.[32] A few studies demonstrate that children and adolescents are able to sense thirst well enough to maintain hydration if they are given the opportunity to consider it (ie, drink breaks).[33,34] It is important for coaches and parents to understand it is their job to help motivate the child to drink in order to maintain hydration.

Fluid loss and dehydration are often associated with heat stress injuries, which is a topic of debate among exercise scientists.[35] While many studies demonstrate the risk for heat injuries are higher in dehydration, poor hydration has not been proven to cause or allow for serious heat injuries; however, high ambient temperatures and thermal strain are common to both conditions. Compared with adults, young athletes have a higher body surface area and produce a higher thermal load for activity.[31] Adult athletes are demonstrated to sweat more than pre-pubertal athletes, while pre-pubertal athletes are better at cooling by radiation because of their greater body surface area. Ambient temperature and humidity are obviously critical factors in hydration. While prior research held that children were not as efficient as adults at thermoregulation, better-controlled research indicates that children do as well as adults when all variables are equal.[36] Regardless of cooling mechanisms, it is prudent to maintain hydration for performance and safety while participating in athletic activities in hot and humid environments. Taking ample time for recovery between practices or events and drinking sufficient amounts to meet the fluid and electrolyte deficit are critical for returning to fluid homeostasis.[36]

Nutrient Timing

The chronic training diet will impact health and performance, but the nutrient manipulation around the time of exercise is the crux of sports nutrition practice with examples provided in Table 17-3. Athletes cannot underestimate the impact on muscle metabolism and fueling from eating throughout the day. Sleep and rest are important parts of recovery when many nutrients are used to heal and grow. Eating breakfast will recover the body from the overnight state of repair to a state of growth. And finally, spreading the calories and nutrients throughout the day keeps the muscle in an anabolic state.

Prior to exercise, the athlete needs to ensure enough energy is on board for the task. The pregame meal is typically taken 2–3 hours before the event to allow time for digestion and individual gastric comfort. The meal should focus on CHOs with a small portion of lean protein with a moderate to lean level of fat.[37] As the time of exercise nears, CHOs become the focus for food or drinks to ensure the athlete has maximized glycogen in the muscle, especially if prior eating has been low in CHOs. Fluids such as sports drinks may work nicely in this period because they facilitate prehydration as well. Athletes need to trial and define the best pregame strategy as an individual to allow maximal fueling, but avoid pregame gastric distress, diarrhea, or crashing blood sugars.

During exercise lasting longer than 60–75 or 90 minutes, athletes might benefit from consumption of a CHO snack or drink to boost blood glucose to the muscle. Child athletes have been documented to use 37% more exogenous CHOs than adults,[18,38] so this could be an important contribution for the serious child competitor. Athletes that undertake high-intensity activity during an extended event or multiple event day, can use CHOs during activity to help delay fatigue. Note that a spectrum of opinions exists on how long the event should be to guide CHO consumption during the event. The best practice is to consume CHOs early in the time frame for longer events and to know one's body well enough to fuel correctly.

After exercise, athletes need to let their muscles recover and prepare them to be anabolic. Standard practice still includes a metabolic window up to about 45–60 minutes after exercise when CHO will be expedited to the muscle for faster glycogen resynthesis.[39] Best practice for adult high-intensity athletes is to consume about 1 g/kg body weight CHO along with 15–20 g of good quality protein.[8,40,41]

Back-to-back tournaments and practices commonly present fueling concerns for parents and athletes alike. When games, matches, or events are continuous and provide limited time between events, food items that are readily available require preplanning. To ensure the adolescent athlete fulfills his or her athletic potential, eating patterns should be supported that integrate the unique needs for

Table 17-3. Examples of Meals and Snacks Used With Timing Around Sport

TIMING	DESCRIPTION	kcal	g CHO	g pro	g fat
Pregame, 2–4 h prior	Target is high CHO, moderate protein, lower in fat				
Pasta meal	2 cups whole wheat pasta with 1 cup sauce and 3 oz lean meat, 1 cup of salad, 1 piece garlic bread, and 1 cup 2% milk	797	120	54	18
Fast food	Wendy's grilled chicken with baked potato with broccoli cheese sauce	790	111	48	18
	Larger athletes might add a small Frosty to above	1130	167	57	27
Pre-event, 20–60 min prior	Target is well-tolerated CHOs				
	1 cup Cheerios with 1 cup skim milk	180	32	11	2
	20 oz sports drink	160	40	0	0
	2 oz pretzels with water	200	47	6	0
	Athletes preferring more sustained or complex CHO:				
	Cup yogurt with ¼ cup granola	303	34	16	7
	½ cup cooked oatmeal with 1.5 oz raisins	293	26	7	4
		kcal	g CHO	g pro	g fat
During event, 4–8 oz every 15–20 min	Sports drink only warranted if longer than 90 min of intense activity (otherwise water is great)				
Per 8 oz	Gatorade G	50	14	110	30
	Gatorade G2 series	25	7	110	30
	Powerade	60	17	55	30
	Powerade Zero	0	0	55	33
	Generation UCAN	110	27	180	130
	Accelerade (including 4 g protein)	80	15	120	15
		kcal	g CHO	g pro	g fat
Recovery, within 45 min	Target is intentional mix of CHO and good-quality protein	Target 200–300	Target 40–60	Target 15–20	Target, low
	1 cup ready to eat cereal (eg, multi-grain Cheerios) with 1 cup skim milk and 1 medium banana	250	50	11	1.5
	Peanut butter (1 TB) and jelly (1 TB) sandwich on 2 slices whole wheat bread with 1 cup milk	368	52	20	10
	Turkey sandwich with 2 slices bread and about 2 oz turkey with 12 oz sports drink	300	50	18	3
	1 cup low-fat chocolate milk with 1 oz pretzels	259	50	11	2.5
	1 mozzarella string cheese stick, 1 cup green grapes, 1 medium orange with water	215	44	10	2
	PowerBar Protein Plus and 8 oz Gatorade	290	46	20	6

CHO, carbohydrate; kcal, calories; TB, tablespoon.

sporting success along with the nutrition considerations for healthy growth and development.[28] Table 17-4 help puts a multiple-event day in nutrient timing perspective for the young athlete.

Sports-Specific Nutrition Needs

Not all sporting activities have the same fueling requirements or nutrition-specific goals. Sports have varying nutrition needs and considerations based on type and inten-

Table 17-4. Fueling Ideas for the Big Day

TIMING	NUTRITION GOALS	EXAMPLE (ALWAYS RELATIVE TO ATHLETE SIZE AND ENERGY NEEDS)
Breakfast at least 2-4 h from event	Balanced meal heavy on the carbohydrate	Whole grain or fruit pancakes with syrup, 8 oz milk, side of fresh fruit, 2 oz lean meat, 16 oz water after meal will begin hydration on right path
Pre-event snack 1-2 h before	High carbohydrate, moderate protein, reduced in fat	12 oz sports drink, piece of fruit or pretzels; if urine is strong, more water
During event if high intensity lasts longer than 60-90 min	Liquid carbohydrate 30-60 g/h	4-8 oz of sports drink every 15-20 min
After event within 45 min if multiple events ("recovery" snack)	Carbohydrate and good-quality protein (3:1 or 4:1 ratio of carbohydrate to protein)	8 oz chocolate milk with peanut butter (limit to 1 TB) and jelly sandwich on whole grain bread
Snacks between meals not as close to event	Carbohydrate with little protein and little fat	Trail mix with 2 TB dried cranberries or raisins, 1 tsp peanuts, and 1 oz mozzarella cheese stick OR Turkey or ham sandwich with 2 oz meat, 2 slices whole grain bread, tomato/lettuce as tolerated, with glass of water
Meals away from the event	Balanced with carbohydrate, adequate protein, and fat	Plate surface divided as ¼ meat, ¼ whole grain, ½ brightly colored fruits and vegetables with glass of milk

TB, tablespoon; tsp, teaspoon.

sity. For example, the estimated energy needs for a football lineman differs greatly from that of a female cross-country runner. Individual athletes should develop their own strategies to ensure they are fueling and hydrating properly. This plan should be individualized for each athlete's own unique sports routine for practice and competitions alike.

Adolescents are generally well adapted to moderate-intensity endurance exercise, but many young adolescent athletes may have a lower capacity to store glycogen compared to adults.[42] In order to maintain adequate energy before and during exercise, it is important to determine a fueling pattern that provides energy from simple CHOs that digest easily. Strength and power sports are defined as repeated bouts of high-intensity or maximal exercise lasting from a few seconds to 3 minutes.[43] It is also essential that these types of athletes ensure they are consuming adequate CHOs for fuel in addition to enough protein for muscle recovery and repair. Intermittent or team sports are generally categorized by recurrent, repeated bouts of high-intensity activity over the course of the competition (30–90 minutes). With team sports, it is important to remember the degree of skill, power, strength, and endurance that are required for optimal performance. Sports that are focused on weight or aesthetic judgment need to be especially mindful of the sensitivity surrounding adequate fueling because the athletes may restrict intake to attain body appearance or weight goals. Athletes who participate in these sports are at a higher risk for eating disorders or disordered eating. A recent review study shows the prevalence of disordered eating and eating disorders vary from 0% to 19% in male athletes and from 6% to 45% in female athletes.[44]

Table 17-5 outlines primary nutrition and performance-related goals for endurance, power/strength, intermittent sprinting (team sports), aesthetic or weight-focused sporting activities, and back-to-back tournaments or practices. Various sports differ in the nutrition strategies according to body type and athlete culture. It is best to be familiar with these goals prior to counseling sport-specific athletes.

Common Nutrition Challenges and Suggestions

Common nutrition-related issues that young athletes may experience are listed in Table 17-6. Young athletes are often serious about their bodies and sports, and a healthcare practitioner's respect and guidance can help them through nutrition-related challenges.

Importance of Parental Involvement

Many parents are eager to be informed about their child's health and sports performance, viewing athletic participation as an opportunity to teach good habits and impact quality of life.[46] Participation in athletic training and events provides many teachable moments. With that in mind and in light of increasing obesity and chronic diseases, additional information could be helpful for families. For instance, national surveys suggest that 2–6-year-olds are consuming more sugary beverages, savory snacks, sweets, and other foods providing an additional 109 kcal/d.[47] Recent U.S. data suggest that while the prevalence of sugar-sweetened bev-

Table 17-5. Sports-Specific Nutrition Goals and Considerations

TYPE OF SPORT	SPORT EXAMPLES	GOALS AND CONSIDERATIONS
Endurance sports	Distance running, swimming, cycling, cross-country skiing	• Maintain energy level to supply working muscles adequate fuel for long bouts of exercise, usually 60 min or more • Avoid overreliance on protein and fat as fuel • Before exercise, optimize glycogen storage and consume adequate carbohydrate • Maintain carbohydrate delivery during competition if needed • Replenish carbohydrate after competition • Ensure proper hydration before and during competition
Strength and power sports	Sprinting, jumping events, power-lifting, track and field events (discus, shot put, javelin), weight-lifting	• Focus on pregame meals with adequate carbohydrate, high-quality protein, and low in fat • Consume adequate (20–30 g), not excessive protein for muscle recovery • Ensure adequate carbohydrate intake in order to avoid reliance on protein for energy
Intermittent sprint sports (team sports)	Football, baseball, softball, hockey, soccer, lacrosse, field hockey, basketball	• Proper fuel for maximal effort in short, high-intensity durations • Maintain adequate hydration before and during competition by utilizing breaks and halftime • Consume meals high in complex carbohydrates, high-quality protein, and low in fat • Eating after competition promotes preservation of lean body mass and muscle recovery
Back-to-back tournaments or practices, 2- or 3-a-days		• Fuel in between games to maintain energy level • Focus on foods that are high in carbohydrate and easily digestible • Fast-food and high-fat food items are unlikely to provide the athlete beneficial fuel • Pack easily digestible food items that provide peace of mind during game or practice • Proper hydration techniques focusing on water and sports drinks • Be aware of food safety issues, keep cold foods cold and warm foods warm; learn more at http://www.foodsafety.gov/keep/index.html
Weight class or aesthetic sports	Gymnastics, dance, diving, swimming, runners, rowing, figure skating, wrestling, boxing, martial arts, horse racing	Consume adequate calories to • Supply fuel for muscles • Proper health and growth • Maintain weight • Optimize body composition versus reduce weight • Prevent catabolism of lean body mass • Encourage a healthy relationship with food • Maintain normal menstrual function (female athletes)

erages increased in children ages 2–11, it declined among adolescents; however, sports beverage consumption tripled in adolescence.[48]

Fully informed, realistic, and practical feeding approaches by parents, guardians, coaches, and trainers would be ideal for supplying food and beverages for young athletes.[49] There are many influential factors, including timing of consumption across the day and around the event(s), portion sizes, nutrient content, food/beverage preferences, and policies about healthy foods within families, schools, or sponsoring organizations.[50] The impact that food/beverage companies have on purchasing by parents, preferences of the athlete, and practices established by the sports' sponsoring organizations has not been well studied, yet it is gaining attention.[51] Some studies show that restricting sponsorship of events by manufacturers of unhealthy foods will limit

Table 17-6. Common Challenges for Athlete Nutrition

ISSUE	POSSIBLE INDICATORS AND CONCERNS	SOLUTIONS
Limited nutrition knowledge related to sports performance	• Cannot describe desirable pre-game meals or recovery eating • Has no hydration plan • Parents do not possess adequate nutrition knowledge to guide young athletes on proper meal planning and food selection • Does not bring food to school • Insufficient calorie intake during the day leads to overconsumption at night • Infrequent eating habits	• Provide reputable Web sites • Suggest easy-to-read books • Prioritize planning to ensure foods and beverages available • Practice having all the foods and beverages needed for sport • Do not try new food/drink items on game days • Encourage fueling throughout the day as a primary habit • Note timing of events and fuel/hydrate accordingly • Note travel impact on eating and hydrating opportunities and on performance • Identify community partners (eg, a Certified Specialist in Sports Dietetics [CSSD]) • Share free resources online from reputable nutrition organizations (Table 17-7)
Picky eater	• Low variety in habitual diet • "Does not like" entire food groups • Not willing to try new food items	• Educate on advantages of diet with varied food groups to include performance advantages of carbohydrate foods • Encourage athlete to bring foods that she or he likes so the athlete is at least fueling • Encourage practice for fuel/hydration • Start with food items the athlete is willing to eat and suggest additional food items based on similar texture, taste, food group, or consistency
Eating on a budget or low income	• Eating 1 or 2 meals per day • Eating little meat and lots of bread and pasta • Eating low amounts of fresh fruits and vegetables • Not eating snacks prior to practices after school • School breakfast or lunch does not always provide optimal food choices	• Discuss planning strategies for foods typically afforded • Buy in bulk and separate/store in pantry/freezer • Help athlete understand correct amount of protein to prevent undernutrition or overspending, educate family on lower cost of mixed plant proteins versus meat products • Cook in bulk and freeze for later access • Buy generic for most foods • Buy fruits and vegetables in season • Determine if family is eligible for federal food assistance program and local food pantry help or connect with social work support • Pack lunch instead of buying if helps optimize food choices
Male athlete with high growth expectations	• Questions about how much protein needed or what supplements will "work" • Usually overt in desire to be bigger, faster, stronger, or leaner • Lack of understanding about growth patterns • Obtaining enough food and nutrients to support growth	• Stress that normal physical activity and adequate nutrition optimize growth • Emphasize importance of adequate calories for proper fueling in order to optimize workout routine • Educate that growth has genetic and environmental components especially in relation to his father's growth patterns • Consider that intense exercise may be associated with delayed growth • Check and reinforce appropriate athlete vs. parent expectations of lean mass accretion; use growth charts • Adolescents have difficulty discerning how short term decisions will affect long-term outcome
Vegetarianism	• Often occurs in young females who want to lose weight • Can be due to perceptions that meat has too much fat and too many calories • Use as means to make or lose weight for competition	• Educate about optimal protein-alternative foods (dairy, legumes, soy products) or how to combine foods to ensure complete proteins • Alert athlete to consume adequate micronutrients such as iron, calcium, and zinc • Inquire about why this lifestyle is appealing to the athlete to ensure answer is consistent with balanced decision • Educate athlete about the roles of macronutrients for an optimal sports diet

Table 17-6. Common Challenges for Athlete Nutrition (continued)

ISSUE	POSSIBLE INDICATORS AND CONCERNS	SOLUTIONS
The Female Athlete Triad; may be called Relative Energy Deficiency in Sport (RED-S)	• A combination of 3 disorders (or spectrums) that includes low energy availability (ie, expend more calories than consume), disordered menstrual pattern, and low bone mineral density • RED-S includes males as well as females outside of menstrual patterns • May be related to disordered eating, poor body image, unrealistic body weight goals, and weight-loss expectations • Could also occur secondary to lack of sports nutrition education • Often undetectable or not considered until stress fracture occurs • Exists in all sports but especially in those with weight or appearance requirements • Critical read for this area of evaluation is International Olympic Committee document[5]	• Encourage eating a diet with a wide variety of foods that will fuel the muscle for optimal performance • When in doubt, suggest evaluation by psychological professional and dietitian • Intervene early to increase chances for recovery • Track menstrual periods each month
Use of performance-enhancing supplements (legal and illegal)	• May be related to athlete's desire to excel but often not supported by evidence • Often used by athlete as a substitute for adequate nutrition • Could be related to peer pressure and media influences • Often linked to lack of proper supplement education and regulation standards • Linked to insufficient calorie intake plus excessive workouts • Not seeing results in weight room • Peers are using supplements	• Pediatric evidence-based clinical trials are lacking on the use or the adverse effects of some supplements (herbals, ergogenic aids, etc.) • Anabolic steroid use ranges from 1% to 11.1% of adolescents surveyed, and creatine use in reviewed studies ranged from 5.6% to 30%[43] • Outside of the possible immediate harm, supplements may act as a gateway to more serious substances and illegal drug use for adolescents • Magazines marketed directly to adolescents contained inaccurate references to supplements and a substantial amount of information with questionable accuracy[7] • Supplements sought frequently for improving speed, decreasing weight, or increasing size/bulk of athlete • Ask questions about particular meals or snacks to ensure eating to support desired changes • Seek advice of CSSD • Table 17-7 provides education resources
Weight control expectations (typically females)	• Secondary sex characteristics not desirable to some female athletes • Underfueling to avoid weight gain; poor performance and health detriments may result • Poor self-esteem and/or self-image • Overt comments about not liking body parts (eg, belly, thighs, hips) • Unhealthy weight control methods (eg, diet pills, smoking, vomiting, laxatives, or starvation)	• Explain puberty progression and risks of stifling puberty • When in doubt, suggest evaluation by psychological professional and dietitian • Early intervention may avoid Female Athlete Triad outcome • Review updates to current DSM V from the American Psychiatric Association for Eating Disorder diagnosis criteria[8]

Table 17-6. Common Challenges for Athlete Nutrition (continued)

ISSUE	POSSIBLE INDICATORS AND CONCERNS	SOLUTIONS
Overweight and obesity epidemic	• Athletes are not exempt from overweight/obesity epidemic • In 2012, more than 1/3 of children and adolescents were overweight or obese[45] • Determine if athlete has un-healthy relationship with food • Athletes with bulimia and binge eating disorder are more likely to be overweight or obese than normal or underweight • Athlete may be limiting intake of certain food items leading to nutrient deficiencies	• High body mass index does not necessarily indicate obesity, consider body composition testing to help athlete set goals realistic to body type • Encourage eating a diet with a wide variety of foods that will fuel the muscle for optimal performance • Encourage high-fat food items and desserts in moderation • Form a healthy relationship with food and exercise • Seek expertise of a dietitian or psychological professional if needed • A "one a day" style multivitamin supplement may be warranted in cases in which eating is not optimal

exposure to these products for the child athletes involved,[52] demonstrating useful models of influence on health policies[53] around restricting unhealthy foods.[49,50]

Preprepared Meal Plans

Families with athletes are incredibly busy and challenged for time. Their ability to be organized and have healthy foods and beverages available as needed is compounded by factors that may be out of their control (traffic, weather, schedule changes). Recent research studying a large urban population of 4800 residents, who tracked nearly 12,000 food-related trips, showed that food is most often purchased while traveling away from home and across these many trips. Essentially this food-travel environment influenced food purchases.[54] Purchasing at grocery stores vs fast food chains or other options and incorporating travel patterns is likely a key factor for having healthy foods and beverages available to the whole family on a daily basis.

Undoubtedly, families who can routinely incorporate to plan, shop, buy, and carryout food/beverage preparations in the days prior to the athletic events and practices will be most successful in meeting recommendations and guidelines. These plans include grocery lists, daily packing lists, and adequate equipment (coolers, ice, etc). Coaches and trainers who offer shopping and packing templates to facilitate this process will empower the athletes and their families in this process of healthy eating. A sample template is provided in Worksheet 17-1.

Family Grocery Store Trips

Some stores provide dietitians to guide grocery store tours and can engage the entire family and team in the process to find optimal foods for health, but sport dietitians (CSSD)

would be the best choice to discuss foods and performance. Point-of-purchase product coding and information demonstrate nutrient content and comparisons so that families can sustain a full pantry of these optimal choices and replenish each time they shop. Standards and policies, especially relating to food groups and away-from-home foods, make food decisions easier and individualized.[53] While it was not designed for the competitive athlete, the U.S. Department of Agriculture Web site http://myplate.gov/ could be a useful tool for daily tips, recipes, shopping, and eating guides for all ages.

Dietary Supplements

The use of dietary supplements in any population is controversial, and performance-enhancing supplements have been formally discouraged for children and adolescents.[55] It may be important to differentiate supplements used for improved health (such as multivitamin) and those used to improve performance or body composition (ergogenic aids). The dietary supplement industry is minimally regulated and contains a spectrum of manufacturers and ingredient suppliers from the conscientious and trustworthy to the unscrupulous. Buyers must be educated and on-guard to avoid dangerous or wasteful products. Table 17-7 provides numerous resources to help educate young athletes about the risks of using dietary supplements as well as resources to tease out efficacy and truth in labeling issues. An appropriate education around the issues of ergogenic supplementation warrants an entire paper dedicated to the risks and realities.[56]

Resources

While this chapter provides young athlete guidance from clinical and practical perspectives, it is helpful to provide pa-

Table 17-7. Nutrition Web Resources

TYPE OF SPORT	RESOURCES

To find a Registered Dietitian (RD) certified to work with athletes; known as a Certified Specialist in Sports Dietetics (CSSD)	• Academy of Nutrition and Dietetics list of RDs
	   http://www.eatright.org
	• Academy Practice Group for Sports, Cardiovascular, and Wellness Nutritionists (SCAN) list of CSSD RDs
	   http://www.scandpg.org
	• Collegiate Professional Sports Dietitians Association (CPSDA)
	   http://www.sportsrd.org

General sports nutrition information	Fact sheets:
	• SCAN free tools http://www.scandpg.org/sports-nutrition/sports-nutrition-fact-sheets/
	Position papers:
	• Academy of Nutrition and Dietetics[8]
	   http://www.eatright.org
	• American College of Sports Medicine[8,30] http://www.acsm.org
	• National Athletic Trainers Association http://www.nata.org/statements/
	• American Academy of Pediatrics
	Books/Web sites:
	• *Sports Nutrition; A Practice Manual for Professionals.* 5th ed. 2012change scandpg.org/sports/
	   nutrition/prof/res.php

Dietary supplement information	• Supplements 411 from U.S. anti-doping agency
	   http://www.supplement411.org/supplement411/
	• Australian Institute of Sport*
	   http://www.ausport.gov.au/ais/nutrition
	• Drug Free Sport*
	   http://www.drugfreesport.com/
	• Office of Dietary Supplements Factsheets
	   http://ods.od.nih.gov/factsheets/list-all/
	• Natural Medicines Database
	   http://www.naturaldatabase.com
	• Consumer Labs third-party quality testing
	   http://www.ConsumerLabs.com
	• Sport use third-party quality testing
	   http://www.nsfsport.com/index.asp
	   http://informed-choice.org

Food assistance starting points	• http://www.fns.usda.gov/snap/supplemental-nutrition-assistance-program-snap • http://www.feedingamerica.org/find-your-local-foodbank/

tients with professional web resources to explore other areas of interest. Table 17-7 can help patients identify local practitioners, current professional consensus (position statements), and fact sheets on many topics to include dietary supplement education and evaluation.

Test Your Knowledge Questions

1. Provide 3 strategies coaches, parents, and athletes can utilize to ensure proper fueling strategies around sport (before, during, after).
2. Provide at least 2 reasons young athletes that are exercising for greater than 60–75 and 90 minutes may benefit from a CHO-rich snack during competition.
3. Provide 3 reasons why parental involvement is crucial to the young athlete's success.
4. Provide 3 strategies coaches, parents, and athletes can utilize to ensure proper hydration and prevention of heat-related illness.

References

1. *Dietary Reference Intakes for Energy, Carbohydrate, Fiber, Fat, Fatty Acids, Cholesterol, Protein, and Amino Acids (Macronutrients).* Washington, DC: The National Academies Press; 2005. http://www.nap.edu/openbook.php?record_id=10490. Accessed August 22, 2014.
2. Thivel D, Chaput JP. Are post-exercise appetite sensations and energy intake coupled in children and adolescents? *Sports Med.* 2014;44(6):735–741.

3. U.S. Department of Agriculture. ChooseMyPlate.gov. http://www.choosemyplate.gov/. Accessed December 30, 2014.

4. Nattiv A, Loucks AB, Manore MM, Sanborn CF, Sundgot-Borgen J, Warren MP; American College of Sports Medicine. American College of Sports Medicine position stand. The female athlete triad. *Med Sci Sports Exerc.* 2007;39(10):1867–1882.

5. Mountjoy M, Sundgot-Borgen J, Burke L, et al. The IOC consensus statement: beyond the female athlete triad—relative energy deficiency in sport (RED-S). *Br J Sports Med.* 2014;48(7):491–497.

6. Loucks AB, Kiens B, Wright HH. Energy availability in athletes. *J Sports Sci.* 2011;29:7–15.

7. Brooks GA, Mercier J. Balance of carbohydrate and lipid utilization during exercise: the "crossover" concept. *J Appl Physiol (1985).* 1994;76(6):2253–2261.

8. Rodriguez NR, Di Marco NM, Langley S. American College of Sports Medicine position stand. Nutrition and athletic performance. *Med Sci Sports Exerc.* 2009;41(3):709–731.

9. Maughan RJ, Shirreffs SM. IOC consensus conference on nutrition in sport, 25–27 October 2010, International Olympic Committee, Lausanne, Switzerland. *J Sports Sci.* 2011;29(suppl 1):S1.

10. Bass S, Inge K. Nutrition for special populations: children and young athletes. In: Burke L, Deakin V, eds. *Clinical Sports Nutrition.* 4th ed. Sydney, Australia: McGraw-Hill Australia; 2010:508–546.

11. Montfort-Steiger V, Williams CA. Carbohydrate intake considerations for young athletes. *J Sports Sci Med.* 2007;6(3):343–352.

12. Aucouturier J, Baker JS, Duché P. Fat and carbohydrate metabolism during submaximal exercise in children. *Sports Med.* 2008;38(3):213–238.

13. Riddell MC. The endocrine response and substrate utilization during exercise in children and adolescents. *J Appl Physiol.* 2008;105(2):725–733.

14. U.S. Department of Agriculture, U.S. Department of Health and Human Services. *Dietary Guidelines for Americans, 2010.* http://www.health.gov/dietaryguidelines/2010.asp. Accessed December 30, 2014.

15. Currell K, Jeukendrup AE. Superior endurance performance with ingestion of multiple transportable carbohydrates. *Med Sci Sports Exerc.* 2008;40(2):275–281.

16. Committee on Nutrition and the Council on Sports Medicine and Fitness. Sports drinks and energy drinks for children and adolescents: are they appropriate? *Pediatrics.* 2011;127:1182–1189.

17. Seifert SM, Schaechter JL, Hershorin ER, Lipshultz SE. Health effects of energy drinks on children, adolescents, and young adults. *Pediatrics.* 2011;127(3):511–528.

18. Timmons BW, Bar-Or O, Riddell MC. Oxidation rate of exogenous carbohydrate during exercise is higher in boys than in men. *J Appl Physiol (1985).* 2003;94(1):278–284.

19. Nybo L. CNS fatigue and prolonged exercise: effect of glucose supplementation. *Med Sci Sports Exerc.* 2003;35(4):589–594.

20. Chambers ES, Bridge MW, Jones DA. Carbohydrate sensing in the human mouth: Effects on exercise performance and brain activity. *J Physiol.* 2009;587(8):1779–1794.

21. Boisseau N, Vermorel M, Rance M, Duche P, Patureau-Mirand P. Protein requirements in male adolescent soccer players. *Eur J Appl Physiol.* 2007;100:27–33.

22. Aerenhouts D, Van Cauwenberg J, Poortmans JR, Hauspie R, Clarys P. Influence of growth rate on nitrogen balance in adolescent sprint athletes. *Int J Sport Nutr Exerc Metab.* 2013;23(4):409–417.

23. Martin WF, Martin WF, Cerundolo LH, et al. Effects of dietary protein intake on indexes of hydration. *J Am Diet Assoc.* 2006;106(4):587–589.

24. Phillips SM, Van Loon LJC. Dietary protein for athletes: from requirements to optimum adaptation. *J Sports Sci.* 2011;29:S29–S38.

25. Deutz NE, Wolfe RR. Is there a maximal anabolic response to protein intake with a meal? *Clin Nutr.* 2013;32(2):309–313.

26. Hawley JA, Gibala MJ, Bermon S. Innovations in athletic preparation: Role of substrate availability to modify training adaptation and performance. *J Sports Sci.* 2007;25:S115–S124.

27. Paoli A, Rubini A, Volek JS, Grimaldi KA. Beyond weight loss: A review of the therapeutic uses of very-low-carbohydrate (ketogenic) diets. *Eur J Clin Nutr.* 2013;67(8):789–796.

28. Desbrow B, McCormack J, Burke LM, et al. Sports Dietitians Australia position statement: sports nutrition for the adolescent athlete. *Int J Sport Nutr Exerc Metab.* 2014;24(5):570–584.

29. Casa DJ, Armstrong LE, Hillman SK, et al. National Athletic Trainers' Association position statement: fluid replacement for athletes. *J Athl Train.* 2000;35(2):212–224.

30. American College of Sports Medicine, Sawka MN, Burke LM, Eichner ER, Maughan RJ, Montain SJ, Stachenfeld NS. American College of Sports Medicine position stand. Exercise and fluid replacement. *Med Sci Sports Exerc.* 2007;39(2):377–390.

31. Climatic heat stress and the exercising child and adolescent. American Academy of Pediatrics. Committee on Sports Medicine and Fitness. *Pediatrics.* 2000;106:158–159.

32. Rowland T. Fluid replacement requirements for child athletes. *Sports Med.* 2011;41(4):279–288.

33. Wilk B, Timmons BW, Bar-Or O. Voluntary fluid intake, hydration status, and aerobic performance of adolescent athletes in the heat. *Appl Physiol Nutr Metab.* 2010;35(6):834–841.

34. Palmer M, Logan H, Spriet L. On-ice sweat rate, voluntary fluid intake, and sodium balance during practice in male junior ice hockey players drinking water or a carbohydrate-electrolyte solution. *Appl Physiol Nutr Metab.* 2010;35:328–335.

35. Wendt D, van Loon LJ, Lichtenbelt WD. Thermoregulation during exercise in the heat: strategies for maintaining health and performance. *Sports Med.* 2007;37(8):669–682.

36. Bergeron MF. Youth sports in the heat: recovery and scheduling considerations for tournament play. *Sports Med.* 2009;39(7):513–522.

37. Berning J, Manore MM, Meyer NL, eds. *Nutrition and Athletic Performance Before, During and After Exercise: Adapting the Joint Position Statement into Practical Guidelines.* Barrington, IL: Gatorade Sports Science Institute; 2010.

38. Timmons B, Bar-Or O, Riddell M. Influence of age and pubertal status on substrate utilization during exercise with and without carbohydrate intake in healthy boys. *Appl Physiol Nutr Metab.* 2007;32:416–425.

39. Ivy JL, Katz AL, Cutler CL, Sherman WM, Coyle EF. Muscle glycogen synthesis after exercise: Effect of time of carbohydrate ingestion. *J Appl Physiol (1985).* 1988;64(4):1480–1485.

40. Bolster DR, Pikosky MA, Gaine PC, et al. Dietary protein intake impacts human skeletal muscle protein fractional synthetic rates after endurance exercise. *Am J Physiol Endocrinol Metab.* 2005;289(4):E678–E683.

41. Ivy JL, Goforth HWJ, Damon BM, McCauley TR, Parsons EC, Price TB. Early postexercise muscle glycogen recovery is enhanced with a carbohydrate-protein supplement. *J Appl Physiol (1985).* 2002;93(4):1337–1344.

42. Boisseau N, Delamarche P. Metabolic and hormonal responses to exercise in children and adolescents. *Sports Med.* 2000;30(6):405–422.

43. Petrie HJ, Stover EA, Horswill CA. Nutritional concerns for the child and adolescent competitor. *Nutrition.* 2004;20(7):620–631.

44. Bratland-Sanda S, Sundgot-Borgen J. Eating disorders in athletes: overview of prevalence, risk factors and recommendations for prevention and treatment. *Eur J Sport Sci.* 2013;13(5):499–508.

45. Centers for Disease Control and Prevention. Adolescent and school health. http://www.cdc.gov/healthyyouth/obesity/facts.htm. Updated December 11, 2014. Accessed June 17, 2013.

46. Vella SA, Cliff DP, Okely AD, Magee CA. Sports participation and parent-reported health-related quality of life in children: longitudinal associations. *J Pediatr.* 2014;164(6):1469–1474.

47. Ford CN, Slining MM, Popkin BM. Trends in dietary intake among US 2- to 6-year-old children, 1989–2008. *J Acad Nutr Diet.* 2013;113(1):35–42.

48. Han E, Powell LM. Consumption patterns of sugar-sweetened beverages in the United States. *J Acad Nutr Diet.* 2013;113(1):43–53.

49. Kelly B, Baur LA, Bauman AE, King L, Chapman K, Smith BJ. Restricting unhealthy food sponsorship: attitudes of the sporting community. *Health Policy.* 2012;104(3):288–295.

50. Merlo CL, Olsen EO, Galic M, Brener ND. The relationship between state policies for competitive foods and school nutrition practices in the united states. *Prev Chronic Dis.* 2014;11:E66.

51. Kelly B, Baur LA, Bauman AE, King L, Chapman K, Smith BJ. "Food company sponsors are kind, generous and cool": (mis)conceptions of junior sports players. *Int J Behav Nutr Phys Act.* 2011;8:95.

52. Carter MA, Signal L, Edwards R, Hoek J, Maher A. Food, fizzy, and football: promoting unhealthy food and beverages through sport—a New Zealand case study. *BMC Public Health.* 2013;13:126.

53. Cohen DA BR. Nutrition standards for away-from-home foods in the USA. *Obes Rev.* 2012;13(7):618–629.

54. Kerr J, Frank L, Sallis JF, Saelens B, Glanz K, Chapman J. Predictors of trips to food destinations. *Int J Behav Nutr Phys Act.* 2012;9:58.

55. Gomez J; American Academy of Pediatrics Committee on Sports Medicine and Fitness. Use of performance-enhancing substances. *Pediatrics.* 2005;115(4):1103–1106.

56. Buell JL, Franks R, Ransone J, Powers ME, Laquale KM, Carlson-Phillips A; National Athletic Trainers' Association. National Athletic Trainers' Association position statement: Evaluation of dietary supplements for performance nutrition. *J Athl Train.* 2013;48(1):124–136.

Test Your Knowledge Answers

1. Provide 3 strategies coaches, parents, and athletes can utilize to ensure proper fueling strategies around sport (before, during, after).
   a. Provide athletes with template planning and shopping list
   b. Plan to pack food needed so it is available, and do not have to rely on fast food or restaurants.
   c. Schedule time in game preparation, during game and in team meetings to allow for appropriate fueling
   d. Educate (direct) and coordinate parents to provide appropriate snacks.

2. Provide at least 2 reasons young athletes that are exercising for greater than 60–75 and 90 minutes may benefit from a CHO-rich snack during competition.
   a. Young athletes may not have same capacity to store glycogen
   b. Athletes of all ages engaged in high intensity exercise benefit from exogenous carbohydrate intake with this timing to delay fatigue

3. Provide 3 reasons why parental involvement is crucial to the young athlete's success.
   a. Money, transportation, knowledge leadership

4. Provide 3 strategies coaches, parents, and athletes can utilize to ensure proper hydration and prevention of heat-related illness
   a. Frequent fluid breaks
   b. Provide appropriate fluids
   c. Adjust practice times as needed when environment is too risky

Worksheet 17-1. Athlete Shopping, Packing, and Eating List

Use this tool to make your shopping, packing, and eating list:
1. Jot down in the food-group columns the foods/beverages you would like to have across your week.
   a. This becomes your grocery list.
   b. See sample below.
2. Notice the level of variety and try to evenly distribute.
3. Circle foods and beverages to pack (your checklist) for practices and games.
   a. Put the list in the cooler with those foods/beverages.
   b. Create new lists to change up your variety.

Grains	Fruits	Proteins	Vegetables	Dairy	Sweets/Junk

Example Form: Your form would have the foods you like to eat!

GRAINS	FRUITS	PROTEINS	VEGETABLES	DAIRY	SWEETS/JUNK OTHERS
Sandwich bread	Apples	Eggs	Baby carrots	Sliced Swiss cheese	Trail mix with nuts, dried fruit, chocolate
Pasta	Dried apricots	White Beans	Salad greens	2% milk	Chocolate chip cookies
Rice	Bananas	Refried beans	Red and yellow peppers	Greek yogurt (fruited only)	Baked chips at lunch
Tortillas	Orange juice	Fish		Ice cream	Pretzels after school
Frosted Mini Wheats	Dried tart cherries or raisins	Chicken		Shredded cheddar (for salads)	Gatorade (berry flavor)
Pretzels					Diet Coke
Wheat Thins					Kool-Aid
					Oreos

EXTRA NOTES: bring cooler and ice for food safety and palatability! Items to PACK ARE CIRCLED.

DISEASE STATES AND NUTRITION

18

Neurological Impairment

Ala K. Shaikhkhalil, MD; and Robin Meyers, MPH, RD, LDN

CONTENTS

Learning Objectives

1. Identify factors that place children with neurological impairment at increased risk for nutrition problems.
2. Assess growth and nutrition in the child with neurological impairment.
3. Understand the approach to provide oral and enteral nutrition support to children with neurological impairment.

Introduction

Children with neurological impairment (NI) experience a variety of disorders characterized primarily by gross and fine motor dysfunction with or without cognitive or speech delay and are at risk for a variety of nutrition-related problems including undernutrition, poor linear growth, excess weight gain, micronutrient deficiencies, and osteopenia.[1-3] This chapter outlines nutrition comorbidities, the approach to nutrition assessment, and various methods of nutrition support in children with NI. Both undernutrition and overweight can result in more hospital admissions and clinic visits and decreased involvement in activities at home and at school.[4,5] Appropriate nutrition support with resultant improvement in nutrition status has beneficial effects on linear growth, weight gain, quality of life, neurological and developmental progress, and wound healing.[6-10] Management from the outset by a multidisciplinary team of physicians, nurses, registered dietitians, feeding therapists, psychologists, and social workers is critical to avoid the negative consequences of poor nutrition in the child with NI. The spectrum of disease varies widely and nutrition assessment and interventions should be tailored to the individual child.

Common Nutrition Problems in Children With Neurological Impairment

Undernutrition, Growth Failure, and Overweight

The true prevalence of nutrition problems in children with NI as a whole is not known. Estimates have been made in individual categories of NI and specific diseases including cerebral palsy (CP), myelodysplasia, spina bifida, spinal cord injury, and Rett's syndrome.[3,11-15] Undernutrition based on weight, weight for length, and triceps skinfold thickness has been documented in varying degrees of frequency in individuals with these disorders, and it is more common in older children and those with more severe neurologic injury.[3,16,17] Linear growth is more affected in children with seizures or spastic quadriplegia and those who are nonambulatory.[3]

Expected height-for-age and weight-for-age of children with NI are generally lower than those of the reference population.[3,11,16,17] Children with CP who have only minimal motor impairment have weight and height similar to age-matched and sex-matched peers without disabilities. Differences in weight and height are more significant with more severe motor impairment and increased feeding difficulties. These differences become more pronounced with age.[16,18] NI may impact linear growth even when the child is receiving appropriate nutrition due to an underlying genetic or medical condition. In these circumstances, nutrition intervention may not resolve the growth failure.[3,19]

Children with NI have various manifestations of altered nutrition status. Some may be underweight due to fat loss while maintaining muscle and visceral stores.[3] Some children continue to maintain linear growth but do not gain weight, and others have progressive muscle atrophy that is refractory to nutrition intervention.[3] Although children with NI may be shorter and weigh less than age-matched peers without disabilities, many are actually overweight using an assessment of weight-for-height or triceps skinfold thickness.[3,12] Weight-for-height monitoring is performed less frequently because of the challenges of obtaining accurate height measurements in these children, and weight gain may not be appreciated in children with small body size or unusual body fat distribution. This can lead to underestimation of the prevalence of overweight in this population.[3]

Pathophysiology of Growth-Related Issues

INAPPROPRIATE DIETARY INTAKE

Inappropriate intake of dietary energy can contribute to undernutrition or growth failure or alternatively to excess weight gain in the child with NI.[20-22] Frequently, they cannot effectively indicate that they are hungry or when they are full. Similarly, they may not be able to communicate food preferences, thus the caregiver must decide what and how much the child should eat.[3] Because poor oral motor function and poor positioning can make the task of feeding difficult and time consuming, the amount of food that is given may be inadequate and children may stop eating before they are full. Increasing energy intake through tube feedings will result in weight gain and linear growth. Careful monitoring is needed to avoid overfeeding and excessive weight gain in these children.[16,23]

ORAL MOTOR DYSFUNCTION

Feeding problems associated with oral motor dysfunction occur frequently in children with NI and have been linked to poor nutrition and health outcomes.[5,24,25] Severe feeding difficulties can sometimes be present before the child is recognized to have CP.[3] Early, persistent, and severe feeding difficulties are correlated with poor health and nutrition outcomes. Common concerns include poor suck, difficulty breastfeeding, and inability to advance to solid foods, difficulty with liquids, problems with biting or chewing solids, and coughing or choking with meals.[24,26]

Oral motor dysfunction can result in frequent spillage of food and prolonged feeding times.[25] Sullivan et al[26] found that more than one quarter of parents spent over 3 hours a day feeding their child, and a few spent twice this much time. Longer mealtimes may not compensate for feeding inefficiency, with these children still not taking in adequate calories. The challenges associated with feeding can make meals stressful and unpleasant for parents;[26] this is a concern because so many children with NI are dependent on a caregiver for feeding.[3]

Oral motor dysfunction generally parallels overall motor impairment in the child with NI and can include inadequate lip closure, drooling, persistent tongue thrusting, poor bolus formation, and delayed swallowing.[3] Difficulty initiating swallowing increases the risk of aspiration, which is greater in those who are unable to lift their head or feed themselves.[25,27] Neurologically impaired children with this degree of oral motor dysfunction have lower body fat and decreased linear growth and weight gain.[3] Gastrostomy tube feedings can help bypass some feeding difficulties.[25]

INCREASED NUTRIENT LOSSES

Children with NI who feed themselves may have poor coordination with resultant loss of food.[3] The use of adaptive utensils may enhance movement performance and minimize food spillage.[28] Gastroesophageal reflux (GER) and delayed gastric emptying, if severe enough to cause vomiting, may result in loss of nutrients.[3]

ABNORMAL ENERGY EXPENDITURE

Energy requirements for children with NI are, for the most part, lower than their able-bodied peers.[12,20,29,30] Ambulatory children and those with athetosis, however, tend to have energy requirements similar to those of their able-bodied peers.[30] Fat-free mass (FFM) appears to be a greater predictor of energy requirement than ambulatory status. Children with NI were found to have a lower FFM, which contributes to lower resting energy expenditure (REE) and energy requirements. However, neurologic injury may impact energy regulation since REE does not correlate well with body mass in some children with NI.[31] Energy requirements can be as low as 50%–61% of the dietary reference intake (DRI) for age and sex in children with spastic quadriplegic CP and myelodysplasia.[12,20,31] REE in children with myelomeningocele is 96% of predicted, but total daily energy expenditure is lower than predicted because of a reduction in physical activity.[32] Children with diplegia, hemiplegia, and spina bifida have higher rates of energy expenditure while walking compared with unaffected children.[33] REE for children with CP who are well-nourished but nonambulatory is lower than that predicted for their healthy counterparts.[31,34] REE × 1.1 may be adequate to meet the energy needs of spastic quadriplegic CP.[20]

The ability to estimate energy requirements in children with NI is complicated by many factors, and it is important to note that many of the formulas used to calculate energy needs in healthy children can result in inaccurate estimates of energy needs in children with NI.[20] Many energy equations include length/height, a measurement that is not easy to obtain in children with NI. An alternative equation for estimating energy needs is provided by the World Health Organization (WHO) and is based on weight and age only.[35] Other factors complicating the ability to estimate dietary energy needs of children with NI include the wide range of clinical features and mobility. Regardless of the method used, individualized monitoring and adjustment of energy needs remain at the cornerstone of nutrition management.

Micronutrient Deficiencies

Children with NI are at risk of developing micronutrient deficiencies. Studies have documented low intake of several micronutrients (iron, folate, vitamin D, and zinc) in cohorts of NI children who are orally or enterally fed.[21,22] Others have demonstrated biochemical evidence of deficiency of several micronutrients including iron, selenium, and essential fatty acids, in addition to vitamins C, D, and E.[36-38] Some children may develop deficiencies because enteral formulas provide adequate amounts of micronutrients based on the age-related DRI for energy; this is more volume of formula than the NI child will receive if their energy needs are lower.[3,38] Children with NI should have their nutrition status evaluated by a registered dietitian (RD) to ascertain sufficient, but not excessive, intake of micronutrients. Replacement therapy should be initiated if deficiencies are present. Excessive intakes should be corrected when necessary.

Osteopenia

Bone growth and bone density represent an important aspect of health, growth, and quality of life. Children with NI are at risk for multiple skeletal problems including poor linear growth, scoliosis, joint subluxation, increased risk of fractures, and reduced bone mineral density (BMD).

BMD is significantly reduced in children with severe CP, with 77% of these children having a BMD z score of <−2. Annual fracture incidence is estimated at 4%. Predictors of low BMD include significant immobilization, stunted growth, previous fractures, and use of anticonvulsants.[39-41]

NI children with these risk factors as well as those who are not ambulatory and those with feeding difficulties should have a BMD evaluation. Dual-energy x-ray absorptiometry scan evaluation remains the standard for evaluating BMD in children.[42] The recommended scanning sites are total body less head and posterior anterior lumbar spine. Other sites (such as proximal femur, lateral distal femur, and forearm) can be used in children in whom the standard measurements are difficult to obtain due to positioning problems or other factors interfering with the ability to get an accurate image (spinal rods, vagal nerve stimulator, etc).[42]

Caregivers need to be cautious to avoid fractures if BMD is low. In this instance, optimization of calcium intake, determination of vitamin D status, and interventions that increase muscle mass are recommended.[40] Research on the use of bisphosphonates in children with NI is limited, and thus clear indications and possible long-term effects on bone remodeling are not known.[3] Henderson et al[43] found that bisphosphonates increased BMD by 89% over 18 months in children with CP. Whether or not this translates to decreased risk of fractures in NI children is not known. [3]

Growth and Anthropometric Measurements

Children who are better nourished and who grow better miss fewer days of school and use less heathcare.[5] Growth measurements reflect a child's nutrition status. Several challenges must be overcome in monitoring the growth of children with NI. First, obtaining reliable measurements of weight, height, and/or length can be difficult. Second, the standards used to interpret growth data are based on children with no disabilities and may not be appropriate.

Whenever possible, measurements of weight and of length or height should be done under the same conditions and with the same equipment. Measurements should be obtained at each visit and documented in the patient's record.

Weight

Weight can be obtained using standardized techniques and equipment. Children should be weighed with little or no clothing. An infant scale should be used for children who cannot stand. Older children should not be weighed on an infant scale.

For older children who are unable to stand, a bed scale, table scale, chair scale, or a wheelchair scale can be used. If none of these are available, a caregiver can stand on the scale and have their weight "zeroed" out. The child can then be given to the caregiver and the resulting weight will be only that of the child. This should only be done if no other method is available.

Length/Height

Length/height should be obtained using standard techniques and equipment. Children under 2 years of age and those who are unable to stand without crouching should be measured on a recumbent length board. Standing height without braces or shoes should be obtained on children above the age of 2 years who are able to stand without crouching.

Alternate Measurements of Stature

Children with NI may have scoliosis or hip, knee, and ankle contractures that can make obtaining an accurate length/height challenging. In this case alternate height measurements can be used. Upper arm length, lower leg length, and knee height can be reliable alternatives.[44] These alternate measurements can be either plotted on corresponding charts or converted to height using corresponding formulas.[44] For children with neuromuscular disorders such as Duchene's muscular dystrophy, an arm board measurement can be used.[45]

Body Mass Index or Weight for Length

Weight-for-length is used for children under the age of 2 years. For children older than 2 years, body mass index (BMI) should be used and can be calculated from height and weight measurements. In theory, lack of a standing height measurement precludes calculation of BMI. However estimates of height derived from upper arm length, lower leg length, and knee height are acceptable surrogates and can be used to derive the BMI for clinical purposes.[3,44]

Upper Arm Anthropometrics

Triceps skinfold (TSF) can be an important tool when assessing a child with NI. According to Samson-Fang and Stevenson,[17] TSF may be a better predictor of nutrition status than weight and height percentiles. They found that weight and height percentiles were poor predictors of nutrition status; TSF was the best predictor in children with NI. The TSF is an easy measure to obtain, the calipers are affordable, and the information is reproducible. Staff involved in doing these measurements should be trained.

A TSF of less than the 10th percentile for age and sex is an indicator that further intervention may be needed. Mid upper arm circumference (MUAC) may also be used to follow nutrition status. WHO reference ranges for MUAC are available for children ages 6–59 months.[33,46] For older children percentile guidelines provided by Frisancho[47] can be used. Serial measurement of MUAC can be useful to track changes in body composition.

Growth Charts

Height, length, weight, BMI, and weight-for-length, when properly measured and plotted on sex-appropriate and age-appropriate growth charts (http://www.cdc.gov/growth charts), can be compared with previous measures and the reference population.

A recumbent length or length proxy for a child age birth to 24 months should be plotted on the WHO birth to

24-month chart. Standing height for children 2–20 years, recumbent length on an older child, or a height proxy should be plotted on the Centers for Disease Control and Prevention (CDC) charts for 2–20 years.[48]

Weight and length/height measurements may also be plotted on condition-specific growth charts. These charts should be used with caution since they are descriptive in nature and represent small cohorts of children.

CP Growth Charts

There have been several versions of growth charts for children with CP.[16,18,33] In 2007, Day et al[18] published charts for children with CP based on a large population of children and adolescents who received services in California. The charts were the first to include children up to the age of 20 years and to separate children by Gross Motor Function Class System (GMFCS).[1] These charts allow children to be plotted based on a population with similar functional disabilities. However, they are still descriptive in nature. In 2011, Brooks et al[16] published new CP charts based on the charts first published in 2007. The 2011 charts have a prescriptive component. Knowing that children who grow better and are better nourished use less healthcare and miss fewer days of social activity, Brooks et al[16] re-examined their data and found that children in GMFCS levels I–V without feeding tubes had lower rates of morbidity and mortality when their weight was above the 20th percentile on the corresponding CP growth chart. For children in GMFCS levels I and II, a weight below the 5th percentile was associated with a higher adjusted hazard ratio. For children in levels III–V, a weight below the 20th percentile was associated with higher rates of morbidity and mortality. Children in the GMFCS level V group who were tube fed were more difficult to assess. These children had lower rates of morbidity when their weight was below the 20th percentile but higher rates of mortality on the corresponding growth chart.[16] Children with a weight that falls below the 20th percentile should be referred for further assessment. The new charts have been published in a format similar to the CDC charts and can be useful in determining the direction of care and nutrition support for children with CP.[16]

Interpretation of Growth

When using the CP charts, weights above the 20th percentile should be considered acceptable. When using the WHO and CDC charts, providers must interpret the growth trends since the reference population does not have NI. A weight or measurement of stature that falls below the 5th percentile or a weight greater than the 95th percentile should raise concerns regarding growth. Children with a weight or length that crosses 2 growth channels upward or downward should also raise concerns. Serial measurements are obtained to determine if the growth pattern is truly abnormal or if the pattern represents constitutional short stature or the rechannelling of the genetic growth potential in children with NI.

BMI-for-age may be used to screen children with NI for underweight and overweight. Children are classified as underweight if their BMI is < 5th percentile, overweight if their BMI-for-age is between the 85th and 95th percentile, and obese if their BMI-for-age is > 95th percentile. A BMI of >50th percentile for child with NI may be too heavy. Clinical judgement should be used when interpreting BMI because its use can be problematic because of decreased muscle mass, increased regional and total body fat, and/or skeletal deformities in children with NI. BMI should serve as one piece of information when determining what nutrition intervention is needed.

Nutrition Assessment

Nutrition assessment of the child with NI includes a comprehensive medical history, careful growth and anthropometric measurements, a complete physical examination, and feeding history, in addition to selected diagnostic studies.[3]

Medical History

It is important to understand the specific type of NI including its manifestations, severity, and prognosis because this relates to nutrition risk and potential nutrition interventions. It is also important to be aware of any comorbid conditions that may affect the child's nutrition status. Periodic review of the medical history for any changes in symptoms, even with a static underlying neurologic injury is indicated.[3]

Medications

A variety of medications may influence the child's eating pattern and nutrition requirements. In turn some medications may enhance the child's ability to take in nutrients. Feeding refusal and gastrointestinal discomfort maybe ameliorated with use of acid-reducing medications if the child has gastroesophageal reflux or laxatives if the child has constipation.[3] Many anticonvulsants can affect appetite both positively and negatively and can also affect level of alertness, which may in turn impact oral motor skills.[3] Some anticonvulsants can affect vitamin D metabolism, further increasing the risk for low BMD. Glycopyrrolate may reduce pooling of oral secretions, but may worsen constipation. Baclofen and trihexyphenidyl may reduce spasticity, and consequently, energy expenditure.

Review of Systems
The review of systems identifies potential problems contributing to feeding difficulties such as reflux, constipation, poor oral health, scoliosis, and contractures among others. It can also identify clues to aspiration (such as chronic cough or recurrent pneumonia) that would affect the type of nutrition intervention prescribed.[3]

Growth History
Previous measures of weight and stature are important for monitoring growth in children with NI. These measurements can be plotted on the WHO (http://www.cdc.gov/growthcharts/who_charts.htm), CDC (http://www.cdc.gov/growthcharts), or CP charts[16] to determine trends. Using serial measurements allows the provider to see if weight gain is slower or faster than expected. Measurements of stature can be difficult to obtain in children with NI (see the Growth and Anthropometric Measurements section, page 254).

Environmental and Social History
The care of the child with NI is time consuming and impacts the family in many ways including work, travel, and leisure activities. When planning nutrition interventions, it is important to take into account whether or not these recommendations are practical given the family's other responsibilities and schedules. Additional considerations include financial and insurance issues, and the nature of home healthcare services available. Nutrition interventions should be thoughtfully integrated into the routine of the family or institution.[3]

Feeding History and Meal Observation
A comprehensive overview of the literature as it relates to prevalence, assessment, and management of feeding difficulties in children with NI is found elsewhere.[17,24,49] Parental and caregiver surveys showed very high prevalence of feeding difficulties in children with NI. Studies have shown that caregivers often overestimate intake and underestimate the time spent feeding the child. Such feeding problems have also been linked to caregiver stress and fatigue, which in turn can worsen the feeding problems.[49] A 24-hour recall of food intake or an actual 3-day diet diary may reflect the adequacy of dietary energy and nutrient intake.[27] Meal observation, with emphasis on the child's ability to feed independently and the efficiency of the feeding process, can

be a key to understanding impediments to adequate nutrition.[3] The child may be given less food or actually consume less food, in part due to food spillage, than was indicated in the food recall. Observation of oral motor skills can detect poor feeding capabilities including inadequate lip closure, drooling, and persistent extrusion reflex, gagging and delayed swallowing, or coughing and choking during meals.[3] Inability to advance texture intake may reflect poor feeding abilities, which can result in decreased intake and thus poor weight gain.[3]

Complementary and Alternative Medicine
Use of complementary and alternative medicine (CAM) has been increasing dramatically in children, especially those with chronic medical conditions or special health needs. The use of CAM has been discussed in detail by an American Academy of Pediatrics (AAP) task force that reviewed different modalities of therapies and developed resources for families and practitioners.[50] A document addressing the use of CAM for children with chronic disease and disability was also published by the AAP.[51] The majority of parents who use CAM for their children do not share that information with their care provider; it is important that providers inquire about the use of CAM and be aware of potential interactions of various supplements with medications or other aspects of care.

Physical Examination
The physical examination can provide additional clues to nutrient deficiencies or excess and can help in determining energy needs. For example, muscle tone, activity level, and the presence or absence of athetoid movement affect energy needs.[3] Head control, truncal tone, contractures, and scoliosis can impact positioning during meals.[3] The skin, hair, mouth, and nails can provide evidence of micronutrient deficiencies.[3]

Diagnostic Studies
Extensive laboratory evaluation for nutrient deficiencies is often not necessary in children with NI, but some laboratory tests may be of value.[36,37,52] Anemia or iron deficiency can be detected with a complete blood count and serum iron parameters. Serum electrolytes and blood urea nitrogen (BUN) are generally markers of hydration, but it should be noted that BUN is often low in children with NI because of reduced protein intake and low muscle mass.[3] Serum albumin and prealbumin are not reliable reflections of nutrition status but were found to be predictors of morbidity and

mortality.[53] Abnormal serum phosphorus, alkaline phosphatase, and 25-hydroxyvitamin D levels may reflect bone mineral status, which should be further evaluated with bone densitometry.[3]

Additional diagnostic studies may be helpful in addressing symptoms and evaluating the need for enteral feeding. The child's risk of aspiration and degree of oral motor dysfunction can be studied by video-fluoroscopic assessment of chewing and swallowing function using different food and beverage textures and various positions.[3] Additional benefits of swallowing function evaluation include detection of silent aspiration and feeding fatigue.[3] Modifying food textures and liquid consistencies with thickening agents may help to reduce the aspiration risk. A pulmonary evaluation is needed if chronic aspiration is suspected. This evaluation, in addition to findings on an impedance study, can help determine if surgical antireflux treatment is indicated, particularly when enteral access is being considered. An impedance study can identify both acid and nonacid reflux.[54] A gastric emptying scan may detect delayed gastric emptying, which may indirectly contribute to GER and aspiration.[3] An upper gastrointestinal series provides information about the anatomy and motility of the upper gastrointestinal tract and can be used to diagnose superior mesenteric artery syndrome.[3] This can also determine the location of the stomach, which can be unusual in children with severe scoliosis, making a gastrostomy placement very difficult and thus potentially altering plans for enteral access.[3]

Nutrition Support

Estimating Nutrition Requirements

As should be evident from the preceding discussion, estimates of energy requirements for children with NI must take into account the degree of neurological disability, mobility, feeding difficulties, altered body composition, and the need for weight gain or weight loss.[3] Several options exist for determining dietary energy needs to use as a starting point, including the DRI standards for basal energy expenditure,[35] indirect calorimetry,[20,55] and the WHO equation (see Table 18-1).[35] Height has been used but is not recommended due to the difficulty in obtaining an accurate height as discussed previously. Each of these methods may overestimate, or possibly underestimate, energy needs in children with NI, so regardless of the method used, it is critical to monitor weight gain or loss as well as linear growth to determine the adequacy of diet.

TABLE 18-1. World Health Organization Equations to Determine Energy Needs

SEX	AGE	ENERGY NEEDS,[a] KCAL/D
Males	0–3	60.9W − 54
	3–10	22.7W + 495
	10–18	17.5W + 651
	18–30	15.3W + 679
Females	0–3	61W − 51
	3–10	22.5W + 499
	10–18	12.2W + 746
	18–30	14.7 + 496

W, weight.
[a]World Health Organization Equations.[35]

When changes to energy intakes are made, it is important to ensure adequate intake of protein and micronutrients.[3] Because evidence-based guidelines specific for children with NI do not exist, protein, vitamins, and minerals should be provided based on the DRIs for healthy children of a similar age.[3] These can be found on the U.S. Department of Agriculture website (http://fnic.nal.usda.gov/dietary-guidance/dietary-reference-intakes/dri-tables). Providing adequate amounts of these nutrients can be a challenge in a tube-fed child who has very low calorie needs and in those who receive only table foods and regular beverages. Multivitamin, mineral, and electrolyte supplementation may be needed to meet their nutrient needs, particularly in relation to the need for improved vitamin D status because intakes can vary greatly from day to day.[56] Evaluation and follow up with an RD is important.

Modes of Nutrition Support

Oral feeding is the preferred method of feeding for children with NI. However, some children may require enteral nutrition support. Enteral tube feeding is necessary in children who cannot meet their energy, fluid, or nutrient needs orally and those who are at risk of aspiration.[57] Evidence of oral motor feeding difficulties, undernutrition, growth failure, overweight, or individual nutrient deficiencies are additional indicators of the need for nutrition intervention.[1]

For orally fed children, many options exist for increasing calorie intake if needed. Caregivers should be encouraged to increase the calorie density of the foods they offer. Modular products are available to increase carbohydrate, protein, and/or fat in foods, but readily available items such as vegetable oils, butter, margarine, dry milk powder, cream, cheese, and gravy may also be added to foods to increase caloric density. Families and caregivers should also be counseled to offer oral supplements. A variety of acceptable nutritionally balanced commercial supplements are available in both a milk and juice base. In the absence of allergy or intolerance, taste is the primary consideration in choosing a supplement. It is essential that the child be evaluated by a RD so an appropriate plan can be developed and the child's weight gain can be monitored.

Positioning and Oral Feeding

Proper positioning is important for feeding, which requires the use of appropriate chairs. A physical therapist can help with equipment such as a feeding chair, standing table, or proper alignment in a wheelchair to help with feeding. Adapted utensils can enhance the success of feeding. The feeding therapist or occupational therapist can assist with correct positioning and use of such utensils, in addition to working on improving oral skills particularly in children under age 5 years.[3] Enhancing oral motor function may not always result in improved feeding efficiency or weight gain. Because of this and the fact that in some instances abilities can decline over time, it is important to reevaluate oral feeding skills as part of routine monitoring to determine if continued oral feeding is appropriate.[3] Another approach to improving oral intake is dedicated behavioral therapy, which to be effective requires a child psychologist who has been specifically trained in such therapy. This has the potential to positively impact several components of oral feeding including the amount of food eaten, how long it takes to complete a feeding, the variety of textures consumed, and importantly the interactions between the caregiver and the child during a meal.[3,58]

Enteral Tube Feeding

Enteral tube feedings should be considered if the child with NI cannot take in enough orally for adequate weight gain, linear growth, and hydration.[3] Additional indications for enteral feeds include risk of aspiration and long mealtimes caused by chewing and swallowing dysfunction.[3] Factors to consider in determining the type of enteral access to recommend include the current nutrition and clinical status of the child, how long enteral feedings are likely to be required, and the type of feeding regimen that may best fit the needs of the child and family.[3]

Enteral Access

Nasogastric (NG) or nasojejunal (NJ) tube feeding is used for short-term nutrition support or in children who are awaiting gastrostomy placement. Long-term use of NG or NJ tubes is not recommended due to discomfort; risk of dislodgement, which can lead to aspiration; and local complications, such as skin and mucosal irritation, nasal congestion, and sinusitis.[3] Most institutions use fluoroscopic assistance for NJ tube placement, which represents an additional barrier for the use of NJ tubes because the family would have to bring the child back to the hospital in case of dislodgement.

A gastrostomy tube or low profile device (button) is preferable for those who need long-term enteral nutrition. Children who receive gastrostomy tube feeds early in the course of their illness have better growth and nutrition outcomes. Children who receive late gastrostomy tube feeding may gain weight but linear growth deficits often persist.[59]

Several options are available for gastrostomy placement, including standard surgical approach, interventional radiology placement, and percutaneous endoscopic gastrostomy (PEG) placement. The latter 2 are minimally invasive nonsurgical procedures, with little postprocedure pain and the ability to use the feeding device within a few hours of placement.[3,60] Surgical gastrostomy placement (typically laparoscopic) is a safe alternative for enteral access in the child with NI. Laparoscopic or open surgical fundoplication may also be required, which can be complicated by postplacement feeding difficulty, gas bloat, or dumping syndrome. The incidence of these complications and the recurrence of acid reflux following fundoplication vary in children with NI.[3] The pros and cons of fundoplication in management of reflux has been reviewed elsewhere.[61] Retching is a particularly distressing symptom that can occur following fundoplication, but it generally can be controlled by slowing the rate of formula administration and also by use of blenderized tube feedings.[62] Less commonly jejunal tube placement is needed, either placement of a gastrojejunal tube through a gastrostomy site or a surgical jejunostomy tube placement. These are reserved for those with poor tolerance of intragastric feeds, severe GER, and aspiration risk, as well as in those who are not good candidates for fundoplication.[3]

The higher morbidity reported in children fed by gastrostomy may reflect the severity of their neurological disability compared with those who are fed orally.[8,63] It may also reflect a tendency to overfeed these children. It may be prudent to evaluate for acid reflux before gastrostomy placement, preferably through pH impedance testing, which has now become the standard of care for diagnosis of acid and nonacid reflux; upper endoscopy with esophageal biopsy is less likely to predict the clinical outcome after PEG placement in children.[3,54] The risk of acid reflux or esophagitis after PEG placement in developmentally impaired children without previous symptoms is increased.[64] Medical, and sometimes surgical, therapy for preexisting acid reflux will often be required after PEG placement.[63]

Enteral Feeding Regimen

There are many ways to administer tube feedings to a child with NI. Regimens typically include a combination of bolus and continuous feeds. Bolus feedings mimic the physiological response to feeding and allow for more convenience and flexibility. If the entire volume of formula cannot be given as boluses during the day, it is reasonable to do some boluses during the day and infuse the remainder as a continuous drip overnight.[3] Children with GER or delayed gastric emptying often do not tolerate bolus feeds. For those who do not tolerate bolus feeds or who receive jejunal feeds, continuous formula infusions are needed. The duration of the continuous drip depends in part on the volume that needs to be infused and what rate of delivery is tolerated. While they allow for more daytime flexibility, night time feeds may interfere with sleep.[3]

Formula Selection

The decision about what formula to use should take into account the child's age, any contributing medical conditions, estimated calorie requirements, and tolerance.[3] Initial selections should include a standard age-appropriate casein-based or whey-based formula. Whey-based formulas may be better tolerated, but if the child has evidence of a milk protein allergy or sensitivity, a protein hydrolysate or amino acid formula can be used.[3] Attention should be given to macronutrient and micronutrient content of formula, especially in children with low energy needs. Addition of supplemental vitamins, minerals, or electrolytes can help avoid or treat deficiencies. Hydration status, protein, and micronutrient intake should be monitored when high energy density (1.2, 1.5, or 2 kcal/mL) formulas are used.[3] Formula with added fiber may help with constipation but can cause gas and bloating.[3]

Home-Prepared Tube Feedings

Home-prepared tube feeding (HPTF) is food that has been liquefied in a blender and is bolus fed through a gastrostomy tube. HPTF was used for many years prior to the development of commercially prepared, sterile, standardized enteral formulas. Families continue to express an interest in using HPTF to replace enteral feeds.[65] The use of home-prepared feeds is rising due to its use in treating gagging and retching associated with fundoplication.[62] Very few peer-reviewed publications address the safe and effective use of homemade feedings except when they have been used for relieving gagging and retching after fundoplication.[62,66] Some families prefer the use of home-prepared formulations, citing lower cost, health benefits of providing a variety of foods, and the psychosocial advantage of their child being able to participate in home-prepared meals.[67]

Contraindications for use of HPTFs include 1) acute illness or severe immunosuppression; 2) having a gastrostomy tube (G tube) size less than 10 French; 3) fluid restrictions or intakes less than 30 oz/d; 4) continuous feedings that require a feeding bag to be left unrefrigerated for more than 2 hours; 5) jejunostomy tube feeding since these require continuous feeds; 6) multiple food allergies/intolerances or special diet restrictions; 7) lack of resources for the family such as no electricity, refrigeration, hot water, or other needed supplies to prepare the formula; and 8) inability to tolerate bolus feedings into a G tube.[65,66] Regardless of the reason for the use of HPTF, the support of an RD is essential to analyze the composition of the mixture for adequacy of all macronutrients and micronutrients. A computer analysis of the formulation is recommended for all tube feedings, especially if they are used as a sole source of nutrition. Energy needs should be met but not exceeded in planning these feedings. Close monitoring for tolerance and growth is needed. Special care and clean technique are very important for all tube feedings but even more important with HPTF.

Feeding Intolerance

Feeding intolerance may present as abdominal distension, discomfort, vomiting or regurgitation, or constipation or diarrhea and may be associated with GER and delayed gastric emptying.[3] The quality and quantity of the feeding regimen requires periodic reevaluation, with particular attention to progression of the neurological disorder, illness, or mechanical obstruction.[3] Interventions to ameliorate feeding intolerance include trying a different feeding schedule (such as smaller more frequent boluses, continuous feeds instead of bolus), adjusting the rate of infusion, changing the concentration of the formula (either increasing the concentration to decrease the volume of feeds or decreasing the concentration if osmolarity is a concern), or trying an alternative formula (such as hydrolyzed or elemental formula).[3] If symptoms persist, attention must be given to possible underlying conditions. In the case of acid reflux or delayed gastric emptying, therapeutic approaches may include use of hydrolyzed formula, acid-suppressing medications, and/or promotility medications as well as consideration of postpyloric feeds. If constipation is thought to be playing a role in feeding intolerance, laxative agents with stool-softening and stimulatory effects can be used.[3] Rectal inertia may require local treatment with suppositories or enemas. In those with severe constipation, antegrade enemas through a surgically created antegrade colonic enema stoma or cecostomy can be used.

Ethical Considerations

The discussion about need for a G tube is often very difficult. Caregivers believe that they have failed to adequately care for the child when physicians suggest G tube placement. Parents of children with G tubes, however, often report higher satisfaction and quality of life.[67,68] Conversations with the family should include discussions of nutrition, quality of life, and meaningful family relationships, and medical recommendations should always take parental wishes into consideration.

Summary and Conclusion

Nutrition support is essential for the care of the child with NI. After a thorough multidisciplinary evaluation, an individualized plan that takes into account the child's nutrition status, feeding ability, and medical condition can be formulated. Assessment of a child with NI includes a thorough medical history, accurate growth and anthropometric measurements, physical examination, feeding history, and selected diagnostic studies. Obtaining the correct anthropometrics and plotting them on the appropriate charts is integral to developing a nutrition plan of care. An individualized plan for nutrition interventions should take into consideration nutrition status, feeding abilities, medical condition, and psychosocial factors. This plan is determined through input from all members of the team and should aim to achieve the child's growth potential and maintain adequate nutrition status as illustrated in Figure 1.

Oral feeding should be maintained in children with adequate oral motor skills and who are at a low risk of aspiration. Nutrition support should be provided by the enteral route when the gastrointestinal tract is functional. Enteral nutrition support should be considered when, after using appropriate growth charts, evidence of malnutrition or growth failure is present or when nutrient deficiencies are found and in children who are at risk of aspiration. When feeding a child with NI by the enteral route, nutrient requirements, type of formula, the method of administration, feeding tolerance, and ethical issues should all be considered. The discussion to use tube feeding can be difficult at times and must be approached with understanding and compassion. Parents may resist starting enteral feeds for a variety of reasons, including lack of control, feelings of failure, or cultural reasons. Continued evaluation of growth and intake is imperative for the health and well-being of children with NI. The frequency of visits depends on the age of the child and their level of health. Young children should be seen at least 3–4 times per year. Older stable children can be seen 1–2 times per year. All children should also be evaluated at times of illness and when feeding issues arise. Using a multidisciplinary team, including physicians, nurses, RDs, psychologists, speech therapists, physical therapists, and occupational therapist, individualized nutrition assessment and support and close monitoring are essential to successful nutrition in children with NI.[69]

Figure 1. Case Study

HH is a male with spastic quadriplegic CP, seizures, and failure to thrive. He is 14 years, 6 months old. At his first visit in CP clinic, he presented for evaluation of feeding ability and nutrition status.

He was at GMFCS V[1,18] and has not had a gastrostomy tube or other means of tube feeding.

Growth parameters:
Weight: 19.1 kg, below 5th percentile on CDC growth chart
Height: 137 cm, below 5th percentile on CDC growth chart (estimated from knee height)
BMI: 10.18 kg/m², below 5th percentile

HH's weight is at the 10th percentile on the CP chart for a non–tube-fed male at the GMFCS V level.[18] This is associated with increased morbidity and mortality. The family reported that he eats puréed foods from all food groups and is fed 3 meals and 1–2 snacks per day. The family prepared puréed food by mixing milk into the food to bring it to the correct texture. The family did not use any calorie boosters at that time. HH frequently coughed with solid food and liquids. He would pause before swallowing and occasionally his father had to massage HH's neck to get him to swallow. HH sat in his stroller or in his father's lap to eat. On further review of symptoms, HH has constipation; he may go 1 week or longer without having a bowel movement. He is not on stool softeners or stimulant laxatives. HH has had no bowel movement in 2 weeks. Medications included lamotrigine and diazepam as needed.

At this first visit, the family was asked to use a 1 kcal/mL commercial nutrition supplement in place of milk and to increase calories in the foods they offer by adding butter or oil to foods. HH was sent for a seating evaluation, and to the feeding team as well as for an evaluation for a gastrostomy tube (G tube). On a speech evaluation, it was deemed safe for HH to receive puréed foods and thickened liquids. Given his degree of malnutrition, it was expected that he would likely require G tube placement. After a few weeks from the first clinic visit, it was found that the initial nutrition interventions resulted in minimal weight gain. HH then underwent placement of a surgical G tube and was started on a 1 kcal/mL nutrition product.

When he left the hospital, HH was tolerating 700 mL, 700 kcal, of formula by continuous feeding overnight and taking some puréed foods by mouth.

Estimated needs were calculated by WHO method:

$$19.1 \times 17.5 + 651 = 985 \text{ kcal/d}$$

The tube feeding regimen provided approximately 70% of his calorie needs.

HH returned to clinic 3 months after his G tube placement.

At that visit, growth parameters were:
Weight: 22 kg, below 5th percentile on CDC chart
Height: 138.5 cm, below 5th percentile on CDC chart (estimated from knee height)
BMI: 11.4 kg/m², below 5th percentile

HH's weight continued to be at the 10th percentile on the CP chart for a tube-fed male at the GMFCS V level.

At that visit, calories were increased by changing to a 1.2 kcal/mL commercial formula given by G tube overnight. He was to take puréed food by mouth with calorie boosters and a 1.0 kcal/mL commercial formula added during the day. After a feeding-focused multidisciplinary evaluation involving speech, physical, and occupational therapists, speech therapists recommended using nectar-thick liquids and provided the family with a commercial thickener. Physical and occupational therapists provided equipment and recommendations to improve seating position during meals. Review of systems showed that HH is now on polyethylene glycol and has had significant improvement in constipation. Medications: polyethylene glycol, Xanthan gum, lamotrigine, and diazepam.

Eight months after his G tube placement, HH was tolerating his tube feeds and taking puréed foods and nectar thick liquids. His growth had improved.

Growth parameters:
Weight: 25.7 kg, below 5th percentile on CDC chart
Height: 140 cm, below 5th percentile on CDC chart (estimated from knee height)
BMI: 13.1 kg/m², below 5th percentile

HH's weight is at the 20th percentile on the CP chart for a tube-fed male at the GMFCS V level. This is associated with lower mortality risk. HH is still followed up regularly for monitoring and adjustment of tube feeding to maintain appropriate weight gain and linear growth.

This case highlights the importance of a multidisciplinary approach to help overcome obstacles faced by families and healthcare providers in providing nutrition to children with NI.

Test Your Knowledge Questions

1. Which anthropometric measurements are most useful to determine nutrition status of the child with neurological impairment?
   A. Height and length
   B. Weight, head circumference, and arm circumference
   C. Head circumference, body mass index, and skinfold thickness
   D. BMI, triceps skinfold, weight, and height

2. What are the most common reasons for poor weight gain in the child with neurological impairment?
   A. Inadequate dietary intake and constipation
   B. Increased basal metabolic rate
   C. Chewing and swallowing dysfunction and inadequate dietary intake
   D. Athetoid or repetitive motor movements and aspiration

3. The best way to determine the adequacy of the diet for children with neurological impairment is to
   A. Calculate energy needs based on WHO equation for estimating needs.
   B. Monitor the rate of weight gain or loss and change in BMI.
   C. Measure hemoglobin concentration and serum albumin levels.
   D. Provide a protein hydrolysate or amino acid formula as the main source of nutrients.

Acknowledgments

The authors of this chapter for the second edition of this text wish to thank Kathleen J. Motil, MD, PhD, for her contributions to the first edition of this text.

References

1. Palisano R, Rosenbaum P, Walter S, Russell D, Wood E, Galuppi B. Development and reliability of a system to classify gross motor function in children with cerebral palsy. *Dev Med Child Neurol*. 1997;39(4):214–223.

2. Thomas AG AA. Technical aspects of feeding the disabled child. *Curr Opin Clin Nutr Metab Care*. 2000;3(3):221–225.

3. Marchand V, Motil KJ. Nutrition support for neurologically impaired children: A clinical report of the North American Society for Pediatric Gastroenterology, Hepatology, and Nutrition. *J Pediatr Gastroenterol Nutr*. 2006;43(1):123–135.

4. Samson-Fang L, Fung E, Stallings VA ea. Relationship of nutritional status to health and societal participation in children with cerebral palsy. *J Pediatr*. 2002;141(5):637–643.

5. Stevenson RD, Conaway M, Chumlea WC, et al. Growth and health in children with moderate-to-severe cerebral palsy. *Pediatrics*. 2006;118(3):1010–1018.

6. Rogers B. Feeding method and health outcomes of children with cerebral palsy. *J Pediatr*. 2004;145(2 suppl):S28–S32.

7. Sleigh G, Brocklehurst P. Gastrostomy feeding in cerebral palsy: a systematic review. *Arch Dis Child*. 2004;89(6):534–539.

8. Samson-Fang L, Butler C, O'Donnell M. Effects of gastrostomy feeding in children with cerebral palsy: AACPDM evidence report. *Dev Med Child Neurol*. 2003;45(6):415–426.

9. Sullivan PB, Juszczak E, AM B. Gastrostomy tube feedings in children with cerebral palsy: a prospective, longitudinal study. *Dev Med Child Neurol*. 2005;47(2):77–85.

10. Craig GM, Carr LJ, H C. Medical, surgical, and health outcomes of gastrostomy feeding. *Dev Med Child Neurol*. 2006;48(5):353–360.

11. Stallings VA, Charney EB, Davies JC, Cronk CE. Nutritional status and growth of children with diplegic or hemiplegic cerebral palsy. *Dev Med Child Neurol*. 1993;35(11):997–1006.

12. Bandini LG, Schoeller DA, Fukagawa NK, Wykes LJ, Dietz WH. Body composition and energy expenditure in adolescents with cerebral palsy or myelodysplasia. *Pediatr Res*. 1991;29(1):70–71.

13. Schultz R, Glaze DG, Motil KJ, et al. The pattern of growth failure in Rett syndrome. *Am J Dis Child*. 1993;147(6):633–637.

14. Stevenson RD, Hayes RP, Carter LV, Blackman JA. Clinical correlates of linear growth in children with cerebral palsy. *Dev Med Child Neurol*. 1994;36(2):135–142.

15. Nelson MD, Widman LM, Abresch RT, et al. Metabolic syndrome in adolescents with spinal cord dysfunction. *J Spinal Cord Med*. 2007;30(suppl 1):S127–S139.

16. Brooks J, Day S, Shavelle R, Strauss D. Low weight, morbidity, and mortality in children with cerebral palsy: new clinical growth charts. *Pediatrics*. 2011;128(2):e299–e307.

17. Samson-Fang LJ, Stevenson RD. Identification of malnutrition in children with cerebral palsy: poor performance of weight-for-height centiles. *Dev Med Child Neurol*. 2000;42(3):162–168.

18. Day SM, Strauss DJ, Vachon PJ, Rosenbloom L, Shavelle RM, Wu YW. Growth patterns in a population of children and adolescents with cerebral palsy. *Dev Med Child Neurol*. 2007;49(3):167–171.

19. Kuperminc MN, Stevenson RD. Growth and nutrition disorders in children with cerebral palsy. *Dev Disabil Res Rev*. 2008;14(2):137–146.

20. Stallings VA, Zemel BS, Davies JC, Cronk CE, Charney EB. Energy expenditure of children and adolescents with severe disabilities: a cerebral palsy model. *Am J Clin Nutr*. 1996;64(4):627–634.

21. Hillesund E, Skranes J, Trygg KU, Bohmer T. Micronutrient status in children with cerebral palsy. *Acta Paediatr*. 2007;96(8):1195–1198.

22. Kilpinen-Loisa P, Pihko H, Vesander U, Paganus A, Ritanen U, Makitie O. Insufficient energy and nutrient intake in children with motor disability. *Acta Paediatr*. 2009;98(8):1329–1333.

23. Sullivan PB, Alder N, Allison ME, et al. Gastrostomy feedings in cerebral palsy: too much of a good thing? *Dev Med Child Neurol*. 2006;48(11):877–882.

24. Arvedson JC. Feeding children with cerebral palsy and swallowing difficulties. *Eur J Clin Nutr.* 2013;67(suppl 2):S9–S12.

25. Fung EB, Samson-Fang L, Stallings VA, et al. Feeding dysfunction is associated with poor growth and health status in children with cerebral palsy. *J Am Diet Assoc.* 2002;102(3):361–373.

26. Sullivan PB, Lambert B, Rose M, Ford-Adams M, Johnson A, Griffiths P. Prevalence and severity of feeding and nutritional problems in children with neurological impairment: Oxford Feeding Study. *Dev Med Child Neurol.* 2000;42(10):674–680.

27. Sullivan PB, Juszczak E, Lambert BR, Rose M, Ford-Adams ME, Johnson A. Impact of feeding problems on nutritional intake and growth: Oxford Feeding Study II. *Dev Med Child Neurol.* 2002;44(7):461–467.

28. van Roon D, Steenbergen B. The use of ergonomic spoons by people, with cerebral palsy: effects on food spilling and movement kinematics. *Dev Med Child Neurol.* 2006;48(11):888–891.

29. Walker JL, Bell KL, Boyd RN, Davies PS. Energy requirements in preschool-age children with cerebral palsy. *Am J Clin Nutr.* 2012;96(6):1309–1315.

30. Becker PJ, Nieman Carney L, Corkins MR, et al. Consensus statement of the Academy of Nutrition and Dietetics/American Society for Parenteral and Enteral Nutrition: indicators recommended for the identification and documentation of pediatric malnutrition (undernutrition). *J Acad Nutr Diet.* 2014;114(12):1988–2000.

31. Azcue MP, Zello GA, Levy LD, Pencharz PB. Energy expenditure and body composition in children with spastic quadriplegic cerebral palsy. *J Pediatr.* 1996;129(6):870–876.

32. van den Berg-Emons HJ, Bussmann JB, Brobbel AS, Roebroeck ME, van Meeteren J, Stam HJ. Everyday physical activity in adolescents and young adults with meningomyelocele as measured with a novel activity monitor. *J Pediatr.* 2001;139(6):880–886.

33. Becker P, Carney LN, Corkins MR, et al. Consensus Statement of the Academy of Nutrition and Dietetics/American Society for Parenteral and Enteral Nutrition: Indicators Recommended for the Identification and Documentation of Pediatric Malnutrition (Undernutrition) [published online ahead of print November 24, 2014]. *Nutr Clin Pract.* 2014;pii: 0884533614557642.

34. Bandini LG, Puelzl-Quinn H, Morelli JA, Fukagawa NK. Estimation of energy requirements in persons with severe central nervous system impairment. *J Pediatr.* 1995;126(5 Pt 1):828–832.

35. Food and Agriculture Organization of the United Nations, United Nations University, World Health Organization. *Human energy requirements: Report of a Joint FAO/WHO/UNU Expert Consultation: Rome, 17–24 October 2001.* Rome: Food and Agricultural Organization of the United Nations; 2004.

36. Jones M, Campbell KA, Duggan C, et al. Multiple micronutrient deficiencies in a child fed an elemental formula. *J Pediatr Gastroenterol Nutr.* 2001;33(5):602–605.

37. Hals J, Bjerve KS, Nilsen H, Svalastog AG, Ek J. Essential fatty acids in the nutrition of severely neurologically disabled children. *Br J Nutr.* 2000;83(3):219–225.

38. Piccoli R, Gelio S, Fratucello A, Valletta E. Risk of low micronutrient intake in neurologically disabled children artificially fed. *J Pediatr Gastroenterol Nutr.* 2002;35(4):583–584.

39. Uddenfeldt Wort U, Nordmark E, Wagner P, Duppe H, Westbom L. Fractures in children with cerebral palsy: a total population study. *Dev Med Child Neurol.* 2013;55(9):821–826.

40. Mergler S, Evenhuis HM, Boot AM, et al. Epidemiology of low bone mineral density and fractures in children with severe cerebral palsy: a systematic review. *Dev Med Child Neurol.* 2009;51(10):773–778.

41. Henderson RC, Kairalla J, Abbas A, Stevenson RD. Predicting low bone density in children and young adults with quadriplegic cerebral palsy. *Dev Med Child Neurol.* 2004;46(6):416–419.

42. Crabtree NJ, Arabi A, Bachrach LK, et al; International Society for Clinical Densitometry. Dual-energy x-ray absorptiometry interpretation and reporting in children and adolescents: the revised 2013 ISCD Pediatric Official Positions. *J Clin Densitom.* 2014;17(2):225–242.

43. Henderson RC, Lark RK, Kecskemethy HH, Miller F, Harcke HT, Bachrach SJ. Bisphosphonates to treat osteopenia in children with quadriplegic cerebral palsy: a randomized, placebo-controlled clinical trial. *J Pediatr.* 2002;141(5):644–651.

44. Stevenson RD. Use of segmental measures to estimate stature in children with cerebral palsy. *Arch Pediatr Adolesc Med.* 1995;149(6):658–662.

45. Miller F, Koreska J. Height measurement of patients with neuromuscular disease and contractures. *Dev Med Child Neurol.* 1992;34(1):55–60.

46. de Onis M, Yip R, Mei Z. The development of MUAC-for-age reference data recommended by a WHO Expert Committee. *Bull World Health Org.* 1997;75(1):11–18.

47. Frisancho AR. New norms of upper limb fat and muscle areas for assessment of nutritional status. *Am J Clin Nutr.* 1981;34(11):2540–2545.

48. Greer FR, Bhatia JJS. CDC: use WHO growth charts for children under 2. *AAP News.* 2010;31(11):1.

49. Rogers B. Feeding method and health outcomes of children with cerebral palsy. *J Pediatr.* 2004;145(2 suppl):S28–S32.

50. Kemper KJ, Vohra S, Walls R; Task Force on Complementary and Alternative Medicine; Provisional Section on Complementary, Holistic, and Integrative Medicine. The use of complementary and alternative medicine in pediatrics. *Pediatrics.* 2008;122(6):1374–1386.

51. Sandler AD, Brazdziunas D, Cooley WC, et al. Counseling families who choose complementary and alternative medicine for their child with chronic illness or disability. *Pediatrics.* 2001;107(3):598–601.

52. Hals J, Ek J, Svalastog AG, Nilsen H. Studies on nutrition in severely neurologically disabled children in an institution. *Acta Paediatr.* 1996;85(12):1469–1475.

53. Fuhrman MP, Charney P, Mueller CM. Hepatic proteins and nutrition assessment. *J Am Diet Assoc.* 2004;104(8):1258–1264.

54. Woodley FW, Mousa H. Acid gastroesophageal reflux reports in infants: a comparison of esophageal pH monitoring

and multichannel intraluminal impedance measurements. *Dig Dis Sci.* 2006;51(11):1910–1916.

55. Krick J, Murphy PE, Markham JF, Shapiro BK. A proposed formula for calculating energy needs of children with cerebral palsy. *Dev Med Child Neurol.* 1992;34(6):481–487.

56. Misra M, Pacaud D, Petryk A, Collett-Solberg PF, Kappy M. Vitamin D deficiency in children and its management: review of current knowledge and recommendations. *Pediatrics.* 2008;122(2):398–417.

57. Axelrod D, Kazmerski K, Iyer K. Pediatric enteral nutrition. *JPEN J Parenter Enteral Nutr.* 2006;30(1 suppl):S21–S26.

58. Linscheid TR. Behavioral treatments for pediatric feeding disorders. *Behav Modif.* 2006;30(1):6–23.

59. Sanders KD, Cox K, Cannon R, et al. Growth response to enteral feeding by children with cerebral palsy. *JPEN J Parenter Enteral Nutr.* 1990;14(1):23–26.

60. Corkins MR, Fitzgerald JF, Gupta SK. Feeding after percutaneous endoscopic gastrostomy in children: early feeding trial. *J Pediatr Gastroenterol Nutr.* 2010;50(6):625–627.

61. Di Lorenzo C, Orenstein S. Fundoplication: friend or foe? *J Pediatr Gastroenterol Nutr.* 2002;34(2):117–124.

62. Cook RC, Blinman TA. Alleviation of retching and feeding intolerance after fundoplication. *Nutr Clin Pract.* 2014;29(3):386–396.

63. Catto-Smith AG, Jimenez S. Morbidity and mortality after percutaneous endoscopic gastrostomy in children with neurological disability. *J Gastroenterol Hepatol.* 2006;21(4):734–738.

64. Sulaeman E, Udall JN, Jr., Brown RF, et al. Gastroesophageal reflux and Nissen fundoplication following percutaneous endoscopic gastrostomy in children. *J Pediatr Gastroenterol Nutr.* 1998;26(3):269–273.

65. Mortensen MJ. Blenderized tube feeding: clinical perspectives on homemade tube feeding. *PNPG Post: A publication of the Pediatric Nutrition Practice Group of the American Dietetic Association.* 2006;17(Fall):104.

66. O'Flaherty T, Santoro K, Pentiuk S. Calculating and preparing a pureed-by-gastrostomy-tube (PBGT) diet for pediatric patients with retching and gagging postfundoplication. *ICAN: Infant, Child, & Adolescent Nutrition.* 2011;3(6):361–364.

67. Adams RA, Gordon C, Spangler AA. Maternal stress in caring for children with feeding disabilities: implications for health care providers. *J Am Diet Assoc.* 1999;99(8):962–966.

68. Ogundele M, Bassi Z. G113(P) A Survey of Carers' Satisfaction with Gastrostomy Tube Feeding from a Tertiary Children's Hospital. *Arch Dis Child.* 2013;98(suppl 1):A53.

69. Van Riper C. Position of the American Dietetic Association: providing nutrition services for people with developmental disabilities and special health care needs. *J Am Diet Assoc.* 2010;110(2):296–307.

Test Your Knowledge Answers

1. The correct answer is **D**. Length and height are difficult to obtain and not always a good representation of nutrition status. Head circumference should not be used given its relation to brain growth.

2. The correct answer is **C**. Inadequate dietary intake related to swallowing dysfunction can be the most important contribution to poor weight gain.

3. The correct answer is **B**. Calculating energy requirements is important, but monitoring response to intervention is important to determine the adequacy of diet for children with NI.

19

Eating Disorders

Mary Pat Turon-Findley, MS, RD, LD

 Podcast

CONTENTS

Learning Objectives

1. Discuss the basic macronutrient and micronutrient needs in the patient with an eating disorder.
2. Determine assessment tools for management of treatment in a patient with an eating disorder or disordered eating.
3. Summarize the rationale for providing oral nutrition vs enteral nutrition or parenteral nutrition in patients with eating disorders.
4. Identify patients at risk for refeeding syndrome and identify key monitoring parameters in its prevention and treatment.
5. Acknowledge that disordered eating can be identified along with or independent of an eating disorder diagnosis with similar criteria, assessment, concerns, and treatment.

Introduction

An eating disorder is an often under-identified disease that afflicts many adolescents and young adults. It can be difficult to detect and can go undiagnosed for extended periods of time, which can greatly affect a young person's growing body as well as the maintenance of health status in adults. An eating disorder diagnosis is categorized under mental health criteria. Unfortunately, eating disorders, specifically anorexia nervosa, have the highest premature fatality rate of all mental illnesses.[1] In the United States alone, more than 10 million females and 1 million males are battling an eating disorder such as anorexia nervosa or bulimia nervosa. Of the females afflicted, approximately 5 million (although numbers vary from different reporting sources in research and articles) are American girls.[2] However, this disease is not specific to the female sex; approximately 10% of those afflicted are males, although this number continues to be on the rise for both sexes. Once thought of as a "white upper-class" disease, eating disorders are seen across all cultures and all socioeconomic classes. Robinson et al[3] found that among the leanest 25% of sixth and seventh grade girls, Hispanics and Asians reported significantly more body dissatisfaction than did Caucasians. A growing number of African Americans have cultural attitude changes associated with altered body image issues leading to an increase in eating disorder cases. Similarly, the increase of Western influence on Hispanic and Asian populations has resulted in increases of eating disorder cases.[4]

This chapter reviews the classification, diagnosis, assessment, and etiology of eating disorders; describes nutrition therapy strategies, interdisciplinary team work, and monitoring interventions for eating disorders; defines and describes the pathogenesis of refeeding syndrome; and discusses prevention and treatment of refeeding syndrome.

Classification and Diagnosis of Eating Disorders

Anorexia nervosa, bulimia nervosa, binge-eating disorder, and eating disorder not otherwise specified are eating disorders with the commonalities of extreme emotion and behaviors around food and body image. The American Psychiatric Association recommends using a multiaxial system in assessing and diagnosing mental disorders and now lists the subcategories Anorexia Nervosa, Bulimia Nervosa, Avoidant/Restrictive Food Intake Disorder, Rumination Disorder, Binge-Eating Disorder, Other Specified Feeding or Eating Disorder, Unspecified Feeding or Eating Disorder, and Pica in its *Diagnostic and Statistical Manual of Mental Disorders* (DSM-V) (Table 19-1).[5] These subcategories are diagnosed and classified on Axis 1 of the multiaxial system.[6] Of note, amenorrhea (ie, the absence of at least 3 consecutive menstrual cycles) is one of the diagnostic criteria for anorexia nervosa listed in DSM-V. However, this may not be useful in the assessment of adolescent patients because healthy adolescent females may normally have episodes of amenorrhea during the first 1–2 years after the onset of menarche.[7] In addition, a variety of disordered eating presentations exist (Table 19-2).

Psychiatric comorbidities, such as obsessive-compulsive disorder and affective disorder, are common and should be treated alongside the eating disorder.[8] Major depression is the most common comorbid disease among persons with anorexia nervosa,[9] and substance abuse prevalence is estimated at 30%–70% in persons with bulimia,[10] although substance abuse is on the rise in all types of eating disorders. Other common comorbid psychiatric diagnoses include

Table 19-1. Eating Disorder/Feeding Disorder Summary From *Diagnostic and Statistical Manual of Mental Disorders*

EATING DISORDER TYPE	CHARACTERISTICS
Anorexia nervosa	Restriction of energy intake or requirements leading to significantly low body weight for age, sex, development trajectory, or physical health; intense fear of weight gains and disturbances in one's body perceptions/false self-evaluations. Types: restricting type (during last 3 mo) and binge-eating/purge type (during the last 3 mo). Ranges of mild, moderate, severe, and extreme are dependent on BMI values.
Bulimia nervosa	Recurrent episodes of binge eating over a discrete period of time and a sense of lacking control over eating during the episode, which is done to prevent weight gain with the use of compensatory behaviors such as self-induced vomiting, misuse of laxatives or diuretics/other medications, fasting, or excessive exercise. Behaviors occur at least weekly for 3 mo, and a dysmorphic body image is present. Ranges of mild, moderate, severe, and extreme based on episodes of compensatory behaviors per week.
Avoidant/restrictive food intake disorder	An eating or feeding disturbance with significant weight loss or failure to achieve expected growth. May be low interest in eating or food; avoidance secondary to sensory issues or reality-altered thoughts on consequences of eating. Sometimes seen with medications or other mental disorders.
Rumination disorder	Characterized by repeating regurgitation or chewing and spitting foods over a period of at least 1 mo. Symptoms may occur in context of another mental disorder or in addition to other eating disorder categories.
Binge-eating disorder	Recurrent episodes of binge eating over a discrete period of time of amounts larger than what most people consume during that period and a sense of lacking control. Eating is more rapid than normal and in large amounts and is accompanied by feelings of being uncomfortably full, embarrassment, loneliness, and guilt/self-disgust. Ranges of mild, moderate, severe, and extreme dependent of binge-eating episodes a week.
Other specified feeding or eating disorder	This category applies to presentations associated with distress or impairment in social, occupational, or other important areas of function over the following designations: atypical anorexia nervosa; bulimia nervosa (low frequency or limited duration); binge-eating disorder (low frequency or limited duration); purging disorder; and night eating syndrome.
Unspecified feeding or eating disorder	Patient may present as having an eating disorder. Due to a variety of signs of clinical distress or impairments of important functional areas in which the patient does not meet full criteria.

BMI, body mass index.

anxiety, attachment disorders (example similar to reactive attachment disorder), sexuality/gender identification, personality disorder, and trauma/posttraumatic stress disorder (including considerations of physical, emotional, sexual, psychological abuse, or neglect). Eating disorders have been observed in patients with psychosis and schizophrenia.[4,5]

Table 19-2. Additional Disordered Eating Presentations

DISORDERED EATING TYPE	CHARACTERISTICS
Diabulimia	Characterized by presentation in type 1, insulin-dependent diabetic, manipulation of or lack of insulin injections as well as possible purging and restricting. Medical issues may include ketones in urine, increase of bacterial infections, and effects on kidneys, vision, and muscle integrity.
Orthrexia	Refers to an obsession with eating healthy food and avoiding unhealthy foods. Perceptions of healthy vs unhealthy food are skewed. This is not recognized as a clinical eating disorder; however, if left untreated, it can progress into an eating disorder.
Muscle dysmorphia (reverse anorexia or bigorexia)	Form of body dysmorphia in which the patient is preoccupied with masculinity, believing their muscles smaller or weak no matter how large they are. Like patients with anorexia, patients' self-perception regarding their bodies is not reality based, and they also develop in a range of eating rituals.
Compensatory	Characterized by a variety of behaviors meant to compensate for or "undo" eating. Behaviors are attempts to relieve guilt associated with eating or enjoyment. After eating, a patient may purge, fast, restrict, use diet pills, chew/spit food, and/or exercise.
Rumination[a]	Now a part of DSM-V. Characterized by repeating regurgitation or chewing and spitting foods.
PANDA	Anorexia nervosa in patients believed to be linked to Group A and β hemolytic *Streptococcus* spp.
Autism spectrum	Patient may present as an eating disorder. Due to a variety of developmental issues as well as obsessive-compulsive disorder or anxiety behaviors. May binge eat, restrict, limit food choices, or purge without a desire to change body or have negative body image.
Psychosis/ schizophrenia	Characterized by fear of food due to auditory or visual hallucinations. May also present as restricting due to paranoid thoughts or general fear of people and surroundings.
Comorbid psychiatric diagnosis	Comorbidity of multiple psychiatric diagnoses may confound eating issues/body image due to cognitive and/or mental status. In some cases medication induced eating issues arise (eg, anorexia with stimulant medications).

DSM-V, *Diagnostic and Statistical Manual of Mental Disorders*; PANDA, pediatric autoimmune neuropsychiatric disorder.

[a]See Table 19-1.

Psychiatric comorbidities or medical problems, such as ongoing dizziness, fatigue, or syncope; unintended weight loss or changes; changes in behavior both in social and physical; prevailing illness or injuries; and isolation, are often presented to the physician prior to the eating disorder detection.[5,11,12]

Binge-eating disorder has been associated with obesity and comorbid anxiety, depression, agitation, and food addiction. Within the assessment for treatment, it is important to clarify triggers for binges and identify self-esteem and self-loathing issues (many patients verbalize this as associated to guilt).[5,13] The treatment often encompasses the addiction to food binging and the feeling of being out of control, which is similar to drugs or alcohol addiction or binging behaviors. The treatment program should be a didactic process that addresses brain and behavioral thought processes.

DSM-V Axis Definitions
Although the updated DSM format does not require Axes I–V, the information is reported within the psychiatric progress note or assessment. This information helps in planning nutrition treatment as well as understanding the individual's needs:

Axis I—Clinical Syndromes: This is what is typically thought of as the DSM diagnosis (example of depression, social phobia, mood, anxiety, posttraumatic stress disorder, eating disorders)

Axis II—Developmental Disorders (including autism and mental retardation with evidence) and Personality Disorders

Axis III—Physical Conditions (especially any that play a role in exacerbation of Axes I and II; examples are side effects of eating disorders, brain injury, HIV infection, AIDS, cancer, diabetes)

Axis IV—Severity of Psychosocial Stressors events in a person's life (such as death of a loved one, college)

Axis V—Highest Level of Functioning (clinicians rate the person's level of functioning known as a Global Assessment of Functioning)[5]

Physical Presentation
The physical presentation of a person with anorexia nervosa includes dehydration, mental/physical lethargy, hair loss, muscle wasting, dry skin, signs of malnutrition in the body, abnormal laboratory values, cyanosis of extremities, bradycardia < 60 beats/min, lanugo-type hair, and cachexia. When anorexia develops in childhood, the first clinical sign may be failure to make weight gain or reduced growth velocity in height (or possibly lack of physical maturation age specific goals) as opposed to documented weight loss. Growth charts should be evaluated for typical growth patterns of the individual.[4,5,14]

Physical signs and symptoms of a person with bulimia nervosa are more difficult to detect but may include parotid gland enlargement, scarring of the hand used to stimulate gag reflux (referred to as Russell's sign), erosion of dental enamel with increased dental caries, and sore red throat secondary to excessive purging.[15] Other signs include swollen or reddened gums, darkened circles under eyes, swollen cheeks, scratches on knuckles or hands, broken nails, and dry skin areas around nose and mouth. Dependent on the degree of purging, or other compensatory behaviors, and whether or not any restriction is utilized, the patient with bulimia nervosa may meet all expected weight gains and track normally along the growth chart percentiles.

Etiology of Eating Disorders

The etiology of eating disorders is complex but appears to originate from not only predisposing genetic factors but also serotonin dysfunction and psychological factors surrounding childhood abuse and/or trauma.[16] A 17-year longitudinal study of 800 children found that eating conflicts, struggles with food, and unpleasant meals were additional risk factors for the development of an eating disorder in this population.[17] The role of heredity is still unclear because twin studies, which are often utilized to differentiate between genetic factors and environment in familial studies, have reported mixed data, with some demonstrating a strong correlation, while others finding little correlation.[18]

Nutrition in Eating Disorders

Although nutrition rehabilitation and weight stabilization are essential components in the treatment of and recovery from eating disorders, research continues to be limited in the affected population. The following recommendations should be used as guidelines and not definitive treatment protocols.

Nutrition Assessment

Establishing trust with a patient is of paramount importance to ascertain information to complete a nutrition assessment and to set parameters for treatment as well as the continuum of care. Often times individuals with eating disorders may have limited cognitive abilities, poor memory due to malnutrition/poor intake, comorbid psychiatric issues, trust issues, and fears of being overfed.

When interviewing a patient (Table 19-3), speak in calm, low tones. Posture should not be threatening; attempt to elevate eye contact needs. Concentrate on open-ended questions. Interactions should be firm but empathetic. Attempt to avoid showing disappointment or surprise with responses. Observe

Table 19-3. Interview Process Template Guide Decision Tree

- Ask patient what brings them into clinical setting (eg, hospital, office)
- If patient responds about eating issue, continue Route A

Route A
- o Ask the patient to describe what is going on
- o Determine how long it has been an issue
- o Inquire when the last time (restricted, purged, etc) occurred
- o Acquire physical parameters, asking about dizziness, headaches, gastrointestinal distress, bowel movements, regular periods, time of last period, sleep patterns
- o Ask the patient to describe any triggers or sentinel event that initiated the practice
- o Acquire any intake recall for a typical day (attempt to get quantities and brand information); eg, when the patient ate, what was eaten, types/amounts of fluids, any food avoidances, food allergies, new diet plans or new diet practices (eg, vegetarian, gluten free)
- o Information on supplements, vitamins, herbs, and medications
- o Inquire about the patient's usual weight and any changes in weight/appetite history
- o Ask the patient how he or she views his or her body: Do you have a negative body image? What do you see in a mirror?
- o Inquire about participation in sports and other activities, including amount of time spent in practice, games, or competition or in exercise
- o Determine the patient's goals for hospitalization/treatment
- o Review any substance use, self-harm, depression, anxiety, suicidal thoughts, or other trauma
- o For patients with posttraumatic stress disorder, consider briefly reviewing the influence of trauma on eating issues

- If patient does not respond about eating issue, but one is suspected, start with Route B

Route B
- o Ask about any recent changes in appetite or weight, and explore the patient's answers
- o Inquire whether the patient's habits about how he or she eats or sees food changed; again, explore the answers
- o Determine whether the patients is able to eat in front of others and explore the parameters
- o Gauge the direction of information before asking if the patient ever restricts, gets sick after eating, or can't stop eating or is addicted to certain foods; explore the responses
- o In cases of binging, inquire about hoarding, triggers, challenging situations, history, and where/when binges occur
- o In cases of purging, inquire about the number of times, history, locations, and triggers
- o In cases of restricting, inquire on trigger, history, challenge foods, and challenge situations
- o Continue with Route A, starting with acquiring physical parameters and continuing to the end

physical attributes during the interview including, but not limited to, posture, signs of malnutrition and dehydration, nonverbal cues, signs of self-harm, and overall cognitive level. Evaluate whether the interview should be one on one as opposed to including family for ascertaining the most accurate information.

In addition to physical, medical, and social information from the medical record/chart, key interview points should include history of eating issues, trauma history, and sentinel events; changes in medical conditions (examples include emesis, changes in bowel habits, sleep pattern, hair loss, dizziness/headache); changes in food acceptance or diet; body image perceptions; intake recall; any comorbid behavioral issues or suicidal ideation; activity levels; and current goals.

Identifying social influences within the assessment can provide critical information for formulating a treatment plan. Teens and those in the developing years can be influenced by external factors, with feelings of insecurity. Factors to explore include genetics/family history, distorted body image, severe family issues/problems, history of abuse (sexual, physical, etc), social pressures from peers or those implied from media, pressure from activities to increase performance, and pressure from coaches, peers, family, parents, or self (see Table 19-4 and Table 19-5 for case studies).

Table 19-4. Eating Disorder Case Study 1

NG, a girl who is 16 years and 5 months old, was admitted with a 15-lb weight loss during the previous 4 weeks due to restrictive intake. She describe a usual day's food intake as follows:

Breakfast: 2–3 fruits, 1 cup vegetables, 8–12 oz of coffee

Snack: vegetables (vague report)

Lunch: cut-up vegetables, 6 oz of low-fat yogurt, fruit, 2 diet pops

Dinner: 6–8 oz of cod with fat-free Butter Spray, salad (no dressing)

Snack: air popped popcorn

Limited fluid intake throughout the day

NG was 68 lb 2 years ago when her eating issues began. At the time, she was active in dance, ballet, and tennis. She currently has dizziness when standing, fatigue, occasional blurred vision, and hair loss. She passed out in the gym last week and notes a "cold that just won't go away." She is cold "all the time." She has dry skin, and her nails appear brittle. Her hair is falling out "a lot." She has not had a period in 2 months (she is not pregnant per urine test). She implies she sometimes gets "sick" (vomits) at home when alone—the last time was a week ago.

NG's admission weight was 37.7 kg (82.94 lb; < 3rd percentile) at 162.5 cm (25th–50th percentile) with a body mass index (BMI) of 14.3 (< 3rd percentile). She does not see herself as "too thin," but people tell her that constantly. She is pale and has a 48-point pulse split. She also has infrequent bowel movements. During the interview, she was incessantly swinging her legs and tapping her feet. Results from her laboratory tests are as follows (with normal ranges for comparison): sodium, 131 mEq/L (135–145 mEq/L); potassium, 3.3 mEq/L (3.6–5.0 mEq/L); blood urea nitrogen, 6 mg/dL (7–20 mg/dL); chloride, 111 mmol/L (98–107 mmol/L); glucose, 117 mg/dL (70–110 mg/dL); hemoglobin, 10.8 g/dL (12.1–15.6 g/dL); and hematocrit, 31% (34%–45%) with elevated liver labs.

NG's mother admits to having a negative body image, and NG's grandmother was hospitalized in her 20s for consistently being ill and having poor bone healing. The mother seemed to think she may have had an eating disorder also.

During the interview:
Using the interview tree, you establish the above information on physical signs and symptoms; NG indicates that her mom and grandmother put pressure on her to excel at both ballet and tennis. Mom also demands good grades, and NG sometimes takes pills to stay awake to do homework. Dad is often out of town for work, and NG worries that he will be disappointed in her for poor grades and not dancing well. Her school work has more difficult lately.

Tentative plan:
- NG has been underweight for age as long as 2 years, and she notes "everyone is very thin in my family."
- Start menu at 1000 calories with 1200 mL of fluids. Suggest 5 feedings a day. If tolerated, food intake increases 200–250 calories per day.
- Take weight daily in morning in gown after void, with NG turned away from scale numbers.
- Monitor at meal time; only allow 20 minutes to eat. Redirect her not to get up or move her legs during meal and snack time.
- Observe her for 1 hour post intake and restrict her from her room and bathroom.
- Note that NG has activity restriction.
- Use a meal/snack supplement replacement if NG does not eat all of her meals/snack/fluids. She has a calorie count, intakes and outputs, orthostatic measures, and reassessment of laboratory values, pulse, and blood pressure each shift. Patient receives a K-Phos packet twice a day.

For the long-term treatment:
Work with NG on food challenges and concerns. Start cognitive and therapeutic interventions as well as working with family during family meetings. Provide support and offer outpatient menu planning for passes and family meal practices. Monitor laboratory values, pulse, blood pressure, weight, and lab values.

Table 19-5. Eating Disorder Case Study 2

ER, a boy who is 15 years and 6 months old, who was admitted with a > 20-lb weight loss over past month due to restricting and excessive exercise. He states his usual day's intake is as follows:

Breakfast: not eaten lately, but sometimes a handful of nuts

Lunch: packed lunch with soy milk and a vegan item (vague)

Snack: sometimes water and another handful of nuts or a fruit

Dinner: sometimes skips; aunt and uncle try to provide a vegetarian entrée and vegetables

Snack: sometimes has protein drink and some soy milk or vegetables

His fluid intake was limited. He noted he adopted a vegan diet about 2 months ago.

He changed his intake to become healthy and get more muscular. He noted he used to be 125 lb. He admits to trying to become muscular and fit after he was "dumped" by a girl at a dance. He is dizzy all the time; has bradycardia, orthostasis, and pallor; and is tired and cold "all the time." Fingernails are down to stubs. Skin is very dry, and he notes his hair falls out. He lives with his aunt and uncle; his dad works 8 hours away and has limited contact, and his mom is in jail.

Admission weight is 48.9 kg (107.8 lb; 10th–25th percentile) at 166 cm (65.4 in; 25th–50th percentile); BMI 17.7 (10th–25th percentile). He doesn't see that he is thin and just wants muscle. Electrolytes were all abnormally low; pulse split was 55 points; glucose was 60 mg/dL; and liver panel laboratory values were abnormal.

Treatment interview intervention:
ER was very guarded and needed to slowly review questions because his cognitive understanding was impaired. He was started on 1200 calories with 1200 mL of fluid for 5 feedings with meal/calorie supplement plan. He had to eat in 20 minutes and was monitored for 1 hour post intake. Calorie count, intakes and outputs, and orthostatic measures were assessed during each shift. His diet advancement goal was 200–250 calories/200 mL daily. Fluid goals were set at 2000–2500 mL/d, and the calorie goal was 2500 calories daily. Weight was measured daily in the morning in a gown, after voiding, with ER turned away from the scale's numbers. Exercise was restricted.

Treatment:
A lot of effort went into keeping the menu plan vegetarian and working with ER's aunt and uncle about parameters to monitor at home. Family meetings included therapy and trauma work around losses and neglect that ER felt. ER worked on coping skills, positive affirmations, and family interventions. He was encouraged to continue outpatient follow-up and started on a behavior medication for mood and sleep as well as a multivitamin with zinc and K-Phos packets twice a day until laboratory values stabilized.

Nutrition Requirements

Macronutrients

ENERGY REQUIREMENTS

Initial energy requirements for anorexia nervosa are 30–40 kcal/kg of current body weight.[6] An elevated diet-induced thermogenesis has been reported in anorexia nervosa.[19] In patients with an elevated diet-induced thermogenesis or in patients who are extremely anxious, energy requirements may be as high as 80–100 kcal/kg before weight gain can be achieved.[6] If higher energy intake appears to be required in a patient with anorexia nervosa due to poor weight gain, the patient should be evaluated for manipulation of intake. In patients with bulimia nervosa or binge-eating disorder, initial energy requirements for weight maintenance may start at 1.2–1.3 times the measured resting energy expenditure for sedentary activity.[20] Avoiding caloric levels that promote weight loss is recommended until the eating pattern is stabilized, because restricting calories in such a patient may trigger a binging episode.

PROTEIN REQUIREMENTS

Recommended protein intake is the recommended dietary allowance in grams per kilogram ideal body weight for age (0.8–1.5 g/kg) or 15%–20% of total calories from a high biologic value source.[6,19] During treatment and follow-up, parameters should be monitored and reassessed.

FAT REQUIREMENTS

Recommended fat intake is 25%–30% of total daily calories from fat, with appropriate sources of essential fatty acids.[6,20]

WATER REQUIREMENTS

See Table 19-6. A patient's pulse values should be monitored from lying, sitting, and standing. If the split is greater than 30 points, he or she requires monitoring for fluid needs and advancement. Monitoring the patient's blood pressure values along with his or her pulse provides orthostatic parameters for fluid advancement.

Micronutrients

A number of micronutrient deficiencies occur in patients with eating disorders. In both anorexia nervosa and buli-

Table 19-6. Timeline for Prevention and Therapy of Refeeding Syndrome[1,26,27,29,30,37,38]

ENERGY/NUTRIENT	DAYS 1–3	DAYS 4–7	DAYS 8–14
Calories	50% of goal, or 15–20 kcal/kg/d	Advance by 200–300 kcal if electrolytes and orthostatic measures are stable	Advance every 3 d by 200–300 kcal if electrolytes and orthostatic measures remain stable
Carbohydrate	2–3 g/kg/d	Advance to meet daily calorie adjustments	Advance to meet daily calorie adjustments
Protein	1–1.5 g/kg/d	1–1.5 g/kg/d	1–1.5 g/kg/d
Fat	1 g/kg/d	1 g/kg/d	1 g/kg/d
Fluid	800–1000 mL/d	Advance with calories if electrolytes stable and no clinical signs of fluid overload	Advance with calories if electrolytes stable and no clinical signs of fluid overload
Phosphorus	0.3–0.6 mmol/kg/d for normal serum levels. Correct low serum levels aggressively with 9–18 mmol over 2–12 h as indicated	0.3–0.6 mmol/kg/d. Continue to correct low serum levels as necessary	0.3–0.6 mmol/kg/d. Continue to correct low serum levels as necessary
Potassium	2–4 mmol/kg/d. Correct low serum levels as necessary	2–4 mmol/kg/d. Correct low serum levels as necessary	2–4 mmol/kg/d. Correct low serum levels as necessary
Magnesium	0.2 mmol/kg/d. Correct moderately low serum levels with 0.5 mmol/kg × 24 h. Correct severely low levels with 24 mmol over 6 h	0.2 mmol/kg/d if stable. 0.25 mmol/kg/d for patients who have been hypomagnesemic	0.2 mmol/kg/d
Thiamin	200–300 mg/d	200–300 mg/d	200–300 mg/d until day 10
Other vitamins/minerals	Multivitamin/mineral supplement daily	Multivitamin/mineral supplement daily	Multivitamin/mineral supplement daily

mia nervosa, zinc deficiency is common and has been documented as resulting from suboptimal intake attributed to severe caloric restriction, avoidance of red meat, and/or the adoption of an inadequate vegetarian lifestyle.[21] Additionally, deficiencies in riboflavin, thiamin, and other B vitamins as well as calcium and magnesium are well documented and are of concern in both anorexia nervosa and bulimia nervosa.[16] Routine screening is recommended with subsequent supplementation for anorectic patients with thiamin and magnesium deficiencies in addition to any other identified deficiencies.[22] At the onset of intervention, providing a 100% recommended dietary allowance multivitamin with minerals is recommended.[20]

Laboratory Assessment

A detailed laboratory assessment is recommended at the time of initial assessment. Although a complete blood count and chemistry profile are recommended, these traditional tests are typically normal and may underestimate the physical damage and degree of malnutrition. More targeted and sensitive tests are recommended, including zinc, iron, prealbumin, transferrin, ferritin, 25-OH vitamin D, thiamin, and complement 3 level.[23] Other laboratory values recommended for review are an electrolyte panel, glucose (for hypoglycemia or hyperglycemia), magnesium, phosphorus, insulin, calcium, and liver panel. Refer to Table 19-7 for a complete recommendation of laboratory tests.

Elevated serum cholesterol and abnormal lipoprotein profiles are often found in an anorectic patient regardless of consumption of extremely low-fat and low-cholesterol diets prior to admission. Arden et al[24] postulated that mild hepatic dysfunction, decreased bile acid secretion, and/or hypothalamic dysfunction may contribute to these abnormalities.

Nutrition Support in Eating Disorders

Milieu Management

The treatment milieu, when it is set up effectively, provides a safe environment and leads to improved outcomes. The milieu includes the following actions:

- Monitor clothing to ensure patients cannot hide food
- Ensure that a room/bathroom precaution (not allowed in room alone) is followed for at least 1 hour post meal or snack; also remove any containers that can hide food or emesis

Table 19-7. Recommended Laboratory Tests

Standard

Complete blood count (CBC) with differential

Urinalysis

Calorie count/intakes and outputs

Complete metabolic profile: sodium, chloride, potassium, glucose, blood urea nitrogen, creatinine, total protein, albumin, globulin, calcium, carbon dioxide, AST, alkaline phosphates, total bilirubin

Serum magnesium

Thyroid screen (triiodothyronine, triiodothyroxine, thyrotropin)

Electrocardiogram

Special Circumstances

15% or more below ideal body weight (IBW)

    Chest x-ray

    Complement 3

    24-h creatinine clearance

    Uric acid

20% or more below IBW or any neurological sign

    Brain scan

    Bone scan

20% or more below IBW or sign of mitral valve prolapse

    Echocardiogram

30% or more below IBW

    Skin testing for immune functioning

Weight loss 15% or more below IBW lasting 6 mo or longer at any time during course of eating disorder

    Dual energy x-ray absorptiometry to assess bone mineral density

    Estradiol level (females)

    Testosterone level (males) .

Adapted from http://www.nationaleatingdisorders.org/suggested-medical-tests. Accessed January 17, 2015.

Copyright © 2008 National Eating Disorders Association. www.nationaleatingdisorders.org.

- Monitor bathroom if indicated
- Monitor for exercise and emesis in room, including showers (emesis, water loading, or exercise in a shower) as well as excessive use of energy such as walking and tensing muscles while sitting/standing
- Monitor for active fears of eating in front of others as well as food challenges/triggers that hamper intake and may increase anxiety

The interdisciplinary team's focal point should be providing a unified treatment plan. The team communication paradigm will guide the continuum of care and support the patient and family. Many teams benefit from having members including, but not limited to, a psychiatrist, medical support specialist, registered nurse, registered dietitian (and registered dietetic technician, as needed), licensed social worker, care manager, teacher, behavioral specialist, occupational therapist, and speech therapist.

Patient observation is an important part of treatment and includes monitoring social interactions, eating requirements, and independent situations. Seeing how the patient interacts and noting his or her responses and triggers lend valuable insights to the severity of the illness as well as other factors to consider for treatment. The goal is to build a treatment tool box that will aid the patient in developing strategies towards remission of symptoms and to treat the mental health aspects of the disorder.

The social aspect and culture of eating disorders should be monitored in the milieu. Sharing of issues during treatment modality has a place, but it should not be encouraged as an avenue for developing additional habits. Often the culture of eating disorders can be the only item the person feels they are good at.[4,5,11,12]

Documentation should be based on evidence and behavior to aid with the advancement of treatment as well to pass insurance reviews. It should include the interventions with family, nutrition education, and cognitive behavioral therapy as well as other therapeutic programs.[4,5]

Nutrition Support Order Set

A general order set depends on hospital policies but should include intakes and outputs (I&O's), calorie count, blind weights in gown after void in morning, restrict activity, monitor lab values, monitor orthostatics, behavior plan on allotted time for eating, monitor at meal/snack time, calorie control plan with advancement plan, vitamin supplements, and supplement replacement plan.

Oral Nutrition and Meal-Planning Guidelines

In all eating disorders, the ultimate nutrition treatment goals include nonrestrictive eating that incorporates variety and nutrition adequacy and an absence of purging or compensatory behaviors.[25] In bulimia, purging efforts are utilized in attempts to lose weight, and patients will often request assistance during treatment to achieve weight-loss goals. Although long-term weight loss may be reasonable and/or recommended, the immediate goal for patients with either bulimia or binge-eating disorder should be interruption of the binge or binge-purge cycle with stabilization of weight.[14]

For all eating disorder types, plan 4–6 eating opportunities per day. Allow no more than 4 hours between eating opportunities in order to prevent hypoglycemia, extreme hunger, and/or the temptation to binge.[25] Each meal and snack should contain a balance of sufficient carbohydrates to prevent craving, adequate protein and fat to promote satiety,[14] and fluids.

For patients with binge-eating disorder or bulimia, the initial meal plan should not include any foods that the patient is unwilling or unable to keep from vomiting. Provide support to the patient during and after meals while encouraging expression of feelings and coping skills. Additionally, encourage the patient to remain out of the bathroom, as well as the bedroom, for up to 1 hour after meal and snack consumption.[25]

In the case of fear of eating in front of others, a behavior plan should be created with an exposure guideline. A similar plan can be developed to offer a challenge of trigger foods as part of the treatment plan.

Enteral Nutrition Support and Route of Feeding

The decision to initiate enteral nutrition (EN) in a person with an eating disorder is a complex one and should take into account not only the patient's immediate physical health but also his or her psychological health. EN support is indicated if a patient is refusing any oral intake, rapid weight loss continues despite improved oral intake, or the patient is hypermetabolic and unable to meet nutrition needs orally. When choosing a route for EN, the nasogastric route is preferred for the relative ease of administration; as part of the eating plan, however, a nasojejunal placement may alleviate discomfort from delayed gastric emptying.[20] If long-term enteral support is needed, the tube ending should be placed in the duodenum to avoid problems with gastric reflux and purging by the patient.[23]

When utilizing EN in a patient with an eating disorder, providing the supplementation in a manner that permits identifying natural hunger cues is encouraged. In a patient with bulimia nervosa, a continuous drip tube feeding is often recommended because a bolus feeding may cause involuntary vomiting and is more easily purged.[20] For the anorectic patient, several options are appropriate: bolus feed appropriate supplemental calories only at mealtimes, bolus feed only uneaten calories to meet mealtime goal, or nighttime continuous feed of uneaten or excessive calories.[25]

When EN is utilized, an isotonic, fiber-containing polymeric formula is usually sufficient for nutrition repletion, unless impaired digestion or absorption indicates use of an elemental-based or peptide-based product. Due to the high risk of refeeding syndrome (discussed in a following section) in an anorectic patient, the initial infusion should not exceed 25–50 mL/h and should be gradually increased 10–25 mL every 8–24 hours as tolerated until goal feeds are achieved.[25] Monitor free water inclusion[1] as well as pulse and blood pressure.

Manipulation behaviors may arise when utilizing EN in an individual with an eating disorder. Precautions need to be taken. Sample behaviors used in tube feeding manipulation include[23]:

- Lowering the delivery rate on the feeding pump
- Using sharp objects to poke holes in the feeding tube
- Filing the tube to reduce thickness, then bending the tube at that point to spill the feeding
- Removing the feeding bag from its hanging pole and swinging it to create air pockets to clog the tube
- Purging through the surgical opening of a percutaneous endoscopic gastrostomy tube
- Placing the nasogastric tube in another place (in a plant, out the window, in the mattress)

Parenteral Nutrition

Parenteral nutrition (PN) is only indicated in cases of digestive inability because it leads to a continued loss of hunger cues in the individual with an eating disorder.[25] When PN is initiated in severely malnourished patients, caution needs to be taken due to the possibility that refeeding syndrome might occur. (Refer to the Refeeding Syndrome section in this chapter for definitions and guidelines.) Monitoring of laboratory values depending on patient treatment plan or hospital policy parameters should be established during treatment.

Monitoring Nutrition Interventions

The anthropometric status of patients with eating disorders should be assessed and monitored regularly. Rehydration and replenished glycogen stores contribute to weight gain during the initial refeeding; thereafter, weight gain results from increased lean and fat stores.[14] In hospitalized patients in whom weight restoration is a goal, 2–3 lb/wk is reasonable.[14]

The hospitalized individual should be weighed daily, gowned, blinded (ie, weighed while turned away from the scale number), preprandial, and postvoid, preferably in the morning/same time. Baseline height and growth history should be obtained and monitored every 1–2 months in patients who still have growth potential. Baseline anthropometric measurements (skinfolds, midarm circumference, and midarm muscle circumference) should be obtained at onset of intervention and monitored as medically indicated.[14,20]

Refeeding Syndrome

Definition and Incidence

Refeeding syndrome can be described as a cascade of potentially fatal complications caused by shifts in fluid and electrolytes as nutrition is reintroduced into the body, taxing wasted and weakened tissues and demanding more nutrients than are readily available.[26,27] The syndrome is manifested in an assemblage of symptoms that result from rapidly and inappropriately refeeding (via an oral, enteral, or parenteral route) individuals who have been malnourished or starved for a period of time, usually exceeding 7–10 days.[28] Additional symptoms of refeeding syndrome include cardiac dysfunction, edema, and neurological changes.[29] Hypophosphatemia is the hallmark clinical sign of refeeding syndrome, but hypomagnesemia and hypokalemia are also common indicators. Glucose intolerance and thiamin deficiency are often present as well.[30]

The exact incidence of refeeding syndrome is unknown, due in part to the lack of a universal definition[26] and also poor recognition of the condition. It is known that 30% to 38% of previously unfed patients receiving PN containing phosphorus experience hypophosphatemia,[31] and 100% of these patients develop hypophosphatemia when no phosphorus has been added to the PN solution. It has also been documented that when patients were vigorously refed, 80% experienced hypokalemia, hypomagnesemia, and/or hypophosphatemia.[32]

Pathophysiology and Characteristics of Starvation and Refeeding

In a normal fed state, glucose and fatty acids are the preferred energy substrates for the human body. During periods of starvation exceeding 3–5 days, the body shifts glucose metabolism to fat and protein metabolism and enters a state of ketosis. The brain switches from glucose to ketones as an energy source. The liver visceral protein stores and vital organs, adipose tissue, and fluids also become depleted. The wasting of muscle affects vital organ function, including both respiratory capacity and cardiac mass and output.[26,29]

During starvation, the kidneys' role is to decrease the excretion of minerals as the body's stores become depleted. Serum electrolyte levels are maintained by decreased excretion through the kidneys and by volume constriction as fluid shifts from extracellular to intracellular spaces.[26] In addition, because electrolytes, especially phosphorus, play a major role in glucose metabolism, electrolyte demands are diminished during ketosis and starvation.[33]

As nutrition is reintroduced to the body, a rapid spike of insulin accompanies the introduction of carbohydrate, which seems to be the driving force of refeeding syndrome.[1] Insulin promotes the uptake of glucose, water, and electrolytes by the cells, and thus glycogen, protein, and fat synthesis resume. Water and sodium are retained causing extracellular fluid overload, which can lead to pulmonary edema and cardiac decompensation.[27] Hyperglycemia may result from excess carbohydrate administration and inadequate insulin output. Hyperglycemic complications include osmotic diuresis, dehydration, metabolic acidosis, and ketoacidosis.[26] Anabolism is triggered by macronutrient intake and places demands on the body for a myriad of other nutrients including phosphorus, potassium, magnesium, and water-soluble vitamins. These nutrients are now in short supply due to their depletion during the prolonged period of fasting, and the body's remaining stores are exhausted quickly.[26] Thus, hypophosphatemia, hypokalemia, hypomagnesemia, and thiamin deficiency may clinically present.

Phosphorous is involved in the intracellular processes and structural integrity of all cells.[26] It is also required for the production of energy in the form of adenosine triphosphate (ATP) and is a structural component of 2,3-diphosphoglycerate (2,3-DPG).[30] Hypophosphatemia may cause clinical symptoms when serum levels reach 1.5 mg/dL, and severe hypophosphatemia ($\leq$ 1 mg/dL) can have devastating effects on multiple systems.[27] Serum phosphorus levels typically reach a nadir around 2–3 days of refeeding.[1] Cardiovascularly, ATP depletion and cardiac atrophy contribute to hypocontractility and ventricular arrhythmia, which is complicated by volume overload. Skeletal muscle weakness and sarcolemmal disruption lead to rhabdomyolysis. Myopathy causes difficulty with ambulation and may additionally contribute to respiratory dysfunction due to accessory muscle and diaphragmatic weakness/catabolism. Hypophosphatemia affects the hemo-immunologic system by inducing bone marrow dysfunction, which can lead to decreased immune function evidenced by hemolytic anemia, thrombocytopenia, hemolysis, and decreased oxygen delivery to peripheral tissue. Hypophosphatemia influences the nervous system via inadequate 2,3-DPG and/or ATP deficiency, which may contribute to the incidence of delirium, coma, hallucinations, seizures, tetany, weakness, and parasthesias.[30]

Hypokalemia may result as anabolism resumes and cells take up potassium during fluid and electrolyte shifts. Serum potassium levels < 2.5 mg/dL may cause devastating paralysis, respiratory dysfunction, rhabdomyolysis, muscle necrosis, and changes in myocardial contraction and signal conduction.[27] Serum magnesium levels < 1 mg/dL can cause electrocardiographic changes, tetany, convulsions, and seizures.[34] All vitamins may be deficient as a result of long-term inadequate nutrition intake. However, due to its role in carbohydrate metabolism, thiamin is of particular importance. Thiamin (vitamin B$_1$) is a structural component of nervous system membranes,[35] and thus its deficiency may present with symptoms of beriberi, such as parasthesia, hypoesthesia, anesthesia, and lower extremity weakness[6]; Wernicke's encephalopathy (ocular abnormalities, ataxia, confusion, hypothermia, coma); or Korsakoff's psychosis (retrograde and anterograde amnesia, confabulation).[36]

Prevention and Therapy

Prevention of refeeding syndrome is the most effective factor in its management; therefore, an awareness and ability to identify high-risk patients is key.[27] Patients with a weight loss of ≥10% within 2–3 months or those at or below 70% ideal body weight are at the greatest risk.[27] Categories of patients who may meet these criteria include those with anorexia nervosa, alcoholism, cancer, uncontrolled diabetes, marasmus, malabsorptive syndrome (eg, pancreatitis, cystic fibrosis, short bowel), prolonged fasting, morbid obesity with profound weight loss, prolonged antacid use (due to binding of phosphorus), and long-term diuretic use (due to electrolyte losses), as well as postoperative patients, the elderly, and patients allowed nothing by mouth for longer than 5–7 days.[26]

If a patient meets the preceding high-risk criteria for refeeding syndrome, several acceptable approaches exist for preventing or treating refeeding (Table 19-6). Importantly, baseline electrolytes (including potassium, phosphorus, magnesium, and calcium) should be obtained and corrected if low prior to the initiation of feeds.[1] Electrolyte monitoring should continue 1–4 times per day depending upon the severity of malnutrition, for the first 3 days.[29] During this time, calories may be introduced at 50% of goal, not to exceed 20–25 kcal/kg/d.[1,26,27,29] Macronutrient distribution should limit carbohydrate intake to 2–3 g/kg/d based on actual body weight. No restriction is necessary for protein or fat intake, and common recommendations for each are 1–1.5 g/kg/d[1,27,29] and 1 g/kg/d, respectively.[1] Fluid should be restricted to 800–1000 mL/d due to the potential risk of fluid overload and cardiac decompensation.[27,29]

During these first few days of renourishment, electrolytes, if low, should be corrected aggressively. Potassium phosphate preferably, or sodium phosphate in the presence of normal serum potassium, can be given intravenously for moderate to severe hypophosphatemia.[30] Different references recommend infusing 9–18 mmol over anywhere from 2 to 12 hours.[26,30,37] For orally fed patients with mild to moderate hypophosphatemia, cow's milk is an excellent source of both phosphorus and potassium[30] and can be used to treat mild electrolyte derangements. Oral sodium phosphate can also be used, at 500 mg 4 times per day until serum phosphorus is stable, then decreased to 250 mg 3 times per day for maintenance.[27] Mild to moderate hypomagnesemia can be treated with an initial dose of 0.5 mmol/kg over a 24-hour infusion, then maintained at 0.25 mmol/kg/d for the next 5 days to maintain serum levels.[26] For severe hypomagnesemia, infuse 24 mmol over 6 hours, then follow with 0.25 mmol/kg/d for the next 5 days as above.[26]

In addition to the attention paid to macronutrients and electrolytes, patients at risk of refeeding should receive a daily multivitamin/mineral supplement. Any signs or symptoms of thiamin deficiency can be treated with 200–300 mg of oral thiamin daily for 10 days to correct deficiency.[26]

After electrolytes have stabilized and the patient has received ≥ 72 hours of nutrition at 50% of goal, calories can gradually be increased every 3 days by 200–300 kcal.[27,29,38] Continue to monitor and correct electrolytes as feedings progress for the duration of the first 2 weeks of feeding.[26]

With awareness and proper monitoring, refeeding syndrome can be prevented or managed appropriately to prevent serious complications and the potential of death. Monitoring and correction of electrolytes, supplementation of nutrients, and conservative administration of carbohydrate and fluid can save lives of those at highest risk for refeeding.

Test Your Knowledge Questions

1. The following are common physical signs and symptoms of anorexia nervosa:
   A. Lanugo-type hair, cyanosis of the extremities, and erosion of the dental enamel
   B. Cyanosis of the extremities, erosion of the dental enamel, and Russell's sign
   C. Cachexia, cyanosis of the extremities, and muscle wasting
   D. Cachexia, Russell's sign, and sore red throat
2. When interviewing an individual with a newly diagnosed eating disorder:
   A. Be judgmental and show no empathy; do not assess physical issues
   B. Be calm, empathic, and nonjudgmental
   C. Establish trust with and offer reassurance to the patient; assess for nonverbal information

D.   Both A and C

E.   Both B and C

3.   In an individual with an eating disorder, PN is only indicated

   A.   If the person is unwilling to consume food orally

   B.   In cases of digestive inability

   C.   If the person is < 75% of ideal body weight

   D.   If the person is manipulating the enteral tube

4.   Persons at greatest risk for refeeding syndrome include:

   A.   Weight loss ≥ 10% within 2–3 months or those at or below 70% ideal body weight

   B.   Weight loss ≥ 10% within 6–8 months or those at or below 70% ideal body weight

   C.   Weight loss ≥ 7% within 2–3 months or those at or below 75% ideal body weight

   D.   Weight loss ≥ 7% within 2–3 months or those at or below 70% ideal body weight

Acknowledgments

The author of this chapter for the second edition of this text wishes to thank Christina Fitzgerald, MD, RD, LDN; and Betsy Hjelmgren, MS, RD, LDN, CSP, for their contributions to the first edition of this text.

References

1.   Skipper A, ed. *Dietitian's Handbook of Enteral and Parenteral Nutrition*. 2nd ed. Gaithersburg, MD: American Society for Parenteral and Enteral Nutrition; 1998.

2.   Crowther JH, Wolf EM, Sherwook N. Epidemiology of bulimia nervosa. In: Crowther M, Tannenbaum DL, Hobfoll SE, Stephens MAP, eds. *The Etiology of Bulimia Nervosa: The Individual and Familial Context*. Washington, DC: Taylor + Francis; 1992:1–26.

3.   Robinson TN, Killen JD, Litt IF, et al. Ethnicity and body dissatisfaction: are Hispanic and Asian girls at increased risk for eating disorders? *J Adolesc Health*. 1996;19(6):384–393.

4.   American Psychiatric Association. *Practice Guideline for the Treatment of Patients With Eating Disorders*. 2nd ed. Washington, DC: APA Press; 2000.

5.   Fisher M, Golden NH, Katzman DK, et al. Eating disorders in adolescents: a background paper. *J Adolesc Health*. 1995;16:420–437.

6.   Carney CP, Andersen AE. Eating disorders. Guide to medical evaluation and complications. *Psychiatr Clin North Am*. 1996;19:657–679.

7.   Herzog DB, Nussbaum KM, Marmor AK. Comorbidity and outcome in eating disorders. *Psychiatr Clin North Am*. 1996;19:843–859.

8.   Vastag B. What's the connection? No easy answers for people with eating disorders and drug abuse. *JAMA*. 2001;285:1006–1007.

9.   Mahan LK, Escott-Stump S. *Krause's Food, Nutrition, & Diet Therapy*. 11th ed. Philadelphia: WB Saunders Co; 2004.

10. Russell GFM. The changing nature of anorexia nervosa. *J Psychiatr Res*. 1985;19:101–109.

11. Patrick L. Eating disorders: a review of the literature with emphasis on medical complications and clinical nutrition—eating disorders. *Altern Med Rev*. 2002;7(3):184–202.

12. Kotler LA, Cohen P, Davies M, Pine DS, Walsh BT. Longitudinal relationships between childhood, adolescent, and adult eating disorders. *J Am Acad Child Adolesc Psychiatry*. 2001;40(12):1434–1440.

13. Fairburn CG, Cowen PJ, Harrison PJ. Twin studies and the etiology of eating disorders. *Int J Eat Disord*. 1999;26:349–358.

14. de Zwaan M, Aslam Z, Mitchell JE. Research on energy expenditure in individuals with eating disorders: a review. *Int J Eating Disord*. 2002;32:127–134.

15. The Royal College of Psychiatrists. Guidelines for the nutritional management of anorexia nervosa. http://www.rcpsych.ac.uk/files/pdfversion/cr130.pdf. Published July 2005. Accessed December 15, 2008.

16. Bakan R, Birminghan CL, Aeberhardt L, Goldner EM. Dietary zinc intake of vegetarian and nonvegetarian patients with anorexia nervosa. *Int J Eating Disord*. 1993;13:229–233.

17. Winston AP, Jamieson CP, Madira W, et al. Prevalence of thiamin deficiency in anorexia nervosa. *Int J Eat Disord*. 2000;28:451–454.

18. Woosley M. *Eating Disorders: A Clinical Guide to Counseling and Treatment*. Chicago, IL: American Dietetic Association; 2002.

19. Arden MR, Weiselberg EC, Nussbaum MP, et al. Effect of weight restoration on the dyslipoproteinemia of anorexia nervosa. *J Adolesc Health*. 1990;11:199–202.

20. Setnick JS. *The Eating Disorders Clinical Pocket Guide: Quick Reference for Healthcare Professionals*. Dallas, TX: Snack Time Press; 2005.

21. Mehanna HM, Moledina J, Travis J. Refeeding syndrome: what it is, and how to prevent and treat it. *BMJ*. 2008;336:1495–1498.

22. Tresley J, Sheean PM. Refeeding syndrome: recognition is the key to prevention and management. *J Am Diet Assoc*. 2008;108:2105–2108.

23. Lagua RT, Claudio VS. *Nutrition and Diet Therapy Reference Dictionary*. 4th ed. New York, NY: Chapman and Hall; 1996.

24. McCray S, Walker S, Parrish CR. Much ado about refeeding. *Pract Gastroenterol*. 2005;23:26–44.

25. Marinella MA. The refeeding syndrome and hypophosphatemia. *Nutr Rev*. 2003;61:320–323.

26. Sacks GS, Walker J, Dickerson RN, et al. Observations of hypophosphatemia and its management in nutrition support. *Nutr Clin Pract*. 1994;9:105–108.

27. Yantis M, Velander R. How to recognize and respond to refeeding syndrome *Nursing*. 2008;38:34–39.

28. Brody T. *Nutritional Biochemistry*. San Diego, CA: Academic Press; 1994.

29. Kraft MD, Btaiche IF, Sacks GS. Review of the refeeding syndrome. *Nutr Clin Pract*. 2005;20:625–633.

30. Itokaiva Y, Schulz RA, Cooper JR. Thiamine in nerve membranes. *Biochem Biophys Acta*. 1972;266:293–299.

31. Reuler JB, Girard DE, Cooney TG. Wernicke's encephalopathy. *N Engl J Med.* 1985;312:1035–1039.

32. Dwyer K, Barone JE, Rogers JF. Severe hypophosphatemia in postoperative patients. *Nutr Clin Pract.* 1992;7:279–283.

33. Klein CJ, Stanek GS, Wiles CE. Overfeeding macronutrients to critically ill adults—metabolic complications. *J Am Diet Assoc.* 1998;98:795–806.

34. National Eating Disorders Association (NEDA). Home page. http://www.nationaleatingdisorders.org. Updated July 25, 2014. Accessed August 5, 2014.

35. American Psychiatric Association. Feeding and eating disorders. In: *Diagnostic and Statistical Manual of Mental Disorders.* 5th ed. Arlington, VA: American Psychiatric Association; 2013:329–354. http://www.psychiatryonline.org

36. Abigail H. Natenshon. *When Your Child Has An Eating Disorder.* San Francisco, CA: Jossey-Bass Inc, Publishers; 1999.

37. Kathryn J. Zerbe. *The Body Betrayed a Deeper Understanding of Women, Eating Disorders, and Treatment.* Carlsbad, CA: Gurze Books; 1995.

38. Volkow N, O'Brien CP. Issues for DSM-V: should obesity be included as a brain disorder? *Am J Psychiatry.* 2007;164:708–710.

Test Your Knowledge Answers

1. The correct answer is **C.** Physical presentation of a person with anorexia nervosa includes lanugo-type hair, muscle wasting, dry skin, cyanosis of extremities, bradycardia less than 60 beats/min, and cachexia. When anorexia develops in childhood, the first clinical sign may be failure to make weight gains while continuing to grow in height as opposed to documented weight loss. Growth charts should be evaluated for typical growth patterns of the individual.

2. The correct answer is **E.** Paramount to good treatment and interventions for a patient with a newly diagnosed eating disorder is gaining trust and assessing cognitive, emotional, and physical parameters in the absence of judgment.

3. The correct answer is **B.** PN is only indicated in cases of digestive inability because it leads to a continued loss of hunger cues in the individual with an eating disorder.

4. The correct answer is **A.** Patients with a weight loss of ≥10% within 2–3 months or those at or below 70% ideal body weight are at the greatest risk. Categories of patients who may meet these criteria include those with anorexia nervosa, alcoholism, cancer, uncontrolled diabetes, marasmus, prolonged fasting, morbid obesity with profound weight loss, malabsorptive syndrome (such as pancreatitis, cystic fibrosis, short bowel), prolonged antacid use (due to binding of phosphorus), or long-term diuretic use (due to electrolyte losses). Additional patient groups include those with no oral intake for longer than 5–7 days, postoperative patients, and the elderly.

20

Food Allergies

Cassandra L.S. Walia, MS, RD, CD, CNSC; **Mary Beth Feuling,** MS, RD, CSP, CD, **Leslie M. Gimenez,** MD; and **Praveen S. Goday,** MBBS, CNSC

 Podcast

CONTENTS

Learning Objectives

1. Understand the epidemiology, pathophysiology, and clinical presentation of pediatric food allergies.
2. Describe the nutrition assessment of children with food allergies.
3. Summarize the nutrition management of children with food allergies.
4. Understand the food and non-food allergy issues that may impact the provision of nutrition support in children with food allergies.

Introduction

Adverse reactions to foods are a rapidly growing public health concern in the Western world. Food allergies are a greater problem in children than in adults, with significant food allergies being associated with poorer nutrition outcomes in children. This chapter discusses the epidemiology, pathophysiology, clinical presentation, management, and prognosis of children with food allergies.

Definitions

Several terms may be used when defining adverse reactions to foods. An abnormal response to a food may include "allergy," "hypersensitivity," or "intolerance." Tolerance usually refers to the ability to consume a food that may have the potential for allergy or a food that previously caused allergy and is now consumed without sequelae.

Adverse reactions to foods may occur within a spectrum of reactions ranging from immune-mediated (IgE or non-IgE) to non–immune-mediated mechanisms. Generally speaking, allergy or hypersensitivity refers to immune-mediated events and intolerance refers to non–immune-mediated events.

Other important definitions that will be used in this chapter are outlined in Table 20-1.

For many clinicians, defining a food reaction as "IgE mediated" or "non–IgE mediated" has great utility. IgE reactions are well understood and chemically described as a cascade of events arising from mast cell or basophil degranulation at mucosal surfaces or the skin. Because IgE can be quantitatively measured, levels of food-specific IgE may aid in the diagnosis of IgE-mediated food allergy, and serial food-specific IgE levels may be followed to help determine the development of clinical tolerance.

Food intolerance is a nonimmunologic reaction due to the effects of other components within food (eg, lactose, seafood toxins, or naturally occurring pharmacologically active compounds such as tyramine). These substances may cause an adverse reaction, but they are differentiated from true food allergy because they do not involve the IgE cascade.

Gastrointestinal diseases related to foods may also be caused by IgE and non-IgE immune-mediated mechanisms. Some diseases such as eosinophilic esophagitis (EoE) may have both an IgE and a non-IgE immune component. These diseases are characterized in Table 20-2.

Table 20-1. Definitions of Common Terms That Are Frequently Used in Association With Food Allergies

TERM	DEFINITION
Adverse food reaction	Any undesired response to a food regardless of mechanism.
Allergen	Substance foreign to the body that interacts with the immune system and causes an allergic reaction.
Anaphylaxis	An acute, often severe, and sometimes fatal immune response that may affect one or more organ systems.
Antibodies	Immunoglobulins produced in response to an antigen or allergen.
Antigen	Any substance (such as a toxin or enzyme) that stimulates an immune response in the body (especially the production of antibodies).
Atopic dermatitis (eczema)	A disease characterized by chronic inflammation of the skin that is atopic, hereditary, and noncontagious.
Atopy	Tendency toward the development of allergic diseases, determined genetically.
Elimination diet	An eating plan that omits one or more foods suspected of causing an adverse food reaction.
Food Allergen Labeling and Consumer Protection Act of 2004 (FALCPA)	The law that governs food allergen labeling in the United States. The 8 most common food allergens must be identified on food products. This includes dietary supplements, infant formulas, and imported food products. Raw agricultural products, medications, lotions, and cosmetics are excluded from this law.
Food allergy (hypersensitivity)	An adverse food reaction that is mediated by an immunologic mechanism; the reaction occurs consistently after consumption of a particular food and causes functional changes in target organs.
Food challenge	Administration of a food in increasing amounts performed in order to establish whether a patient is orally tolerant. This may be performed in an open, single-blind, or double-blind fashion.
Food and symptom diary	A subjective tool for recording food and drink consumed and onset, intensity, and duration of symptoms.
Food intolerance	An adverse reaction to a food caused by toxic, pharmacologic, metabolic, or idiosyncratic reactions to the food or chemical substances in the food.
Mast cells	Tissue cells that release histamine and other mediators that cause allergic symptoms.
Skin prick test	A test in which an antigen is applied directly to the skin and is pricked with a specifically designed device. The localized histamine and mediator release correlates to the presence of allergen-specific IgE.
Tolerance	Ability to consume a food that may have the potential for allergy or a food that previously caused allergy and is now consumed without sequelae.

Table 20-2. Clinical Food Allergy Syndromes Associated With IgE or Non-IgE Immune-Mediated Mechanisms

IgE-MEDIATED SYNDROMES	MIXED IgE AND NON-IgE IMMUNE-MEDIATED SYNDROMES	NON-IgE IMMUNE-MEDIATED SYNDROMES
Oral allergy syndrome	Eosinophilic esophagitis	Protein-induced enterocolitis
Anaphylaxis	Eosinophilic gastritis	Protein-induced enteropathy
Urticaria	Eosinophilic gastroenteritis	Food protein–induced enterocolitis syndrome
Angioedema	Atopic dermatitis	Dermatitis herpetiformis, celiac disease

Epidemiology

Adverse reactions to foods have been reported in up to 15%–20% of the population, with the highest prevalence in infancy and childhood. A comprehensive review of the literature found that food allergy affects more than 1%–2% but < 10% of the population.[1] The most recent National Health and Nutrition Examination Surveys (NHANES) performed from 2007 to 2010 suggests a food allergy prevalence of 7.6%.[2] Studies evaluating the proportion of food allergies associated with anaphylaxis varied between 13% and 65%, with the lowest percentages being from studies using more stringent diagnostic criteria.[3] A more recent analysis of children hospitalized for food-induced anaphylaxis reported the rate more than doubled from 2000 to 2009.[4]

A significant rise in atopic conditions has occurred in westernized countries during the past 20 years. Results from the NHANES III study, which measured the prevalence of positive skin prick test (SPT) responses to common food and nonfood allergens in the U.S. population from 1988 to 1994, showed a significant rise in allergy SPT reactivity from the NHANES II study of 1976–1980.[5] In 2007, the reported food allergy rate among all children younger than 18 years was 18% higher than in 1997. In 2013, the Centers for Disease Control and Prevention (CDC) reported the prevalence of food allergies increased in children under 18 years from 3.4% in 1997–1999 to 5.1% in 2009–2011. Hispanic children had a lower prevalence of food allergy (3.6%) compared with non-Hispanic white and non-Hispanic black children.[6] During the 10-year period of 1997–2006, food allergy rates increased significantly among both preschoolers and older children. In addition, from 2004 to 2006, approximately 9500 hospital discharges per year were associated with a diagnosis related to food allergy among children under age 18 years.[7]

Most studies suggest that 6%–8% of the pediatric population and up to 1%–3% of adults may have true food allergy based on SPTs. The true prevalence in the population is probably lower because SPTs can yield false-positive results.[8] Telephone surveys tend to find a lower prevalence; the prevalence of peanut and tree nut allergy was found to be 0.7% in adults and 0.4% in children in a New York telephone survey.[8,9] In 2010, a study examining the data from the NHANES 2005–2006 found the prevalence estimate of clinical allergy to peanut, milk, egg, and/or shrimp was 2.5%. The highest food allergy rates were in children (4.2%, 1–5 years; 3.8%, 6–19 years), and the lowest in older adults (1.3%, ≥60 years).[10]

Children with food allergies are more likely to have other allergic conditions, including asthma and atopic dermatitis, compared to children without food allergies. Asthma has been reported in 29% of children with food allergies (12% in children without food allergies); respiratory allergy is noted in over 30% vs 9% without food allergies, while eczema is seen in 27% as compared with 8% of children without food allergies.[5] Patients with a peanut allergy have asthma and atopic dermatitis prevalence rates of 46% and 50%, respectively.[11] Moreover, several studies have indicated that having food allergy may be a risk for problematic asthma, and having asthma may be a risk for severe/fatal food allergy.[12] A recent study found that 30.4% of children with reported food allergy have multiple food allergies.[13]

Other risk factors for food allergy have been reported and offer new insights. The 2005–2006 NHANES found that vitamin D levels of <15 ng/mL compared with >30 ng/mL were associated with an increased risk of peanut sensitization. However, not all studies support this theory.[14] In addition, this survey also found increased risk among black subjects, males, and children.[10,12] Other proposed risk factors include increased affluence, obesity, reduced consumption of antioxidants, increased use of antacids, and delayed introduction of foods.[12,14]

Pathophysiology

The production of IgE antibodies may occur in the genetically predisposed individual through mechanisms that involve multiple factors. Once allergen-specific IgE is produced, binding to the high-affinity IgE receptor that is present on mast cells and basophils occurs. Low-affinity

IgE receptors are present on eosinophils, monocytes, and macrophages.[15]

Multiple host, antigen, and allergen factors may be involved in the IgE-sensitization cascade, which may result in the subsequent development of clinical allergy. These factors include the genetics of the host, immunologic competence at the mucosal level, and allergen presentation by intact antigen-processing cells, as well as the route of exposure to the allergen. Sensitization may occur via ingestion, inhalation of airborne residue (eg, steam droplets carrying antigen), or by skin contact. Sensitization through skin exposure may be especially important in those with atopic dermatitis, in which a breakdown in the epithelial barrier occurs.[16] The allergenic properties of foods may be affected by product processing (eg, heating or enzymatic digestion), which may alter the antigenic epitope conformation. This alteration may render a food more or less allergenic. Recent studies observed 73% of children with cow's milk allergy were able to tolerate baked cow's milk and 64% of children allergic to egg could tolerate baked egg.[17,18] The allergen threshold dose, which is the dose that triggers a systemic allergic reaction in the host, involves many factors and is an area of current research interest.

IgE-mediated degranulation of effector cells occurs after the food allergen contacts the food-specific IgE antibodies. Cross-linking of the IgE antibodies present on the surface of these cells results in mediator release of histamine, leukotrienes, and prostaglandins. These mediators cause the clinical manifestations of immediate hypersensitivity reactions including pruritus, vasodilatation, smooth muscle contraction, mucus production, and inflammatory cell recruitment to tissues.[6]

Major Food Allergens

Almost every major food allergen identified is a protein or glycoprotein. These allergens tend to resist denaturation by heat or acid and may be more or less common depending on the society or ethnicity of the population observed. In the United States, milk, soy, egg, wheat, peanut, tree nut, fish, and shellfish are the most common allergens noted and are considered the top 8 allergens. However, other legumes, sesame, poppy seed, sunflower seed, pine nuts, and spices are allergens of increasing importance.

Clinical Presentation

IgE-Mediated Diseases

The major IgE-mediated allergic diseases are oral allergy syndrome, anaphylaxis, urticaria, and angioedema.

The pollen-associated **oral allergy syndrome**, or pollen food allergy syndrome, presents with pruritus of the lips, palate, tongue, and oropharynx following oral mucosal contact with fresh fruits and vegetables. The reaction usually does not occur following a cooking process because the cross-reactive allergen is very heat sensitive. These symptoms usually resolve without treatment and generally do not become systemic. Cross-reactivity between plant pollens and fruits is responsible for the clinical syndrome. Specifically, patients with ragweed sensitivity may have these symptoms after ingesting watermelon, cantaloupe, banana, or honeydew melon while patients sensitive to birch pollen may notice symptoms with apple, pear, celery, carrot, or peach.

Food-induced **anaphylaxis** is the most severe form of immediate hypersensitivity reaction. Symptoms may include hypotension, urticaria, angioedema, respiratory compromise including laryngeal edema, and gastrointestinal symptoms of pain, vomiting, and diarrhea; however, food-induced anaphylaxis can occur without any skin manifestations. Near-fatal and fatal reactions often occur in the teenage to 35-year age range and are associated with a patient history of asthma, an accidental ingestion of a known allergen, and the delayed administration of epinephrine. The foods implicated are usually peanut, tree nut, or seafood.[19]

Recently, a new food allergy to mammalian meat (ie, beef, pork, lamb) has been described. Allergic symptoms, including anaphylaxis, occur hours after the meat is ingested instead of immediately afterward. Food allergy to mammalian meat has been linked to IgE sensitization to the carbohydrate galactose-α-1,3-galactose. The route of sensitization appears to be from tick bites.[14]

Mixed IgE and Non-IgE Immune-Mediated Diseases

The gastrointestinal eosinophilic disorders listed in Table 20-2 have features that may best be described as mixed IgE and non-IgE disorders. Evidence of IgE may be present (eg, positive SPTs or serologic in vitro IgE to the offending food), but other mechanisms may be involved. These disorders are characterized by eosinophilic infiltration of the esophageal, gastric, or intestinal mucosa. These patients often present with vomiting, abdominal pain, weight loss, or failure to thrive. Diagnosis is confirmed by endoscopic examination and biopsy. EoE is discussed later in this chapter.

Non-IgE Immune-Mediated Diseases

Efforts to define the mechanisms underlying the non-IgE immune-mediated diseases listed in Table 20-2 have shown varying results. These conditions are thought to be caused by other immunologic mechanisms not involving IgE. Typical symptoms may include recurrent vomiting or diarrhea. In infancy, this is most commonly related to cow's milk or soy protein. This condition, called **food protein–induced enterocolitis syndrome** (FPIES), is discussed in detail later in this chapter.

Allergy Testing

Allergy skin prick testing is commonly used by the practicing allergist-immunologist to determine the presence of IgE to specific foods. Clinical correlation of the patient's history to the testing results is important. The skin prick technique is highly reproducible, and extracts for these tests are commercially available for hundreds of airborne and food allergens. These tests are performed by applying the extracts by a prick or puncture technique to the palmar surface of the forearm or to the upper back. The allergy prick test is actually a localized mediator-release phenomenon that occurs following allergen presentation to skin mast cells. The reaction is a nearly immediate wheal and flare reaction characteristic of IgE-mediated allergy. The test is read within 20 minutes and correlates closely with the presence of specific IgE to the suspected allergen. Positive tests indicate the presence of IgE but not clinical reactivity, with an estimated false-positive rate of approximately 50% if used for screening or with a low pretest probability of IgE food allergy based on clinical history. In children with a history of previous reaction, mean wheal size cutoffs with a 95% positive predictive value have been established for peanut, egg, milk, and fish.[3] A negative test has high negative predictive value of nearly 95%, thus excluding the role of IgE.[20]

In vitro radioallergosorbent tests (RASTs) are blood tests for determining allergen-specific IgE (sIgE) with close correlation to skin prick testing results. Like skin prick testing, a positive sIgE indicates sensitization or presence of IgE but not clinical reactivity, with similar false-positive rates if used for screening. The ImmunoCAP system (fluorometric enzyme immunoassay), was studied with food challenge results and yielded a >95% predictive value for reactions to peanut, egg, and milk for children with a previous reaction. A small number of false-negative ImmunoCAP tests occurred for peanuts. Clinicians can use established values to determine when a food challenge may be safe to perform in the patient with IgE-mediated food allergy.[21]

A newer diagnostic test, termed component testing, is a major area of investigation. Researchers are trying to use this test to better distinguish sensitization to food from clin-

ical allergy.[10,12] In component testing, IgE binding to various, specific protein components of an allergen is measured. Studies have addressed the utility of component testing for allergies to egg, milk, wheat, soy, fruits, hazelnut, and peanut.[22] Peanut allergy has had the most attention. Studies testing sIgE against whole peanut, followed by sIgE to Ara h 2, are assessing whether this approach can minimize the need for oral food challenges.[23]

Management

Currently no cure is available for food allergies. Strict avoidance of the allergy-causing food is the only way to prevent a reaction. Future treatment horizons may include anti-IgE monoclonal antibody, which has already been trialed in peanut allergy, as well as newer forms of allergen immunotherapy.[24] Immunotherapy involves gradual increments of exposure to the allergenic food in an attempt to develop tolerance. The 3 major forms of immunotherapy under investigation are oral, sublingual, and epicutaneous. Trials in oral desensitization have been recently published and have shown efficacy in inducing tolerance.[25] Combining oral immunotherapy with anti-IgE monoclonal antibody may further facilitate desensitization.[22] Additional trials evaluating efficacy and safety are needed before instituting immunotherapy in clinical practice.

Exclusion of foods may lead to nutrition problems that require the expertise of a qualified dietitian. All patients with anaphylaxis to foods (or other allergens) and patients with severe food allergies should be educated regarding the use of injectable epinephrine, which may be lifesaving in the event of accidental exposure. All children with multiple food allergies should be co-managed by an allergist and a dietitian as recommended by the national guidelines for the management of food allergy in the United States.[26]

Because avoidance is the only proven treatment,[27] children with food allergies need to avoid the foods to which they are allergic. The goals of the dietitian are 2-fold: to provide families and patients with guidelines, education, and suggestions for avoiding the allergenic foods and to monitor the child to ensure a nutritionally adequate diet that will promote appropriate weight gain and growth. There must be a multidisciplinary approach that is adopted in conjunction with the allergist with accurate diagnosis of causative foods, assessment of nutrition status, institution of a diet that eliminates the offending foods (elimination diet), prevention of adverse reactions, development of proper emergency treatment with an "action plan" in place, and treatment of associated atopic disorders. There should be ongoing care by both the allergist who periodically determines whether the child has developed tolerance to any of the offending foods and the dietitian who continues to monitor the nutrition status and growth of the child. An algorithm for the management of the food-allergic child is proposed in Figure 20-1.

Preventing the development of food allergy is a topic of great interest. The Adverse Reactions to Foods Committee of the American Academy of Asthma, Allergy, and Immunology established guidelines about the primary prevention of allergic diseases through nutritional interventions.[28] Due to insufficient evidence, restricting maternal diet during pregnancy or lactation is not recommended. Infants should be exclusively breastfed for at least 4–6 months. If exclusive breastfeeding for the first 4–6 months is not possible, then use of a hydrolyzed formula for high-risk infants (at least one first degree relative, parent or sibling, with allergic disease) is endorsed. Complementary foods can be started at 4–6 months, including potentially highly allergenic foods. Once a few typical complementary foods have been tolerated, it is suggested that highly allergenic foods be introduced one at a time at home.

Nutrition Assessment

Restriction of a child's diet due to the diagnosis of food allergies may have a severe impact on his or her nutrition intake. This section provides a practical approach to identifying the

Figure 20-1. Algorithm for the Evaluation of Suspected Food Reactions

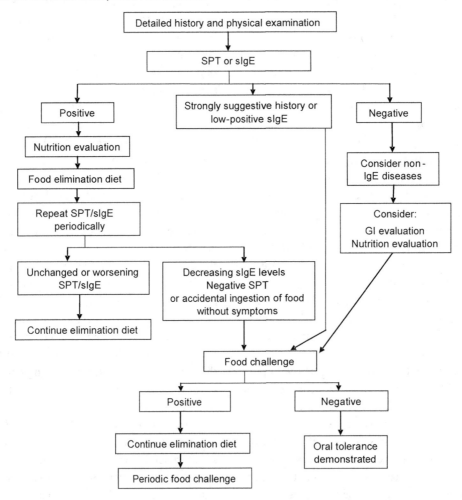

Key:
GI = gastroenterology
sIgE = allergen-specific IgE
SPT = skin prick test'

risk factors that can lead to nutrition deficiencies, undernutrition, and poor growth, while providing guidelines for a comprehensive nutrition assessment.

Because strict avoidance of the causative food is necessary, clearly defining the avoidance list is critical. The nutrition risk increases as the number of foods to be avoided increases, which compounds the challenge for providing a nutritionally complete diet. Any additional problems associated with feeding further exacerbate the risk. It is crucial for the dietitian to collaborate with the allergist and the family to clearly define the foods to be avoided and prevent any unnecessary restrictions. The degree of nutrition risk can be ascertained by methods outlined in Table 20-3.

Table 20-3. Questions That Need to Be Asked to Determine the Degree of Nutrition Risk in Children With Food Allergies

HOW MANY FOODS NEED TO BE AVOIDED?

Risk increases with more foods being/needing to be avoided

WHAT IS THE IMPACT ON NUTRIENTS?

Risk increases with more of the following nutrients being impacted or fewer nutrients being severely impacted
- Calories
- Protein
- Fat
- Micronutrients

ARE THERE OTHER CONCERNS ABOUT FOOD INTAKE?

Risk increases with other medical and psychological diagnoses affecting intake
- Swallowing/chewing difficulties
- Psychological diagnoses affecting intake
- Feeding disorder associated with concurrent medical condition, sensory food aversion, or lack of appetite, which results in low volume and/or limited variety of food intake

When a diagnosis of food allergy has been made, medical nutrition therapy with scheduled follow-up visits can provide a way to monitor the overall health effects of food elimination. Identifying individuals at risk may protect and possibly improve the patient's nutrition and overall health status. Medical nutrition therapy that provides appropriate food substitutions and resources gives the patient with food allergies the specific focus needed for improved nutrition self-care and food allergen avoidance.[29] Referrals to other specialists may be necessary to address concerns related to food intake. Specialists such as a speech-language pathologist, gastroenterologist, psychologist, and occupational therapist may provide intervention independently or through interdisciplinary care to improve food intake.

Table 20-4 provides a case scenario in which 3 toddler diets are presented. The first diet is a typical unrestricted diet. Once the toddler is diagnosed with food allergies to milk, egg, and peanut, the second diet that needs to be followed puts him or her at a high risk for malnutrition and micronutrient deficiencies. The third diet provides the vital food substitutions (for the foods that the child must avoid) to ensure adequate nutrition.

Nutrient intake needs change over time throughout the life cycle. These changes include macronutrient, micronutrient, and fluid needs, all of which play a key role in a developing child. Intake guidelines are presented in other chapters of this book. Nutrient requirements for infants and children with food allergies are the same as the requirements for healthy children. Occasionally they will require increased caloric intake to provide catch-up growth due to poor growth often associated with allergen restriction. In addition, children with moderate to severe atopic dermatitis may have higher caloric and protein needs based on the degree of skin involvement. The more medically complex allergic child may have other nutrition needs due to his or her other medical diagnoses, and these are discussed elsewhere in this book.

Clinical and Laboratory Assessment

Studies have shown that nutrient intake and growth are affected in children with food allergies. Children with food allergies have lower height and weight than children without food allergies.[31] Children with more than 2 food allergies have a lower height, weight, and body mass index than those with 1 food allergy.[32] Children with 3 or more food allergies are smaller than children with 2 or fewer food allergies.[31] Diagnosis of food allergies often results in poor growth due to lack of caregiver knowledge, inadequate intake due to lack of guidance for substitutions to meet nutrition needs, and increased anxiety associated with feeding. Failure to achieve normal growth rates or growth velocity definitely suggests the need for medical nutrition therapy. A multidisciplinary approach involving a dietitian at the time of diagnosis of food allergy may prevent or attenuate problems associated with growth. Accurate anthropometric data and use of growth charts are critical to the evaluation of these children.

Based on the diet and feeding history, the clinician must review the risk of micronutrient deficiency. Table 20-5 summarizes the micronutrients provided by the top 8 allergens and provides the most common food alternatives that can be used when these foods need to be avoided.

Many children with multiple food allergies are at high risk for inadequate intake of essential amino acids and essen-

Table 20-4. Case Scenario

DIET 1			DIET 2ᵃ			DIET 3		
BREAKFAST	LUNCH	DINNER	BREAKFAST	LUNCH	DINNER	BREAKFAST	LUNCH	DINNER
Whole milk	Whole milk	Whole milk	~~Whole milk~~	~~Whole milk~~	~~Whole milk~~	Enriched soy milk	Enriched soy milk	Enriched soy milk
Fortified breakfast cereal	Peanut butter and jelly sandwich	Meatloaf	Fortified breakfast cereal	~~Peanut butter and jelly sandwich~~	~~Meatloaf~~	Fortified breakfast cereal	Sunflower seed butter and jelly sandwich	Milk-free, egg-free meatloaf
Banana	Cooked carrots with butter	Peas	Banana	Cooked carrots ~~with butter~~	Peas	Banana	Cooked carrots with milk-free margarine	Peas
	Strawberries	Mashed potatoes		Strawberries	~~Mashed potatoes~~		Strawberries	Mashed potatoes made with chicken broth
		Roll with butter			~~Roll with butter~~			Milk-free roll with milk-free margarine
SNACK	SNACK	SNACK	SNACK	SNACK	SNACK	SNACK	SNACK	SNACK
Granola bar	Yogurt drink	Ice cream	~~Granola Bar~~	~~Yogurt drink~~	~~Ice cream~~	Teddy Grahams	Soy yogurt	Soy ice cream
Juice	Chocolate chip cookie	400 IU vitamin D	Juice	~~Chocolate chip cookie~~	400 IU vitamin D	Juice	Milk-free, egg-free, and peanut-free chocolate chip cookie	400 IU vitamin D

NUTRITIONAL ANALYSIS OF DIET 1			NUTRITIONAL ANALYSIS OF DIET 2			NUTRITIONAL ANALYSIS OF DIET 3		
NUTRIENT		% GOALᵇ	NUTRIENT		% GOALᵇ	NUTRIENT		% GOALᵇ
Calories	1420 kcal	>100	Calories	232 kcal	25	Calories	1425 kcal	>100
Protein	46 g	>100	Protein	5 g	41	Protein	43 g	>100
Fat	52 g	32% of total calories	Fat	2 g	6% of total calories	Fat	51 g	32% of total calories
Calcium	955 mg	136	Calcium	94 mg	13	Calcium	920 mg	132
Vitamin D	615 IU	103	Vitamin D	420 IU	70	Vitamin D	547 IU	91
Iron	10 mg	146	Iron	6 mg	89	Iron	12 mg	181
Zinc	6.4 mg	213	Zinc	3 mg	100	Zinc	4.9 mg	165

ᵃStrikethrough text indicates that these foods are eliminated because of the child's allergies.
ᵇBased on RDA for age.[30]
Diet 1: Sample menu for an 18-month-old child prior to diagnosis of food allergy.
Diet 2: Nutritionally depleted sample menu for the same child who has been diagnosed with milk, egg, and peanut allergies.
Diet 3: Revised nutritionally adequate menu with acceptable food substitutions for the child.

Table 20-5. Key Micronutrients Provided by the Most Common Food Allergens and Alternative Food Sources That Can Serve As Food Substitutes for the Allergenic Foods

ALLERGENIC FOODS	MICRONUTRIENTS PROVIDED	APPROPRIATE FOOD SUBSTITUTES
Milk[33]	Vitamin A, vitamin B_1, vitamin B_2 (riboflavin), vitamin B_{12}, vitamin D, vitamin B_5 (pantothenic acid), calcium, magnesium, selenium, zinc, potassium, phosphorus	Meats, legumes, whole grains, nuts, mushrooms, fortified foods/beverages (fortified with B vitamins, calcium, and vitamin D), fish, bright yellow and orange vegetables
Egg	Vitamin B_{12}, vitamin B_2 (riboflavin), vitamin B_5 (pantothenic acid), biotin, selenium, iron, folic acid, vitamin E, chromium	Meats, legumes, beans, lentils, whole grains, nuts, leafy green vegetables, fish, dried fruit
Soy	Thiamin, vitamin B_2 (riboflavin), pyridoxine, folic acid, calcium, phosphorus, magnesium, iron, zinc	Meats, legumes, enriched whole grain bread products, egg, nuts, peas, seeds, milk, dried fruit
Wheat	Thiamin, vitamin B_2 (riboflavin), niacin, iron, zinc, selenium, chromium, folic acid if fortified	Alternative fortified grains (barley, rice, oat, corn, rye, quinoa, amaranth, farina), soybean, legumes, egg, milk, nuts, seeds, apples, banana, spinach, potatoes
Peanut/tree nut	Vitamin E, biotin, copper, folic acid, niacin, magnesium, manganese, chromium	Whole grains, vegetable oils, soybean, egg, other legumes
Fish/shellfish	Vitamin B_6, vitamin E, niacin, phosphorus, selenium, omega-3 fatty acids, folic acid, copper, zinc, potassium, vitamin A	Fortified whole grains, meats, oils, soybean, seeds, nuts, milk, egg

tial fatty acids. Refer to Chapter 5 (Protein) and Chapter 4 (Fats) for a complete discussion of the goals for the pediatric population. Often protein hydrolysate–based and/or amino acid–based (elemental) formulas can be used to supplement the diet to meet these nutrition needs. Patients who present after being on prolonged significantly restricted diets without concomitant multivitamin-multimineral use and patients who present with significant malnutrition should be considered for laboratory tests of micronutrient adequacy. The clinical scenario should guide which laboratory tests are obtained (eg, a vegetarian child who is sustained on rice milk should be tested for anemia, zinc deficiency, essential fatty acid deficiency, and vitamin D deficiency if the rice milk is not enriched). Most patients in the United States with minimal dietary restrictions can be managed through judicious use of a multivitamin-multimineral supplement and careful food/beverage intake goals without laboratory testing.

Nutrition Intervention

Education provides a family and patient the pathway for success with an elimination diet. This education includes information on dietary avoidance and consideration of nutrition deficiencies that may result. In addition, it encompasses the nutrition goals for the patient in order to avoid nutrition consequences of food allergies. The family and patient must also be educated about resources for obtaining further information regarding living with food allergies (eg, how to prepare allergen-free foods, support groups, local retail es-

tablishments that sell allergen-free foods, tips for management at daycare and schools, cookbooks, food labeling laws, and other helpful tips for the elimination diet). A list of food allergy resources is provided in Table 20-6. Each caregiver of a child with food allergies must be given a list of food substitutions to be successful with strict avoidance of the food allergens. In addition, a nutritionally complete formula or beverage, if possible, should be recommended. This type of information assists the patient and family/caregivers in living a normal and well-nourished life despite the patient's food allergies. Without education, the recommendation of an elimination diet can be overwhelming and unsuccessful as families struggle to find accurate and useful information, and it may result in unnecessary medical consequences.

With the changing practice of managing cow's milk and egg allergy, evaluating patients to determine if they can tolerate baked products with cow's milk or egg as an ingredient has become more common. Nutrition counseling for this recommendation has been challenging and is a critical part of the care. Guidelines to incorporate baked milk and baked egg into the diet have been published and should be considered when providing education to patients and their families.[34] This practice may or may not increase the number of allowed foods, depending on the preferences for food consumed.

Nutritionally Complete Formulas

Identification of formulas depends on the known food allergens. Most standard formulas are free of wheat, egg, peanut,

Table 20-6. Food Allergy Resources

RESOURCE	WEBSITE
Food Allergy Research and Education	http://www.foodallergy.org
American Academy of Allergy, Asthma, and Immunology	http://www.aaaai.org
Academy of Nutrition and Dietetics	http://www.eatright.org
Asthma and Allergy Foundation of America	http://www.aafa.org
American Partnership for Eosinophilic Disorders	http://www.apfed.org
American College of Allergy, Asthma, and Immunology	http://www.acaai.org
Consortium of Food Allergy Research	http://cofargroup.org
Food Allergy Research and Resource Program	http://farrp.unl.edu
National Institute of Allergy and Infectious Diseases	http://www.niaid.nih.gov
National Association of School Nurses	https://www.nasn.org/ToolsResources/FoodAllergyandAnaphylaxis
Centers for Disease Control and Prevention	http://www.cdc.gov/healthyyouth/foodallergies/publications.htm
U.S. Food and Drug Administration	http://www.fda.gov/Food/IngredientsPackagingLabeling/FoodAllergens/default.htm

tree nut, fish, and shellfish. Careful review of ingredients of any standard formula is critical prior to the recommendation of use. It is common to substitute a soy protein–based formula for the patient allergic to cow's milk protein. In patients who are allergic to both cow's milk and soy, a protein hydrolysate or elemental formula is recommended. These formulas exploit the concept that intact proteins are allergenic and with increasing breakdown of the intact protein, the allergenicity can be reduced. Protein hydrolysates are made by hydrolysis of proteins into mostly dipeptides and tripeptides and can be tolerated by the vast majority (~90%) of patients with allergies to milk and soy.[35,36] Elemental formulas are made up of individual amino acids and are tolerated by the small fraction of children who are also allergic to the protein hydrolysates.[37] Both of these types of formulas are generally less palatable than standard formulas and are considerably more expensive. Significant advances in the flavor and acceptability of these formulas have been made, which has improved the adherence to incorporating them as supplemental nutrition. The major categories of formulas are enumerated in Table 20-7. Increasing use of homemade whole-food tube feedings to replace formulas should be used cautiously in children with food allergies. The degree of complete nutrition will vary based on allowed foods and recipes used for tube feeding preparation. This should be done with close nutrition monitoring and in conjunction with a dietitian familiar with the preparation of the whole-food tube feedings.

Most children with food allergies can be managed through judicious food substitutions. When faced with an

Table 20-7. Major Pediatric Formulas

FORMULA	PROTEIN	EXAMPLES	
		Infant formulas	Formulas for older children
Cow's Milk	Casein, whey	Similac Advancea Enfamil Infant	PediaSure PediaSmart
Lactose-free		Similac Sensitivea Gerber Good Start Gentle Gerber Good Start Soothe	PediaSure PediaSmart
Soy	Soy	Enfamil Prosobee Similac Soy Isomila Gerber Good Start Soy	Bright Beginnings Soy Pediatric Drink Parents Choice Soy Pediatric Drink PediaSmart Soy Organic Nutritional Beverage
Hydrolysate	Peptides, amino acids	Enfamil Nutramigen with EnfloraLGG Similac Expert Care Alimentum	Pediasure Peptide Peptamen Junior
Elemental	Amino acids	Neocate Infant DHA/ARA EleCare for Infants PurAmino	Neocate Junior EleCare Jr. EO28 Splash

aDenotes formulas that are available as 19 cal/oz when made in the standard manner.

extensive array of food allergies that span multiple food groups, protein hydrolysate and elemental formulas become the primary option. Infants under the age of 4–6 months usually accept these less-palatable formulas without difficulty, but with increasing age, acceptability of these formulas becomes a problem. In toddlers or preschool children, when elemental formulas are the sole or major source of nutrition and the patient will not consume enough to sustain nutrition, tube feeding may become necessary.

Patients who are extremely malnourished at presentation may need to be admitted to the hospital to monitor for refeeding syndrome (Chapter 19); otherwise, most patients with food allergies can be managed in the outpatient setting.

Milk Substitutes/Beverages

Milk substitutes/beverages must be used in combination with nutrition assessment and monitoring. Many different "milk" products are in the marketplace and provide alternatives for the allergic patient. However, each product should only be used with careful consideration of its nutritional quality. Many provide adequate micronutrients such as vitamin D, calcium, and B vitamins; however, most provide

minimal fat and protein. Children under the age of 2 are at high risk for malnutrition if one of the incomplete milk substitutes is used in place of whole cow's milk. See Table 20-8 for a list of the nutritional constituents of various milk substitutes.

When evaluating a milk substitute for a patient, it is important to read the food label of the exact product that will be consumed by the patient. The nutrient content of milk substitutes varies not only by the type (food source) of "milk" (see Table 20-8), but also by brand and versions within the brand. Milk substitutes with added flavors may have higher calorie contents than unflavored versions, and some milk substitutes are not enriched. Nonenriched products often contain < 100 mg calcium per 8 oz (~240 mL) serving and do not contain vitamin D.

Food Allergy Education and Labeling

The diagnosis of food allergy impacts the patient and family/caregivers in many different ways, including grocery shopping, cooking, socializing, travel/vacations, eating out, and family relationships. Providing education on all of these topics is essential. One of the cornerstones of management

Table 20-8. Nutrient Comparison of Enriched Unflavored Milk Substitutes/Beverages[a]

NUTRIENTS PER 8 OZ	COCONUT MILK	ALMOND MILK	RICE MILK	SOY MILK	WHOLE MILK	PEDIASURE	HEMP MILK	ALMOND COCONUT BLEND	COCONUT, ALMOND, AND CHIA BLEND
Calories	70–80	60–70	120	80–130	150	240	70	50	70
Protein (g)	0[b]	1–5[b]	1[b]	7–11	8	7	2–3[b]	<1[b]	<1[b]
Carbohydrate (g)	7–8	7–8	23	7–13	11	33	1	5	8
Fat (g)	4–5	2–4	2.5	2.5–4.5	8	9	5–6	3	4
Saturated fat (g)	4–5	0	0	0–0.5	5	1	0.5	1	2.5
Calcium (mg)	100–450	100–450	300	200–450	294	250	300	450	300
Iron (mg)	0.4–0.7	0.4–0.7	0.7	0.7–1.8	0.1	2.7	1.1–1.8	0.4	0.4
Vitamin A (IU)	500	500	500	500–1500	300	500	500	500	500
Vitamin D (IU)	100–120	100–120	100	40–140	100	160	100–120	100	100

[a] These are typical nutritional values for various milk substitutes/beverages using enriched, unflavored versions. Individual brands may have varying amounts of nutrients.
[b] Protein source is not a complete protein.

is education about reading food labels.[38] Labels must be read every time a food product is purchased because the ingredients may change without warning. Labels must also be read for supplements, medications, bath products, lotions, pet foods, and cosmetics because young children may accidentally or voluntarily consume these products.

The Food Allergen and Consumer Protection Act of 2004 (FALCPA) is an amendment to the Food, Drug, and Cosmetic Act and requires that a food that contains an ingredient that is 1 of the 8 major food allergens (or contains a protein of these allergens) is declared on the food label.[39] This requirement includes the presence of the 8 major food allergens in spices, flavorings, and other ingredients. The law applies to all food regulated by the Food and Drug Administration (FDA), including many packaged food products, dietary supplements, and infant formula. The U.S. Department of Agriculture (USDA) in collaboration with the Federal Safety and Inspection Service (FSIS) regulates food products that primarily consist of meat, poultry, and egg. FSIS supports the voluntary addition of allergen statements (eg, "contains" statements) on meat, poultry, and egg product labels.[40] FALCPA does not apply to medications, cosmetics, or lotions. Consumers should read the ingredient list of all products carefully to ensure that they are allergen free.

Voluntary allergen advisories or "may contain" statements are appearing on an increasing number of products.[41] Food processing companies elect when to use these statements and what language to use. The allergen advisories are used by some food processors to indicate a possible risk of cross-contact with an allergen from another product. Recent efforts to increase public awareness and strides made in labeling of food products are encouraging. However, concern also exists that food processors may choose to make voluntary allergen advisories regarding cross-contact in an attempt to avoid accidental exposures to allergens. If this practice does occur, it may decrease food choices for patients with food allergies. Table 20-9 provides some examples of "hidden" food allergens in common foods.

The FDA issued a regulation that defines the term "gluten-free" for food labeling.[42] This law standardizes the definition of what a "gluten-free" claim on a label means. The FDA set the gluten limit as <20 parts per million for foods labeled "gluten-free," "no gluten," "free of gluten," or "without gluten." Because the use of the "gluten-free" claim is voluntary, it may not appear on a food label even if the food is, in fact, gluten free.

Micronutrient Supplementation

The benefit of early nutrition intervention is to avoid micronutrient deficiency by recommending adequate substitutions and supplementation. The dietary reference intakes for vitamins, minerals, and trace elements can be used for children with food allergies because the vast majority of these children are healthy except for their food allergies and atopic problems.[30] Chapter 6 (Minerals), Chapter 7 (Water-Soluble Essential Micronutrients), and Chapter 8 (Fat-Soluble Vitamins) discuss these topics. Recommendations for supplements should be made based on foods that need to be eliminated and the patient's nutrition status. Several hypoallergenic multivitamin-multimineral supplements are

Table 20-9. Common Sources of Hidden Food Allergens

EGG	MILK	NUTS	SOY	WHEAT	RICE
Pasta	Cakes/muffins	Breakfast cereals/ granola bars	Bread/bread crumbs	Cereals	Baby food
Bread/bread crumbs	Breakfast cereals	Egg rolls	Waffles	Oatmeal cookie	Bread/bread crumbs
Egg Beaters	Frozen desserts	Cakes/cookies	Crackers	Chicken hot dogs/low-fat beef franks	Cake/muffin mixes
Candy/chocolate	Candy/chocolate	Frozen desserts	Chicken hot dogs/ low-fat beef franks	Soy sauce	Waffles
Marshmallows	Canned tuna	Nut butters	Cakes/muffins	Barbecue-flavored potato chips	Soups
Waffles	Processed meats	Sauces/chili	Bouillon cubes	Modified food starch	Food marketed as free of the 8 most common food allergens

appropriate for children with food allergies (Table 20-10). Two of the most common micronutrient supplements recommended for children with food allergies are calcium and vitamin D (Table 20-11).

Table 20-10. Allergen-Free Multivitamins[a]

FOR CHILDREN	FOR TEENAGERS AND YOUNG ADULTS
Garden of Life Vitamin Code Kids[b,c]	One A Day Teen Advantage for Him or Her Multivitamin[b]
Vitaflo FruitiVits Powder Multivitamin[b,d]	Nature's Plus Source of Life Power Teen Multivitamin
Flintstones Complete-Children's Chewable Multivitamin	Active Health Teen Multivitamin from RainbowLight
NanoVM powder (1–3 y and 4–8 y)[b,d] Multivitamin	
Nature's Plus Animal Parade Gold Children's Liquid Multivitamin[b]	
Nature's Plus Animal Parade Sugar Free Children's Chewable Multivitamin	

[a]All of these products are free of milk, soy, egg, wheat, peanut, tree nut, fish, and shellfish; however, it should be noted that products can change at any time, and labels should be read before use. Store and generic brands may also be allergen free.
[b]This allergen-free vitamin contains selenium.
[c]This product does not contain iron.
[d]This product is only available online.

Table 20-11. Allergen-Free Calcium and Vitamin D Supplements

SUPPLEMENT NAME[a]	SERVING SIZE	CALCIUM (mg)	VITAMIN D (IU)
Lil' Critters Calcium with Vitamin D	2 gummy bears	200	220
Cal EZ Packets	1 packet/day	1000	1000
Tums Regular Strength	1 tablet	200	0
D-Vi-Sol	1 mL daily	0	400
Nature Made Kids Chewable Vitamin D3	1 tablet	0	400
Rainbow Light Vitamin D3 400 IU Sunny Gummies	1 gummy	0	400

[a]All of these products are free of milk, soy, egg, wheat, peanut, tree nut, fish, and shellfish; however, it should be noted that products can change at any time, and labels should be read before use.

Special Scenarios

Cow's Milk-Protein Allergy

Cow's milk-protein allergy (CMPA) is the most common food allergy in early childhood, with an incidence of 2%–3% in the first year of life.[43] Most infants with CMPA develop symptoms before 1 month of age, often within a week after introduction of cow's milk–based formula. The majority have 2 or more symptoms with symptoms from 2 or more organ systems: cutaneous symptoms (urticarial rash, atopic eczema), gastrointestinal symptoms (blood in the stool, diarrhea, vomiting, protein-losing enteropathy), and respiratory symptoms (cough and wheeze).[44] This condition can also develop when an infant is exclusively breastfed, through the passage of the offending antigens from food consumed by the mother through the breast milk.

The diagnosis is usually made through the history of clinical symptoms in young infants that develop soon after birth or shortly after they start consuming cow's milk–based formula. A family history of atopy is often present. If the reaction is IgE-mediated, then the specific IgE levels may be elevated.

Up to 90% of these infants will do well with a protein hydrolysate and the rest will require an elemental formula.[45] In breastfed infants, the mother should initially avoid cow's milk; if no improvement is seen, she may also need to exclude other common food allergens.

These children, particularly infants with gastrointestinal symptoms, have a good prognosis. Approximately 50% of infants are able to tolerate cow's milk by the age of 1 year and the vast majority remit by the age of 3 years.[44]

Eosinophilic Esophagitis

EoE is a disorder of the esophagus characterized by upper gastrointestinal tract symptoms in association with esophageal mucosal eosinophilia.[46] EoE tends to be a chronic disease with persistent or relapsing symptoms and appears to be becoming more prevalent.

Children under the age of 5 years commonly present with food refusal, regurgitation, and emesis. Abdominal pain and failure to thrive may also be seen. Dysphagia and food impaction tend to be increasingly common with age. A strong association exists between EoE and allergic rhinitis, asthma, and eczema as well as food allergies. All patients with EoE must be managed with coordinated care between a gastroenterologist, allergist, and dietitian.

Systemic and topical corticosteroids effectively resolve acute features of EoE; however, when they are discontinued, the disease generally recurs. Despite this, EoE can be maintained in remission in a vast majority of patients with the use of topical corticosteroids. Nutrition intervention can be used as an adjunct to corticosteroid therapy or as the sole therapy for EoE. Three types of nutrition intervention have met with varying degrees of success in EoE. First, specific food elimination can be based on allergy testing and clinical history.[47] Even when allergy testing does not reveal specific food allergens, elimination diets can be used. Simply removing the 8 most common allergenic foods (milk, soy, egg, wheat, peanut, tree nut, fish, and shellfish) from the diet has significant efficacy.[48] Foods with baked milk can be tolerated in a subset of patients with milk-induced EoE.[49] While one study suggested that up to 65% of patients with EoE can be treated with milk elimination alone,[50] Spergel et al[51] found only a 30% response rate in a milk only elimination diet. Finally, a 100% amino acid–based formula diet can be utilized, thus removing all potential food allergens; this approach has been extremely effective.[52,53]

Hence, medical nutrition therapy should be considered as an effective treatment in all children diagnosed with EoE. When deciding on the use of a specific nutrition therapy, the patient's lifestyle and family resources also need to be considered. This requires comprehensive education and nutrition monitoring by a dietitian.[54]

Food Protein–Induced Enterocolitis Syndrome

FPIES is classified as a non–IgE-mediated allergic disorder, triggered by the ingestion of certain food proteins.[55] Children usually present at <12 months of age with delayed vomiting and/or diarrhea in about 2–4 hours of ingestion of the causative food. These patients do not present with urticaria, angioedema, or respiratory compromise. Some children present in a moribund state, with shock and metabolic acidosis secondary to their gastrointestinal symptoms.[56] These symptoms typically resolve within 48–72 hours after removal of the suspected antigen.[57] Typically, the offending food is either cow's milk, soy, or rice,[58,59,60] although other grains, poultry, fruits, and vegetables have also been implicated.[56] Tests for food-specific IgE by either skin prick testing or serologic in vitro methods are negative in patients with FPIES.[61] Awareness of the entity is important because the clinical presentation can be confused with other life-threatening conditions. Multiple presentations before the true diagnosis is established are the norm. Early diagnosis should be based on the clinical history and presentation, and removal of the offending food antigen serves as a simple and effective therapy. The age at which oral tolerance develops varies.

Medical nutrition therapy for FPIES is similar to that for food allergies. The dietitian should seek advice from the physician as to which foods should be avoided and which foods should be introduced. The dietitian can help the physician focus on specific food groups that will provide necessary nutrients based on the nutrition assessment. Breastfeeding is recommended because reactions to breast milk are rare; however, reactions to breast milk have been reported.[62,63] For formula-fed patients that do not tolerate milk, soy formula may be tolerated, but a food challenge should be considered because there is a high incidence of concomitant milk and soy FPIES.[60] FPIES patients may tolerate extensively hydrolyzed formula; however, up to 20% of patients require amino acid–based formula.[60] Infants and toddlers with a history of reactions to solid foods may lead to delayed introduction of solid foods, which may lead to the development of feeding difficulties. Practitioners must pay careful attention to this interruption of a sensitive time period for the development of feeding and provide strategies for enhancing feeding skills to avoid development of a more severe feeding disorder.

Prognosis and Follow-Up

A good possibility exists that many young children diagnosed with allergies to foods such as milk, egg, wheat, and soy will outgrow the sensitivity after several years.[64] Non–IgE-mediated milk allergy tends to be outgrown more quickly than IgE-mediated allergy, with both forms of the allergy having a good prognosis.[64] Resolution of an IgE-mediated milk allergy is thought to occur in about 80% of patients by 5 years of age. More recent studies suggest a slower rate of resolution. Wood et al[65] observed about half of infants diagnosed with milk allergy at age 3–15 months had a resolution of it at a median age of about 5 years. A similarly slow resolution has been found for egg allergy. In a cohort of infants diagnosed with egg allergy at age 3–15 months, the allergy resolved at a median age of 6 years in 49% of the cohort.[66] Factors associated with outgrowing an IgE allergy include a mild to moderate reaction history, being allergic to only 1 food, eczema as the sole allergy symptom, and white compared with black race.[67] Studies looking at the natural history of egg and milk allergy also found that baseline sIgE, SPT wheal size, and severity of eczema were important predictors of the likelihood of resolution.[65,66] Children who develop a food allergy after 3 years of age are less likely to lose the food reactivity over a period of several years.[25] Peanut allergy is a lifelong disorder for most, but not all patients.[31] A recent study found that 21% of children with a peanut allergy may tolerate peanut later in life.[68] A smaller percentage of those with tree nut allergy seem to develop tolerance.[69] While data for individuals with allergies to fish are unavailable, seafood allergies appear to be permanent.[34] The ages at which tolerances are likely to develop for common food allergens are shown in Table 20-12.

Table 20-12. Ages at Which Tolerance May Be Expected to Common Food Allergens

FOOD[a]	AGE (Y)	TOLERANCE (%)	REFERENCES
Milk	4	19	65,70
	5	52.6	
	12	64	
	16	79	
Egg	4	12	66,71
	6	37, 49.3	
	10	68	
Wheat	4	29	72
	8	56	
	12	65	
Soy	4	25	73
	6	45	
	10	69	
Peanut	5	21[b]	68
Tree nuts		9[c]	69

[a]Natural history data for fish allergy are unavailable and shellfish allergy is considered to be persistent. [26]
[b]Predictors of persistent allergy: skin prick test wheal size > 6 mm and allergen-specific IgE (sIgE) > 3 kUA/L before age 2 years.
[c]The percentage is 63% with sIgE < 2 kUA/L and passed oral challenge.

Follow-up visits with the allergist-immunologist are important for the management of food allergies. Because pediatric patients have the potential for outgrowing a food allergy, the follow-up visits can reassess the allergic status and determine if any food allergens may be reintroduced. Reintroduction of a food allergen should only be considered if managed and directed by the allergist. Introduction of previously avoided allergens may increase food options, decrease cost if the patient is drinking a specialty formula and/or eating specialty allergen-free foods, and decrease the stress around preparing meals for the child.

Food Allergies and Nutrition Support

Two scenarios are possible wherein food allergies are associated with nutrition support. The first is when a child with known food allergies requires nutrition support and the second is where allergies to formula or parenteral nutrition (PN) components become apparent only after the commencement of nutrition support.

Enteral Nutrition

Enteral nutrition support of children presenting with food allergies can be straightforward. Because most enteral formulas contain cow's milk protein, children with CMPA can be managed with soy-based, protein hydrolysate, or elemental formula using the principles outlined earlier in this chapter.

Some of the formula intolerances that occur in young children receiving nutrition support are probably secondary to food allergies and are usually not recognized at the first instance. Since one of the management strategies for formula intolerances during nutrition support includes a transition to a protein hydrolysate/elemental formula, the acute situation usually resolves. Often, food allergy is diagnosed retrospectively when the child cannot be transitioned back to a more standard formula.

Parenteral Nutrition

Minimal data are available on PN support in children with documented allergies to foods. Egg allergy can be a cause for concern because these proteins are found in intravenous (IV) fat emulsions. In patients with documented allergies to eggs, several options could be considered—consultation with an allergist who may or may not do an SPT, fat-free PN, the use of a fish oil–based lipid emulsion, Omegaven (which does contain some egg and is not approved for use in the United States), or the use of Liposyn II (which does contain some egg).[74] A risk exists for extremely soy-allergic patients needing PN. Patients may tolerate IV soy-based fat emulsion, but the first 2 options outlined above should be considered. With regard to soy allergy and PN, 2 case reports present directly opposing views. The first found no detectable soy allergen in the 20% Intralipid emulsion preparation.[75] In the second report, a patient with soy allergy developed systemic signs of anaphylaxis upon being given a test dose of the Intralipid.[76] This patient was successfully maintained on the fish oil–based lipid emulsion as the sole source of fat for 45 days.[76]

A variety of allergies to PN have been described through case reports in the literature.[74,77–82] As with other allergies, they appear to be more common in children.[77,78,80] Skin rashes appear to be the most common manifestation. However, they can present with dyspnea, cyanosis, nausea, vomiting, headache, flushing, fever, and chest pain. Anaphylaxis can occur.[78,80,83] All of these reactions can occur at the first administration, after several days of administration, or after reinstitution following a hiatus.

These reactions have been attributed to IV fat emulsions,[74,82] crystalline amino acid solutions,[80] and multivitamin mixtures (either due to stabilizers and emulsifiers in the M.V.I. Pediatric or due to thiamine, vitamin B complex, or vitamin K).[77,80,81,83,84] A neonate presented with allergic manifestations with Trophamine amino acid solution containing PN, but the symptoms did not occur with the use of Premasol amino acid solution. The reaction was presumed to be due to bisulfite, which is present in the former but not in the latter solution.[85] Finally, latex allergy (from the latex stopper on the IV fat emulsion) can present with allergic manifestations each time PN is commenced.[86]

When these reactions occur, PN needs to be stopped and appropriate drug treatment for the allergic reaction started. If the reaction is severe and the patient is going to continue to require PN, a multidisciplinary approach utilizing an allergist, pharmacist, nutrition-support physician, and/ or dietitian should be pursued. Two approaches may be considered when the reaction is mild and resolves after PN is discontinued. The first is to have skin prick testing of the fat emulsion, multivitamin, and amino acid components and removal of the offending agent(s) before PN is restarted. The other approach has been to identify the offending agent through trial and error. In severe reactions, an approach using IV desensitization in the intensive care unit has been described; it is unclear if this method actually worked.[75]

One micronutrient that may be added to PN solutions and cause significant allergic reactions is IV iron. All 3 parenteral iron compounds—iron dextran, sodium ferric gluconate complex in sucrose, and iron sucrose—can be associated with allergic reactions.[87,88] Iron sucrose appears to be associated with the lowest risk of allergy.[41,87] Iron dextran is the least expensive preparation, and a test dose should always be given with the thought of routinely pretreating patients with diphenhydramine and acetaminophen to minimize adverse events. Both sodium ferric gluconate and iron sucrose offer safe alternatives to patients intolerant of iron dextran, but at a higher cost.[87,88] Iron dextran–sensitive patients and patients with multiple allergies who receive one of the newer preparations should receive test doses prior to therapy.

Test Your Knowledge Questions

1. A 7-year-old boy with an enterocutaneous fistula develops an urticarial rash the day that he is started on parenteral nutrition. All of the following constituents of his parenteral nutrition could cause the rash EXCEPT:
   A. Intravenous fat emulsion
   B. Amino acid solution
   C. Pediatric multivitamin solution
   D. Dextrose

2. An 18-month-old vegetarian girl with presumed milk and soy protein allergy is drinking 32 ounces of enriched rice milk per day. She also eats rice, wheat, corn, fruits, and vegetables but does not consume any egg or meat products. She does not receive any vitamin or mineral supplementation. You are concerned about her intake of all of the following EXCEPT:
   A. Fat
   B. Vitamin D
   C. Energy
   D. Zinc

3. A 6-year-old Asian boy is seen by a dietitian for follow-up nutrition assessment and education. His parents report he is allergic to milk, soy, and peanuts. He has a history of anaphylaxis while eating peanut butter 1 year ago. His current intake includes tofu stir-fry and milk chocolate candy bars. Parents report he eats these foods at least once a week without any problems. He does not drink a milk substitute. All of the following must be done or considered at this visit EXCEPT:
   A. Assessment of growth and nutrient intake
   B. Suggesting an age-appropriate beverage
   C. Recommending follow-up with allergist as patient is tolerating milk and soy
   D. Suggesting food challenge of peanut butter at home

4. A 6-month-old breastfed infant has significant vomiting and diarrhea within hours of being given a bottle of cow's milk–based formula. His mother reports that this has happened each time he has been fed the formula. She denies any skin rashes. A RAST for IgE directed against cow's milk protein is negative. All of the following are true about this child EXCEPT:
   A. This is consistent with IgE-mediated anaphylaxis.
   B. This is most likely food protein-induced enterocolitis syndrome.
   C. Cow's milk protein must be eliminated from the child's diet.
   D. In addition to breastfeeding, a protein hydrolysate formula may be appropriate.

Acknowledgments

The authors of this chapter for the second edition of this text wish to thank Michael Levy, MD, for his contributions to the first edition of this text.

References

1. Chafen JJ, Newberry SJ, Riedl MA, et al. Diagnosing and managing common food allergies: a systematic review. *JAMA*. 2010;303(18):1848–1856.

2. McGowan EC, Keet CA. Prevalence of self-reported food allergy in the National Health and Nutrition Examination Survey (NHANES) 2007-2010. *J Allergy Clin Immunol*. 2013;132(5):1216–1219.e5.

3. Sampson HA, Aceves S, Bock SA, et al. Food allergy: a practice parameter update-2014. *J Allergy Clin Immunol*. 2014;pii: S0091-6749(14)00672-1.

4. Rudders SA, Arias SA, Camargo CA Jr. Trends in hospitalizations for food-induced anaphylaxis in US children, 2000-2009. *J Allergy Clin Immunol*. 2014;134(4):960-962.e3.

5. Arbes SJ Jr, Gergen PJ, Elliott L, Zeldin DC. Prevalences of positive skin test responses to 10 common allergens in the US population: results from the third National Health and Nutrition Examination Survey. *J Allergy Clin Immunol*. 2005;116(2):377–383.

6. Jackson KD, Howie LD, Akinbami LJ. Trends in allergic conditions among children: United States, 1997-2011. *NCHS Data Brief*. 2013;(121):1–8.

7. Branum AM, Lukacs SL. Food allergy among U.S. children: trends in prevalence and hospitalizations. *NCHS Data Brief*. 2008;(10):1–8.

8. Sicherer SH, Muñoz-Furlong A, Burks AW, Sampson HA. Prevalence of peanut and tree nut allergy in the US determined by a random digit dial telephone survey. *J Allergy Clin Immunol*. 1999;103(4):559–562.

9. Sicherer SH, Muñoz-Furlong A, Sampson HA. Prevalence of seafood allergy in the United States determined by a random telephone survey. *J Allergy Clin Immunol*. 2004;114(1):159–165.

10. Liu AH, Jaramillo R, Sicherer SH, et al. National prevalence and risk factors for food allergy and relationship to asthma: results from the National Health and Nutrition Examination Survey 2005-2006. *J Allergy Clin Immunol*. 2010;126(4):798–806.e713.

11. Sicherer SH, Furlong TJ, Muñoz-Furlong A, Burks AW, Sampson HA. A voluntary registry for peanut and tree nut allergy: characteristics of the first 5149 registrants. *J Allergy Clin Immunol*. 2001;108(1):128–132.

12. Sicherer SH. Epidemiology of food allergy. *J Allergy Clin Immunol*. 2011;127(3):594–602.

13. Gupta RS, Springston EE, Warrier MR, et al. The prevalence, severity, and distribution of childhood food allergy in the United States. *Pediatrics*. 2011;128(1):e9–e17.

14. Sicherer SH, Sampson HA. Food allergy: epidemiology, pathogenesis, diagnosis, and treatment. *J Allergy Clin Immunol*. 2014;133(2):291–307; quiz 308.

15. Sampson HA, Burks AW. Mechanisms of food allergy. *Annu Rev Nutr*. 1996;16:161–177.

16. Asai Y, Greenwood C, Hull PR, et al. Filaggrin gene mutation associations with peanut allergy persist despite variations in peanut allergy diagnostic criteria or asthma status. *J Allergy Clin Immunol*. 2013;132(1):239–242.

17. Mehr S, Turner PJ, Joshi P, Wong M, Campbell DE. Safety and clinical predictors of reacting to extensively heated cow's milk challenge in cow's milk-allergic children. *Ann Allergy Asthma Immunol*. 2014;113(4):425–429.

18. Turner PJ, Mehr S, Joshi P, et al. Safety of food challenges to extensively heated egg in egg-allergic children: a prospective cohort study. *Pediatr Allergy Immunol*. 2013;24(5):450–455.

19. Bock SA, Muñoz-Furlong A, Sampson HA. Fatalities due to anaphylactic reactions to foods. *J Allergy Clin Immunol*. 2001;107(1):191–193.

20. Bock SA, Lee WY, Remigio L, Holst A, May CD. Appraisal of skin tests with food extracts for diagnosis of food hypersensitivity. *Clin Allergy*. 1978;8(6):559–564.

21. Sampson HA. Utility of food-specific IgE concentrations in predicting symptomatic food allergy. *J Allergy Clin Immunol*. 2001;107(5):891–896.

22. Sicherer SH, Leung DY. Advances in allergic skin disease, anaphylaxis, and hypersensitivity reactions to foods, drugs, and insects in 2013. *J Allergy Clin Immunol*. 2014;133(2):324–334.

23. Renz H. Advances in in vitro diagnostics in allergy, asthma, and immunology in 2012. *J Allergy Clin Immunol*. 2013;132(6):1287–1292.

24. Burks W, Bannon G, Lehrer SB. Classic specific immunotherapy and new perspectives in specific immunotherapy for food allergy. *Allergy*. 2001;56(Suppl 67):121–124.

25. Jones SM, Pons L, Roberts JL, et al. Clinical efficacy and immune regulation with peanut oral immunotherapy. *J Allergy Clin Immunol*. 2009;124(2):292–300, 300.e1–97.

26. Panel NI-SE, Boyce JA, Assa'ad A, et al. Guidelines for the diagnosis and management of food allergy in the United States: report of the NIAID-sponsored expert panel. *J Allergy Clin Immunol*. 2010;126(6 Suppl):S1–S58.

27. Sicherer SH. Diagnosis and management of childhood food allergy. *Curr Probl Pediatr*. 2001;31(2):35–57.

28. Fleischer DM, Spergel JM, Assa'ad AH, Pongracic JA. Primary prevention of allergic disease through nutritional interventions. *J Allergy Clin Immunol Pract*. 2013;1(1):29–36.

29. Hubbard S. Nutrition and food allergies: the dietitian's role. *Ann Allergy Asthma Immunol*. 2003;90(6 Suppl 3):115–116.

30. Institute of Medicine. Dietary reference intakes (DRIs): recommended dietary allowances and adequate intakes, vitamins. http://iom.edu/Activities/Nutrition/Summary-DRIs/~/media/Files/Activity%20Files/Nutrition/DRIs/RDA%20and%20AIs_Vitamin%20and%20Elements.pdf. Published 2011. Accessed June 28, 2014.

31. Flammarion S, Santos C, Guimber D, et al. Diet and nutritional status of children with food allergies. *Pediatr Allergy Immunol*. 2011;22(2):161–165.

32. Christie L, Hine RJ, Parker JG, Burks W. Food allergies in children affect nutrient intake and growth. *J Am Diet Assoc*. 2002;102(11):1648–1651.

33. Gaucheron F. Milk and dairy products: a unique micronutrient combination. *J Am Coll Nutr*. 2011;30(5 Suppl 1):400S–409S.

34. Groetch M, Nowak-Wegrzyn A. Practical approach to nutrition and dietary intervention in pediatric food allergy. *Pediatr Allergy Immunol*. 2013;24(3):212–221.

35. Antigen-reduced infant formulae. ESPGAN Committee on Nutrition. *Acta Paediatr.* 1993;82(12):1087–1088.

36. Sampson HA, Bernhisel-Broadbent J, Yang E, Scanlon SM. Safety of casein hydrolysate formula in children with cow milk allergy. *J Pediatr.* 1991;118(4 Pt 1):520–525.

37. de Boissieu D, Matarazzo P, Dupont C. Allergy to extensively hydrolyzed cow milk proteins in infants: identification and treatment with an amino acid-based formula. *J Pediatr.* 1997;131(5):744–747.

38. Joshi P, Mofidi S, Sicherer SH. Interpretation of commercial food ingredient labels by parents of food-allergic children. *J Allergy Clin Immunol.* Jun 2002;109(6):1019–1021.

39. U.S. Food and Drug Administration. Food allergen labeling and Consumer Protection Act of 2004. http://www.fda.gov/food/guidanceregulation/guidancedocumentsregulatoryinformation/allergens/ucm106187.htm. Updated February 27, 2013. Accessed September 25, 2014.

40. Food Safety and Inspection Service. FSIS compliance guidelines: allergens and ingredients of public health concern: identification, prevention and control, and declaration through labeling. http://www.fsis.usda.gov/wps/wcm/connect/f9cbb0e9-6b4d-4132-ae27-53e0b52e840e/Allergens-Ingredients.pdf?MOD=AJPERES. Published April 2014. Accessed September 25, 2014.

41. Food Allergy Issues Alliance. *Food Allergen Labeling Guidelines.* Washington, DC: National Food Processors Association; 2001.

42. U.S. Food and Drug Administration. Food labeling; gluten-free labeling of foods. https://www.federalregister.gov/articles/2013/08/05/2013-18813/food-labeling-gluten-free-labeling-of-foods. Published August 5, 2013. Accessed June 29, 2014.

43. Host A. Frequency of cow's milk allergy in childhood. *Ann Allergy Asthma Immunol.* 2002;89(6 Suppl 1):33–37.

44. Host A. Cow's milk protein allergy and intolerance in infancy. Some clinical, epidemiological and immunological aspects. *Pediatr Allergy Immunol.* 1994;5(5 Suppl):1–36.

45. Atkins D. Food allergy: diagnosis and management. *Prim Care.* 2008;35(1):119–140, vii.

46. Furuta GT, Liacouras CA, Collins MH, et al. Eosinophilic esophagitis in children and adults: a systematic review and consensus recommendations for diagnosis and treatment. *Gastroenterology.* 2007;133(4):1342–1363.

47. Spergel JM, Andrews T, Brown-Whitehorn TF, Beausoleil JL, Liacouras CA. Treatment of eosinophilic esophagitis with specific food elimination diet directed by a combination of skin prick and patch tests. *Ann Allergy Asthma Immunol.* 2005;95(4):336–343.

48. Kagalwalla AF, Sentongo TA, Ritz S, et al. Effect of six-food elimination diet on clinical and histologic outcomes in eosinophilic esophagitis. *Clin Gastroenterol Hepatol.* 2006;4(9):1097–1102.

49. Leung J, Hundal NV, Katz AJ, et al. Tolerance of baked milk in patients with cow's milk-mediated eosinophilic esophagitis. *J Allergy Clin Immunol.* 2013;132(5):1215–1216.e1.

50. Kagalwalla AF, Amsden K, Shah A, et al. Cow's milk elimination: a novel dietary approach to treat eosinophilic esophagitis. *J Pediatr Gastroenterol Nutr.* 2012;55(6):711–716.

51. Spergel JM, Brown-Whitehorn TF, Cianferoni A, et al. Identification of causative foods in children with eosinophilic esophagitis treated with an elimination diet. *J Allergy Clin Immunol.* 2012;130(2):461–467.e5.

52. Kelly KJ, Lazenby AJ, Rowe PC, Yardley JH, Perman JA, Sampson HA. Eosinophilic esophagitis attributed to gastroesophageal reflux: improvement with an amino acid-based formula. *Gastroenterology.* 1995;109(5):1503–1512.

53. Markowitz JE, Spergel JM, Ruchelli E, Liacouras CA. Elemental diet is an effective treatment for eosinophilic esophagitis in children and adolescents. *Am J Gastroenterol.* 2003;98(4):777–782.

54. Feuling MB, Noel RJ. Medical and nutrition management of eosinophilic esophagitis in children. *Nutr Clin Pract.* 2010;25(2):166–174.

55. Sicherer SH. Food protein-induced enterocolitis syndrome: clinical perspectives. *J Pediatr Gastroenterol Nutr.* 2000;30(Suppl):S45–S49.

56. Sicherer SH, Eigenmann PA, Sampson HA. Clinical features of food protein-induced enterocolitis syndrome. *J Pediatr.* 1998;133(2):214–219.

57. Maloney J, Nowak-Wegrzyn A. Educational clinical case series for pediatric allergy and immunology: allergic proctocolitis, food protein-induced enterocolitis syndrome and allergic eosinophilic gastroenteritis with protein-losing gastroenteropathy as manifestations of non-IgE-mediated cow's milk allergy. *Pediatr Allergy Immunol.* 2007;18(4):360–367.

58. Burks AW, Casteel HB, Fiedorek SC, Williams LW, Pumphrey CL. Prospective oral food challenge study of two soybean protein isolates in patients with possible milk or soy protein enterocolitis. *Pediatr Allergy Immunol.* 1994;5(1):40–45.

59. Powell GK. Milk- and soy-induced enterocolitis of infancy. Clinical features and standardization of challenge. *J Pediatr.* 1978;93(4):553–560.

60. Leonard SA, Nowak-Wegrzyn A. Clinical diagnosis and management of food protein-induced enterocolitis syndrome. *Curr Opin Pediatr.* 2012;24(6):739–745.

61. Nowak-Wegrzyn A, Sampson HA, Wood RA, Sicherer SH. Food protein-induced enterocolitis syndrome caused by solid food proteins. *Pediatrics.* 2003;111(4 Pt 1):829–835.

62. Monti G, Castagno E, Liguori SA, et al. Food protein-induced enterocolitis syndrome by cow's milk proteins passed through breast milk. *J Allergy Clin Immunol.* 2011;127(3):679–680.

63. Tan J, Campbell D, Mehr S. Food protein-induced enterocolitis syndrome in an exclusively breast-fed infant—an uncommon entity. *J Allergy Clin Immunol.* 2012;129(3):873, author reply 873–874.

64. Wood RA. The natural history of food allergy. *Pediatrics.* 2003;111(6 Pt 3):1631–1637.

65. Wood RA, Sicherer SH, Vickery BP, et al. The natural history of milk allergy in an observational cohort. *J Allergy Clin Immunol.* 2013;131(3):805–812.

66. Sicherer SH, Wood RA, Vickery BP, et al. The natural history of egg allergy in an observational cohort. *J Allergy Clin Immunol.* 2014;133(2):492–499.

67. Gupta RS, Lau CH, Sita EE, Smith B, Greenhawt MJ. Factors associated with reported food allergy tolerance among

US children. *Ann Allergy Asthma Immunol.* 2013;111(3):194-198 e194.

68. Ho MH, Wong WH, Heine RG, Hosking CS, Hill DJ, Allen KJ. Early clinical predictors of remission of peanut allergy in children. *J Allergy Clin Immunol.* 2008;121(3):731–736.

69. Fleischer DM, Conover-Walker MK, Matsui EC, Wood RA. The natural history of tree nut allergy. *J Allergy Clin Immunol.* 2005;116(5):1087–1093.

70. Skripak JM, Matsui EC, Mudd K, Wood RA. The natural history of IgE-mediated cow's milk allergy. *J Allergy Clin Immunol.* 2007;120(5):1172–1177.

71. Savage JH, Matsui EC, Skripak JM, Wood RA. The natural history of egg allergy. *J Allergy Clin Immunol.* 2007;120(6):1413–1417.

72. Keet CA, Matsui EC, Dhillon G, Lenehan P, Paterakis M, Wood RA. The natural history of wheat allergy. *Ann Allergy Asthma Immunol.* 2009;102(5):410–415.

73. Savage JH, Kaeding AJ, Matsui EC, Wood RA. The natural history of soy allergy. *J Allergy Clin Immunol.* 2010;125(3):683–686.

74. Buchman AL, Ament ME. Comparative hypersensitivity in intravenous lipid emulsions. *JPEN J Parenter Enteral Nutr.* 1991;15(3):345–346.

75. Nicklas RA. Lack of allergenic soy in intralipid for total parenteral nutrition. *Ann Allergy Asthma Immunol.* 2013;111(5):423.

76. Gura KM, Parsons SK, Bechard LJ, et al. Use of a fish oil-based lipid emulsion to treat essential fatty acid deficiency in a soy allergic patient receiving parenteral nutrition. *Clin Nutr.* 2005;24(5):839–847.

77. Bullock L, Etchason E, Fitzgerald JF, McGuire WA. Case report of an allergic reaction to parenteral nutrition in a pediatric patient. *JPEN J Parenter Enteral Nutr.* 1990;14(1):98–100.

78. Market AD, Lew DB, Schropp KP, Hak EB. Parenteral nutrition-associated anaphylaxis in a 4-year-old child. *J Pediatr Gastroenterol Nutr.* 1998;26(2):229–231.

79. Nagata MJ. Hypersensitivity reactions associated with parenteral nutrition: case report and review of the literature. *Ann Pharmacother.* 1993;27(2):174–177.

80. Pomeranz S, Gimmon Z, Ben Zvi A, Katz S. Parenteral nutrition-induced anaphylaxis. *JPEN J Parenter Enteral Nutr.* 1987;11(3):314–315.

81. Scolapio JS, Ferrone M, Gillham RA. Urticaria associated with parenteral nutrition. *JPEN J Parenter Enteral Nutr.* 2005;29(6):451–453.

82. Weidmann B, Lepique C, Heider A, Schmitz A, Niederle N. Hypersensitivity reactions to parenteral lipid solutions. *Support Care Cancer.* 1997;5(6):504–505.

83. Andersen HL, Nissen I. Presumed anaphylactic shock after infusion of Lipofundin [in Danish]. *Ugeskr Laeger.* 1993;155(28):2210–2211.

84. Wu SF, Chen W. Hypersensitivity to vitamin preparation in parenteral nutrition: report of one case. *Acta Paediatr Taiwan.* 2002;43(5):285–287.

85. Huston RK, Baxter LM, Larrabee PB. Neonatal parenteral nutrition hypersensitivity: a case report implicating bisulfite sensitivity in a newborn infant. *JPEN J Parenter Enteral Nutr.* 2009;33(6):691–693.

86. Wynn RJ, Boneberg A, Lakshminrusimha S. Unexpected source of latex sensitization in a neonatal intensive care unit. *J Perinatol.* 2007;27(9):586–588.

87. Bailie GR, Clark JA, Lane CE, Lane PL. Hypersensitivity reactions and deaths associated with intravenous iron preparations. *Nephrol Dial Transplant.* 2005;20(7):1443–1449.

88. Silverstein SB, Rodgers GM. Parenteral iron therapy options. *Am J Hematol.* 2004;76(1):74–78.

Test Your Knowledge Answers

1. The correct answer is **D**. Allergens are usually proteins or glycoproteins. Except for galactose-α-1,3-galactose sensitization in allergic reactions specific to meat, allergies do not develop to carbohydrates. Allergies to intravenous fat emulsion, amino acid solution, and the multivitamin solution have all been described.

2. The correct answer is **B**. Children under 2 years of age and avoiding milk and soy protein are at increased risk of consuming insufficient fat, protein, calcium, vitamin D, zinc, iron, and total energy. Enriched rice milk provides adequate vitamin D and calcium but does not provide appropriate fat, protein, and energy intake. Appropriate substitute for liquid intake would be a hydrolysate formula or if that is not tolerated, an elemental formula.

3. The correct answer is **D**. In a patient with a history of anaphylaxis to a food, a food challenge at home should never be recommended. Follow-up with an allergist is the only safe way to assess if a patient has "outgrown" or developed tolerance to the food. Annual follow-up assessment with an allergist is recommended for children with food allergies. The nutrition assessment of a these children should always review growth and nutrient intake. By obtaining a 24-hour recall and reviewing common foods consumed, exposures to food allergens can be identified. If a patient is tolerating exposures to foods that were allergenic, again the patient must follow up with the allergist to clarify the allergen list. Liberalizing a patient's diet will provide more options for improving the overall nutrition intake.

4. The correct answer is **A**. In IgE-mediated anaphylaxis, cutaneous signs such as an urticarial rash are typical. The absence of cow's milk–specific IgE on RAST makes an IgE-mediated mechanism unlikely. This clinical scenario is consistent with food protein–induced enterocolitis syndrome and avoidance of cow's milk is the most important therapy. A protein hydrolysate formula would be an effective substitute and if not tolerated, an elemental formula.

$$21$$

Diabetes Mellitus and Other Endocrine Disorders

Alaa Al Nofal, MD; and **W. Frederick Schwenk II,** MD

 Podcast

CONTENTS

Learning Objectives

1. Define the common types of diabetes mellitus that occur in childhood.
2. Relate how to create a parenteral formulation or choose an enteral formula in a child with diabetes mellitus receiving nutrition support.
3. Report the optimal way to administer insulin in a child with diabetes on parenteral or enteral nutrition support.
4. State how to prevent hyponatremia or hypernatremia in a child with central diabetes insipidus on nutrition support.

Diabetes Mellitus

Diabetes mellitus is one of the most common chronic illnesses in the pediatric-aged population. It results from an absolute or relative lack of insulin, with or without insulin resistance. While several different causes exist for diabetes in children, all forms of diabetes mellitus are associated with elevated plasma glucose and most (all but cystic fibrosis [CF]-related diabetes) are associated with dyslipidemia. In this chapter we will focus on the most common types of diabetes. The less common types of diabetes are beyond the scope of this book.

Definitions

Type 1 Diabetes Mellitus

Type 1 diabetes remains the most common form of diabetes in children.[1] This disorder is usually an autoimmune destruction of the β cells of the pancreas, resulting in an absolute deficiency of insulin.[2-4] The presence of genetic predisposition to type I diabetes has been proposed, which could explain the increased risk of type I diabetes in siblings of patients with this disease.[5] The incidence of type 1 diabetes mellitus in the United States and other Western countries has been increasing. In the United States, the prevalence of type 1 diabetes mellitus in children younger than 18 years of age is 2–3 per 1000.[6] In addition, the incidence of type 1 diabetes mellitus is higher in non-Hispanic white children compared to other ethnicities in the United States.[1] Children with type 1 diabetes mellitus are at risk for developing ketoacidosis and require insulin to prevent hyperglycemia.[3] Because of a risk for developing low blood glucose concentrations, current recommendations from the American Diabetes Association (ADA) are to keep target blood glucose goal ranges in children somewhat higher than what is recommended for adults.[2,4]

Type 2 Diabetes Mellitus

An epidemic of childhood obesity has occurred in the last few decades in developed countries.[7] Associated with this increase in childhood obesity has been a marked increase in the incidence of children with type 2 diabetes mellitus.[1,8] The natural history of type 2 diabetes remains to be defined, but appears to be caused by a relative insufficiency of insulin secretion by the pancreas in addition to insulin resistance at the tissue level.[9,10] In the United States, in 2008–2009, type 2 diabetes accounted for 22% of all newly diagnosed cases of childhood diabetes.[1] In contrast to adults with type II diabetes, children with this type of diabetes might present with diabetic ketoacidosis.[11] Optimal treatment of children with type 2 diabetes mellitus remains controversial.[12] Long-term therapy generally consists of lifestyle modifications (diet changes and increased physical activity) in addition to oral hypoglycemic agents, insulin therapy, or both. In hospital settings, it is unclear whether hypocaloric feeding should be utilized. The incidence of type 2 diabetes mellitus varies by ethnic groups, with higher rates (in order) in Native Americans, African Americans, Hispanic Americans, Pacific Islanders/Asian children, and whites.[1,12]

CF-Related Diabetes Mellitus

Children with CF and pancreatic insufficiency are at increased risk of developing CF-related diabetes.[13,14] The prevalence of this condition in adolescents with CF has been reported to be close to 20%, while in similar adults the prevalence may be as high as 40%–50%.[15] CF-related diabetes is primarily caused by reduced insulin secretion due to impairment in pancreatic endocrine function.[16] Children with CF-related diabetes do not typically develop ketoacidosis

and may have increased insulin resistance, particularly at the time of an intercurrent illness.[17] Children with CF-related diabetes may be asymptomatic for years[18] and not exhibit the classic symptoms of polyuria and polydipsia associated with other types of diabetes mellitus.[19] Patients with CF-related diabetes have increased risk for microvascular disease, worse pulmonary function, and increased mortality (see also Chapter 28, Pulmonary Disorders).[15,20]

Consequences of Hyperglycemia and Hypoglycemia in the Critically Ill Child

Hyperglycemia appears to be common in pediatric intensive care units (ICUs) regardless of whether a child has known diabetes mellitus.[21,22] In one retrospective study involving 152 children in a pediatric ICU, blood glucose concentrations > 125 mg/dL were observed in over half of the patients within 24 hours of admission and in almost 90% of the patients sometime during the admission.[23] In a second retrospective study, almost 70% of 192 critically ill children had blood glucose concentrations > 120 mg/dL within 24 hours of admission to a pediatric ICU.[24]

Whether tight glycemic control is linked with better outcomes in critically ill patients is controversial. In a study of 184 children < 1 year of age who had undergone cardiac surgery, hyperglycemia in the postoperative period was associated with increased mortality and morbidity.[22] While one recent randomized, prospective study of intensive insulin therapy in critically ill children did show improved morbidity and mortality in a subgroup of patients,[25] another recent large randomized control trial reported no change in mortality was noticed between patients receiving tight glycemic control vs conventional glycemic control. However, the tight glycemic control group needed less electrolyte replacement during hospitalization but experienced more serious hypoglycemic reactions compared to the other group.[26]

In theory, many reasons exist that might explain why hyperglycemia could affect mortality and morbidity in critically ill patients. In vitro, high glucose concentrations have been shown to cause abnormalities in several aspects of immune function, including intracellular killing, complement function, granulocyte adhesion, chemotaxis, phagocytosis, and respiratory burst function.[27] Glucose attaches itself to the third component of complement, affecting this component's ability to attach itself to microbes and impairing opsonization of the microbe.[28] However, the recurrent hypoglycemia may increase the risk of morbidity and mortality in patients receiving tight glycemic control in the ICU.

Glucose Control in Healthy Children With Diabetes

Short-Term Implications

The current recommendations of the ADA are that target blood glucose concentrations be individualized for each child with diabetes.[4] In general, children < 7 years old often have a form of "hypoglycemic unawareness" due to limited cognitive understanding and developmental stage as well as the immature counter-regulation, making them more susceptible to severe hypoglycemia.[4] Children < 5 years of age appear to be at risk for permanent cognitive impairment after episodes of severe hypoglycemia.[29,30] In addition, severe hypoglycemia occurs in younger children most frequently during sleep.[31] Consequently, blood glucose targets for younger children are usually higher than for adolescents or adults.[4]

Diabetic ketoacidosis is a concern in undiagnosed children with type 1 diabetes mellitus, as well as in children with known diabetes during times of stress (illness or trauma) if the insulin dose is not adjusted, or in patients who receive an inadequate amount of insulin.[30] Overall, the incidence of short-term adverse events in children, such as hospitalization and severe hypoglycemia, is high.[32]

Long-Term Complications

In contrast to some older children with type 2 diabetes, children with type 1 diabetes rarely have complications at the time of diagnosis.[33] A large prospective, randomized study called the Diabetes Control and Complications Trial found that intensive diabetes treatment significantly reduced the risk of diabetes retinopathy, nephropathy, and neuropathy.[34] A follow-up to this study demonstrated that intensive diabetes therapy had a favorable long-term, sustained effect in cardiovascular risk in patients with insulin-dependent diabetes.[35] However, despite marked improvement in treatment options, > 50% of patients with type 1 diabetes develop complications or comorbidities.[36] Persistently high blood glucose levels over time also appear to increase the risk of macrovascular complications, but these rarely occur in childhood.

Glucose Control in Children With Diabetes Mellitus on Enteral Nutrition

Choice of Formula

The use of enteral formulas designed for patients with diabetes has not been studied in children with diabetes. Therefore, the current recommendations are to use a standard age-appropriate formula.[37] Experts suggest carbohydrates and monounsaturated fat should provide 60%–70% of calorie intake, taking into consideration the metabolic profile and whether weight loss is needed.[37]

Administration of Insulin

Blood glucose concentrations in children with diabetes on enteral nutrition (EN) support can usually be adequately controlled by using subcutaneous injections of insulin. Guidelines for adults have been published for the administration of insulin at the initiation of tube feedings, as the rate of tube feedings increases, and for continuous intermittent and nocturnal feeding schedules.[38] By dosing the insulin on a per kilogram body weight basis, these recommendations can also be utilized in children. Of course, careful monitoring of blood glucose concentrations is required. Wesorick et al[38] suggest a starting dose of 40% of the usual total daily dose of insulin, which could be adjusted based on the frequent glucose measurements. Although no consensus exists in regard to optimal insulin doses in children, use of a similar approach would be reasonable.

Glucose Control in Children With Diabetes Mellitus on Parenteral Nutrition

Choice of Dextrose Solution

No data suggest that children with diabetes require a special formulation for parenteral nutrition (PN). The composition of the PN solution should be determined independent of whether the patient has diabetes. This includes the choice of the final concentration of dextrose. However, it should be noted that many children with diabetes have dyslipidemia,[39] so the triglyceride levels in children with diabetes on PN need to be monitored carefully.

Use of an Insulin Infusion

When an intravenous (IV) infusion containing a high concentration of dextrose is given to a child (or adult) with diabetes, blood glucose concentrations are most safely controlled using a separate IV insulin infusion.[40,41] If insulin is given intravenously, the infusion can easily be changed if the rate of IV glucose administration is changed. In adults, insulin is often directly added to the PN, beginning with a dose of 0.1 U of regular insulin per gram of dextrose in the infusate (eg, 10 U/L of 10% dextrose; 20 U/L of 20% dextrose).[40] Additional subcutaneous regular insulin or an IV insulin infusion may be needed to supplement the insulin in the PN. This ratio of insulin to dextrose is unlikely to cause hypoglycemia and minimizes the need to discard a bag of PN because it contains too much insulin.[40]

While a similar protocol may be used in children, a strong case can be made for controlling blood glucose concentrations using a separate infusion of insulin. Using a syringe pump, the insulin infusion can be directly "piggy-backed" into the IV line. A reasonable rate to begin such an infusion would be 0.02–0.05 U of regular insulin per kilogram body weight per hour, taking into consideration the patient's clinical status and the presence of urine ketones. The rate of insulin administration can be changed to optimize blood glucose control.

As mentioned previously, no consensus has been reached as to how tightly the plasma glucose concentration should be controlled in a critically ill child, with or without a previous diagnosis of diabetes. However, blood glucose concentrations between 110 and 180 mg/dL might be a reasonable goal, preventing both hypoglycemia and ketoacidosis.[42]

Whatever method is chosen to administer the IV insulin, blood glucose concentrations need to be checked frequently. Such checks are often done at least hourly in children on an insulin infusion until blood glucose concentrations appear to be stable. Blood glucose concentrations are easiest to control if the PN is given as a continuous infusion, rather than being cycled. It should also be mentioned that even if the IV infusion of dextrose is stopped, patients with type 1 diabetes mellitus will continue to need some insulin to inhibit hepatic gluconeogenesis and prevent the child from developing ketoacidosis.

Addition of Insulin to PN Solutions

If a separate IV insulin infusion is used to control blood glucose concentrations and both the rate of insulin infusion and blood glucose concentrations have remained stable for 24 hours, the separate insulin infusion can be discontinued and insulin added directly to the PN. In such cases, one can easily calculate the amount of insulin that is required to control blood glucose concentrations during the administration of the PN by totaling the amount of insulin infused with the separate infusion.

Nutrition Support in CF-Related Diabetes

Choice of Formula

PN support is rarely required in children with CF.[43] If EN support is being considered, no enteral formulation has been shown to be superior to another.[44] Some data in adults suggest that patients who develop CF-related diabetes have

lower body mass indices and are more likely to require enteral feedings from 2 years prior to CF-related diabetes diagnosis compared to adults who do not develop CF-related diabetes.[45]

Control of Blood Glucose

Blood glucose concentrations in children with CF and CF-related diabetes receiving EN support can usually be managed with subcutaneous insulin. However, with intercurrent illness, children with CF have increased insulin resistance, requiring larger doses of insulin (2-fold to 4-fold) than the usual dose they require when they are at their baseline health status.[17] In addition, patients with CF-related diabetes are often placed on systemic steroids during illness, which can worsen hyperglycemia.

Nutrition Support in Other Endocrine Conditions

Central Diabetes Insipidus

Central or neurogenic diabetes insipidus is a relatively rare condition in children and results from an inability to secrete active vasopressin from the posterior pituitary gland.[46] While genetic defects in vasopressin synthesis have been described, the usual etiology of this condition is a hypothalamic or posterior pituitary lesion.[46] Multiple potential causes underlie this condition including tumors, inflammatory lesions, vascular diseases, and cranial malformations.[46]

Outpatient treatment for this condition in children with intact thirst sensation involves giving an analogue of vasopressin either orally or intranasally. These children are allowed to drink to thirst. Fluid intake in children without an intact thirst mechanism must be monitored carefully to prevent hyponatremia or hypernatremia. Infants with central diabetes insipidus are at higher risk for electrolyte abnormalities when they receive vasopressin analogs because their calorie intake is fluid based and their lack of access to free water. Many of these patients are managed with low solute formula and the use of thiazide diuretics.[47]

There do not appear to be any published guidelines on managing nutrition support in a child with central diabetes insipidus who might require PN. Because of the large volumes of fluid associated with such therapy, the child is at risk for both hyponatremia and hypernatremia.

One option for managing these patients is to use a low-dose IV infusion of aqueous vasopressin, as has been described for children who are receiving additional fluid as part of a chemotherapy regimen.[48] To maintain adequate hydration and serum sodium concentrations, a dilute infusion of aqueous vasopressin is given at a starting rate of 0.08–0.1 mU/kg/h. During the infusion, fluid intake, urine output, body weight, urine specific gravity, and serum electrolyte concentrations are monitored carefully.

Panhypopituitarism

Another relatively uncommon endocrine condition that might affect nutrition support is panhypopituitarism. Again, no guidelines exist for how to manage nutrition support in such patients. Children with panhypopituitarism are unable to secrete several anterior pituitary hormones, including growth hormone and corticotropin. This condition can be the result of intracranial surgery, but can also be idiopathic.

Neonates with this condition often present with hypoglycemia and are at continuing risk for low blood sugars. The hypoglycemia arises from the pituitary gland being unable to secrete the counter-regulatory hormones during fasting.[49] To prevent hypoglycemia in a critically ill child with this condition, additional glucocorticoids are administered. In such patients, a strong case can also be made for administering nutrition support as a constant infusion, rather than giving enteral feeds as boluses or cycled PN.

Future Research

Research in children is difficult, not only because they cannot give informed consent, but also because mortality is quite low and large numbers of patients are needed to do outcome studies. Consequently, many of the existing recommendations are extrapolated from adult recommendations. Future studies will hopefully define the optimal blood glucose concentration for a critically ill child. It is also hoped that new strategies will be developed to help children with diabetes mellitus achieve improved blood glucose control when they are receiving PN or EN.

Test Your Knowledge Questions

1. When a parenteral formulation is created for use in a child with diabetes mellitus, the dextrose concentration should be
   A. Kept to a minimum
   B. No greater than 15%
   C. At least 20%
   D. Chosen without regard to whether the child has diabetes mellitus

2. To prevent hyperglycemia, hospitalized children with CF-related diabetes mellitus and acute infections may require

   A. An increased amount of insulin
   B. A decreased amount of insulin
   C. Their usual doses of insulin
   C. Frequent doses of short-acting insulin

3. In children with diabetes mellitus on EN, insulin should usually be
   A. Discontinued
   B. Given parenterally
   C. Given subcutaneously
   D. Given enterally

4. Serum sodium concentrations can be safely maintained in a child with diabetes insipidus on PN support by
   A. Limiting oral fluids
   B. Administering a vasopressin analogue orally
   C. Doubling the patient's usual dose of a vasopressin analogue
   D. Using an intravenous drip of aqueous vasopressin

Acknowledgments

The authors of this chapter for the second edition of this text wish to thank Diane Olson, RD, CNSD, CSP, LD, for her contributions to the first edition of this text.

References

1. Blackman NJ. Systematic reviews of evaluations of diagnostic and screening tests. Odds ratio is not independent of prevalence. *BMJ.* 2011;323:1188.

2. American Diabetes Association. Standards of medical care in diabetes—2012. *Diabetes Care.* 2012;35(suppl 1):S11–S63.

3. Hanas R, Donaghue KC, Klingensmith G, Swift PG. 2009 ISPAD clinical practice consensus guidelines 2009 compendium. Introduction. *Pediatr Diabetes.* 2009;10(suppl 12):1–2.

4. Kunz W, Mismar A, Wille G, Ahmad R, Materazzi G, Miccoli P. Preoperative prediction of the risk of malignancy in thyroid nodules. *Acta Med Mediterr.* 2014;30:329–334.

5. Gillespie KM, Gale EA, Bingley PJ. High familial risk and genetic susceptibility in early onset childhood diabetes. *Diabetes.* 2002;51:210–214.

6. Cooke DW, Plotnick L. Type 1 diabetes mellitus in pediatrics. *Pediatr Rev.* 2008;29:374–384; quiz 385.

7. Orsi CM, Hale DE, Lynch JL. Pediatric obesity epidemiology. *Curr Opin Endocrinol Diabetes Obes.* 2011;18:14–22.

8. Sinha R, Fisch G, Teague B, et al. Prevalence of impaired glucose tolerance among children and adolescents with marked obesity. *N Engl J Med.* 2002;346:802–810.

9. Cree-Green M, Triolo TM, Nadeau KJ. Etiology of insulin resistance in youth with type 2 diabetes. *Curr Diab Rep.* 2013;13:81–88.

10. Taylor R. Pathogenesis of type 2 diabetes: tracing the reverse route from cure to cause. *Diabetologia.* 2008;51:1781–1789.

11. Dean H, Sellers E, Kesselman M. Acute hyperglycemic emergencies in children with type 2 diabetes. *Paediatr Child Health.* 2007;12:43–44.

12. Kaufman FR, Shaw J. Type 2 diabetes in youth: rates, antecedents, treatment, problems and prevention. *Pediatr Diabetes.* 2007;8(suppl 9):4–6.
13. Moran A, Hardin D, Rodman D, et al. Diagnosis, screening and management of cystic fibrosis related diabetes mellitus: a consensus conference report. *Diabetes Res Clin Pract.* 1999;45:61–73.
14. Moran A, Doherty L, Wang X, Thomas W. Abnormal glucose metabolism in cystic fibrosis. *J Pediatr.* 1998;133:10–17.
15. Moran A, Dunitz J, Nathan B, Saeed A, Holme B, Thomas W. Cystic fibrosis-related diabetes: current trends in prevalence, incidence, and mortality. *Diabetes Care.* 2009;32:1626–1631.
16. Brennan AL, Geddes DM, Gyi KM, Baker EH. Clinical importance of cystic fibrosis-related diabetes. *J Cyst Fibros.* 2004;3:209–222.
17. Moran A, Brunzell C, Cohen RC, et al; CFRD Guidelines Committee. Clinical care guidelines for cystic fibrosis-related diabetes: a position statement of the American Diabetes Association and a clinical practice guideline of the Cystic Fibrosis Foundation, endorsed by the Pediatric Endocrine Society. *Diabetes Care.* 2010;33:2697–2708.
18. O'Riordan SM, Robinson PD, Donaghue KC, Moran A. Management of cystic fibrosis-related diabetes in children and adolescents. *Pediatr Diabetes.* 2009;10(suppl 12):43–50.
19. Jabeen S, Ujala B. Frequency of agreement between ultrasound and FNAC in differentiating benign and malignant thyroid neoplasm. *Pak J Med Health Sci.* 2014;8:212–214.
20. Schwarzenberg SJ, Thomas W, Olsen TW, et al. Microvascular complications in cystic fibrosis-related diabetes. *Diabetes Care.* 2007;30:1056–1061.
21. Yung M, Wilkins B, Norton L, Slater A. Glucose control, organ failure, and mortality in pediatric intensive care. *Pediatr Crit Care Med.* 2008;9:147–152.
22. Yates AR, Dyke PC 2nd, Taeed R, et al. Hyperglycemia is a marker for poor outcome in the postoperative pediatric cardiac patient. *Pediatr Crit Care Med.* 2006;7:351–355.
23. Srinivasan V, Spinella PC, Drott HR, Roth CL, Helfaer MA, Nadkarni V. Association of timing, duration, and intensity of hyperglycemia with intensive care unit mortality in critically ill children. *Pediatr Crit Care Med.* 2004;5:329–336.
24. Faustino EV, Apkon M. Persistent hyperglycemia in critically ill children. *J Pediatr.* 2005;146:30–34.
25. Vlasselaers D, Milants I, Desmet L, et al. Intensive insulin therapy for patients in paediatric intensive care: a prospective, randomised controlled study. *Lancet.* 2009;373:547–556.
26. Macrae D, Grieve R, Allen E, et al. A randomized trial of hyperglycemic control in pediatric intensive care. *N Engl J Med.* 2014;370:107–118.
27. van den Berghe G, Wouters P, Weekers F, et al. Intensive insulin therapy in critically ill patients. *N Engl J Med.* 2001;345:1359–1367.
28. McMahon MM, Bistrian BR. Host defenses and susceptibility to infection in patients with diabetes mellitus. *Infect Dis Clin North Am.* 1995;9:1–9.
29. Bjorgaas M, Gimse R, Vik T, Sand T. Cognitive function in type 1 diabetic children with and without episodes of severe hypoglycaemia. *Acta Paediatr.* 1997;86:148–153.
30. Rovet J, Alvarez M. Attentional functioning in children and adolescents with IDDM. *Diabetes Care.* 1997;20:803–810.
31. Ryan C, Gurtunca N, Becker D. Hypoglycemia: a complication of diabetes therapy in children. *Pediatr Clin North Am.* 2005;52:1705–1733.
32. Levine BS, Anderson BJ, Butler DA, Antisdel JE, Brackett J, Laffel LMB. Predictors of glycemic control and short-term adverse outcomes in youth with type 1 diabetes. *J Pediatr.* 2001;139:197–203.
33. Gallego PH, Wiltshire E, Donaghue KC. Identifying children at particular risk of long-term diabetes complications. *Pediatr Diabetes.* 2007;8:40–48.
34. The effect of intensive treatment of diabetes on the development and progression of long-term complications in insulin-dependent diabetes mellitus. The Diabetes Control and Complications Trial Research Group. *N Engl J Med.* 1993;329:977–986.
35. Nathan DM, Cleary PA, Backlund JY, et al. Intensive diabetes treatment and cardiovascular disease in patients with type 1 diabetes. *N Engl J Med.* 2005;353:2643–2653.
36. Srbova L, Gabalec F, Ryska A, Cap J. Results of retrospective classification of thyroid FNAs according to the Bethesda system: would this have improved accuracy [published online ahead of print July 30, 2014]? *Cytopathology.* doi:10.1111/cyt.12171.
37. Franz MJ, Bantle JP, Beebe CA, et al. Nutrition principles and recommendations in diabetes. *Diabetes Care.* 2004;27(suppl 1):S36–S46.
38. Wesorick D, O'Malley C, Rushakoff R, Larsen K, Magee M. Management of diabetes and hyperglycemia in the hospital: a practical guide to subcutaneous insulin use in the non-critically ill, adult patient. *J Hosp Med.* 2008;3:17–28.
39. American Diabetes Association. Management of dyslipidemia in children and adolescents with diabetes. *Diabetes Care.* 2003;26:2194–2197.
40. Taghipour Zahir S, Binesh F, Mirouliaei M, Khajeh E, Noshad S. Malignancy risk assessment in patients with thyroid nodules using classification and regression trees. *J Thyroid Res.* 2013;2013:983953.
41. Gosmanov AR, Umpierrez GE. Medical nutrition therapy in hospitalized patients with diabetes. *Curr Diab Rep.* 2012;12:93–100.
42. Umpierrez GE, Hellman R, Korytkowski MT, et al. Management of hyperglycemia in hospitalized patients in non-critical care setting: an endocrine society clinical practice guideline. *J Clin Endocrinol Metab.* 2012;97:16–38.
43. Jelalian E, Stark LJ, Reynolds L, Seifer R. Nutrition intervention for weight gain in cystic fibrosis: a meta analysis. *J Pediatr.* 1998;132:486–492.
44. Erskine JM, Lingard C, Sontag M. Update on enteral nutrition support for cystic fibrosis. *Nutr Clin Pract.* 2007;22:223–232.
45. White H, Pollard K, Etherington C, et al. Nutritional decline in cystic fibrosis related diabetes: the effect of intensive nutritional intervention. *J Cyst Fibros.* 2009;8:179–185.
46. Ghirardello S, Garre ML, Rossi A, Maghnie M. The diagnosis of children with central diabetes insipidus. *J Pediatr Endocr Metab.* 2007;20:359–375.

47. Rivkees SA, Dunbar N, Wilson TA. The management of central diabetes insipidus in infancy: desmopressin, low renal solute load formula, thiazide diuretics. *J Pediatr Endocrinol Metab.* 2007;20:459–469.

48. Bryant WP, Omarcaigh AS, Ledger GA, Zimmerman D. Aqueous vasopressin infusion during chemotherapy in patients with diabetes-insipidus. *Cancer.* 1994;74:2589–2592.

49. Bolli GB, Fanelli CG. Physiology of glucose counterregulation to hypoglycemia. *Endocrin Metab Clin.* 1999;28:467–493.

Test Your Knowledge Answers

1. The correct answer is **D**. The concentration of dextrose used in the PN should be chosen based on the optimal formulation of the PN, rather than on the fact that the child has diabetes mellitus.

2. The correct answer is **A**. The hospitalized child with CF-related diabetes mellitus often has increased insulin resistance and therefore requires a larger amount of insulin to control blood glucose excursions.

3. The correct answer is **C**. Acceptable blood glucose control in children with diabetes mellitus on EN can usually be obtained by using subcutaneous insulin. Insulin is usually not administered enterally.

4. The correct answer is **D**. Acceptable serum sodium concentrations in a child with diabetes insipidus on nutrition support can usually be obtained by using an intravenous drip of aqueous vasopressin.

22

Inborn Errors of Metabolism

Sandy van Calcar, PhD, RD, LD

 Podcast

Learning Objectives

1. Understand the basic principles of treating inborn errors of metabolism.
2. Understand the biochemistry and medical nutrition therapy for phenylketonuria.
3. Understand the biochemistry and medical nutrition therapy for methylmalonic acidemia.
4. Understand the biochemistry and medical nutrition therapy for ornithine transcarbamylase deficiency.
5. Understand the biochemistry and medical nutrition therapy for very long-chain acyl-CoA dehydrogenase deficiency.
6. Understand the biochemistry and medical nutrition therapy for classical galactosemia.
7. Understand the biochemistry and medical nutrition therapy for disorders of mitochondrial metabolism.

Background

Inborn errors of metabolism (IEM) are inherited disorders caused by mutations in the genes responsible for the synthesis of proteins that function as enzymes, coenzymes, and transporters necessary for the metabolism of carbohydrates, lipids, or amino acids. Abnormal production or function of these proteins results in both accumulation and deficiency of metabolites that can cause detrimental symptoms (Table 22-1). Presentation of disease varies greatly depending on the specific IEM and the degree of enzyme, coenzyme, or transporter deficiency; thus, many IEM can present at any age with a wide range of symptom severity. Severe forms of some disorders can present with overwhelming illness in the newborn period, including poor feeding, hypotonia, seizures, and eventually coma and death without prompt and

Table 22-1. Various Signs and Symptoms of Inborn Errors of Metabolism

Overwhelming illness in the newborn period
Recurrent vomiting
Poor growth
Failure to thrive
Developmental delay
Mental retardation
Loss of previously acquired skills
Hypotonia
Ataxia
Seizures or infantile spasms
Unusual odor
Episodes of rhabdomyolysis with intense exercise
Cardiomyopathy
Ophthalmoplegia
Cataracts
Neuropsychiatric symptoms

aggressive treatment. Some disorders do not present with overt illness but rather with symptoms such as intellectual disability that develop more gradually over time.

Many IEM can be detected in the neonate by newborn screening, which facilitates early diagnosis and initiation of treatment.[1,2] Newborn screening was initiated in the 1960s with detection of elevated phenylalanine (Phe) as a marker of phenylketonuria (PKU). PKU is often referred to as the model for newborn screening because the methodology is reliable and cost-effective, and early intervention with medical nutrition therapy yields clear benefits. In the 1990s, screening by tandem mass spectrometry (MS/MS) was introduced, and now more than 30 IEM can be detected from dried blood spots collected from newborns 24–48 hours after birth.[1-3] Since the initiation of screening by MS/MS, the overall prevalence of some IEM has been found to be greater than originally believed because the range of phenotypes that can be detected has increased to include not only those with classical forms of these disorders, but milder variants as well.[3]

Any infant found with an abnormal screen suggestive of an IEM is referred to a specialized metabolic clinic for prompt clinical evaluation, biochemical and molecular confirmatory testing, and appropriate medical and nutrition management. The overall goal of treatment for IEM is to achieve and maintain improved metabolic homeostasis, while allowing appropriate growth and development. Med-

ical nutrition therapy plays a large role in accomplishing these goals. The basic principles of nutrition management of IEM include prevention of catabolism with adequate energy intake, restriction of the offending substrate, supplementation of deficient products, and/or supplementation with the enzyme's cofactor (Figure 22-1).[4-7]

To meet nutrient needs but prevent excessive intake of substrates, specialized formulas, termed "medical foods," have been developed for treatment of numerous IEM. Medical foods do not contain the substrate or substrates that cannot be metabolized. For instance, a medical food designed for an amino acidopathy will be devoid of the amino acids that cannot be completely metabolized, but will provide all other amino acids, sources of carbohydrate and fat, and micronutrients.[4,5] If the blocked substrate is an essential amino acid, a limited but sufficient quantity of substrate must be provided to allow for protein anabolism. In infants, this is accomplished by providing a source of intact protein from a limited amount of regular infant formula or, for some disorders, breast milk. As the patient ages, the intact protein will be provided by limited quantities of lower protein foods. Careful laboratory, clinical, and developmental monitoring and ongoing nutrition education are essential to manage individuals with IEM.[4,5]

To illustrate the diversity of IEM and their nutrition management, this chapter provides a basic overview of 6 IEM: PKU, methylmalonic acidemia (MMA), ornithine transcarbamylase (OTC) deficiency, very long-chain acyl-CoA dehydrogenase

Figure 22-1. Basic Principles of Nutrition Management of Inborn Errors of Metabolism

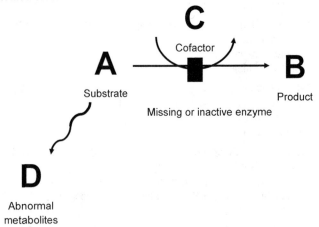

Restrict the amount of substrate (**A**)

Supplement the product (**B**) to prevent deficiency

Supplement the cofactor (**C**) to increase residual enzyme activity

Use adjunct therapies to remove abnormal metabolites (**D**)

deficiency (VLCADD), galactosemia, and the mitochondria disorder mitochondrial encephalomyelopathy, lactic acidosis, and stroke-like episodes (MELAS). All of these disorders can be detected by newborn screening, except for OTC deficiency (although other disorders of the urea cycle are included in the screening panel) and MELAS; screening is not yet available for any of the mitochondrial disorders. Various references are available that can provide further detail about the biochemistry and treatment of the wide range of IEM.[5-7]

Phenylketonuria

Natural History

PKU is an inborn error of Phe metabolism caused by a deficiency of the hepatic enzyme phenylalanine hydroxylase (PAH), which catalyzes the hydroxylation of Phe to tyrosine (Tyr) (Figure 22-2). PKU is an autosomal recessive disorder with an incidence of approximately 1 in 10,000–15,000 births and a carrier frequency of approximately 1 in 50 in those of European ancestry. Over 800 mutations have been identified in the PAH gene, but genotype-phenotype correlations have not proven to always predict outcome.[8]

PKU is often classified based on the degree to which blood Phe concentrations are elevated prior to initiation of treatment. Individuals with classical PKU show blood Phe elevations > 1200 μmol/L (20 mg/dL) compared to Phe concentrations < 120 μmol/L (2 mg/dL) in individuals without PKU. Individuals with untreated classical PKU are at risk for profound intellectual disability, seizures, and

Figure 22-2. Phenylketonuria results from a deficiency of phenylalanine hydroxylase (PAH), with elevated phenylalanine concentrations and tyrosine deficiency. PAH requires the cofactor tetrahydrobiopterin.

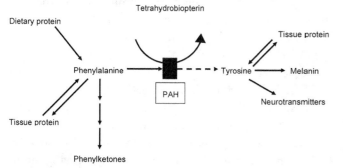

Adapted with permission from van Calcar SC and Ney DM. Food products made with glycomacropeptide, a low-phenylalanine whey protein, provide a new alternative to amino acid-based medical foods for nutrition management of phenylketonuria. *J. Acad. Nutr. Diet.* 112(8):1201-1210. Copyright 2012, with permission from Academy of Nutrition and Dietetics.

autistic-like behavior. Adequate treatment with a Phe-restricted diet ameliorates this outcome, and individuals with classical PKU can have similar IQ and developmental potential as their unaffected siblings.[9] On the other end of the spectrum, Phe elevations in those with mild hyperphenylalaninemia remain < 360 μmol/L (6 mg/dL) and may not require any diet modification.[4,5]

Treatment recommendations for PKU have evolved since diet therapy was first described in the 1950s.[10] Initially, metabolic specialists discontinued the Phe-restricted diet in early childhood since it was felt that brain development was complete and continuation of the diet could cause nutritional deficiencies.[11] This practice was formally evaluated in the National PKU Collaborative Study (1968–1984) in which 211 subjects with classical PKU were randomized at age 6 years to continue or discontinue the PKU diet.[9] Results from this study demonstrated that individuals with PKU who discontinued the diet developed significant reductions in IQ and academic performance by age 12 years.[9,12] A follow-up study of 70 adults who participated in the PKU Collaborative Study found significantly fewer adverse medical, cognitive, and psychological outcomes in those who were randomized to remain on diet compared with those who stopped diet treatment.[13] Conclusions from these and other studies led to the recommendation of lifelong treatment for PKU.[12,14-17]

Maternal Phenylketonuria

Phe is a known teratogen, and in utero exposure to elevated blood Phe interferes with embryonic development.[18] Infants born to women with elevated Phe throughout pregnancy are at risk for low birth weight, microcephaly, intellectual disability, cardiac defects, and other congenital abnormalities. The National Maternal PKU Collaborative Study (1984–2000) found that these detrimental effects to the fetus could be prevented if maternal plasma Phe concentrations remained below 360 μmol/L (6 mg/L) prior to conception and throughout pregnancy.[19,20] Education about the risks of elevated Phe concentrations during pregnancy should begin early in adolescence for all females with PKU. Over-restriction of dietary Phe also needs to be avoided during pregnancy since poor fetal growth has been noted in infants born to women with excessively low blood Phe during pregnancy.[21]

Acute Management

Initial Presentation

When an infant with PKU is identified by newborn screening, treatment should be initiated as soon as possible. Depending on the degree of elevation in blood concentrations, dietary Phe is eliminated or greatly reduced in the diet until blood Phe decreases below 360 μmol/L (6 mg/dL).[4,5] This can be accomplished by exclusively feeding a Phe-free, but otherwise nutritionally complete, medical food. Once plasma Phe concentrations are reduced, a limited quantity of an intact protein provided by a standard infant formula or breast milk is added to the medical food to meet minimum Phe needs for growth and protein anabolism (Table 22-2).[4,5,14,17]

Chronic Management

The primary goal of chronic management for PKU is restriction of dietary Phe to maintain blood Phe within the recommended treatment range of 120–360 μmol/L (2–6 mg/dL) for all ages.[14,16,17] Additional treatment goals include supporting normal growth and development, preventing protein deficiency, and achieving adequate macronutrient and micronutrient status.[4,5,14,17]

Table 22-2. Recommended Daily Nutrient Intakes for Phenylketonuria

Age	Nutrient			
	PHE (mg/kg)	TYR (mg/kg)	Protein[a] (g/kg)	Energy (kcal/kg)
Infants[b]				
0 to <3 mo[c]	25–70	300–350	3.50–3.00	120 (145–95)
3 to <6 mo	20–45	300–350	3.50–3.00	120 (145–95)
6 to <9 mo	15–35	250–300	3.00–2.50	110 (135–80)
9 to <12 mo	10–35	250–300	3.00–2.50	105 (135–80)
Girls and boys[b]	(mg/d)	(mg/d)	(g/d)	(kcal/d)
1 to <4 y	200–320	2800–3500	≥30	EER estimate
After early childhood				
>4 y to adult[d]	200–1100	4000–6000	120%–140% RDA for age	EER estimate

Data from Acosta and Yannicelli,[4] Acosta,[5] and Singh et al.[17]

EER, estimated energy requirement; Phe, phenylalanine; RDA, recommended dietary allowance; Tyr, tyrosine.

[a]Protein recommendations are greater than dietary reference intake estimates because of faster absorption and utilization of amino acids compared to intact protein.

[b]Recommended intakes for individuals < 4 years old apply to those with classical phenylketonuria treated with diet only.

[c]Requirements for premature infants may be higher.

[d]Recommended intakes for individuals > 4 years old apply to the entire spectrum of phenotypes (mild to classical).

Energy requirements for those with PKU are not different than that for the general population and standard dietary reference intake estimates can be utilized.[5,22] However, total protein needs for those with PKU may be greater than those for the general population because amino acids are more rapidly absorbed and utilized when free amino acids rather than an intact protein are given as the source of protein.[23] Medical food continues to provide the primary source of protein for all ages.

Phe needs vary between individuals and change with age, weight, and growth velocity (Table 22-2). In infancy, the Phe requirement is met by a standard infant formula or breast milk (Figure 22-3). Adjustments in dietary Phe are based on frequent monitoring of blood Phe concentrations. If blood Phe is elevated above the treatment range, the amount of intact protein is incrementally decreased.[4,5,14,17] Breastfeeding is possible in the treatment of PKU; metabolic control in infants allowed to breastfeed is similar to those consuming a regular infant formula as their Phe source.[24] The average Phe concentration of mature breast milk is approximately 1 mg/mL; it is somewhat higher in colostrum.[4,25]

An individual's Phe requirement is the same regardless of the source of intact protein consumed (formula, breast milk, or solid food). When an infant transitions to solids, the infant formula or breast milk is decreased and replaced by an equivalent amount of Phe from foods. Caregivers are instructed to "count" milligrams of Phe or use an exchange system (1 exchange = 15 mg Phe).[4,5,17]

Meat, legumes, nuts, and dairy products are too high in Phe and are not allowed in the Phe-restricted diet. All grains, fruits, and vegetables are weighed or measured, and the Phe content is calculated to ensure optimal blood Phe control (Table 22-3).[26,27] Low-protein grain products, made primarily from wheat starch instead of wheat flour, are available to increase variety and meet the energy needs of individuals with PKU.[28,29] For the PKU diet, "free" foods and beverages are those that contain no protein (and no Phe) such as sugars and fats.[26,27] Aspartame (Nutrasweet) is a dipeptide derived from aspartic acid and Phe; all foods and medications containing this sweetener need to be avoided.[30]

Recent studies have suggested that all fruits and vegetables containing less than 50 mg Phe/100 g serving can be considered "free" foods without adversely affecting metabolic control.[31] References are available that list the Phe and protein content of various foods and beverages.[4,26,27]

In PKU, decreased PAH activity reduces the production of Tyr. Thus, Tyr becomes a conditionally essential amino

Figure 22-3. Calculating a Low Phenylalanine (Phe) Formula

An infant weighing 3.6 kg is diagnosed with phenylketonuria (PKU) with an initial blood Phe concentration of 15 mg/dL. Determine an appropriate formula for this infant.

Answer

Provide a Phe-free medical food until Phe concentrations are less than 6 mg/dL. Then add an intact protein source to meet nutrition needs.

DETERMINE NEEDS

1) *Determine Phe Requirement using Table 22-2*
   3.6 kg × 45 mg of Phe*/kg = 162 mg of Phe per day
   *Phe requirements range from 25 to 70 mg/kg. Given the moderate elevation in blood Phe of 15 mg/dL, Phe requirements are estimated at 45 mg/kg.

2) *Determine Tyrosine (Tyr) Requirement*
   3.6 kg × 325 mg of Tyr/kg = 1170 mg

3) *Determine Protein Requirement*
   3.6 kg × 3.2 g of pro/kg ≈ 11–12 g of protein

4) *Determine Calorie (kcal) Requirement*
   3.6 kg × ~120 kcal/kg ≈ 430–450 kcal

CALCULATE FORMULA

1) *Determine the Amount of Infant Formula (the Source of Intact Protein) Needed to Meet Phe Needs*
   Infant formula A contains 330 mg of Phe in 100 g

$$\frac{162 \text{ mg of Phe needed per day} \times 100 \text{ g of infant formula}}{330 \text{ mg of Phe}} = 49 \text{ g of infant formula A needed}$$

2) *Determine Amount of Calories and Protein in Infant Formula*
   Infant formula A contains 10.8 g of protein and 518 kcal in 100 g

$$\frac{49 \text{ g infant formula A} \times 10.8 \text{ g protein}}{100 \text{ g of infant formula}} = 5.3 \text{ g of protein}$$

$$\frac{49 \text{ g of infant formula A} \times 518 \text{ kcal}}{100 \text{ g of infant formula}} = 254 \text{ kcal}$$

3) *Determine Amount of Phe-Free Medical Food B Needed to Meet Protein Needs*
   Phe-free medical food B contains 15 g of protein in 100 g
   11.5 g total protein needs − 5.3 g of protein from Infant formula A = 6.2 or ~6 g of protein needed

$$\frac{6 \text{ g of protein needed} \times 100 \text{ g of medical food B}}{15 \text{ g of protein}} = 40 \text{ g of Phe-free medical food}$$

4) *Determine Calories from Phe-Free Medical Food B*

$$\frac{40 \text{ g of medical food B} \times 480 \text{ kcal}}{100 \text{ g of Phe-free medical food}} = 192 \text{ kcal}$$

FINAL RECIPE

PRODUCT	AMOUNT (g)	PHE (mg)	PROTEIN (g)	CALORIES (kcal)
Infant formula A	49	162	5	254
Phe-free medical food B	40	0	6	192
Total	–	162	11	446

Volume required at 20 kcal/oz = 22 fluid ounces (625 mL)

Table 22-3. Example of a Daily Meal Plan for Classical Phenylketonuria

Age: 3 years, 9 months

Weight: 15.2 kg

Height: 101 cm

Sex: Female

Medical food prescription: 125 g of Phenex-2 unflavored + 18 fluid ounces of water = 20 fluid ounces total volume

Daily phenylalanine (Phe) prescription from foods: 200 mg

Estimated needs: Protein: >30 g/d   Kilocalories: 900–1800 kcal/d

MEAL	FOOD OR LIQUID OFFERED	AMOUNT EATEN	PHE	PROTEIN	CALORIES
Breakfast	Medical food	6 oz	0 mg	11 g	154 kcal
	Froot Loops	6 g	17 mg	0.4 g	25 kcal
	Crackles low protein cereal	30 g	7 mg	0.2 g	120 kcal
	Blueberries, fresh	32 g	8 mg	0.2 g	18 kcal
Lunch	Medical food	7 oz	0 mg	13 g	179 kcal
	French fries, Ore-Ida Golden Fries	56 g	50 mg	1.4 g	80 kcal
	Broccoli, cooked	28 g	14 mg	0.6 g	6.0 kcal
	Thousand island dressing	16 g	6 mg	0.1 g	59 kcal
	Peaches, canned	57 g	8 mg	0.3 g	42 kcal
Snack	Cantaloupe, fresh	27 g	8 mg	0.2 g	9 kcal
Dinner	Medical food	7 oz	0 mg	13 g	179 kcal
	Sweet potato, fresh, with skin, cooked	22 g	25 mg	0.4 g	23 kcal
	Green beans, canned	28 g	14 mg	0.4 g	6 kcal
	Pears, canned	90 g	8 mg	0.2 g	66 kcal
Snack	Zoo animal crackers, Farley's	22 g	20 mg	1.6 g	94 kcal
	Sorbet, strawberry	122 g	15 mg	0.4 g	119 kcal
Total			200 mg	43.4 g	1179 kcal
% from medical food			0%	85.3%	43.4%

acid for this population, and all medical foods for PKU are supplemented with this amino acid. Additional Tyr supplementation is indicated only if the combination of intact protein and medical food does not meet Tyr requirements. Plasma Tyr concentrations should be routinely monitored in individuals with PKU.[5,16,17]

Some micronutrients may be insufficient in the low Phe diet, particularly for individuals consuming a suboptimal amount of medical food. Inadequate intake of iron, folate, vitamin B12, calcium, vitamin D, and essential fatty acids has been reported.[32-36] Dietary intake should be analyzed for micronutrient content and additional supplementation prescribed, as needed.[17,33] Additionally, reduced bone mineral density and bone mineral content have been found in some individuals with PKU.[37,38] Whether this finding is related to various nutritional factors or is an effect of PAH deficiency itself remains unclear.

Large neutral amino acids (LNAA): Phe and other LNAA (leucine [Leu], valine [Val], isoleucine [Ile], methionine [Met], Tyr, tryptophan [Trp], and threonine [Thr]) share common transporters at the blood-brain barrier and intestinal mucosa. In PKU, competitive inhibition from high concentrations of Phe reduces the transport of other LNAA into cerebral cells, thus reducing synthesis of various neurotransmitters.[39] Supplementation with high doses of LNAA can reduce both blood and brain concentrations of Phe and may improve executive function skills in individuals who have not been successful maintaining good dietary control.[40,41] Several LNAA medical foods are now commercially available.

Cofactor supplementation: A newer therapy for the treatment of PKU is supplementation with sapropterin dihydrochloride (Kuvan), a synthetic form of tetrahydrobiopterin, the cofactor for the PAH enzyme.[42-45] In a phase III randomized, placebo-controlled, double-blind study, 44% of participants taking sapropterin for 6 weeks showed a reduced Phe concentration of 30% or greater.[42] Response to sapropterin needs to be individually assessed because not all individuals with PKU will respond to supplementation, and the degree of response to the drug varies. Individuals with milder forms of PKU are most likely to respond to sapropterin[44]; however, supplementation rarely allows for complete liberalization of the low Phe diet or eliminates the need for medical food.[45] The reduced need for a medical food may adversely affect the sapropterin-responsive patient's overall nutritional status if other sources of essential nutrients such as fats, vitamins, and minerals are not provided.[46]

Methylmalonic Acidemia

Natural History

MMA is an inborn error of Ile, Met, Thr, Val, and odd-chain fatty acid metabolism caused by a deficiency of the enzyme methylmalonyl-CoA mutase responsible for converting methylmalonyl CoA to succinyl-CoA, which is eventually oxidized in the citric acid cycle (Figure 22-4).[6,7] In MMA, methylmalonyl CoA is not metabolized, leading to accumulation of various methylmalonate intermediates. The degree of deficiency in the mutase enzyme affects the clinical outcome of this disorder.[47-49] Those classified with mut– deficiency have some residual activity and often a less severe clinical course than those with mut0 deficiency who have < 2% residual enzyme activity.[47-49] Methylmalonyl-CoA mutase requires the cofactor 5-dehydroxyadenosylcobalamin, which is derived from vitamin B12. Defects in the production of the cobalamin cofactor, such as cobalamin (cbl) A or cbl B deficiency, can also cause MMA. The estimated prevalence of all forms of MMA is 1 in 80,000 births.[50]

Infants with classical MMA caused by a severe deficiency of the mutase enzyme often present in the first week of life with overwhelming illness. Symptoms include poor feeding, failure to thrive, hypotonia, vomiting, and dehydration with ketosis, acidosis, hyperammonemia, and hypoglycemia.[47-49,51,52] Acute episodes are often fatal without aggressive medical and nutrition management. Despite treatment, individuals with severe mutase deficiency often have developmental delays, progressive renal failure, and other medical complications.[48,51,52] Screening for MMA is included in the MS/MS screening panel, leading to earlier diagnosis and improved clinical outcomes of this disorder, although infants with severe forms of this disorder may have significant illness before screening results become available.[53]

For patients with MMA caused by a mild late-onset mut– deficiency or a defect in cofactor production, supplementation with high doses of vitamin B12 may be sufficient to achieve metabolic control. This is particularly true for patients with cbl A defects.[47] Other cofactor deficiencies, such as cbl B and cbl C, can have a more complicated clinical course and require both medical nutrition therapy and vitamin B12 supplementation.[47,54]

Liver and/or renal transplantation is now an option for treatment of this disorder, particularly for individuals with severe mutase deficiency.[55-59] Although transplantation can greatly reduce the incidence of metabolic episodes and improve the clinical outcome, it is not curative, and continued medical nutrition therapy is typically required.[59]

Figure 22-4. Methylmalonic acidemia is caused by a defect in methylmalonyl CoA mutase. Cobalamin (cbl) A and cbl B are 2 of 6 known cbl cofactor synthesis defects, which also cause methylmalonic acidemia.

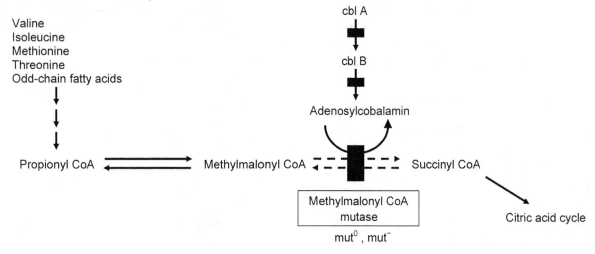

Adapted with permission from Nyhan WL, Barshop BA, Ozand PT. *Atlas of Metabolic Diseases.* 2nd ed. New York, NY: Oxford University Press Inc; 2005.

Acute Management

Initial Presentation

Infants with MMA presenting in an acute episode require immediate medical attention to control acidosis, hyperammonemia, and hypoglycemia.[47,52,60,61] Nutrition management during the acute phase of illness concentrates on delivery of nonprotein energy sources to help slow catabolism. Typically, intravenous (IV) dextrose at the maximum glucose infusion rate (GIR) with additional lipid is provided to achieve maximal energy intake.[52,60,61] Insulin may be required to maintain normoglycemia when delivery of a high GIR is required. Intravenous L-carnitine may also be indicated.[6,52,60–62]

A source of protein needs to be added within 24–48 hours to prevent further catabolism.[5,52,60,61] Enteral feedings of a medical food containing all amino acids except Ile, Met, Thr, and Val can be initiated; if it is poorly tolerated, specialized parenteral solutions without the offending amino acids are available.[5,52,61] As metabolic control improves, a standard infant formula or parenteral amino acid solution is incrementally added to provide a source of protein to meet the infant's Met, Val, Ile, and Thr needs.[4,5] Frequent monitoring of ammonia, prealbumin, bicarbonate, and plasma amino acids is necessary to adjust the dietary prescription to achieve optimal metabolic control.

Illness

Any illness, significant injury, or surgery can lead to catabolism of protein stores. In MMA, the offending amino acids cannot be utilized, and a metabolic episode, with symptoms similar to those observed during the initial episode in infancy, can develop. A metabolic crisis can occur at any age and can be life-threatening if not managed aggressively.[51,52,60,61]

For management of a nonacute illness at home, a "sick day" diet can be prescribed to increase energy intake and reduce intact protein by 50%–100%, depending on the severity of the illness.[52] If tolerated, medical food is continued to provide adequate amino acids and energy to promote protein anabolism.[5,63] Fasting times need to be reduced to prevent hypoglycemia and reduce protein catabolism. For any illness causing the inability to tolerate oral intake, aggressive medical intervention is required.[6,52,60,61] Caretakers need to be educated about the signs of metabolic decompensation and provided with an emergency protocol that includes contact information for the metabolic team.[61]

Chronic Management

Long-term medical nutrition therapy for individuals with mutase deficiency includes restriction of the amino acids Ile, Met, Thr, and Val with adequate energy intake to prevent catabolism.[4,5,52,63] Often 50% of total protein needs are provided by a medical food and 50% from intact protein sources; however, the tolerance for the offending amino acids can vary greatly between patients.[52,63,64] Individuals with MMA may have significant deviations in growth and body composition, resulting in lower energy expenditure than that predicted by standard equations. Adjusting predicted resting energy expenditure by a patient's fat-free mass may provide a more accurate assessment of energy requirements[64].

In infants, a standard infant formula or expressed breast milk provides the source of Ile, Val, Thr, and Met. When the child is developmentally ready for solid foods, low-protein foods replace the intact protein from these sources.[4,5,52] However, for infants with developmental delay and poor feeding skills, gastrostomy-tube feedings may be required.

For individuals responding to vitamin B12 supplementation, the initial dose is 1000 mcg/d given via intramuscular injection; further dose adjustments are based on monitoring serum MMA and other metabolite concentrations.[52,65] For some patients, high doses of oral vitamin B12 may be sufficient to maintain adequate metabolic control.[65] The preferred source of vitamin B12 for these disorders is hydroxocobalamin rather than the standard cyanocobalamin formulation.[66]

L-carnitine is often deficient in individuals with MMA.[62] Carnitine binds to the intermediate metabolites that accumulate in this disorder; thus, individuals with MMA can have a higher requirement for this nutrient. Supplementation with prescription strength L-carnitine (Carnitor) is a common practice, especially if low levels of free carnitine are observed. Doses for carnitine supplementation range from 50 to 200 mg/kg/d depending on serum carnitine concentrations.[6,52] Side effects from excessive carnitine intake include diarrhea, stomach upset, and a fishy odor.

Frequent laboratory, clinical, and developmental monitoring is required to assess metabolic status and determine dietary prescription changes. Biochemical testing typically includes amino acids, carnitine, acylcarnitine profile, and methylmalonic acid in plasma or serum and organic acids in urine.[52,63,64,67] In addition, labs to assess general nutrition status including iron indices, calcium, vitamin D, essential fatty acids, and albumin/prealbumin concentrations should be routinely conducted.[5]

Ornithine Transcarbamylase Deficiency

Natural History

The most common inborn error of the urea cycle is deficiency of OTC. OTC deficiency results in hyperammonemia because conversion of ammonia to nontoxic urea is impaired. Production of arginine is decreased, and arginine becomes a conditionally essential amino acid in this disorder (Figure 22-5).[6,7] OTC deficiency is an X-linked disorder; therefore, males are often more severely affected than females. How-

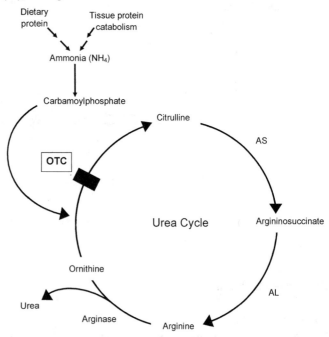

Figure 22-5. Nitrogen metabolism in the urea cycle. Ornithine transcarbamylase (OTC) deficiency results in hyperammonemia, elevated glutamine concentrations and deficiency of arginine. Other enzymes in the urea cycle include argininosuccinate synthetase (AS), argininosuccinate lyase (AL), and arginase.

Adapted from Wijburg FA, Nassogne MC. Disorders of the urea cycle and related enzymes. In: Saudubray JM, van den Berghe G, Walter JH, eds. *Inborn Metabolic Diseases: Diagnosis and Treatment.* Heidelberg, Germany: Springer Medizin; 2012:297–310. With kind permission from Springer Science and Business Media.

ever, a wide range of clinical presentations exist, including childhood or adult-onset OTC deficiency, especially in females who are carriers for this disorder.[68]

The severe form of the disease is characterized by overwhelming hyperammonemia in the newborn period causing recurrent vomiting, lethargy, irritability, and seizures, which can quickly lead to coma and death if not treated aggressively to rapidly decrease ammonia concentrations.[69] Intellectual and developmental disabilities are common in those surviving the initial episode.[68,69] Milder forms of the disorder may not present until later in life often precipitated by a severe illness or other catabolic stress. Histories of vomiting episodes, aversion to dietary protein, and psychiatric complications have been reported in late-onset OTC deficiency.[68] At this time, OTC deficiency is not included in the newborn screening panel, so diagnosis relies on recognition of this wide range of clinical presentations. Long-term outcome varies greatly and often depends on the ability to prevent further episodes of hyperammonemia. Liver transplantation is now an option for treatment of this disorder.[70,71]

Acute Management

Acute management may be necessary at the time of initial presentation or with any intercurrent illness or injury. The goal of acute management of OTC deficiency is to slow protein catabolism and thus reduce ammonia production by providing a protein-free, high-calorie nutrition source via enteral and/or parenteral nutrition.[60,61,72,73] Acute medical management often includes use of nitrogen-scavenger drugs, which are available in both oral (Buphenyl or Ravicti) and IV forms (Ammunol).[74,75]

A protein source should be initiated within 48–72 hours to prevent catabolism of lean muscle mass, which can contribute to ammonia production.[72,73] A medical food containing only essential amino acids as the protein source is incrementally added as ammonia concentrations decrease. If the patient is unable to tolerate enteral feedings, a standard parenteral amino acid solution can be added. Providing essential amino acids promotes protein anabolism, yet restricts intake of the nonessential amino acids that can contribute to the nitrogen load.[72,73] As clinical status continues to improve, an intact protein source is initiated to provide approximately 50% of total protein needs.[5,73]

Since arginine is a conditionally essential amino acid in OTC deficiency, supplementation with IV L-arginine is often indicated during illness.[72,73] Arginine bypasses the enzymatic block to allow for production of urea rather than further ammonia production.[6,7]

Chronic Management

Given the wide range of clinical phenotypes in OTC deficiency, chronic management needs to be individualized, but typically includes dietary restriction of total protein with approximately 50% from intact sources and 50% from a medical food providing essential amino acids.[5,72,73,76] The total protein prescription for OTC deficiency may be lower than the protein requirements outlined in the dietary reference intakes.[5,73] Sufficient total energy with addition of fat and/or carbohydrate-based medical foods or dietary sources is needed to promote anabolism.

In infancy, the intact protein source can be provided by a standard infant formula or expressed breast milk with transition to lower protein foods when the patient is developmentally ready for oral feeding. The use of specialty low-protein food products may be necessary to meet energy needs, increase satiety, and provide variety in the diet.[5,28] In individuals with more severe forms of this disorder, gastrostomy feedings of a medical food is often necessary to provide adequate energy and appropriate sources of protein. In addition, L-citrulline is routinely supplemented at an initial dose of 100–170 mg/kg because it is the precursor for arginine and utilizes additional nitrogen via aspartate in the urea cycle.[5,72,73]

To assess metabolic control, frequent monitoring of ammonia and plasma amino acids is necessary. Of particular interest are concentrations of citrulline and arginine to evaluate L-citrulline supplementation and glutamine, which increases with excessive protein intake and/or inadequate energy intake.[77] Additionally, monitoring concentrations of the branched-chain amino acids Leu, Val, and Ile is necessary since chronic use of a nitrogen-scavenging medication can increase their oxidation. This can lead to deficient concentrations of these amino acids despite adequate total protein intake, and additional supplementation may be indicated.[78] Routine monitoring of albumin, prealbumin, and other indices of nutrition status is also recommended.[5,72,73]

Very Long-Chain Acyl-CoA Dehydrogenase Deficiency

Natural History

VLCADD is an inborn error in the first step of mitochondrial β-oxidation of long-chain fatty acids (14–20 carbons in length), resulting in disturbed energy production with hypoglycemia, reduced ketone production, and accumulation of fatty acid intermediates (Figure 22-6).[6,7] Severe forms of this disorder can present in early infancy with hypoglycemia, liver dysfunction, cardiomyopathy, and myopathy and can be fatal without medical intervention. Milder forms of this disorder may present during early childhood with episodes of hypoglycemic encephalopathy or in adolescents and adults with episodes of muscle pain and rhabdomyolysis, especially after intense and/or prolonged exercise.[79,80] Even in individuals with more severe forms of VLCADD, long-term development and outcome for those diagnosed and treated early can be favorable.[80,81]

With MS/MS screening, VLCADD appears to be more prevalent than earlier estimates since screening is identifying milder forms of this disorder that may not have presented clinically in the past.[82] Consensus is lacking about the necessity and degree of treatment required during infancy for individuals with phenotypes that may not present until later in life.[81,83] Research continues to establish evidence to predict the long-term phenotype based on newborn screening values and/or genotype.[84]

Figure 22-6. Fatty Acid Oxidation and Very Long-Chain Acyl-CoA Dehydrogenase (VLCAD) Deficiency

Fatty acid oxidation requires entry of long-chain fatty acids (LCFAs) into the mitochondria. This process requires carnitine. Carnitine cycle enzymes include acyl-CoA synthetase (AS), carnitine palmitoyltransferase I and II (CPT I and CPT II), and acylcarnitine/carnitine translocase (CT). Once in the mitochondria, the β-oxidation spiral sequentially oxidizes the fatty acyl-CoA to the 2-carbon unit acetyl-CoA. Oxidation of LCFAs requires VLCAD and a trifunctional protein, which includes 3 enzyme activities.

In treatment of VLCAD deficiency, supplementation with medium-chain triglycerides (MCTs) bypasses the LCFA enzymes and utilizes enzymes that oxidize medium-chain and short-chain fatty acids, including medium-chain acyl-CoA dehydrogenase (MCAD) and short-chain acyl-CoA dehydrogenase (SCAD) enzymes.

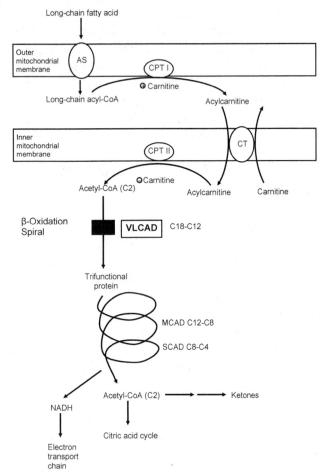

Adapted with permission from Nyhan WL, Barshop BA, Ozand PT. *Atlas of Metabolic Diseases.* 2nd ed. New York, NY: Oxford University Press Inc; 2005.

Acute Management

The primary goal of acute management of VLCADD is to provide sufficient energy to prevent hypoglycemia and slow catabolism of fat stores.[6,7] Typically, IV dextrose with a minimum 10% concentration is infused at the upper threshold of the GIR for the patient's age and weight.[61,81,85] Intralipid is contraindicated in VLCADD since it is a source of long-chain fatty acids. As enteral feeding becomes possible, sources of glucose and medium-chain triglycerides (MCTs) are provided to meet energy demands. Medical foods providing the majority of total fat as MCTs, but containing sufficient long-chain fat sources to meet essential fatty acid needs are available.

Even for those with mild VLCADD who remain asymptomatic during infancy, any illness or other catabolic event can trigger an acute metabolic crisis.[86] Glucose polymer solutions can be used for home treatment,[87] but caregivers need to understand signs of decompensation and have an emergency protocol in place.

Chronic Management

Long-term nutrition management of VLCADD includes prevention of fasting, restriction of long-chain fatty acid intake, and supplementation with MCTs.[81,88,89] Prevention of fasting, especially in infancy when energy stores are limited, is imperative to prevent acute decompensation. Fasting guidelines need to be individualized, but fasting is typically limited to a maximum of 4 hours for infants up to 4 months of age.[81,88-90] Longer periods of fasting can be allowed as the infant ages, but often a feeding during the night is recommended during the first year.[88] In severe VLCADD, continuous overnight feedings may be needed.

Depending on the severity of the disorder and age of the patient, long-chain fat intake may need to be reduced to 15 to 20% of total energy.[5,81,88,89,91] The remaining energy provided by fat is supplied by MCTs, which include fatty acids of 8–12 carbons in length and thus can bypass the enzymatic block in long-chain fatty acid oxidation (Figure 22-6).

In infancy, MCT-based medical foods are prescribed. Limited breastfeeding may be allowed in milder forms of this disorder.[81,88,89] In older children, continued restriction of dietary fat and supplementation of low-fat or nonfat foods and beverages with MCTs from an oil, powder, or emulsified liquid source are necessary to maintain metabolic control.[5,81,88,89] With intense exercise, consuming MCTs and carbohydrates prior to activity may be beneficial as an energy source during activity.[92]

Addition of raw cornstarch to night-time feedings may be indicated in some children with VLCADD. Cornstarch provides a slowly digested source of glucose and is employed in the treatment of glycogen storage disease to prevent hypoglycemia.[93] Cornstarch supplementation may be helpful in fatty acid oxidation disorders to prevent low glucose concentrations and reduce production of abnormal fat metabolites during overnight fasting.[85,88] Because of poor digestion, cornstarch is contraindicated before 9 months of age.[93]

With the restriction in long-chain fat, it is important to assess the intake of the essential fatty acids linoleic acid and α-linolenic acid. An essential fatty acid profile, measured in red cells rather than plasma, needs to be routinely monitored.[88,94] Supplementation with walnut, flax, and/or safflower oil may be necessary to meet linoleic acid and α-linolenic acid needs unless the child is prescribed a medical food supplemented with arachidonic acid and docosahexaenoic acid.[88,95] Other parameters to monitor typically include fasting serum glucose, creatine phosphokinase, plasma carnitine, and acylcarnitine profile.[5,94,96]

Galactosemia

Natural History

Classical galactosemia, with an incidence of approximately 1 in 60,000 births, is an autosomal recessive disorder caused by the enzymatic deficiency of galactose-1-phosphate uridyl transferase (GALT). Abnormal elevations of galactose-1-phosphate (gal-1-P), galactitol, and galactonate are present (Figure 22-7).[6,7] Over 250 mutations have been identified in the GALT gene.[97,98] In the white population, a common mutation is c.Q188R; homozygosity of this mutation results in a severe phenotype, often with no residual enzyme activity.[97] The c.S135L mutation, prevalent in the African American population, results in a milder clinical course.[99] Another prevalent form of galactosemia is the Duarte variant, which results in a mild phenotype that may not require dietary intervention.[100]

Infants with classical galactosemia can present within the first few days of life with jaundice, poor feeding, and vomiting. If not treated, symptoms can progress to liver failure and risk of *Escherichia coli* sepsis, which can be fatal. Galactosemia is detected by newborn screening, which has reduced the incidence of severe illness during the neonatal period.[98]

Treatment of classical galactosemia requires a lifelong galactose-restricted diet. Despite nutrition management, long-term complications can include cognitive delays, neurological abnormalities, speech delay, and premature ovarian failure in females.[101–103] The etiology of these complications remains unknown, although endogenous production

Figure 22-7. Classical galactosemia is caused by a deficiency of galactose-1-phosphate uridyltransferase (GALT). Elevations in galactose-1-phosphate, galactose, galactitol, and galactonate are present in this disorder. Other enzymes involved in this pathway include galactokinase (GALK) and UDP galactose-4-epimerase (GALE). UDP galactose is used as a substrate for production of various glycoconjugates, such as glycoproteins and galactolipids.

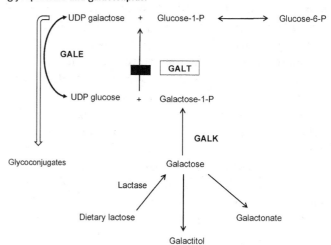

Adapted from Berry GT, Walter JH. Disorders of galactose metabolism. In: Saudubray JM, van den Berghe G, Walter JH, eds. *Inborn Metabolic Diseases: Diagnosis and Treatment.* Heidelberg, Germany: Springer Medizen; 2012:141–150. With kind permission from Springer Science and Business Media.

of galactose and/or abnormal glycosylation of glycoproteins have been implicated.[104,105]

Acute Management

Infants identified with classical galactosemia should be immediately placed on a soy-based medical food containing soy protein isolate as the protein source. These formulas contain minimal galactose compared to cow's milk–based formulas or breast milk.[98,106] If an infant does not tolerate enteral feeds, standard parenteral nutrition (PN) may be used. Efforts should be made to choose medications that are free of lactose fillers. Unlike some disorders of amino acid and fat metabolism, those with galactosemia do not develop further metabolic episodes associated with illness or other catabolic processes.[6,7]

Chronic Management

Long-term management of classical galactosemia requires dietary restriction of galactose. Lactose is the primary source of galactose and most dairy-based products are eliminated. Throughout infancy, a soy-based formula is provided and breastfeeding or milk-based infant formulas are contraindicated.[106] Elemental formulas devoid of galactose have been used to treat some infants with classical galactosemia who have erythrocyte gal-1-P concentrations that are slow to decrease into the treatment range.[107,108] Whether routine use of elemental formulas could lead to a more rapid reduction in gal-1-P concentrations or whether this reduction could reduce or prevent long-term complications remains unknown.[106] Since soy-based formulas are not recommended for premature infants, an elemental formula needs to be considered for premature infants with classical galactosemia.[109]

When starting infants on solids, caregivers are instructed to check food labels for foods and ingredients that contain lactose or galactose (Table 22-4). Restricted foods and ingredients are primarily dairy based; however, negligible galactose has been found in some aged cheeses and the additives calcium and sodium caseinate. These products are allowed in the diet for classical galactosemia.[106,110] Many fruits, vegetables, and legumes contain

Table 22-4. Foods and Ingredients That Contain Lactose and/or Galactose and Are Eliminated in the Diet for Classical Galactosemia

Milk	Casein
Milk solids	Lactose
Nonfat dry milk	Hydrolyzed whey protein
Nonfat dry milk solids	Hydrolyzed casein protein
Dry milk and dry milk solids	Whey and whey solids
Butter	Lactalbumin
Buttermilk and buttermilk solids	Lactoglobulin
Cream	Milk chocolate
Organ meats	Sour cream
Meat byproducts	Yogurt
Ice cream	Fermented soy products[b]
Sherbet	Fermented soy sauce[c]
Cheese, except those listed below[a]	

[a]Allowed aged cheeses include Jarlsberg, Emmentaler, Swiss, Gruyere, Tilsiter, Parmesan aged > 10 months, 100% Parmesan cheese powder, and sharp Cheddar cheese.

[b]Includes miso, tempeh, natto, sufu, and similar products.

[c]Unfermented soy sauce is made from hydrolyzed soy protein and is allowed.

Adapted from van Calcar SC, Bernstein LE, Rohr FJ, Scaman CH, Yannicelli S, Berry GT. A re-evaluation of life-long severe galactose restriction for the nutrition management of classic galactosemia. *Mol. Genet. Metab.* 3(7):191–197. Copyright 2014, with permission from Elsevier.

small amounts of free galactose,[111-113] but guidelines are no longer recommending elimination of these minor sources of galactose.[106]

Erythrocyte gal-1-P is the primary metabolite monitored in galactosemia and concentrations below 4 mg/dL are considered optimal, although some individuals maintain higher gal-1-P concentrations even with strict dietary management. Gal-1-P is not a sensitive measure of treatment compliance; however, a significant increase above a patient's typical gal-1-P concentrations should be investigated for possible dietary indiscretions.[114]

Osteoporosis and abnormal concentrations of various measures of bone metabolism have been described in this population.[115] Recommendations suggest monitoring serum total 25-OH vitamin D [116] and initiating dual-energy X-ray absorptiometry scans as early as age 4 years with repeat scans every year if the Z-score is ≤ 2 SD and every 2 years if above this score.[117] While the mechanism of decreased bone density in patients with galactosemia is not well understood, ensuring adequate intake of calcium, vitamin D, and other nutrients associated with bone metabolism can prevent deficiencies that could exacerbate the development of these problems.[115,117]

Mitochondrial Disorders

Natural History

The first mitochondrial disorder was initially described over 30 years ago, but the number of known disorders has increased greatly since that time; the estimated incidence is now 1 in 8500 births.[118] Disorders have been described in the synthesis, transport, assembly, or maintenance of mitochondrial proteins.[6,7]

These disorders can be inherited by defects in encoded genes in either mitochondrial DNA or nuclear DNA. The inheritance pattern is typically autosomal recessive or autosomal dominant for disorders stemming from nuclear DNA and maternal inheritance for disorders stemming from mitochondrial DNA.[118] Mitochondrial disorders ultimately affect functioning of the electron transport chain (ETC), which is composed of 5 complexes with 70 protein subunits (Figure 22-8).[6,7] Disorders can either directly affect production of one or more of the complexes or cause secondary reductions in their activity.[118]

Mitochondrial disorders can present at any point in the lifespan and the same disorder can have a wide range of phenotypes, even in members of the same family (Table 22-5).[118] Often mitochondrial disorders affect more than one organ system and all of the potential findings listed

Figure 22-8. The electron transport chain (ETC) produces ATP from ADP by oxidative phosphorylation. The ETC is composed of 5 multiprotein enzyme complexes: complex 1 = NADH:ubiquinone oxidoreductase; complex II = succinate:ubiquinone; complex III = cytochrome bc; complex IV = cytochrome c oxidase; and complex V = ATP synthetase. There are 2 electron carriers, coenzyme Q-10 and cytochrome C. The figure indicates the entry point of electrons from various macronutrients. Electrons from carbohydrate and amino acid sources enter via complexes I and II. Fatty acids, choline, branched chain amino acids, lysine, and tryptophan enter via the electron transfer flavoprotein (ETF). Nutritional supplements such as coenzyme Q-10 or various B-vitamins are prescribed as precursors to ETC substrates or cofactors.

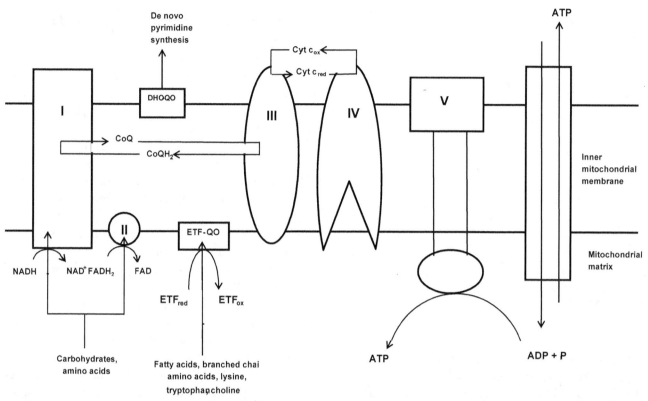

Adapted with permission from Nyhan WL, Barshop BA, Ozand PT. *Atlas of Metabolic Diseases*. 2nd ed. New York, NY: Oxford University Press Inc; 2005.

in Table 22-1 have been described in one or more of these disorders. Typically, the earlier the onset, the more severe the disorder; neonatal and infant presentations are often eventually fatal. Once the diagnosis is clinically suspected, molecular testing is used to confirm the disorder. Newer

Table 22-5. Names of Some Common Mitochondrial Myopathies

- MELAS = Mitochondrial enchephalomyopathy, lactic acidosis, and stroke-like episodes
- MERFF = Myoclonic epilepsy and ragged red fiber disease
- NARP = Neurodegeneration, ataxia, and retinitis pigmentosa
- Kearns-Sayre syndrome
- Pearson Syndrome
- Mitochondrial DNA depletion syndrome
- MNGIE = mitochondrial neurogastrointestinal encephalopathy
- Respiratory chain enzyme deficiencies (complex I deficiency, others)

techniques, such as mitochondrial DNA sequencing or whole genome sequencing are improving diagnosis.[118–120]

Acute and Chronic Management

Few mitochondrial disorders present as an acute event; most are slowly progressing over time. A specific treatment does not exist for any mitochondrial disorder, and care is primarily supportive.[118,121] Infants and children with mitochondrial disorders are often clinically fragile and have a difficult time recovering from illness or other stress. To prevent catabolism, nutrition support should be initiated at an early stage of disease.[121,122] Infants and children may have severe developmental delays and are often unable to consume adequate nutrition by mouth. Many require gastrostomy or jejunostomy-tube feedings on a chronic basis.

Gastrointestinal dysfunction and dysmotility are common symptoms of mitochondrial disorders and can be se-

Table 22-6. Some Common Nutritional Supplements Prescribed for Various Mitochondrial Disorders[121,123-125]

NAME OF SUPPLEMENT	EXAMPLE DAILY DOSE IN PEDIATRIC CASES
Co-enzyme Q-10 (ubiquinone)	2–15 mg/kg
B vitamins	
Niacin	50 mg
Riboflavin	50–400 mg
Thiamin	50–300 mg
Combination therapy	Vitamin B-50 or B-100 complex
L-carnitine	50–100 mg/kg
α-Lipoic acid	300–600 mg/d
Vitamin C	5 mg/kg
Vitamin E	1–2 IU/kg
Creatine	100 mg/kg
L-arginine	For MELAS only
	Acute: IV 500 mg/kg every 6 h for 1–3 d
	Chronic: Oral 150–300 mg/kg

IV, intravenous; MELAS, mitochondrial enchephalomyopathy, lactic acidosis, and stroke-like episodes.

vere enough to make enteral feeding impossible.[122] In these cases, PN may be required on a chronic basis. Of note, use of IV lipid may need to be limited due to impaired fatty acid oxidation associated with mitochondrial disorders.[121] For disorders causing an isolated deficiency of complex I, a ketogenic or a high-fat diet (>50% of total kilocalories) may be beneficial; however, feedings emphasizing carbohydrate may be more appropriate for disorders affecting other complexes.[6,121]

High doses of various vitamins and nutritional supplements that serve as antioxidants, ETC substrates, and/or ETC cofactors have been prescribed to augment the production and utilization of ATP. Few of these therapies have been evaluated in randomized clinical trials, and most reported success is from single cases or case series. These therapies are used in various combinations, and dosing recommendations are typically not standardized (Table 22-6).[121,123-125] Of those listed, coenzyme Q-10 (also called ubiquinone) is the most widely prescribed because of its well-documented role in transporting electrons from complexes I and II to complex III in the ETC. Reported benefits of coenzyme Q-10 supplementation include improved cardiac conduction and neurological function, increased eye movements, and improved muscle strength with improved exercise tolerance.[121] However, sustained clinical benefit has not been noted. Research continues to find more effective nutritional and pharmaceutical options.[126]

Mitochondrial Encephalomyopathy, Lactic Acidosis, and Stroke-Like Episodes

MELAS is one of the most common mitochondrial disorders and is caused by a mutation in mitochondrial genes encoding for transfer RNA resulting in a severe reduction in activity of complex I and to a lesser extent, complexes III and IV.[121] Although MELAS can present in infancy, symptoms often do not develop until 4–15 years of age with onset of severe progressive encephalomyopathy. Increasing number and severity of episodes with vomiting, headache, convulsions, and visual abnormalities are reported. A subsequent computed tomography or magnetic resonance imaging scan will be consistent with an infarction. These events are called "stroke-like" episodes because the vascular changes or inflammation typically associated with stroke are not present.[118]

Over time, MELAS develops into a multisystem disorder with seizures, dementia, migraines, sensorineural deafness, ophthalmoplegia, and/or intestinal dysfunction, often with renal and cardiac involvement. A unique symptom associated with MELAS is development of type 2 diabetes mellitus. The syndrome carries a high morbidity and mortality rate with a reported mean survival time of approximately 6.5 years from disease onset.[121]

After the initial presentation, individuals with MELAS are at risk for developing further stroke-like episodes. As a vasodilator, L-arginine has been shown to reduce the frequency and severity of these episodes if administered soon after the development of symptoms. The initial recommended dose is 500 mg/kg in 5%–10% dextrose at 1.25–1.5 times the patient's maintenance fluid rate.[121,127] Repeated doses are administered every 6 hours for 1–3 days until symptoms resolve. Hydration status and acid-base balance need frequent monitoring. This treatment is specific for MELAS and is not advocated for other mitochondrial disorders. Following an episode, oral L-arginine at a dose of 150–300 mg/kg/d has been shown to reduce the frequency and severity of symptoms associated with future episodes.[121,127] Some of the therapies listed in Table 22-6 are also recommended; riboflavin and coenzyme Q-10 have been specifically mentioned as beneficial in this disorder.[6]

Conclusion

Management of those with an IEM is complex and often requires lifelong medical and nutrition therapy. For any IEM, medical nutrition therapy can vary greatly depending on the severity of the disorder and the patient's age, growth parameters, development, and other clinical factors. Thus, care by a team specializing in treatment of IEM, including a medical geneticist and metabolic dietitian trained to manage these disorders, is imperative for successful outcomes.

Test Your Knowledge Questions

1. PKU is often referred to as the model for newborn screening because
   A. Screening is economically feasible and results are reliable.
   B. Early medical nutrition therapy is available.
   C. Nutrition therapy prevents mental retardation associated with untreated PKU.
   D. All of the above.

2. When PN is indicated for an individual with MMA:
   A. Standard PN solutions should never be given to patients with this disorder.
   B. Only specialty PN solutions containing no Ile, Met, Thr, and Val should be provided.
   C. Depending on a patient's clinical status, a combination of specialty PN and standard PN can be provided.
   D. PN is always contraindicated in this disorder.

3. In VLCADD, _____ is/are contraindicated because _____:
   A. MCTs; they cannot be metabolized
   B. Intralipid; of its long-chain fat content
   C. Carbohydrates; they interfere with oxidation of fatty acids
   D. Cornstarch; it helps prevent hypoglycemia and rhabdomyolysis

4. Which of the following statements is FALSE?
   A. IV dextrose infusions are often used during acute episodes of metabolic decompensation in several types of IEM.
   B. During acute episodes, parenteral solutions should never contain more than a 5% dextrose concentration because of the high risk of hyperglycemia in these disorders.
   C. Often, dextrose solutions are infused at the high end of the recommended GIR for the patient's age and weight to help promote anabolism.
   D. Both statements B and C are false.

5. Which of the following statements best describe the mitochondrial disorder MELAS?
   A. MELAS typically presents as an acute episode with hypoglycemia and reduced ketone production in early infancy.
   B. Coenzyme Q-10 (ubiquinone) in doses of 4–10 g/d is often prescribed for patients with MELAS because of its documented long-term benefit.
   C. High doses of the IV form of L-alanine given at the first sign of a stroke-like episode can reduce the severity of symptoms.
   D. Oral doses of L-arginine at 150–300 mg/kg/d may reduce the severity of stroke-like episodes in patients with MELAS.

Acknowledgments

The author of this chapter for the second edition of this text wish to thank Bridget Reineking, MS, RD, CD, for her contributions to the first edition of this text.

References

1. Garg U, Dasouki M. Expanded newborn screening of inherited metabolic disorders by tandem mass spectrometry: clinical and laboratory aspects. *Clin Biochem.* 2006;39:315–332.

2. Watson AS, Mann MY, Lloyd-Puryear MA, Rinaldo P, Howell RR. Newborn screening: toward a uniform panel and system. Executive summary. *Genet Med.* 2006;8:S1–11.

3. Mak CM, Lee HC, Chan AY, Lam CW. Inborn errors of metabolism and expanded newborn screening: review and update. *Crit Rev Clin Lab Sci.* 2013;50:142–162.

4. Acosta PB, Yannicelli S. *The Ross Metabolic Formula System Nutrition Support Protocols.* 4th ed. Columbus, OH: Ross Products Division/Abbott Laboratories; 2001.

5. Acosta PB, ed. *Nutrition Management of Patients With Inherited Metabolic Disorders.* Sudbury MA: Jones & Bartlett; 2009.

6. Nyhan WL, Barshop BA, Ozand PT. *Atlas of Metabolic Diseases.* 2nd ed. New York, NY: Oxford University Press Inc; 2005.

7. Scriver CR, Beaudet AL, Sly WS, Valle D, eds. *The Online Metabolic & Molecular Bases of Inherited Disease.* New York, NY: McGraw-Hill, 2007. Available from http://www.ommbid.com. Accessed May 10, 2014

8. Sarkissan CN, Gamez A, Scott P, et al. Chaperone-like therapy with tetrahydrobiopterin in clinical trials for phenylketonuria: is genotype a predictor of response? *JIMD Rep.* 2012;5:59–70.

9. Koch R, Azen C, Friedman EG, et al. Paired comparisons between early treated PKU children and their matched sibling controls on intelligence and school achievement test results at eight years of age. *J Inherit Metab Dis.* 1984;7:86–90.

10. Bickel H, Gerrard J, Hickmans EM. The influence of phenylalanine intake on phenylketonuria. *Lancet.* 1953; 265:812–813.

11. Berry HK, Wright S. Conference on treatment of phenylke-tonuria. *J Pediatr.* 1967;70:142–147.

12. Azen CG, Koch R, Friedman EG, et al. Intellectual development in 12-year-old children treated for phenylketonuria. *Am J Dis Child.* 1991;145:35–39.

13. Koch R, Burton B, Hoganson G, et al. Phenylketonuria in adulthood: a collaborative study. *J Inherit Metab Dis.* 2002;25:333–346.

14. Camp KM, Parisi MA, Acosta PB, et al. Phenylketonuria Scientific Review Conference: state of the science and future research needs. *Mol Genet Metab.* 2014;112:87–122.

15. Waisbren SE, Noel K, Fahrbach K, et al. Phenylalanine blood levels and clinical outcomes in phenylketonuria: a systematic literature review and meta-analysis. *Mol Genet Metab.* 2007;92:63–70.

16. Vockley J, Andersson HC, Antshel KM, et al. Phenylalanine hydroxylase deficiency: diagnosis and management guideline. *Genet Med.* 2014;16:188–200.

17. Singh RH, Rohr F, Frazier D, et al. Recommendations for the nutrition management of phenylalanine hydroxylase deficiency. *Genet Med.* 2014;16:121–131.

18. Levy H, Ghavami M. Maternal phenylketonuria: a metabolic teratogen. *Teratology.* 1996;53:176–184.

19. Waisbren SE, Hanley W, Levy HL, et al. Outcomes at age 4 years in offspring of women with maternal phenylketonuria: the Maternal PKU Collaborative Study. *JAMA.* 2000;283:756–762.

20. Waisbren SE, Azen C. Cognitive and behavioral development in maternal phenylketonuria offspring. *Pediatrics.* 2003;112:1544–1547.

21. Teissier R, Nowak E, Assoun M, et al. Maternal phenylketonuria: low phenylalanine might increase the risk of intrauterine growth retardation. *J Inherit Metab Dis.* 2012;35:993–999.

22. Otten JJ, Helwig JP, Meyers LD. *Dietary Reference Intakes: The Essential Guide to Nutrient Requirements.* Washington, DC: National Academies Press; 2006.

23. Dangin M, Boirie Y, Garcia-Rodenas C, et al. The digestion rate of protein is an independent regulating factor of post-prandial protein retention. *Am J Physiol Endocrinol Metab.* 2001;280:E340–E248.

24. Van Rijn M, Bekhof J, Dijkstra T, Smit PG, Moddermam P, van Spronsen FJ. A different approach to breast-feeding of the infant with phenylketonuria. *Eur J Pediatr.* 2003; 162:323–326.

25. Leamons JA, Reyman D, Moye L. Amino acid composition of preterm and term breast milk during early lactation. *Early Hum Dev.* 1983;8:323–329.

26. Singh R, Lesperance E, Crawford K. *PKU Food List.* 2nd ed. Atlanta, GA: Emory University, Department of Human Genetics, Division of Medical Genetics; 2006.

27. Schuett V. *Low Protein Food List for PKU.* 3rd ed. Seattle, WA: National PKU News; 2010.

28. Schuett V. *Low Protein Cookery for PKU.* 4th ed. Madison, WI: The University of Wisconsin Press; 1997.

29. Schuett V, Corry D. *Apples to Zucchini—A Collection of Favorite Low Protein Recipes.* 1st ed. Seattle, WA: National PKU News; 2005.

30. Yagasaki M, Hashimoto S. Synthesis and application of dipeptides; current status and perspectives. *Appl Microbiol Biotechnol.* 2008;81:13–22.

31. Rohde C, Mütze U, Schulz S, et al. Unrestricted fruits and vegetables in the PKU diet: a 1-year follow-up. *Eur J Clin Nutr.* 2014;68:401–403.

32. Acosta PB, Yannicelli S, Singh RH, Elsas LJ, Mofidi S, Steiner RD. Iron status of children with phenylketonuria undergoing nutrition therapy assessed by transferrin receptors. *Genet Med.* 2004;6:96–101.

33. Acosta PB, Yannicelli S. Plasma micronutrient concentrations in infants undergoing therapy for phenylketonuria. *Biol Trace Elem Res.* 1999;67:75–84.

34. Hvas AM, Nexo E, Nielsen JB. Vitamin B12 and vitamin B6 supplementation is needed among adults with phenylketonuria (PKU). *J Inherit Metab Dis.* 2006;29:47–53.

35. Moseley K, Koch R, Moser AB. Lipid status and long-chain polyunsaturated fatty acid concentrations in adults and adolescents with phenylketonuria on phenylalanine-restricted diet. *J Inherit Metab.* 2002;25:56–64.

36. Koletzko B, Beblo S, Demmelmair H, Hanebutt FL. Omega-3 LC-PUFA supply and neurological outcomes in children with phenylketonuria (PKU). *J Pediatr Gastroenterol Nutr.* 2009;48:S2–S7.

37. Mendes AB, Martins FF, Cruz WM, da Silva LE, Abadesso CB, Boaventura GT. Bone development in children and adolescents with PKU. *J Inherit Metab Dis.* 2012;35:425–430.

38. Ney DM, Blank RD, Hansen KE. Advances in the nutritional and pharmacological management of phenylketonuria. *Curr Opin Clin Nutr Metab Care.* 2014;17:61–68.

39. Puglisi-Allegra S, Cabib S, Pascucci T, et al. Dramatic brain aminergic deficit in a genetic mouse model of phenylketonuria. *Neuroreport.* 2000;11:1361–1364.

40. Matalon R, Michals-Matalon K, Bhatia G, et al. Double blind placebo control trial of large neutral amino acids in treatment of PKU: effect on blood phenylalanine. *J Inherit Metab Dis.* 2007;30:153–158.

41. Schindeler S, Ghosh-Jerath S, Thompson S, et al. The effects of large neutral amino acid supplements in PKU: an MRS and neuropsychological study. *Mol Genet Metab.* 2007;91:48–54.

42. Levy HL, Milanowski A, Chakrapani A, et al. Efficacy of sapropterin dihydrochloride (tetrahydrobiopterin, 6R-BH4) for reduction of phenylalanine concentrations in patients with phenylketonuria: a phase III randomized placebo-controlled study. *Lancet.* 2007;370:504–510.

43. Burton BK, Grànge DK, Milanowski A, et al. The response of patients with phenylketonuria and elevated serum phenylalanine to treatment with oral sapropterin dihydrochloride (6R-tetrahydrobiopterin): a phase II, multicentre, open-label, screening study. *J Inherit Metab Dis.* 2007;30:700–707.

44. Keil S, Anjema K, van Spronsen J, et al. Long-term follow-up and outcome of phenylketonuria patients on saproterin: a retrospective study. *Pediatrics.* 2013;131:e1881–e1888.

45. Cunningham A, Bausell H, Brown M, et al. Recommendations for the use of sapropterin in phenylketonuria. *Mol Genet Metab.* 2012;106:269–276.

46. Thiele AG, Weigel JF, Ziesch B, et al. Nutritional changes and micronutrient supply in patients with phenylketonuria under therapy with tetrahydrobiopterin (BH₄). *JIMD Rep.* 2013;9:31–40.

47. Merinero B, Pérez C, Pérez-Cerdá A, et al. Methylmalonic acidaemia: examination of genotype and biochemical data in 32 patients belonging to mut, cbIA or cbIB complementation group. *J Inherit Metab Dis.* 2008;31:55–66.

48. Knerr I, Weinhold N, Vockley J, Gibson KM. Advances and challenges in the treatment of branched-chain amino/keto acid metabolic defects. *J Inherit Metab Dis.* 2012;35:29–40.

49. Manoli I, Venditti CP. Methylmalonic acidemia. In: Pagon RA, Adam MP, Ardinger HH, et al, eds. *GeneReviews.* Seattle, WA: University of Washington, Seattle; 2010. http://www.ncbi.nlm.gov/pubmed/2031409. Accessed October 10, 2014.

50. Chace D, DiPerna J, Kalas T, Johnson R, Naylor E. Rapid diagnosis of methylmalonic and propionic acidemias: quantitative tandem mass spectrometric analysis of propionylcarnitine in filter-paper blood specimens obtained from newborns. *Clin Chem.* 2001;47:2040–2044.

51. de Baulny HO, Benoist JF, Rigal O, Touati G, Rabier D, Saudubray JM. Methylmalonic and propionic acidaemias: management and outcome. *J Inherit Metab Dis.* 2005;28:415–423.

52. Baumgartner MR, Hörster F, Assoun M, et al. Proposed guidelines for the diagnosis and management of methylmalonic and propionic acidemia. *Orphanet J Rare Dis.* 2014;9:130.

53. Dionisi-Vici C, Deodato F, Röschinger W, Rhead W, Wilcken B. 'Classical' organic acidurias, propionic aciduria, methylmalonic aciduria and isovaleric aciduria: long-term outcome and effects of expanded newborn screening using tandem mass spectrometry. *J Inherit Metab Dis.* 2006;29:383–389.

54. Weisfield-Adams JD, Bender HA, Miley-Akerstedt A, et al. Neurological and neurodevelopmental phenotypes in young children with early-treated combined methylmalonic acidemia and homocysteinuria, cobalamin C type. *Mol Genet Metab.* 2013;110:241–247.

55. Nyhan WL, Gargus JJ, Boyle K, Selby R, Koch R. Progressive neurologic disability in methylmalonic acidemia despite transplantation of the liver. *Eur J Pediatr.* 2002;161:377–379.

56. Morioka D, Kasahara M, Horikawa R, Yokoyama S, Fukuda A, Nakagawa A. Efficacy of living donor transplantation for patients with methylmalonic acidemia. *Am J Transplant.* 2007;7:2782–2787.

57. McGuire PJ, Lim-Melia E, Diaz GA, et al. Combined liver-kidney transplant for the management of methylmalonic aciduria: a case report and review of the literature. *Mol Genet Metab.* 2008;93:22–29.

58. Brassier A, Boyer O, Valayannopoulos V, et al. Renal transplantation in four patients with methylmalonic acidemia: a cell therapy for metabolic disease. *Mol Genet Metab.* 2013;110:106–110.

59. Clothier JC, Chakrapani A, Preece MA, et al. Renal transplantation in a boy with methylmalonic acidemia. *J Inherit Metab Dis.* 2011;34:695–700.

60. Prietsch V, Lindner M, Zschocke J, Nyhan WL, Hoffmann GF. Emergency management of inherited metabolic diseases. *J Inherit Metab Dis.* 2002;25:531–546.

61. New England Consortium of Metabolic Programs. Acute illness protocols for healthcare professionals. http://newenglandconsortium.org/for-professionals/acute-illness-protocols. Updated September 16, 2013. Accessed October 15, 2014.

62. Chalmers RA, Roe CR, Stacey TE, Hoppel CL. Urinary excretion of L-carnitine and acylcarnitines by patients with disorders of organic acid metabolism: evidence for secondary insufficiency of L-carnitine. *Pediatr Res.* 1984;18:1325–1328.

63. Yannicelli S. Nutrition therapy of organic acidaemias with amino acid-based formulas: emphasis on methylmalonic and propionic acidaemia. *J Inherit Metab Dis.* 2006;29:281–287.

64. Hauser NS, Manoli I, Graf JC, Sloan J, Venditti CP. Variable dietary management of methylmalonic acidemia: metabolic and energetic correlations. *Am J Clin Nutr.* 2011;93:47–56.

65. Wedel U, deBaulny HO. Branched-chain organic acidurias/acidemias. In: Fernandes J, Saudubray JM, van den Berghe G, Walter JH, eds. *Inborn Metabolic Diseases: Diagnosis and Treatment.* 4th ed. Heidelberg, Germany: Springer Medizen Verlag; 2006:245–260.

66. Andersson HC, Shapira E. Biochemical and clinical response to hydroxocobalamin versus cyanocobalamin treatment in patients with methylmalonic acidemia and homocystinuria (cblC). *J Pediatr.* 1998;132:121–124.

67. Lee NC, Chien YH, Peng SF, et al. Brain damage by mild metabolic derangements in methylmalonic acidemia. *Pediatr Neurol.* 2008;39:325–329.

68. Tuchman M, Lee B, Lichter-Koenecki U, et al. Cross-sectional multicenter study of patients with urea cycle disorders in the United States. *Mol Genet Metab.* 2008;94:397–402.

69. Maestri N, Clissold D, Brusilow S. Neonatal onset ornithine transcarbamylase deficiency: a retrospective analysis. *J Peds.* 1999;134:255–256.

70. McBride K, Miller G, Carter S, et al. Developmental outcomes with early orthotopic liver transplantation for infants with neonatal-onset urea cycle defects and a female patient with late-onset ornithine transcarbamylase deficiency. *Pediatrics.* 2004;114:523–526.

71. Puppi J, Tan N, Mitry RR, et al. Hepatocyte transplantation followed by auxiliary liver transplantation—a novel treatment for ornithine transcarbamylase deficiency. *Am J Transplant.* 2008;8:452–457.

72. Leonard JV. The nutritional management of urea cycle disorders. *J Pediatr.* 2001;138(suppl):S40–S45.

73. Singh RH. Nutritional management of patients with urea cycle disorders. *J Inherit Metab Dis.* 2007;30:880–887.

74. Scaglia F, Carter S, O'Brien W, Lee B. Effect of alternative pathway therapy on branched chain amino acid metabolism in urea cycle disorder patients. *Mol Genet Metab.* 2004;81:79–85.

75. Batshaw ML, MacArthur RB, Tuchman M. Alternative pathway therapy for urea cycle disorders: twenty years later. *J Pediatr.* 2001;138:S46–S54.

76. Acosta PB, Yannicelli S, Ryan AS, et al. Nutritional therapy improves growth and protein status of children with a urea cycle enzyme defect. *Mol Genet Metab.* 2005;86:448–455.

77. Wilson CJ, Lee PJ, Leonard JV. Plasma glutamine and ammonia concentrations in ornithine carbamyltransferase deficiency and citrullinaemia. *J Inherit Metab Dis.* 2001;24:691–695.

78. Scaglia F. New insights in nutritional management and amino acid supplementation in urea cycle disorders. *Mol Genet Metab.* 2010;100:S72–S76.

79. Pons R, Cavadini P, Baratt S, et al. Clinical and molecular heterogeneity in very-long chain acyl-coenzyme A dehydrogenase deficiency. *Pediatr Neurol.* 2000;22:98–105.

80. Spiekerkoetter U, Lindner M, Santer R, et al. Management and outcome in 75 individuals with long-chain fatty acid oxidation defects: results from a workshop. *J Inherit Metab Dis.* 2009;32:488–497.

81. Spiekerkoetter U, Lindner M, Santer R, et al. Treatment recommendations in long-chain fatty acid oxidation defects: consensus from a workshop. *J Inherit Metab Dis.* 2009;32:498–505.

82. Liebig M, Schymik I, Mueller M, et al. Neonatal screening for very-long chain acyl-CoA dehydrogenase deficiency: enzymatic and molecular evaluation of neonates with elevated C14:1-carnitine levels. *Pediatrics.* 2006;118:1065–1069.

83. Potter BK, Little J, Chakraborty P, et al. Variability in the clinical management of fatty acid oxidation disorders: results of a survey of Canadian metabolic physicians. *J Inherit Metab Dis.* 2012;35:115–123.

84. Merritt JL, Vedal S, Abdenur JE, et al. Infants suspected to have very-long chain acyl-CoA dehydrogenase deficiency from newborn screening. *Mol Genet Metab.* 2014;111:484–492.

85. Vockley J, Singh RH, Whiteman DA. Diagnosis and management of defects of mitochondrial beta-oxidation. *Curr Opin Clin Nutr Metab Care.* 2002;5:601–609.

86. Coughlin CR, Ficicioglu C. Genotype-phenotype correlations: sudden death in an infant with very-long-chain acyl-CoA dehydrogenase deficiency. *J Inherit Metab Dis.* 2010;33:S129–S131.

87. Van Hove JL, Myers S, Kerckhove KV, Freehauf C, Bernstein L. Acute nutrition management in the prevention of metabolic illness: a practical approach with glucose polymers. *Mol Genet Metab.* 2009;97:1–3.

88. Rohr F, van Calcar S. Very-long acyl-CoA dehydrogenase deficiency (VLCADD). Genetic Metabolic Dietitians International. http://www.gmdi.org/guidelines/. 2008. Accessed May 10, 2014.

89. Arnold GL, Van Hove J, Freedenberg D, et al. A Delphi clinical practice protocol for the management of very-long chain acyl-CoA dehydrogenase deficiency. *Mol Genet Metab.* 2009;96:85–90.

90. Walter J. Tolerance to fast: rational and practical evaluation in children with hypoketonaemia. *J Inherit Metab Dis.* 2009;32:214–217.

91. Gillingham M, Connor W, Matern D, et al. Optimal dietary therapy of long-chain 3-hydroxyacyl-CoA dehydrogenase deficiency. *Mol Gen Metab.* 2003;79:114–123.

92. Gillingham MB, Scott B, Elliott D, Harding CO. Metabolic control during exercise with and without medium chain triglycerides (MCT) in children with long-chain

93. 3-hydroxyacyl-CoA dehydrogenase (LCHAD) or trifunctional protein (TFP) deficiency. *Mol Genet Metab.* 2006;89:58–63.

93. Shah KK, O'Dell SD. Effect of dietary interventions in the maintenance of normoglycemia in glycogen storage disease type 1a: a systematic review and meta-analysis. *J Hum Nutr Diet.* 2013;26:329–339.

94. Lund AM, Skovby F, Vestergaard H, Christensen M, Christensen E. Clinical and biochemical monitoring of patients with fatty acid oxidation disorders. *J Inherit Metab Dis.* 2010;33:495–500.

95. Roe CR, Roe DS, Wallace M. Garritson B. Choice of oils for essential fat supplements can enhance production of abnormal metabolites in fat oxidation disorders. *Mol Genet Metab.* 2007;92:346–350.

96. Spiekerkotter U, Schwahn B, Korall H, Trefz FK, Andresen BS, Wendel U. Very-long-chain acyl-coenzyme A dehydrogenase (VLCAD) deficiency: monitoring of treatment by carnitine/acylcarnitine analysis in blood spots. *Acta Paediatr.* 2000;89:492–495.

97. McCorvie T, Timson DJ. Structural and molecular biology of type I galactosemia: disease-associated mutations. *IUBMB Life.* 2011;63:949–954.

98. Berry GT. Galactosemia: when is it a newborn screening emergency? *Mol Genet Metab.* 2012;106:7–11.

99. Lai K, Langley SD, Singh RH, Dembure PP, Hjelm LN, Elsas LJ. A prevalent mutation for galactosemia among black Americans. *J Pediatr.* 1996;128:89–95.

100. Ficicioglu C, Thomas N, Yager C, et al. Duarte (DG) galactosemia: a pilot study of biochemical and neurodevelopmental assessment in children detected by newborn screening. *Mol Genet Metab.* 2008;95:206–212.

101. Waggoner DD, Buist NMR, Donnell GN. Long-term prognosis in galactosemia: results of a survey of 350 cases. *J Inherit Metab Dis.* 1990;13:802–818.

102. Ridel KR, Leslie ND, Gilbert DL. An updated review of the long-term neurological effects of galactosemia. *Pediatr Neurol.* 2005;33:153–161.

103. Waisbren SE, Potter NL, Gordon CM, et al. The adult galactosemic phenotype. *J Inherit Metab Dis.* 2012;35:279–286.

104. Berry GT, Moate PJ, Reynolds RA, et al. The rate of de-novo galactose synthesis in patients with galactose-1-phosphate uridyltransferase deficiency. *Mol Genet Metab.* 2004;81:22–30.

105. Liu Y, Xia B, Gleason TJ, et al. N- and O-linked glycosylation of total plasma glycoproteins in galactosemia. *Mol Genet Metab.* 2012;106:442–454.

106. Van Calcar SC, Bernstein LE, Rohr FJ, Scaman CH, Yannicelli S, Berry GT. A re-evaluation of life-long severe galactose restriction for the nutrition management of classic galactosemia. *Mol Genet Metab.* 2014;112:191–197.

107. Ficicioglu C, Hussa C, Yager C, Segal S. Effect of galactose-free formula on galactose-1-phosphate in two infants with classical galactosemia. *Eur J Pediatr.* 2008;167:595–596.

108. Zlatunich CO, Packman S. Galactosaemia: early treatment with an elemental formula. *J Inherit Metab Dis.* 2005;28:163–168.

109. Bhatia J, Greer F; Committee on Nutrition, American Academy of Pediatrics. Use of soy-protein based formulas in infant feeding. *Pediatrics.* 2008;121:1062–1068.

110. Van Calcar SC, Bernstein LE, Rohr FJ, Yannicelli S, Berry GT, Scaman CH. Galactose content of legumes, caseinates, and some hard cheeses: implications for diet treatment of classic galactosemia. *J Agric Food Chem.* 2014;62:1397–1402.

111. Acosta PB, Gross K. Hidden sources of galactose in the environment. *Eur J Pediatr.* 1995;154:S1–S6.

112. Scaman C, Jim VJ, Hartnett C. Free galactose concentrations in fresh and stored apples (*Malus domestica*) and processed apple products. *J Agric Food Chem.* 2004;52:511–517.

113. Kim H, Hartnett C, Scaman CH. Free galactose content in selected fresh fruits and vegetables and soy beverages. *J Agric Food Chem.* 2007;55:8133–8137.

114. Hutchesson AC, Murdoch-Davis C, Green A, et al. Biochemical monitoring of treatment for galactosaemia: biological variability in metabolic concentrations. *J Inherit Metab Dis.* 1999;22:139–148.

115. Batey LA, Welt CK, Rohr A, et al. Skeletal health in adult patients with classical galactosemia. *Osteoporos Int.* 2013;24:501–509.

116. Pramyothin P, Holick MF. Vitamin D supplementation: guidelines and evidence for subclinical deficiency. *Curr Opin Gastroenterol.* 2012;28:139–150.

117. van Erven B, Römers MM, Rubio-Gonzalbo ME. Revised proposal for the prevention of low bone mass in patients with classic galactosemia. *JIMD Rep.* 2014;17:41–46.

118. Chinnery PF. Mitochondrial disorders overview. In: Pagon RA, Adam MP, Ardinger HH, et al, eds. *Gene Reviews.* Seattle, WA: University of Washington; 2010. http://www.ncbi.nlm.nih.gov/books/NBK1224. Accessed May 15, 2014.

119. Milone M, Wong LJ. Diagnosis of mitochondrial myopathies. *Mol Genet Metab.* 2013;110:35–41.

120. Menezes MJ, Riley LG, Christodoulou J. Mitochondrial respiratory chain disorders in childhood: insights into diagnosis and management in the new era of genomic medicine. *Biochim Biophys Acta.* 2014;1840:1368–1379.

121. Santa KM. Treatment options for mitochondrial myopathy, encephalopathy, lactic acidosis, and stroke-like episodes (MELAS) syndrome. *Pharmacotherapy.* 2010;30:1179–1196.

122. Rahman S. Gastrointestinal and hepatic manifestations of mitochondrial disorders. *J Inherit Metab Dis.* 2013;36:659–673.

123. Pfeffer G, Chinnery PF. Diagnosis of treatment of mitochondrial myopathies. *Ann Med.* 2013;45:4–16.

124. Avula S, Parikh S, Demarest S, Kurz J, Gropman A. Treatment of mitochondrial disorders. *Curr Treat Options Neurol.* 2014;16:292.

125. Tarnopolsky MA. The mitochondrial cocktail: rationale for combined nutraceutical therapy in mitochondrial cytopathies. *Adv Drug Deliv Rev.* 2008;60:1561–1567.

126. Goldstein A, Wolfe LA. The elusive magic pill: finding effective therapies for mitochondrial disorders. *Neurotherapeutics.* 2013;10:320–328.

127. Yoneda M, Ikawa M, Arakawa K, et al. In vivo functional brain imaging and a therapeutic trial of L-arginine in MELAS patients. *Biochim Biophys Acta.* 2012;1820:615–618.

128. van Calcar SC, Ney DM. Food products made with glycomacropeptide, a low-phenylalanine whey protein, provide a new alternative to amino acid-based medical foods for the nutrition management of phenylketonuria. *J Acad Nutr Diet.* 2012;112:1201–1210.

129. Saudubray JM, van den Berghe G, Walter JH et al, eds. *Inborn Metabolic Diseases: Diagnosis and Treatment.* Heidelberg, Germany: Springer Medizin; 2012.

Test Your Knowledge Answers

1. The correct answer is **D.** Disorders selected for newborn screening programs must be cost-effective and reliably detected by population-based screening methods. Realistic and effective treatment modalities should be available for the disorder to prevent severe sequelae of the disease.

2. The correct answer is **C.** Specialty PN solutions for MMA provide all essential amino acids except Met, Val, Ile, and Thr. As metabolic control improves, standard PN may need to be added in limited quantities to prevent protein deficiency if enteral feeding is not possible.

3. The correct answer is **B.** Individuals with VLCADD cannot metabolize long-chain fats effectively and Intralipid is a long-chain fat source. Answer A is incorrect since MCTs provide a source of fat that can be metabolized to meet calorie needs. Answer C is incorrect since carbohydrates provide an energy source that can be utilized without fatty acid oxidation. Answer D is incorrect since cornstarch is a slowly digested carbohydrate source that can be effective in preventing low glucose concentrations during fasting.

4. The correct answer is **B.** In IEM, higher concentrations of dextrose (usually 10% by peripheral parenteral nutrition or higher concentrations if central access is available) are used to slow catabolism and prevent hypoglycemia, which is more common in IEM than hyperglycemia.

5. The correct answer is **D.** Answer A is incorrect since MELAS typically presents later in childhood with a slower onset of symptoms. Answer B is incorrect since coenzyme Q-10 is prescribed in milligram quantities, not gram quantities; also the long-term benefit of coenzyme Q-10 supplementation is not well documented. Answer C is incorrect since the amino acid administered in MELAS is L-arginine rather than L-alanine.

23

Cardiac Disease

Janice Antino, RD, MS, CNSC; Mindy Freudenberg, RD, MS, CNSC; and Anupama Chawla, MD, DCH (UK), CNSC

 Podcast

CONTENTS

Learning Objectives

1. Identify factors contributing to growth failure in children with congenital heart disease.
2. Summarize the components of nutrition assessment and optimal methods of nutrient delivery in children with congenital heart disease.
3. Recognize and manage postoperative complications and prescribe appropriate nutrition therapy.
4. Identify interventions for cardiovascular disease risk reduction through pediatric screening.

Congenital Heart Disease

Congenital heart diseases (CHDs) are abnormalities in the heart structure that are present at birth. Approximately 8 out of every 1,000 infants are born with a CHD. Congenital heart disease can be classified into 2 major categories: cyanotic and acyanotic (Table 23-1).[1]

With acyanotic heart defects, shunting of blood occurs from the left side of the heart to the right side of the heart. The development of congestive heart failure (CHF) is a major concern in acyanotic heart disease. In cyanotic heart defects, oxygen-poor blood mixes with oxygen-rich blood. The main concern with cyanotic heart disease is hypoxia. The tissues do not receive fully oxygenated blood, which is apparent from the bluish tint, or cyanosis, of the skin, lips, and nail beds.

This population is presented with unique challenges in meeting their energy requirements for optimal growth and development. Depending on the severity of the defect, a child with CHD may face feeding difficulties and malnutrition during a critical developmental period.

Table 23-1. Two Major Categories of Congenital Heart Disease

ACYANOTIC	CYANOTIC
Atrial septal defect	Interrupted aortic arch
Ventricular septal defect	Pulmonary atresia
Patent ductus arteriosus	Ebstein's anomaly
Common A-V canal	
Pulmonary stenosis[a]	
Coarctation of aorta[a]	
Aortic stenosis	
Tetralogy of Fallot[a]	
Transposition of the great vessels[a]	
Total anomalous pulmonary venous return[a]	
Truncus arteriosus[a]	
Tricuspid atresia[a]	
Hypoplastic left heart syndrome[a]	

[a]These conditions may present as cyanotic congenital heart disease or as acyanotic congenital heart disease that transitions to the cyanotic state.

Nutrition Assessment and Malnutrition

Failure to thrive and malnutrition are well documented in infants and children with CHD. The severity of malnutrition can range from mild to severe, with the potential for both acute and chronic health implications. The degree of impact on an infant's nutrition status varies with the type of cardiac malformation and tends to be the most severe in cardiac conditions associated with increased pulmonary blood flow, severe cyanosis, and pulmonary hypertension.[2]

Acute and chronic malnutrition is of particular concern for infants and children with cyanotic heart disease due to their chronic hypoxic state and the prolonged course until final surgical correction. Cameron et al[3] reported the prevalence of acute and chronic malnutrition to be as high as 33% and 64%, respectively. Although malnutrition is more likely with cyanosis and CHF, it can be encountered with any cardiac defect with or without cyanosis.[4]

CHDs associated with significant rates of morbidity and mortality are hypoplastic left heart syndrome (HLHS) and other single ventricle defect variants. These infants typically undergo a series of palliative surgical procedures and have difficulty achieving adequate growth between surgical stages.[5] They are particularly at risk for malnutrition between neonatal surgical palliation, the Norwood procedure, and the second surgical stage, the bidirectional Glenn procedure (BDG), typically performed at 4–6 months of age. The time between these 2 procedures is commonly referred to as the interstage period, during which weight gain is often suboptimal.[6,7] Kelleher et al[5] evaluated the growth of 50 infants with HLHS during the interstage period. From initial discharge and subsequent readmission for BDG shunt surgery, infants experienced a significant drop in weight age z score (WAZ), with a median WAZ of –2.0, suggesting that 50% of infants were severely underweight at the time of major cardiac surgery. Anderson and colleagues[6] also identified lower WAZ in a group of infants who underwent BDG. Infants with lower WAZ tended to experience longer duration of mechanical ventilation, prolonged hospitalization, additional days in the intensive care unit, and more frequent postoperative complications.[5,6]

The interstage period is a critical time for infants with CHD and presents unique challenges to the practitioner providing nutrition care. To address the challenges these infants face, the National Pediatric Cardiology Quality Improvement Collaborative (NPC-QIC) was formed with the mission to improve outcomes of children with cardiovascular disease (CVD). The NPC-QIC is the first multicenter quality improvement collaborative within pediatric cardiology. Nutrition is a major focus of this group, which aims to improve survival and quality of life during the interstage period.

Significant variations in nutrition practices exist between different surgical cardiac centers; however, the NPC-QIC demonstrated that if energy goals are met and children are closely monitored during the interstage phase, adequate growth can be achieved.[6-8] Early identification of children with growth and feeding difficulties leading to early intervention results in improved growth outcomes and reduced mortality. Considering these facts, the Feeding Work Group (FWG) of the NPC-QIC was formed to develop consensus recommendations for feeding and nutrition for infants with single ventricle heart disease. The algorithms are presented as Figures 23-1, 23-2, 23-3, and 23-4. Recommendations for feeding preoperative, postoperative, and after hospital discharge are summarized below.[9]

1. Preoperative (Figure 23-1)
   a. Due to the high risk for malnutrition, parenteral nutrition (PN) should be initiated early and advanced to full calorie and protein goals until enteral feeding goals can be achieved.
   b. Provide enteral nutrition (EN) as long as the infant is hemodynamically stable. With appropriate monitoring, EN can be achieved safely.
   c. Preoperative oral feeding should be encouraged but may become a challenge. Nasogastric (NG) tube

feeds have been a widely accepted practice used adjunctively to oral feeds. Therefore, NG tube feeding support should be considered preoperatively.

d. Patients with umbilical arterial catheters may be fed enterally without increased adverse outcome based on a number of case studies and observational studies.

e. Prostaglandin infusions increase concern for gastrointestinal complications, systemic vasodilation, respiratory depression, edema, and increased secretions. Despite these concerns, enteral feedings in this scenario have been used safely, and these infusions are not a contraindication to enteral feeding.

f. Human milk is the preferred option for initiation of enteral feeds due to its immunologic benefits and high biological value protein, but when it is unavailable it is reasonable to use a standard infant formula.

2. <u>Postoperative Enteral Feeding</u> (Figures 23-2 and 23-3)

a. Postoperative PN should be used to achieve energy goals initially. When the infant is hemodynamically stable and as soon as gut function returns, enteral feeding should be initiated.

b. Due to the high incidence of vocal cord injury and oral motor dysfunction, a feeding evaluation should

Figure 23-1. Recommendations for preoperative feeding.

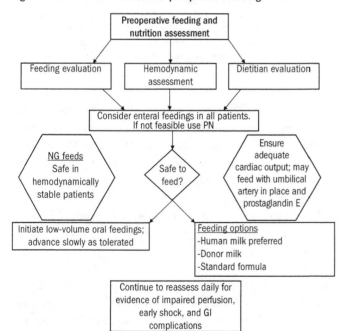

Adapted from Slicker J, Hehir AD, Horsley M, et al; Feeding Work Group of the National Pediatric Cardiology Quality Improvement Collaborative. Nutrition algorithms for infants with hypoplastic left heart syndrome: birth through the first interstage period. Congenit Heart Dis. 2013; 8(2):89–102. GI, gastrointestinal; IL, Intralipds; NG, nasogastric; PN, parenteral nutrition.

Figure 23-2. Recommendations for postoperative enteral feeding.

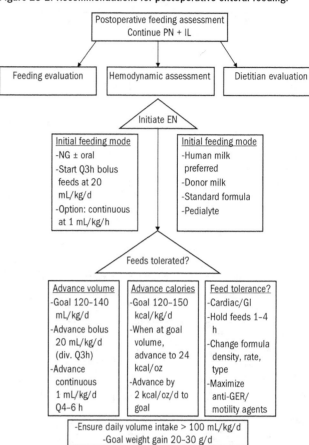

Adapted from Slicker J, Hehir AD, Horsley M, et al; Feeding Work Group of the National Pediatric Cardiology Quality Improvement Collaborative. Nutrition algorithms for infants with hypoplastic left heart syndrome: birth through the first interstage period. Congenit Heart Dis. 2013; 8(2):89–102. EN, enteral nutrition; GER, gastroesophageal reflux; GI, gastrointestinal; IL, Intralipds; NG, nasogastric; Q3; Q4–6; PN, parenteral nutrition.

be conducted to evaluate aspiration risk and safety of providing oral feeds.

c. During the feeding advance, close monitoring for gastrointestinal and cardiac complications is required.

3. <u>Interstage Feeding Guidelines</u> (Figure 23-4)

a. During the interstage period, close monitoring of weight changes is critical to modify the feeding regimen to promote growth.

b. Oral aversions must be addressed in this stage, and referral to speech and occupational therapy should be considered to improve oral–motor skills.

c. For symptoms of vomiting and intolerance to feeds, medications should be reviewed, taking into account their side effects and toxicity.

Figure 23-3. Transition to postoperative oral feeding.

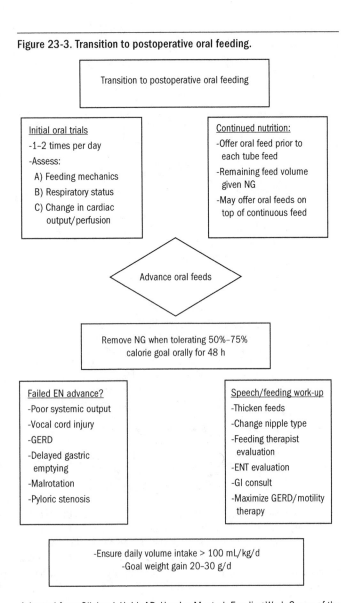

Adapted from Slicker J, Hehir AD, Horsley M, et al; Feeding Work Group of the National Pediatric Cardiology Quality Improvement Collaborative. Nutrition algorithms for infants with hypoplastic left heart syndrome: birth through the first interstage period. Congenit Heart Dis. 2013; 8(2):89–102. EN, enteral nutrition; ENT, ear, nose and throat specialist; GERD, gastroesophageal reflux disease; GI, gastrointestinal; NG, nasogastric.

Figure 23-4. Interstage feeding guidelines.

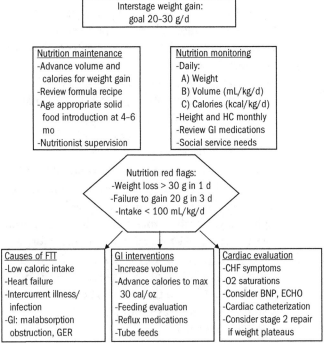

Consider admission for severe or concerning red flags

Adapted from Slicker J, Hehir AD, Horsley M, et al; Feeding Work Group of the National Pediatric Cardiology Quality Improvement Collaborative. Nutrition algorithms for infants with hypoplastic left heart syndrome: birth through the first interstage period. Congenit Heart Dis. 2013; 8(2):89–102. BNP, B-type natriuretic peptide; CHF, congestive heart failure; ECHO, echocardiogram; FTT, failure to thrive; GER, gastroesophageal reflux; GI, gastrointestinal; HC, head circumference.

Etiology of Growth Impairment

Many published reports support the high prevalence of malnutrition among infants with CHD; however, whether malnutrition is a result of high metabolic demands, poor feeding, hypoxia, or all 3 factors remains unclear. All factors are interdependent; for example, hypoxia leads to an increased respiratory effort, resulting in increased metabolic demands. Hypoxia and increased respiratory rate also result in an infant easily becoming fatigued, which leads to poor feeding effort. The exact etiology of documented energy deficit, whether arising from decreased intake or increased energy expenditure, is difficult to determine and is often multifactorial, with the complexity of the congenital anomalies, comorbidities, age, and aggressiveness of nutrition support playing roles.[10]

The factors that have been identified as contributing to growth failure in this population are listed in Table 23-2.

Energy Expenditure

Increased metabolic demands have been proposed as a factor contributing to malnutrition in infants with CHD. Cyanosis has been implicated as an important factor determining the basal metabolic rate. Cyanosis is associated with increased myocardial lactate levels, suggesting that these infants may have increased metabolic demands because they have a greater dependence on anaerobic metabolism for ATP production in the setting of reduced oxygen availability.[11] An increased re-

Table 23-2. Factors Contributing to Growth Failure in Congenital Heart Disease

ETIOLOGY	SIGNS AND SYMPTOMS
Increased energy requirements	Tachypnea and tachycardia can increase metabolic demands
Decreased energy intake	Anorexia, dysphagia, reflux, fatigue during feeding
Increased nutrient losses	Protein-losing enteropathy, renal electrolyte losses
Insufficient utilization of nutrients	Acidosis, hypoxia
Malabsorption	Gut edema

liance on anaerobic metabolism in these patients may be less energy efficient and thereby increase energy demands.[10]

Several studies have been performed to evaluate the energy needs of infants with CHD and to identify factors contributing to alterations in the metabolic rate. Avitzur et al[12] measured the metabolic rate using indirect calorimetry of 29 children with cyanotic or noncyanotic heart disease to determine if cyanosis contributes to increased metabolic rate. No differences between resting energy expenditure (REE) were found before or 5 days after open heart surgery using indirect calorimetry. In contrast, Nydegger et al[13] observed an increased REE in 108 infants with CHD by using indirect calorimetry and found that it normalized within 1 week after corrective surgery. Both studies cautioned against use of predictive equations because their results showed a high rate of variability and did not correlate to measurements by indirect calorimetry.

Leitch et al[10] failed to identify a difference in REE but did detect increased total energy expenditure (TEE). The authors measured REE by using indirect calorimetry and TEE by using the double-labeled water technique in 12 infants with uncorrected cyanotic CHD and compared them to a group of age-matched controls at 2 weeks and again at 3 months of age. No significant differences in REE were identified at either time. However, a significant increase in TEE was identified at 3 months of age.[10] Therefore, an increased TEE but not an increased REE may be the primary factor in the reduced growth of infants with cyanotic CHD. This finding suggests that TEE should not be extrapolated from REE, and that caloric recommendations determined by indirect calorimetry may significantly underestimate the actual energy needs of patients.

Nutrition Assessment

A thorough and accurate nutrition assessment is the primary step for early recognition of feeding difficulties and growth delay in children with CHD. Identifying infants at nutrition risk early allows intervention by a dietitian or feeding specialist to address inadequate intake and feeding difficulties. Known risk factors for infants with CHD have been identified and are outlined in the infant malnutrition and feeding checklist for CHD (Table 23-3). Early identification of infants with known risk factors can facilitate a nutrition care plan that promotes better outcomes for the infant with CHD.[15]

The primary step in the nutrition care process is a thorough and accurate nutrition assessment, which includes factors such as obtaining an accurate feeding history, conducting a visual assessment and anthropometric evaluation, and evaluating biochemical indices. Using the checklist outlined in Table 23-3 will help identify children with CHD who are at risk for malnutrition and feeding difficulties. Standard growth charts are used for monitoring children with CHD without any underlying syndrome. However, CHD may be present in conjunction with an underlying chromosomal abnormality or syndrome. In these conditions, anthropometric data can be evaluated using specialized growth charts as available for children with trisomy 21, trisomy 18, Turner syndrome, and infants born preterm (see Chapter 32).

Biochemical evaluation should include prealbumin, serum albumin, and serum electrolytes as well as calcium, magnesium, and phosphorus. Serum albumin results must be interpreted with caution because these are highly sensitive to the patient's hydration status. Prealbumin is influenced by infection, sepsis, inflammation, and operative course, and it should be evaluated with consideration of non-nutrition factors. Fluid overload secondary to CHF or dehydration secondary to diuretics can alter fluid and electrolyte balance and may affect renal function. If the serum albumin is low, then protein-losing enteropathy (PLE) is a consideration, and stool for α-1-antitrypsin and total lymphocyte count should be obtained to assess for PLE.

Recent data support the use of B-type natriuretic peptide (BNP) as a useful adjunct prognostic and disease-severity marker in children undergoing cardiac surgery. Both preoperative values and postsurgical variations in BNP should be interpreted first according to age and disease severity and only secondarily as the consequence of additional factors, including malnutrition and body fat mass. An inverse correlation exists between total body fat mass and BNP levels.[16] Infants and children with heart disease that causes significant pressure or volume overload of the right or the left ventricle have elevated BNP levels. Perioperative BNP levels have been found to predict outcome, specifically longer duration of mechanical ventilation and longer intensive care unit stay after surgery for CHD.

Table 23-3. Infant Feeding and Nutrition Checklist for Congenital Heart Disease[a]

		YES	NOT SURE	NO
Fast track: If *yes* or *not sure* for any item, initiate a referral to the dietitian and OT	The following cardiac diagnoses: interrupted aortic arch, hypoplastic left heart, coarctation of the aorta, truncus arteriosus			
	The following known/suspected chromosomal or other abnormalities:			
	• DiGeorge (22q11 del), trisomy 18/13, CHARGE, VACTERL			
	• Brain injury			
	• Vocal cord paresis			
Nutrition: If *yes* or *not sure* to any item, initiate a referral to the dietitian	Weight (any of the following): • < 3rd percentile • Dropped 2 major percentile groups			
	Diet • Fortified breast milk or hypercaloric formula			
	Feeding tube			
	GI tolerance: • Vomiting			
Feeding: If *yes* or *not sure* for any item, initiate a referral to the OT	Physiological status: • RR > 65 bpm • Increased WOB • Tachycardia • Desaturations			
	Vocal cords: • Stridor, hoarse voice, or wheezy cry			
	During feeds: • Coughing, choking, or gagging • Congestion/upper airway sounds • Poor sucking • Not taking full feeds orally			

CHARGE, coloboma, heart defects, atresia of the choanae, retardation of growth and development, genital and urinary abnormalities, ear abnormalities and/or hearing loss; CHD, congenital heart disease; GI, gastrointestinal; OT, occupational therapist; RR, respiratory rate; VACTERL, vertebral, anal atresia, cardiac, trachea, esophageal, renal, and limb defects; WOB, work of breathing.

[a]The checklist should be completed for all babies with CHD admitted/transferred into a unit.

Reprinted from the *Journal of Pediatric Nursing*, vol. 25(5), St. Pierre A, Khattra P, Johnson M, Cender L, Manzano S, Holsti L, Content Validation of the Infant Malnutrition and Feeding Checklist for Congenital Heart Disease: A Tool to Identify Risk of Malnutrition and Feed Difficulties in Infants with Congenital Heart Disease, pages 367–374, Copyright 2010, with permission from Elsevier.

Nutrition Management

Adequate nutrition intake is not always easily achieved in infants and children with CHD. These infants require increased energy intakes to achieve significant growth but are often unable to achieve their nutrition goal due to anorexia and increased fatigue during feeding.

Nutrient Delivery

The primary goal is to maximize oral energy intake. When oral intake alone fails to support growth and development, alternative methods of nutrition delivery are indicated and should be initiated relatively early. Tube feedings should be considered to supplement inadequate oral intake (Figures 23-1 to 23-4).

To maintain the infant's hunger and satiety cycle, intermittent bolus tube feeds may be used to supplement oral nutrition intake. To preserve the infant's oral motor function and desire to eat, supplemental feeds should be delivered after allowing the infant to feed orally for 10–15 minutes at each feed time.

Infants and children with CHF often need to be fluid restricted. Concentrating formula helps provide adequate calories, while limiting fluid intake. Increasing the formula concentration from 20 kcal/oz to 24 or 27 kcal/oz can be achieved by the addition of modular components or by reducing the water to powder ratio. If intermittent bolus feeds are not tolerated because of compromised motility, reflux, or concomitant respiratory distress, then continuous feeds should be considered. Continuous feeds allow delivery of daily requirements with smaller hourly volumes with decreased energy expenditure.[17] Continuous 24-hour nasogastric feedings are a safe and effective method of achieving increased nutrient intake resulting in improved overall nutrition status. If the infant is anticipated to require supplemental feeds for a prolonged duration (for longer than 8 weeks), then placing a gastrostomy tube should be considered. A gastrostomy tube is better accepted socially and also decreases the risks associated with prolonged NG tube feeds, which include dislodgement of the tube, stenting open the lower esophageal sphincter with resultant increased reflux, sinusitis, and nasal skin and cartilage breakdown.[18]

Infants and children who are unable to meet their nutrition needs via the enteral route should be considered for PN, which can be initiated preoperatively or postoperatively, with a therapeutic goal of restoring or maintaining nutrition status and inducing somatic growth. In view of the relatively high prevalence of malnutrition in infants and children with CHD, aggressive nutrition support via PN is an appropriate approach to prevent a further decline in their nutrition status. Almost all children can be nourished enterally after corrective surgery. However, during the preoperative and perioperative period PN support may be indicated. PN formulation in children with CHD requires close electrolyte monitoring, especially in patients on diuretics and digoxin therapy.

Significant caloric intake not only considerably impacts the surgical outcomes but also the ultimate growth and development in children with CHD.

Complications After Congenital Heart Disease Surgery

Feeding Difficulties

Feeding difficulties and intolerances are common during the first year of life in infants with CHD. Vomiting occurs frequently in this population and has been identified as the most common feeding intolerance.[19,20] Suboptimal intake and loss of nutrients from vomiting can further decrease the amount of energy available for growth. Vomiting after feeding has been estimated to result in a loss of up to 12% of the infant's energy intake.[20] Utilization of nutrients is compromised in the setting of chronic hypoxia and acidosis and is often seen in infants with CHD.

Increased risk-adjusted congenital heart surgery score, prolonged intubation, and intraoperative transesophageal echocardiography have been identified as risk factors associated with feeding difficulties after surgery among infants and children with CHD. Problems encountered may include a prolonged time to reach feeding goals, prolonged transition to oral feeds requiring tube feeding at discharge, and aspiration and/or reflux.[21] Postoperative vocal cord dysfunction is also a clinically important complication following cardiac surgery and may increase the risk of aspiration due to an impaired airway protection. In a study by Sachdeva et al,[22] patients whose surgery involved manipulation of the laryngeal nerves were at greater risk for vocal cord injury, with the presumed cause being injury to the vagus nerve. In an infant or child with vocal cord dysfunction, a swallowing evaluation is highly recommended to identify the presence of aspiration.[22,23] Although only 1.7% of patients were identified as having vocal cord dysfunction in this particular study, 100% of those patients had abnormal swallowing study results. Most of these patients required modified oral feeds and nutrition support.

Patients who undergo cardiac surgery with the use of transesophageal echocardiography often have symptoms of dysphagia. Transesophageal echocardiography has been identified to cause airway obstruction, common pulmonary vein compression, vascular compression, tracheal extubation, esophageal perforation, gastric perforation, and dental injury. Transesophageal echocardiography probe size in relation to the patient's weight was identified as a risk factor for dysphagia. In infants weighing < 3 kg, transesophageal echocardiography should be used cautiously.[23]

Protein-Losing Enteropathy

PLE is an abnormal loss of protein from the digestive tract or the inability of the digestive tract to absorb protein. The prevalence of PLE in infants and children with CHD seems to be most prominent after the Fontan procedure (anastomosis of the inferior vena cava to the pulmonary artery, which is the preferred surgical correction for tricuspid atresia, HLHS, and other single ventricle physiology). PLE can be a life-threatening complication, with onset of the disease occurring from 2 months to 10 years postoperatively.[24] Within 10 years of a Fontan procedure, approximately 13% of patients will develop PLE. 46 percent of PLE patients develop significant morbidity and mortality within 5 years.[24] Children with PLE have changes in bowel habits, abdominal discomfort, and diarrhea. With ongoing protein loss in the stool, the concentrations of serum protein can become severely depleted over time, resulting in hypoproteinemia and especially hypoalbuminemia and hypogammaglobulinemia. Hypocalcemia and lymphocytopenia are often seen in this condition as well. The loss of serum proteins decreases the vascular oncotic pressure and promotes the development of edema, ascites, and pleural as well as pericardial effusion. Edema of the intestinal wall secondary to chronic hypoalbuminemia may result in poor absorption of nutrients and promote worsening of the diarrhea.[25]

Nutrition management of infants and children with PLE should be tailored to the severity of bowel dysfunction, diarrhea, and malabsorption. Dietary changes should include increasing protein intake and transition from long-chain triglycerides (LCTs), which once absorbed must travel through the lymphatic circulation, to a medium-chain triglyceride (MCT)–based diet. The use of a MCT–enriched diet is based on the understanding that enterocytes absorb MCTs directly into the portal circulation, allowing delivery of adequate calories while reducing lymphatic flow to allow for healing. MCTs are rapidly absorbed and reduce the amount of high-protein lymph fluid moving through the vessels within the intestines, thereby reducing the quantity of protein loss. Specialized nutrition support with the use of formulas with very high MCT levels (80%–90% of the total fat content; Tables 23-4 and 23-5) should be provided to infants and children with intractable diarrhea who are unable to maintain their nutrition status with standard formula.[26] With long-term use of these formulas, essential fatty acids should be monitored due to the risk of developing deficiency. In severe cases, the use of PN may be implemented to allow complete enteric rest to minimize lymphatic flow and promote healing.

Medical therapies have been studied. Several reports exist on the efficacy of heparin therapy and beneficial ef-

Table 23-4. Medium-Chain Triglyceride Content of Formulas for Infants and Children < 1 Year of Age

MCT FORMULAS (MANUFACTURER)	MCT TO LCT RATIO
Pregestemil (Mead Johnson)	55:45
Alimentum (Abbott)	33:67
Portagen (Mead Johnson)	87:13
Monogen (Nutricia)	88:12
Neocate (Nutricia)	33:67
EleCare (Abbott)	33:67
Enfaport (Enfamil)	84:16

LCT, long-chain triglyceride; MCT, medium-chain triglyceride.

Table 23-5. Medium-Chain Triglyceride Formula for Children > 1 Year of Age

FORMULA (MANUFACTURER)	MCT TO LCT RATIO
Vivonex Pediatric (Nestlé Nutrition)	70:30
Peptamen Junior (Nestlé Nutrition)	60:40
Pediasure Peptide (Abbott)	50:50
Neocate Junior (Nutricia)	35:67
Pepdite Junior (Nutricia)	35:65

LCT, long-chain triglyceride; MCT, medium-chain triglyceride.

fects of corticosteroids in patients with PLE, although the precise mechanism by which they work in this setting is unclear. In a recent small study, oral budesonide was found to be beneficial in patients with PLE following a Fontan procedure.[27] Sildenafil has been used in these children to address increased pulmonary vascular reactivity, with improvement in the mesenteric arterial flow and in serum albumin after 6 weeks of therapy.[28]

Octreotide, a somatostatin analogue, has also been used with some success in patients with PLE following Fontan surgery.[29] Octreotide decreases lymphatic flow and is mainly recommended as an adjunct in a treatment regimen that targets cardiac and other intestinal etiologies.

Surgical interventions carry a high risk of mortality but Fontan revisions with conversion of older-style Fontans to that of an extra cardiac or lateral tunnel, surgical relief of obstruction to the pulmonary venous return, and cardiac transplantation have all been reported as potential treatment strategies.[30]

Chylothorax

Chylothorax, a known complication of pediatric cardiac surgery, requires special nutrition support considerations. Chylothorax is the accumulation of chyle within the pleural space. The chyle leak can be the result of injury to the thoracic duct, disruption of accessory lymphatics, or from an increased systemic venous pressure exceeding that in the thoracic duct.[31–34] Studies have suggested that the increase in postoperative chylothorax complications from 1% or less in the 1970s and 1980s to 2.5%–4.7% currently may be due to the increased complexity of the surgeries performed and possibly to the earlier initiation of enteral feeds.[31] Chan et al reported an incidence of 3.8% from 2000 to 2002, with a higher percentage occurring after heart transplant and the Fontan procedure.[31]

The challenge in managing chylothorax is in maintaining fluids and electrolytes while minimizing the lymphatic leak. Chylothorax can be corrected surgically, but the results are not always favorable and not always feasible for children who are already compromised after having had congenital heart surgery. Adverse effects of chylothorax include immunosuppression, the need for long-term chest tubes and intravenous access, and prolonged hospitalization.[32] Postoperative length of stay is reported to be significantly longer, with a median of 22 vs 8 days if a chylous leak develops.[33] Conservative management is usually attempted prior to surgery for the resolution of the leak.

Conservative management includes pleural space evacuation, the use of low-fat diets with MCTs, or PN for complete enteric rest. As in PLE, the use of a MCT–enriched diet is based on the understanding that MCTs are readily absorbed by the enterocytes into circulation, providing adequate calories and minimizing lymphatic flow to allow for healing.[33] For formula feedings, a high-MCT/low-LCT formula may be used (Table 23-4). To prevent essential fatty acid deficiency, 2%–4% of total calories should be in the form of linoleic acid, with 0.25%–0.5% from linolenic acid. If patients are on oral feedings and adequate calories can be consumed, a low-fat diet may be sufficient. In the study by Chan et al,[33] 34 of 48 patients (71%) had resolution with changes to their enteral diet.

Octreotide has been used as a treatment for chylothorax drainage that did not respond to dietary manipulations alone. In a study conducted from 1981 to 2004, 83% of patients receiving octreotide responded with complete resolution of their chylothorax after approximately 15 days of treatment, and no side effects from the octreotide therapy were noted after 2 weeks of treatment.[31] In an extensive analysis of a large multi-institution database, octreotide therapy was found to be beneficial as adjunct therapy.[35]

The early diagnosis and treatment of chylothorax can reduce the length of the chylous leak. At present, dietary management is the mainstay of treatment when managing these patients conservatively.

Pediatric Cardiomyopathy

Cardiomyopathy refers to a chronic disease of the heart muscle in which the myocardium is abnormally enlarged, thickened, and/or stiffened. Eventually, the weakened heart loses the ability to pump blood effectively and arrhythmias or dysthymia may occur. According to the national pediatric cardiomyopathy registry, 1 in every 100,000 children in the United States is diagnosed with primary cardiomyopathy.

Cardiomyopathy is a common cause of heart failure in children and is the most common cause of heart transplantation in children older than 1 year of age. Nearly 40% of children who present with symptomatic cardiomyopathy receive a heart transplant or die within the first 2 years of diagnosis.[36]

Pediatric cardiomyopathies are generally classified as nonischemic and predominately involve the heart's abnormal structure and function. Due to varying clinical features and therapies, the disease is separated into 4 categories: dilated (or congestive), hypertrophic, restrictive, and arrythmogenic right ventricular (Table 23-6). Each form is determined by the nature of muscle damage, and dilated cardiomyopathy is the most common.

Children with CHD and/or cardiomyopathy often do not grow along expected standards for age, making it especially important for these children to receive adequate energy intake. Optimal intake of macronutrients promoting an anabolic state can help improve cardiac function. In addition, several specific nutrients have been shown to correct abnormalities that often occur with cardiomyopathy and heart failure. In particular, antioxidants can protect against free radical damage, which is also common in the context of heart failure. Nutrients that augment myocardial energy production are important therapies that have been primarily explored in adults with cardiomyopathies (Table 23-7). As a general rule, food factors that trigger the acute phase response should be avoided (eg, excess carbohydrates and saturated fats). Foods that counteract inflammatory processes such as foods with ω-3 fatty acids have been shown to have possible favorable effects on ventricular function and should be recommended.[37]

Table 23-6. Types of Pediatric Cardiomyopathies

TYPE	DESCRIPTION
Dilated cardiomyopathy	The heart muscle fibers stretch, causing a chamber of the heart to enlarge, thus weakening the heart's ability to pump blood.
Hypertrophic cardiomyopathy	A functional type of cardiomyopathy that occurs among older children and adults in which the growth or arrangement of muscle fibers is abnormal, leading to a thickening of the heart walls, a reduction in size of the chambers, and possible restriction of blood flow.
Restrictive cardiomyopathy	The walls of the ventricles stiffen and lose their flexibility.
Arrythmogenic right ventricular cardiomyopathy	Myocytes in the right ventricle are replaced with fatty, fibrous tissue.

Table 23-7. Nutrients That Augment Myocardial Energy Production in Adults

ANTIOXIDANTS AND NUTRIENTS THAT MAY HAVE AN EFFECT ON CARDIAC FUNCTION IN HEART FAILURE	NUTRIENTS THAT MAY IMPROVE MYO-CARDIAL ENERGY PRODUCTION
Vitamin A	Thiamine
Vitamin E	L-carnitine
Vitamin C	Creatine
Taurine	Zinc
Coenzyme Q10	Magnesium
	Selenium

Coenzyme Q10 and selenium are 2 nutrients of special interest in cardiomyopathy. Coenzyme Q10, also known as ubiquinone, is an oil-soluble, vitamin-like substance present in most eukaryotic cells, primarily in the mitochondria. A component of the electron transport chain, it participates in aerobic cellular respiration, generating energy in the form of ATP. The clinical evidence for a potential role of coenzyme Q10 in cardiomyopathy is based primarily on adult patients with heart failure. The primary biochemical basis for the use of coenzyme Q10 in the treatment of various types of cardiomyopathy in adults centers on the critical role of coenzyme Q10 in mitochondrial bioenergetics; the underlying pathophysiology involves defective bioenergetics, specifically the availability of ATP, which plays a central role in regulating myocardial contractility. Evidence supports that coenzyme Q10 acts at the mitochondrial level to improve the efficiency of energy production in heart tissue. The antioxidant properties of coenzyme Q10 also have an important role in protecting the mitochondria from free radical damage and thus maintain its integrity and function.[37,38]

Due to endogenous production, coenzyme Q10 is not considered a vitamin, and no recommended dietary allowance has been established. Deficiency of this coenzyme may be caused by impaired biosynthesis, insufficient dietary intake, poor gastrointestinal absorption, and/or excessive utilization of coenzyme Q10. Exogenous sources of coenzyme Q10 include animal products, such as beef, pork, and chicken, and plant products, such as broccoli, spinach, and soy and palm oils.[38]

The referenced data are derived from small heterogeneous trials. However, a 2014 Cochrane Collaboration meta-analysis of 7 studies found "no convincing evidence to support or refute" the use of coenzyme Q10 for the treatment of heart failure. More clinical trials and testing need to be completed, especially in the pediatric population, before recommendations regarding coenzyme Q10 and cardiomyopathy can be made responsibly.[39]

Selenium is an essential trace mineral with established recommended dietary allowances. Deficiency has been associated with congestive cardiomyopathy (Keshan disease), skeletal myopathy, osteoarthropathy (Kashin-Beck disease), anemia, and immune system alterations. Selenium's most significant role is its action as a cofactor for the antioxidant enzyme glutathione peroxidase, which removes hydrogen peroxide and the deleterious lipid hydroperoxides generated by oxygen-derived species. Glutathione peroxidase deficiency contributes to endothelial dysfunction, a major contributing factor in heart failure.[37]

Heart Transplant

Failure to thrive is common in patients with CHD with end-stage heart failure leading to heart transplant. These patients have had multiple interventions, poor feeding tolerance and absorption, increased energy needs, and inadequate provision of energy.[40] Heart transplantation is a widely accepted treatment for end-stage heart disease in pediatric patients. Evidence exists for suboptimal outcomes in underweight patients post-transplant, such as decreased overall graft survival compared with normal weight patients.

It is crucial to maximize the child's nutrition status prior to transplant. Anthropometric measurements are easily obtained, and age-specific standards are available for comparison. Growth measurements such as weight, length, weight for length, and head circumference, if < 3 years old, should be measured over time.[41]

Calorie and protein requirements of children on enteral/oral feedings are based on the dietary reference intakes for age with adjustments to promote growth. The requirements of patients who are supported with EN or PN are estimated at 5%–10% less than the estimated for oral/enteral alone.[41] It is important to correct malnutrition prior to transplant. Malnutrition places the patient at an increased risk for infection, impaired wound healing, and extended rehabilitation after transplant. Laboratory values should be obtained to determine if macronutrient and micronutrient intake is sufficient or if additional supplementation is warranted.[41]

Hypertension, hyperglycemia, and weight gain are common in post-transplant pediatric heart recipients.[42] The goals for post-transplant patients are to maintain ideal body weight, limit sweets and foods high in cholesterol and fat, and limit salt intake.[42] Calcineurin inhibitors commonly used in post-transplant patients may cause elevated lipid levels. These inhibitors, along with pretransplant nutrition status and steroids, can result in decreased calcium absorption and bone formation, and osteoporosis is a common problem in heart transplant recipients.[43] Supplemental vitamin D (400–800 IU) and calcium (1200–1500 mg) are recommended.

Survival rates for patients with heart transplants are approximately 85%.[44] Growth and development are important determinants of quality of life. Great strides have been made in nutrition management in recent decades, including the identification, treatment, and prevention of nutrition issues leading up to transplant and continuing afterward, and have had positive influences on outcomes.

Cardiovascular Disease in the Pediatric Patient

Atherosclerosis is the buildup of fat and cholesterol on the arterial walls. Atherosclerosis increases the risk of CVDs, including heart attack and stroke. Although secondary effects of atherosclerosis are not common in children because the narrowing of the arteries takes years to develop, the process begins in childhood. Risk factors for developing early atherosclerosis include obesity, high blood pressure, family history of CVD, exposure to cigarette smoke, and underlying medical conditions such as diabetes, chronic kidney disease, and treatment for cancer during childhood.

Children should be screened for cholesterol initially at 9–11 years of age and again at age 17–21. Children 2 years of age or older who have a family history or medical diseases associated with CVD and children who are overweight with high blood pressure should be screened as well (Table 23-8).[45]

Table 23-8. Classification of Total and LDL Cholesterol Levels in Children and Adolescents From Families With Hypercholesterolemia or Premature Cardiovascular Disease

CATEGORY	TOTAL CHOLESTEROL, MG/DL	LDL CHOLESTEROL, MG/DL
Acceptable	< 170	< 110
Borderline	170-199	110-129
High	> 200	> 200

Adapted with permission from American Academy of Pediatrics Committee on Nutrition. Cholesterol in childhood. *Pediatrics.* 1998;101(1):141–147. LDL, low-density lipoprotein.

The National Cholesterol Education Program (NCEP) discusses the effects of early elevated lipid levels on adult atherosclerosis and coronary heart disease risk. The program focuses on prevention and lowering of lipids in children and adolescents. Eating behavior and genetics affect cholesterol levels. Behavioral changes require intervention at several levels. An individual approach by itself is less effective. The key to success requires both population and individualized approaches.

One approach for lowering cholesterol levels in children and adolescents is through changing eating behaviors on a population-wide basis. The recommendations of the NCEP as well as the guidelines of the American Heart Association have been adopted by the American Academy for Pediatrics.[46] These recommendations include consuming a variety of food and adequate calories to support growth and maintain an ideal body weight while keeping fat intakes at an acceptable level.

To support their efforts for population-wide changes, the NCEP also provides recommendations for organizations that influence the eating behaviors of children, such as schools, health professionals, government agencies, and the food industry.

The individualized approach aims to identify and treat children and adolescents who are at the greatest risk of CVD. This approach aims at screening children who are from families with a history of premature CVD or who have at least one parent with high cholesterol. Universal screening is not cost effective and may impose an unnecessary stigma on a child.[47] Reis et al[47] looked at risk factors in children and investigated whether families at risk for CVD can be identified. The authors looked at children to see if identification of risk factors in them would help predict risk factors in their parents. This population was targeted because children are more likely to receive regular primary care than adults. The participants underwent assessment of cardiovascular risk factors: obesity, hypertension, dyslipidemia, and metabolic syndrome. Parent–child association was strong for body mass index, waist circumference, systolic blood pressure, triglyceride, and total cholesterol. Risk factors in children were found to be significant predictors for the same risk factors for their parents. This study suggests that CVD risk factors in children can predict elevated CVD risk factors in parents.

Children identified with an elevated cholesterol level at an early age should be treated. Initial therapy should always be diet modification accompanied by lifestyle changes, such as minimizing sedentary habits and promoting physical activity. The step I diet mimics the recommendations of the population approach. The step I diet limits saturated fat to <10% of total calories, total fat intake to ≤30% of total calories, and cholesterol to <300 mg/d. If LDL levels remain elevated after 3 months of adhering to the step I diet, the step II diet should be initiated. The step II diet reduces saturated fat to <7% of calories and cholesterol to <200 mg/d. Drug therapy is suggested in children 10 years or older if diet fails after 6–12 months for those with LDL levels > 190 mg/dL or > 160 mg/dL if other risk factors are also present.[48,49]

The American Academy of Pediatrics released a policy statement on cardiovascular risk reduction in high-risk pediatric populations. This policy outlines CVD risk stratification based on existing comorbidities and assesses cardiovascular risk factors to stratify patients into at-risk, moderate-risk, and high-risk categories. Lifestyle changes to include diet, exercise, and cessation of smoking as well as disease-specific management are the basis of its recommendations in all 3 groups.[49] Pharmacologic intervention is recommended only if goals are not met.[45,46]

Obesity, hypertension, insulin resistance, and dyslipidemia, also known as the metabolic syndrome or syndrome X (Chapter 14), are risk factors for childhood CVD.

Metabolic syndrome often requires adjunct pharmacotherapy in addition to aggressive diet and exercise regimen.

Studies suggest that obese children with risk factors for CVD become obese adults with increased risk of morbidity from CVD. Prevention and early intervention should be a primary goal of health professionals and government agencies. The NCEP has reported on these issues and implemented recommendations for dietary changes, screening, and treatment of children and adolescents who are identified as at risk for CVD and for developing into an adult with CVD.[47]

Summary

Children with CHD often have difficulty achieving adequate caloric intake to support their growth and development. A child should be provided with nutrition support to maximize growth and development prior to corrective surgery. The interstage period has been recognized as a critical time for infants with CHD and presents unique challenges to the practitioner providing nutrition care. Suboptimal weight gain often occurs during this interstage period. If energy goals are met and children are closely monitored during the interstage phase, adequate growth can be achieved with significantly improved surgical outcomes.[2–4]

Postsurgical complications may occur depending on the complexity of the defect and surgical intervention. Complications that may arise postoperatively include PLE and chylothorax, which require specialized nutrition modifications.

Pediatric cardiac disease over the past 2 decades has extended to include CVD. Prevention and early intervention in these children holds promise of impacting CVD and its complications in the adult population.

Test Your Knowledge Questions

1. The potential for growth and nutrition recovery in children with CHD seems to be most affected by
   A. Degree of growth impairment
   B. Feeding difficulties
   C. Energy intake/expenditure
   D. Age and timing of corrective surgery
2. To assess risk of CVD, children should have their blood cholesterol levels screened at what age?
   A. Annually
   B. At birth and every 5 years
   C. At 9–11 years and again at 17–21 years old
   D. Children should only be screened if their body mass index suggests obesity.
3. Failure to thrive in infants with CHD is secondary to
   A. Poor caloric intake
   B. Increased energy expenditure
   C. Hypoxia
   D. All of the above
4. When selecting a formula for treatment of infants with a chylous leak, the following characteristics should be considered:
   A. Only LCTs
   B. Only MCTs
   C. Fat blend (high MCT and low LCT)
   D. Fat blend (high LCT and low MCT)

References

1. Go AS, Mozaffarian D, Roger VL, et al. American Heart Association Statistics Committee and Stroke Statistics Subcommittee. Heart disease and stroke statistics—2013 update: a report from the American Heart Association. *Circulation.* 2013;127:e6–e245.
2. Toole BJ, Toole LE, Kyle UG, Cabrera AG, Orellna RA, Coss-Bu JA. Perioperative nutritional support and malnutrition in infants and children with congenital heart disease. *Congenit Heart Dis.* 2014;9(1):15–25.
3. Cameron JW, Rosenthal A, Olsen AD. Malnutrition in hospitalized children with congenital heart disease. *Arch Pediatr Adolesc Med.* 1995;149(10):1098–1102.

4. Mitchell IM, Logen RW, Pollock JCS, Jamieson MPG. Nutritional status of children with congenital heart disease. *Br Heart J*. 1995;73:277–283.

5. Kelleher KD, Laussen P, Teixeira-Pinto A, Duggan C. Growth and correlates of nutritional status among infants with hypoplastic left heart syndrome (HLHS) after stage I Norwood procedure. *Nutrition*. 2006;22:237–244.

6. Anderson BJ, Beekman HR 3rd, Border LW, et al. Lower weight age z-score adversely affects hospital length of stay after the bidirectional Glenn procedures in infants with single ventricle. *J Thorac Cardiovasc Surg*. 2009;138(2):397–404.

7. Menon SC, McCandless RT, Mack GK, et al. Clinical outcomes and resource use for infants with hypoplastic left heart syndrome during bidirectional Glenn: summary from the Joint Council for Congenital Heart Disease National Cardiology Quality Improvement Collaborative registry. *Pediatr Cardiol*. 2013;34:143–148.

8. Hill GD, Hehir AD, Bartz PJ, et al. Effect of feeding modality on interstage growth after stage I palliation: a report from the National Pediatric Cardiology Quality Improvement Collaborative. *J Thorac Cardiovasc Surg*. 2014;148(4):1534–1539.

9. Slicker J, Hehir AD, Horsley M, et al; Feeding Work Group of the National Pediatric Cardiology Quality Improvement Collaborative. Nutrition algorithms for infants with hypoplastic left heart syndrome: birth through the first interstage period. *Congenit Heart Dis*. 2013;8(2):89–102.

10. Leitch C, Karn C, Peppard R, et al. Increased energy expenditure in infants with cyanotic congenital heart disease. *J Pediatr*. 1998;133(6):755–760.

11. Modi P, Suleiman MS, Reeves BC, et al. Basal metabolic rate of heart patients with cyanosis age, and pathology. *Ann Thorac Surg*. 2004;78:1710–1716.

12. Avitzur Y, Singer P, Dagan O, et al. Resting energy expenditure in children with cyanotic and non-cyanotic congenital heart disease before and after open heart surgery. *JPEN J Parenter Enter Nutr*. 2003;27(1);47–51.

13. Nydegger A, Bines JE. Energy metabolism in infants with congenital heart disease. *Nutrition*. 2006;22(7–8):697–704.

14. Leitch C. Growth, nutrition and energy expenditure in pediatric heart failure. *Prog Pediatr Cardiol*. 2000;11:195–202.

15. St Pierre A, Khattra P, Johnson M, Cender L, Manzano S, Holsti L. Content validation of the infant malnutrition and feeding checklist for congenital heart disease: a toll to identify risk of malnutrition and feeding difficulties in infants with congenital heart disease. *J Pediatr Nurs*. 2010;25(5):367–374.

16. Radman M, Mack R, Barnoya J, et al. The effect of preoperative nutritional status on postoperative outcomes in children undergoing surgery for congenital heart defects in San Francisco (UCSF) and Guatemala City (UNICAR). *J Thorac Cardiovasc Surg*. 2014;147(1):441–450.

17. Schwartz MS, Gewitz HM, See CC, et al. Enteral nutrition in infants with congenital heart disease and growth failure. *Pediatrics*. 1990;86(3):368–373.

18. Durai R, Venkatraman R, Ng P. Nasogastric tubes 2: risks and guidance on avoiding and dealing with complications. *Nurs Times*. 2009;105(17):14–16.

19. da Silva VM, de Oliveira Lopes MV, de Araujo TL. Growth and nutritional status of children with congenital heart disease. *J Cardiovasc Nurs*. 2007;22(5):390–396.

20. van der Kuip M, Hoos MB, Forget PP, Westerterp KR, Gemke RJ, de Meer K. Energy expenditure in infants with congenital heart disease, including a meta-analysis. *Acta Paediatr*. 2003;92:921–927.

21. Kogon BE, Ramaswamy V, Todd K, et al. Feeding difficulty in newborns following congenital heart surgery. *Congenit Heart Dis*. 2007;2(5):332–337.

22. Sachdeva R, Hussain E, Moss M, et al. Vocal cord dysfunction and feeding difficulties after pediatric cardiovascular surgery. *J Pediatr*. 2007;151:312–315.

23. Kohr LM, Dargan M, Hague A, et al. The incidence of dysphagia in pediatric patients after open heart procedures with transesophageal echocardiography. *Ann Thorac Surg*. 2003;76:1450–1456.

24. Feldt RH, Driscoll DJ, Offord KP, et al. Protein-losing enteropathy after the Fontan procedure. *J Thorac Cardiovasc Surg*. 1996;112:672–680.

25. Ostrow MA, Hudsen F, Rychik J. Protein-losing enteropathy after Fontan operation: investigations into possible pathophysiologic mechanisms. *Ann Thorac Surg*. 2006;83(2):695–700.

26. Parrish RC, Krenitky J, Willcutts K, Radigan A. Gastrointestinal disease. In: Gottschlich MM, DeLegge MH, Mattox T, Mueller C, Worthington P, eds. *The A.S.P.E.N. Nutrition Support Core Curriculum: A Case-Based Approach—The Adult Patient*. Silver Spring, MD: American Society for Parenteral and Enteral Nutrition; 2007:524–525.

27. Gursu HA, Erdogan I, Varan B, et al. Oral budesonide as a therapy for protein-losing enteropathy in children after the Fontan operation. *J Card Surg*. 2014;3:712–716.

28. Uzun O, Wong JK, Bhole V, Stumper O. Resolution of protein-losing enteropathy and normalization of mesenteric Doppler flow with sildenafil after Fontan. *Ann Thorac Surg*. 2006;82(6):e39–e40.

29. John AS, Johnson JA, Khan M, et al. Clinical outcomes and improved survival in patients with protein-losing enteropathy after the Fontan operation. *J Am Coll Cardiol*. 2014;64(1):54-62.

30. Meadows J, Jenkins K. Protein-losing enteropathy: integrating a new disease paradigm into recommendations for prevention and treatment. *Cardiol Young*. 2011;21(4):363–377.

31. Chan S, Lau W, Wong W, et al. Chylothorax in children after congenital heart surgery. *Ann Thorac Surg*. 2006;82:1650–1656.

32. Pelletier GJ. Invited commentary. *Ann Thorac Surg*. 2005;80:1870–1871.

33. Chan EH, Russell JL, Williams WG, et al. Postoperative chylothorax after cardiothoracic surgery in children. *Ann Thorac Surg*. 2005;80(5):1864–1879.

34. Hise M, Brown C. Lipids. In: Gottschlich MM, DeLegge MH, Mattox T, Mueller C, Worthington P, eds. *The A.S.P.E.N. Nutrition Support Core Curriculum: A Case-Based Approach—The Adult Patient*. Silver Spring, MD: American Society for Parenteral and Enteral Nutrition; 2007:48–70

35. Mery CM, Moffett BS, Khan MS, et al. Incidence and treatment of chylothorax after cardiac surgery in children: analysis of a large multi-institution database. *J Thorac Cardiovasc Surg.* 2014;147(2):678–686.

36. Liphultz E, Steven MD, Sleeper A, et al. The incidence of pediatric cardiomyopathy in two regions of United States. *N Engl J Med.* 2003;328:1647–1655.

37. Miller TL, Neri D, Extein J, Somarriba G, Strickman-Stein N. Nutrition in cardiomyopathy. *Progr Pediatr Cardiol.* 2007;24(1):59–71.

38. Bhagavan HN, Chopra RK. Potential role of ubiquinone (coenzyme Q10) in pediatric cardiomyopathy. *Clin Nutr.* 2005;24(3):331–338.

39. Madmani ME, Yusuf Solaiman A, Tamr Agha K, et al. Coenzyme Q10 for heart failure. *Cochrane Database Syst Rev.* 2014;6:CD008684.

40. Bannister L, Manlhiot C, Pollock-BarZiv S, Stone T, McCrindle BW, Dipchand AI. Anthropometric growth and utilization of enteral feeding support in pediatric heart transplant recipients. *Pediatr Transplant.* 2010;14(7):879–886.

41. Nucci A, Strohm S, Katyal N. Organ transplantation. In: Corkins MR, ed. *The A.S.P.E.N Pediatric Nutrition Support Core Curriculum.* Silver Spring, MD: American Society for Parenteral and Enteral Nutrition; 2010:337–348.

42. Chin C, Rosenthal D, Bernstein D. Lipoprotein abnormalities are highly prevalent in pediatric heart transplant recipients. *Pediatr Transplant.* 2000;4(3):193–199.

43. Blume E. Current status of heart transplantation in children: update 2003. *Pediatr Clin North Am.* 2003;50(6):1375–1391.

44. Sudan D, Bacha EA, John E, Bartholomew A. What's new in childhood organ transplantation. *Pediatr Rev.* 2007;28(12):439–452.

45. Expert Panel on Integrated Guidelines for Cardiovascular Health and Risk Reduction in Children and Adolescents; National Heart, Lung, and Blood Institute. Expert panel on integrated guidelines for cardiovascular health and risk reduction in children and adolescents: summary report. *Pediatrics.* 2011;128(suppl 5):S213–S256.

46. National Cholesterol Education Program (NCEP): highlights of the report of the Expert Panel on Blood Cholesterol Levels in Children and Adolescents. *Pediatrics.* 1992;89:495–501.

47. Reis EC, Kip KE, Marroquin OC, et al. Screening children to identify families at increased risk for cardiovascular disease. *Pediatrics.* 2006;118(6):e1789–e1797.

48. American Academy of Pediatrics Committee on Nutrition. Cholesterol in childhood. *Pediatrics.*1998;101(1):141–147.

49. American Academy of Pediatrics. Cardiovascular risk reduction in high-risk pediatric populations. *Pediatrics.* 2007;119(3):618–621.

Test Your Knowledge Answers

1. The correct answer is **D**. Surgical correction has emerged as the most efficient method to improve the nutrition status of these infants. Surgical correction eliminates the cardiac factors contributing to malnutrition.

2. The correct answer is **C**. Children should be screened for cholesterol initially at 9–11 years of age and again at age 17–21. Children 2 years or older who have a family history or medical diseases associated with CVD and children who are overweight with high blood pressure should be screened as well.[35]

3. The correct answer is **D**. The exact etiology for growth impairment in children with CHD remains unclear. Many factors have been identified as contributing to growth failure in this population.

4. The correct answer is **C**. The use of an MCT–enriched diet is based on the understanding that enterocytes directly absorb MCTs into circulation, allowing adequate calories while reducing lymphatic flow to allow for healing. At least 3%–4% of fat calories should come from LCTs to prevent essential fatty acid deficiency.

24

Renal Disease

Christina L. Nelms, MS, RD, CSP, LMNT; **Marisa Juarez**, MPH, RD, LD; and **Bradley A. Warady**, MD

 Podcast

CONTENTS

Learning Objectives

1. Describe normal kidney physiology and causes of pediatric renal failure.
2. Discuss nutrition care for pediatric patients with chronic kidney disease and acute kidney injury and following kidney transplantation.
3. Review nutrition needs and specifications for infants, children, and adolescents receiving supplemental enteral and parenteral nutrition.
4. Discuss specific nutrition needs for other kidney disorders in pediatrics, including nephrotic syndrome, nephrolithiasis, and renal tubular disorders.

Background

Chronic kidney disease (CKD) in children, as well as adults, is classified by the National Kidney Foundation's Kidney Disease Outcomes Quality Initiative (K/DOQI) staging schema in 5 stages, with stage 5 CKD being at or near end-stage disease and requiring dialysis or transplantation to sustain life.[1] CKD is more common in black children and males, with congenital disorders such as posterior urethral valves, prune belly syndrome, and renal dysplasia being major contributors.[1] On occasion, CKD may present acutely at an advanced stage, with children exhibiting only mild symptoms such as fatigue or flu-type illness until substantial progression of kidney damage has occurred. End-stage kidney disease (ESKD) in children (0–19 years of age) is much less common than in the adult population. Less than 2% of the total world ESKD population (dialysis and transplantation) is composed of children. However, as in adult populations, the incidence of ESKD continues to increase, albeit at a slower pace. The prevalence in children in the United States is about 82 per million of the age-related population. Although hard to quantify, earlier stages of CKD account for much larger numbers than the end-stage disease.

Children may also have sudden onset of new disease, called acute kidney injury (AKI) from a variety of causes including dehydration, the use of nephrotoxic medications, or severe infections giving rise to multisystem organ failure. In some cases, those patients who experience AKI go on to have CKD.

This chapter will discuss unique nutrition challenges of CKD and AKI as well as other kidney-related conditions in children, including nephrotic syndrome, nephrolithiasis, and renal tubular disorders.

Irrespective of the cause of kidney injury, patients with impaired kidney function typically have a variety of nutrition issues that should be addressed for optimal patient management. Nutritional issues are almost universally common for patients with impaired kidney function. Young children and infants have great metabolic and nutrition demands to promote normal growth and cognitive development. Inadequate intake related to anorexia is a common problem associated with CKD in children, and altered feeding regimens, such as fortified and nutrient-altered breast milk and formulas and tube feedings, are frequently required. Adolescents often have challenges related to puberty, high-calorie needs, and adherence issues. Nearly all infants, children, and adolescents with kidney disease or other kidney-related conditions have altered micronutrient needs and often have altered fluid needs.[2,3] Protein-energy malnutrition or the more recently described protein-energy wasting produces profound effects on growth and development and may be associated with increased risk of hospitalization and mortality in children on dialysis.[4–6] This chapter reviews those issues for the clinician.

Kidney Development and Function

Human kidney development, or nephrogenesis, begins during week 5 of gestation. The first functioning nephrons are formed by week 9, and the entire process is completed by 32–34 weeks of gestation. Once nephrogenesis has been completed, the kidney is unable to respond to injury by de novo generation of nephrons. Key components of nephrogenesis include formation of the pelvicalyceal system, renal tubular development, and glomerulogenesis. Urine production begins at about 10 weeks of gestation, and by 20 weeks it accounts for approximately 90% of amniotic fluid.[7] The fraction of cardiac output received by the kidneys is only 2.5% during late gestation. It increases to nearly 20% during the initial 6 weeks of life.[8] Kidney function, as measured by creatinine clearance, doubles during the first 2 weeks of life in term infants and reaches adult values by 2 years of age.[9] Normal serum creatinine values also increase with age.[10] Most important from the clinical perspective is the fact that the kidney is key to a variety of functions that, if impaired, may significantly alter body homeostasis. These functions influence solute removal; fluid and electrolyte regulation; calcium, phosphorus, and vitamin D metabolism; erythropoietin production; acid-base balance; and blood pressure regulation. All of these factors must be addressed medically if kidney function is decreased on an acute or chronic basis.

Acute Kidney Injury Physiology

Acute renal failure, now more accurately called AKI, is commonly characterized by an abrupt (hours to weeks) and prolonged loss of kidney function that is reversible in most cases.[11] It is typically accompanied by a change in creatinine clearance and possibly urine output. The causes of AKI are divided into

3 categories: prerenal, renal, and postrenal. The categories localize the predominant site of injury and help describe the mechanism of injury. For example, prerenal AKI primarily includes the state of reduced renal blood flow that might result from diarrhea and vomiting, burns, bleeding, or congestive heart failure. Insults to the renal glomeruli or tubules can give rise to so-called renal or intrinsic AKI. Sources of injury include glomerulonephritis (eg, postinfection, systemic lupus erythematosus, membranoproliferative diseases, and Henoch-Schönlein purpura), nephrotoxins (eg, aminoglycosides, amphotericin B, and heavy metals), interstitial nephritis, hemolytic-uremic syndrome, or acute tubular necrosis. Finally, postrenal or obstructive AKI can be the sequela of disorders such as nephrolithiasis, neurogenic bladder, hemorrhage, renal tumors, or posterior urethral valves in newborns. Strict attention to the etiology of AKI and prompt therapeutic intervention often result in a return to baseline kidney function.

Chronic Kidney Disease Physiology

While AKI is often reversible, CKD is characterized by an irreversible renal injury that is often progressive in nature. The National Kidney Foundation Kidney Disease Outcomes Quality Initiative (NKF KDOQI) guidelines classify CKD in children > 2 years of age, adolescents, and adults by the presence of kidney damage and the level of estimated glomerular filtration rate (GFR) (Table 24-1).[12] A GFR of 90 mL/min/1.73 m² or greater is considered normal. Stage 1 CKD is a GFR of >90 with evidence of kidney damage, such as protein in the urine. Additional clinical signs of impaired kidney function occur as GFR decreases. At stage 5, defined by a GFR of <15 mL/min/1.73 m², the child typically requires the initiation of renal replacement therapy (dialysis or transplantation). A modification of this staging schema

has recently been published by the Kidney Disease Improving Global Outcomes (KDIGO) initiative.[13]

A variety of disorders are associated with the development of CKD in pediatrics, as reflected by data from more than 7000 patients enrolled in the North American Pediatric Renal Trials and Collaborative Studies (NAPRTCS) registry as of 2008 (Table 24-2).[14] The 2 most common diagnoses are congeni-

Table 24-1. NKF KDOQI Classification of the Stages of Chronic Kidney Disease[12]

STAGE	GFR (mL/min/1.73 m²)	DESCRIPTION
1	> 90	Kidney damage with normal or increased GFR
2	60–89	Kidney damage with mild reduction of GFR
3	30–59	Moderate reduction of GFR
4	15–29	Severe reduction of GFR
5	< 15 (or dialysis)	Kidney failure

GFR, glomerular filtration rate; NKF KDOQI, National Kidney Foundation Kidney Disease Outcomes Quality Initiative.

Table 24-2. Chronic Kidney Disease Primary Diagnosis[14]

PRIMARY DIAGNOSIS	ALL PATIENTS[a] N	%
Obstructive uropathy	1454	20.7
Aplastic/hypoplastic/dysplastic kidney	1220	17.3
Focal segmental glomerulosclerosis	613	8.7
Reflux nephropathy	594	8.4
Polycystic disease	278	4.0
Prune belly	193	2.7
Renal infarct	158	2.2
Hemolytic uremic syndrome	141	2.0
SLE nephritis	114	1.6
Familial nephritis	111	1.6
Cystinosis	104	1.5
Pyelo/interstitial nephritis	99	1.4
Medullary cystic disease	90	1.3
Chronic glomerulonephritis	82	1.2
Congenital nephrotic syndrome	75	1.1
Membranoproliferative glomerulonephritis, type I	75	1.1
Berger's (IgA) nephritis	66	0.9
Idiopathic crescentic glomerulonephritis	47	0.7
Henoch-Schönlein nephritis	43	0.6
Membranous nephropathy	37	0.5
Wilms's tumor	32	0.5
Membranoproliferative glomerulonephritis, type II	30	0.4
Other systemic immunologic disease	26	0.4
Wegener's granulomatosis	25	0.4
Sickle cell nephropathy	14	0.2
Diabetic glomerulonephritis	11	0.2
Oxalosis	7	0.1
Drash's syndrome	6	0.1
Other	1110	15.8
Unknown	182	2.6

SLE, systemic lupus erythematosus.

[a]Percentages based on the total number of patients (N = 7037).

tal obstructive uropathy and aplastic/hypoplastic/dysplastic kidneys, while focal segmental glomerulosclerosis is the most common acquired cause. Clear evidence from clinical studies shows that both hypertension (HTN) and proteinuria play a key role in the progression of CKD to ESKD.[15,16] The ESCAPE Trial Group demonstrated that tight blood pressure control with values in the low range of normal and decreasing proteinuria were significant factors in delaying progression of renal disease and preserving renal function. Pharmacological means to tightly control blood pressure should be pursued if needed.[17] The developmental abnormalities of the urinary tract that account for the largest percentage of patients with CKD stages 2–4 logically account for the largest (eg, 30%–50%) proportion of children with ESKD (stage 5 CKD), resulting in the affected children having a life-long experience with their respective kidney disorders and the requirement for long-term medical and nutrition intervention.[14]

Chronic Kidney Disease

Dialysis in Children

Hemodialysis

Hemodialysis (HD) is a form of renal replacement therapy in which soluble substances and water are removed from the blood by diffusion through a semipermeable membrane. Access to the patient's blood is achieved either through a surgically constructed arteriovenous fistula or with a central venous catheter. A single session of HD typically lasts 3–4 hours and occurs 3 times per week in most pediatric patients. Young patients who receive the majority of their nutrition as formula often require HD more often because of the substantial fluid gains that take place on a daily basis. Alternatives to thrice weekly in-center HD include frequent home HD and nocturnal HD, both of which are practiced in a minority of pediatric dialysis programs.[18–20]

Peritoneal Dialysis

Peritoneal dialysis (PD) is typically prescribed for infants, toddlers, children, and approximately 50% of adolescents needing dialysis treatment.[14] It is usually a nightly process that makes use of an automated cycling machine. PD involves the infusion of a glucose-based solution through a catheter that is surgically inserted into the peritoneal cavity. Diffusion across the peritoneal membrane allows for waste products (eg, urea nitrogen, creatinine) and water to cross from the patient into the dialysis solution, prior to being drained from the body through the catheter. Fresh dialy-

sis fluid is then infused and a defined number of cycles of fluid occur during the dialysis session. In most children, this process occurs over 10–12 hours while they sleep. Some patients also maintain dialysis fluid in their peritoneal cavity throughout the day to permit additional dialysis, called a daytime dwell or last fill.

Characterization of the rate of movement of glucose and creatinine across the peritoneal membrane can be determined by conducting the peritoneal equilibration test (PET). Patients may be classified as high, high-average, low-average, or low transporters depending on how rapidly solute (eg, creatinine, glucose) moves across the peritoneal membrane during a 4-hour test. High transporters tend to have more porous peritoneal membranes and thus rapidly remove waste products along with significant amounts of potassium and protein. The rapid absorption of glucose from the dialysate in these patients decreases the osmotic gradient that is generated by glucose and results in less fluid removal from them. In contrast, low transporters tend to have less kidney waste removes, but also lose less protein and potassium and remove fluid well. The nutrition prescription for the PD patient is, in turn, often influenced by the transport capacity of the patient's peritoneal membrane.

Growth and CKD

Poor growth is a common manifestation of CKD in children. Growth velocity suffers as GFR declines. Many factors contribute to growth failure, including decreased appetite with poor energy intake, acidosis, reduced residual kidney function, excessive urinary sodium losses, renal osteodystrophy, and abnormalities of the growth hormone (GH)–insulin-like growth factor (IGF) axis.[3,21] Birth abnormalities such as premature birth and small for gestational age, as well as many of the comorbidities/syndromes that accompany CKD are also associated with poor growth. Parental short stature and steroid usage are additional independent risk factors.[21,22] Over the past 25–30 years, final adult heights have improved in pediatric CKD patients; however, much improvement is still needed because 35%–50% of children with CKD continue to be adults of small stature. One factor may be late referral to pediatric renal specialists.[18,21] Note that poor growth is associated with an impaired quality of life and an increased risk of hospitalizations and mortality in children with CKD.[18]

Linear Growth and Growth Hormone

In all cases of impaired growth associated with CKD, adequacy of nutrition should be assessed prior to consideration of GH therapy (Figure 24-1).[2,23] Evidence suggests that aggressive dialysis, as reflected by better solute clearance, along with caloric and protein intake at or above the recommended intake for age, helps prevent growth failure.[24] Nutrition support, primarily supplemental enteral nutrition (EN), may be needed to meet nutrition needs. Increasing evidence suggests that daily HD may improve linear growth, not only by providing a more physiologic pattern of solute removal, but also by facilitating a reduction of cachexia and, in turn, an improved nutrition intake.[25,26] Finally, in children with renal disorders such as obstructive uropathy (eg, posterior urethral valves) or renal dysplasia, supplementation of water

Figure 24-1. Growth Evaluation and Recombinant Human Growth Hormone Initiation and Monitoring, Including the Essential Assessment of Nutrition Parameters Prior to its Initiation

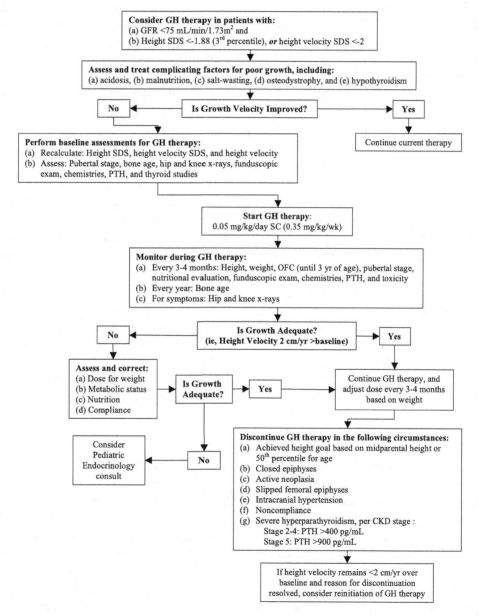

Reprinted from Mahan JD, Warady BA. Assessment and treatment of short stature in pediatric patients with chronic kidney disease: a consensus statement. *Pediatr Nephrol.* 2006;21:917-930 with kind permission of Springer Science+Business Media.

CKD, chronic kidney disease; GH, growth hormone; OFC, oral food challenge; PTH, parathyroid hormone; SC, subcutaneous; SDS, standard deviation score.

and 2–4 mEq of sodium (as chloride, bicarbonate, or both) per 100 mL of formula is recommended.[27] NKF KDOQI pediatric nutrition guidelines also recommend correcting the serum bicarbonate level to at least 22 mmol/L.[12,28]

GH insensitivity/resistance and alterations in the somatotropic hormone axis are significant factors influencing the growth of children with CKD. Typically, growth occurs as a result of the action of IGF-1, a product released from the liver following stimulation by endogenous GH. In children with CKD, serum levels of IGF-1–binding proteins may be increased 7-fold to 10-fold due to a reduction in their renal clearance. The increase in IGF-1–binding proteins decreases the free or bioactive levels of IGF-1 and consequently limits growth despite normal or elevated levels of circulating GH. Additionally, inadequate protein or caloric intake may impair GH's ability to stimulate IGF-1. In this situation, therapeutic doses of recombinant human growth hormone (rhGH) may be given to patients with CKD, resulting in improved height velocity.[27] The NKF KDOQI Clinical Practice Guideline for Nutrition in Children with CKD indicates that children with CKD (including transplant patients) and a height or height velocity standard deviation score (SDS) < –1.88 or height-for-age < 3rd percentile qualify for treatment with rhGH.[2]

A Cochrane review[29] of studies assessing the use of rhGH in children with CKD, including predialysis, dialysis, and transplant patients, indicates that treated children had a significant increase in height SDS and height velocity at 1 year after starting therapy. Potential side effects include slipped capital femoral epiphysis and abnormal bone development if the patient's metabolic status (eg, parathyroid hormone [PTH] level, serum bicarbonate) is not well controlled. Despite the safety and efficacy of the therapy, rhGH is currently used in only a minority of growth-retarded children with CKD, which is especially concerning for those who could benefit the most—young children and those in the early stages of CKD. Some of the reasons for the underutilization of rhGH include family refusal, secondary hyperparathyroidism, financial reasons, and concerns about nonadherence, as reported by Greenbaum et al.[23] Most importantly, the early initiation of rhGH therapy may result in a more optimal final adult height as well as an improved psycho-social status.

Although kidney transplantation may improve the growth of younger children, many older children do not achieve adequate catch-up growth with transplantation alone. The use of a steroid-free immunosuppressive regimen or the introduction of rhGH > 1 year after transplant has been associated with improved posttransplantation growth. Figure 24-1 reviews the process of growth evaluation and rhGH initiation and monitoring, including the essential assessment of nutrition parameters prior to its initiation.[28] A dosage of 0.35 mg/kg/wk is suggested for children with renal disease.

Adequacy of Weight Gain

Weight gain should be monitored often, with the most frequent assessments occurring with infants and toddlers who have CKD. Dry weight should be used when assessing weight parameters (see following text). If poor weight gain occurs, contributing factors should be sought, identified, and corrected. Many patients with CKD have a dietary intake that is compromised, restricted, or both, and in these cases nutrition supplements are required to meet age-appropriate nutrition goals. Oral supplements should be provided first, followed by tube feeding (nasogastric or gastrostomy) if deemed necessary. Infants with advanced CKD typically demonstrate delays in feeding and often require enteral tube-feeding support for an extended period of time.[5] In fact, tube feeding may also provide relief to parents and caretakers concerned about their child's poor intake. Some children may require more aggressive nutrition therapy to help reverse a catabolic state (see Intradialytic Parenteral Nutrition section). It is important to recognize that all infants receiving a substantial portion of their daily nutrition needs by a nonoral route need continued oral stimulation to promote normal oral motor development. As with linear growth, some preliminary evidence suggests intensified and daily HD may be associated with improved weight gain and nutrition status.[24,30,31]

Recent studies have investigated the roles of ghrelin and leptin in the pathogenesis of protein-energy wasting, inflammation, and cardiovascular manifestations in CKD.[32,33] Ghrelin is a peptide hormone that induces appetite and promotes gastric motility. It also has anti-inflammatory properties and reduces oxidative stress, showing beneficial cardiac effects. Leptin is an anorexigenic hormone produced in adipose tissues. It suppresses food intake. Low levels of ghrelin and high levels of leptin have been found in patients with CKD. This is mainly thought to be due to the decreased renal clearance of leptin and other anorexic hormones without a compensatory increase in ghrelin and other orexigenic hormones.[32] Consequently, CKD patients are at an increased risk for an imbalance of these hormones and their protein-energy wasting effects. More research is needed to investigate the use of supplementing ghrelin in patients with CKD to reverse these effects.

Nutrition Assessment

No single measurement adequately defines nutrition status in patients with CKD.[3,5] It is challenging to assess this population due to the metabolic and growth complexities that are present. Early nutrition intervention may be critical in optimizing growth and development. NKF KDOQI recommends routine monitoring of the following parameters in children with CKD.[2] The recommended frequency of assessment can be found in the NKF KDOQI guidelines. A table including NKF KDOQI guidelines and recent updates are included as follows.

- *Dry weight*: Dry weight is the patient's weight at a euvolemic state. Dry weight should be assessed regularly and used when assessing growth, including weight-for-age, and body mass index (BMI)-for-age. In oliguric or anuric patients who receive chronic dialysis, fluid overload will influence weight as well as other anthropometric measures such as head circumference and mid-arm circumference. Fluid overload is the most common source of error in measuring anthropometric data in this population.[34] In other renal diseases in which urine-concentrating capacity is impaired and volume depletion is common, dry weight is equally important in assessing growth. World Health Organization (WHO) growth charts should be used to plot patients < 2 years of age, and Centers for Disease Control and Prevention (CDC) for patients > 2 years of age. In addition, z scores should be included in assessment to better track growth below the normal distribution.

- *Length/height*: Length or height should be regularly measured. Length-for-age and height-for-age trends are a reflection of the chronic nutrition status. Height velocity can be assessed using reference data from the Fels Longitudinal Study.[34] This can be assessed at 6-month intervals. As with dry weight, WHO and CDC charts should be used as appropriate for age, and z scores provide additional assessment for outliers.

- *Weight-for-length*: This calculation is used for children < 2 years to assess weight-to-length proportion using the WHO growth charts. For assessment of those outside of the typical weight/length distribution range, z scores may be used. BMI for age should be used in children > 2 years old.

- *BMI-for-age*: BMI should be used in patients with kidney disease as in part of the assessment of the healthy pediatric population. Dry weight should be used when calculating BMI-for-age. Because a predisposition for stunted growth and developmental delays accompanies

CKD, BMI-for-height age (the age at which height is at the 50th percentile) may be more appropriate in assessing BMI and ideal body weight. Using chronological age to assess BMI and ideal body weight may actually overestimate ideal body weight.[35] Studies have shown a U-shaped curve in BMI-for-age vs mortality risk, meaning that both very high and very low BMIs are associated with an increased risk of mortality in pediatric patients with kidney disease.[36]

- *Head circumference*: As described in the nutrition assessment chapter, regular measurements should be taken through 3 years of age and plotted on the 2006 WHO head circumference-for-age curve.[2] Any variance not associated with a comorbidity, in which large or small head size is expected, should be noted, including z score.

- *Dietary intake*: Dietary intake should be assessed regularly. A 3-day food diary or three 24-hour diet recalls with at least 1 weekend day are acceptable methods to measure intake. Both have limitations, but they can be useful in gaining a better understanding of actual intake patterns and eating behaviors.[2]

- *Serum albumin*: The 2000 NKF KDOQI pediatric nutrition guidelines include serum albumin as a marker of nutrition status.[2] However, recent studies and the 2009 nutrition guidelines highlight the limitations of using serum albumin in this manner because of its long half-life and the dilutional effect of excess fluid. Also, lower levels are often a manifestation of inflammation.[2,37] Therefore, serum albumin may be used as a nutrition status marker, but with caution and recognition of its limitations.[35]

- *Normalized protein catabolic rate (nPCR)*: The 2009 NKF KDOQI nutrition guidelines[2] include recommendations on monitoring nPCR for children on HD. The primary biochemical marker of nutrition status has historically been albumin. However, nPCR has been shown to be a superior marker of nutrition status in children on maintenance HD compared to albumin.[5,38,39] These studies show serum albumin to be a poor indicator of nutrition status. A nPCR of <1 g/kg/d is a strong predictor of weight loss in adolescent patients.[39]

The nPCR is a specific renal marker and involves calculation. The protein catabolic rate (PCR) is a measure of protein intake. The nPCR is the PCR normalized to a function of body weight, measured in grams of protein per kilogram per day. New evidence suggests that a 3-point nPCR measurement is a superior method of calculating nPCR.[40] This method, however, requires a computer algorithm to measure and may not be feasible or accessible to a clinician.

In this case, the calculation below is appropriate. nPCR is determined by first calculating the urea generation rate (G):

$$G \text{ (mg/min)} = [(C_2 \times V_2) - (C_1 \times V_1)]/t$$

where

C_2 = predialysis blood urea nitrogen (BUN) (mg/dL)
C_1 = postdialysis BUN
V_2 = predialysis total body water (dL; V_2 = 5.8 dL/kg × predialysis weight in kg)
V_1 = postdialysis total body water (dL; V_1 = 5.8 dL × postdialysis weight in kg)
 t = time (minutes) from end of the dialysis treatment to the beginning of next treatment.

Then, using a modified Borah equation, nPCR is calculated:

$$\text{nPCR (g/kg/d)} = 5.43 \times \text{est } G/V_1 + 0.17$$

where

V_1 = postdialysis total body water (L; V_1 = 0.58 × postdialysis weight in kg)

Similar to nPCR in HD, protein equivalent of nitrogen appearance (PNA) has been recommended to assess dietary protein intake in adults receiving PD. In adults, PNA is calculated by measuring urea nitrogen content of both urine and dialysate and then multiplying the result by 6.25; the same calculation, but with a modification, is used for pediatrics. However, it is only valid when the patient is not anabolic or catabolic and can have great variability.[2] Protein metabolism is age dependent, with younger children having greater differences. Due to these factors and limited pediatric data, PNA is not routinely performed in pediatric patients.[41]

Specifics on nutrition assessment (Table 24-3) are included in the chapter on nutrition assessment (Chapter 32). Unless specifically described, the calculation and assessment of these measurements apply to patients with renal disease as well as other populations.

Nutrition Requirements

Macronutrients

ENERGY

According to the 2009 NKF KDOQI Clinical Practice Guideline for Nutrition in Children with CKD, the energy requirements for CKD stages 3–5 should be the estimated energy requirements, with an adjustment for physical activ-

Table 24-3. Nutrition Assessment[2,34–36]

CATEGORIES OF ASSESSMENT	FACTORS
Anthropometrics	• Dry (target) weight and weight-for-age percentile • Length-for-age or height-for-age percentile • Length-for-age or height velocity-for-age percentile • Weight/length percentile (for <2 y) • BMI-for-age percentile (for ≥2 y)[a] • Ideal body weight[a] • Head circumference-for-age percentile (for <3 y)
Medical history	• Assess for conditions relevant to nutrition status and care • Psychological and social factors affecting nutrition
Intake assessment tools	• Food diary for 3 d • Diet recall: 24-h recall for 3 d
Laboratory tests	• Electrolytes: Na, K, Cl, bicarbonate • Minerals: Ca, Phos, Mg • Glucose • Lipids: triglycerides, cholesterol • Renal function: BUN, Cr ○ For ESKD, Kt/V for adequacy of dialysis • Malnutrition signs: nPCR (HD), ↑CRP, proteinuria
Fluid status	• Blood pressure • Urine output • I/O • HD: noninvasive monitoring, intradialytic weight gain • Bioimpedance
Medications	• Assess for medications that may influence nutrition parameters

BMI, body mass index; BUN, blood urea nitrogen; Cr, creatinine; CRP, C-reactive protein; ESKD, end-stage kidney disease; HD, hemodialysis; I/O, input/output; Kt/V, K is dialyzer clearance of urea, t is dialysis time, V is volume of urea distribution; nPCR, normalized protein catabolic rate.
[a]BMI-for-height age percentile and ideal weight based on BMI-for-height age may be more appropriate.

ity and body size.[2] No evidence exists to suggest that patients with CKD stages 3–5 have higher energy needs compared to healthy controls. However, these patients need regular assessments to adjust for inappropriate weight gain or loss. If energy needs cannot be met with regular solid food intake, consider oral supplementation with a product that meets electrolyte, mineral, and/or fluid restrictions. Supplementation can include modulars of glucose polymers, protein, or fat if necessary to meet nutrition needs. A balance of calories from all 3 macronutrients—carbohydrate, protein, and fat—is desirable.

Children receiving PD typically have a poor energy intake, often taking in <75% of needs.[42] Clinical practice indicates that children on HD also often have a deficient energy intake. Even after glucose calories derived from the dialysis fluid are accounted for, energy intake is still often insufficient. Additionally, malnutrition has been found to be common in pediatric PD patients as well as the more recently described phenomenon of protein-energy wasting, which involves loss of lean body mass with normal or elevated fat mass, high basal metabolic rate, and poor nutrition response. This situation may be related to multiple factors, including patients' sense of fullness from PD fluids, delayed gastric emptying, hormonal imbalance, altered macronutrient intake, variation in peritoneal toxin removal, and inability to reach full dialysate prescription.[43]

The recommended range of 45%–65% of energy from carbohydrate and 20%–35% from fat (25%–40% for infants and young children) as set by the Institute of Medicine is acceptable for children with CKD. Because cardiovascular disease (CVD) is a significant and frequent complication of CKD in children, carbohydrate and fat sources should be closely monitored and altered in the setting of dyslipidemia. Diet management of dyslipidemia should include heart-healthy fats such as monounsaturated and polyunsaturated fats rather than saturated or *trans* fats.[44,45] Complex carbohydrates should replace simple sugars. If carbohydrate and fat modulars are needed to increase calories to promote growth while conforming to fluid restrictions, they should be added proportionally to keep the macronutrient content consistent with the base/standard formula. (See Cardiovascular Disease and Lipid Management section for further discussion.)

PROTEIN

Children with CKD may demonstrate a lower dietary protein intake compared to healthy children. If children are unable to consume adequate amounts of protein to meet their needs, protein modulars or concentrated formula may be used. In contrast, if protein intake is high, it may be beneficial to restrict dietary protein intake to 100%–140% of the dietary reference intake (DRI) in children with CKD stage 3 and 100%–120% of the DRI in CKD stages 4 and 5.[2] By restricting protein, phosphorus is also restricted, which may prove beneficial in terms of preventing CVD and helping to control renal osteodystrophy, addressing the so-called chronic kidney disease–mineral bone disorder (CKD-MBD). Because CVD increases mortality and an abnormal calcium and phosphorus balance is a risk factor for CVD (see section on Cardiovascular Disease), regular evaluation of dietary protein intake as a source of excessive phosphorus intake is recommended.

As for the dialysis population, patients on HD may only require 0.1 g/kg/d more than the DRI for protein to account for dialytic losses. PD patients may require 0.15–0.3 g/kg/d more than the DRI to account for losses across the peritoneum during dialysis.[2] Other factors, such as inflammation or recent infection, which may contribute to protein catabolism, should also be considered when making recommendations on protein needs.

Although adequacy of protein intake is important to consider in PD patients because of peritoneal losses, studies show that unlike caloric intake, protein intake is typically adequate in this population. Reduced height, weight, and muscle mass are common findings, although the reduced weight and muscle mass for age may be consistent with overall short stature and size because these patients are often proportional. Many plasma proteins, including albumin, total protein, transferrin, and individual amino acids, are found to be decreased in patients undergoing PD. Although these patients do lose about 7%–10% of protein intake (depending on body surface area) into the dialysis effluent, inadequate caloric intake or uremia can affect amino acid and protein profiles.[42,46] Infants on PD have twice the protein losses per square meter of body surface area than "adult-sized" adolescents[47] and thus may need greater protein supplementation per kilogram. However, it is important not to provide excessive protein intake. Excess protein has been shown to increase body acidity, creating poor bone mineralization. Sometimes patients may have extreme protein losses in urine or through the peritoneum. Increasing protein far above the DRI may just exacerbate further protein loss in these patients and create a high acid load. Use clinical judgment when assessing protein-related laboratory values to determine if added protein will benefit hypoalbuminemic patients. In summary, adequate, but not excessive, amounts of protein are important in this population.[48]

Micronutrients

Children with CKD are at risk for micronutrient deficiencies due to poor intake, poor absorption, abnormal renal metabolism, medication interactions, and dialysis losses. Adequate intake of fat-soluble and water-soluble vitamins, zinc, and copper should be encouraged. Growth and overall health are at risk if these micronutrients are deficient. Supplementation of these vitamins and minerals is necessary if dietary intake is low or if clinical evidence shows a deficiency and/or low blood levels. Because excess losses of water-soluble vitamins are possible during the dialysis procedure, all children with stage 5D CKD (eg, dialysis patients) should take a water-soluble vitamin supplement.[2]

FAT-SOLUBLE VITAMINS

Both dialysis and predialysis patients with significant renal impairment have high retinol levels, despite having a normal intake of vitamin A. This may be because of increased retinol-binding protein levels that are present in patients with CKD. Although elevated retinol levels are not found to be toxic to these patients, supplemental vitamin A is not recommended for patients with renal impairment because long-term elevated levels may lead to eventual liver damage.[49–51]

Vitamin D has a significant and unique role when discussed in the context of CKD. It is well known that vitamin D synthesis from the inactive to active form takes place in the kidney, and patients with CKD typically need supplementation with the active form of vitamin D, calcitriol. As GFR declines, plasma concentrations of 1,25-dihydroxyvitamin D $(1,25-(OH)_2D)$ decline concurrently. There usually is a concurrent increase in the PTH level, inducing secondary hyperparathyroidism.[52] Limitation of dietary phosphorus can improve $1,25-(OH)_2D$ levels, as will be discussed later.[53]

Recent research indicates that dietary or "inactive" vitamin D (25-hydroxyvitamin D) may also have an important role in bone metabolism and prevention of inflammation and CVD in patients with CKD. Low plasma 25-hydroxyvitamin D is an independent and major risk factor for infection and autoimmune diseases, even in healthy children.[54–57] Multiple studies have previously shown that 25-hydroxyvitamin D is often deficient in children with CKD and supplementation may help reduce the incidence of secondary hyperparathyroidism.[2,58] As a result, the NKF KDOQI Clinical Practice Guideline for Nutrition in Children with CKD suggests measuring serum 25-hydroxyvitamin D levels at least once per year and supplementing with vitamin D_2 (ergocalciferol) or vitamin D_3 (cholecalciferol) if levels are < 30 ng/mL.[2] Once levels are replete, a maintenance daily supplement of up to 800 IU and yearly assessment of serum levels are appropriate.[2] Work by Dibas and Warady[59] support this recommendation, noting that 78% of 51 pediatric dialysis patients reviewed had low 25-hydroxyvitamin D levels. Older children, longer length of dialysis, and non-Caucasian patients were more likely to be associated with low levels. Sixty percent of these patients had improved to normal vitamin D levels after given a monthly high-dose ergocalciferol treatment for 3 months and then continued on maintenance doses.

Serum vitamin E levels are often elevated in CKD, and vitamin E is not cleared well by dialysis.[51] However, recent evidence suggests that vitamin E may be beneficial in the treatment of anemia. In a single center study of 10 children on HD, patients given 15 mg/kg/d of vitamin E and erythropoietic stimulating agent (ESA) therapy had improved hemoglobin and hematocrit values in comparison to control patients receiving an ESA alone. Vitamin E therapy was also found to reduce oxidative stress and insult. Accordingly, vitamin E supplementation may be beneficial for patients who are anemic,[60] but excessive vitamin E intake is not recommended due to poor renal clearance.

Vitamin K is synthesized by the intestine, and no evidence exists for dialysis losses. Unless a patient is receiving long-term antibiotic therapy, vitamin K supplementation is not needed in children with CKD.[2]

WATER-SOLUBLE VITAMINS

A water-soluble vitamin supplement may be appropriate for children with CKD stages 3–5 if dietary intake and/or laboratory values are low. Low intakes of many water-soluble vitamins are common in patients with CKD, often because of dietary phosphorus restrictions and poor intake due to uremia. Supplementation is recommended for CKD stage 5D due to potential dialysis losses. Adult patients who receive continuous ambulatory peritoneal dialysis have been documented to have low serum levels of vitamin B_1 (thiamin), vitamin B_6 (pyridoxine), folic acid, and vitamin C.[61] Vitamin B_{12} (cyanocobalamin) and B_2 (riboflavin) levels were normal. Low oral intakes of vitamins B_1, B_6, and B_{12} were also noted. Supplementation of water-soluble vitamins produced increased levels of B_6, folic acid, and vitamin C. Similar vitamin losses have been noted in HD patients, with low levels of B12 reported in children on HD.[62] Vitamin C and folic acid levels, while low, have been easily corrected with low-dose supplementation. Vitamin B_6 and vitamin B_1 are typically low, requiring supplementation as well.[61]

Hyperhomocysteinemia is common in children with CKD. However, only a small percentage of these patients have low folate levels, and a smaller percentage have low vitamin B_{12} levels.[63] Treatment with 1 mg of folic acid has been shown to improve homocysteine levels significantly and to increase serum folic acid levels in pediatric patients.[64] Whether decreased morbidity and mortality occur as a result of this therapy is unknown. In fact, a large study of adult patients treated with high-dose folic acid, vitamin B_6, and vitamin B_{12} did demonstrate resultant lower serum homocysteine levels, but no evidence was found of decreased cardiovascular morbidity or mortality. These study results were consistent with studies in the general population regarding cardiovascular risk and homocysteine. High doses of folic acid can potentially mask a vitamin B_{12} deficiency.[65]

Another consideration for folic acid supplementation is to improve erythropoietin-resistant anemia. Five milligrams of folic acid has been found to improve hemoglobin and reduce ESA requirements in pediatric and adolescent HD patients.[66] In light of this evidence, folic acid supplementation is likely beneficial to pediatric patients in moderate doses as part of a standard renal multivitamin supplement.

Although vitamin B_6 losses are minimal in children on PD, intake is typically limited due to poor appetite and dietary restrictions, resulting in low serum levels. One study suggests supplementation of 2 mg/d, but further research would be beneficial.[67]

Intake of vitamin C, like the B vitamins noted above, is often poor in CKD. Vitamin C is also lost through dialysis. Supplementation of vitamin C, as part of a water-soluble vitamin supplement, is recommended for patients with CKD stages 3–5 who are at risk for deficiency and for all patients with CKD stage 5D. However, excess amounts of vitamin C may be detrimental. Ascorbic acid and amino acids are precursors to oxalate. High doses of vitamin C may contribute to higher blood oxalate levels that, along with the reduced oxalate clearance common in advanced CKD/dialysis patients, can contribute to secondary oxalosis. Therefore, it is key to assess predialysis patients for adequate vitamin C intake to determine the need for supplementation. For dialysis patients, supplementation to the DRI or slightly higher is recommended, taking into account dialysis losses.[2,68]

Currently no pediatric renal vitamins are available on the market in the United States. However, many adult-formulated vitamins are appropriate for older children and adolescent patients. The goal is to find a vitamin with a content that is close to or slightly above the DRI for age for the patient in question. Adult preparations of liquid renal vitamins are also available and smaller doses can be titrated to more closely meet the DRI requirements for younger children and infants.[2] Many "adult" renal vitamins provide much more than the DRI for younger children, and supplemented children may consequently have normal or above-normal serum concentrations of vitamins, including thiamin, riboflavin, vitamin B_6, and folic acid. Because these vitamins are water soluble, they are not likely to cause harm.[49,69] Infants may receive more vitamins and minerals than older children due to the use of infant formula.[60] Older children on dialysis who receive nutrition supplementation also have been shown to achieve B vitamin intakes that are more than adequate.[62]

MINERALS

An inadequate intake of zinc and copper is frequently found in patients with CKD due to diet restrictions, dialysis losses, and poor oral intake. Altered zinc metabolism has been noted in chronic renal disease and nephrotic syndrome with low serum levels, especially in the face of proteinuria and uremia.[70] Zinc deficiency can cause impaired wound healing, skin changes, anemia, taste changes, and growth retardation, among other problems. Children on PD have been found to have losses of zinc across the peritoneum with resultant low serum levels. These levels improve with supplementation of zinc.[71] In adult patients, supplementation of zinc not only improves serum levels, but is also associated with reduced oxidative stress.[72] A small, single-center study also found that copper levels may be low in patients with CKD stage 5D due to medication interactions.[73] Thus, assessing both zinc and copper levels on a regular basis (semi-annually) in dialysis patients is suggested. Supplementation to the DRI if low or to therapeutic levels if severely low is recommended.[2] Nondialysis CKD patients should have zinc levels checked if they present with poor dietary intake or show clinical symptoms of zinc deficiency.

Abnormalities of selenium metabolism have also been noted in patients with CKD. In a study of adult HD patients, plasma selenium levels were found to be significantly lower than controls but could be corrected with supplementation.[74] Selenium is involved with the regulation of thyroid function, and low thyrotropin levels and increased triiodothyronine levels were found in these patients. However, there have been no studies of selenium in children with CKD and supplementation is not recommended at this time.[2]

Iron deficiency, which often complicates anemia management, is frequently present in patients with CKD. Poor dietary intake and blood loss from medical procedures can contribute to low serum iron levels.[75] Specific titration of iron supplementation as well as erythropoiesis, which is needed to utilize iron, is outside the scope of this chapter but can be reviewed in NKF KDOQI or KDIGO guidelines. Of note, the practice of pica has been reported in 46% of patients on dialysis, more commonly on HD, and can be related to iron deficiency. The majority of this practice is "soft pica" or chewing on ice, but 13% engage in "hard" pica—eating of items like chalk or dirt.[76]

OTHER ELECTROLYTES OF CONCERN

Magnesium metabolism is often altered in patients with CKD resulting in low ionized levels and high total circulating levels.[77] Typically, serum magnesium levels will be elevated or high-normal in dialysis patients. Symptomatic hypermagnesemia is rare. A recent study looking at adult HD patients determined that elevated serum magnesium levels were consistent with high dietary magnesium intake, notably when magnesium intake exceeded recommended intakes. A high-protein or high-lactose diet, as well as the use of vitamin B_6 supplementation, may increase magnesium absorption in the gut. Some phosphate binders contain magnesium and can be considered safe in the absence of hypermagnesemia.[78]

Other minerals of concern are those that may be impacted by ongoing dialysis treatments. Minerals such as lead, mercury, and cadmium have been noted to be elevated in long-term dialysis patients. Contamination of dialysis fluids may contribute to these mineral abnormalities.[79]

Aluminum has been found to be very harmful to patients with renal impairment, and toxicity has caused severe bone disease and encephalopathy in patients with severe impairment of kidney function. Prevention of excess aluminum intake by choosing non–aluminum-based phosphate binders and avoiding aluminum contamination of dialysate or parenteral solutions is critical.

Fluid and Electrolyte Balance

Fluid and electrolyte restrictions will vary among individuals according to urine output, stage of CKD, primary disease, and serum levels. In patients on dialysis, sodium and fluid control is particularly important to help control blood pressure and decrease the risk for CVD.

Sodium

Sodium is often restricted to help control volume overload and blood pressure. According to the 2005 Dietary Guidelines for Americans older than 2 years, all individuals with HTN should limit sodium intake to ≤1500 mg/d.[80] This is complicated by the environmental cues and peer pressures that promote high sodium intake, especially where fast food is concerned. Stringent sodium restrictions are challenging. A more reasonable sodium restriction of 2000–3000 mg/d may be better accepted and hence adhered to in older children or adolescents. The amount of sodium restriction needed should be based on individual patient parameters such as blood pressure, fluid gains, and nutrition intake. Most sodium in the diet comes from pro-

cessed foods. Therefore, an increased intake of fresh food vs processed or canned foods will decrease dietary sodium intake. Using natural herbs and spices to season foods vs table salt is extremely helpful in reducing sodium content in foods. It is important to educate patients not only on low-sodium foods but also on how to read nutrition facts labels. According to the U.S. Department of Agriculture, foods with <5 mg of sodium per serving are considered sodium or salt free. Foods with <35 mg of sodium per serving are considered very low sodium, and foods with <140 mg of sodium per serving are low sodium.[80] The use of salt substitutes is often contraindicated in CKD patients because potassium chloride is typically substituted for sodium chloride. Potassium chloride can cause hyperkalemia in those at risk for the condition.

In patients with polyuria and salt wasting, adequate hydration and supplementation is crucial to prevent growth retardation. Parekh et al[81] described an intervention of supplementing volume and salt in patients in patients with chronic volume depletion and a negative sodium balance while maintaining normal macronutrient intake to obtain normal linear growth in the treatment group. Salt depletion in infants on PD can also result in hypotension and severe central nervous system–related complications (eg, blindness) necessitating substantial supplementation.[82]

Potassium

Dietary potassium is often restricted in patients with CKD to prevent hyperkalemia, since the ability to excrete potassium is decreased as kidney failure progresses. Hyperkalemia can, in turn, lead to impaired muscle function, including the heart, resulting in cardiac death. When dietary management is not sufficient to keep serum potassium levels acceptable, medication may be necessary to prevent or treat hyperkalemia. It is important to remember that certain medications, such as steroids, nonsteroidal anti-inflammatory drugs, angiotensin-converting enzyme (ACE) inhibitors, and β-blockers, have a drug-nutrient interaction that can result in hyperkalemia. Other medical conditions such as hypoaldosteronism, constipation, acidosis, and rhabdomyolysis may also cause hyperkalemia.[83] Some PD patients may not need to limit potassium and may even need to supplement if they experience high dialysis losses.

Adult patients are typically advised to limit potassium to 2000–3000 mg/d. No direct evidence is available for appropriate amounts for children. However, an extrapolation of the adult recommendation to children is < 30–40 mg/kg/d or 0.8–1 mmol/kg/d. However, for infants and young children, 1–3 mmol/kg/d may be an appropriate place to start.[2] Restriction can be adjusted based on individual tolerance and serum laboratory values.

Bone Mineral Management

Phosphorus

Elevated phosphorus values are well known to be associated with increased PTH levels as early as stage 3 CKD. Elevated PTH levels lead to high bone turnover, increasing risk for bone calcium loss and consequent calcium deposition in organs and small vessels (CKD-MBD) and poor growth. A low intake of dietary phosphorous can help control serum phosphorus and PTH levels. Even when phosphorus levels are normal in the earlier stages of CKD, limiting phosphorus intake can improve PTH values and increase 25-hydroxyvitamin D levels.[53] Supplementation with active vitamin D (calcitriol) is necessary to increase calcium uptake by the gut and further suppress the PTH level to prevent calcium bone loss. The downside of vitamin D therapy is that it also increases phosphorus absorption, typically increasing serum phosphorus levels and fibroblast growth factor 23 (FGF 23) levels.[58,84] Recently, calcimimetic drugs have been used in adult populations to lower PTH levels. These medications have been used in pediatric populations, notably adolescents, with some success, but substantial research is still needed to determine if they are safe for some or all pediatric patients with CKD and elevated PTH levels.[58]

Consequences of excess phosphorus intake in patients with advanced stages of CKD include increased cardiovascular morbidity and mortality. An elevated calcium and phosphorus product can result in calcification of soft tissues and small vessels. In adult patients, a phosphorus level > 6.5 mg/dL is correlated with an increased risk of death.[67] The NKF KDOQI Clinical Practice Guidelines for Bone Metabolism and Disease in Children With Chronic Kidney Disease[85] recommend that serum phosphorus levels should be maintained within age-appropriate reference ranges for CKD stages 1–4, and between 4 and 6 mg/dL for ages 1–2 years and 3.5–5.5 mg/dL for adolescents for CKD stage 5 and 5D. The NKF KDOQI Nutrition guidelines[2] recommend normal values for age, but this may be difficult to achieve without the risk of inadequate caloric intake in anuric patients. In contrast to the situation with elevated phosphorus levels, hypophosphatemia can also arise, most commonly due to phosphate wasting disorders or overcorrection of high levels. This too should be addressed as hypophosphatemia can be associated with bone abnormalities and poor growth.

The 2005 NKF KDOQI pediatric bone guidelines, supported by the 2009 nutrition guidelines suggest that when PTH levels are elevated for the given stage of CKD, dietary phosphorus should be limited to the DRI for age. When phosphorus values and PTH values exceed reference ranges for age and stage of CKD, phosphorus should be limited to 80% of the DRI.[2,85] However, this recommendation can equate to a low phosphorus intake in children younger than age 8. It should be noted that < 500 mg of phosphorus, even in young children, may not allow for adequate caloric intake. The exception are children who get a controlled amount of phosphorus via a set amount of enteral formula by mouth or feeding tube. Overrestriction of protein-rich foods in an effort to control serum phosphorus levels may also lead to protein-energy wasting.[86]

Limiting phosphorus in the pediatric diet may be a challenge, especially because fast food and convenience food increases with age in the usual diet of children and adolescents. Foods high in protein typically contribute the most phosphorus in a natural diet, with dairy and meats, including fish, providing 20%–30% each of the usual daily intake. These numbers are increasing as more instant and processed foods and colas, all of which have phosphate additives, are on the market. Foods made with phosphate additives are characterized by almost 100% absorption of their phosphate content. Foods with phosphate additives are nearly 70% higher in phosphorus than the same "natural" food product of equal size.[87] The differences in these products are not accounted for in standard nutrition databases.[88] Estimates are that these foods could additionally contribute to dietary phosphorus intake by about 1 g/d, even with unchanged protein and calcium intakes.[89] This, coupled with the great variation of phosphorus content between products, makes it difficult to estimate phosphorus content of foods and to advise patients who need to limit dietary phosphorus. Despite the challenge associated with the increase in processed foods with phosphate additives on the market as it relates to controlling the phosphorus intake, evidence suggests that intensified education regarding phosphorus management does increase knowledge of phosphate-containing foods in patients and their families.[90]

A common treatment for elevated serum phosphate levels in addition to dietary modification is the use of phosphorus binders. These medications induce excretion of phosphorus through fecal elimination when taken with food and formula. Frequently used phosphorus binders include calcium-based binders, notably calcium carbonate (Tums, Calcarb, or others) and calcium acetate (Phoslo), and non–calcium-based binders including sevelamer carbonate (Renvela) and lanthanum carbonate (Fosrenol). Lanthanum carbonate is not recommended for pediatric patients at this time. Sevelamer has been shown to be as effective as calcium-based binders, and because it does not contribute to calcium intake, it is much less likely to result in increased serum calcium levels.[91] The NKF KDOQI guidelines[2] recommend that phosphorus binders should be used when the serum phosphorus level is elevated and does not normalize with dietary restriction alone. The guidelines also recommend that calcium-based binders should be the initial therapy in infants and young children, but non–calcium-based binders (eg, sevelamer) may be used if further correction of hyperphosphatemia is needed, especially if serum calcium levels are elevated.[85] Either type of binder may be used in adolescents. Calcium acetate has a higher binding capacity than calcium carbonate. Forty-five milligrams of phosphorus is bound by 667 mg of calcium acetate as opposed to 39 mg of phosphorus per 1250 mg of calcium carbonate. Twenty-five percent of calcium is absorbed from calcium acetate vs 40% from calcium carbonate, resulting in a lower calcium load from calcium acetate.[92]

Adherence to binder use is often poor in children, especially in adolescents. A novel approach to manage adherence to binder therapy focuses on patient empowerment. Children and adolescents who are taught binder self-management, which includes adjusting the dose to the estimated amount of phosphorus consumed, may demonstrate greater adherence levels and consequently improved phosphorus values.[93]

Factors such as residual kidney function and dialysis also play a large role in determining serum phosphorus levels. If serum creatinine levels are higher, patients typically have less phosphorus losses through urine and dialysis. High transporters receiving PD also enjoy greater phosphorus clearance than patients who are low or average transporters.[94] Increased dialysis time also improves phosphorus clearance. Patients receiving nocturnal HD, which is typically 6–10 hours nightly while they sleep, typically have twice the phosphorus clearance of patients who receive standard 3 times per week HD.[95]

FGF 23 is a newly discovered hormone that has received recent attention in the CKD population because it may be elevated as early as CKD stage 2 in association with impaired phosphorus excretion. A large study involving 464 children in the Chronic Kidney Disease in Children (CKiD) study demonstrated this because FGF 23 values increased as CKD progressed. However, FGF 23 levels were elevated in earlier stages of CKD compared to PTH levels and especially serum phosphorus values.[96] This early marker may aid with early dietary intervention and the prevention or delay of associated renal damage. Early intervention may be important; a recent pediatric study including 16 pediatric patients receiving chronic HD showed that increased FGF 23 levels were associated with increased coronary calcification.[97] Phosphate binders may help reduce FGF 23 levels, as they would serum phosphorus levels.[58]

Calcium

Insufficient dietary calcium intake may result in poor bone mineralization. However, excess intake may contribute to an increased risk for CVD. Consequently, close monitoring of the intake of calcium is important for children with CKD. Although at least 100% of the DRI for age is recommended for children with CKD, many sources may contribute to calcium intake and thus increase the risk for the ingestion of an excessive amount. The total elemental calcium intake derived from dietary intake, enteral supplementation, and calcium-based phosphorus binders should not provide more than 200% of the DRI for calcium, or 2500 mg for adolescents in which twice the DRI would slightly exceed 2500 mg.[85]

If intake is inadequate because of poor appetite and dietary restrictions, calcium supplementation is recommended. A supplement should be offered away from mealtime and iron supplements to allow for maximum calcium absorption. Calcium gluconate, lactate, acetate, or carbonate are all reasonable alternatives and should be given in doses ≤ 500 mg elemental calcium at a time for best absorption. As already noted, calcium carbonate (Tums or others) and calcium acetate (Phoslo) are often used as phosphorus binders in children with CKD. Research indicates that use of calcium-based binders may contribute to hypercalcemia and, as mentioned previously, may contribute to the development of soft tissue calcification with organ and small vessel damage. Also as already noted, some calcium-containing binders have less calcium than others and should be considered if calcium load needs to be decreased.

Calcium citrate should not be given because it can increase aluminum absorption. Calcium chloride should also be avoided because it can contribute to metabolic acidosis.[2] If patients are hypocalcemic (< 8.8 mg/dL, corrected calcium value), combined calcium and vitamin D therapy should be considered.[81] Intestinal calcium absorption is suboptimal in patients with CKD, especially as renal failure advances, due to low levels of 1,25-(OH)$_2$D. Higher doses of active vitamin D can decrease the patient's need for calcium supplements.[2] At the same time, the NKF KDOQI pediatric bone guidelines[85] indicate that serum calcium levels should not exceed the norms for age in CKD, and should be on the lower end of normal in ESKD patients.

Elevated serum calcium levels are also a concern. If the serum calcium is elevated and the PTH level is low, bone is not turning over at a rate necessary for proper growth and bone maintenance, a state known as adynamic bone disease. In this case, excessive calcium and vitamin D should be discouraged as calcium is not being incorporated into bone appropriately.[85,98]

Cardiovascular Disease and Lipid Management

CVD is a major cause of mortality contributing to ~40% of patients with CKD, accounting for about 20%–30% of deaths directly.[99,100] Children with ESKD have a 1000-fold higher risk of cardiac death compared to children without ESKD.[99] Additionally, children with CKD are among the American Heart Association's (AHA's) list of high-risk pediatric populations.[45] Traditional risk factors including HTN, left ventricular hypertrophy (LVH), and dyslipidemia are highly prevalent in adult CKD patients. However, recent data show that nontraditional markers or uremic factors are also contributing to CVD in pediatric patients. These factors include abnormal calcium and phosphorus levels, secondary hyperparathyroidism, vascular injury due to vascular calcifications and arteriosclerosis, inflammation, anemia, fluid overload, hyperhomocysteinemia, and proteinuria.[101] CVD risk factors increase in prevalence 2-fold to 4-fold with decreasing GFR. For example, a ~16% prevalence of LVH exists in patients with GFR < 30. Adolescents are at higher risk for CVD than younger children with CKD.

Uncontrolled HTN increases the progression of CKD and is exacerbated by decreased renal function. HTN appears to be the main risk factor for CVD and LVH. The AHA statement recommends the use of ambulatory blood pressure monitoring (ABPM) to verify/validate the diagnosis of HTN.[102] ABPM has been shown to be the superior method of evaluating HTN, identifying target-organ damage, and tailoring antihypertensive medication dosages in pediatrics.[102] Volume and pressure overload contribute to the HTN and LVH present in many children and if uncontrolled, LVH may lead to cardiomyopathy and cardiac failure. Therefore, blood pressure and volume control are needed to help reduce the manifestations of CVD.

Dyslipidemia also occurs in association with the development and progression of CKD. The CKiD study has shown a significant association between dyslipidemia and both lower GFR and nephrotic range proteinuria.[103] Triglyceride levels were also shown to be increased by 8% for every 10 mL/min/1.73 m² decrease in GFR. Increased levels of non–high-density lipoprotein cholesterol and reduced high-density lipoprotein cholesterol were also associated with lower GFR. Elevated triglyceride levels are also associated with increased age and obesity. According to the AHA, treatment of dyslipidemia starts with lifestyle changes consisting of dietary modification and exercise.[44] The NKF KDOQI guidelines do not recommend dietary intervention for dyslipidemia in malnourished children with CKD. However, in well-nourished children, a change to a diet characterized by heart-healthy fat, increased fiber, and a limitation in sugar intake is recommended.[2,45] Pharmacological agents have not proven effective in reducing mortality in this patient population. Research in this area is ongoing.

PD patients are notably at risk because serum triglycerides and cholesterol are often elevated in this population, likely due to dextrose infusion of PD. Younger children (< 10 years of age) often have more lipid abnormalities than older children despite greater CVD risk in adolescents.[42]

Obesity, especially in the posttransplant population, contributes to CVD risk and the development of other risk factors for CVD including dyslipidemia, HTN, and diabetes mellitus. Therefore, weight management is a key component of the nutrition intervention (see Renal Transplant section). Evidence also exists for reverse epidemiology for low serum cholesterol levels, low serum homocysteine levels, and low BMI, suggesting that malnutrition is also a risk factor for CVD.[36,101]

As mentioned previously, a nontraditional risk factor for CVD is abnormal calcium and phosphorus metabolism. Calcifications form in the vessels and soft tissues, including the heart. As many as 60% of pediatric patients on dialysis have soft-tissue calcifications at the time of death (see Phosphorus and Calcium sections).[104]

Inflammation is another nontraditional risk factor that appears to contribute to CVD risk. Systemic inflammation is often characterized by elevated serum C-reactive protein (CRP) levels. Evidence suggests an elevated CRP level is associated with cardiac morbidity and mortality in CKD patients.[105] Causes of inflammation include the presence of uremic toxins increasing oxidative stress, chronic infections, increased presence of proinflammatory cytokines, and abnormal calcium and phosphorus metabolism.[106]

Finally, a syndrome known as MIA (malnutrition, inflammation, and atherosclerosis syndrome) is thought to be one of the main causes of mortality in adults. This syndrome is based on evidence of a strong link between these 3 factors and an increased risk of mortality in CKD patients.[105] Recent pediatric studies suggest MIA may contribute to cardiac calcifications and hence, greater CVD risk[107]; however, more studies in this area are needed.

Renal Transplant

The ultimate medical goal for children with ESKD is renal transplantation, either from a living or a deceased organ donor. However, transplantation is considered a treatment modality and not a cure for CKD. Children who have received a renal transplant are still considered to have CKD. Unfortunately, until advances in medicine provide improved medication treatment or alternatives to human organs, slow deterioration of a renal transplant is probable. Close attention to the nutrition and overall health care of the transplant recipient is often paramount to the longevity of the transplanted kidney.

General Issues of Concern

CVD is not only a significant risk for morbidity and mortality in pediatric and young adult ESKD patients, but it is also more prevalent in kidney transplant patients than in the general population. Whereas the reduction of many risks for CVD, infection, and psychosocial issues compared to patients on dialysis typically makes transplant the more desirable alternative for renal replacement therapy, continued or new risks such as hyperlipidemia, hyperhomocysteinemia, inflammation, malnutrition, anemia, and hyperglycemia or insulin resistance can all occur in the transplant patient. These are factors that may contribute to the development or continuation of CVD in this population.

Several medications used for immunosuppression are associated with potential side effects that can be damaging to the kidney and to the overall health of the transplant recipient. Although many centers have developed protocols that minimize corticosteroid usage, these medications are still frequently used in transplant recipients and are well known to adversely impact growth, bone health, lipid and glycemic control, and blood pressure. Additional adverse effects of corticosteroids include increased appetite leading to weight gain, peptic ulcer disease, osteoporosis, muscle wasting, and an increased risk of infection. Calcineurin inhibitors such as cyclosporine and tacrolimus can cause hy-

perglycemia, hypomagnesemia, hyperkalemia, HTN, and nephrotoxicity. T-cell receptor (mTOR) inhibitors such as sirolimus have additional potential side effects, including hypertriglyceridemia, hypercholesterolemia, diarrhea, delayed wound healing, and mouth ulcers. The use of antiproliferative agents such as mycophenolate mofetil and azathioprine may result in gastrointestinal (GI) side effects such as nausea and diarrhea, sore throat, or altered taste acuity.[108] A clinician must be aware of these potential side effects and work with the patient to minimize the medication-related complications as part of the strategy to optimize the nutrition management. NKF KDOQI guidelines[2] provide a more extensive review of immunosuppressive medication side effects.

Since transplant patients are immunosuppressed, food safety and hygiene are especially important for this patient population. Foods such as nonheated lunch meat, which carries a listeria risk, or the consumption of food items containing raw eggs and consequently a risk of salmonella are potentially dangerous, despite the commonality of their consumption in the general population. Not only are many transplant patients on medications that lower gastric pH to treat GI reflux and related conditions, which reduces natural resistance to food-borne pathogens, but symptoms of food-borne illness can interfere with critical anti-rejection medication absorption or administration. In turn, education about food safety practices is important, especially during those times when patients are receiving the highest doses of immunosuppressive therapy.[2]

Of note, some practitioners may be caring for the kidney donor when living donation takes place. Although no specific nutrition regimen is recommended for organ donors, the donor should be aware of the positive impact that proper nutrition has on healing. In the long term, kidney donors should ideally limit dietary sodium intake to help prevent future HTN. Their diet should also be characterized by moderate protein intake, adequate fluid intake, and adequate micronutrients and fiber. They should also strive to maintain a healthy weight because being overweight or obese can contribute to future kidney disease.[109]

Growth

Although growth may improve posttransplant, pediatric transplant recipients should undergo frequent growth assessment followed by intervention as deemed appropriate. The KDIGO transplant guidelines recommend monitoring at intervals of at least every 3 months for weight, length, and head circumference for children younger than age 3 and at least every 6 months for weight, height, and BMI for children aged 3 or older.[110]

rhGH is approved for and appropriate to treat slow growth post transplant if the impaired growth persists despite the provision of adequate nutrition, the correction of acidosis or salt depletion, and minimization of the dosages of medications associated with poor growth velocity (eg, corticosteroids, sirolimus). A very small concern exists for greater rejection risk with rhGH use in patients who have had multiple prior rejection episodes.[111,112]

Rapid weight gain and obesity are common post transplant. Although transplant medications such as tacrolimus and especially corticosteroids may increase appetite and encourage weight gain, other factors have been speculated as contributors as well, including relaxation of dietary restrictions, improved appetite, and reduced feelings of malaise. Although some patients continue to exhibit a poor appetite and struggle to gain adequate weight, the majority reach or exceed an appropriate weight and/or rate of weight gain post transplant. Dietary counseling should focus on a healthy diet with appropriate caloric intake,[2] and a weight reduction program should be offered to all obese patients.[110] Historically, concern has existed that supplemental tube feedings initiated prior to transplant might contribute to obesity in the posttransplant period. A recent study discredited this notion, finding that tube-fed children had no greater rates of obesity post transplant than their non–tube-fed counterparts.[113]

Because obesity is so prevalent post transplant, metabolic syndrome is a significant concern for this population. It has been estimated that as many as 38% of posttransplant adolescents may have metabolic syndrome. Weight loss, reduced caloric intake, sugar reduction (specifically, decreased fructose intake), and increased physical activity, focusing on aerobic activity, are recommended treatments to combat metabolic syndrome. Although medications can be effective, diet and lifestyle changes are considered the most effective treatments.[114] Regular screening for diabetes is also recommended in the group of patients.[110]

Concerns for protection of the transplanted kidney may limit involvement in sports or similar activities. Patients may also have a history of lethargy and malaise from CKD and/or dialysis. Consequently, physical inactivity is common. However, physical activity and achieving appropriate muscle mass are important for the transplant patient, especially given higher risks for CVD, obesity, and HTN and thus should be encouraged and monitored.[115]

Macronutrient Needs

NKF KDOQI nutrition guidelines[2] recommend that pediatric transplant recipients have macronutrient intakes consistent with the acceptable macronutrient distribution ranges for the general population, including a balance of carbohydrates, fats, and proteins. However, a focus on healthy fats and carbohydrates is emphasized.[2]

Transplant patients should be advised to limit concentrated sweets, especially when immunosuppressive medication dosages are highest, such as soon after transplant or when treating transplant rejection. Unless patients are underweight, water and other fluids low in calories and simple sugars are recommended to control weight gain, limit hyperglycemia, and promote good dental health.

In the setting of prevalent cardiovascular risk, a diet low in saturated and *trans* fat is recommended.[2] Hyperlipidemia can be treated with diet modification (eg, increase in polyunsaturated fats and decrease in saturated fat) and medication. The use of 3–4 g of ω-3 fatty acids daily or at least 2 servings of fatty fish weekly may also lower triglyceride and cholesterol levels.[110,116]

Although no definitive evidence supports limiting dietary protein post transplant, it is prudent to avoid high-protein diets and to discourage protein supplements beyond protein needs for age, given the concerns regarding the long-term viability of the transplanted kidney. At the same time, adequate protein intake is important for healing immediately following the transplant procedure.[2]

Micronutrient Needs

Subsequent to receiving a kidney transplant, patients often need to continue to limit their dietary sodium intake to prevent or control HTN. Intakes below the upper limit for age are appropriate, with adjustment as needed based on blood pressure response and kidney function. Measuring blood pressure at every clinic visit is recommended.[110] Infants who receive an adult transplanted kidney may require additional salt to optimize kidney function. Correction of abnormal mineral or electrolyte concentrations is also recommended.[2]

Dietary inclusion of foods containing high magnesium and limitation of foods containing high potassium may be warranted if laboratory values dictate. However, pharmacological management may be necessary, with treatment of hypomagnesemia with magnesium oxide or less frequently gluconate-based magnesium preparations. Persistent or severe hyperkalemia can be treated with medications such as fludrocortisone or with Kayexalate-treated formula for the infant or tube-fed patient.

Adequate intake of calcium is important for bone health, not only because of the potential for transplant medication-related side effects such as osteoporosis but also due to high likeliness of preexisting bone damage. Calcium and vitamin D intakes of at least 100% of the DRI are typically suggested. However, if transplant function has deteriorated such that serum phosphorus and PTH levels are elevated, total elemental calcium intake should not exceed 200% of the DRI, as indicated for other CKD patients at a similar stage.[2] Hypophosphatemia is common post transplant, with approximately 46% of patients needing phosphate supplements within the first 6 months of transplant. This need is thought to be related to elevated PTH levels pretransplant and the function of FGF 23. PTH levels are slow to change, with 69% of patients having elevated PTH values at transplant, 59% at 6 months post transplant, and 47% at 1 year. This situation exacerbates calcium loss from the bone and into the urine, along with phosphorus. Supplementation of calcium is important for bone health especially if dietary intake is limited.[117] As with any other CKD patient, as function of the transplanted kidney declines over time, limiting phosphorus may be necessary and is indicated by laboratory values of phosphorus and PTH.

Some transplant patients may experience issues with iron deficiency and anemia, which mandates treatment similar to other children with CKD. In most cases, vitamin and mineral supplements are not required in the posttransplant population, until transplant kidney function has deteriorated significantly or if the diet is significantly limited. The clinician should regularly assess for dietary adequacy, and supplement to 100% of the DRI for any given vitamin or mineral found to be inadequate.[2]

Fluid Needs

Fluid intake is key for the transplant recipient to ensure adequate perfusion of the transplanted kidney. In pediatric patients, this intake is typically 1.5–4 L/d depending on the size and activity of the child.[118] A recommended intake of 2–3 L is typical for adult-sized adolescents. In young children, including infants and toddlers, adequate fluid intake may be especially important to prevent acute tubular necrosis, graft thrombosis, and graft nonfunction. Transplant success in this age group is best when adult-sized donor kidneys are used. However, due to a child's small heart, blood volume, and blood vessels, meeting the kidney's requirement for a large blood flow may be difficult, resulting in loss of kidney function. One center's experience has indicated that a total daily fluid intake (enteral formula and water orally and via tube feeding) of 2500 mL per body surface area (2500 mL/m²/d) and a sodium intake of 8–10 mEq/kg/d prevented these complications.[119,120] This type of protocol may be necessary for 6 months to 1 year after transplant in the youngest patients.[119]

Acute Kidney Injury

AKI, formerly referred to as acute renal failure, is a temporary condition of kidney dysfunction typically characterized by electrolyte imbalances, an increase in BUN and serum creatinine, and a decrease in urine output.[121] (For further discussion of physiology, refer to the section on Kidney Development and Function.) Although kidney function is usually restored once the etiology of AKI is eliminated or corrected, supportive therapy is required in the interim. Therapy may or may not include temporary dialysis. If dialysis is required, PD, HD, or continuous renal replacement therapy (CRRT) may be used, the specific choice being dependent on specific patient characteristics, clinical status, and the resources of the treatment center. CRRT is chosen by an increasing number of pediatric centers because of the safety and efficacy of the technique, even in patients who are experiencing hemodynamic instability.[121,122]

Nutrition assessment and planning for patients with AKI typically follow the same guidelines as for patients with CKD stage 5D and critical illness. No definitive standards exist for estimating caloric and protein needs in the setting of AKI, either with or without the use of dialysis. Nutrition needs are based on the age-related requirements of the patients, in addition to modifications based on comorbid medical conditions such as sepsis. Hypercatabolism and alterations in metabolism are common in AKI. Some of the alterations of metabolism that occur include decreased protein synthesis, inefficient cellular utilization of protein, altered amino acid pools, hyperglycemia secondary to insulin resistance, lipid alterations caused by impaired lipolysis, acidosis, and electrolyte imbalances. The primary goal of nutrition therapy in patients with AKI is to prevent catabolism as much as possible. Unfortunately, underfeeding is prevalent in this population, due to concerns of fluid and electrolyte balance, especially when renal replacement therapy is not used, delayed, or insufficient. Inadequate protein intake is especially common, which can lead to increased risk of morbidity and mortality in this compromised group of patients.[123] Use of indirect calorimetry is recommended in this population, given the many variables affecting energy needs.[124]

The patient with AKI and not on dialysis may need more rigid electrolyte and fluid restrictions. If a nutrition supplement is required, use of a renal supplement such as Suplena or Nepro, which is nutrient dense and has a low renal solute load, is recommended. For infants, Similac PM 60/40 is usually the most appropriate choice. Once renal function is restored, a regular diet and/or supplement is appropriate. However, when dialysis is performed, depending on the modality, restrictions may vary (see sections on Continuous Renal Replacement Therapy, Hemodialysis, and Peritoneal Dialysis). Fluid and electrolyte concerns as well as prevention of catabolism take priority in the setting of AKI to more long-term concerns associated with CKD, such as CVD, growth, and renal osteodystrophy that are addressed in the CKD nutrition guidelines.

Continuous Renal Replacement Therapy

CRRT is an umbrella term that includes a variety of continuous therapies including continuous arteriovenous hemofiltration (CAVH), continuous venovenous hemofiltration (CVVH), slow continuous ultrafiltration (SCUF), continuous arteriovenous hemodiafiltration (CAVHDF), continuous venovenous hemodiafiltration (CVVHDF), continuous arteriovenous hemodialysis (CAVHD), and continuous venovenous hemodialysis (CVVHD). CRRT replaces kidney function on a continuous or nearly continuous basis in terms of solute and fluid removal and has been found to increase survival in critically ill children and even infants < 10 kg.[125] Because CRRT is a relatively new technology, little literature exists regarding associated nutrition needs, especially in children.

Consistent with adult studies, EN is the first choice for the route of nutrition support in children receiving CRRT. Because CRRT improves clearance of solutes, phosphorus, potassium, and sodium, these dietary components typically do not need to be limited; in fact, they may need to be supplemented. A renal formula may increase GI complications, such as diarrhea or emesis, due to its high osmolality. A standard tube-feeding formula started at a slow, continuous rate and monitored for tolerance is optimal, even for children on vasoactive and sedative drugs. Gastric emptying can be problematic in patients with renal failure and may be alleviated by using transpyloric feeding.[126]

Caloric needs related to the primary condition should in large part determine caloric needs associated with the use of CRRT. AKI itself is typically not thought to increase caloric needs. Oftentimes CRRT is used to support patients with AKI secondary to conditions such as burns or sepsis in which caloric requirements may be markedly increased. Although dialysis may cause some inaccuracies in measure-

ment of caloric needs due to carbon dioxide removal by the dialysis membrane, indirect calorimetry is still considered the "gold standard" and has been used in studies to determine caloric needs of pediatric patients receiving CRRT.[127]

Protein losses may be very high in patients receiving CRRT. Maxvold et al[127] attempted to assess nitrogen balance and amino acid loss in pediatric patients. In this study, children receiving 120%–130% of indirect calorimetry–predicted resting energy expenditure and 1.5 g/kg protein were in negative nitrogen balance, results that suggested the need for an even greater protein intake. A recent study with adult patients indicated that at least 2.5 g/kg protein may be necessary to achieve a positive nitrogen balance.[128] Thus, protein needs for children receiving CRRT are likely to be at least as high, if not higher because the baseline per kilogram protein needs are greater in children than adults. Studies in both adults and pediatrics demonstrate a 10%–25% loss of amino acids in CRRT via the dialysis filter.[129]

Minimal published studies have assessed the micronutrient needs for children receiving CRRT. However, adult studies indicate micronutrient loss is high in this patient population. A single pediatric study did demonstrate hypophosphatemia in two-thirds of pediatric CRRT patients, and supplementation in replacement or dialysis fluids is safe and efficacious.[130] In general, high losses of trace elements and vitamins, such as selenium, copper, and thiamin, are common. It is speculated that other water-soluble vitamins are lost in a similar fashion.[131,132] Experts recommend doubling the standard trace element preparations for adult patients receiving CRRT plus an additional 100 mg of thiamin and 100 mcg of selenium supplementation.[133] It is likely that additional micronutrient supplementation, proportional to the DRI for age, would also be appropriate for children.

Neonatal Issues

AKI is common in the neonatal intensive care unit and may be of primary origin, such as in the case of congenital renal disease, or secondary to conditions such as sepsis, drug toxicity, obstruction, hypoxia, or respiratory distress.[134] Many of these patients will continue to be treated for CKD.[21,22] Twenty percent of new dialysis cases are reported to be in newborns.[134] Mortality is high (46%) in neonates and low-birth-weight infants with AKI.[135] Dialysis, including PD, CRRT, or less commonly HD, may be used to maintain fluid, acid-base, and electrolyte balance, as well as to remove toxins in the short or long term. It is important to remember that serum laboratory values, such as phosphorus and potassium, may have higher normal limits for neonates than for older infants and children. Strict attention to fluid balance is important because patients may exhibit an exceptionally high urine output due to sodium and fluid-wasting renal disorders, stomas, repeated emesis, or suction. This may necessitate a high fluid intake, consisting of replacing losses and providing maintenance needs. Poor urine output or additional sources of fluids, such as medication drips, may lead to the need for fluid restriction and the need to concentrate formula with additives.[136] Oliguric and anuric infants typically should receive only 25–30 mL/kg/d, with infants < 26 weeks gestational age possibly needing more.[137]

Controlling HTN and edema in this population is important, and maintenance fluid needs are a good starting point, with adjustment based on clinical conditions.[138] Children with high fluid and sodium losses often require sodium supplementation of 1–3 mEq/kg/d.[137] Correction of acidosis with sodium bicarbonate is often necessary,[134] and sodium bicarbonate supplementation of 1–2 mEq/kg/d may be needed to prevent hyperkalemia. If serum potassium levels are high, potassium intake should be limited to 1–2 mEq/kg/d.[137]

It is important to be aware of medications that may affect nutrition in this patient population. Pressors or narcotics may decrease gastric motility and may affect tolerance to enteral feeding. Continuous jejunal or transpyloric feedings may be better tolerated than nasogastric feedings when this occurs. Antihypertensive agents, specifically ACE inhibitors and angiotensin II receptor blockers, can increase serum potassium levels. Diuretics may cause potassium and chloride losses that need to be replaced. Antibiotic therapy may result in the need for vitamin K supplementation, especially because gut flora and vitamin K production may not be established in the neonate.[136]

The energy and protein needs for a neonate with AKI are estimated to be 120 kcal/kg/d and 2.5 g/kg/d, respectively.[136] Another proposed guideline has been 8–12 kcal/cm/d.[137] It is important to provide adequate, but not excessive protein and calorie intake to not only children with AKI, but premature infants in general because inadequate nutrition has been associated with chronic renal damage later in life.[138] Patients on PD may receive some carbohydrate calories from the dialysate solution, whereas the same patient[137] may need greater amounts of protein because of urine and dialysate protein losses. Although the protein-related recommendations are a good starting place, the quantity of protein administered may need to be adjusted based on laboratory values and individual needs. For example, a child with poor urine output not receiving renal replacement therapy will need reduced amounts of protein in contrast to the child receiving continuous dialysis therapy.[136]

Oral intake alone is commonly unable to meet nutrition needs, and tube feeding is a frequently used alternative route to meet nutrition demands. It should be emphasized that neonates who are tube fed should still be encouraged to take at least a portion of their feedings by mouth. Breast milk is the optimal choice and partial breastfeeding or bottle-fed breast milk should be considered. If oral intake is not well tolerated, regular oral stimulation is necessary. If breast milk is not an option, a whey-based formula, especially a low-electrolyte, low-aluminum, and low vitamin A formula, is the next best option. Caloric density of breast milk or formula can be gradually increased from 20 kcal/oz to more than 30 kcal/oz as needed due to volume intolerance or restriction. Typically, this is accomplished with glucose polymers or fat modulars as opposed to volume concentration, to reduce the renal solute load.[136] Some concentration of formula may be acceptable in premature infants with increased needs for calcium and phosphorus for bone accretion, especially if serum phosphate levels are appropriate. However, phosphate retention related to renal failure should be kept in mind. Calcium needs should be closely assessed and supplementation may be needed.[137] However, calcium-based medications and vitamin D that patients with kidney disease may be receiving may increase calcium uptake. Consequently, the need for calcium supplementation may be less compared to what other premature infants need. Increasing formula concentration may not be appropriate even if higher phosphate and calcium load is needed because aluminum and other solute concentrations also increase. If a non–renal-preferred product is used, this may be a greater risk.

Feeding tolerance should be closely monitored. Reflux and delayed gastric emptying are common in patients with renal impairment and should be treated if they are contributing to a suboptimal nutrition status. Treatment options include decreasing concentration of the formula with a slow increase back to the desired concentration, slowing the rate of delivery by using continuous feeds, considering postpyloric feeding access, and possibly adding medications to enhance gastric motility.[136] Bolus feeds, if tolerated, are the most physiologic. Some infants may do best with a combination of bolus feeds during the day and continuous feeds overnight.

In some cases, oral and/or tube feeding cannot meet the nutrition needs of the neonate, mandating the use of parenteral nutrition (PN) support. Glucose monitoring with PN is mandatory, with consideration for the use of an insulin drip if needed to provide adequate carbohydrate calories, while keeping serum glucose levels normal. Use of a neonatal amino acid solution, such as TrophAmine, is appropriate, as is the use of 20% intralipids to provide energy and essential fatty acids. Intravenous fat emulsions (IVFE) are started at 1 g/kg and are then increased to increase caloric intake, but typically not to an amount > 3 g/kg. Triglycerides should be monitored, and IVFE should be advanced only if triglyceride values are < 250 mg/dL. If triglyceride values are > 300 mg/dL, IVFE should be reduced or stopped,[136] although some clinical guidelines would indicate 400 mg/dL as an upper limit. Parenteral solution additives, particularly micronutrients that are cleared by the kidney, should be based on an individual patient's response. Small amounts of potassium in the parenteral solution, especially if the patient is on dialysis, is often appropriate. It is best to start with half the standard amounts or less for neonates without renal impairment. Likewise, the reduction of magnesium and phosphorus in PN to one-third or one-half the normal amount may be wise to decrease the risk of toxicity and still prevent low serum levels. Selenium, chromium, and molybdenum may need to be intermittently given or avoided due to impaired renal clearance. Zinc and copper intakes should remain standard, unless liver impairment is present, in which case copper may need to be limited. In high-output renal failure, additional zinc may be needed and assessing serum values may be beneficial.[134,137] Providing water-soluble vitamins separately, daily, while limiting the quantity of fat-soluble vitamins is most appropriate[136] (see discussion on micronutrients in Chronic Kidney Disease section).

Close follow-up of a neonate with previous or ongoing renal impairment is important, and growth and feeding tolerance should be monitored post discharge. Easy-to-read formula mixing instructions in household measurements, as well as demonstration of mixing is important.[136] Preterm or low-birth-weight infants who experienced AKI may be at particular risk for medical complications later in life, likely due to the loss of renal mass from the early insult or as a result of failure to complete glomerulogenesis.[135] Problems that may occur include high blood pressure and proteinuria associated with a low GFR. Height and weight gains tend to be impaired in these patients and mandate close monitoring/supervision of their nutrition status. Growth goals are the same as for other neonates.

Enteral Nutrition

Inadequate intake is common in children with CKD. Gastroesophageal reflux, medication taste, and uremia, as well as thirst for water instead of formula, may contribute to this problem. Gastroesophageal reflux and delayed gastric emptying can contribute to vomiting, which has been associated with as much as one-third of feedings being lost. Many children also need water and salt supplementation, which may be difficult to achieve completely by means of the oral route.[139] The NKF KDOQI Clinical Practice Guidelines for Nutrition for Children indicate that supplemental nutrition support should be considered in CKD stages 3–5 or 5D to meet energy needs if the child is not growing or gaining weight well. Additionally, although oral intake of an energy-dense diet and/or supplements is the preferred source of nutrition support, it should be followed by tube feeding, if energy needs are not met orally.[2]

The majority of infants and young children who receive PD as treatment for ESKD require supplemental enteral feedings to help achieve adequate growth. Some concern exists that placement/use of a gastrostomy tube may be a risk factor for the development of peritonitis. Peritonitis is the most significant complication of PD and can permanently damage or alter a patient's peritoneal membrane and limit the use of this dialysis modality in the future. Consequently, most experts recommend placement of a percutaneous gastrostomy or an open gastrostomy prior to the initiation of PD, if possible. If a gastrostomy is needed after initiating dialysis, an open gastrostomy, along with antibiotic/antifungal prophylaxis, is associated with a lower risk of peritonitis than a percutaneous gastrostomy placement.[139]

When supplemental feedings are given via tube feeding, intake needs can typically be met in young children. In one study, both caloric and protein needs were met or exceeded in infants and young children receiving gastrostomy feeding, with 61% of needs coming from supplemental feeding.[136] However, whether intake from supplemental feedings, even if meeting estimated nutrition needs, improves height or even weight standard deviation scores in children on dialysis remains controversial.[140,141]

Infant and Toddler Feeding

Frequent nutrition assessment and revision of plan of care is essential for optimal management of the infant and young child with CKD or on dialysis. One dialysis center reported that dietetic contacts, including direct, phone, and patient-related activities such as school or daycare contacts, averaged about 6 per month for children < 5 years of age, as opposed to about 3 per month for children > 5 years of age.[142]

Breast milk, which is low in phosphorus, calcium, and other minerals, is an optimal food source for infants with

CKD. As a second choice, a whey-based formula is most appropriate for this population. Of note, the potential for aluminum toxicity is an important concern for patients with kidney impairment. Breast milk has the lowest content of aluminum, and infants fed breast milk have the lowest serum aluminum levels.[143] Whey-based formulas have the next-lowest aluminum concentration, followed by whey-based formula fortified with carbohydrate and lipid modulars. Preterm formulas are higher in aluminum followed by casein hydrolysate formulas. Consequently, soy and casein hydrolysate formulas are not recommended for children with renal impairment.

As noted in the discussion of neonates, concentrating formula with a reduction of the water to formula ratio is not an ideal approach for patients with CKD due to the electrolyte and renal solute load. Adding fat and carbohydrate modulars as well as protein modulars as needed based upon the protein needs of the infant is the most appropriate way to increase caloric intake or to concentrate the formula density in this population.

Infants often require supplemental tube feeding to meet nutrition needs, as already discussed. Infants may benefit from continuous overnight feeding and bolus feedings during the day.[2,144] Renal wasting disorders such as renal dysplasia are a common cause of renal impairment in this age group, and sodium supplementation using sodium bicarbonate or sodium chloride is often needed.[145] Phosphate additives are also sometimes needed to correct serum phosphate levels in patients who use a low-phosphorus formula.

Introducing solids at age-appropriate times is important, limiting but not avoiding foods that are high in electrolytes or protein, based on the child's underlying renal condition.[2] It is important to offer a wide array of foods, increasing texture gradually and allowing infants to experience food exploration and other good feeding habits such as family mealtimes. Children with CKD may have oral hypersensitivity and exhibit food-aversive behavior, and speech, occupational, or child psychology therapists may aid normal feeding skill advancement. The need for intervention should be identified in a timely manner to prevent more lengthy feeding delays. Even for children who are tube fed, oral stimulation, including nonthreatening contact with food or pacifier use, helps encourage oral development. Oral feeding acceptance should be positively reinforced, while feeding refusal should be ignored. Gradual introduction of oral feeding in children with food aversion is preferred, in contrast to rapidly stopping tube feeding to promote growth

and adequate intake. Many children advance to an oral diet after transplantation, when factors such as uremia, excess thirst, or GI reflux may be reduced.[2,139,144] The latter problem may occur in as many as 70% or more of infants with chronic renal disease and may result in impaired intake, increased feeding refusal, and excess emesis. The potential need for standard reflux precautions, medication, or even surgical intervention (fundoplication) should be assessed in this situation.[146]

Infants and toddlers with severe renal impairment often experience high potassium levels. One method to reduce potassium content of the formula is to treat it with sodium polystyrene sulfonate (Kayexalate). Work by Bunchman et al[147] indicates that adding Kayexalate to formula, allowing it to precipitate for 30 minutes in a refrigerator, and then pouring off the formula from the residue that has settled to the bottom of the container, is an effective way to reduce potassium content of liquid beverages including breast milk and formula. Although potassium content reduces significantly (and calcium and magnesium to lesser degrees), sodium content of the treated formula greatly increases because of the exchange of sodium for potassium. In related experiments, sodium content of the treated liquids increased by an average of 234%. The greatest removal of potassium coupled with the lowest addition of sodium was found to be at the 30-minute time point. This sodium exchange may be of benefit in the infant with wasting disorders and should be taken into account. A recent study validated this technique by assessing the effect on serum potassium in infants given these treated formulas. A 24% reduction in patients' serum potassium levels was demonstrated within 48 hours.[148] Bunchman and colleagues[147] used Kayexalate in the amount of 1 g/mEq of potassium in the formula; however, this approach may overcorrect serum potassium levels if potassium is only moderately elevated. As such, the dose should be adjusted on an individualized basis per patient tolerance and requirement. Another technique to reduce the potassium intake of infants and toddlers is to use an adult renal formula, which typically has a high caloric content compared to the potassium content. Although found to be effective in decreasing the amount of potassium delivered via total amount of formula, concerns with tolerance as reflected by emesis, diarrhea, and reduced intake have been reported.[148,149]

Fewer infants and young children experience elevated serum phosphorus levels. However, for those who do, some data suggest that treating formula or other beverages with Sevelamer or calcium carbonate can effectively lower phosphorus content.[150]

Tube Feeding for Older Children

Older children and adolescents may benefit from tube feeding as well to meet their nutrition needs, but social and cosmetic reasons often prevent initiation of tube feedings in this age group. However, some children who were infants or toddlers with CKD or on dialysis remain on tube feeding past toddler years because of parent and patient desires or when inadequate intake is an issue. In this situation, it may be best to only provide tube feeding overnight to allow for hunger during daytime hours to help advance feeding skills and transition to a completely oral feeding regimen.[2]

Parenteral Nutrition

Malnutrition is caused by multiple factors including anorexia, poor food intake, the catabolic effects of dialysis, and the demands of growth.[5,151] Because of these issues, meeting the needs for catch-up growth can be challenging with oral and enteral supplementation alone. Network 14 data suggest that 4.5%–7.5% of the adult dialysis population has malnutrition to a degree that requires greater nutrition intervention than nutrition counseling, diet liberation, and oral or enteral supplementation can provide.[152]

In the case of mild to severe intolerance of oral or enteral supplements due to GI dysfunction, PN may be necessary to ensure the provision of adequate nutrition. Patients with CKD stage 5 often have a fluid restriction. Hence, this approach to therapy requires central venous access to accommodate the concentrated high osmolar parenteral solutions that are often used.

These guidelines provide general recommendations for patients with CKD or AKI. For specific recommendations for PN for neonates or in association with CRRT, see sections on Neonatal Issues and Continuous Renal Replacement Therapy.

Intradialytic Parenteral Nutrition

Intradialytic parenteral nutrition (IDPN) is a noninvasive method of providing carbohydrate, protein, and lipids to undernourished patients during HD via venous access. It is supplemental to other forms of nutrition, including PN. The main goals of this therapy are to replace nutrients lost during HD, increase dry body weight, prevent further muscle wasting, improve the patient's appetite and strength, increase albumin and nPCR, and decrease hospital admissions.

IDPN is typically composed of a concentrated dextrose and amino acid solution and a separate IVFE.[153] The solution must be formulated based on the patient's needs and tolerance. Concentrated dextrose is used to mini-

mize the amount of free water given but to keep the glucose infusion rate at 5–9 mg/kg/min. While the energy provided may seem minimal, its purpose is to maximize protein utilization. Serum glucose levels must be monitored because of the potential for hyperglycemia. Serum glucose levels should be maintained at <200 mg/dL, using insulin if needed. Because of increased insulin levels, a potential exists for hypokalemia and hypophosphatemia; therefore, serum potassium and phosphorus levels should be monitored as well. Amino acids typically provide about 1.3 g protein per kilogram per treatment. IVFE are given as a 20% intralipid solution. Triglycerides must be monitored before and after the initial IVFE infusion to assure tolerance. If levels increase 50% above the baseline, there may be inadequate clearance of fat, and IVFE should be discontinued.

IDPN has been shown to be an effective and safe treatment for adults on chronic HD with protein-energy malnutrition.[129,152,154,155] The NKF KDOQI nutrition guidelines provide recommendations for its use in children.[2] Intraperitoneal nutrition during PD is another treatment that may be considered, but minimal data support its use, especially in pediatrics.

Nephrotic Syndrome

Nephrotic syndrome (NS) is a combination of symptoms occurring in association with various renal and systemic disorders rather than a single disease. NS is characterized by proteinuria, hypoalbuminemia, hyperlipidemia, anasarca, and oliguria. It is defined by KDIGO as having edema, urine protein ≥ 300 mg/dL or 3+ protein on urine dipstick, and hypoalbuminemia or a serum albumin ≤ 2.5 g/dL.[156] Most children with NS have a renal disorder known as minimal change disease. The cause of minimal change disease is unknown. Whereas most patients will have more than one episode of severe proteinuria, the majority of patients with minimal change disease will outgrow it and not develop permanent kidney damage.[157]

The main treatment goals are to decrease/correct proteinuria and minimize fluid retention. The DRI for age based on ideal body weight is the appropriate standard to be used for energy and protein needs. Although proteinuria and hypoalbuminemia may be present, a high-protein diet is not recommended because it can contribute to further kidney damage. Edema and diuretic therapy make the patient's weight parameters unreliable. Patients are usually sodium and fluid restricted to control edema. As a guide to sodium restriction, a sodium content of 1–2 mEq/kg is used in most circumstances (Table 24-4). Fluids are restricted if a patient is fluid overloaded.[157]

Hyperlipidemia is also commonly present and is secondary to the increased hepatic synthesis of cholesterol, triglycerides, and lipoprotein with concurrent decreased catabolism of lipoproteins and lipase activity. Lipid levels typically return to normal once NS resolves, and diet therapy is not indicated unless the hyperlipidemia persists.

Corticosteroids are the primary medications used to treat NS that is secondary to minimal change disease. From a nutrition perspective, it is important to consider the effects of prolonged corticosteroid use such as growth delay, HTN, obesity, impaired glucose tolerance, and decreased bone mineral density. It is also important to be mindful of drug-nutrient interactions that warrant education.

Table 24-4. General Nutrition Management of Renal Dysfunction

	NEPHROTIC SYNDROME	AKI, NO DIALYSIS	AKI, PD OR HD	AKI, CRRT	CKD (STAGES 3–5)	CKD5, HD	CKD5, PD
Energy[a]	EER for age	EER for age or original disease state	EER for age or original disease state	EER for age or original disease state	EER for age	EER for age	EER for age
Protein	DRI—do not supplement to replace urinary losses	DRI or less per BUN monitoring	DRI with 0.2 g/kg increases for HD, 0.4 g/kg increases for PD	At least 2.5 g/kg or greater	Stage 3: 100%–140% × DRI/kg IBW Stages 4–5: 100%–120% × DRI/kg IBW	DRI + 0.1[b] g/kg IBW	DRI + 0.15–0.3[b] g/kg IBW (dependent on age)
Sodium	1–3 mEq/kg; will vary according to edema or HTN	Will vary; consult with renal/primary team to determine	Will vary; consult with renal/primary team to determine	Typically no restriction; may need electrolyte supplementation	1–3 mEq/kg will vary according to edema or HTN unless sodium wasting	1–3 mEq/kg will vary according to edema or HTN unless sodium wasting	1–3 mEq/kg will vary according to edema or HTN unless sodium wasting
Potassium	Restriction not needed	Tightly limit	Limit		Most will tolerate > 3 mEq/kg/d	1–3 mEq/kg but will vary according to serum levels and age	Generally unrestricted unless low transporter; will need to be monitored
Phosphorus	Restriction not needed	Tightly limit	Limit		Limit to 80%–100% × DRI to keep serum levels WNL		
Fluids	Will vary according to UOP; consult with renal team to determine	Will vary according to UOP; consult with renal team to determine	Will vary according to UOP; consult with renal team to determine.	May need additional replacement fluids	Generally unrestricted	Replace UOP, insensible losses, + UF	Replace UOP, insensible losses, + ~1 L/d
Micronutrients[c]	DRI	Tightly limit fat-soluble vitamins	Limit fat-soluble vitamins	May need supplementation especially selenium and thiamin	100% DRI; supplement water-soluble vitamins if needed	100% DRI. Water-soluble vitamin supplement is recommended.	

AKI, acute kidney injury; BUN, blood urea nitrogen; CKD, chronic kidney disease; CKD5, chronic kidney disease stage 5; CRRT, continuous renal replacement therapy; DRI, dietary reference intake; EER, estimated energy requirement; HD, hemodialysis; HTN, hypertension; IBW, ideal body weight; PD, peritoneal dialysis; UF, ultrafiltration; UOP, urinary output; WNL, within normal limits.

[a]Energy requirements may need to be adjusted for physical activity level and/or based on rate of weight gain or loss.

[b]Protein requirements may need to be adjusted according to dialytic protein and amino acid losses.

[c]DRI typically appropriate unless otherwise noted.

Patients who have steroid-resistant NS may actually have an disease process that is more serious causing the nephrotic syndrome, such as focal segmental glomerulosclerosis, which may progress to ESKD, thus further medical investigation may be needed for patients with steroid-resistant NS. Post transplant, these patients have an increased risk of recurrence of disease.[156]

Congenital Nephrotic Syndrome

Congenital nephrotic syndrome (CNS) is a rare kidney disorder characterized by heavy proteinuria in the first 3 months of life. It may be diagnosed prenatally by amniocentesis. Other characteristics include hypoproteinemia, hyperlipidemia, and edema. The majority of cases are genetic in origin. Most of these cases are due to a podocyte gene mutation such as with CNS of the Finnish type, focal segmental glomerulosclerosis, Pierson's syndrome, and Wilms's tumor. Nongenetic forms are mostly caused by infections such as congenital syphilis, congenital rubella, human immunodeficiency virus, or hepatitis B. Genetic testing is the best method of diagnosing the etiology of CNS. The nutrition management goal, irrespective of the etiology of CNS, is to promote age-appropriate growth and maintain normal electrolyte, mineral, and protein levels. In turn, nutrition management typically includes a hypercaloric diet, a dietary protein intake up to 4 g/kg/d, and calcium and magnesium supplementation. Supplemental vitamins A, D, and E and water-soluble vitamins may also be required. Infant fluid needs are 100–130 mL/kg/d. Most infants have difficulty meeting their nutrition and fluid requirements by mouth alone, and the provision of supplements may be taxing on parents; therefore, supplemental gastric or nasogastric tube feeding is often required.

Edema caused by proteinuria in these patients is often inadequately treated by enteral protein supplements alone. Albumin infusions are often a necessary part of the treatment. Treatment may include a unilateral or bilateral nephrectomy to resolve the problem. However, some centers choose to delay nephrectomies until the child is bigger, ~7–10 kg, to make dialysis and transplant more medically feasible.[158,159]

Nephrolithiasis

Nephrolithiasis refers to kidney stones or calculi within the urinary tract. Calcium and oxalate are the primary components of the most common (50%–75%) kind of stone in all age groups, followed by uric acid stones (10%–20%), struvite (ammonium-magnesium phosphate) stones (5%–10%), and cystine stones (1%–2%). Nephrolithiasis is most common in Caucasians and males. Being overweight, having HTN, and living in a warm climate are additional risk factors for stone formation. Although the majority of stones are primary and idiopathic in nature, a variety of kidney or urinary tract disorders can be associated with the development of stones; they include medullary sponge kidney, distal tubular acidosis, secondary hyperuricemia, and obstructive uropathy. Other disorders such as sarcoidosis, Crohn's disease, thyroid or parathyroid disease, disorders of calcium or vitamin D metabolism, short bowel syndrome, and drug ingestion may contribute to stone formation as well. Nephrolithiasis may lead to CKD with some conditions, such as infection stones and primary hyperoxaluria.[160,161]

Renal stone disease appears to be increasing in pediatric patients. In one center, the overall incidence of kidney stones increased more than 4-fold from the 1990s to the 2000s, with the most significant increase present in children younger than age 10 years. There was a distinct familial tendency for stone formation, and obese children composed 31% of the patients with stones.[152] A more recent study assessed children with hypercalciuric kidney stones and reported that 77% of the population was either at risk for obesity or obese, with 74% having an increased percentage of body fat.[162] However, another recent study has suggested that malnutrition is not uncommon in this population, noting about a 10% incidence of it in association with factors such as stomach pain or other GI symptoms contributing to poor nutrition intake. Malnutrition was more common in younger children.[163]

Hypercalciuria and hypocitraturia are commonly found in pediatric stone formers.[164,165] Changing societal and environmental dietary habits in children, such as increased sodium and animal protein intake, as well as a decreased fruit and vegetable intake, may play a role. Such habits reduce potassium and citrate and increase sodium and acid load in the typical childhood diet. Children who form kidney stones are likely to have repeat kidney stones. However, proper nutrition care is paramount in treatment and may significantly reduce or eliminate recurrence of stone formation (Table 24-5).[160,164]

Fluid intake is an especially important preventive measure for all types of kidney stones. Adequate fluid intake has been shown to almost eliminate supersaturation of stone-forming agents.[165] Urine output, and thus fluid intake, appears to be inadequate in more than half of pediatric patients, based on one center's experience. A urine output of 1 mL/kg/h has been suggested to be adequate to avoid satu-

Table 24-5. Nutrition for Kidney Stone Management[160,161,164–167,169–170]

	INCREASE FLUID (AT LEAST 1 oz/kg)	INCREASE FRUIT AND VEGETABLE INTAKE	LIMIT ACID-BASED FOODS	LIMIT MEATS AND PROTEIN	LIMIT OXALATE	LIMIT SODIUM	DRI CALCIUM INTAKE[a]
Calcium-based stones	X	X	X	X		X	X
Oxalosis or hyperoxaluria with calcium-based stones	X	X	X	X	X	X	X
Uric acid stones	X	X	X	DRI, especially limit purines			
Cystine stones	X	X	X	X		X	
Struvite stones	X						
Other kidney stones	X	?	?	X		?	

DRI, dietary reference intake.

[a]Although DRI calcium intake is appropriate general medical management for general pediatric health, including patients with a variety of kidney stone disorders, avoidance of excessive or inadequate intakes of calcium are especially important with the types of kidney stones noted.

ration of stone components in the urine, thus limiting stone formation.[165] Other recommendations are that the urine output should be as high as 35 mL/kg/d. The 1 mL/kg/h rule can be equated, for practical purposes and taking insensible losses into consideration, to a recommendation of 1 oz/kg of body weight or more per day.[165] Another guideline for fluid intake is 2 L or more for adults or adult-sized adolescents.[167] A more general qualitative guideline is that a child or teen should be encouraged to consume enough fluid so that their urine is nearly colorless.[159,164]

Hypercalciuria and Calcium-Based Stones

Hypercalciuria, or an excessive loss of calcium in the urine, predisposes a patient to calcium-based kidney stones. Hypercalciuria is thought to be both familial and related to environmental factors.[161] In this type of stone disease, calcium typically combines with oxalate or phosphate. Preventing the loss of calcium in the urine is key to reducing the incidence of kidney stone formation. Acid may contribute to this kind of stone formation. Diets high in animal protein can reduce urine citrate and increase the acid load, predisposing bones to calcium loss and to an increase in urinary calcium. Some patients who form calcium-based stones and have hypocitraturia have a higher risk of stones because citrate typically increases the solubility of urine calcium.[166,167] Fruit and vegetable intake has an integral role in addressing some of the risk factors associated with stone disease. Research indicates that increasing fruit and vegetable intake not only increases potassium intake, an important protective factor, but also increases citrate in-

take. Additionally, fruits and vegetables confer an alkali load, reducing the risk of calcium loss and subsequent stone formation.

A high sodium intake is another important risk factor for stone formation. Sodium increases urinary calcium losses and may lower urinary citrate. It may also interfere with the actions of some medications used to treat hypercalciuria.[167] Of interest, although excessive calcium intake is not advised, restriction of calcium can be detrimental to stone-formers. Patients with hypercalciuria have bone calcium loss, and limiting calcium intake can put patients at further risk for poor bone status and limited bone density into adulthood. In fact, low bone mineral density is commonly reported in pediatric stone-formers.[168] Additionally, many calcium-rich foods are high in potassium. Finally, limiting calcium may increase the presence of the stone-forming factor oxalate in the urine, due to decreased availability of calcium to bind with oxalate.[167,169] Potassium citrate may be recommended as a medication if compliance with diet is poor. A high magnesium intake may also be a protective.[160]

Reducing protein intake may also be helpful to prevent these type of kidney stones, but it does not seem to be as critical as a high fluid and potassium intake and a limited dietary sodium intake. Although limiting meat intake may be difficult for some, discouraging a particularly high-protein intake is a minimal goal.[160]

In summary, practical dietary recommendations for hypercalciuria would indicate the need to limit sodium to 2000–2400 mg/d; provide 100% of the DRI for potassium with at least 5 fruits and vegetables, particularly those high in potassium; provide 100% of the DRI for calcium; and provide adequate fluid intake for size and age.

Oxalate

Primary hyperoxaluria is rare and will be discussed further below. However, secondary hyperoxaluria may result from fat malabsorption or idiopathic increased absorption of oxalate. Oxalate intake needs to be restricted in hyperoxaluric stone formers.[167] Hyperoxaluria is rare, reported to be present in only 6% of stone-formers in one pediatric study. Therefore, even though oxalate is part of many hypercalciuric or other types of stones, limiting it does not seem beneficial to the prevention of these type of stones.[165] In fact, limiting oxalate in hypercalcuric patients has not been shown to reduce stone formation in a study of adult patients.[169]

Cystinuria

Cystinuria is an autosomal-recessive disorder and is the cause of about 10% of kidney stones in children. The disorder is related to impaired transport of the amino acids cystine, ornithine, lysine, and arginine. Of these amino acids, cystine is insoluble in the urine, and thus it can cause stone formation. Recurrent stone formation is common without medical management; however, adherence may be poor due to side effects, such as GI intolerance, and lack of treatment efficacy. Cystinuria often leads to renal insufficiency, including ESKD, due to recurrent stone formation. Male patients tend to be more severely affected. In addition to medications, dietary interventions such as a high fluid intake, low-sodium diet, and foods high in alkali, such as fruits and vegetables, and limiting excess protein intake may also be beneficial. A fluid intake of 3 L/d of neutral or alkali beverages is recommended, and ideally, individuals should drink frequently during the day, prior to bedtime, upon waking, and also waking once or twice at night. A 2-g sodium intake has been shown to reduce cystine stone formation. Additionally, limiting protein to the DRI also limits intake of methionine, which is metabolized to cystine. The limitation of protein-rich foods including meat, fish, eggs, soy, and wheat can reduce methionine intake and thus urinary cystine excretion. However, strict protein restriction is not advised in children. Unfortunately, adherence to a low-sodium and lower-protein diet may be poor. High vitamin C intake is controversial in children. In addition, cystinuric patients often produce other types of kidney stones, and excess ascorbic acid may increase oxalate production. In the absence of other types of stones, 3 g of vitamin C has been recommended for adolescents with cystinuria who require this additional therapy.[170]

Other Kidney Stones

Uric acid stones, found in 2%–4% of pediatric stone-formers, are often a consequence of a high purine load. Limitation of animal protein and other high-purine foods should be considered. Meat, including fish, should be reduced to the DRI for protein. Other foods that should be limited include meat extracts such as boullion, meat gravies, cocoa, mushrooms, high-yeast products, peas, and beans. Organ meat should be avoided.[160,167]

Struvite calculi consist of magnesium ammonium phosphate or a calcium phosphorus mix and are often called "infection stones" because they frequently result from urinary tract infections. Unlike other stone diseases, these stones form in an alkali environment and increasing urine acidity may help prevent them. Ascorbic acid is suggested as a treatment.[160]

Other stones include 2,8-dihydroxyadenine calculi, which should be treated with purine restriction, and xanthine stones, which should be treated with an increased fluid intake.[160]

Renal Tubular Disorders

Renal Tubular Acidosis

Renal tubular acidosis (RTA), subtyped as being distal or proximal, can be a primary condition, or secondary as a consequence of another condition such as posterior urethral values (PUV). It is characterized by an inability to acidify urine, and if it is left untreated, growth impairment is common as are nephrolithiasis and nephrocalcinosis (calcium deposits in the kidney). Typical treatment of this condition is alkali therapy.[171] In clinical practice, monitoring for failure to thrive and for renal stone disease is imperative. Metabolic bone disease and bone calcium loss may require nutrition monitoring as well.[160]

Bartter's Syndrome

Bartter's syndrome is an autosomal-recessive disorder with symptoms of poor growth, hypokalemia, and metabolic alkalosis. Gitelman syndrome resembles Bartter's syndrome but is a milder disorder. Some mixed forms of Gitelman syndrome and Bartter's syndrome may result in hypomagnesemia. Lack of sodium, chloride, and water reabsorption causes high urine losses. Chloride loss causes alkalosis and increased potassium wasting. On occasion, calcium absorption is impaired and results in hypercalciuria. Treatment includes replacement of sodium, chloride, potassium, and often magnesium. Monitoring for growth failure is important.[160,172]

Nephrogenic Diabetes Insipidus

Nephrogenic diabetes insipidus (NDI) is typically an X-linked or autosomal-recessive disorder in which impaired water reabsorption occurs in the kidney. It manifests as vomiting, anorexia, failure to thrive, and constipation in young infants. Hypernatremia is common, and aggressive water supplementation is needed. Infants will often need overnight tube feedings to meet fluid and calorie needs because the amount of fluid needed may inhibit adequacy of oral caloric intake. Growth is typically poor, with both weight and linear growth suffering from poor intake and possibly repeated dehydration.[173] Growth and dietary intake should be carefully monitored in this population.[160] The NDI Foundation recommends a sodium intake of 500 mg/d and a potential benefit from a low-protein diet. The goal of this diet is to reduce solute load on the kidneys and thus the amount of urine the kidneys must excrete.[174] The sodium allowance should be adjusted according to the patient's tolerance, growth, and clinical picture, but should be limited as much as possible. In infants, breast milk is ideal because it has a low sodium and protein load and is typically much better tolerated than infant formula.[174]

Other Renal Dysfunction

Oxalosis

Primary hyperoxaluria (type 1) is an autosomal-recessive disorder characterized by a deficiency in glyoxalate aminotransferase. Oxalosis is the final stage of primary hyperoxaluria in which calcium oxalate accumulates in the blood and tissues due to an abundance of oxalate production. Oxalate crystals deposit in the kidneys, and this accumulation, known as nephrocalcinosis, causes progressive renal failure. As renal failure progresses, oxalate accumulates because of the continued excessive production and the impaired renal excretion. While frequent HD can help clear oxalate and attempt to control oxalate deposition, success is often limited and further buildup in the tissues can occur. Oxalate can deposit in the bones, eyes, heart, vessels, and nerves. The optimal treatment is a combined liver-kidney transplant because the defect that results in excessive oxalate production resides in the liver.[175] A kidney transplant alone is not recommended because the liver continues to produce oxalate and can cause renal failure in the transplanted kidney. Typically, treatment during the immediate posttransplantation period will include hyperdilution or hyperdiuresis through superhydration methods to keep the concentration of urine crystals at low levels. A low-oxalate diet is also recommended.

As for secondary causes of oxalosis, excessive vitamin C intake may increase the risk of oxalate stone formation and should be avoided. Secondary hyperoxaluria can also occur in the context of fat malabsorption because unabsorbed fat binds with calcium making it unavailable to bind oxalate. A low-fat diet with an increased calcium intake is recommended. A high fluid intake is important for urine oxalate removal. Potassium citrate, pyridoxine, magnesium citrate, and other medications may be helpful.[160]

Hemolytic Uremic Syndrome and Atypical Hemolytic Uremic Syndrome

Hemolytic uremic syndrome (HUS) is defined as the combination of hemolytic anemia, thrombocytopenia, and AKI.[176,177] Two types of HUS exist: epidemic/postinfection and hereditary. Epidemic HUS, or D+ HUS, is the more common type and is the most common type of AKI in otherwise healthy children, especially those < 4 years old. It is typically preceded by watery or bloody diarrhea. It is usually the result of exposure to a toxin such as *Escherichia coli* or *Shigella dysenteriae* from the consumption of raw/undercooked beef, unpasteurized milk, or contaminated water. Very few affected patients have long-term unfavorable outcomes with epidemic HUS.

The second type of HUS is known as D- HUS, hereditary HUS, or atypical HUS. It is characterized by a variety of different genetic defects in the complement system. The onset of the disease is typically preceded by an event such as an infection or pregnancy that triggers the complement defect. It may occur at any age. In contrast to epidemic HUS, atypical HUS is associated with unfavorable outcomes. Many patients will progress to CKD and possibly ESKD. Recurrence of the disease is common, even posttransplantation. The main treatments for atypical HUS are plasmapheresis and eculizumab. The use of eculizumab to prevent recurrence after transplant has proven to be very successful in children and adults with atypical HUS.[177]

The renal manifestations that occur in either type of HUS can include oligouria or anuria, fluid and electrolyte imbalances, metabolic acidosis, HTN, and tissue catabolism. Dialysis may be required acutely to manage complications. Nutrition should be optimized and adjusted based on renal function and enteral tolerance.

Other

Many other rare renal disorders exist, including phosphate metabolism disorders, cystinosis, Fanconi's syndrome, Liddle syndrome, Gordon syndrome, and others that are too numerous to discuss in this context. These other disorders may be primary renal disorders or renal disease secondary to a systemic disease. In either case, the nutrition needs of these patients should routinely be assessed because of the impact that they have on the growth and development of these children. Close attention to electrolytes and growth are often the primary role of nutrition care in these diseases.

Most causes of kidney disease require the typical monitoring of macronutrient and micronutrient intake for growth and normal laboratory parameters. However, some disease processes do not follow the same pattern. It is important to assess for these special cases to ensure that appropriate nutrition therapy is provided. Table 24-6 summarizes some of the specific concerns. It is important to remember that as kidney disease progresses or urine output decreases, needs may change.

Test Your Knowledge Questions

1. What is the optimal feeding route for children in AKI receiving CRRT who need supplemental nutrition?
   A. Parenteral nutrition
   B. Nasogastric feeding of a "renal" formula
   C. Transpyloric feeding of a standard tube-feeding formula
   D. Nasogastric feeding of a standard tube-feeding formula

Table 24-6. Summary of Nutritional Needs for Common Kidney Conditions[a]

CONDITIONS	ENERGY	PROTEIN	FLUIDS	SODIUM	POTASSIUM	PHOSPHORUS	OTHER
Obstructive uropathy			High	High, salt wasting common			Proteinuria common
Dysplasia	DRI baseline, high needs likely	High needs likely	High	High, salt wasting common			Proteinuria common
FSGS			Restrict when NS occurs				Proteinuria common
Polycystic disease	Low volume, high concentration needed due to volume intolerance						Volume tolerance improved with nephrectomies
Cystinuria			High, polyuria	High, Na wasting	High, K+ wasting	High	High Mg
Congenital NS	High	High	High + IV albumin				Mineral (Ca, Mg) supplements may be needed
Urinary tract anomalies (posterior urethral valves, prune belly, reflux)			High, polyuria common	High, salt wasting common in infants and young children			
Fanconi's syndrome			High, polyuria common	High, Na wasting	High, K+ wasting	High	Mineral supplements may be needed
Bartter's syndrome	High-poor growth common			High-Na wasting	High, K+ wasting		High Mg, high Cl
HUS (post infection)			High	If AKI requiring dialysis, treat per modality			Present with watery diarrhea
Atypical HUS (hereditary)				Treat per symptoms upon presentation and relapses			

AKI, acute kidney injury; DRI, dietary reference intake; HUS, hemolytic uremic syndrome; IV, intravenous; NS, nephrotic syndrome.

[a]Open cells indicate no disease-specific guidelines for that specific nutrition parameter.

2. Which of the following vitamins or minerals may be beneficial to supplement to pediatric patients receiving dialysis treatments?
   A. Vitamin B_6
   B. 25-Hydroxyvitamin D
   C. Folic acid
   D. All of these
3. Which of the following comorbid diseases is responsible for 20%–30% of deaths in CKD patients?
   A. ESKD
   B. Respiratory arrest
   C. CVD
   D. Diabetes mellitus
4. Which of the following statements regarding nPCR is false?
   A. Recent studies show that serum albumin is a better nutrition marker than nPCR.
   B. NKF KDOQI recommends monitoring nPCR in chronic pediatric HD patients.
   C. It is a measure of protein intake in g/kg/d.
   D. nPCR is an algebraic equation.

References

1. Warady BA, Chadha V. Chronic kidney disease in children: the global perspective. *Pediatr Nephrol.* 2007;22:1999–2009.
2. National Kidney Foundation. KDOQI Clinical Practice Guideline for Nutrition in Children with CKD: 2008 update. *Am J Kidney Dis.* 2009;53(suppl 2):S1–S124.
3. Rees L, Shaw V. Nutrition in children with CRF and on dialysis. *Pediatr Nephrol.* 2007;22:1689–1702.
4. Goldstein SL, Baronette S, Gambrell TV, Currier H, Brewer ED. nPCR assessment and IDPN treatment of malnutrition in pediatric hemodialysis patients. *Pediatr Nephrol.* 2002;17:531–534.
5. Brewer ED. Pediatric experience with intradialytic parenteral nutrition and supplemental tube feeding. *Am J Kidney Dis.* 1999;33:205–207.
6. Krause I, Shamir R, Davidovits M, et al. Intradialytic parenteral nutrition in malnourished children treated with hemodialysis. *J Ren Nutr.* 2002;12:55–59.
7. Vanderheyden T, Kumar S, Fisk NM. Fetal renal impairment. *Semin Neonatol.* 2003;8(4):279–289.
8. Paton JB, Fisher DE, DeLannoy CW, Behrman RE. Umbilical blood flow, cardiac output, and organ blood flow in the immature baboon fetus. *Am J Obstet Gynecol.* 1973;117(4):560–566.
9. Bueva A, Guignard JP. Renal function in preterm neonates. *Pediatr Res.* 1994;36(5):572–577.
10. Ceriotti F, Boyd JC, Klein G, et al; IFCC Committee on Reference Intervals and Decision Limits (C-RIDL). Reference intervals for serum creatinine concentrations: assessment of available data for global application [erratum in *Clin Chem.* 2008;54(7):1261]. *Clin Chem.* 2008;54(3):559–566.
11. Lameire N, Van Biesen W, Vanholder R. Acute renal failure. *Lancet.* 2005;365(9457):417–430.
12. National Kidney Foundation. K/DOQI clinical practice guidelines for chronic kidney disease: evaluation, classification and stratification. *Am J Kidney Dis.* 2002;39(2 suppl 1):S1–S266.
13. Kidney Disease Improving Global Outcomes. KDIGO 2012 clinical practice guideline for the evaluation and management of chronic kidney disease. *Kid Int Suppl.* 2013;3(1):S1–S164.
14. North American Pediatric Renal Trials and Collaborative Studies. NAPRTCS 2008 annual report. https://web.emmes.com/study/ped/annlrept/Annual%20Report%20-2008.pdf. Published 2008. Accessed February 2009.
15. Wong CS, Pierce CB, Cole SR, et al; CKiD Investigators. Association of proteinuria with race, cause of chronic kidney disease, and glomerular filtration rate in the Chronic Kidney Disease in Children Study. *Clin J Am Soc Nephrol.* 2009;4(4):812–819.
16. Flynn JT, Mitsnefes M, Pierce C, et al; Chronic Kidney Disease in Children Study Group. Blood pressure in children with chronic kidney disease: report from the Chronic Kidney Disease in Children Study. *Hypertension.* 2009;52(4):631–637.
17. ESCAPE Trial Group; Wuhl E, Trivelli A, Picca S, et al. Strict blood-pressure control and progression of renal failure in children. *N Engl J Med.* 2009;361(17):1639–1650.
18. Fischbach M, Fothergill H, Seuge L, Zaloszyc A. Dialysis strategies to improve growth in children with chronic kidney disease. *J Ren Nutr.* 2011;21(1):43–46.
19. Lacson E Jr, Weiling W, Lester K, Ofsthun N, Lazarus JM, Hakim RM. Outcomes associated with in-center nocturnal hemodialysis from a large multicenter program. *Clin J Am Soc Nephrol.* 2010;5:220–226.
20. Querfeld U, Muller D. A hospital-based intermittent nocturnal hemodialysis program for children and adolescents. *J Pediatr.* 2011;158:95–99.
21. Rees L, Jones H. Nutritional management and growth in children with chronic kidney disease. *Pediatr Nephrol.* 2013;28:527–536.
22. Franke D, Alakan H, Pavičić L, et al. Birth parameters and parenteral height predict growth outcome in children with chronic kidney disease. *Pediatr Nephrol.* 2013;28:2335–2341.
23. Greenbaum LA, Hidalgo G, Chand D, et al. Obstacles to the prescribing of growth hormone in children with chronic kidney disease. *Pediatr Nephrol.* 2008;23:1531–1535.
24. Tom A, McCauley L, Bell L, et al. Growth during maintenance hemodialysis: impact of enhanced nutrition and clearance. *J Pediatr.* 1999;134:464–471.
25. de Carmargo MFC, Henriques CL, Vieira S, Komi S, Leão ER, Nogueira PC. Growth of children with end-stage renal disease undergoing daily hemodialysis. *Pediatr Nephrol.* 2014;29:439–444.
26. Fischbach M, Fothergill H, Seuge L, Zaloszyc A. Dialysis strategies to improve growth in children with chronic renal disease. *J Ren Nutr.* 2011;21(1):43–46.

27. Tonshoff B, Kiepe D, Ciarmatori S. Growth hormone/insulin-like growth factor system in children with chronic renal failure. *Pediatr Nephrol.* 2005;20:279–289.

28. Mahan JD, Warady BA. Assessment and treatment of short stature in pediatric patients with chronic kidney disease: a consensus statement. *Pediatr Nephrol.* 2006;21:917–930.

29. Vimalachandra D, Hodson EM, Willis NS, Craig JC, Cowell C, Knight JF. Growth hormone for children with chronic kidney disease. *Cochrane Database Syst Rev.* 2006;3:CD003264. pub003262.

30. Fischbach M, Terzic J, Menouer S, et al. Intensified and daily hemodialysis in children might improve statural growth. *Pediatr Nephrol.* 2006;21:1746–1752.

31. Hoppe A, von Puttkamer C, Linke U, et al. A hospital-based intermittent nocturnal hemodialysis program for children and adolescents *J Pediatr.* 2011;158(1):95–99.

32. Gunta S, Mak RH. Ghrelin and leptin pathophysiology in chronic kidney disease. *Pediatr Nephrol.* 2013;28:611–616.

33. Suzuki H, Asakawa A, Amitani H, Nakamura N, Inui A. Ghrelin and cachexia in chronic kidney disease. *Pediatr Nephrol.* 2013;28:521–526.

34. Baumgartner RN, Roche AF, Himes JH. Incremental growth tables: supplementary to previously published charts. *Am J Clin Nutr.* 1986;43:711–722.

35. Foster BJ, Leonard MB. Measuring nutritional status in children with chronic kidney disease. *Am J Clin Nutr.* 2004;80:801–814.

36. Wong CS, Gipson DS, Gillen DL, et al. Anthropometric measures and risk of death in children with end-stage renal disease. *Am J Kidney Dis.* 2000;36:811–819.

37. Wong CS, Hingorani S, Gillen DL, et al. Hypoalbuminemia and risk of death in pediatric patients with end-stage renal disease. *Kidney Int.* 2001;61:630–637.

38. Orellana P, Juarez-Congelosi M, Goldstein SL. Intradialytic parenteral nutrition treatment and biochemical marker assessment for malnutrition in adolescent maintenance hemodialysis patients. *J Ren Nutr.* 2005;15:312–317.

39. Juarez-Congelosi M, Orellana P, Goldstein SL. Normalized protein catabolic rate versus serum albumin as a nutrition status marker in pediatric patients receiving hemodialysis. *J Ren Nutr.* 2007;17:269–274.

40. Srivaths PR, Sutherland S, Alexander S, Goldstein SL. Two-point normalized protein catabolic rate overestimates nPCR in pediatric hemodialysis patients. *Pediatr Nephrol.* 2013;28(5):797–801.

41. Mendley SR, Majkowski NL. Urea and nitrogen excretion in pediatric peritoneal dialysis patients. *Kidney Int.* 2000;58:2564–2570.

42. Salusky IB, Fine RN, Nelson P, Blumenkrantz MJ, Kopple JD. Nutritional status of children undergoing continuous ambulatory peritoneal dialysis. *Am J Clin Nutr.* 1983;38:599–611.

43. Paglialonga F, Edefonti A. Nutrition assessment and management in children on peritoneal dialysis. *Pediatr Nephrol.* 2009;24:721–734.

44. Kavey RE, Allada V, Daniels SR, et al; American Heart Association Expert Panel on Population and Prevention Science; American Heart Association Council on Cardiovascular Disease in the Young; American Heart Association Council on Epidemiology and Prevention; American Heart Association Council on Nutrition, Physical Activity and Metabolism; American Heart Association Council on High Blood Pressure Research; American Heart Association Council on Cardiovascular Nursing; American Heart Association Council on the Kidney in Heart Disease; Interdisciplinary Working Group on Quality of Care and Outcomes Research. Cardiovascular risk reduction in high-risk pediatric patients: a scientific statement from the American Heart Association Expert Panel on Population and Prevention Science; the Councils on Cardiovascular Disease in the Young, Epidemiology and Prevention, Nutrition, Physical Activity and Metabolism, High Blood Pressure Research, Cardiovascular Nursing, and the Kidney in Heart Outcomes Research: endorsed by the American Academy of Pediatrics. *Circulation.* 2006;114:2710–2738.

45. American Academy of Pediatrics. Cardiovascular risk reduction in high-risk pediatric populations. *J Pediatr.* 2007;119:618–621.

46. Kaiser BA, Polinsky MS, Stover J, Morgenstern BZ, Baluarte HJ. Growth of children following the initiation of dialysis: a comparison of three dialysis modalities. *Pediatr Nephrol.* 1994;8:733–738.

47. Quan A, Baum M. Protein losses in children on continuous cycler peritoneal dialysis. *Pediatr Nephrol.* 1996;10:728–731.

48. Azocar MA, Cano FJ, Marin V, Delucchi MA, Rodrigues EE. Body composition in children on peritoneal dialysis. *Adv Perit Dial.* 2004;20:231–236.

49. Vannucchi MTI, Vannucchi H, Humphreys M. Serum levels of vitamin A and retinol binding protein in chronic renal patients treated by continuous ambulatorial peritoneal dialysis. *Int J Vitam Nutr Res.* 1992;62:107–112.

50. Kriley M, Warady BA. Vitamin status of pediatric patients receiving long-term peritoneal dialysis. *Am J Clin Nutr.* 1991;53:1476–1479.

51. Blumberg A, Hanck A, Sander G. Vitamin nutrition in patients on continuous ambulatory peritoneal dialysis (CAPD). *Clin Nephrol.* 1983;20(5):244–250.

52. Portale AA, Booth BE, Tsai HC, Morris RC Jr. Reduced plasma concentration of 1,25-dihydroxyvitamin D in children with moderate renal insufficiency. *Kidney Int.* 1982;21:627–632.

53. Portale AA, Booth BE, Halloran BP, Morris RC Jr. Effect of dietary phosphorus on circulating concentrations of 1,25-dihydroxyvitamin D and immunoreactive parathyroid hormone in children with moderate renal insufficiency. *J Clin Invest.* 1984;73:1580–1589.

54. Ghazali A, Fardellone P, Pruna A. Is low plasma 25-(OH) vitamin D a major risk factor for hyperparathyroidism and Looser's zones independent of calcitriol? *Kidney Int.* 1999;55:2169–2177.

55. Wagner CL, Greer FR. Prevention of rickets and vitamin D deficiency in infants, children, and adolescents. *Pediatrics.* 2008;122:1142–1152.

56. Querfeld U. Vitamin D and inflammation. *Pediatr Nephrol.* 2013;28:605–610.

57. Patange AR, Valentini RP, Du W, Pettersen MD. *Pediatr Cardiol.* 2012;33:122–128.

58. Wesseling-Perry K, Salusky IB. Phosphate binders, vitamin D and calcimimetics in the management of chronic kidney disease-mineral bone disorders (CKD-MBD) in children. *Pediatr Nephrol.* 2013;28:617–625.

59. Dibas BI, Warady BA. Vitamin D status of children receiving chronic dialysis. *Pediatr Nephrol.* 2012;27:1967–1973.

60. Nemeth I, Turi S, Haszon I, Bereczki C. Vitamin E alleviates the oxidative stress of erythropoietin in uremic children on hemodialysis. *Pediatr Nephrol.* 2000;14:13–17.

61. Descombes E, Hanck AB, Fellay G. Water soluble vitamins in chronic hemodialysis patients and need for supplementation. *Kidney Int.* 1993;1319–1328.

62. Don T, Friedlander S, Wong W. Dietary intakes and biochemical status of B vitamins in a group of children receiving dialysis. *J Ren Nutr.* 2010;20:23–28.

63. Canepa A, Carrea A, Caridi G, et al. Homocysteine, folate, vitamin B12 levels, and C677T MTHFR mutation in children with renal failure. *Pediatr Nephrol.* 2003;18:225–229.

64. Kang HG, Lee BS, Hahn H, et al. Reduction of plasma homocysteine by folic acid in children with chronic renal failure. *Pediatr Nephrol.* 2002;17:511–514.

65. Sunder-Plassmann G, Winkelmayer WC, Fodinger M. Approaching the end of the homocysteine hype? *Am J Kidney Dis.* 2008;51(4):549–553.

66. Bamgbola OF, Kaskel F. Role of folate deficiency on erythropoietin resistance in pediatric and adolescent patients on chronic dialysis. *Pediatr Nephrol.* 2005;20:1622–1629.

67. Stockberger RA, Parrott KA, Alexander SR, Miller LT, Leklem JE, Jenkins RD. Vitamin B-6 status of children undergoing continuous ambulatory peritoneal dialysis. *Nutr Res.* 1987;7:1021–1030.

68. Rolton HA, McConnell KM, Modi KS, Macdougall AI. The effect of vitamin C intake on plasma oxalate in patients on regular haemodialysis. *Nephrol Dial Transplant.* 1991;6:440–443.

69. Warady BA, Kriley M, Alon U, Hellerstein S. Vitamin status of infants receiving long-term peritoneal dialysis. *Pediatr Nephrol.* 1994;8:354–356.

70. Mahajan SK. Zinc in kidney disease. *J Am Coll Nutr.* 1989;8(4):296–304.

71. Tamura T, Vaughn WH, Waldo FB, Kohaut EC. Zinc and copper balance in children on continuous ambulatory peritoneal dialysis. *Pediatr Nephrol.* 1989;3:309–313.

72. Mazami M, Argani H, Rashtchizadeh N, et al. Effects of zinc supplementation on antioxidant status and lipid peroxidation in hemodialysis patients. *J Ren Nutr.* 2013;23:180–184.

73. Warady BA, Nelms C, Jennings J, Johnson S. Copper deficiency: a common cause of erythropoietin (rHuEPO) resistant anemia in children on hemodialysis? *Hemodial Int.* 2005;9(1):99.

74. Napolitano G, Bonomini M, Bomba G, et al. Thyroid function and plasma selenium in chronic uremic patients on hemodialysis treatment. *Biol Trace Elem Res.* 1996;55:221–230.

75. National Kidney Foundation. K/DOQI clinical practice guidelines and clinical practice recommendations for anemia in chronic kidney disease. *Am J Kidney Dis.* 2006;47(Suppl 3):S1–S146

76. Katsoufis CP, Kertis M, McCullough J, et al. Pica: an important and unrecognized problem in pediatric dialysis patients. *J Ren Nutr.* 2012;22:567–571.

77. Pedrozzi NE, Truttman AC, Faraone R, et al. Circulating ionized and total magnesium in end-stage kidney disease. *Nephron.* 2002;92(3):616–621.

78. Wyskida K, Witkowicz J, Chudek J, Wiecek A. Daily magnesium intake and hypermagnesemia in hemodialysis patients with chronic kidney disease. *J Ren Nutr.* 2012;22:19–26.

79. Skarupskiene I, Kuzminskis V, Bumblyte IA, et al. Changes of trace elements in blood of patients with chronic renal failure. *Dial Transplant.* 2005;34(12):870–880.

80. U.S. Department of Health and Human Services, U.S. Department of Agriculture. *Dietary Guidelines for Americans 2005.* 6th ed. Washington, DC: U.S. Government Printing Office; 2005. http://www.health.gov/DietaryGuidelines/. Accessed December 9, 2008.

81. Parekh RS, Flynn JT, Smoyer WE, et al. Improved growth in young children with severe chronic renal insufficiency who use specified nutritional therapy. *J Am Soc Nephrol.* 2001;12: 2418–2436.

82. Rodriguez-Soriano J, Arant BS. Fluid and electrolyte imbalances in children with chronic renal failure. *Am J Kidney Dis.* 1986;7:268–274.

83. Beto J, Bansal VK. Hyperkalemia: evaluating dietary and nondietary etiology. *J Ren Nutr.* 1992;2(1):28–29.

84. Combe C, Aparicio M. Phosphorus and protein restriction and parathyroid function in chronic renal failure. *Kidney Int.* 1994;46:1381–1386.

85. National Kidney Foundation. Kidney Disease Outcomes Quality Initiative. Clinical practice guidelines for bone metabolism and disease in children with chronic kidney disease. *Am J Kidney Dis.* 2003;42(4 suppl 3):S1–S201.

86. Shinaberger CS, Greenland S, Kopple JD, et al. Is controlling phosphorus by decreasing dietary protein intake beneficial or harmful in persons with chronic kidney disease? *Am J Clin Nutr.* 2008;88:1511–1518.

87. Benini O, D'Alessandro C, Gianfaldoni D, Cupisti A. Extra-phosphate load from food additives in commonly eaten foods: a real and insidious danger for renal patients. *J Ren Nutr.* 2011;21:303–308.

88. Sullivan CM, Leon JB, Sehgal AR. Phosphorus-containing food additives and the accuracy of nutrient databases: implications for renal patients. *J Ren Nutr.* 2007;17(5):350–354.

89. Uribarri J, Calvo MS. Hidden sources of phosphorus in the typical American diet: does it matter in nephrology? *Semin Dial.* 2003;16(3):186–188.

90. Abercrombie EL, Greenbaum LA, Baxter DH, Hopkins BH. Effect of intensified diet education on serum phosphorus and knowledge of pediatric peritoneal dialysis patients. *J Ren Nutr.* 2010;20(3):193–198.

91. Chertow GM, Burke SK, Raggi P. Sevelamer attenuates the progression of coronary and aortic calcification in hemodialysis patients. *Kidney Int.* 2002;62:245–252.

92. Wallot M, Klaus-Eugen B, Winter A, Georger B, Lettgen B, Bald M. Calcium acetate versus calcium carbonate as oral phosphate binder in pediatric and adolescent hemodialysis patients. *Pediatr Nephrol.* 1996;10:625–630.

93. Ahlenstiel T, Pape L, Ehrich JHH, Kuhlmann MK. Self-adjustment of phosphate binder dose to meal phosphorus content improves management of hyperphosphataemia in children with chronic kidney disease. *Nephrol Dial Transplant.* 2010;25:3241–3249.

94. Sedlacek M, Dimaano F, Uribarri J. Relationship between phosphorus and creatinine clearance in peritoneal dialysis: clinical implications. *Am J Kidney Dis.* 2000;36(5):1020–1024.

95. Koolenga L. Phosphorus balance with daily dialysis. *Semin Dial.* 2007;20(4):342–345.

96. Portale AA, Wolf M, Juppner H, et al. Disordered FGF23 and mineral metabolism in children with CKD. *Clin J Am Soc Nephrol.* 2014;9:344–353.

97. Srivaths PR, Goldstein SL, Krishnamurthy R, Silverstein DM. High serum phosphorus and FGF 23 levels are associated with progression of coronary calcifications. *Pediatr Nephrol.* 2014;29:103–109.

98. Kurz P, Monier-Faugere MC, Bognar B, et al. Evidence for abnormal calcium homeostasis in patients with adynamic bone disease. *Kidney Int.* 1994;46:855–561.

99. Parekh RS, Carroll CE, Wolfe RA, Port FK. Cardiovascular mortality in children and young adults with end-stage renal disease. *J Pediatr.* 2002;141:191–197.

100. Lilien MR, Groothoff JW. Cardiovascular disease in children with CKD or ESRD. *Nat Rev Nephrol.* 2009;5:229–235.

101. Mitnefes MM. Cardiovascular complications of pediatric chronic kidney disease. *Pediatr Nephrol.* 2008;23:27–39.

102. Flynn JT, Daniels SR, Hayman LL, et al; American Heart Association Atherosclerosis, Hypertension and Obesity in Youth Committee of the Council on Cardiovascular Disease in the Young. Update: ambulatory blood pressure monitoring in children and adolescents: a scientific statement from the American Heart Association. *Hypertension.* 2014;63(5):1116–1135.

103. Saland J, Pierce CB, Mitsnefes MM, et al; CKiD Investigators. Dysplipidemia in children with chronic kidney disease. *Kid Int.* 2010;78:1154–1164.

104. Milliner DS, Morgenstern BZ, Murphy M, Gonyea J, Steriofff S. Lipid levels following renal transplantation in pediatric recipients. *Transplant Proc.* 1994;26:112–114.

105. Stenvinkel P, Heimbürger O, Paultre F, et al. Strong association between malnutrition, inflammation, and atherosclerosis in chronic renal failure. *Kidney Int.* 1999;55:1899–1911.

106. Sylvestre LC, Fonseca KP, Stinghen AE, Pereira AM, Meneses RP, Pecoits-Filho R. The malnutrition and inflammation axis in pediatric patients with chronic kidney disease. *Pediatr Nephrol.* 2007;22:864–873.

107. Srivaths P, Silverstein DM, Leung J, Krishnamurthy R, Goldstein SL. Malnutrition-inflammation-coronary calcification in pediatric patients receiving chronic hemodialysis. *Hemodial Int.* 2010; 14:263–269.

108. McPartland KJ, Pomposelli JJ. Update on immunosuppressive drugs used in solid-organ transplantation and their nutrition implications. *Nutr Clin Pract.* 2007;22:467–473.

109. Phillips S, DeMello S. Nutrition and the kidney donor. *J Ren Nutr.* 2014;24(2):e15–e17.

110. Kasiske BL, Zeier MG, Chapman JR, et al. KDIGO clinical practice guideline for the care of kidney transplant recipients: a summary. *Kidney Int.* 2010;77:299–311.

111. Wu Y, Cheng W, Yang X, Xiang B. Growth hormone improves growth in pediatric renal transplant recipients—a systemic review and meta-analysis of randomized controlled trials. *Pediatr Nephrol.* 2013;28:129–133.

112. Mehls O, Fine RN. Growth hormone treatment after renal transplantation: a promising but underused chance to improve growth. *Pediatr Nephrol.* 2013;28:1–4.

113. Sienna JL, Saqan R, Teh JC, et al. Body size in children with chronic kidney disease after gastrostomy tube feeding. *Pediatr Nephrol.* 2010;25:2115–2121.

114. Litwin M, Niemirska A. Metabolic syndrome in children with chronic kidney disease and after renal transplantation. *Pediatr Nephrol.* 2014;29:203–216.

115. Hoppe B, Schaar B. The impact of nutrition and physical activity on long-term survival after pediatric solid organ transplantation. *Pediatr Transplant.* 2012;16:675–677.

116. Filler G, Weiglein G, Gharib MT, Casier S. Omega three fatty acids may reduce hyperlipidemia in pediatric renal transplant recipients. *Pediatr Transplant.* 2012;16:835–839.

117. Guzzo I, Di Zazzo G, Laurenzi C, et al. Parathyroid hormone levels in long-term renal transplant children and adolescents. *Pediatr Nephrol.* 2011;26:2051–2057.

118. Fine RN, Webber SA, Olthoff KM, Kelly DA, Harmon WE, eds. *Pediatric Solid Organ Transplantation.* 2nd ed. Oxford, UK: Blackwell Publishing; 2007.

119. Salvatierra O Jr, Singh T, Shifrin R, et al. Successful transplantation of adult-sized kidneys into infants requires maintenance of high aortic blood flow. *Transplantation.* 1998;66:819–823.

120. Salvatierra O Jr, Millan M, Concepcion W. Pediatric renal transplantation with considerations for successful outcomes. *Semin Pediatr Surg.* 2006;15:208–217.

121. Andreoli SP. Acute renal failure. *Pediatrics.* 2002;14:183–188.

122. Star RA. Treatment of acute renal failure. *Kidney Int.* 1998;54:1817–1831.

123. Kyle UG, Akcan-Arikan A, Orellana RA, Coss-Bu JA. Nutrition support among critically ill children with AKI. *Clin J Am Soc Nephrol.* 2013;8:568–574.

124. Basu RK, Devarajan P, Wong H, Wheeler DS. An update and review of acute kidney injury in pediatrics. *Pediatr Crit Care Med.* 2011;12(3):339–347.

125. Symons JM, Brophy PD, Gregory MJ, et al. Continuous renal replacement therapy in children up to 10 kg. *Am J Kidney Dis.* 2003;41(5):984–989.

126. López-Herce J, Sánchez C, Carrillo A, et al. Transpyloric enteral nutrition in the critically ill child with renal failure. *Intensive Care Med.* 2006;32:1599–1605.

127. Maxvold NJ, Smoyer WE, Custer JR, Bunchman TE. Amino acid loss and nitrogen balance in critically ill children with

acute renal failure: a prospective comparison between classic hemofiltration and hemofiltration with dialysis. *Crit Care Med.* 2000;28(4):1161–1165.

128. Scheinkestel F, Adams F, Mahony L, et al. Impact of increasing parenteral protein loads on amino acid levels and balance in critically ill anuric patients on continuous renal replacement therapy. *Nutrition.* 2003;19:733–740.

129. Zappitelli M, Goldstein SL, Symons JM, et al; Prospective Pediatric Continuous Renal Replacement Therapy Registry Group. Protein and calorie prescription for children and young adults receiving continuous renal replacement therapy: a report from the Prospective Pediatric Continuous Renal Replacement Therapy Registry Group. *Pediatr Crit Care Med.* 2008;36:3239–3245.

130. Santiago MJ, López-Herce J, Urbano J, Bellón JM, del Castillo J, Carillo A. Hypophosphatemia and phosphate supplementation during continuous renal replacement therapy in children. *Kidney Int.* 2009;75:312–316.

131. Nakamura AT, Btaiche IF, Pasko DA, Jain JC, Mueller BA. In vitro clearance of trace elements via continuous renal replacement therapy. *J Ren Nutr.* 2004;14(4):214–219.

132. Berger MM, Shenkin A, Revelly JP, et al. Copper, selenium, zinc, and thiamine balances during continuous venovenous hemodiafiltration in critically ill patients. *Am J Clin Nutr.* 2004;80:410.

133. Chioléro R, Berger M. Nutritional support during renal replacement therapy. *Acute Kidney Inj.* 2007;156:267–274.

134. Moghal NE, Embleton ND. Management of acute renal failure in the newborn. *Semin Fetal Neonatal Med.* 2006;11:207–213.

135. Abitbol CL, Bauer CR, Montane B, Chandar J, Duara S, Zilleruelo G. Long-term follow-up of extremely low birth weight infants with neonatal renal failure. *Pediatr Nephrol.* 2003;18:887–893.

136. Spinozzi NS, Nelson P. Nutrition support in the newborn intensive care unit. *J Ren Nutr.* 1996;6(4):188–197.

137. Groh-Wargo S, Thompson M, Hovasi Cox J, eds. *ADA Pocket Guide to Neonatal Nutrition.* Chicago: American Dietetic Association; 2009.

138. Carmody JB, Charlton JR. Short-term gestation, long-term risk: prematurity and chronic kidney disease. *Pediatrics.* 2013;131:1168–1179.

139. Rees L, Brandt ML. Tube feeding in children with chronic kidney disease: technical and practical issues. *Pediatr Nephrol.* 2010;25:699–704.

140. Coleman JE, Watson AR, Rance CH, Moore E. Gastrostomy buttons for nutritional support on chronic dialysis. *Nephrol Dial Transplant.* 1998;13:2041–2046.

141. Ellis EN, Yiu V, Harley F, et al. The impact of supplemental feeding in young children on dialysis: a report of the North American Pediatric Renal Transplant Cooperative Study. *Pediatr Nephrol.* 2001;16:404–408.

142. Coleman JE, Norman LJ, Watson AR. Provision of dietetic care in children on chronic peritoneal dialysis. *J Ren Nutr.* 1999;9(3):145–148.

143. Hawkins NM, Coffey S, Lawson MS, Delves HT. Potential aluminum toxicity in infants fed special infant formula. *J Pediatr Gastroenterol Nutr.* 1994;19:377–381.

144. Warady BA, Kriley M, Belden B, Hellerstein S, Alon U. Nutritional and behavioural aspects of nasogastric tube feeding in infants receiving chronic peritoneal dialysis. *Adv Perit Dial.* 1990;6:265–268.

145. Rodriguez-Soriano J, Arant BS, Brodehl J, Norman ME. Fluid and electrolyte imbalances in children with chronic renal failure. *Am J Kidney Dis.* 1986;7(4):268–274.

146. Ruley EJ, Bock GH, Kerzner B, Abbott AW, Majd M, Chatoor I. Feeding disorders and gastroesophageal reflux in infants with chronic renal failure. *Pediatr Nephrol.* 1989;3:424–429.

147. Bunchman TE, Wood EG, Schenck MH, Weaver KA, Klein BL, Lynch RE. Pretreatment of formula with sodium polystyrene sulfonate to reduce dietary potassium intake. *Pediatr Nephrol.* 1991;5:29–32.

148. Thompson K, Flynn J, Okamura D, Zhou L. Pretreatment of formula or expressed breast milk with sodium polystyrene sulfonate (kayexalate) as a treatment for hyperkalemia in infants with acute or chronic insufficiency. *J Ren Nutr.* 2013;23(5):333–339.

149. Hobbs DJ, Gast TR, Ferguson KB, Bunchman TE, Barletta GM. Nutritional management of hyperkalemic infants with chronic kidney disease, using adult renal formulas. *J Ren Nutr.* 2010;20(2):121–126.

150. Raaijmakers R, Willems J, Houkes B, Heuval CS, Monnens LA. Pretreatment of various dairy products with sevelamer: effective P reduction but also a rise in pH. *Perit Dial Int.* 2008;29:S15A.

151. Wolfson M. Management of protein and energy intake in dialysis patients. *J Am Soc Nephrol.* 1999;10:2244–2247.

152. Kopple JD, Foulks CJ, Piraino B, Beto JA, Goldstein J. Proposed Health Care Financing Administration guidelines for reimbursement of enteral and parenteral nutrition. *Am J Kidney Dis.* 1995;26:995–997.

153. Council on Renal Nutrition of New England. Intradialytic parenteral nutrition. In: *Renal Nutrition Handbook for Renal Dietitians.* Norwood, MA: National Kidney Foundation; 1993:86–98.

154. Cherry N, Shalansky K. Efficacy of intradialytic parenteral nutrition in malnourished hemodialysis patients. *Am J Health Syst Pharm.* 2002;15:1736–1741.

155. Chertow GM, Ling J, Lew NL, Lazaras JM, Lowrie EG. The association of intradialytic parenteral nutrition administration with survival in hemodialysis patients. *Am J Kidney Dis.* 1994;24:912–920.

156. Kidney Disease: Improving Global Outcomes (KDIGO) Glomerulonephritis Work Group. KDIGO clinical practice guidelines for glomerulonephritis. *Kidney Int Suppl.* 2012;2(2):139–274.

157. National Kidney Foundation. Childhood nephrotic syndrome. http://www.kidney.org/atoz/atozItem.cfm. Accessed November 6, 2008.

158. Kovacevic L, Reid CJ, Rigden SP. Management of congenital nephrotic syndrome. *Pediatr Nephrol.* 2003;18:426–430.

159. Jalanko H. Congenital nephrotic syndrome. *Pediatr Nephrol.* 2009;24:2121–2128.

160. Kher KK, Schnaper HW, Makker SP, eds. *Clinical Pediatric Nephrology.* 2nd ed. London: Informa Healthcare; 2007.

161. Ramello A, Vitale C, Marangella M. Epidemiology of nephrolithiasis. *J Nephrol.* 2000;13(3):S45–S50.

162. Ayoob R, Wang W, Schwaderer A. Body fat composition and occurrence of kidney stones in hypercalciuric children. *Pediatr Nephrol.* 2011;26:2173–2178.

163. Selimoğlu MA, Menekşe E, Tabel Y. Is urolithiasis in children associated with obesity or malnutrition? *J Ren Nutr.* 2013;23(2):119–122.

164. VanDervoort K, Wiesen J, Frank R, et al. Urolithiasis in pediatric patients: a single center study of incidence, clinical presentation and outcome. *J Urol.* 2007;177:2300–2305.

165. Lande MB, Varade W, Erkan E, Niederbracht Y, Schwartz GJ. Role of urinary supersaturation in the evaluation of children with urolithiasis. *Pediatr Nephrol.* 2005;20:491–494.

166. Meschi T, Maggiore U, Fiaccadori E, et al. The effect of fruits and vegetables on urinary stone risk factors. *Kidney Int.* 2004;66:2402–2410.

167. Pak CYC. Medical management of urinary stone disease. *Nephron Clin Pract.* 2004;98:49–53.

168. Schwaderer AL, Kusumi K, Ayoob RM. Pediatric nephrolithiasis and the link to bone metabolism. *Curr Opin Pediatr.* 2014;26:207–214.

169. Bataille P, Pruna A, Gregoire I, et al. Critical role of oxalate restriction in association with calcium restriction to decrease the probability of being a stone former: insufficient effect in idiopathic hypercalciuria. *Nephron.* 1985;39:321–324.

170. Knoll T, Zollner A, Wendt-Nordahl G, Michel MS, Alken P. Cystinuria in childhood and adolescence: recommendations for diagnosis, treatment and follow-up. *Pediatr Nephrol.* 2005;20:19–24.

171. Caldas A, Broyer M, Dechaux M, Kleinknecht C. Primary distal tubular acidosis in childhood: clinical study and long-term follow-up of 28 patients. *J Pediatr.* 1992;121:233–241.

172. Favero M, Calò LA, Schiavon F, Punzi L. Bartter's and Gitelman's diseases. *Best Pract Res Clin Rheumatol.* 2011;25:637–648.

173. Wesche D, Deen PMT, Knoers NVAM. Congenital nephrogenic diabetes insipidus: the current state of affairs. *Pediatr Nephrol.* 2012;27:2183–2204.

174. NDI Foundation. Diagnosis and treatment of NDI. http://www.ndif.org/pages/6-Diagnosis_Treatment. Accessed December 9, 2008.

175. Strobele B, Loveland L, Britz R, Gottlich E, Welthagen A, Botha J. Combined paediatric liver-kidney transplantation: analysis of our experience and literature review. *S Afr Med J.* 2013;103(12):925–929.

176. Corrigan JJ Jr, Boineau FG. Hemolytic-uremic syndrome. *Pediatr Rev.* 2001;22(11):365–369.

177. Greenbaum LA. Atypical hemolytic uremic syndrome. *Adv Pediatr.* 2014;61:335–356.

Test Your Knowledge Answers

1. The correct answer is **C**. The use of CRRT provides greater solute clearance, and thus electrolytes typically do not need to be limited and are often supplemented. Therefore, use of a regular formula as opposed to a low-electrolyte renal formula is appropriate. Additionally, enteral products designed for renal patients often are more concentrated, which can cause GI discomfort. GI side effects are common in this population and use of transpyloric feeding improves tolerance. Only if continued tolerance problems or poor gut perfusion/function is suspected should PN be considered.

2. The correct answer is **D**. Although dialysis losses may be minimal, vitamin B_6 intake is often inadequate, likely due to restriction of high-protein foods to limit excess intake of phosphorus and potassium. Recent studies indicate that 25-hydroxyvitamin D may have a role, in addition to the well-known 1,25-$(OH)_2$D, in bone metabolism and prevention of hyperparathyroidism. Supplementation of 1,25-$(OH)_2$D to keep serum levels in the appropriate reference range is recommended. Folic acid, although controversial in its role with homocysteine reduction and cardiovascular implications, has a role with anemia management.

3. The correct answer is **C**. CVD is the major cause of mortality in patients with CKD. Not only do CKD patients typically have traditional risk factors, including HTN, dyslipidemia, and LVH, but they also have nontraditional markers or uremic factors that can contribute to CVD. These factors include inflammation, anemia, fluid overload, proteinuria, abnormal calcium and phosphorus levels, dyslipidemia, and vascular injury.

4. The correct answer is **A**. Recent studies indicate nPCR is a superior marker of nutrition status in adolescent children on maintenance HD. In these studies, serum albumin was a poor indicator of nutrition status. An nPCR of <1 g/kg/d was a strong predictor of weight loss in adolescent patients. However, increased risk of mortality has also been associated with hypoalbuminemia. Therefore, serum albumin may be used as a nutrition status marker as well, with recognition of its limitations in the setting of inflammation or hypervolemia when low values of albumin may result.

25

Gastrointestinal Disease

Donald George, MD; **Elizabeth Bobo**, MS, RD, LDN, CNSC; and **Jill Dorsey**, MD, MS

 Podcast

CONTENTS

Learning Objectives

1. Enumerate the mechanisms leading to nutrition deficiency in gastrointestinal diseases.
2. List several common gastrointestinal diseases in children and review the pathophysiology as it applies to nutrition.
3. Describe the role of nutrition support as primary treatment of inflammatory bowel disease, celiac disease, and functional gastrointestinal disorders.

Introduction

The tasks of ingesting, processing, digesting, and absorbing nutrients are coordinated through a complex network of cellular, neural, and hormonal factors that help direct the function of the gastrointestinal (GI) tract. GI diseases may cause malnutrition by affecting nutrient intake, nutrient digestion, or absorption or by altering nutrient requirements. When dealing with a patient who has a GI disease, the clinician must determine if the patient is malnourished, whether nutrition deficiencies are likely to occur, and whether the patient would benefit from nutrition therapy.

Mechanisms of Nutrition Deficiency

Mechanisms responsible for nutrition deficiency are summarized in Table 25-1. They include the following:

Disordered Ingestion

Disordered ingestion may result from refusal to feed or difficulty swallowing or from being presented an inadequate diet. Refusal to feed may be related to pain with swallowing or abdominal pain with eating.

Table 25-1. Mechanisms of Nutrition Deficiency

MECHANISM	EXAMPLES
Disordered ingestion	Anorexia Dental disease Dysphagia of any cause Esophagitis Foreign body Inadequate access to food
Failure of digestion	Pancreatic enzyme deficiency Sucrase-isomaltase deficiency Cholestasis with failure of bile salt secretion
Failure of absorption	Short bowel syndrome due to surgery Celiac disease Inflammatory bowel disease Liver disease Motility disorders
Increased needs	Fever Work of breathing Certain medications

Difficulty swallowing can be related to oral, neurological, or esophageal diseases. Inability to chew or produce saliva also interferes with the ability to swallow. In addition, a number of behavioral problems (eg, food aversion, depression, and eating disorders) influence the ability to ingest nutrients. GI inflammation or vomiting of any cause will limit the ability to eat.

Failure of Digestion

Failure of digestion occurs in diseases that affect the production of digestive enzymes secreted from the stomach (pepsin), pancreas (lipase, amylase, proteases), or the surface of the GI tract (lactase or sucrase-isomaltase). In addition, bile acids are important in the solubilization of fat, and patients with cholestasis of any cause will have impaired digestion.

Failure of Absorption

Failure of absorption occurs if an inadequate surface area is available due to either mucosal injury or surgical shortening of the GI tract. There may be failure of systems involved in particular nutrient absorption (eg, pernicious anemia, glucose-galactose malabsorption). Lack of luminal factors such as biliary secretions impairs absorption, especially of lipids. Deficiency of luminal bile salts occurs in liver disease, gallbladder disease, or disease of the biliary ducts.

In rare instances, absorption may not occur despite an adequate surface area. Congenital disorders such as microvillus inclusion disease preclude normal absorption, while motility problems such as pseudoobstruction may interfere with absorption by inhibiting movement of the food bolus.

Increased Needs

A hypermetabolic state resulting in increased energy needs can occur in diseases with fever, increased work of breathing, or because of certain medications needed for treatment.

Nutrition deficiency usually involves multiple mechanisms. For example, a patient with Crohn's disease may have a poor appetite or be unable to eat because of pain or oral ulcers. In addition, there may be small bowel involvement or intestinal resection that affects absorption (eg, vitamin B_{12} in the terminal ileum). Some patients with Crohn's disease will have lactase deficiency. Further, the presence of fever or underlying inflammation may increase needs for energy and protein.

Nutrition Assessment

Nutrition assessment is an essential component of the evaluation of all children. It cannot be assumed that all children eat normally, and a detailed diet history is important. Monitoring of growth should be part of each routine well-child examination. Assessment of both linear and ponderal growth of the child or adolescent is central to evaluation of nutrition status. Alterations in patterns of linear growth and weight gain (both inadequate as well as excessive weight gain) may be the earliest manifestation of disease. Malnutrition is commonly diagnosed in hospitalized patients and is also a common comorbidity in patients with GI disease.[1,2] Malnutrition during illness may complicate the response to therapies or impair recovery (Table 25-2). Thus, nutrition assessment is an integral part of both the initial and ongoing evaluation of all children with acute and/or chronic disease and is of crucial importance in the evaluation of the child with GI disease.[3,4]

The initial nutrition evaluation includes both subjective and objective assessment of the patient's current nutrition status and projected nutrition requirements. The subjective assessment includes the presence and duration of GI symptoms, fever, frequent infections, fatigue, food aversion, allergies to particular foods, or feeding intolerance. Specific attention is paid to previous growth, detailed diet history, changes in body weight and dietary intake, GI symptoms (eg, abdominal pain, diarrhea, and vomiting), and anorexia. The objective assessment should include data from clinical,

Table 25-2. Gastrointestinal Nutrient Deficiencies[4-6]

NUTRIENT	SIGNS/SYMPTOMS OF DEFICIENCY	LABORATORY MARKERS
Iron	Fatigue Microcytic anemia	↓ Hemoglobin ↓ Hematocrit ↓ MCV ↑ RDW ↓ % TIBC ↓ Ferritin ↓ Serum iron
Folate	Megaloblastic anemia Glossitis Diarrhea Forgetfulness	↓ Serum folate ↓ Red blood cell folate ↑ MCV
Vitamin B$_{12}$	Megaloblastic anemia Ataxia Diarrhea Mental status changes Paresthesias Glossitis	↑ MCV ↓ Hemoglobin ↓ Serum vitamin B$_{12}$
Calcium	Osteopenia Osteoporosis Tetany	↓ Serum total calcium ↓ Serum ionized calcium
Vitamin D	Bone pain Muscle weakness Tetany Osteomalacia Rickets	↑ Serum alkaline phosphatase ↓ 25-Hydroxyvitamin D ↑ PTH
Vitamin A	Night blindness Decreased appetite Decreased immune function Hyperkeratosis	↓ Plasma vitamin A
Vitamin K	Bleeding Bruising	↑ PT
Vitamin E	Hemolytic anemia Truncal ataxia Hyporeflexia or areflexia	↓ Serum creatinine; creatinuria ↓ Serum vitamin E to total serum lipid ratio
Zinc	Diarrhea Dry skin Skin sloughing on palms Mental status changes Hair loss Growth stunting Anorexia	↓ Serum alkaline phosphatase ↓ Serum zinc[a] ↓ Urinary zinc[b]
Magnesium	Muscle cramps Bone pain Nausea Seizures	↓ Serum magnesium

MCV, mean corpuscular volume; PT, prothrombin time; PTH, parathyroid hormone; RDW, red cell distribution width; TIBC, total iron binding capacity.

[a]Zinc binds to serum proteins, which can make levels appear low if protein levels are depleted.
[b]Associated with disease status.

anthropometric, and laboratory evaluations (Table 25-3). Clinical data include the diagnosis, current medical or surgical problems, allergies, and medications that may affect nutrition support options. Objective measures of nutrition status include growth indices (both previous and current), current weight, and Tanner stage. The determination of body mass index (BMI) for children > 3 years of age provides important information regarding the nutrition status. In children < 2 years of age, weight-for-length is used. In children between the ages of 2 and 3, BMI is used when a standing height is obtained while weight-for-length is used when a recumbent length is obtained. Refer to chapter 32 on nutrition assessment for more detailed information.

Careful examination of the child is the initial step in evaluation.[7] Obesity and wasting are obvious. Edema, dehydration, excess fat, or decreased muscle mass can be appreciable. Anthropometric measurements, including mid-upper arm circumference and skinfold thickness determinations, are useful. It is standard practice to measure these parameters in patients at risk for chronic malnutrition such as those with pancreatic insufficiency, inflammatory bowel disease, celiac disease, or short bowel syndrome in which maldigestion or malabsorption may be prominent. It is rare to find many specific stigmata of severe malnutrition in children. Most often wasting, sometimes accompanied by edema, is seen. The clinician, however, should have special concern for micronutrient deficiencies, especially in children with inflammatory disorders or disorders of absorption.

Table 25-3. Nutrition Assessment

ASSESSMENT CATEGORY	FACTORS
History	Gastrointestinal symptoms (diarrhea, vomiting) Feeding tolerance Allergies/aversion Developmental feeding skills Recent changes in growth or intake
Clinical data	Diagnosis Medications Anthropometry (height, weight, Tanner stage) Laboratory • Blood: electrolytes, CRP, albumin, prealbumin, CBC, vitamin levels, minerals (eg, iron and zinc) • Stool: pH and reducing substances (carbohydrate malabsorption) Quantitative fat Body composition: DEXA, bioelectric impedance

CBC, complete blood count; CRP, C-reactive protein; DEXA, dual energy x-ray absorptiometry.

Specific attention is paid to examination of the abdomen. Abdominal tenderness, abdominal distention, and the presence of bowel sounds not only provide helpful clues to the nature of the disease process but also influence treatment decisions. There may be other findings that suggest nutrient deficiency. Careful examination of the hair noting both texture and distribution may suggest specific deficiency of biotin. Angular stomatitis and dermatitis may suggest riboflavin deficiency. Dry cracked skin in areas exposed to sunlight suggests niacin deficiency. Dystrophic nails, spooning of the nails, or pallor of the conjunctiva or skin may suggest iron deficiency. Peripheral neuropathy can be seen with a number of vitamin deficiencies including thiamin, B_6, B_{12}, and niacin. Zinc deficiency is often manifested by alopecia and perioral or perianal rash. Bowing of the legs, tetany, or rickets suggest vitamin D deficiency. Petechiae, bruising of the skin, or bleeding gums may indicate vitamin K deficiency as may be seen in liver disease.

Gastroesophageal Reflux

Gastroesophageal reflux (GER) is the passage of gastric contents into the esophagus with or without regurgitation. It can occur several times a day in healthy infants, children, and adults.[8–10] Regurgitation occurs daily in 40% of healthy infants and usually resolves spontaneously by 12–24 months of age.[11–13] However, regurgitation occurs at least weekly in 12%–15% of children ages 3–17 years (Table 25-4).[9] Gastroesophageal reflux disease (GERD) refers to reflux-associated tissue damage (eg, esophagitis) or symptoms severe enough to impair quality of life.[14]

The genesis of reflux-related injury and reflux symptoms is not the same. Each relates to a combination of factors that lead to an excessive number of reflux events, impaired clearance of material from the esophagus, increased acidity, or decreased buffering of the refluxed material or impaired protection of the esophageal or supraesophageal mucosa.[15] The most important mechanism causing GER is transient lower esophageal sphincter relaxations.[16] Delayed gastric emptying, increased intra-abdominal pressure, and chronically reduced lower esophageal sphincter resting pressure have also been implicated.[17] Studies of stomach function have demonstrated that gastric emptying is related to both the composition and caloric density of the feedings. Higher fat diets or diets of higher caloric density will slow the emptying and thereby promote reflux.

GER and GERD have a variety of presentations that vary with age. Regurgitation associated with poor growth, irritability, or airway compromise are common reasons for evaluation in infancy. Heartburn and epigastric abdominal pain are more common complaints in older children and adolescents. Abnormal posturing (Sandifer's syndrome) and acute life-threatening events are typical manifestations in the infant with GERD but are rarely seen in older children or adults (Table 25-5).

Regurgitation in infancy is rarely serious. Most instances of infantile GER resolve spontaneously. However, a minority of infants may have severe or prolonged problems that lead to caloric insufficiency and malnutrition. Some severe cases result in failure to thrive, which may be due to persistent vomiting, difficulty feeding (coughing or gagging), and/or feeding aversion with subsequent lack of intake. In these cases specialized nutrition support may be needed. This may be accomplished orally with the use of specialized formulas or supplements. In some patients with complicated GER or GERD, alternate enteral access may be

Table 25-4. Incidence of Regurgitation

AGE GROUP (FREQUENCY)	AGE	%*
Infancy (daily GERD)	3 mo 6 mo 12 mo	40% 30% 15%
Children (weekly)	3–9 y 10–17 y	12% 15%

GERD, gastroesophageal reflux disease.

*Refers to percentage of infants with GER requiring medical attention.

Table 25-5. Common Presentation of Gastroesophageal Reflux Disease

AGE GROUP	EXAMPLES
Infant	Regurgitation Vomiting Feeding difficulties (acute) Unexplained crying Failure to thrive Posturing
Child	Vomiting Cough Abdominal pain Sore throat Respiratory difficulties
Adolescent	Hoarseness Regurgitation Chest pain Heartburn Epigastric pain Dysphagia

needed. Factors that influence this decision include aspiration risk, degree of malnutrition, the age of the child, and associated anatomic or neurological problems.

Disordered ingestion or nutrient losses due to vomiting or regurgitation dominate the clinical picture. In children who have poor weight gain, or weight loss, attention is paid to modalities to increase calories. Insufficient oral intake can be related to pain associated with eating, food aversion due to vomiting, or dysphagia associated with esophagitis.

Treatments to reduce emesis in infants with regurgitation include smaller feedings, thickening the formula with cereal or using a prethickened formula, and positioning. Smaller, more frequent feeds are often suggested but are sometimes impractical and poorly tolerated by babies and parents.[18] In neonates with dysphagia the frequency of GER events is reduced if feeds are given over a longer duration.[19] Feeding in an upright position and maintaining the infant with the head elevated for a period after eating is often recommended although data demonstrating effectiveness are sparse. Because of the risk of sudden infant death syndrome, prone positioning is acceptable only if the infant is awake and carefully observed.[18,20]

Thickening of feedings has been shown to reduce symptomatic GER. Agents commonly used to thicken formula include rice cereal, guar gum, carob bean gum, locust bean gum, pectin, pregelatinized waxy rice starch, and soy polysaccharides.[21,22] Thickened formulas lessen the frequency of emesis but may contribute to some undesirable side effects. Despite a reduced number of episodes of obvious reflux and emesis, pH probe studies do not indicate a reduction in exposure to acid in the esophagus.[23,24] Thickening of feeds does not reduce apnea events in preterm infants.[25] Further, studies found increased postprandial coughing in infants fed thickened formula, suggesting continued reflux despite improvement in emesis.[26] Thickening infant formulas is relatively free of major side effects.[27] However, there have been reports of necrotizing enterocolitis in some premature infants given specific thickening agents.[28]

Also of concern is the effect of thickened formulas on the macronutrient content of formula, as well as the micronutrient absorption. Thickening of formulas with rice cereal alters the macronutrient composition of the formula by providing additional calories and protein. Importantly, indigestible carbohydrate thickening agents, such as locust bean gum, have been linked with decreased bioavailability of calcium, zinc, and iron. Conversely, digestible carbohydrate thickening agents, such as pregelatinized waxy rice starch, have not been linked with decreased nutrient absorption.[29]

Due to lack of definite data regarding the efficacy of thickened formulas, it is recommended that they only be used under medical supervision.[20]

Milk protein intolerance may have a clinical presentation that mimics GERD. A 2–4 week trial of an extensively hydrolyzed protein or an amino acid–based formula may be beneficial. For the breastfed infant, a 2–4 week trial of a maternal exclusion diet that restricts dairy and possibly egg protein is recommended. [20,30]

In older children with GER, the nutrition therapy is dependent on individual tolerance to various foods. Obesity and exposure to alcohol and tobacco smoke may worsen GER. Sparse evidence supports avoidance of caffeine (coffee in particular), peppermint, spearmint, chocolate, and spicy foods.[31–33] The fat content of a meal does not have an effect on esophageal reflux except in the presence of delayed gastric emptying.[34,35] Nutritional rehabilitation can improve symptoms of GER. Data suggest that GER is reduced in malnourished, neurologically hindered children when they are nutritionally repleted.[36]

Medications commonly used in the treatment of GERD include antacids, proton pump inhibitors (PPIs), and H2 histamine receptor antagonists. These medications are associated with various nutrition-related side effects (Table 25-6). Also worthy of mention is the decreased absorption of supplemental iron associated with PPI usage. Possible infection risks from long-term use of PPIs are additional concerns.[37,38]

Prokinetic medications are often suggested to improve gastric emptying. Metoclopramide is often prescribed, although evidence supporting its effectiveness is scant. It reduces symptoms, but it is also associated with many side effects that limit its use. It is now rarely used in children.[20,39]

Table 25-6. Potential Effects of Medications Used for Gastroesophageal Reflux Disease[31]

SIDE EFFECT	PROTON PUMP INHIBITOR	H2 HISTAMINE RECEPTOR ANTAGONIST
Diarrhea	X	X
Constipation	X	X
Abdominal pain	X	X
Nausea/vomiting	X	X
Anorexia	X	
Anemia	X	
Weight gain/loss	X	
Hepatotoxicity		X

Erythromycin has prokinetic activity and improves gastric emptying, although it has not been shown to improve GER symptoms. These medications are most commonly used in patients with weight loss or failure to gain related to GERD.

Clinical outcome in GERD can be measured in a variety of ways. Lower esophageal pH recording is accepted as a valid measure of GER; however, serial recordings are rarely used in clinical practice. Symptom reduction (usually frequency of vomiting in infants or episodes of heartburn in older children and adolescents) can be monitored by recall or the use of diaries with symptom severity and frequency estimates. For GERD causing poor weight gain, improvement in weight gain over time is the accepted measure.

Celiac Disease

Celiac disease is a chronic T-cell–mediated autoimmune inflammatory disorder. It is characterized by damage to the small intestinal mucosa in genetically susceptible individuals and is due to abnormal reactions to the gliadin fraction of wheat gluten and similar peptides present in barley and rye. A specific peptide fragment of gliadin, comprising 33 amino acids, is resistant to degradation by pancreatic, gastric, or small intestinal enzymes. This peptide can pass through the epithelial barrier and interact with immune cells of the intestine. Immune responses affecting both the adaptive and innate immunity promote an inflammatory reaction in the lamina propria of the intestinal wall leading to villus atrophy. The genetic factors are linked to the human leukocyte antigen system, which regulates the immune response.

The availability of serologic testing for celiac disease has changed our understanding of both the prevalence and presentation of the disease. Previously celiac disease was thought to be uncommon and was diagnosed mainly in patients who had typical symptoms (Table 25-7). Screening studies using serologic markers now suggest that celiac disease occurs in roughly 1% of the population. Little difference exists in the rates in Europe compared with North America, North Africa, or the Middle East.[40]

The typical presentations of celiac disease usually occur in the first few years of life and manifest as diarrhea with growth failure and anemia. It is now recognized that celiac disease can present at any age following inclusion of gluten in the diet and has a variety of manifestations, many of which are extraintestinal in nature. Indeed, with the development and implementation of screening of patients "at risk" (Table 25-8), it is clear that some patients with celiac disease are asymptomatic despite significant intestinal mucosal injury.

Table 25-7. Presentation of Celiac Disease

TYPE OF PRESENTATION	SIGNS AND SYMPTOMS
Typical (usually young)	Weight loss Failure to grow Vomiting Diarrhea Bloating Anorexia Abdominal pain
Atypical (adolescent or young adult)	Constipation Short stature Dermatitis Herpetiformis Osteopenia Elevated liver enzymes Arthritis Iron deficiency Anemia Dental enamel defects
Silent (any age)	No obvious signs or symptoms; patient identified when tested because of risk factors and on biopsy has typical enteropathy
Latent (any age)	Mild or nonspecific symptoms identified by screening; positive serology but normal biopsy. May develop typical disease at a later time.

Further, patients may have symptoms that do not immediately call to mind intestinal disease. Older children and adolescents may present with constitutional symptoms such as fatigue or lassitude. GI symptoms may be mild or even absent. Patients with celiac disease often have derangements of bone and mineral metabolism and idiopathic osteopenia may be the sole clinical feature.[41,42]

The mainstay of diagnosis of celiac disease remains the small intestinal biopsy with demonstration of the typical features of enteropathy. Serologic tests are a valuable adjunct in the diagnosis and are often the initial diagnostic

Table 25-8. Groups at Risk for Celiac Disease

Relative of patient with celiac disease
Diabetes mellitus (type 1)
Down syndrome
Thyroiditis
Turner syndrome
Williams syndrome
Other autoimmune diseases

tool in patients with unexplained GI symptoms, anemia, or poor growth. Further, they are used to screen high-risk groups and to aid in monitoring compliance with diet. Serologic tests available include the tissue transglutaminase (tTG) IgG and IgA and anti-endomysial antibodies. Antireticulin antibodies are rarely used because the more sensitive and specific tests are commonly available. Recently, serology using antibodies to deamidated gliadin have become available. These appear to have sensitivity and specificity similar to those of the tTG antibodies and can sometimes be helpful in children < 2 years of age when other celiac disease–specific antibodies are negative.

Because of the recognition of atypical presentations of celiac disease, screening with serology is offered to patients with growth failure or short stature, recurrent abdominal pain, irritable bowel syndrome (IBS), unexplained diarrhea or iron deficiency, or delayed puberty. In addition, serologic testing is indicated in children with type 1 diabetes mellitus, Down syndrome, Turner syndrome, Williams syndrome, or autoimmune thyroid or liver disease. First-degree relatives of patients with celiac disease should be screened.[43]

The effects of celiac disease on nutrition status can be profound. A patient may have linear and/or ponderal growth failure. Diarrhea and weight loss may also be present. In addition, vitamin and mineral deficiencies may be present at the time of diagnosis. A thorough physical assessment of the patient and assessment of laboratory values when indicated are necessary to identify such deficiencies. Attention is paid to growth, bony abnormalities, and pigmentary changes. Laboratory investigation, including serology, is often revealing. In particular microcytic or macrocytic anemia may be present due to impaired absorption of iron or folic acid in the proximal intestine[44] or B_{12} in the distal small bowel. Other nutrients of concern include, but are not limited to, fat-soluble vitamins (A, D, E, and K), zinc, and calcium. Special attention is paid to vitamin D. Calcium supplementation may also be needed. Inadequate calcium may be due to malabsorption or poor dietary intake. Lactose intolerance is common in untreated patients due to damage to the villi. Most often this improves with treatment; however, "adult-type" lactase deficiency, not associated with intestinal injury, may complicate the clinical picture.

The primary nutrition management of celiac disease includes complete avoidance of all gluten and correction of any vitamin/mineral deficiencies. The fundamental basis of the gluten-free (GF) diet includes avoidance of wheat, barley, and rye.[45] Oats that are specifically labeled as being GF may be consumed in the diet; however, general commercial oats

should not be consumed secondary to cross-contamination with wheat, rye, or barley in processing.[5] It is recommended that patients introducing pure, uncontaminated oats into their diet be monitored for clinical symptoms as abdominal discomfort (often a product of increased dietary fiber) or an allergy can develop. Addition of a moderate amount (¼ cup dry rolled oats per day) is generally thought to be appropriate for children following a GF diet.[46] Refer to Table 25-9 for a list of gluten-containing and GF grains. The diet is more cumbersome than simply avoiding the grains listed as containing gluten because there may be secondary hidden sources of gluten in processed foods in the form of additives. Detailed patient instruction on label reading and avoiding cross-contamination is crucial for proper adherence to the GF diet. When replenishing vitamin/mineral stores with dietary supplements, it is important to read the label for the presence of gluten because many dietary supplements are not GF.

The GF diet should be considered only after thorough evaluation of the possibility of celiac disease. Placing a patient on a GF diet before celiac disease is excluded or confirmed may be detrimental because this can interfere with the ability to make a clear-cut diagnosis, which is essential since the GF diet for celiac disease is strict, lifelong, and of-

Table 25-9. Grains and Gluten[a]

GLUTEN CONTAINING	GLUTEN FREE
Barley	Amaranth
Bulgur	Arrowroot
Couscous	Buckwheat
Dinkle (spelt)	Corn
Durum	Flaxseed
Einkorn	Rice
Emmer	Millet
Farina	Milo
Fu	Potato flour
Graham flour	Quinoa
Kamut	Sorghum
Seitan	Soy
Semolina	Tapioca
Rye	Tef
Wheat	Taro flour
Triticale	Urd

[a]This is not an all-inclusive list.

ten cumbersome, and consuming gluten later can result in significant illness. GF diets are sometimes recommended for the treatment of other conditions, not celiac disease. Evaluation for celiac disease prior to the initiation of the diet is necessary.[43]

Removal of gluten from the diet usually results in clinical and histological recovery. Specialized oral feedings or enteral feedings are rarely necessary in a patient with celiac disease. Parenteral feedings are not used unless some other indication exists for that therapy.

When the diagnosis of celiac disease is confirmed, routine nutrition follow-up of the child is necessary to monitor growth parameters, promote adherence to the diet, and ensure proper nutrition, particularly because many of the GF products are not fortified. Ongoing monitoring of vitamins (especially A, D, B_{12}, and folate), as well as assessment of anemia and markers of bone health, is suggested.[47] Fortunately, with proper nutrition and adherence to the GF diet, bone density in children returns to normal 1 year post initiation of the diet.[48]

Clinical outcome is measured by resumption of normal growth and weight gain and by monitoring of serologic markers, especially tTG IgA. Failure of tTG IgG and IgA levels to return to normal values after adherence to a GF diet for 6–12 months warrants further inspection of the child's diet for inadvertent gluten consumption.

Inflammatory Bowel Disease

Inflammatory bowel disease (IBD) refers to chronic inflammation anywhere along the GI tract. The term includes Crohn's disease, ulcerative colitis, and indeterminate colitis (ie, IBD with features that do not allow clear distinction between Crohn's disease and ulcerative colitis). The incidence of Crohn's disease seems to be increasing in childhood, while the rates of ulcerative colitis are steady. IBD may present at any age. Ulcerative colitis is more common in younger children. Peak age of incidence of Crohn's disease is in the second decade of life. The most important risk factor for developing IBD is a positive family history.

Inflammation of the bowel leads to a number of derangements that culminate in diarrhea, GI bleeding, and abdominal pain. Other symptoms depend on the location of inflammation within the GI tract. For example, vomiting is more prominent in patients with gastric or small bowel disease. The most common presentation is a patient with abdominal pain and diarrhea. Stools may be bloody. Weight loss is common, especially in patients with Crohn's disease. However, nonspecific manifestations of the disease may be the initial presentation and failure to recognize their importance may lead to delay in the diagnosis. Joint pain and swelling, skin rashes, muscle pain, elevated liver enzymes, or eye changes (uveitis, iritis, or episcleritis) may be present prior to any specific GI manifestation. Oral ulcerations can range from painless to severe pain with bleeding. It is well recognized that deterioration of linear and ponderal growth may precede the development of more specific symptoms.

The effect of IBD on nutrition status is multifaceted. Growth, bone health, and macronutrient and micronutrient stores are commonly affected and malnutrition is common.[49] Nutrition assessment of children with IBD includes measurements of weight, height, and calculation of BMI. These values should be plotted and followed serially on appropriate growth charts.[50] The importance of tracking these measurements is emphasized by the fact that upon diagnosis the majority of children with IBD will have growth failure.[51] In fact, reduced linear growth velocity may precede GI manifestations of IBD by months or even years.[52–54] Criteria for defining growth failure include a height velocity < 3rd percentile, height < 3rd percentile, height-for-age z score of –2.0 or lower, or a bone age less than the chronological age by 2 or more standard deviations. Males may be more susceptible to growth failure, but all children with IBD are at risk.[55] Factors affecting risk include malnutrition, treatment modality, and the extent and severity of intestinal inflammation.

Malnutrition in IBD patients is multifactorial and includes energy losses, increased requirements, malabsorption, and decreased energy intake due to diarrhea, abdominal pain, and other disease-related side effects.[56] Further contributing to malnutrition is poor appetite related cytokine activity in the inflammatory process.[57] Inflammatory cytokines have also been shown to reduce insulin-like growth factor 1 (IGF-1).[6] Children with active Crohn's disease often have lower serum IGF-1 levels than controls. In addition, chronic usage of corticosteroids as treatment can suppress IGF-1 and also decrease osteoblast activity.[58] Data indicates that nutrition therapy in comparison to corticosteroid usage is beneficial in the treatment of Crohn's disease and spares linear growth.[59–61]

Assessment of nutrition status includes sufficiency of vitamin and mineral stores. Analyses of dietary records and/or 24-hour food recall, as well as laboratory values are helpful in assessing micronutrient status. Commonly deficient nutrients include iron, folate, vitamin B_{12}, vitamin D, calcium, zinc, and magnesium.[62] Refer to Table 25-2 for information regarding deficiency signs/symptoms and laboratory markers. Reduced iron stores are due to decreased intake, reduced absorption, and increased losses (ie, blood loss). Often, iron supplementation is required along with a diet rich in iron and vitamin C to correct the deficiency. Laboratory values to monitor iron status include hemoglobin, reticulocyte count, mean corpuscular volume, red blood cell distribution width, ferritin, transferrin saturation, and iron. However, one should use caution in interpreting the ferritin since it is an acute-phase respondent and can be elevated during episodes of acute inflammation.

Folate stores may be affected by insufficient intake, because many good sources of folate (eg, leafy green vegetables) are often not tolerated by the child with active inflammation. In addition, medications used in disease treatment such as methotrexate and sulfasalazine have direct and deleterious effects on folate metabolism. Children on these medications need folate supplementation.[50]

Vitamin B_{12} deficiency may occur in children with involvement of the stomach and terminal ileum and in cases of bacterial overgrowth. Notably, deficiency may be masked by supplementation of folate. Deficiency is corrected by intramuscular injection, oral supplementation, or nasal gel.[62]

Maintenance of adequate calcium and vitamin D stores is imperative in children with IBD, particularly in those receiving steroid therapy due to the relationship of steroid usage and decreased bone mineral density. Lactose intolerance often limits consumption of milk and dairy products rich in these nutrients.[62] Supplementation may be required to obtain values within normal limits. Research suggests that supplementation of vitamin D above the standard recommendation may be necessary to achieve an appropriate 25-hydroxyvitamin D level.[63] Children with Crohn's disease of the upper intestine and children with darker complexions may have an increased need for vitamin D supplementation.[64] The winter season may also dictate increased need. Vitamin D replacement guidelines for children with IBD recommend a cumulative dose at least 400,000 IU if the 25-hydroxy vitamin D level is < 20 ng/mL (= 50,000 IU/wk for 8 weeks), and a minimum of 250,000 IU if the level is between 20 and 31 ng/mL.[65]

Zinc and magnesium deficiencies are associated with increased stool output and may require supplementation. Treatment is usually given empirically as interpretation of serum zinc levels is sometimes difficult. Oral magnesium supplementation is important, but it can worsen diarrhea if it is administered at increased doses over a short time frame.

Energy and protein needs of the child with IBD are based on collected anthropometric data as well as disease status. In the adequately nourished child with IBD, resting energy expenditure is no different than in healthy children.[50] However, in children with insufficient energy stores and increased inflammation, energy needs may be elevated 5%–35% above estimated needs. Protein supplementation has no guidelines. However, it may be prudent to increase protein delivery in a child with inflammation or infection or postoperatively.[62] Enteral nutrition (EN) is the recommended route of nutrition support in IBD when needs cannot be met through oral intake alone. Parenteral nutrition (PN) may be indicated if the enteral route is not feasible or is insufficient to completely meet nutrient needs. Furthermore, PN may be indicated preoperatively and/or postoperatively or in the patient with fistulas. Refer to the chapter on pediatric surgery (Chapter 31) for more information regarding PN and surgery.

Evidence suggests that nutrition therapy is as effective in inducing disease remission as corticosteroid usage in children with active Crohn's disease.[66,67] This method of treatment may be particularly beneficial in children with ileal or ileocolonic Crohn's disease. With EN as primary therapy, 100% of the child's needs are met with a formula, either orally or with tube feedings, for approximately 8–12 weeks.[59] The caloric provision is initially based on the child's estimated energy requirement if indirect calorimetry is not available. Weight gain and reports of hunger should be monitored to indicate if an increase in the calorie goal is indicated. Additional fluid sources will likely be needed to meet maintenance fluid requirements. Outcomes are not significantly different for patients receiving a polymeric, semi-elemental, or elemental diet.[68,69] If a child is significantly malnourished it is prudent to monitor for refeeding syndrome when initiating EN therapy. If an improvement in clinical status is not seen within 3–4 weeks of starting nutrition therapy, a different course of treatment may need to be considered. After the initial phase of treatment, solids are gradually reintroduced as the formula is concurrently reduced. No definitive guidelines exist on the most effective way to introduce solids. However, one method is to add in 1 meal every 2–3 days, while decreasing the amount of formula. Nutrition therapy has a role in maintaining disease remission.[70–72] Research indicates that individuals who incorporate EN therapy along with a regular diet are less likely to relapse than those who follow a regular diet alone after remission of Crohn's has been achieved.[73] Standardized guidelines on how to continue EN therapy after achieving disease remission are not currently available. However, some have advocated using either a schedule of 1 week a month, or 1 month every 3 months, for the formula-only diet.

Decreased bone mineral density, as determined by dual energy x-ray absorptiometry scan, is an unfortunate side effect of IBD. Osteopenia may result from malnutrition, inadequate calcium intake or malabsorption, vitamin D deficiency, physical inactivity, corticosteroid use, or it may be related to cytokines released as part of the inflammatory disease. Children receiving 7.5 mg/d of steroids, a lifetime dose of 5 g, or 12 months of exposure are particularly at increased risk and should be monitored closely.[74]

Diarrhea

Worldwide, diarrheal disease is a major cause of morbidity and mortality in children. Despite improvements in sanitation, aggressive use of oral rehydration therapy, and early refeeding, diarrhea remains a significant cause of undernutrition and malnutrition in both developed and developing countries.[75]

Diarrhea is defined as the excessive loss of fluid and electrolytes in the stool. This loss may also be associated with nutrient loss. Acute diarrhea (ie, diarrhea of sudden onset) is most often related to infection or specific food intolerance. Chronic diarrhea (diarrhea that lasts more than 2 weeks without obvious cause) has a number of possible etiologies. It is beyond the scope of this chapter to discuss in detail the many different causes of diarrhea. Emphasis here is on the general principles guiding nutrition therapy in patents with the symptoms.

The basis for diarrhea is impaired transport of intestinal content including nutrients, electrolytes, and other solutes. Water movement across the intestinal mucosa depends on the active and passive fluxes of solute. Diarrhea encompasses 4 mechanisms that often overlap. Each mechanism may present a unique nutrition challenge (Table 25-10). In addition, patients with diarrhea often do not ingest adequate amounts of nutrients due to associated nausea and vomiting or discomfort.[76]

Osmotic diarrhea happens when a nonabsorbed material, often carbohydrates, creates an osmotic load in the distal bowel and produces increased fluid losses. This can be due to either congenital or acquired disease. A common example is diarrhea associated with lactose intolerance. Excessive sugar intake by children, either juices or sodas, may contribute to osmotic diarrhea. Ingestion of nonabsorbable materials such as sorbitol or xylitol, used in some candies,

Table 25-10. Pathophysiology of Diarrhea

TYPE	CAUSE
Osmotic	Increased osmotic load due to failure to absorb carbohydrates
Secretory	Net intestinal secretion of fluid and electrolytes
Motility	Rapid transit with failure to reabsorb water
Inflammatory	Combination of the above with added exudative loss of protein
Medication	Antibiotics (eg, amoxicillin/clavulanic acid) Antacids containing magnesium Laxatives

will cause diarrhea as well. This type of diarrhea will stop with fasting or the removal of the offending solute.

Secretory diarrhea occurs when the intestinal surface cells secrete fluid into the lumen of the bowel. This may be due to congenital disorders, such as congenital chloridorrhea, or acquired. Toxins may induce fluid and electrolyte secretion. This is seen with cholera and some other infections. Also some tumors may produce hormones that induce secretion. Secretory diarrhea does not stop with fasting.

Children with motility-type diarrhea often have normal absorption and digestion; however, they have rapid transit with resultant looseness and fluidity of stools. This mechanism predominates in toddler's diarrhea or irritable bowel syndrome.

Intestinal inflammation is associated with diarrhea. It often involves elements of the other 3 mechanisms. In addition, there may be increased loss of blood and protein. Infectious enteritis, celiac disease, IBD, eosinophilic disease of the GI tract, and certain medications can cause intestinal inflammation.

Diarrhea can affect nutrition status in numerous ways. Reduced and/or altered dietary intake, fecal loses of macronutrients and micronutrients, fluid losses, and malabsorption of ingested nutrients are all factors that can compromise the child with diarrhea. Prolonged diarrhea coupled with insufficient dietary intake may result in growth failure.[77,78] Malnutrition is an independent risk factor for development of diarrhea. Thus, correction of diarrhea-associated malnutrition is not only crucial for assuring proper growth of the child but also for prevention of future diarrheal episodes. Impaired absorption and/or increased losses of carbohydrates, particularly lactose, protein, fat, and fluids, are associated with acute and chronic diarrhea episodes.[79,80] In cases of acute diarrhea the degree of malabsorption and/or loss is dependent upon the type and severity of infection.[79]

Guidelines for treatment for acute diarrhea have been established.[80,81] Acute diarrhea is often related to infection. A common occurrence during infectious diarrhea is the development of dehydration. Subsequently, acidosis secondary to high output of bicarbonate may occur.

Central to the treatment of acute diarrhea is the use of reduced osmolarity oral rehydration solution (ORS) with a sodium concentration of 50–60 nmol/L. Many products are available. It has efficacy comparable with intravenous (IV) rehydration. In most situations use of ORS will eliminate the need for IV therapy.

Following correction of dehydration, maintenance fluids may be given. If dehydration is mild, oral fluids may be given using an ORS containing sodium, chloride, bicarbonate, and potassium at a dosage of 50–120 mL/kg over 4–6 hours, then followed by maintenance fluids. Fluids with a high osmotic load, such as sodas or fruit juices, should not be given because they may worsen the diarrhea.[76,82] Breastfeeding should be continued during rehydration.

After initial rehydration, rapid reintroduction of feeding is recommended. In the absence of vomiting, feeding of a regular diet (ie, breast milk, infant formula, and/or solids) should begin after rehydration commences to reduce or prevent malnutrition and subsequent growth stunting.[81,82] Caloric intake enhances recovery.[80] Some evidence indicates that use of lactose-free foods can decrease the duration of diarrhea, but if they are not available, then lactose-containing foods/formulas can be used. Diluted formulas do not reduce the duration of diarrhea. BRAT diets (banana, rice, apple, toast) are often recommended; however, the efficacy of the diet has not been studied, and it carries a risk of inadequate nutrient intake if used for more than a few days.

IV rehydration is used in cases in which shock, altered level of consciousness, deterioration despite oral therapy, persistent vomiting, or ileus occurs. To correct severe dehydration ($\geq$ 10% loss in body weight), children may receive 20 mL/kg/h of 0.9% saline, or lactated Ringer's solution, for 2–4 hours. Once fluid volume has been restored, glucose can be added to IV fluids. The amount of sodium then depends on the type of dehydration.

Congenital sucrase-isomaltase deficiency is the most common of the congenital disaccharidase deficiencies. This condition usually presents when juices, formula, or solids containing sucrose, such as baby food fruits, are introduced to the infant's diet.[83] Absence of enzyme prevents breakdown and absorption of the sucrose disaccharide, which in turn results in osmotic diarrhea.[84] Other symptoms include, but are not limited to, failure to thrive, colic, abdominal dis-

tention, gassiness, and diaper rash.[85] Congenital sucrase-isomaltase deficiency is identified by analysis of disaccharidases (lactase, sucrase, isomaltase, maltase) obtained from an intestinal biopsy. The management strategy is avoidance or significant limitation of dietary sucrose, maltose, and starch due to a reduction or absence of the enzymes needed to break down these disaccharides on the intestinal surface.[85] Initially, foods and beverages containing sucrose and starch are removed from the diet, while nutrition needs to support growth and development are provided. Once symptoms have abated and the child is stable, foods/beverages containing low amounts ($\leq$ 2%) of sucrose are introduced. Foods are gradually introduced over time and the amount of sucrose allowed is increased as tolerated as per the direction of the medical team. In some instances, the usage of an oral enzyme preparation (sacrosidase) may be beneficial to improve dietary sucrose tolerance. Once the tolerance level for sucrose has been established, starch can be introduced into the diet. Tolerance to starch is variable and dependent on the child's enzyme levels.[86] A registered dietitian/nutritionist should counsel caregivers regarding label reading and provide resources regarding sucrose and starch presence in foods and beverages in order to achieve optimal results.

Similarly, individuals with chronic lactose intolerance also may present with abdominal distention, gassiness, and diarrhea. Lactose intolerance is a result of absence of the lactase enzyme to break down the dairy carbohydrate lactose. Management of this condition involves avoidance or limited consumption of lactose-containing foods and beverages depending on the lactase level. Lactose-free formula and milk substitutes are available. Older children with lactose intolerance can supplement with lactase pills prior to ingestion of lactose-containing foods.

Fructose intolerance is yet another source of diarrhea and abdominal pain observed in children.[87] Fructose is found in the diet as a monosaccharide, as a component of the disaccharide sucrose, and in a polymeric form (fructans). Free fructose has limited absorption in the small intestine. Fructose is absorbed by passive diffusion; it is not actively transported. Fructans are neither digested nor absorbed. Fructose malabsorption contributes to osmotic load. In addition, it provides substrate for bacterial fermentation and may affect GI motility, all leading to diarrhea. Malabsorption may contribute to abdominal pain. Fructose intolerance can be evaluated using a breath hydrogen test. Treatment is dietary restriction of foods rich in fructose, foods with a high fructose to glucose ratio, and foods high in sorbitol.

In both acute and chronic diarrhea, various micronutrients may be compromised either due to failure of absorption or increased losses in the stool. Losses commonly associated with diarrhea include zinc, copper, folate, magnesium, vitamin A, vitamin B_{12}, and trace elements, particularly selenium.[88,89] The clinician should be mindful of signs of deficiency of these nutrients and conduct laboratory screening as appropriate.

Supplementation of probiotics, particularly of *Lactobacillus GG* and *Saccharomyces boulardii*, may be beneficial in the management of diarrhea.[90,91] In controlled studies the duration of diarrhea was reduced about one day. The effects are strain specific, and safety and efficacy of each should be established. Currently, no standard guidelines exist for using probiotics in the management of pediatric diarrhea. In areas where zinc deficiency is common, zinc supplementation has been beneficial in reducing the duration of diarrhea.

Chronic diarrhea has many causes and detailed evaluation is necessary. The approach to management of chronic diarrhea depends on the etiology of the condition.

Pancreatic Insufficiency

The pancreas plays an integral role in the digestion of complex carbohydrates, proteins, and fats. This organ is composed of endocrine cells that secrete hormones, exocrine cells that make digestive enzymes, and duct cells that secrete bicarbonate and water. The endocrine pancreas only makes up approximately 2% of the pancreatic cell mass. It is primarily in the form of islet of Langerhans cells that produce and secrete the hormones insulin and glucagon, which are central to glucose homeostasis. The exocrine pancreas, on the other hand, consists of cells organized into acini and a ductal system that provides a pathway to the small intestine. The pancreas secretes approximately 1.5 L of an enzyme-rich alkaline fluid each day. Pancreatic juice is clear, colorless, and isotonic. Even though this juice is continuously secreted, the composition changes depending on hormonal and neuronal mechanisms. For example, in response to acid in the duodenum from a meal, the duodenal endocrine cells release secretin into the bloodstream. Secretin stimulates the pancreatic duct cells to release bicarbonate and water to neutralize the acid, thus achieving the optimal environment for digestion of gastric chyme. Furthermore, in response to the presence of proteins and fats in the proximal intestine, cholecystokinin is released from gut endocrine cells. This regulatory hormone stimulates pancreatic acinar cells to release digestive proenzymes through vagal afferents. These acinar cells secrete inactivated forms (zymogens) of the pro-

teolytic digestive enzymes (trypsin, chymotrypsin, elastase, etc) to prevent autodigestion of the pancreas. Other pancreatic enzymes are secreted in their active forms. After transportation to the duodenum via the ductal system, the inactivated trypsin is converted to its active form by enterokinase, which is produced from the duodenal mucosa. The activated trypsin, then activates other zymogens. Autodigesion of the pancreas is further prevented by trypsin inhibitors (for example, SPINK1) that are produced by the exocrine pancreas. Furthermore, trypsin can cleave and thus inactivate itself, which limits the amount of active trypsin.

When the normal mechanisms are disrupted, then pancreatic exocrine dysfunction results in the malabsorption of nutrients. Pancreatic insufficiency exists when the amount of digestive enzymes delivered to the intestine is inadequate for nutrient digestion. Overt steatorrhea, the presence of excess fat in the stool, occurs when 90% of the glandular function has been lost. Children may present with growth failure, weight loss, foul-smelling stools, edema, or diarrhea. Parents of children who are toilet-trained may report that the stools appear to be floating (due to the high fat content of the stool). It is possible that with mild pancreatic insufficiency, stools appear normal. Pancreatic insufficiency may result from congenital or acquired disease.

Cystic fibrosis (Chapter 28) is the most common cause of pancreatic insufficiency in childhood; approximately 90% of children with cystic fibrosis will develop pancreatic insufficiency by 1 year of age.[92] Other causes of pancreatic insufficiency in childhood are uncommon (Table 25-11).

Shwachman-Diamond syndrome (SDS) is the second most common cause of pancreatic insufficiency in children. It is estimated to occur in 1 in 77,000 live births. In the majority of patients with SDS, a mutation on the Shwachman-Bodian-Diamond syndrome (*SBDS*) gene, located on chromosome 7, can be found[93] Children will classically present with pancreatic insufficiency, hematologic abnormalities (especially variable neutropenia), and bone abnor-

Table 25-11. Pancreatic Insufficiency Not Cystic Fibrosis

TYPE	EXAMPLES
Congenital	Shwachman-Diamond syndrome Pearson syndrome Johanson-Blizzard syndrome Specific enzyme defects
Acquired	Chronic pancreatitis Common duct obstructions

malities (especially metaphyseal dysostosis). The pancreatic insufficiency found in children with SDS results from severe depletion of acinar cells. The normal tissue is replaced with fat.[94,95] Interestingly, the ductal tissue remains intact.

The most sensitive noninvasive measures to identify pancreatic dysfunction in SDS are serum trypsinogen and pancreatic isoamylase.[96] The response to pancreatic enzyme supplementation for pancreatic insufficiency is usually excellent in this population. However, children should be monitored intermittently for the need for enzyme replacement; approximately 50% of children can stop their replacement therapy by four years of age.[97] Clinical consensus guidelines for the diagnosis and treatment of SDS were published in 2011.[98]

Johanson-Blizzard syndrome is a rare disorder first described in 1971.[99] This autosomal recessive disorder is the result of mutations in the *UBR1* gene located on chromosome 15.[100] A history of parental consanguinity can often be found. No gender-based difference has been noted. The most consistent features of this syndrome are a small beak-like nose due to aplasia of the alae nasi and exocrine pancreatic insufficiency. However, other possible clinical features include dental anomalies, congenital scalp defects, sensorineural hearing loss, hypothyroidism, imperforate anus, and genitourinary anomalies.[101]

Even rarer is Pearson syndrome, which is exocrine pancreatic insufficiency associated with sideroblastic anemia.[102] It results from defects in mitochondrial DNA.[103] Because it is a mitochondrial disease, multiple organs can be involved.

In addition, isolated congenital deficiencies of the exocrine pancreas (lipase, colipase, amylase, and trypsinogen) have been described but are exceedingly rare. Enterokinase deficiency has also been described. As previously mentioned, enterokinase is produced by the intestinal mucosa and activates trypsin. These deficiencies are treated with enzyme replacement therapy.

Chronic pancreatitis can also cause pancreatic insufficiency over time due to chronic inflammation leading to fibrosis and destruction of exocrine and endocrine tissue. Unfortunately, this damage is irreversible.

Evaluation of pancreatic insufficiency is typically made by direct or indirect testing. Direct testing requires stimulation of the pancreas (with secretin, cholecystokinin, or both) and collection of pancreatic fluid to analyze the pancreatic enzyme content. However, these tests are invasive given that they require tube placement or an endoscopic procedure to accomplish the testing. In children who require long-term follow-up for their pancreatic insufficiency, repetitive test-ing is not feasible. Indirect tests are noninvasive and less expensive. However, in mild pancreatic exocrine dysfunction, indirect testing is less sensitive and specific.[104] In contrast, direct stimulation of the pancreas with secretin has high sensitivity and specificity in identifying pancreatic insufficiency in general, as well as isolated pancreatic enzyme deficiencies.[105]

The most widely used of the indirect tests is fecal elastase-1. This test is the most specific for the human pancreas and resistant to intestinal breakdown.[106] Children do not have to stop pancreatic enzyme supplementation to complete this test. However, false positives can be found in children with villous atrophy (as in celiac disease) or acute episodes of diarrhea.[107,108] The ordering clinician should be aware of the limitations of indirect testing and consider direct pancreatic exocrine testing if clinical suspicion remains high for pancreatic insufficiency.

Pancreatic insufficiency can lead to poor growth and nutritional deficiencies. Children with pancreatic insufficiency can develop deficiencies in fat-soluble vitamins (A, D, E, and K). Symptoms may include impaired night vision, metabolic bone disease, sensory or motor neuropathy, hemolysis, and easy bleeding or bruising. Children with documented pancreatic insufficiency should be screened with serum vitamin A, 25-hydroxyvitamin D, α-tocopherol (this value divided by cholesterol plus triglycerides; desired ratio is > 0.8 mg of α-tocopherol per gram of total lipids), and prothrombin time (PT). Based upon the results, individual supplementation can be prescribed. Deficiency of B_{12} is thought to be due to the decreased intestinal pH interfering with the transfer of vitamin B_{12} from R protein to intrinsic factor.[109]

A low-fat diet used to be advised in the past, but current recommendations are to optimize pancreatic enzyme supplementation instead so as not to promote further weight loss.[110] Research indicates that individuals with pancreatic insufficiency have a higher resting energy requirement than individuals with pancreatic sufficiency.[111] Thus, calories will likely need to be provided at > 100% of estimated needs.[112] In 1991, the U.S. Food and Drug Administration mandated that all pancreatic enzymes must be approved. Currently, 6 approved products are available (Zenpep, Creon, Pancreaze, Viokase, Ultresa, and Pertzye). Viokase is the only pancreatic enzyme preparation that is not enteric-coated, and it is only approved for adults. The remaining pancreatic enzymes are approved for children (although Ultresa and Pertzye are approved for > 12 months plus a weight requirement). Dosing is based on the lipase component. Enzyme dosage should not exceed 2500 lipase units/kg per meal or 4000 lipase units/g fat per day to avoid fibrosing colonopathy.[113]

Pancreatitis

Pancreatitis is an inflammatory process of the pancreas with variable involvement of other organs and tissues. Exposure to a causal factor initiates a cascade of events in which trypsinogen is converted to trypsin in quantities that overwhelm the innate protective mechanisms. Causes of pancreatitis include trauma, infection, drugs or toxins, multisystem disease, and congenital abnormalities of the pancreatic or biliary ductal system. Many cases do not have a clear trigger identified. In children, most cases are either acute and isolated or recurrent acute attacks. Chronic pancreatitis is seen more commonly in adults. In children it is most often related to structural malformation or a specific gene defect as seen in hereditary pancreatitis.

The incidence of acute pancreatitis in childhood is uncertain. Though not rare, it accounts for a small proportion of pediatric admissions.[114,115] Likewise, the incidence of chronic pancreatitis in children is not clear.

Pancreatitis is diagnosed by the combination of abdominal pain with elevation of the levels of amylase and lipase in the serum. The levels of the enzymes do not predict the severity of pancreatitis. No scoring systems are applicable to children, in contrast to adults. Clinical features suggestive of more severe disease include hypotension, renal failure, altered sensorium, and hemorrhage.

Initial management of children with acute pancreatitis is analgesia and IV fluids. If vomiting is present, a nasogastric tube is used to decompress the stomach. In patients with mild disease, enteral feedings are withheld for a short period. Reinitiation of feedings is based on resolution of abdominal pain, ileus, and vomiting. Most patients with mild disease recover quickly without complications.

Patients with severe pancreatitis often show signs of hemodynamic instability and are at risk for multiple complications including severe nutrition depletion. Nutrition support is important in these patients once they are hemodynamically stable and is considered an active therapeutic intervention.[116] Patients can be fed enterally by nasogastric or nasojejunal tube or by the IV route. Although a number of studies have been done in adults, data concerning nutrition support in pediatric patients with pancreatitis are scarce. Adult studies suggest a trend to fewer adverse outcomes in patients who receive enteral as opposed to parenteral feedings; however, the effect on outcome is not clear.[117] There does not seem to be a difference in feedings of polymeric vs semi-elemental or "immune-enhancing" formulas.[118] A study in children with severe acute pancreatitis found little difference between EN and PN in length of stay, infection, mortality, or need for surgery.[119]

Chronic pancreatitis is a condition in which continued inflammation of the pancreas produces irreversible changes in the gland. In some cases it is related to continued recurrent injury from acute attacks. Often the etiology is not clear even when risk factors are present. In adults, repeated exposure to toxins (eg, alcohol) is often implicated. In children, hereditary factors such as mutation of the trypsinogen molecule, or mutations of the cystic fibrosis transmembrane regulator (CFTR) gene or trypsin inhibitor genes are often sought. Autoimmune disorders, both isolated autoimmune pancreatitis as well as systemic autoimmune diseases, are seen. Patients with recurrent acute pancreatitis are at risk for developing chronic pancreatitis.[120]

Treatment of chronic pancreatitis revolves around several concerns: chronic pain, development of diabetes due to islet cell destruction, and pancreatic insufficiency due to acinar cell destruction. Pain impacts ability to ingest nutrients. The treatment of chronic pain is beyond the scope of this chapter. In addition, the treatment of diabetes mellitus is discussed elsewhere (Chapter 21). Digestive enzyme insufficiency is a late complication of chronic pancreatitis. The treatment for pancreatic digestive enzyme insufficiency is enzyme replacement. The goal is to provide enzyme supplements enough to restore digestive function. The dose of pancreatic enzyme is calculated according to the lipase content. A usual dose of enzyme is 1000 to 2500 U of lipase per kilogram of body weight per meal. This is often altered based on the estimated fat content of the meal. This is discussed in more detail in Chapter 28. Both polymeric as well as elemental dietary supplements have been used for nutrition support, and scant data have evaluated the effectiveness in children. It deserves to be restated that a major goal of nutrition support in these patients is maintenance of normal growth.

Disorders of Chyle Loss

Chyle is a creamy fluid consisting of fat, protein, electrolytes, and lymphocytes, and it is an important aspect of the metabolism of fat. Triglycerides are broken down in the intestinal lumen to fatty acids and mono-acyl glycerols, which are then absorbed into the intestinal epithelial cells. This process is aided by the action of bile salts mixing with the fatty acids, forming micelles that enhance the transport of the molecules. Within the enterocytes, the absorbed fatty acids are re-esterified to glycerol, and the resultant lipid is complexed with proteins (forming chylomicrons) and transported through the lymphatic system of the GI tract and abdomen, ultimately into the thoracic duct, and then into the bloodstream. Disorders of chyle loss are rare, with the most common disorders being chylothorax or chylous ascites. Chylothorax is defined by pooling of lymphatic fluid, chyle, in mediastinal or pleural cavities. Chylous ascites occurs when lymphatic disruption is present in the abdominal cavity with resultant pooling of chyle in the abdomen. This condition is usually seen as a complication of surgery,[121] although congenital defects of lymph flow are also described. For more detailed information refer to the chapter on cardiac disease (Chapter 23). A less common disorder of chyle is that of intestinal lymphangiectasia. This condition results from failure of lymph flow often related to inflammation, causing enlargement of intestinal lymph vessels, which causes breakage of the lacteals and spillage of chyle into the intestinal lumen.[122] As a result, protein-losing enteropathy leading to hypoalbuminemia and edema may result. Hypogammaglobulinemia is often present. Edema of the intestinal mucosa causes malabsorption. Steatorrhea is typically seen.[123] Even more rare are the disorders of chylomicron formation such as abetalipoproteinemia in which a defect exists in the ability to complex the lipids with carrier proteins, and the lipid is therefore not carried into the lymphatic system.

Regardless of the specific disorder of chyle processing, the nutrition approach is similar. The initial treatment is restriction of dietary fat. A low-fat, high-protein diet is recommended because associated protein loss usually occurs in the GI tract. Because medium-chain length fatty acids and triglycerides can be metabolized without entry into the lymphatic system, dietary fats should be primarily from medium-chain triglycerides (MCTs), often by using a specialized formula that is high in MCTs but low in long-chain triglycerides (LCTs).[122] The rationale for this diet is twofold. One, the decreased amount of fat lowers the amount of circulating chyle. This reduction lowers the risk of lacteals becoming dilated and releasing chyle. Two, MCTs are directly transported via the portal system, which reduces lymphatic circulation.[123] Most often, this diet is needed for 4–8 weeks[121] If an infant or child is on formula, one should be cautious about supplying sufficient amounts of essential fatty acids, linoleic and linolenic acids, to prevent deficiency; not all high-MCT oil-containing formulas contain sufficient quantities of these nutrients. The American Academy of Pediatrics recommends that a minimum of 3% of calories should come from these essential fatty acids. Also depending on which formula is used, chromium, molybdenum, and selenium need to be supplemented if the child is on formula for an extended period of time. PN may be initiated in instances when EN is not adequate to meet nutrient needs or not indicated for other reasons. Lipids in PN are not absorbed via the lymphatic system and have no effect on the condition so can be used without modification.

Functional Disorders

The functional disorders are a diverse group of conditions in which symptoms persist for a prolonged period and no specific tissue change is associated with the symptom.[124] These include recurrent and/or chronic abdominal pain, chronic nonspecific diarrhea, gastroparesis, cyclic vomiting syndrome, and constipation. Because the underlying pathophysiology is unclear, both the evaluation and treatment are related to the predominant symptom. Malnutrition is rare in these patients and, if present, suggests an alternative diagnosis. Frequently, dietary interventions are suggested for symptom control. These include increasing fiber, reducing fermentable carbohydrate, and altering the fat content of the diet. These interventions are often recommended and frequently reported to be helpful though data documenting effectiveness are lacking.[125]

Chronic abdominal pain is a common symptom in children and adolescents, and it is estimated to affect 10%–15% of the population at some time. The etiology and pathogenesis are unknown, and no specific diagnostic markers have been identified to help in diagnosis. The clinical presentation and careful history and physical examination will often suggest that the diagnosis is functional abdominal pain. A few laboratory or x-ray studies may assist in the evaluation and are remarkable for their normality.

The role of dietary modifications in the management of the functional abdominal pain disorders is not established. If symptoms are mainly post prandial or include the sensation of bloating, a low-fat diet is sometimes recommended. If diarrhea or constipation is prominently associated with the pain, an increase in the amount of fiber in the diet is considered. Poor absorption of ingested carbohydrate may trigger symptoms in susceptible individuals. Therefore, restrictions of lactose (milk), fructose (eg, carbonated beverages and certain fruits), or dietary starches (eg, corn, wheat, oat, and potato) are sometimes tried. Restriction of nonabsorbable sugar alcohols, often used as artificial sweeteners (eg, sorbitol, xylitol), is advised. It is important to avoid multiple restrictive diets because they may lead to nutrition insufficiency. GF diets should be instituted only after appropriate evaluation for celiac disease.

Gastroparesis

Gastroparesis is the delay of emptying of the stomach in the absence of a mechanical obstruction. Multiple causes exist (Table 25-12). Disorders of the intestinal muscula-ture (myopathic) and the intestinal nervous system (neu-ropathic), both congenital and acquired, are described. Common causes are immaturity (especially in premature infants), viral infections, systemic diseases, and drugs. Gastroparesis often complicates the management of type 1 diabetes mellitus. Evaluation should include assessment of gastric anatomy and function (eg, upper GI series x-ray or gastric emptying study) as well as a search for and treat-ment of any underlying condition and bacterial overgrowth. Importantly, malnutrition may be both a cause as well as a result of gastroparesis.

Gastroparesis has many symptoms, including nausea, vomiting, bloating, upper abdominal discomfort, early sati-ety, heartburn, esophageal reflux, and decreased appetite.[126] These symptoms may lead to malnutrition and the need for nutrition support. Initial treatment of gastroparesis should include maximizing the therapy of treatable systemic illness (eg, optimizing glycemic control in the diabetic patient) and eliminating causes such as medications.

The nutrition assessment of a child with gastroparesis should include a dietary recall and/or dietary record, eval-uation of changes in weight over time, laboratory studies, description of symptoms, and listing of medications as well as nutrition supplements.[127] The dietary recall and record provide important information regarding both symptoms and intake. Factors to consider are meal volume tolerance, preference of liquids over solids, and fiber and fat tolerance. Because early satiety is commonly seen in gastroparesis, small frequent meals may be better tolerated than 3 large meals. Liquids are often better tolerated than solids, with the exception of carbonated beverages, which may worsen symptoms.[128] Thus, a diet of liquids and/or purees may be more effective in delivering ample nutrition than a conven-tional solid-based diet. Avoidance of a high-fiber and high-fat diet, with the exception of fat in liquid nutrition, is also often beneficial in delivering nutrition because both of these nutrients delay gastric emptying. Dietary osmolality is less an issue in managing gastroparesis.[127]

Laboratory markers commonly monitored include fer-ritin, glucose, and hemoglobin A_{1C}. Iron-deficiency anemia is common in this cohort of patients, in part due to symptom

Table 25-12. Conditions Associated With Gastroparesis

TYPE	EXAMPLES
Infection	Postviral illness (eg, rotavirus)
Neurological disease	Mitochondrial disorders Familial dysautonomia
Systemic disease	Diabetes Malnutrition Connective tissue disorders

management. Usage of acid-reducing medications to man-age reflux and heartburn decreases the gastric acid needed to convert dietary iron to its more absorbable form. Further, use of jejunal tube feeds to control vomiting and promote weight gain can increase the risk of iron-deficiency anemia because the duodenum is the main area of iron absorption. Ferritin is a more appropriate marker to screen for iron-de-ficiency anemia than hemoglobin and hematocrit. However, it is important to remember that ferritin is an acute phase respondent and will not be accurate during acute inflamma-tion.[129] Other laboratory markers may require monitoring if indicated by the nutrition assessment (see Chapter 32).

Constipation

Constipation is a common symptom among humans of all ages and is often especially troubling in infants and young children. It is most often both self-limited and short lived. However, a substantial number of patients have symptoms that persist for six months or more. Constipation may be related to inadequate intake of fluid or fiber, side effects of medication, inactivity, or disordered bowel motility. Most cases are idiopathic and fulfill the definitions of functional constipation. Although most recognize a role for diet in both the etiology and the treatment of constipation, little data identify specific foods as either causal or beneficial.

It has long been suggested that cow's milk consumption contributes to constipation.[130] Evidence suggests a role of cow's milk protein sensitivity in constipation.[131,132] In addi-tion, it is known that the fat content of milk may also be as-sociated with harder or more difficult-to-pass stools.

Historically, a high-fiber diet has been recommended for children with constipation. However, few studies doc-ument benefit.[133,134] Additionally, no conclusive evidence exists that fiber supplements or a lactose-free diet is bene-ficial in alleviating recurrent abdominal pain in children. However, in some children it may be beneficial to undergo a trial of a high-fiber diet (0.75 g soluble fiber per year of age) or based on recommendations for age outlined in the 2010 Dietary Guidelines for Americans.[135]

Cyclic Vomiting Syndrome

Although increasingly recognized in children, the pathogenesis of cyclic vomiting syndrome remains unknown. The clinical features overlap with those of abdominal migraine. The distinguishing characteristic is a repeated pattern of stereotypical episodes of severe vomiting often associated with pallor, lethargy, and abdominal pain. The episodes are similar in onset and usually duration. A prodrome of variable duration often occurs. An important feature is that the children return to baseline health in between episodes.

In cyclic vomiting syndrome the primary nutrition concern is management of any fluid and electrolyte disturbances that may arise because dietary interventions to prevent onset or reduce duration of the condition are unknown.[124] Diets used to prevent migraines have been tried. It is recommended to avoid prolonged fasting because that may trigger vomiting.

Irritable Bowel Syndrome

In IBS no clear evidence exists to suggest that diet causes the condition; however, diet modification is frequently recommended.[136] It may be prudent to undergo an elimination trial of foods containing lactose, fructose, and/or sorbitol because intolerance to these foods manifests as abdominal pain.[137] Specifically, the low FODMAP (fermentable, oligosaccharides, disaccharides, monosaccharides, and polyols) diet has been beneficial in managing abdominal pain in adults with IBS (see Table 25-13).[138,139] This diet eliminates and/or restricts the consumption of certain fermentable short-chain carbohydrates, which can exacerbate GI symptoms such as gas production. The diet consists of an elimination phase of FODMAPs and then a gradual introduction of one category at a time, while monitoring for disease symptoms. It may be prudent to have a breath hydrogen test prior to starting the diet to determine if lactose or fructose malabsorption is present. Depending on the results, foods and beverages within these groups may or may not need to be restricted as part of the diet.[140]

The role of dietary fiber, particularly soluble fiber, in symptom management, especially of constipation, is debatable. Soluble fiber is found in fruits, vegetables, and whole grains. When ingested, fiber helps to give the stool a gel-like consistency and serves as a fuel source for colonic bacteria. The end result is a reduction in gut transit time and a subsequent reduction in constipation and intracolonic pres-

Table 25-13. Low FODMAP (Fermentable Oligosaccharides, Disaccharides, Monosaccharides and Polyols) Diet[138]

FERMENTABLE SHORT-CHAIN CARBOHYDRATES	EXAMPLES
Oligosaccharides	Fructans (eg, wheat products, inulins, some vegetables, and fructo-oligosaccharides) and galacto-oligosaccharides (eg, legumes)
Disaccharides	Lactose (eg, cow, sheep and goat milk)
Monosaccharides	Fructose (eg, fruits, high-fructose corn syrup, honey, certain vegetables and grains)
Polyols	Mannitol, maltitol, xylitol, sorbitol, polydextrose, isomalt

sure.[120,141] However, increased fiber consumption can also exacerbate bloating and flatulence, which are undesirable side effects and can limit adherence to a high-fiber diet.[142] To date, no definitive conclusions exist as to the benefit of fiber in IBS symptom management.[143] Similarly, no definitive recommendations have been proposed for the usage of probiotics in the management of IBS. More research is needed regarding which strains or combinations of strains are most beneficial before guidelines can be established.[139] Nutrition counseling should be individualized based on the patient's reported food-symptom correlations.[144] The suspected offending food should be removed from the diet for 2–3 weeks. If no relief in symptoms is observed, the food may be added back to the diet.

Eosinophilic Conditions of the Gut

Eosinophilic gastroenteritis is a condition characterized by either patchy or diffuse infiltration of eosinophils anywhere in the GI tract. Damage to the GI tract is due to both the infiltration and degranulation of eosinophils. The triggering process is not clear. Both IgE-mediated and non–IgE-mediated sensitivities are described. Many patients (especially older patients) have conditions such as a high eosinophil count, asthma, allergic rhinitis, or eczema suggesting underlying atopy. Allergies to food or inhalants are sometimes implicated. In addition, atopy often appears in the family history. It may affect children of any age.

The signs and symptoms are nonspecific, and the presentation varies by location, depth, and extent of the eosinophilic infiltration (Table 25-14). There may be involvement of the mucosal, muscular, or serosal layers. Mucosal disease presents as nausea and vomiting, diarrhea (often bloody), malabsorption, and weight loss. When the muscular layers

Table 25-14. Presentation Characteristics of Eosinophilic Gastroenteritis by Tissue

TISSUE TYPE	SIGNS AND SYMPTOMS
Mucosal	Diarrhea, gastrointestinal bleeding, vomiting, abdominal pain
Muscular	Vomiting, colicky, abdominal pain
Serosal	Ascites, abdominal pain

are involved, signs and symptoms of obstruction are present. If serosal involvement occurs, there may be ascites. The most common symptom is colicky abdominal pain.

The most frequently seen form of eosinophilic gastroenteritis is proctitis in infants, often referred to as allergic colitis. The disorder is characterized by the bloody diarrhea in an infant < 2 months of age.

Cases of food-induced eosinophilic proctocolitis are reported regardless of the infant being breastfed or formula fed. Infants presenting with this condition usually have normal linear and ponderal growth. The infants will have diarrhea, usually accompanied by mucous and/or blood, and often with pain or straining at the time of bowel motion. Biopsy of the rectal mucosa will show eosinophilic infiltration of the mucosa. Frequently the diagnosis is made on clinical presentation alone. The dietary management of this condition involves elimination of the offending protein until approximately 9–12 months of age. If an infant is breastfed then the offending protein should be removed from the mother's diet. Earlier reintroduction of the protein will usually result in bleeding.[145]

In older children with eosinophilic conditions of the gut symptoms include, but are not limited to, vomiting, abdominal pain, diarrhea, hematochezia, poor growth/weight gain, and iron-deficiency anemia.[146] The recommended dietary treatment is avoidance of the offending allergens. Particular attention should be paid to the quality of the diet as malnutrition may develop if numerous foods are eliminated. For some children, use of an amino acid–based formula may be appropriate. For more information regarding eosinophilic conditions of the gut please refer to the Chapter on Allergic Diseases.

Summary

Because of the central role of the digestive system in maintaining normal nutrition, disease of the GI tract, liver, or pancreas has a profound influence on growth and development of children. Provision of adequate nutrition support can not only improve nutrition parameters and growth but also in

many cases can treat the underlying disease. Careful evaluation of the child with assessment of nutrition needs is the initial step in effective management. The clinical examination and judiciously applied laboratory investigation will identify nutrition deficiencies. With understanding of the underlying disease process, appropriate nutrition management can improve growth, quality of life, and outcomes of these patients.

Test Your Knowledge Questions

A 15-year-old boy is admitted to the hospital because of diarrhea and abdominal pain. He has had unintentional weight loss of 15 lb in the last 3 months. Laboratory evaluation reveals the following:

- Albumin, 3.1 gm/dL
- Total protein, 6.2 gm/dL
- Hemoglobin/hematocrit, 9.3gm/dL/27%
- MCV, 71 fL (normal > 79 fL)
- WBC, 11,500 K/microL

Radiology studies demonstrated inflammation of the ileum and cecum.

1. Diet therapy should include:
   A. A polymeric defined formula diet
   B. A semi-elemental defined formula diet
   C. An elemental defined formula diet
   D. Any of A, B, or C
   E. A clear liquid diet
2. His medical therapy includes methotrexate and sulfasalazine. Supplementation should include:
   A. Folate, B_{12}, and iron
   B. Pyridoxine, thiamin, and magnesium
   C. B_{12}, vitamin C, and manganese
   D. Folate, vitamin C, and copper
3. In a patient with celiac disease, a GF diet should be maintained:
   A. Until diarrhea subsides
   B. Until normal linear growth is established
   C. Until new and as yet undiscovered treatments are available
   D. Until bone mineral density has returned to normal
   E. A GF diet is not necessary
4. Your patient has just been diagnosed with pancreatic insufficiency. Which lab tests are appropriate?
   A. Vitamin A, 25-hydroxyvitamin D, iron panel
   B. 25-hydroxyvitamin D, folate, iron panel
   C. Vitamin A, folate, PT
   D. Vitamin A, 25-hydroxyvitamin D, α-tocopherol/total lipids, PT

5. Which of the following recommendations is not appropriate to make for this patient with pancreatic insufficiency?

A. Start pancreatic enzymes at a dose < 2500 lipase units/kg per meal.

B. Your patient should start a low-fat diet.

C. Your patient's actual caloric needs will likely be > 100% of their estimated needs.

D. Your patient should take the prescribed pancreatic enzymes prior to all meals and snacks.

References

1. Gibbons T, Fuchs GJ. Malnutrition: a hidden problem in hospitalized children. *Clin Pediatr.* 2009;48:356–361.

2. Motil KJ, Phillips SM, Conkin CA. Nutritional assessment. In: Wyllie R, Hyams JS, Kay M, eds. *Pediatric Gastrointestinal and Liver Disease. Pathophysiology, Diagnosis, Management.* 3rd ed. London: Saunders Elsevier; 2011:948–956.

3. Pacheco-Acosta JC, Gomez-Correa AC, Flores ID, et al. Incidence of nutrition deterioration in nonseriously ill hospitalized children younger then 5 years [published online ahead of print June 2, 2014]. *Nutr Clin Pract.* 2014;29(5):692–697.

4. Groleau V, Thibault M, Doyon M, et al. Malnutrition in hospitalized children: prevalence, impact and management. *Can J Diet Pract Res.* 2014;75(1):29–34.

5. Gatti S, Caporelli N, Galeazzi T, et al. Oats in the diet of children with celiac disease: preliminary results of a double-blind, randomized, placebo-controlled multicenter Italian study. *Nutrients.* 2013;5:4653–4664.

6. Motil KJ, Grand RJ, Davis-Kraft L, Ferlic LL, O'Brian Smith E. Growth failure in children with inflammatory bowel disease: a prospective study. *Gastroenterology.* 1993;105:681–691.

7. Baker SS, Baker RD, Davis AM. *Pediatric Nutrition Support.* Sudbury, MA: Jones and Bartlett Publishers; 2007:459–475.

8. Shay S, Tutian R, Sifrim D, et al. Twenty-four hour ambulatory simultaneous impedance and pH monitoring: a multicenter report of normal values from 60 healthy volunteers. *Am J Gastroenterol.* 2004;99:1037–1043.

9. Nelson SP, Chen EH, Syniar GM, et al. Prevalence of symptoms of gastroesophageal reflux during childhood: a pediatric practice-based survey. *Arch Pediatric Adol Med.* 2000;154:150–154.

10. Vandenplas Y, Goyvaerts H, Helven R, Sacre L. Gastroesophageal reflux, as measured by 24-hour pH monitoring, in 509 healthy infants screened for risk of sudden infant death syndrome. *Pediatrics.* 1991;88:834–890.

11. Martin AJ, Pratt N, Kennedy JD, et al. Natural history and familial relationships of infant spilling to 9 years of age. *Pediatrics.* 2002;109:1061–1067.

12. Nelson SP, Chen EH, Syniar GM, et al. Prevalence of symptoms of gastroesophageal reflux during infancy: a pediatric practice-based survey. *Arch Pediatr Adolesc Med.* 1997;151:569–572.

13. Nelson SP, Chen EH, Syniar GM, Christoffel KK. One year follow up of symptoms of gastroesophageal reflux during infancy. Pediatric Practice Research Group. *Pediatrics.* 1998;102:e67.

14. Vandenplas Y. Gastroesophageal reflux. In: Wyllie R, Hyams JS, Kay M, eds. *Pediatric Gastrointestinal and Liver Disease. Pathophysiology, Diagnosis, Management.* 4th ed. London: Saunders Elsevier; 2011:242–247.

15. Pandolfino JE, Kwiatek MA, Kahrilas PJ. The pathophysiologic basis for epidemiologic trends in gastroesophageal reflux disease. *Gastroenterol Clin North Am.* 2008;37:827–843.

16. Vandenplas Y, Hassall E. Mechanics of gastroesophageal reflux and gastroesophageal reflux disease. *J Pediatr Gastroenterol Nutr.* 2002;35:119–136.

17. Kawahara H, Dent J, Davidson G. Mechanics responsible for gastroesophageal reflux in children. *Gastroenterology.* 1997;113:399–408.

18. Lightdale JR, Gremse DA; Section on Gastroenterology, Hepatology, and Nutrition. Gastroesophageal reflux: management guidance for the pediatrician. *Pediatrics.* 2013;131:e1684–e1695.

19. Jadcherla SR, Chan CY, Moore R, et al. Impact of feeding strategies on the frequency and clearance of acid and nonacid gastroesophageal reflux events in dysphagic neonates. *JPEN J Parenter Enter Nutr.* 2012;36(4):449–455.

20. Vandenplas Y, Rudolph CD, Di Lorenzo C, et al; , North American Society for Pediatric Gastroenterology Hepatology and Nutrition, European Society for Pediatric Gastroenterology Hepatology and Nutrition. Pediatric gastroesophagela reflux clinical practice guidelines: joint recommendations of the North American Society for Pediatric Gastroenterology, Hepatology, and Nutrition (NASPGHAN) and the European Society for Pediatric Gastroenterology, Hepatology, and Nutrition (ESPGHAN). *J Pediatr Gastroenterol Nutr.* 2009;49(4):498–547.

21. Vanderhoof JA, Moran JR, Harris CL, Merkel KL, Orenstein SR. Efficacy of a pre-thickened infant formula: a multicenter, double-blind, randomized, placebo-controlled parallel group trial in 104 infants with symptomatic gastroesophageal reflux. *Clin Pediatr.* 2003;42:483–495.

22. Aggett PJ, Agostoni C, Axelsson I, et al. Antireflux or antiregurgitation milk products for infants and young children: a commentary by the ESPGHAN Committee on Nutrition. *J Pediatr Gastroenterol Nutr.* 2002;394:496–498.

23. Vandenplas Y, De Wolf D, Sacre L. Influence of xanthines on gastroesophageal reflux in infants at risk for sudden infant death syndrome. *Pediatrics.* 1986;77:807–810.

24. Wenzl TG, Schneider S, Scheele F, Silny J, Heimann G, Skopnik H. Effects of thickened feeding on gastroesophageal reflux in infants: a placebo-controlled crossover study using intraluminal impedance. *Pediatrics.* 2003;111(4 Pt 1):e355–e359.

25. Corvaglia l, Spizzichino M, Aceti A, et al. A thickened formula does not reduce apneas related to gastroesophageal reflux in preterm infants. *Neonatology.* 2013;103:98–102.22.

26. Orenstein SR, Shalaby TM, Putnam PE. Thickened feedings as a cause of increased coughing when used as therapy for gastroesophageal reflux in infants. *J Pediatr.* 1992;121:913-915.

27. Huang RC, Forbes DA, Davies MW. Feed thickener for newborn infants with gastro-oesophageal reflux. *Cochrane Database Syst Rev.* 2009; (4): CD003211.DOI:10.1002/14651858. CD003211

28. Woods CW, Lewis OT, Yang Q. Development of necrotizing enterocolitis in premature infants receiving thickened feeds using SimplyThick. *J Perinatol.* 2012;322:150–152.

29. Bosscher D, Van Caillie-Bertrand M, Van Dyck K, Robberecht H, Van Cauwenbergh R, Deelstra H. Thickening infant formula with digestible and indigestible carbohydrate: availability of calcium, iron, and zinc in vitro. *J Pediatr Gastroenterol Nutr.* 2000;30:373–378.

30. Corvaglia L, Mariani E, Aceti A, et al. Extensively hydrolysed protein formula reduces acid gastro-esophageal reflux in symptomatic preterm infants. *Early Hum Dev.* 2013;89(7):453–455.

31. Hills JM, Aaronson PI. The mechanism of action of peppermint oil on gastrointestinal smooth muscle. *Gastroenterology.* 1991;101:55–65.

32. Wendl B, Pfeiffer A, Pehl C, Schmidt T, Kaess H. Effect of decaffeination of coffee or tea on gastro-oesophageal reflux. *Aliment Pharmacol Ther.* 1994;8:283–287.

33. Pehl C, Pfeiffer A, Wendl B, Kaess H. The effect of decaffeination of coffee on gastroesophageal reflux in patients with reflux disease. *Aliment Pharmacol Ther.* 1997;11:483–486.

34. Bulat R, Fachnie E, Chauhan U, Chen Y, Tougas G. Lack of effect of spearmint on lower esophageal sphincter function and acid reflux in healthy volunteers. *Aliment Pharmacol Ther.* 1999;13:805–812.

35. Penagini R, Mangano M, Bianchi PA. Effect of increasing the fat content but not the energy load of a meal on gastro-oesophageal reflux and lower oesophageal sphincter motor function. *Gut.* 1998;42:330–333.

36. Lewis D, Khoshoo V, Pencharz PB, Golladay ES. Impact of nutritional rehabilitation on gastroesophageal reflux in neurologically impaired children. *J Pediatr Surg.* 1994;29:167–169.

37. Herzig SJ, Howell MD, Ngo LH, Marcantonio GR. Acid-suppressive medication use and the risk for hospital-acquired pneumonia. *JAMA.* 2009;301(20):2120–2188.

38. Canani RB, Cirillo P, Roggero P, et al; Working Group on Intestinal Infections of the Italian Society of Pediatric Gastroenterology, Hepatology and Nutrition (SIGENP). Therapy with gastric acid inhibitors increases the risk of acute gastroenteritis and community-acquired pneumonia in children. *Pediatrics.* 2006;117(5):e817–e820.

39. Tighe M, Afzal NA, Bevan A, Hayen A, Munro A, Beatie RM Pharmacological treatment of children with gastro-oesopheal reflux *Cochrane Database Syst Rev.* 2014 (11): CD008550.DOI:10:1002/1465158.CD008550.pub2

40. Green PHR, Collier C. Celiac disease. *N Engl J Med.* 2007;357:1731–1743.

41. D'Amico MA, Holmes J, Stavropoulos SN, et al. Presentation of celiac disease in the United States: prominent effect of breast feeding. *Clin Pediatr (Phila).* 2005;44:249–258.

42. Rampertab SD, Poorfan N, Baur P, Singh P, et al. Trends in the presentation of celiac disease. *Am J Med.* 2006;119(4):355. e9–355.e14.

43. Husby S, Koletzko S, Korponay-Szabó IR, et al; ESPGHAN Working Group on Coeliac Disease Diagnosis; ESPGHAN Gastroenterology Committee; European Society for Pediatric Gastroenterology, Hepatology, and Nutrition. European Society for Pediatric Gastroenterology, Hepatology, and Nutrition guidelines for the diagnosis of coeliac disease. *J Pediatr Gasteroenterol Nutr.* 2012;54(1):136–160.

44. Haapalahti M, Kulmala P, Karttunen TJ, et al. Nutritional status in adolescents and young adults with screen-detected celiac disease. *J Pediatr Gastroenterol Nutr.* 2005;40:566–570.42.

45. See J, Murray JA. Gluten-free diet: the medical and nutrition management of celiac disease. *Nutr Clin Pract.* 2006;21:1–15.

46. Butzner J. Pure oats and the gluten-free diet: are they safe? *JPEN J Parenter Enteral Nutr.* 2011;35:447–448.

47. Hallert C, Grant C, Grehn S, et al. Evidence of poor vitamin status in celiac patients on a gluten-free diet for 10 years. *Aliment Pharmacol Ther.* 2002;16:1333–1339.

48. Mora S, Barera G, Beccio S, et al. A prospective, longitudinal study of the long-term effect of treatment on bone density in children with celiac disease. *J Pediatr.* 2001;139(4):473–475.

49. Shamir R. Nutritional aspects in inflammatory bowel disease. *J Pediatr Gastroenterol Nutr.* 2009;48:586–588.

50. Kleinman RE, Baldassano RN, Caplan A, et al. Nutrition support for pediatric patients with inflammatory bowel disease: a clinical report of the North American Society for Pediatric Gastroenterology, Hepatology and Nutrition. *J Pediatr Gastroenterol Nutr.* 2004;39:15–27.

51. Seidman E, LeLeiko N, Ament M, et al. Nutritional issues in pediatric inflammatory bowel disease. *J Pediatr Gastroenterol Nutr.* 1991;12:424–438.

52. Kanof ME, Lake AM, Bayless TM. Decreased height velocity in children and adolescents before the diagnosis of Crohn's disease. *Gastroenterology.* 1988;95:1523–1527.

53. Saha MT, Ruuska T, Laippala P, Lenko HL. Growth of prepubertal children with inflammatory bowel disease. *J Pediatr Gastroenterol Nutr.* 1998;26:310–314.

54. Markowitz J, Grancher K, Rosa J, Aiges H, Daum F. Growth failure in pediatric inflammatory bowel disease. *J Pediatr Gastroenterol Nutr.* 1993;16:373–380.

55. Sentongo TA, Semeao EJ, Piccoli DA, Stallings VA, Zemel BS. Growth, body composition and nutritional status in children and adolescents with Crohn's disease. *J Pediatr Gastroenterol Nutr.* 2000;31:33–40.

56. Mamula P, Markowitz JE, Baldassano RN. Inflammatory bowel disease in early childhood and adolescence: special considerations. *Gastroenterol Clin North Am.* 2003;32:967–995.

57. Wiskin AE, Wootton SA, Beattie RM. Nutrition issues in pediatric Crohn's disease. *Nutr Clin Pract.* 2007;22:214–222.

58. Navarro FA, Hanauer SB, Kirschner BS. Effect of long-term low-dose prednisone on height velocity and disease activity in pediatric and adolescent patients with Crohn disease. *J Pediatr Gastroenterol Nutr.* 2007;45:312–318.

59. Critch J, Day A, Otley A, et al. Use of enteral nutrition for the control of intestinal inflammation in pediatric Crohn disease. *J Pediatr Gastroenterol Nutr.* 2012;54:298–305.

60. Sanderson IR, Udeen S, Davies PS, Savage MO, Walker-Smith JA. Remission induced by an elemental diet in small bowel Crohn's disease. *Arch Dis Child.* 1987;61:123–127.

61. Borrelli O, Cordischi L, Cirulli M, et al. Polymeric diet alone versus corticosteroids in the treatment of active pediatric Crohn's disease: a randomized controlled open-label trial. *Clin Gastroenterol Hepatol.* 2006;4:744–753.

62. Eiden KA. Nutritional considerations in inflammatory bowel disease. *Practical Gastroenterol.* 2003;27:33–54.

63. Sentongo TA, Semaeo EJ, Stettler N, Piccoli DA, Stallings VA, Zemel BS. Vitamin D status in children, adolescents and young adults with Crohn disease. *Am J Clin Nutr.* 2002;76:1077–1081.

64. Pappa HM, Gordon CM, Saslowsky TM, et al. Vitamin D status in children and young adults with inflammatory bowel disease. *Pediatrics.* 2006;118:1950–1961.

65. Pappa H, Thayu S, Leonard F, et al. Skeletal health of children and adolescents with inflammatory bowel disease. *J Pediatr Gastroenterol Nutr.* 2011;53:11–25.

66. Canani RB, Terrin G, Borrelli O, et al. Short- and long-term therapeutic efficacy of nutritional therapy and corticosteroids in pediatric Crohn's disease. *Dig Liver Dis.* 2006;38:381–387.

67. Lochs H, Dejong C, Hammarqvist F, et al; ESPEN (European Society for Parenteral and Enteral Nutrition). ESPEN Guidelines on Enteral Nutrition: Gastroenterology. *Clin Nutr.* 2006;25:260–274.

68. Zachos M, Tondeur M, Griffiths AM. Enteral nutritional therapy for induction of remission in Crohn's disease. *Cochrane Database Syst Rev.* 2007;(1):CD000542.

69. Griffiths AM, Ohlsson A, Sherman PM, Sutherland LR. Meta-analysis of enteral nutrition as a primary treatment of active Crohn's disease. *Gastroenterology.* 1995;108:1056–1067.

70. Akobeng AK, Thomas AG. Enteral nutrition for maintenance of remission in Crohn's disease. *Cochrane Database Syst Rev.* 2007;(3):CD005984.

71. Takagi S, Utsunomiya K, Kuriyama S, et al. Effectiveness of an 'half elemental diet' as maintenance therapy for Crohn's disease: a randomized-controlled trial. *Aliment Pharmacol Ther.* 2006;24:1333–1340.

72. Wilschanski M, Sherman P, Pencharz P, Davis L, Corey M, Griffiths A. Supplementary enteral nutrition maintains remission in pediatric Crohn's disease. *Gut.* 1996;38:543–548.

73. Verma S, Kirkwood B, Brown S. Oral nutritional supplementation is effective in the maintenance of remission in Crohn's disease. *Digest Liver Dis.* 2000;32:769–774.

74. Levine A, Milo T, Buller H, Markowitz J. Consensus and controversy in the management of pediatric Crohn's disease: an international survey. *J Pediatr Gastroenterol Nutr.* 2003;36:464–469.

75. Lanata CF, Fischer-Walker CL, Olascoaga AC, et al. Global causes of diarrheal disease mortality in children <5 years of age: a systematic review. *PLoS One.* 2013;8:e72788.

76. Gracey M. Nutritional effects and management of diarrhea in infancy. *Acta Paediatr Suppl.* 1999;430:110–126.

77. Lutter CK, Habicht JP, Rivera JA, Martorell R. The relationship between energy intake and diarrhoeal disease in their effects on child growth: biological model, evidence,

78. Rosenberg IH, Solomons NW, Schneider RE. Malabsorption associated with diarrhea and intestinal infections. *Am J Clin Nutr.* 1977;30:1248–1253.

79. Molla A, Molla AM, Rahim A. Intake and absorption of nutrients in children with cholera and rotavirus infection during acute diarrhea and after recovery. *Nutr Res.* 1982;2:233–242.

80. Islam M, Roy SK, Begum M, Chisti MJ. Dietary intake and clinical response of hospitalized patients with acute diarrhea. *Food Nutr Bull.* 2008;29:25–31.

81. Guarino A, Winter H, Sandhu B, et al. Acute gastroenteritis disease: report of the FISPGHAN Working Group. *J Pediatr Gastroenterol Nutr.* 2012;55:621–626.

82. Guarino A, Ashkenazi S, Gendrel D, Lo Vecchio A, Shamir R, Szajewska H. European Society for Pediatric Gastroenterology, Hepatology, and Nutrition/European Society for Pediatric Infectious Diseases evidence-based guidelines for the management of acute gastroenteritis in children in Europe: update 2014. *J Pediatr Gastroenterol Nutr.* 2014;59:132–152.

83. Treem W. Clinical aspects and treatment of congenital sucrase-isomaltase deficiency. *J Pediatr Gastroenterol Nutr.* 2012;55(suppl 2):S7–S13.

84. Belmont JW, Reid B, Taylor W, et al. Congenital sucrase-isomaltase deficiency presenting with failure to thrive, hypercalcemia and nephrocalcinosis. *BMC Pediatr.* 2002;2:4.

85. Treem WR, McAdams L, Stanford L, Kastoff G, Justinich C, Hyams J. Sacrosidase therapy for congenital sucrase-isomaltase deficiency. *J Pediatr Gastroenterol Nutr.* 1999;28:137–142.

86. McMeans A. Congenital sucrase-isomaltase deficiency: diet assessment and education guidelines. *J Pediatr Gastroenterol Nutr.* 2012;55(suppl 2):S37–S39.

87. Escobar MA Jr, Lustig D, Pflugeisen B, et al. Fructose intolerance/malabsorption and recurrent abdominal pain in children. *J Pediatr Gastroenterol Nutr.* 2014;58:498–501.

88. Castillo-Duran C, Vial P, Uauy R. Trace mineral balance during acute diarrhea in infants. *J Pediatr.* 1988;113:452–457.

89. Matoth Y, Zamir R, Bar-Shani S, Grossowicz N. Studies in folic acid in infancy. II. Folic and folinic acid blood levels in infants with diarrhea, malnutrition, and infection. *Pediatrics.* 1964;33:694–699.

90. Guandalini S. Probiotics for children with diarrhea. *J Clin Gasteroenterol.* 2008;42:S53–S57.

91. Wallace B. Clinical use of probiotics in the pediatric population. *Nutr Clin Pract.* 2009;24:50–59.

92. Bronstein MN, Sokol RJ, Abman SH, et al. Pancreatic insufficiency, growth, and nutrition in infants identified by newborn screening as having cystic fibrosis. *J Pediatr.* 1992;120(4 Pt 1):533–540.

93. Boocock GR, Morrison JA, Popovic M, et al. Mutations in SBDS are associated with Shwachman-Diamond syndrome. *Nat Genet.* 2003;33:97–101.

94. Bodian M, Sheldon W, Lightwood R. Congenital hypoplasia of the exocrine pancreas. *Acta Pediatr.* 1964;53:282–293.

95. Shwachman H, Diamond LK, Oski FA, Khan KT. The syndrome of pancreatic insufficiency and bone marrow dysfunction. *J Pediatr.* 1964;65:645–663.

96. Myers KC, Davies SM, Shimamura A. Clinical and molecular pathophysiology of Shwachman-Diamond Syndrome. *Hematol Oncol Clin North Am.* 2013; 27(1):117–128.

97. Mack DR, Forstner GG, Wilschanski M, Freedman MH, Durie PR. Shwachman syndrome: exocrine pancreatic dysfunction and variable phenotypic expression. *Gastroenterology.* 1996;111:1593–1602.

98. Dror Y, Donadieu, J, Koglmeier J, et al. Draft consensus guidelines for diagnosis and treatment of Shwachman-Diamond syndrome. *Ann NY Acad Sci.* 2011;1242:40–55.

99. Johanson AJ, Blizzard RM. A syndrome of congenital hypoplasia of the alae nasi, deafness, hypothyroidism, dwarfism, absent permanent teeth and malabsorption. *J Pediatr.* 1971;79:982–987.

100. Zenker M, Mayerle J, Lerch MM, et al. Deficiency of UBR1, a ubiquitin ligase of the N-end rule pathway, causes pancreatic dysfunction, malformations and mental retardation (Johanson-Blizzard syndrome). *Nat Genet.* 2005;37:1345–1350.

101. Almshraki N, Abdulnabee MZ, Sukalo M, et al. Johanson-Blizzard syndrome. *World J Gastroenterol.* 2011;17(37):4247–4250.

102. Pearson HA, Lobel JS, Kochshis SA, et al. A new syndrome of refractory sideroblastic anemia with vacuolization of marrow precursors and exocrine pancreatic dysfunction. *J Pediatr.* 1979;95:976–984.

103. Rotig A, Cormier V, Knoll F, et al. Site-specific deletions of the mitochondrial genome in the Pearson marrow-pancreas syndrome. *Genomics.* 1991;10:502–504.

104. Walkowiak J, Cichy WK, Herzig KH. Comparison of fecal elastase-1 determination with the secretin-cholecystokinin test in patients with cystic fibrosis. *Scand J Gastroenterol.* 1999;34:202–207.

105. Wali PD, Loveridge-Lenza B, He Z, Horvath K. Comparison of fecal elastase-1 and pancreatic function testing in children. *J Pediatr Gastroenterol Nutr.* 2012;54(2):277–280.

106. Sziegoleit A, Krause E, Klör HU, Kanacher L, Linder D. Elastase 1 and chymotrypsin B in pancreatic juice and feces. *Clin Biochem.* 1989;22:85–89.

107. Walkowiak J, Herzig KH. Fecal elastase-1 is decreased in villous atrophy regardless of the underlying disease. *Eur J Clin Invest.* 2001;31:425–430.

108. Salvatore S, Finazzi S, Barassi A, et al. Low fecal elastase: potentially related to transient small bowel damage resulting from enteric pathogens. *J Pediatr Gastroenterol Nutr.* 2003;36:392–396.

109. Chen WL, Morishita R, Eguchi T, et al. Clinical usefulness of dual-label Schilling test for pancreatic exocrine function. *Gastroenterology.* 1989;96(5 Pt 1):1337–1345.

110. Lindkvist B. Diagnosis and treatment of pancreatic exocrine insufficiency. *World J Gastroenterol.* 2013;19(42):7258–7266.

111. Moudiou T, Galli-Tsinopoulou A, Nousia-Arvanitakis S. Effect of exocrine pancreatic function on resting energy expenditure in cystic fibrosis. *Acta Paediatr.* 2007;96:1521–1525.

112. Stallings VA, Stark LJ, Robinson KA, Feranchak AP, Quinton H. Evidence-based practice recommendations for nutrition-related management of children and adults with cystic fibrosis and pancreatic insufficiency: results of a systematic review. *J Am Diet Assoc.* 2008;108:832–839.

113. Borowitz D, Baker RD, Stallings V. Consensus report on nutrition for pediatric patients with cystic fibrosis. *J Pediatr Gastroenterol Nutr.* 2002;35:246–259.

114. Lopez MJ. The changing incidence of acute pancreatitis in children: a single institution perspective. *J Pediatr.* 2002;140:622–624.

115. Park A, Latif SU, Shah AU, et al. Changing referral trends of acute pancreatitis in children: a 12-year single center analysis. *J Pediatr Gastroenterol Nutr.* 2009;49:316–322.

116. March PC. What is the best way to feed patients with pancreatitis. *Curr Opin Crit Care.* 2009;15:131–138.

117. Al-Omran M, AlBalawi ZH, Tashkandi MF, Al-Ansary LA. Enteral versus parenteral nutrition for acute pancreatitis. *Cochrane Database Syst Rev.* 2010;(1):CD002837.

118. Petrov MS, Loveday BP, Pylypchuk RD, McIlroy K, Phillips AR, Windsor JA. Systematic review and meta-analysis of enteral nutrition formulations in acute pancreatitis. *Br J Surg.* 2009;96:1243–1252.

119. Doley RP, Yadav TD, Wig JD, et al. Enteral nutrition in severe acute pancreatitis. *JOP.* 2009;10:157–162.

120. Werlin SL, Kugathasan S, Frautschy BC. Pancreatitis in children. *J Pediatr Gastroenterol Nutr.* 2003;12:47–52.

121. Suddaby EC, Schiller S. Management of chylothorax in children. *Pediatr Nurs.* 2004;30:290–295.

122. McDonald KQ, Bears CM. A preterm infant with intestinal lymphangiectasia: a diagnostic dilemma. *Neonatal Netw.* 2009;28:29–36.

123. Bliss CM, Schroy PC. Primary intestinal lymphangiectasia. *Curr Treat Options Gastroenterol.* 2004;7:3–6.

124. Hyams J, Colletti R, Faure C, et al. Functional gastrointestinal disorders: Working Group Report of the First World Congress of Pediatric Gastroenterology, Hepatology and Nutrition. *J Pediatr Gastroenterol Nutr.* 2002;35(suppl 2):S110–117.

125. Whitfield KL, Shulman RJ. Treatment options for functional gastrointestinal disorders: from empiric to complementary approaches. *Pediatr Ann.* 2009;38:288–294.

126. Parkman HP, Hasler WL, Fisher RD. American Gastroenterological Association technical review on the diagnosis and treatment of gastroparesis. *Gastroenterology.* 2004;127:1592–1622.

127. Parrish CR, Yoshida CM. Nutrition intervention for the patient with gastroparesis: an update. *Pract Gastroenterol.* 2005;30:29–66.

128. Bouras E, Vazquez Roque M, Aranda-Michel J. Gastroparesis: from concepts to management. *Nutr Clin Pract.* 2013;28:437–447.

129. Gabay C, Kushner I. Acute-phase proteins and other systemic responses to inflammation. *New Engl J Med.* 1999;320:448–454.

130. Clein NW. Cow's milk allergy in infants. *Pediatr Clin North Am.* 1954;25:949–962.

131. Iacono G, Cavataio F, Montalto G, et al. Intolerance of cow's milk and chronic constipation in children. *N Engl J Med.* 1998;339:1100–1104.

132. Dahr S, Tahan S, Sole D, et al. Cow's milk protein intolerance and chronic constipation in children. *Pediatr Allergy Immunol.* 2001;12:339–342.

133. Guimãres EV, Goulart EM, Penna FJ. Dietary fiber intake, stool frequency and colonic transit time in chronic functional constipation in children. *Braz J Med Biol Res.* 2001;34:1147–1153.

134. Pipers MA, Tabbers MM, Benninga MA, et al. Currently recommended treatments of childhood constipation are not evidence based: a systematic literature review on the effect of laxative treatment and dietary measures. *Arch Dis Child.* 2009;94:117–131.

135. Office of Disease Prevention and Health Promotion. Dietary guidelines. http://www.dietaryguidelines.gov. Accessed January 13, 2015.

136. Huertas-Ceballos AA, Logan S, Bennett C, Macarthur C. Dietary interventions for recurrent abdominal pain (RAP) and irritable bowel syndrome (IBS) in childhood. *Cochrane Database Syst Rev.* 2009;(1):CD003019.134.

137. Sood MR. Treatment approaches to irritable bowel syndrome. *Pediatr Ann.* 2009;38:272–276.

138. Halmos E, Power V, Shepherd S. A diet low in FODMAPs reduces symptoms of irritable bowel syndrome. *Gastroenterology.* 2014;146:67–75.

139. Vanuytsel T, Tack J, Boeckxstaens G. Treatment of abdominal pain in irritable bowel syndrome. *J Gastroenterol.* 2014;49:1193–1205.

140. Fernández-Bañares F, Esteve-Pardo M, de Leon R, et al. Sugar malabsorption in functional bowel disease: clinical implications. *Am J Gastroenterol.* 1993;88:2044–2050.

141. Shen YA, Nahas R. Complementary and alternative medicine for treatment of irritable bowel syndrome. *Can Fam Physician.* 2009;55:143–148.

142. Bijkerk CJ, Muris JWM, Knottnerus JA, Hoes AW, de Wit NJ. Systematic review: the role of different types of fibre in the treatment of irritable bowel syndrome. *Aliment Pharmacol Ther.* 2004;19:245–251.

143. Quartero AO, Meineche Schmidt V, Muris J, Rubin G, de Wit N. Bulking agents, antispasmodic and antidepressant medication for the treatment of irritable bowel syndrome. *Cochrane Database of Syst Rev.* 2005;(2):CD003460.

144. Torii A, Toda G. Management of irritable bowel syndrome. *Intern Med.* 2004;43:353–358.

145. Talley NJ. Gut eosinophilia in food allergy and systemic and autoimmune diseases. *Gastroenterol Clin North Am.* 2008;37:307–332.

146. Salvatore S, Hauser B, Devreker T, Arrigo S, Vandenplas Y. Chronic enteropathy and feeding in children: an update. *Nutrition.* 2008;24:1205–1216.

147. AGA Institute. AGA Institute medical position statement on the diagnosis and management of celiac disease. *Gastroenterology.* 2006;131:1977–1980.

148. Sollid LM, Khosla C. Future therapeutic options for celiac disease. *Nat Clin Pract Gastroenterol Hepatol.* 2005;2:140–145.

Test Your Knowledge Answers

1. The correct answer is **D**. This patient has Crohn's disease. Diet therapy is effective in the treatment of Crohn's disease. No difference exists in the effectiveness of the polymeric vs elemental diets. A clear liquid diet is inadequate.

2. The correct answer is **A**. Patients with IBD often have deficits of several nutrients. This patient has disease of the ileum and is therefore at greater risk of B_{12} malabsorption. The combination of anemia and low MCV are suggestive of iron deficiency. Both sulfasalazine and methotrexate interfere with folate metabolism and therefore routine supplementation with folate is recommended. It should be mentioned that patients with inflammatory bowel disease are also at risk for bone disease and vitamin D and calcium may also be considered.

3. The correct answer is **C**. Currently a strictly GF diet is the sole recommended treatment for celiac disease and it should be maintained lifelong.[147] Research is ongoing to discover alternative treatments including enzyme therapy and immune agents, but as yet none are recommended.[148] It should be emphasized that the GF diet should be continued even after all symptoms have abated.

4. The correct answer is **D**. Pancreatic insufficiency can lead to malabsorption of fat soluble vitamins if not adequately treated. Direct measurement of Vitamin A, D, E, and K is therefore recommended.

5. The correct answer is **B**. Individuals with pancreatic insufficiency have a higher resting energy requirement then individuals with pancreatic sufficiency. Rather then a low fat diet, pancreatic enzyme replacement therapy should be optimized. Folate and iron absorption are not directly effected by pancreatic insufficiency.

26

Hepatic Disease

Samuel A. Kocoshis, MD; **Renee A. Wieman**, RD, LD, CNSC; and **Monique L. Goldschmidt**, MD

 Podcast

CONTENTS

Learning Objectives

1. Outline the underlying mechanisms associated with pediatric liver disease and the risk factors for nutritional deficiencies.
2. Describe supplementation with fat and fat-soluble vitamins in cholestatic liver disease.
3. Understand the macronutrient and micronutrient requirements for infants and children with liver disease.
4. Identify common nutritional problems after liver transplantation.

Introduction

All children stressed by chronic illness are at greater risk than adults for becoming malnourished. In adults, nutritional intake, digestion, and assimilation need only provide adequate energy to maintain bodily functions, but children require energy over and above maintenance requirements to facilitate growth, development, and maturation. Thus, any chronically ill child is at risk for irreversible complications such as linear growth failure, metabolic bone disease, and neurodevelopmental impairment.

Children with liver disease also face an additional nutritional impediment because the liver is so crucial for maintaining homeostasis. The liver is responsible for the synthesis, storage, and metabolism of carbohydrate, protein, and fat. Additionally, major growth factors such as insulin-like growth factor-1 (IGF-1) and its binding proteins are directly synthesized by the liver; pediatric patients with severe liver dysfunction become growth hormone–resistant.[1] Pediatric patients with chronic liver disease are also prone to hypoglycemia, because a malfunctioning liver has reduced glycogen stores. Protein synthesis may be directly impaired and amino acid utilization for energy may be accelerated in the face of reduced glycogen stores.[2] Furthermore, detoxification of ammonia and synthesis of clotting proteins may also be impeded. Finally, the synthesis of cholesterol and high-density lipoproteins may be faulty, as may the uptake, hydrolysis, and transport of triglycerides.[3] These changes frequently result in hypertriglyceridemia and hypocholesterolemia under conditions of severe hepatic dysfunction.

The nutritional management of infants and children with liver disease is a critical component of the overall care required for optimal interventions and metabolic control of these patients. It is best accomplished using a team approach, with the team composed of multiple medical disciplines, including hepatologists, nurses, dietitians, pharmacists, social workers, speech therapists, occupational therapists, and physical therapists.

Nutritional requirements are dependent on the disease being treated, the anticipated disease course, and the likelihood that liver transplantation will be necessary. Acute diseases such as viral or toxin-induced hepatitis typically require supportive therapy alone, whereas nutritional therapy is the definitive treatment for some metabolic disorders.

Causes of Malnutrition

Malnutrition is common in pediatric liver disease and adversely affects survival both before and after liver transplantation.[4,5] Beyond the impaired intermediate metabolism of carbohydrate, protein, and fat, a variety of factors account for malnutrition in the context of primary hepatic disease. Most studies exploring mechanisms of malnutrition in liver disease have been performed in adults, but it is known that malnutrition can occur both before and after liver transplantation in children.[4,5] Even though the mechanisms of malnutrition in liver disease have not been as fully investigated in pediatric patients, it is quite likely that they are identical.

Inadequate Intake

A foremost concern among both adult and pediatric liver patients is inadequate dietary intake. A simple reason that intake might be inadequate is that these patients are frequently offered low-protein, low-sodium diets that are unappetizing and unappealing. This practice may result not only in suboptimal oral intake but also a diet of poor caloric quality. Secondly, many forms of liver disease result in anorexia. One potential mechanism for anorexia is elevation of both serum and tissue leptin levels.[6] Leptin, an appetite-suppressing hormone, is probably cleared via enterohepatic circulation, and serum levels are elevated in patients with hepatic fibrosis and other forms of liver disease. However, the role of leptin in producing anorexia among patients with liver disease remains controversial, specifically because leptin levels are consistently normal in some forms of liver disease (such as primary biliary cirrhosis) and are consistently elevated in other forms (such as Laennec's, or alcoholic, cirrhosis).[6] A third factor accounting for anorexia is hepatic encephalopathy. Anorexia has long been recognized as a major symptom of encephalopathy, and it is remarkably difficult to treat without successfully treating the underlying cause of the liver disease. Among children with inflammatory hepatitides, proinflammatory cytokines are released, predictably resulting in anorexia.[7] While the phenomenon of hyperinsulinemia and insulin resistance has not been established in children with chronic liver disease, it has been confirmed in adults and may also contribute to anorexia.[8] Yet another factor potentially contributing to anorexia is zinc deficiency, which is known to be quite common among patients with chronic liver disease.[9] Finally, the gastric capacity of children with either massive hepatosplenomegaly or ascites may be so restricted (due gastric compression by viscera or ascitic fluid) that adequate oral intake becomes impossible.

Iatrogenic Factors

The effect of iatrogenic factors on the nutritional state of pediatric liver patients should not be minimized. Excessive restriction of sodium in the absence of hyperaldosteronism will result in salt depletion syndrome, and may actually induce a secondary hyperaldosteronism that would not have been present otherwise. This factor can clearly lead to both malnutrition and growth failure. Unwarranted protein restriction can also result in deficiencies of both somatic and visceral proteins, with subsequent malnutrition. Therefore, clinicians caring for children with liver dysfunction should refrain from restricting either salt or protein in the absence of ascites or encephalopathy refractory to pharmacotherapy.

Known to be relatively safe, large-volume paracentesis has been a popular therapy for adults with ascites, but it has been relatively unpopular in the pediatric setting because of concerns about large, rapid fluid shifts.[10] This potential complication notwithstanding, the practice now has advocates in the pediatric hepatology community. If large-volume paracentesis is used in pediatric patients, the loss of plasma proteins can be prodigious, rendering the patient deficient in both visceral and somatic proteins. Hence, for patients undergoing paracentesis, albumin infusions are advisable during paracentesis to maintain adequate circulating blood volume. Adequate protein intake should be maintained in the absence of overt encephalopathy.

Many of the medications administered to children with hepatic disease may also negatively impact their nutritional state. Diuretics, if administered overzealously, may salt-deplete the child. Broad-spectrum systemic or enteral antibiotics may eliminate vitamin K–synthesizing enteric flora, resulting in vitamin K deficiency among cholestatic patients. Additionally, neomycin, commonly administered for hepatic encephalopathy, is believed to produce villous atrophy, reduced intestinal surface area, and malabsorption of multiple nutrients. Administration of lactulose for encephalopathy may speed intestinal transit enough to result in malabsorption as well. Finally, cholestyramine, an anion exchange resin used to treat the pruritus of cholestasis by binding bile acids, may be so efficient that the intraluminal bile acid concentration may fall below the critical micellar concentration, resulting in malabsorption of fat and fat-soluble vitamins.[11] Because cholestyramine exchanges organic anions for chloride, hyperchloremic metabolic acidosis with resultant growth failure and malnutrition may occur in children on this medication.

Malabsorption

Pediatric patients with liver disease are more likely to have cholestatic disease than their adult counterparts. In cholestatic patients, bile acids are retained in the liver and excreted very poorly into bile. Therefore, intraduodenal primary bile acid concentrations customarily fall below the critical micellar concentration necessary for efficient solubilization and transport of fat and fat-soluble vitamins across the unstirred water layer and into the enterocyte. Malabsorption is very common and requires enteral administration of large quantities of fat-soluble vitamins, as well as an enteral "cocktail" of medium-chain triglycerides (MCTs) and long-chain triglycerides (LCTs) in food or formula. Patients must receive enough long-chain fat to prevent essential fatty acid deficiency, and they must receive enough medium-chain fat to optimize their enteric fat balance. Arachidonic, linoleic, and linolenic acids, all essential fatty acids, are long-chain fats that can only be derived from dietary LCTs. MCT formulas that were designed during the late 1960s for cholestatic patients were deficient in LCTs, commonly resulting in essential fatty acid deficiency among this population.[12]

Malabsorption may occur in select cases of pediatric cholestasis, not only from intraluminal bile acid deficiency but also from exocrine pancreatic insufficiency. Both cystic fibrosis and Shwachman-Diamond syndrome, systemic disorders characterized by exocrine pancreatic insufficiency, may present during the neonatal period with cholestasis. Exocrine pancreatic insufficiency is also a less recognized feature of 2 childhood disorders characterized by severe cholestasis: progressive familial intrahepatic cholestasis, type 1 (PFIC 1) and Alagille syndrome. PFIC 1, previously known as Byler disease, is due to a mutation in the *ATP8B1* gene, previously known as the FIC1 gene. *ATP8B1* mutations result in reduced activity of the Farnesoid X nuclear receptor (FXR), which maintains intra-hepatocyte bile acid homeostasis as well as reduced activity of the cystic fibrosis transporter. As a result, patients with PFIC 1 frequently experience diarrhea, malabsorption, recurrent pancreatitis, and pancreatic fibrosis, leading to exocrine pancreatic insufficiency.[13] Alagille syndrome arises due to mutations in the Jagged1 chromosome, which participates in the notch signaling pathway.[14] These mutations result in bile duct malformations, leading to intrahepatic bile duct paucity. The syndrome is also characterized by butterfly vertebrae; right-sided cardiac disease, such as pulmonary artery atresia or tetralogy of Fallot; posterior embryotoxon of the eye; and facies typified by a long nose, deep-set eyes, a prominent frontal ridge, and a pointed chin. People with Alagille syndrome frequently have steatorrhea disproportionate to their degree of cholestasis. Studies in humans have documented pancreatic insufficiency in Alagille syndrome due to pancreatic ductal and acinar malformations. Similar pancreatic histology is seen in Jagged1 knockout animals, whose pancreatic ductules and acini are malformed in a fashion similar to bile ductules.[15] It is notable that any form of chronic liver disease, whether cholestatic or noncholestatic, may be associated with exocrine pancreatic insufficiency. Longstanding cirrhosis and portal hypertension occasionally result in exocrine pancreatic insufficiency, due to either pancreatic fibrosis because of venous congestion or the absence of hepatic regulatory mechanisms for satisfactory pancreatic enzyme secretion in response to dietary stimulus.[16] Patients suspected of having pancreatic insufficiency because of fatty stools or poor weight gain should undergo testing of pancreatic function, either by formal pancreozymin-secretin testing or by fecal elastase measurement. Documentation of exocrine pancreatic insufficiency mandates treatment with pancreatic enzymes.

Intestinal function itself may become impaired in children with chronic liver disease. Portal hypertension with or without cholestasis may be so severe as to result in protein-losing enteropathy. In addition, the elevated serum bile acid concentrations observed in cholestasis may have a deleterious effect on small intestine function. In studies performed among dogs with surgically created Thiry-Villa loops, exposure of the mesenteric artery to bile acids at concentrations of 8 to 22 micromoles results in impaired transport of water and electrolytes.[17]

Hypermetabolism

The prevalence of hypermetabolism is unknown in children with liver disease, but at least 30% of cirrhotic adults are hypermetabolic.[2] Even though some cirrhotic adults are normometabolic and a few are hypometabolic, those who are hypermetabolic display a measured resting energy expenditure of 20% or more above predicted levels. Hypermetabolism in cirrhotic adults is closely associated with suboptimal total body mass and total body protein. One documented mechanism for this phenomenon is increased adrenal tone, presumably because of reduced hepatic catecholamine metabolism. Patients with documented hypermetabolism express a starvation pattern when their respiratory quotient is measured: they have respiratory quotients approaching 0.6, documenting that they begin using fat for energy quite early after a fast and suggesting a reduction in glycogen stores. Under these conditions, gluconeogenesis is increased and protein catabolism is accelerated. Thus, hypermetabolic patients with cirrhosis are best served by taking 4 or 5 meals per day and receiving adequate dietary protein, even in the face of encephalopathy. For this reason, pharmacologic management of encephalopathy should be attempted prior to reduction of protein in cirrhotic patients.

Specific Pediatric Liver Disorders

Neonatal Cholestasis

Infantile liver disease is quite commonly cholestatic in nature.[18] Extrahepatic biliary atresia is responsible for approximately half of cases among infants with cholestasis; the rest result from a wide variety of infectious and metabolic disorders. As molecular medicine has advanced, disorders previously lumped into the "wastebasket" diagnosis of "neonatal hepatitis" are now being recognized as discrete entities. Alagille syndrome, neonatal iron storage disease, PFIC1, PFIC2, PFIC3, citrin deficiency, Niemann-Pick type C, type I tyrosinemia, galactosemia, hereditary fructose intolerance, and type IV glycogenosis are a few of the many infantile disorders characterized by cholestasis at the time of presentation. In addition, while cholestasis is far from universally present in α-1-antitrypsin deficiency or cystic fibro-

sis, it may be the dominant symptom for selected patients with these disorders.

Nutritional strategies may be the definitive therapy for some of these disorders. For example, elimination of dietary galactose for galactosemia and fructose for hereditary fructose intolerance are curative. For other disorders, such as tyrosinemia, reduction of dietary tyrosine is helpful, but not curative. Because the block in tyrosine metabolism results in an overabundance of toxic intermediates such as succinylacetone, succinylacetoacetate, fumarylacetoacetate, and maleylacetoacetate, upstream inhibition of tyrosine metabolism with 2-(2-nitro-4-trifluoromethylbenzoyl)-1,3-cyclohexanedione (NTBC) has been lifesaving, insofar as metabolism is shunted to nontoxic intermediates such as parahydroxy-phenylpyruvate.[19] Neonatal iron storage disease (now also called gestational alloimmune liver disease) appears to be an alloimmune disorder, with maternal antibodies affecting the fetal liver.[20] Iron storage may thus be secondary rather than primary. Unlike therapy for adult-onset hemochromatosis associated with mutations in the HFE gene, treatment of neonatal iron storage probably should not include chelation, which can theoretically render infants susceptible to bloodstream infections due to siderophagic bacteria. Still, administration of intravenous immunoglobulin may be beneficial to provide "blocking antibodies" to the infant.[20]

Whatever the cause of neonatal cholestasis, the basic nutritional strategy should be to provide ample quantities of fat-soluble vitamins (vitamins A, D, K, and E) and to monitor vitamin levels and/or coagulation studies frequently to prevent fat-soluble vitamin deficiency. Because some element of fat malabsorption nearly always occurs during cholestatic periods, a substantial percentage of fat calories should be given in the form of MCTs, which do not require micellar solubilization before absorption into the portal circulation. However, infants should not be overloaded with MCTs, because MCTs cannot be stored and must be immediately oxidized, putting infants at risk for metabolic acidosis from short-chain fatty acid oxidation products.[21] Furthermore, MCTs are less calorically dense than LCTs because of the reduced number of carbon atoms in their skeleton. Finally, in the 1980s, overenthusiastic efforts to provide MCTs to cholestatic infants resulted in diets that were inadequate in essential fatty acids, leading to essential fatty acid deficiency. At worst, with complete biliary diversion, about 50% of long-chain fats can be absorbed without full solubilization. Therefore, infants with cholestasis should receive a mixture of MCTs and LCTs.[21] Formulas with a 1:1 mix of the 2 types of fat tend to result in optimal fat balance for infants with cholestasis.

Noncholestatic Liver Disease

Some pediatric liver disorders result in cholestasis only intermittently. Among these disorders are viral hepatides, autoimmune hepatitis, α-1-antitrypsin deficiency, the glycogenoses, mitochondrial hepatopathies, Wilson's disease, and nonalcoholic steatohepatitis. When the patient is not cholestatic, absorption is customarily normal and specialized formulas may be unnecessary, but it is imperative to provide adequate calorie and protein intake. It is also important to recognize the underlying metabolic abnormalities that impede adequate assimilation of calories and design nutritional regimens that maximize energy availability. Providing 150% of the estimated caloric and protein requirement to cirrhotic patients is quite reasonable based on adult data suggesting hypermetabolism.[2] Additionally, patients with primary mitochondrial disorders or glycogenoses should be advised to avoid prolonged fasting, because incomplete beta oxidation in mitochondrial disease and absent glycogenolysis results in hypoglycemia and/or the production of toxins, such as ketoacids.

Nutrition as Primary Therapy for Select Liver Disorders

Glycogen Storage Disease

The glycogen storage diseases, also known as glycogenoses, are a group of disorders whereby enzyme deficiencies adversely affect glycogen degradation or glycogen synthesis. There are at least 10 of these disorders, affecting the liver, muscle, or both. Dietary therapy is variably effective for these disorders.[22] For example, the only effective therapy for type IV glycogen storage disease is liver transplantation. Among those for which dietary therapy is beneficial, types II and VI have shown only modest responses to high-protein diets; the only definitive therapy for type II is enzyme replacement. The greatest dietary advances have been made for type I. This disorder, caused by impaired movement of glucose-6-phosphatase into or out of the endoplasmic reticulum, is characterized by fasting hypoglycemia, hyperuricemia, lactic acidosis, and hyperlipidemia. Type IB is also characterized by neutrophil dysfunction, and frequently, inflammatory bowel disease. Late complications include hepatic adenomas, pulmonary hypertension, and renal hyperfiltration. Initial trials in the 1980s of continuous enteral glucose or polycose infusions to prevent hypoglycemia had the unexpected benefit of totally or partially reversing lactic acidosis, hyperuricemia, and hyperlipidemia. Glucose infusion rates of 8 mg/kg/min for infants, 6 mg/kg/min for children, and 4 mg/kg/minute for adults were empirically noted to be beneficial. More recently, raw cornstarch has been used in preference to glucose polymers because of its longer duration of action, obviating the need for a nasogastric tube or gastrostomy tube. It is important that the cornstarch be uncooked, because cooking partially hydrolyzes it and produces a glucose tolerance curve similar to that of glucose. A dose of 1.75–2.75 g/kg will deliver about 5–7 mg/kg/minute of glucose for approximately 6 hours.[22]

Wilson's Disease

Wilson's disease is due to a mutation in a p-type adenosine triphosphatase (ATPase) responsible for transporting copper across membranes to permit formation of metallothionein and biliary excretion of copper.[23] Defective copper excretion results in excessive hepatic copper stores, leading to hepatic dysfunction. Excessive brain and renal copper stores are responsible for central nervous system and renal manifestations. Wilson's disease, if not allowed to progress too far, can be treated with copper chelators. Hepatic manifestations vary from mild transaminase elevation to fulminant hepatic failure. Customarily, when the total body copper level is elevated, there is a reciprocal deficiency in zinc because copper and zinc share a common intestinal transporter; excessive copper absorption results in inadequate zinc absorption. Zinc is a cofactor for alkaline phosphatase synthesis, so in Wilson's disease, the alkaline phosphatase level is disproportionally low in the face of severe liver dysfunction. Chelation is employed to increase copper excretion or to decrease copper absorption. D-penicillamine has been used for years, but trientene is just as effective, with a lower risk of complications. Zinc can also be used to prevent copper absorption by competitive inhibition of intestinal transporters. A newer agent, tetrahydromolybdenate, shows great promise insofar as it complexes with copper in the intestinal lumen, rendering copper unabsorbable, and it is absorbed itself, complexing with serum copper and albumin, preventing cellular uptake of copper. Beyond chelation, dietary therapy is important (especially in the early phases of treatment). Foods high in copper, such as shellfish, nuts, gelatin, mushrooms, liver, and soy products, should be avoided. In addition, the copper content of the patient's major water supply should be analyzed if well water is consumed.

Nonalcoholic Fatty Liver Disease

It is ironic that overnutrition should be the etiology of a liver disease that is seen in pandemic proportions throughout the world. Approximately 20% of the population of the United States is obese, and 75% of obese individuals have some degree of fatty liver.[24] Nonalcoholic fatty liver disease may range in severity from simple fatty infiltrate on one end of the spectrum to steatohepatitis on the other.[24] By definition, steatohepatitis is characterized by both fat and inflammation, and its prognosis is far worse than that of fatty liver alone. Natural progression or a second hepatic insult of any sort may result in fibrosis and eventually cirrhosis. The factors governing the progression of nonalcoholic fatty liver disease to steatohepatitis are not fully understood, but oxidative stress seems to play a role. Therapy should target comorbid conditions such as type 2 diabetes mellitus and hypertriglyceridemia and should emphasize weight reduction. In addition, treatment with betaine, n-acetylcysteine, vitamin E, or ursodeoxycholic acid may lower liver enzyme levels.[24] Oral hypoglycemics such as gemfibril or metformin may decrease hepatic steatosis and improve enzymes, but clofibrate seems to be ineffective.[24] Ultimately, the most reliable therapy is a sensible weight loss regimen. The optimal rate of loss should be < 0.9 kg/week because too rapid a rate may result in excessive lipid peroxidation and more rapid progression to fibrosis.[25]

Assessment of Nutritional State

Protein-energy malnutrition is the most common comorbidity associated with chronic liver disease in children. Because malnutrition is directly linked to unsatisfactory patient and graft survival following pediatric liver transplantation, optimization of nutritional status is of paramount importance.[4]

An initial comprehensive nutritional assessment should be conducted when patients first present with liver insufficiency. Evaluations of formula selection, feeding frequency, daily intakes, vitamin and mineral supplementation, and anthropometric status—including the assessment of lean body mass (LBM)—is essential to initiate early interventions that will optimize nutritional status and minimize some complications. The usual markers of nutritional status, such as weight and body mass index, are very unreliable in the face of advanced liver disease, because body weight is significantly impacted by ascites, edema, and organomegaly. LBM assessment is best evaluated by serial upper arm measurement of mid-arm muscle circumference and triceps skin folds. These measurements are a simple, noninvasive way to

detect early deterioration in nutritional status for which aggressive nutritional interventions are required.[25-27]

Specific Nutrient Requirements

Energy

Recommended caloric intakes for infants and children with end-stage liver disease are estimated to be approximately 130%–150% of the recommended daily allowance (RDA) for age, based on ideal body weight or actual dry weight. This computes to about 130–150 kcal/kg/d in infants and 90–120 kcal/kg/d in children.[28]

Protein

Goals for age are generally provided unless encephalopathy with fulminant hepatic failure and an elevated ammonia level are observed. Enough protein must be provided to preserve LBM and prevent catabolism with the breakdown of endogenous protein stores, but not contribute to hyperammonemia and encephalopathy. Infants generally require 3–4 g/kg/d.[28] The use of branched-chain amino acid (BCAA) formulas or supplements in infants and children improves nitrogen balance but has fallen out of favor because the cost/benefit ratio remains low. Still, BCAA-enriched nutrition is a safe and effective therapy, and further clinical application may be beneficial.[29]

Fat

Formula or oral supplements providing > 50% of dietary fat as MCTs are recommended to optimize fat absorption. However, a balance must be struck to provide appropriate lipid sources, an appropriate MCT:LCT ratio, and a palatable diet.[12] Infant formulas that contain MCT oil (preferably those highest in MCT oil) should be progressively calorie-concentrated up to a goal of 30 kcal/oz with a balance of concentrated infant formula base and modular additives of glucose polymers and/or MCT oil. Children greater than 1 year of age should be trialed on oral MCT oil-containing pediatric formulas and modular additives mixed with food items for additional calories. These formulas generally contain at least 60% MCT oil and will enhance fat absorption.

In some cases when infant formulas are concentrated to 30 kcal/oz, it may be advisable to consider changing to a semi-elemental toddler/pediatric formula that is flavored to encourage better oral intake of an MCT oil-containing beverage. Some manufacturers have recently developed tasteless MCT oil powder and liquid supplements that can easily be added to foods or beverages.[30]

Fluids

Infants and children with liver disease require adequate fluid volume to ensure appropriate caloric and protein intake to maintain LBM. Because maintenance of good nutrition is more important than is restriction of fluid, diuretics may be required to minimize ascites and edema.[30]

Vitamins

The intestinal absorption of vitamins A, D, E, and K is strongly dependent on adequate hepatic secretion of bile acids into the intestinal lumen. Therefore, children with chronic liver disease and hepatic dysfunction are at risk of fat-soluble vitamin deficiency. It is imperative that proper monitoring of blood levels and appropriate supplementation is upheld. Table 26-1 summarizes the doses of fat-soluble vitamin supplements described below:

- The recommended oral supplementation of vitamin A ranges from 5000 to 25,000 IU of water-miscible preparations of vitamin A per day.[31]
- Vitamin E is indicated for all infants and children who are cholestatic and should be dosed at 25–50 IU/kg/d of a water-soluble preparation (tocopherol polyethylene glycol succinate, or TPGS).
- Vitamin D[32] supplementation in children with liver disease is essential, especially if there is a potential to progress to transplantation, because preexisting bone loss can be further aggravated during the early post-transplant period by the use of corticoid steroids. Vitamin D should be administered in a daily dose of ergocalciferol (D2) or cholecalciferol (D3), 3 to 10 times the RDA for age. Depending on the vitamin D level, either of these agents can be given in a dose of 800–8000 IU/d. While oral cholecalciferol tends to be more bioavailable than oral ergocalciferol, cholecalciferol requires sun exposure for conversion to ergocalciferol, and in the winter, sun exposure may be reduced. Another reason for giving ergocalciferol is that most high-concentration liquid pediatric vitamin D preparations are composed of ergocalciferol rather than cholecalciferol. Mixing the water-soluble form of vitamin E (TPGS) with vitamin D has been shown to improve vitamin D absorption in children with cholestasis.[33]
- Oral vitamin K[34] supplementation of 2.5–5.0 mg daily should be administered to all infants and children who have chronic cholestasis. Parenteral administration may be required during illness and bleeding because of the poor absorption of enteral vitamin K.

Children should generally be first started on a commercially available multivitamin fat-soluble supplement.

Table 26-1. Fat-Soluble Vitamin Recommendations

VITAMIN	AMOUNT GIVEN
Vitamin A (aqueous)	5000 IU/d up to a maximum of 25 000 IU/d
Vitamin E	25–50 IU/kg/d as TPGS
25-OH vitamin D	800–8000 IU/d of vitamin D2 or D3
Vitamin K	2.5–5.0 mg/d, 3 times per week

TPGS, tocopherol polyethylene glycol succinate.

AquADEK will usually maintain fat-soluble vitamins in a normal range, but if normal levels cannot be achieved, additional individual supplementation must be added.[34]

Minerals

Supplementation with calcium, zinc, and sometimes iron may be required. Calcium absorption is not significantly impaired in children with chronic cholestatic liver disease compared with controls, but it can be improved by vitamin D administration. Supplementation will improve calcium intake and allow for positive calcium balance. Calcium-fortified foods such as orange juice and waffles, or palatable agents such as Tums and Viactiv, can also be used for calcium supplementation in children.

The repletion of magnesium levels in cholestatic children may also improve bone mineral density.

Zinc deficiency is fairly common in this population, but zinc is required for the crucial enzymatic processes that affect liver metabolism. The usual dose of zinc for supplementation is 1–2 mg/kg/d of elemental zinc.

Because of the malnutrition associated with pediatric liver disease and recurrent gastrointestinal bleeding, these patients may be predisposed to iron deficiency; iron supplementation may be required.

Copper, on the other hand, is excreted into the intestinal tract via the biliary route; thus, in patients with cholestatic disease, copper may be retained in potentially toxic amounts.[30,35]

Enteral Nutrition

When patients are unable to consume adequate calories to maintain appropriate LBM, supplemental enteral tube feeding should be initiated. Many proprietary formulas are available for individuals with liver disease; these are summarized in Tables 26-2, 26-3, and 26-4. Nasogastric tubes are the preferred route of administration because of their easy placement and are useful if patients can tolerate adequate formula volume in their stomachs to achieve goals. However, in many

Table 26-2. Elemental and Semi-Elemental Formulas for Infants[a]

FORMULA	NUTRIENT SOURCE			kcal/cc	g/cc			mOsm/kg H₂O	% H₂0	COMMENTS
	PROTEIN	FAT	CHO		PROTEIN	FAT	CHO			
Similac Expert Care Alimentum (Abbott)	Hydrolyzed casein, free amino acids	33% MCT oil, safflower oil, soy oil	Modified tapioca starch, sucrose	0.67	0.019	0.037	0.069	320	90	• For severe food allergies, protein maldigestion, or fat malabsorption • Contains hydrolyzed milk proteins • Ready-to-feed only
Pregestimil (Mead Johnson)	Hydrolyzed casein, free amino acids	55% MCT oil, corn oil, soy oil, high oleic safflower or sunflower oil	Corn syrup solids, dextrose, modified cornstarch	0.67	0.019	0.037	0.068	320	89	• For severe or multiple food allergies (sensitive to milk protein) • For fat malabsorption • Hypoallergenic, isotonic formula • Contains hydrolyzed milk protein
Elecare Infant (Abbott)	100% free amino acids	High oleic safflower oil, MCT and soy oil, DHA and ARA, 33% MCT oil	Corn syrup solids	0.67	0.021	0.032	0.072	350	88	• Hypoallergenic formula for infants with intact protein intolerance or malabsorption
Enfaport (Mead Johnson)	Calcium and sodium caseinates (from milk)	MCT and soy oil, DHA, ARA 84% MCT oil	Corn syrup solids	1	0.036	0.055	0.103	280	84	• For infants with chylothorax or long-chain fatty acid deficiency • Ready-to-feed
Neocate Infant (Nutricia)	100% free amino acids	Refined vegetable oil, MCT, sunflower and canola oil, DHA, ARA	Corn syrup solids	0.67	0.019	0.034	0.072	340	87	• Hypoallergenic • For infants intolerant of intact protein hydrolysates or who have had gut resections

AHA, arachidonic acid; CHO, carbohydrate; DHA, docosahexaenoic acid; MCT, medium-chain triglyceride.

[a]For infants with protein maldigestion or fat malabsorption. Data from "Nutrition Handbook, 2008" Nutrition Therapy Department, Cincinnati Children's Hospital Medical Center, Cincinnati, OH and "Pediatric Nutrition Reference Guide (10th edition), 2013," Texas Children's Hospital, Houston, TX.

instances nasojejunal placement of feeding tubes must be used because of emesis from medications and volume intolerance secondary to abdominal distension with ascites and/or organomegaly. Nocturnal drip feedings are commonly used so that oral feeding skills can be maintained during the day. This feeding schedule allows for supplementation during the normal hours of fasting and may also be beneficial in patients with end-stage liver disease who are unable to maintain fasting glucose levels overnight. In many instances, these patients progress to 24-hour continuous tube-feeding infusions to achieve the increased intakes required to maintain nutritional status. Attempting to maintain oral motor function is essential during pretransplant care to ensure appropriate and op-

portune transition to normal feedings post-transplantation. In many instances, enteral tube feeding supplementation may be required for a short duration post-transplant until adequate oral intake can be achieved. As post-transplant patients are able to normalize their daily schedules, pain subsides, and the added effect of appetite stimulation from higher-dose steroids is seen, oral intake can quickly achieve and sometimes even surpass goals.[30,35]

Parenteral Nutrition

Parenteral nutrition may be required when complications such as severe varices, gastrointestinal bleeding, excessive emesis, or recurrent complications make it impossible to

Table 26-3. Elemental and Semi-elemental Pediatric Enteral Products[a]

FORMULA	NUTRIENT SOURCE			kcal/cc	g/cc			mOsm/kg H₂0	% H₂0	COMMENTS
	PROTEIN	FAT	CHO		PROTEIN	FAT	CHO			
Peptamen Junior (Nestle)	Enzymatically hydrolyzed whey	60% MCT oil, soy oil, canola oil	Maltodextrin, cornstarch	1	0.03	0.038	0.136	260–400 Depending on flavor	85	• Ready-to-feed and powder available • Contains glutamine • Vanilla, chocolate, strawberry, and unflavored
Pediasure Peptide (Abbott)	Whey protein hydrolysate, hydrolyzed sodium caseinate	Structured lipids, MCT, canola oil 50% MCT oil	Corn maltodextrin, short chain fructo-oligo-saccharides					250–390 Depending on flavor	84	• Ready-to-feed • Peptide-based pediatric formula for malabsorption • Vanilla, strawberry, and unflavored
Vivonex Pediatric (Nestle)	100% free amino acids	70% MCT oil, soybean oil	Maltodextrin, modified cornstarch	0.8	0.024	0.023	0.126	360	88	• Powder • Standard 24 cal/oz concentration • Can be concentrated up to 30 cal/oz • Contains glutamine and arginine
Neocate Junior (Nutricia)	100% free amino acids	Fractionated coconut oil, canola oil, high oleic safflower oil, 35% MCT, 65% LCT	Corn syrup solids	1	0.033	0.05	0.104	550–650 Depending on flavor	80	• Protein hypersensitivity and allergy • Powder for oral or tube feeding • Contains free glutamine • unflavored, tropical, and chocolate
Elecare Junior (Abbott)	100% free L-amino acids	33% MCT oil, high oleic safflower oil, soy oil	Corn syrup solids	1	0.031	0.049	0.107	590	84	• Free amino acids • Powder only • Unflavored, vanilla
EO 28 Splash (Nutricia)	100% free amino acids	Fractionated coconut oil, canola, high oleic sunflower and palm oil, 35% MCT oil	Maltodextrin, sugar	1	0.025	0.035	0.146	820	80	• Elemental, hypoallergenic ready-to-feed formula • Orange-pineapple, grape, and tropical fruit

CHO, carbohydrate; LCT, long-chain triglyceride; MCT, medium-chain triglyceride.

[a]Designed for children with significantly impaired gastrointestinal function ages 1–13 years. Data from "Nutrition Handbook, 2008" Nutrition Therapy Department, Cincinnati Children's Hospital Medical Center, Cincinnati, OH and "Pediatric Nutrition Reference Guide (10th edition), 2013," Texas Children's Hospital, Houston, TX.

safely provide feeding enterally, or when adjunctive nutritional therapy is needed in patients who are severely malnourished and cannot achieve full enteral nutritional support. Parenteral nutrition solutions should include a balance among standard amino acids, dextrose, lipids, electrolytes, and minerals designed to meet nutritional needs while minimizing metabolic complications. In many instances this route of nutritional support is reserved as a last resort because of its known deleterious effect on the liver, but parenteral nutrition has also been touted by some to successfully maintain and build LBM before orthotopic liver transplant.[36]

Table 26-4. Adult Elemental and Semi-elemental Enteral Products[a]

FORMULA	NUTRIENT SOURCE			kcal/cc	g/cc			mOsm/kg H₂O	% H₂O	COMMENTS
	PROTEIN	FAT	CHO		PROTEIN	FAT	CHO			
Peptamen (Nestle)	Enzymatically hydrolyzed whey protein	70% MCT oil, soy oil	Maltodextrin, cornstarch	1	0.04	0.039	0.128	270–380	85	• Peptide-based for patients with impaired GI function • Contains glutamine • Vanilla flavor • Ready-to-feed
Peptamen 1.5 (Nestle)	Enzymatically hydrolyzed whey protein	70% MCT oil, soy oil	Maltodextrin, cornstarch	1.5	0.068	0.056	0.184	550	77	• Higher calories than standard Peptamen • Contains glutamine • Vanilla flavor • Ready-to-feed
Tolerex (Nestle)	100% free amino acids	Safflower oil	Corn maltodextrin, modified corn starch	1	0.021	0.002	0.23	550	84	• Elemental minimal fat formula • Supplemental fat recommended for long-term use • Powder packets
Vital (Abbott)	Partially hydrogenated protein blend, whey protein hydrolysate free amino acids	Structured lipids to promote absorption of fatty acids, 47% MCT oil	Corn maltodextrin, sucrose	1	0.40	0.0375	0.128	390	84	• Peptide-based, semi-elemental formula for impaired GI function • Ready-to-feed

CHO, carbohydrate; LCT, long-chain triglyceride; MCT, medium-chain triglyceride.

[a]Designed for children ages >13 years with significantly impaired gastrointestinal function. Data from "Nutrition Handbook, 2008" Nutrition Therapy Department, Cincinnati Children's Hospital Medical Center, Cincinnati, OH and "Pediatric Nutrition Reference Guide (10th edition), 2013," Texas Children's Hospital, Houston, TX.

Whatever modality of nutritional support is used pretransplant, serial anthropometric measurements are recommended to follow the effects and adequacy of nutritional interventions once deficiencies have been identified.[26]

Nutrition After Liver Transplantation

Protein energy malnutrition and growth failure are observed in 60% of infants and children with chronic liver disease.[5]

To prevent rapid deterioration of nutritional status and the profound complications of end-stage liver disease, liver transplantation should be performed in a timely manner.[37] The goals of nutritional support prior to transplant should be focused on prevention of any further liver injury, minimization of nutrient depletion, conservation of growth, maintenance of LBM, and control of disease-related complications. One valuable recommendation is that pediatric patients with arm muscle circumferences below the fifth percentile be initiated on aggressive nutritional support regimens before transplantation.[26]

In the immediate post-transplant period, clinicians should strive to manage the catabolic effect of the surgery, facilitate weaning from the ventilator, minimize infection risk, ensure wound healing, and anticipate metabolic/electrolyte issues associated with liver regeneration, medications administration, and malnutrition.[37] Refeeding syndrome is a serious complication associated with the aggressive nutritional rehabilitation of malnourished patients and is seen frequently after liver transplant. It is characterized by metabolic disturbance in potassium, magnesium, and phosphate levels; glucose and fluid intolerance; and possible cardiac and pulmonary dysfunction.[38] These metabolic issues are further complicated by the energy required for and the electrolyte shifts engendered by regeneration of hepatocyte function.[37]

Parenteral nutrition via a central venous catheter is typically initiated within 24–48 hours post-transplant, after hemostasis is achieved. In most instances, substantial potassium, phosphorus, and magnesium replacements are required to cope with these refeeding and regeneration requirements. Additional magnesium can also be required to address the renal losses seen with tacrolimus administration. Parenteral nutrition is maintained until the patient is able to take 50%–75% of his or her total caloric requirements enterally (orally or via feeding tube).[37] The intermittent shortages of some parenteral nutrition constituents have made parenteral replacement challenging; sometimes early use of enteral mineral replacements with phosphorus, calcium and magnesium is required.[39]

Oral enteral feeding should be reinstituted as soon as gut function is restored. If patients are unable to achieve nutritional goals with oral feeding and the use of high-calorie oral supplements or fortified standard infant formulas, supplemental tube feeding support should be initiated to facilitate weaning from parenteral nutrition support. Patients can be given standard infant or pediatric supplements after liver transplant, as long-chain fats can again be absorbed. As oral intake improves, patients can be weaned from tube-feeding supplementation. Most children will resume a normal diet before discharge from the hospital after transplantation, although some may require additional oral supplements to achieve catch-up goals. Some children and infants, particularly those with behavioral feeding issues from pretransplant tube feeding, may require supplemental nocturnal enteral feedings for several months to 2 years post-transplant. Some infants and younger children who have received enteral tube feeding supplementation pretransplant may have never developed normal feeding practices, because they have missed their normal developmental milestones for chewing and swallowing. These feeding problems can contribute to persistent growth failure during this post-transplant period, because of lack of adequate caloric intake. Data have shown that behavioral feeding problems are fairly common in children who were tube-fed pretransplant, and are a major cause of growth failure in 10% of children. However, most children who survive liver transplantation will achieve normal growth patterns within 1 year post-transplant.[40]

Post-transplant maintenance goals need to address issues surrounding quality of life. Long-term goals are focused on maximizing linear growth potential and developing optimal cognitive, physical, and emotional states. Optimal nutritional support can improve quality of life in pediatric patients by reducing or avoiding linear growth failure, rickets from osteomalacia with related pathologic fractures, and neurodevelopmental delay. Reaching a normal height is an important aspect of quality of life for children who undergo transplantation, because it impacts their social reintegration and self-esteem. The causes of poor growth after liver transplantation can be summarized as stemming from pretransplant growth failure, those associated with poor graft function, and those due to iatrogenic causes, such as the use of medications that impact the metabolic and nutritional status of patients who undergo transplantation.

Iatrogenic Factors

One of the primary goals post-transplantation is to decrease the complications associated with the chronic use of immunosuppressive drugs while optimizing graft survival.

The cornerstone of most post-transplant immunosuppressive regimens is Tacrolimus (Prograf), a calcineurin inhibitor (CNI) discovered in 1984 that suppresses T-lymphocyte activation and prevents allograft rejection after transplantation. Prograf-based immunosuppression is accompanied by a number of inherent side effects, ranging from hypertension and abnormal renal function to nausea and abdominal pain. Metabolic and nutritional effects often include hypomagnesemia secondary to renal wasting of magnesium; hyperkalemia or hypokalemia due to altered renal handling of potassium; diabetes mellitus from the inhibitory effect on insulin production by islet cells;[41] and dyslipidemia. CNIs may also be linked to deficiency of pyridoxine levels after intestinal transplantation, possibly secondary to accelerated catabolism of this vitamin by the drugs themselves.[42]

CNIs have also been associated with increased incidence of post-transplant eosinophilic enteritis after solid organ transplantation. While the exact mechanism is unknown, the differential inhibition of cytokine elaboration by tacrolimus might alter the balance between Th1 and Th2 T-cell subsets, facilitating an altered pattern of reaction to antigenic exposure.[43]

As the predecessor to tacrolimus, the CNI cyclosporine (Csa) was introduced as an effective immunosuppressive agent following liver transplantation in 1982. It is considered inferior to tacrolimus due to a greater incidence of steroid-resistant rejection following induction.[44,45] While it has a similar toxicity profile to tacrolimus, cyclosporine is less frequently associated with new-onset diabetes mellitus and more associated with gingival hyperplasia and hirsutism.[45,46]

Corticosteroids play a vital role in most immunosuppressive protocols. Unfortunately, their benefit to allograft survival comes with a price. In addition to augmenting the diabetogenic, lipidemic, and hypertensive effects of other immunosuppressive medications, children on steroid-inclusive immunosuppressive regimens are often challenged by sodium and fluid retention, poor growth, osteoporosis, muscle weakness, pancreatitis, suppression of the pituitary-adrenal axis, and impaired wound healing.[47,48] Of all immunosuppressives, steroids have the most profound negative effect on growth. If steroids can be weaned satisfactorily, those growth-stunting effects can be minimized.

Azathioprine and mycophenolic acid are similar antimetabolite agents that are important adjuncts to combination immunosuppressive therapy. They both work by impeding lymphocyte proliferation. While the therapeutic range of the active azathioprine metabolite 6-thioguanine has been established for treatment of inflammatory bowel disease, the range necessary to prevent rejection remains uncertain. Even though it has a mechanism of action similar to azathioprine, mycophenolic acid has been the preferred agent in many immunosuppressive protocols because it has been associated with a lower incidence of acute cellular rejection in and liver toxicity in liver transplantation.[49] Unfortunately, the commonplace gastrointestinal toxicity associated with mycophenolic acid may mandate the substitution of azathioprine. Among patients undergoing *en bloc* liver-intestinal transplantation, histologic patterns of mycophenolic acid–induced enteropathy may be difficult to differentiate from acute allograft rejection.[50] In the event that dose-dependent gastrointestinal side effects ensue during therapy with mycophenolic acid—including anorexia, vomiting, diarrhea, and gastrointestinal hemorrhage from mucosal ulceration—compensation for calorie, protein, fluid, electrolyte, and mineral losses is mandatory.

Sirolimus, a mammalian target of rapamycin (mTOR) inhibitor, is another immunosuppressive agent that has facilitated CNI-sparing immunosuppressive regimens for liver transplant patients. Sirolimus used in conjunction with tacrolimus, for example, allows for lower doses of tacrolimus and reduced severity or occurrence of CNI-induced side effects, such as tacrolimus-induced renal insufficiency. In many cases, sirolimus can substitute for tacrolimus to prevent allograft rejection. While this strategy spares the adverse effects associated with calcineurin use, another set of adverse effects may be induced by sirolimus, including hyperlipidemia, hypercholesterolemia, gastrointestinal ulcers, impaired wound healing, peripheral edema, and myelosuppression.[51] Sirolimus-associated impaired wound healing has prompted many programs to eschew its use for at least 6 weeks after transplantation. However, once wound healing has occurred in the late post-transplant period, sirolimus appears to be a valuable tacrolimus-sparing agent. Reducing drug doses is key to minimizing their long-term complications. Besides employing calcineurin-sparing agents, early steroid weaning has been employed by many transplantation programs.[52]

Complications

Osteopenia

Multiple factors contribute to the development of osteopenia in pediatric patients receiving liver transplants, including immobility, malnutrition, poor muscle mass, poor renal function, and chronic cholestasis pretransplant and post-transplant; high-dose corticosteroids have long been identified as the main cause of bone loss. In a retrospective study of children with end-stage liver disease who underwent orthotopic liver transplantation, 16% had bone fractures in the postoperative period. Regardless of postoperative bone density, most liver transplant recipients lose bone mass for up to 3–6 months after transplantation, but by 6 months, the bone loss typically ends in patients with normal allograft function and then begins to stabilize and increase. Adequate calcium and vitamin D supplementation during the pretransplant and post-transplant phases, as well as promoting physical activity and minimizing the use of osteopenia-producing medications, will help preserve bone mass during the early post-transplant phase.[32,53–55]

Nephrotoxicity

Nephrotoxicity, defined as a decreased glomerular filtration rate, has been associated with the long-term use of CNIs such as cyclosporine and tacrolimus; nephrotoxic antibiotics; rejection episodes; and hypertension.[56–58] Hypertension occurs in approximately one-third of all children at any given time post-transplant, and remains a serious post-transplant complication, with 10%–30% of children requiring long-term antihypertensive treatment. Blood pressure should be routinely monitored during postoperative medical follow-ups.

Hyperlipidemia

The use of cyclosporine, sirolimus, and high-dose corticosteroids, as well as obesity and diabetes mellitus, are all associated with post-transplant hyperlipidemia. Severe hypertriglyceridemia is particularly common among patients receiving sirolimus. Among pediatric patients undergoing liver transplant, dyslipidemia is more common in patients approaching puberty. Familial predisposition to hyperlipidemia can also be a contributing factor. In comparison with sirolimus, tacrolimus exerts a relatively minor effect on serum lipid levels. One of the major focuses of treatment for hyperlipidemia is dietary intervention. Patient and family education on proper food purchasing, low-fat substitutions, preparation techniques, menu planning, and lifestyle modifications that include an exercise regimen are essential.[59,60]

Post-Transplant Diabetes Mellitus

The most significant factor that influences the development of post-transplant diabetes mellitus is the use of diabetogenic immunosuppressive medications, such as corticosteroids and CNIs. Hyperglycemia may occur in some children on tacrolimus alone or in combination with high-dose corticosteroids. When hyperglycemia is associated with corticosteroid use, it usually resolves when corticosteroid doses are reduced. When hyperglycemia is sustained, treatment with insulin is required. Detailed diabetes education on dietary modifications (carbohydrate counting), monitoring, and insulin therapy should be implemented upon diagnosis. Patients with a family history of diabetes mellitus or a diagnosis of an autoimmune liver disease appear to have a greater risk of developing diabetes mellitus in the postoperative period.[61]

Obesity

Obesity after liver transplantation is seen more frequently in adult patients, but it can affect adolescent patients and children who receive a transplant during the prepubertal period. The goal of treatment should focus on lifestyle change and behavior modification rather than on calorie-restricted diets, as the tendency for weight gain will be present throughout their life.[62–66]

Linear Growth Failure

Up to 20% of pediatric patients who have undergone orthotopic liver transplant experience impairment in linear growth. The impairment is more prevalent in boys than in girls, and height z scores are characteristically lower than predicted midparental z scores. While linear growth impairment is more prevalent in the prepubertal and pubertal period, 11% of Tanner stage V adolescents remain growth-impaired.[67] Not only does chronic undernutrition result in nutritional growth failure, but the use of sirolimus may produce vascular compromise to the growth plate of long bones.[68] Whether growth hormone deficiency can be documented or not, children who are growth-impaired after transplantation consistently improve their linear growth velocity on recombinant growth hormone therapy, and they do not seem to be excessively prone to acute or chronic rejection.[69,70] Hence, growth hormone therapy appears to be warranted when the post-transplantation linear growth velocity is suboptimal.

Optimal Nutritional Management

Providing nutritional support to pediatric patients with liver disease who are listed for liver transplantation requires a concerted medical team effort. Pretransplant goals are to preserve LBM and medically manage the complications associated with the disease process. Post-transplant goals should focus primarily on ensuring quality of life; developing cognitive, physical, and emotional states; and minimizing the side effects associated with post-transplant medications. Rigorous attention to metabolic management and aggressive nutritional support during all phases of disease are essential for optimizing transplantation outcomes.

Conclusion

The goals of nutrition for pediatric patients with liver disease are to optimize the potential for normal growth and development, prevent further liver injury, prevent worsening of the patient's nutritional status, minimize the risk of infection, avoid vitamin and mineral deficiency, and improve quality of life. Achievement of these goals requires detailed attention to all of the components of nutritional support by caregivers, the patient, and the patient's family—working as a team to provide optimal care.

Test Your Knowledge Questions

1. What is the best serial marker of nutritional status in pediatric patients with liver disease?
    A. Fat-soluble vitamin levels
    B. Upper extremity anthropometric measurements
    C. Prealbumin
    D. Weight/length or body mass index
    E. A and D
2. Which of the following liver disorders is most likely to be associated with exocrine pancreatic insufficiency?
    A. Hepatitis C
    B. Alagille syndrome
    C. Autoimmune hepatitis
    D. Extrahepatic biliary atresia

3. In the nutritional therapy of Wilson's disease, which should be avoided?
   A. Grapefruit
   B. Red meat
   C. Endive
   D. Lobster

4. Which of the following has been used for the nutritional therapy of glycogen storage disease, type I?
   A. Subcutaneous octreotide
   B. Glucagon infusions
   C. Cooked cornstarch
   D. Metformin
   E. Raw cornstarch

5. Hypomagnesemia in liver transplant patients is most likely associated with which antirejection therapy?
   A. Tacrolimus
   B. Antithymocyte globulin
   C. Sirolimus
   D. Methylprednisolone

6. Which of the following is a complication associated with sirolimus use?
   A. Hypertriglyceridemia
   B. Impaired wound healing
   C. Opportunistic infection
   D. All of the above

References

1. Bucuvalas JC, Horn JA, Chernausek SD. Resistance to growth hormone in children with chronic liver disease. *Pediatr. Transplant.* 1997;1:73–79.

2. Merli O, Riggio M, Leonetti F, et al. Impaired nonoxidative glucose metabolism in patients with liver cirrhosis. Effects of two insulin doses. *Metabolism.* 1997;46:840–843.

3. Muller P, Felin R, Lambrecht J, et al. Hypertriglyceridaemia secondary to liver disease. *Eur J Clin Invest.* 1974;4:419–428.

4. Shepherd RW, Chin SE, Cleghorn GJ, et al. Malnutrition in children with chronic liver disease accepted for liver transplantation: clinical profile and effects on outcome. *J Paediatr Child Health.* 1991;27:595.

5. Heubi JE, Heyman MB, Shulman RJ. The impact of liver disease on growth and nutrition. *J Pediatr Gastroenterol Nutr.* 2002;35(suppl 1):S55–S59.

6. Ben-Ari Z, Schafer Z, Sulkes J, et al. Alterations in serum leptin in chronic liver disease. *Dig Disease Sci.* 2002;47:183–189.

7. Plata-Salamán CR. Cytokines and anorexia: a brief overview. *Semin Oncol.* 1998;251(suppl 1):64–72.

8. Selberg O, Burchert W, Van Der Hoff J. Insulin resistance in liver cirrhosis. Positron-emission tomography scan analysis of skeletal muscle glucose metabolism. *J Clin Invest.* 1993;91:1897–1903.

9. Saner G, Süoglu OD, Yigitba M, et al. Zinc nutrition in children with chronic liver disease. *J Trace Elements Exp Med.* 2000;13:271–276.

10. Gines P, Arroyo V. Is there still a need for albumin infusions to treat patients with liver disease? *Gut.* 2000;46:588–590.

11. West RJ, Lloyd JK. The effect of cholestyramine on intestinal absorption. *Gut.* 1975;16:93–8.

12. Pettei MJ, Daftary S, Levine JJ. Essential fatty acid deficiency associated with the use of a medium-chain-triglyceride infant formula in pediatric hepatobiliary disease. *Am J Clin Nutr.* 1991;53:1217–1221.

13. Knisely AS. Progressive familial intrahepatic cholestasis: a personal perspective. *Pediatr Dev Pathol.* 2000;3:113–125.

14. Piccoli DA, Spinner NB. Alagille syndrome and the Jagged1 gene. *Semin Liver Dis.* 2001;21:525–534.

15. Golson ML, Loomes KM, Oakey R, et al. Ductal malformation and pancreatitis in mice caused by conditional Jag1 deletion. *Gastroenterology.* 2009;136:1761–1771.e1.

16. Lee SP, Lai KS. Exocrine pancreatic function in hepatic cirrhosis. *Am J Gastroenterol.* 1976;65:244–248.

17. Berant M, Diamond E, Alon U, et al. Effect of infusion of bile salts into the mesenteric artery in situ on jejunal mucosal transport function in dogs. *J Pediatr Gastroenterol Nutr.* 1988;7:588–593.

18. Bezerra JA, Balistreri WF. Cholestatic syndromes of infancy and childhood. *Semin Gastrointest Dis.* 2001;12:54–65.

19. Masurel-Paulet A, Poggi-Bach J, Rolland MO, et al. NTBC treatment in tyrosinaemia type I: long-term outcome in French patients. *J Inherit Metab Dis.* 2008;31:81–87.

20. Whitington PF. Gestational alloimmune liver disease and neonatal hemochromatosis. *Semin Liv Dis.* 2012;32:325–332.

21. Wanten GJ, Naber AH. Cellular and physiological effects of medium-chain triglycerides. *Mini Rev Med Chem.* 2004;4:847–857.

22. Heller S, Worona L, Consuelo A. Nutritional therapy for glycogen storage diseases. *J Pediatr Gastroenterol Nutr.* 2008;47(suppl 1):515–521.

23. Pfeil S, Lynn DJ. Wilson's disease: copper unfettered. *J Clin Gastroenterol.* 1999;29:22–31.

24. McCullough AJ. Update on nonalcoholic fatty liver disease. *J Clin Gastroenterol.* 2002;34:255–262.

25. Merli M, Romiti A, Riggio O, et al. Optimal nutritional indexes in chronic liver disease. *JPEN J Parenter Enteral Nutr.* 1987;11(5 suppl):130S–134S.

26. Zamberlan P, Leone C, Tannuri U, et al, Nutritional risk and anthropometric evaluation in pediatric liver transplantation. *Clinics (Sao Paulo).* 2012;67:1387–1392.

27. Sokol, RJ, Stall C Anthropometric evaluation of children with chronic liver disease. *Am J Clin Nutr.* 1990;52:203–208.

28. Mouzaki M, Ng V, Kamath BM, et al. Enteral energy and macronutrients in end-stage liver disease. *JPEN J Parenter Enteral Nutr.* 2014;38:673–681.

29. Shu X, Kang K, Zhong J, et al. Meta-analysis of branched chain amino acid-enriched nutrition to improve hepatic function in patients undergoing hepatic operation. *Zhonghua Gan Zang Bing Za Zhi* 2014:22:43–47.

30. Nightingale S, Ng VL. Optimizing nutritional management in children with chronic liver disease. *Pediatr Clin North Am.* 2009;56:1161–1183.

31. Feranchak AP, Gralla J, King R, et al. Comparison of indices of vitamin A status in children with chronic liver disease. *Hepatology.* 2005;42:782–792.

32. D'Antiga L, Ballan D, Luisetto G, et al. Long-term outcome of bone mineral density in children who underwent a successful liver transplantation. *Transplantation.* 2004;78:899–903.

33. Argao EA, Heubi J, Hollis BW, et al. d-Alpha-tocopheryl polyethylene glycol-1000 succinate enhances the absorption of vitamin D in chronic cholestatic liver disease of infancy and childhood. *Pediatr Res.* 1992;31:146–150.

34. Sathe MN, Patel AS. Update in pediatrics: focus on fat-soluble vitamins. *Nutr Clin Pract.* 2010;25:340–346.

35. Kelly DA, Bucuvalas JC, Alonso EM, et al. Long-term medical management of the pediatric patient after liver transplantation: 2013 practice guideline by the American Association for the Study of Liver Diseases and the American Society of Transplantation. *Liver Transpl.* 2013;19:798–825.

36. Sullivan JS, Sundaram SS, Pan Z, et al. Parenteral nutrition supplementation in biliary atresia patients listed for liver transplantation. *Liver Transpl.* 2012;18:120–128.

37. Hammad A, Kaito T, Uemoto S. Perioperative nutritional therapy in liver transplantation. *Surg Today.* 2014 [epub ahead of publication].

38. Dunn RL, Stettler N, Mascarenhas MR. Refeeding syndrome in hospitalized pediatric patients. *Nutr Clin Pract.* 2003;18:327–332.

39. Guenter P, Holcombe B, Mirtallo JM, et al. Parenteral nutrition utilization: response to drug shortages. *JPEN J Parenter Enteral Nutr.* 2014;38:11–12.

40. Alonso EM. Growth and developmental considerations in pediatric liver transplantation. *Liver Transpl.* 2008;14:585–591.

41. Oetjen E, Baun D, Beimesche S, et al. Inhibition of human insulin gene transcription by the immunosuppressive drugs cyclosporin A and tacrolimus in primary, mature islets of transgenic mice. *Mol Pharmacol.* 2003;63:1289–1295.

42. Matarese LE, Dvorchik I, Costa G, et al. Pyridoxal-5'-phosphate deficiency after intestinal and multivisceral transplantation. *Am J Clin Nutr.* 2009;89:204–209.

43. Saeed SA, Integlia MJ, Pleskow RG, et al. Tacrolimus-associated eosinophilic gastroenterocolitis in pediatric liver transplant recipients: role of potential food allergies in pathogenesis. *Pediatr Transplant.* 2006;10:730–735.

44. Collins RH. Tacrolimus (FK506) versus cyclosporin in prevention of liver allograft rejection. *Lancet.* 1994;344:949.

45. McAlister VC, Haddad E, Renouf E, et al. Cyclosporin versus tacrolimus as primary immunosuppressant after liver transplantation: a meta-analysis. *Am J Transplant.* 2006;6:1578–1585.

46. Heisel O, Heisel R, Balshaw R, et al. New onset diabetes mellitus in patients receiving calcineurin inhibitors: a systematic review and meta-analysis. *Am J Transplant.* 2004;4:583–595.

47. Mukherjee S, Botha JF, Mukherjee U. Immunosuppression in liver transplantation. *Curr Drug Targets.* 2009;10:557–574.

48. Tredger JM, Brown NW, Dhawan A. Immunosuppression in pediatric solid organ transplantation: opportunities, risks, and management. *Pediatr Transplant.* 2006;10:879–892.

49. Wiesner R, Rabkin J, Klintmalm G, et al. A randomized double-blind comparative study of mycophenolate mofetil and azathioprine in combination with cyclosporine and corticosteroids in primary liver transplant recipients. *Liver Transpl.* 2001;7:442–450.

50. Delacruz V, Weppler D, Island E, et al. Mycophenolate mofetil-related gastrointestinal mucosal injury in multivisceral transplantation. *Transplant Proc.* 2010;42:82–84.

51. Montalbano M, Neff GW, Yamashiki N, et al. A retrospective review of liver transplant patients treated with sirolimus from a single center: an analysis of sirolimus-related complications. *Transplantation.* 2004;78:264–268.

52. McPartland KJ, Pomposelli JJ. Update on immunosuppressive drugs used in solid-organ transplantation and their nutrition implications. *Nutr Clin Pract.* 2007;22:467–473.

53. Ebeling PR. Approach to the patient with transplantation-related bone loss. *J Clin Endocrinol Metab.* 2009;94:1483–1490.

54. Guthery SL, et al. Bone mineral density in long-term survivors following pediatric liver transplantation. *Liver Transpl.* 2003;9:365–370.

55. Okajima H, Shigeno C, Inomata Y, et al. Long-term effects of liver transplantation on bone mineral density in children with end-stage liver disease: a 2-year prospective study. *Liver Transpl.* 2003;9:360–364.

56. Matloff RG, Arnon R, Saland JM. The kidney in pediatric liver transplantation: an updated perspective. *Pediatr Transplant.* 2012;16:818–828.

57. Anastaze Stell K, Belli DC, Parvex P, et al. Glomerular and tubular function following orthotopic liver transplantation in children treated with tacrolimus. *Pediatr Transplant.* 2012;16:250–256.

58. Campbell K, Ng V, Martin S, et al. Glomerular filtration rate following pediatric liver transplantation—the SPLIT experience. *Am J Transplant.* 2010;10:2673–2682.

59. Kniepeiss D, Iberer F, Schaffellner S, et al. Dyslipidemia during sirolimus therapy in patients after liver transplantation. *Clin Transplant.* 2004;18:642–646.

60. Fellstrom B. Impact and management of hyperlipidemia posttransplantation. *Transplantation.* 2000;70(suppl):S51–57.

61. Obayashi PA. Posttransplant diabetes mellitus: cause, impact, and treatment options. *Nutr Clin Pract.* 2004;19:165–171.

62. Perito ER, Rhee S, Glidden D, et al. Overweight and obesity in pediatric liver transplant recipients: prevalence and predictors before and after transplant, United Network for Organ Sharing Data, 1987–2010. *Pediatr Transplant.* 2012;16:41–49.

63. Rothbaum Perito E, Lau A, Rhee S, et al. Posttransplant metabolic syndrome in children and adolescents after liver transplantation: a systematic review. *Liver Transpl.* 2012;18:1009–1028.

64. Dick AA, Perkins JD, Spitzer AL, et al. Impact of obesity on children undergoing liver transplantation. *Liver Transpl.* 2010;16:1296–1302.

65. Pagadala M, Dasaratha S, Eghtesad B, et al. Posttransplant metabolic syndrome: an epidemic waiting to happen. *Liver Transpl.* 2009;15:1662–1670.

66. Sundaram SS, Alonso EM, Zeitler P, et al. Obesity after pediatric liver transplantation: prevalence and risk factors. *J Pediatr Gastroenterol Nutr.* 2012;55:657–662.

67. Muhammed S, Grimberg A, Rand E, et al. Long-term linear growth and puberty in pediatric liver transplant recipients. *J Pediatr.* 2013;163:1354–1360.

68. Alvarez-García O, García-López E, Loredo V, et al. Rapamycin induces growth retardation by disrupting angiogensis in the growth plate. *Kidney Int.* 2010;78:561–568.

69. Puustinen L, Jalanko H, Holmberg C. Recombinant human growth hormone treatment after liver transplantation in childhood: the 5 year outcome. *Transplantation.* 2005;79:1241–1246.

70. Fuqua JS. Growth after organ transplantation. *Semin Pediatr Surg.* 2006;15:162–169.

Test Your Knowledge Answers

1. The correct answer is **B**.
2. The correct answer is **B**.
3. The correct answer is **D**.
4. The correct answer is **E**.
5. The correct answer is **A**.
6. The correct answer is **D**.

27

Intestinal Failure

Robert H. Squires, MD, and **Kishore R. Iyer,** MBBS, FRCS (Eng), FACS

Podcast

CONTENTS

Learning Objectives

1. Understand that while intestinal length is important, it is not the only factor that determines a child's ability to reach enteral autonomy.
2. Understand that the intestinal adaptive process takes months and even years before enteral autonomy can, if ever, be achieved.
3. Describe why enteral nutrition is necessary for intestinal adaptation to occur.
4. Explain how lipid-lowering strategies for soy-based lipid preparations or substitution with a fish oil–based lipid can improve serum aminotransferase levels and reduce serum bilirubin.

Introduction

Intestinal failure (IF) in infants and children is a devastating condition that can be broadly defined as the inability of the intestinal tract to sustain life without supplemental parenteral nutrition (PN).[1,2] Prior to PN, many infants died as a consequence of insufficient bowel length or function. Infants found to have an "abdominal catastrophe" at laparotomy for conditions such as necrotizing enterocolitis (NEC), volvulus, or gastroschisis simply had their abdomen closed and were made comfortable to await the natural course of their tragic circumstance. However, with the development of safe PN, central line placement and care, improved medical and surgical management, including intestinal transplantation, infants with IF have an opportunity to survive with a satisfactory or even excellent quality of life. Although, the clinical course for the child can, at times, be challenging and frustrating to the family, as well as those who provide medical care and support. Intestinal adaptation associated with full enteral feeding and satisfactory weight gain and growth accompanied by discontinuation of PN can require months or years to achieve.[3] Along the way, the child is at risk for episodes of dehydration, electrolyte imbalance, and macronutrient and micronutrient deficiencies. More importantly, life-threatening complications such as sepsis, end-stage liver disease, and vascular thrombosis may occur.

Management of children with IF is best provided by an experienced multidisciplinary team that includes experts in pediatric gastroenterology, surgery, nutrition, nursing, social work, and feeding techniques.[4] Most management strategies have not been rigorously investigated, leaving much to experience, tradition, trial and error, or "art" as most would prefer. The great majority of studies of children with IF are single-site experiences, with small numbers of patients collected over many decades.[5-8] Goals of this brief chapter are to review the topic of IF and outline some strategies that might be useful in the care and management of infants and children with IF.

Definition of Intestinal Failure

The small intestine almost doubles in length during the last trimester, with the normal full-term infant having a small intestine length of 210–350 cm at birth.[9] While the literature attempts to define short bowel syndrome (SBS) as the remnant intestine measuring < 75 cm, a better approach was put forward by Teitelbaum and colleagues.[8] They proposed incorporating gestational age into the assessment and suggested that infants with < 10% of their expected bowel length are at increased risk of death than those with a longer residual bowel length.

IF is a functional description independent of bowel length and better reflects the nature of the clinical condition encountered in practice. It identifies a child whose loss of intestinal length or competence is below the minimal amount necessary to maintain normal digestion and absorption of nutrients and fluids for weight gain and growth in children independent of PN. Such a definition acknowledges children with conditions such as immune-mediated enteropathy, enteric myopathy, mitochondrial disorders, intestinal pseudoobstruction, tufting enteropathy, and microvillus inclusion disease who have a normal length of intestine but inadequate function to sustain life without PN.

Scope of the Problem

Surprisingly, neither the incidence nor prevalence of IF/SBS in the United States is well known.[10] In 1992, Wallander et al[11] estimated the incidence of extreme SBS to be 3–5 per 100,000 births per year. However, improvements in neonatal intensive care, anesthesia, and surgical techniques have improved survival of children who would have previously died, thus it is likely that the incidence and prevalence has increased in recent years.[12] Other estimates suggest that at least 16,000 children are on home PN (HPN) in the United States, but the precise number on PN for management of IF/SBS is unknown.[13] More importantly, we have no estimate of the number of children with SBS who have been weaned from PN but remain at risk for various nutrition and growth abnormalities as a consequence of their altered intestinal anatomy. A decade ago, the annual costs for managing a PN–dependent patient with IF/SBS were estimated to range between $100,000 and $150,000 with a mortality rate of approximately 30% at 5 years for those who cannot be weaned from PN.[12] More recently, patient outcomes have improved with advances in care by multidisciplinary intestinal rehabilitation programs.[4,14-19]

Etiology of Intestinal Failure

Conditions associated with IF in infants and children are generally due to surgical SBS, motility disorders, or enterocyte abnormalities (Table 27-1).[1] SBS is the underlying cause in the majority of these patients, and its etiology may be congenital abnormalities such as gastroschisis, intestinal atresia, malrotation with volvulus, or acquired causes such as NEC, vascular thrombosis, or trauma. Less commonly seen are motility disorders such as total intestinal aganglionosis and chronic intestinal pseudoobstruction or enterocyte abnormalities such as microvillus inclusion disease and tufting enteropathy.

Intestinal Adaptation

Intestinal adaptation is a complex and incompletely understood process that ensues following significant bowel resection to compensate for the loss of intestinal surface area. It is characterized by both functional and morphologic changes in the remnant bowel.[20,21] Enteral nutrition (EN) is necessary for adaptation. Clinical features associated with patients who are eventually weaned from PN include the absence of jaundice or cholestasis, the presence of the ileocecal valve, an intact colon, small bowel length > 15 cm, and placement of the small intestine in continuity with the colon.[7] The underlying physiologic mechanisms by which these clinical factors might directly impact the adaptive process in the human are incompletely understood. For instance, it is not clear whether the ileocecal valve must be

Table 27-1. Causes of Intestinal Failure in Children

LIFE STAGE	CAUSE OF INTESTINAL FAILURE
Prenatal	Gastroschisis/omphalocele
	Intestinal atresia
	Total intestinal or very long-segment Hirschsprung's disease

	Constitutive enterocyte disorders
	    Tufting enteropathy
	    Microvillus inclusion disease

	Megacystis microcolon hypoperistalsis syndrome
	Malrotation/volvulus
	Bladder extrophy
Neonatal	Necrotizing enterocolitis
	Enteric anendocrinosis
	Vascular thrombosis
	Desquamative enteropathy (Intracellular β4 integrin mutation)
	Malrotation/volvulus
Postnatal	Complicated intussusception

	Trauma
	    Seat belt injury
	    Suction evisceration (eg, swimming pool drain)
	    Riding lawn mower injury

	Extensive vascular anomaly

	Autoimmune/immune-mediated enteropathy
	    IPEX[a]
	    Autoimmune polyglandular syndrome

	Tumor
	    Fibroma
	    Desmoid

	Sclerosing encapsulating peritonitis (abdominal cocoon)
	Munchausen syndrome by proxy
	Protracted diarrhea of infancy

	Intestinal motility disorders
	    Mitochondrial defects/mutations
	    Intestinal pseudoobstruction

[a]Immune dysregulation, polyendocrinaopthy, enteropathy, X-linked.

physically present or whether its presence merely serves as a "marker" for a long colon segment. Over time, the residual bowel lengthens and dilates, which are changes thought to be positive signs of adaptation. However, excessive intestinal dilatation may be associated with altered intestinal motility resulting in stasis of luminal contents and bacterial overgrowth (BO), which can negatively impact adaptation. Surgical techniques aimed to improve intestinal function by reducing bowel diameter and incidentally increasing bowel length include the Bianchi procedure (longitudinal intestinal lengthening and tailoring [LILT]) and serial transverse enteroplasty (STEP).[22,23]

The adaptive process occurs over many months or years.[7,24] Increased enteral intake, or hyperphagia, is associated with intestinal adaptation in adults.[25] The impact of luminal nutrients upon intestinal adaptation is complex, but it likely involves a direct trophic effect on intestinal epithelium, as well as stimulation of trophic hormones and pancreaticobiliary secretions.[26] In animal models, it appears that a more complex nutrient enhances adaptation better than one that is simple or more "processed." For example, disaccharides enhance adaptation more effectively than monosaccharides,[27] and whole proteins are more adaptogenic than protein hydrolysates.[28] Testing these findings in the human have not been undertaken in a rigorous fashion. Hormones and growth factors such as growth hormone, glucagon-like peptide 2, glutamine, cholecystokinin, gastrin, insulin, peptide YY, and enteroglucagon, as well as dietary fiber and short-chain fatty acids have been shown to be involved in the adaptive process, but their clinical significance in humans remains unclear.[26] The functional capabilities of the remnant intestine also impact adaptation. For instance, complete absence of the ileum precludes absorption of bile acids and vitamin B_{12}. The absence of the ileocecal valve appears to have a negative impact on intestinal adaptation for some, but not all patients.[5-7,29,30] However, it is possible that the presence of a sufficient length of colon may be just as, if not more, important than the presence or absence of the ileocecal valve.[31,32] A biomarker for intestinal adaptation, such as citrulline,[33] would ideally reflect the quality and quantity of intestinal function, but its clinical usefulness is uncertain. Markers of hepatic function in patients with IF have not been evaluated. Valid biomarkers are urgently needed so that successful rehabilitation regimens can be objectively identified, and adaptation failure can be recognized earlier. Translational studies to identify potential genetic susceptibilities that would favor or impede intestinal adaptation have not been performed.[34]

Management

Enteral Nutrition

Enteral feeding is essential if intestinal adaptation is to occur.[35] The 2 initial considerations are the type of formula used and the manner in which it is provided. Breast milk is preferred, and its use has been associated with decreased duration of PN.[5] The beneficial effects of breast milk are attributable to its immunoprotective properties, effect on postnatal development of intestinal flora, and its nutrient composition that includes long-chain triglycerides, free amino acids, nucleotides, and growth factors, as well as complex protein and fat.[36] When breast milk is unavailable, however, formula choice is complicated by a variety of options that reflect differences in the desired complexity of protein, fat, and carbohydrate. Complex nutrients, such as polysaccharides and whole protein, increase the functional workload of the intestine, and as a result, may stimulate adaptation.[37] Despite this, some experts favor the use of amino acid–based formulas with the view that these have been associated with improved outcomes.[38] Studies to identify the ideal enteral protein[39-41] and lipid[42] have been plagued by insufficient numbers of patients or have been extrapolated from animal models. In addition, energy expenditure is variable among children with IF, making estimates of caloric needs for individual patients difficult.[43]

A variety of methods can deliver enteral feedings to the intestinal lumen and include oral, gastric as bolus or continuous, or jejunal, which should only be given as a continuous feeding. Advantages of early oral feeding include stimulation of oral digestive enzymes and maintenance of oral feeding skills to prevent oral aversion.[44] If the patient is capable of oral feeding, but is incapable of taking sufficient calories or if oral feedings result in excess stool output, supplemental direct enteral feeding is possible via a nasogastric tube, gastrostomy, or direct jejunal feeding. Continuous enteral infusion was found to be more beneficial in very low birth weight infants,[45] but studies in piglets suggest that bolus feedings are more advantageous.[46] Continuous vs bolus feedings have not been thoroughly studied in older infants and children.

Clinical decisions to adjust the enteral feeding regimen are determined by a number of factors, primarily stool or ostomy output, evidence of malabsorption, and other less objective symptoms such as abdominal fullness, irritability, and regurgitation. Currently, decisions related to advancing enteral feeding, weaning PN, and long-term monitoring of patients at risk for growth failure are based almost completely upon experience, tradition, and art rather than evidence-based algorithms. However, the understanding of the relative importance of these factors, how they are incorporated into daily management, and how they impact adaptation in patients with IF/SBS is critical if management of infants with IF/SBS is to move beyond art and tradition and into an evidence-based practice of medicine.

Parenteral Nutrition

PN, first introduced in the late 1960s, is now an established life-saving treatment for children with IF/SBS.[47-49]

Components of PN include glucose, amino acids, lipids, electrolytes, vitamins, minerals, trace elements, and water. Glucose is the primary source of energy in PN, but glucose oxidation varies depending upon age and diagnosis.[50,51] Glucose infusion rates that are in excess of the patients' oxidative capacity will promote fat deposition.[41] While glucose infusion rates vary, an intake > 10 mg/kg/min may result in the conversion of glucose to fat.[42] However, anecdotally, glucose infusion rates up to 15 mg/kg/min appear to be well tolerated in infants and young children. An amino acid solution, ranging from 3 to 4 g/kg/d for preterm infants to 0.75 g/kg/d for adolescents, is administered to support protein metabolism.[54] Amino acids are best utilized when balanced with a proper proportion of nonnitrogen calories. The ideal ratio of nitrogen to nonnitrogen calories is estimated to be between 1:150 and 1:400.[55] The lipid source currently available in the United States is soy based. It is administered to prevent essential fatty acid deficiency and to provide an efficient, high-density caloric source. An estimated 0.5 g/kg/d of intravenous (IV) lipid is the minimal requirement to prevent deficiency.[56] An IV lipid preparation containing ω-3 fatty acids, not currently approved by the U.S. Food and Drug Administration (FDA) in the United States, has been reported to reduce the incidence of PN–related biochemical cholestasis,[57,58,59] but it has not been rigorously studied in children and persistent hepatic fibrosis has been reported despite normalization of bilirubin.[60-62] Similar reductions in serum bilirubin have been achieved by limiting soy-derived lipid to 1 g/kg/d or less.[63] Serum electrolytes are monitored on a regular basis and adjustments in electrolyte concentration are based on individual needs of the patient. Guidelines for pediatric vitamin, mineral, and trace element supplementation are available, but they are supported by a paucity of data.[48] In addition, deficiencies, such as vitamin D deficiency, have been reported even in individuals receiving PN with vitamins, so monitoring and supplementation as needed are warranted.[64] While PN is lifesaving in children with IF/SBS, long-term use of PN is often complicated by sepsis and liver disease, which can become life threatening.

Given the host of potential complications associated with PN and IF/SBS, careful longitudinal monitoring should be implemented to reduce complications and improve outcome. The frequency of monitoring will depend upon patient age, duration of PN, and acute changes in the clinical condition. Growth parameters (eg, height or length, weight, head circumference) should be checked at each clinical visit. For infants and young children, monthly visits are typical. For older children, on stable PN, visit frequency can be extended to every 3–4 months. Please see Chapter 36 for more information on evaluation and monitoring.

Fluid Management

In addition to PN, children may also require supplemental fluid management to maintain satisfactory hydration. This is particularly important for children with an ileostomy or those whose intestine is in continuity, but with a short length of colon. These children are at increased risk of developing sodium and water depletion and should be monitored carefully.[65,66] In particular, sodium depletion, which may only be evident based on a low urine sodium, can result in poor weight gain. Unless the child's fluid and electrolyte requirements are very consistent day to day and week to week, supplemental fluids should be calculated and administered separately from PN because this allows for more rapid and less expensive adjustments in fluid and electrolyte administration.

Medications

A variety of medications are used to manage symptoms and complications associated with IF/SBS. It is important to know that none of them have been studied in a randomized fashion in an adequately powered study.

Intestinal dysmotility is common in children with IF/SBS. Antimotility agents (eg, loperamide) are used in an attempt to slow intestinal transit in hopes of providing a longer duration of contact between the intestinal mucosa and luminal nutrients. Children with gastroschisis are more likely to have problems with delayed gastric emptying and nonpropulsive intestinal motility. In this setting, promotility agents (eg, metoclopramide, erythromycin, or amoxicillin-clavulanic acid) have been used to improve intestinal motility.[67] Cisapride was removed from the market in the United States due to its association with cardiac arrhythmias. Metoclopramide now has a black box warning due to its association with tardive dyskinesia.

Antisecretory agents are used to reduce fluid secretion and stool output. Histamine-2 blockers and proton pump inhibitors might be useful during the early months following massive intestinal resection. However, continued use, in the absence of clear benefit, may place the child at increased risk for BO or candida esophagitis as gastric acid serves a useful function in limiting fungal and bacterial growth.

Bile acid–binding resins (eg, cholestyramine) have been tried in patients with little or no ileum when increased stool output is thought to be related to bile acid malabsorption. These agents are not easily administered, have little or no palatability, and their efficacy in this clinical setting has not been tested.

A variety of novel therapies are being developed with the hope of improving the adaptive process.[68] Exogenous growth factors such as glucagon-like peptide-2 (GLP-2) and epidermal growth factor (EGF) have shown promising results in animal studies. GLP-2 appears to reduce the duration of PN in adults with SBS[69] and has recently been approved by the FDA for use in adults with SBS/IF[70]; it is currently being studied in children.

Nontransplant Surgery

Half of children with SBS will have more than one abdominal operation.[71] Following the initial surgical intervention, subsequent surgeries often address complications such as stricture, intestinal dilation, and placement of invasive feeding devices which are all considered standard of care.[72]

LILT and STEP represent advanced techniques that both taper dilated segments of bowel and increase intestinal length. Digestive function may improve not only because aboral flow is facilitated by a normalized luminal caliber, but also because subsequent adaptation may lead to increased intestinal surface area. LILT was first described in 1980 by Bianchi,[23] and has since been used at many centers.[1] Criteria for using LILT vary, but generally require > 20 cm of symmetrically dilated intestine in the context of residual intestinal length of >40 cm.[1] Standardized indications, contraindications, and surgical guidelines have not been developed, which may explain inconsistent results reported in the literature.[73] STEP involves the application of a stapling device incompletely across a dilated loop of intestine in serial fashion to create a zig-zag pattern that results in a lumen that is both narrower and longer. Since its description by Kim et al[74] in 2003, it has become an accepted technique at many IF centers.[75] A recent report from the International STEP Data Registry identified 13 participants who underwent a STEP procedure as a primary procedure and found it to be feasible and safe.[76] However, its full impact and usefulness has yet to be determined.

While a growing literature describes individual experiences with nontransplant surgery for children with IF/SBS, the relatively small numbers of patients, retrospective nature of data collection spanning many years, and heterogeneous definitions and patient characteristics have limited the ability to promulgate data-driven indications and timing for these techniques.

General Principles

With the understanding that management of IF is highly individualized and that evidence-based practice supported by randomized, controlled trials is lacking, the following outline might serve as a "principled guide" to the management of IF in children:

1. PN:
    A. Glucose infusion rate: < 15 mg/kg/min for the duration of infusion.
    B. Protein: ≤ 4 g/kg/d, with higher amounts in neonates and lower for older children.
    C. Fat: In the first month, may need 1–2 g/kg/d; but after that, with an eye on the degree of cholestasis and total caloric needs, would consider different strategies.
        i. 1 g/kg/d given every other day; or Monday/Wednesday/Friday or Monday/Thursday.
        ii. Lipid reduction presumes that some enteral feeding is possible.
        iii. Follow essential fatty acids every 3 months.
    D. Fluid: Based on needs, it is hard to provide sufficient calories with a fluid rate < 125 mL/kg/d, unless a very high glucose concentration is used; may need additional salt and water to support losses.
2. Enteral feeds:
    A. Use oral feeds if at all possible to maintain oral skills and stimulate EGF, even if the child has a gastrostomy tube; 3–5 mL per feed and then gradually increase as one can.
    B. Breast milk is preferred and a formula containing casein hydrolysate/medium-chain triglyceride is the author's fallback, assuming that intestinal adaptation is favored by a more complex enteral diet; use of an amino acid–containing formula can be reserved for protein allergy.
    C. Jejunal tubes should be used rarely because they further shorten the length of useable bowel length.
3. Advancing feeds/reducing PN:
    A. Tolerance of enteral feeds is ill-defined and difficult to assess.
        i. Stool volume can only be estimated in diapered children because urine and stool are often "mixed." Stool number is often confounded by "squirts" that are frequent but low volume. For example, 10 stools per day may be "okay" if only 3–4 or so are big enough to fill the diaper, the perianal area is not excoriated, the family is comfortable, and hydration is maintained.
        ii. Aim for a rate of weight gain that is adjusted for prematurity and for infants who were small for gestational age and also takes into account the child's residual bowel length and function.

Efforts to achieve weight gain that follows the 50th percentile may be unrealistic. The goal is to find the minimal amount of PN and maximal amount of enteral feeding to support reasonable weight gain and growth.
    B. Once on <25% total calories from PN, consider efforts to transition from PN to IV fluids. If tolerance of enteral feedings and minimal PN is accompanied by satisfactory weight gain and growth, transitioning from PN to IV fluids will maintain hydration, while calories derived from enteral feeding can be determined to be sufficient to support the child. With continued weight gain on full enteral feeds, transitioning off IV fluids before the central line is pulled can be considered.
4. Nontransplant surgery:
    A. When to consider in a child with SBS
        i. A sufficient length of small bowel is dilated to at least 3–5 cm and
            1. Enteral feedings cannot be advanced.
            2. The child is experiencing poor weight gain and/or growth.
    B. What type of surgery?
        i. May be surgeon specific; a learning curve is needed for both the STEP and Bianchi, but more so for the Bianchi.
        ii. One can STEP a STEP, and STEP a Bianchi, but one cannot Bianchi a STEP.

Complications

Nutrition Deficiencies

Deficiencies in vitamins, minerals, and trace elements are associated with IF/SBS.[77] Malabsorption of fat-soluble vitamins A, D, E, and K may result from an insufficient intraluminal concentration of bile acids secondary to excess fecal loss.[78] Surgical resections of the duodenum or ileum, which have unique absorptive functions, add to the risk of developing nutrition deficiencies. The duodenum is a primary site for iron and folate absorption and its resection can result in these micronutrient deficiencies. Absence of the ileum, with its unique ability to absorb vitamin B_{12} and bile acids, places the patient at risk for fat-soluble vitamin and vitamin B_{12} deficiency. Calcium and magnesium deficiencies can result from binding to intraluminal long-chain fatty acids.[79,80] Deficiencies of other minerals and trace elements such as zinc, riboflavin, thiamin, biotin, and also selenium can occur.[81] In addition, nutrient deficiencies hinder intestinal adaptation, further compounding the clinical impact.[82]

Functional and Metabolic Complications

Following massive bowel resection that alters normal intestinal physiology, a number of acute and chronic medical complications develop that prompt an effort for medical interventions. Unfortunately, many interventions and treatments have not been adequately studied with sufficient numbers of patients.

Hypergastinemia develops shortly after small bowel resection and can reduce nutrient absorption by inactivating pancreatic enzymes and precipitating bile salts, thus leading to diarrhea as well as nausea and vomiting.[83-85] Small case series have reported mixed benefits of acid reduction to improve absorption.[86-89] However, no large trials demonstrate a benefit to the use of these medications in children with IF/SBS. Indiscriminate use of these medications may predispose patients to small bowel BO, calcium and iron malabsorption, or a heightened risk of Candida esophagitis or sepsis.[90] Bile acid malabsorption as a consequence of ileal resection can result in a secretory diarrhea that complicates fat and fat-soluble vitamin absorption.[91] Rapid intestinal transit occurs following small bowel resection[92,93] and is often managed with the use of antimotility agents such as loperamide, which have mixed effects on water and salt balance.[94,95] Nephrolithiasis, when it occurs in the setting of IF/SBS, is typically due to either uric acid or calcium oxalate stones.[96]

Alterations in gastrointestinal motility, along with the use of acid blocking agents, may increase the bacterial content in the small intestine, resulting in BO. BO can result in deconjugation of luminal bile acids, making them ineffective in micellar formation, and can be associated with mucosal inflammation, nutrient deficiencies (notably vitamin B_{12}), D-lactic acidosis as well as cramps, diarrhea, gastrointestinal bleeding, and arthritis. The relationship between small bowel BO and systemic sepsis is not well understood.[97-100] BO is most often treated empirically with intermittent oral or enteral doses of broad-spectrum antibiotics, and in some cases probiotics, but many varying practices exist for the frequency and duration of administration, with no data available to evaluate relative efficacies.

D-lactic acidosis is a unique feature of patients with IF/SBS and was first described in children in 1983.[101] The combination of a high anion gap acidosis and altered mental status that develops after a high carbohydrate enteral feeding should prompt the clinical suspicion of d-lactic acidosis. Treatment involves discontinuation of enteral feeding,

selective bowel decontamination, and, if needed, a surgical procedure aimed at decreasing intestinal diameter and reducing BO.[102,103] Frequent antibiotic therapy may, paradoxically, place the patient at risk for D-lactic acidosis by creating a selective advantage for D-lactate producing bacteria.[104]

Liver Disease

Liver disease is the most frequent complication of long-term PN, with consequences that include cirrhosis, end-stage liver disease, and even death.[105] Historically, the incidence of IF/SBS-associated liver disease (IFALD) is as high as 50% in infants who receive PN for 2 months, with end-stage liver disease developing in 90% of premature infants on PN for > 3 months.[106] However, this development is becoming less frequent with care by multidisciplinary teams and careful approaches to PN, enteral feeding, and surgical techniques. Elevated serum transaminase and bilirubin levels are commonly observed in infants on PN, but these levels can normalize and jaundice resolve with intestinal adaptation and PN withdrawal. The long-term outcome of IFALD in patients who adapt is unknown. The population currently thought to be at greatest risk for IFALD is premature infants with a birth weight < 1 kg and those with IF/SBS resulting from surgical resection.[107-109] The etiology of IFALD remains unknown but is likely multifactorial with prematurity, multiple abdominal surgeries, lack of enterally stimulated bile flow, bacterial sepsis, and components or deficiencies of PN infusates, all potential contributors.

Treatment of PN–associated liver disease is empiric and imperfect. Current strategies to avert liver disease associated with long-term PN include employing a choleretic such as ursodeoxycholic acid,[110] bowel "decontamination" to treat BO,[108,110] vigilant daily catheter care,[111] and modifying PN formulations. Infusing PN calories over < 24 hours, casually referred to as "cycling" PN, is thought to improve cholestasis.[112] The underlying mechanism for this action and effect is not clearly understood but may involve providing a metabolic "rest" from the continuous infusion of calories, protein, and/or carbohydrate. Administration of pediatric formulations of PN that include specific "targeted" amino acids including taurine[113] and limiting the infusion of dextrose so as to potentially decrease steatosis have also been utilized.[114] Decreasing the aluminum and manganese content in PN may decrease hepatotoxicity.[115,116] Decreasing the amount or altering the type of lipids administered may improve serum transaminase levels, reverse PN–associated liver disease, or reduce lipid peroxidation.[57,117,118] As already noted, use of a fish oil–based IV lipid source was found to be associated with improvement of serum bilirubin in 2 children,[57] although its long-term use in an animal model was associated with increased fibrosis.[119] Unfortunately, most of these interventions to reduce or prevent IFALD are employed empirically and lack significant clinical confirmation in large pediatric trials. Once end-stage liver disease develops, portal hypertension, variceal and stomal bleeding, infection, hypoglycemia, and hyperammonemia occur, making a combined liver-intestinal transplant the only remaining lifesaving measure for patients unable to be weaned from PN. Disappointingly, hepatic fibrosis and steatosis persist for some children despite resolution of cholestasis and achieving enteral autonomy.[120] A clinical guideline on the support of pediatric patients with IF/SBS at risk for PN–associated liver disease was recently published.[121]

Central Line Complications

Maintaining central venous catheter (CVC) access is critical in the long-term management of IF/SBS. Loss of vascular access can be fatal in this population and is an indication for intestinal transplantation. As a result, salvage of the CVC line is a strategy employed to preserve vascular access. In addition, the advancement of newer approaches such as recanalization of a thrombosed vessel has been employed in selected patients when vascular sites are limited.[122,123] The threshold for removing CVC lines and referral to centers that perform recanalization is likely variable from both an institutional and physician standpoint. A greater understanding of the source of this variability will allow standardization to a best practice model and allow centers participating in this collaborative to preserve access sites and better equip patients for long-term survival.

Sepsis is an important cause of death in children with IF/SBS. Accordingly, multiple factors contribute to the management of suspected sepsis in the patient with IF/SBS including age and presence of a CVC. Catheter-associated bloodstream infections (CABSIs) are responsible for a majority of the infectious morbidity. While the true incidence of CABSIs is unknown, IF/SBS patients constitute a high-risk group within the CVC population. Potential risk factors include the proximity of fecal material to line entry sites and connections, frequent line access for laboratory tests, and intestinal bacterial translocation. While translocation occurs in animal models, its proof in human populations is elusive.[124] At the same time, several lines of evidence suggest a role for bacterial translocation in IF/SBS. Enteric organisms are more frequently isolated in cultures from these patients compared with other populations with CVC lines.[125] Furthermore, a comparison of CVC isolates with fecal flora and mesenteric lymph node cultures were highly concordant.[126] Finally, the incidence of infection has been demonstrated to be increased while advancing enteral feeds.[127] Treatment strategies to manage and prevent CABSIs are expanding[128] and include ethanol[129] and antibiotic locks of central catheters and antibiotic-impregnated catheters.[130]

While CABSIs are of the greatest concern, patients with IF/SBS are also subject to numerous other central line–related complications. Of these, thrombosis and line breakage are the 2 most frequent. Fortunately, the salvage rate is high, and treatment with thrombolytics or CVC repair has been shown to result in a high CVC salvage rate.[131] The development of consensus guidelines based upon the accrual of data across the population of individuals with IF/SBS is predicted to reduce CVC-associated complications as well as lengthen the life span of each individual catheter and preserve access sites critical to survival and potential transplantation.

Outcomes

Growth and Development

Infants and children must digest and absorb sufficient calories, vitamins, minerals, and trace elements to gain weight, grow, and develop. Children with IF/SBS are incapable of sustaining adequate growth and development without supplemental PN. Successful intestinal adaptation implies complete independence from PN, while continuing to demonstrate satisfactory linear growth and weight gain that is commensurate with the capabilities of the residual small bowel and colon. The expected weight gain and growth of patients with IF/SBS weaned from prolonged PN is not known. Well-designed prospective studies are needed to address long-term growth and development in children with IF/SBS following PN withdrawal. A recent retrospective study of 87 children identified over a period of 16 years provides some insight into the long-term problems that children with IF/SBS may face.[24] The authors found that in those children who achieved enteral autonomy, maximum weight gain and growth was achieved during the first 4 years after weaning PN. However, between 4 and 8 years post PN, weight gain and growth, expressed as a z score, appeared to decline with the weight z score 8 years post PN almost identical to the weight at the time of weaning and height z score slightly lower than the score at the time of weaning. Interestingly, 21 children were noted to enter puberty at an age similar to their peers.

Quality of Life

Studies in adult patients have identified reduced quality of life (QOL) scores in patients with SBS, which were further reduced if the patient was on HPN. Interestingly, the presence of a stoma did not appear to influence their quality of life.[132] Similarly detailed studies that address QOL and school performance have not been performed in children; however, children on HPN appear to fare better than those hospitalized for PN.[133,134]

Intestinal Transplant

Intestinal transplant is reserved as the final lifesaving procedure for patients with irreversible IF/SBS and life-threatening complications associated with PN administration. In 1994, very few intestinal transplants were performed in the pediatric population worldwide (approximately 25 according to the Intestinal Transplant Registry), with unsatisfactory outcomes in these early years.[1] With advances in posttransplant care and immunosuppression protocols, these outcomes have dramatically improved.[2] More than 2500 intestinal transplants have now been performed in all age groups worldwide, with more than 1400 in the pediatric population.[2,5,135] Five-year patient survival rates exceed 50% worldwide.[6] Unfortunately, the indications for intestinal transplant are broad and subject to a significant degree of interpretation. Evidence-based parameters are needed that would improve the selection of patients for intestinal transplant and determine optimal timing for transplant to maximize outcomes and minimize the need for combined organ transplantation.

At the present time, intestinal transplantation is reserved for patients who have refractory PN–dependence and fail PN as defined by Centers for Medicare and Medicaid Services. In principle, PN failure may be defined as the onset of potential life-threatening complications of PN in the form of progressive IFALD or catheter-related complications including recurrent life-threatening sepsis or even a single episode of fungal sepsis, or loss of central venous access. Additional indications that may be more contentious include nonresectable tumors at the root of the mesentery, nonreconstructible gastrointestinal tract due to complex entero-cutaneous fistulae or recurrent or life-threatening metabolic and fluid-electrolyte derangements that become unmanageable on PN.

The goal of intestinal transplantation is to achieve autonomy from PN, with removal of the CVC becoming a major milestone—this milestone is achieved typically within a month of transplant in the majority of cases. Nutritional management of the post–intestinal transplant patient is complex, often punctuated by transplant-related complications and is best viewed as a form of IF with the potential of rapid intestinal adaptation. An important early nutrition complication following intestinal transplantation is the occurrence of chylous ascites in a small percentage of cases. This complication occurs because no attempt is made at lymphatic reconstitution during the intestinal transplant procedure. The risk of this complication decreases to almost zero at 4–6 weeks as the abdominal and diaphragmatic lymphatics appear to reconstitute in the first few weeks. This complication can be avoided by the use of fat-free diets for the first 2–4 weeks after transplant and the cautious introduction of small amounts of dietary fat thereafter. It is customary to place a gastrostomy or jejunostomy feeding tube at the time of transplant as a means to achieve rapid weaning from PN in the first month after transplant. The enteral access device provides a means for supplementary enteral feedings if needed, and more importantly at a time that the allograft bowel may still be recovering from ischemia-reperfusion, provides an important means for enteral delivery of appropriate glucose-saline solutions such as oral rehydration solution or pedialyte, to prevent renal dysfunction secondary to dehydration. The majority of patients are able to accomplish full oral feedings and dispense with an enteral access device typically within 6 months of transplant.

A subset of patients with IF/SBS and associated liver disease may benefit from an isolated liver transplant.[136–138] It has been postulated that IFALD may hinder bowel adaptation and delay progression toward enteral feeding tolerance.[8] In fact, various authors have reported remarkable bowel adaptation and feeding tolerance after isolated liver transplant for severe IFALD.[6,7,136]

Test Your Knowledge Questions

1. A 30-week infant with 35 cm of small bowel, an ileocecal valve, and an intact colon has an advantage over a full-term infant with the same anatomy because:
   A. Etiologies for short bowel syndrome are different between the 2 groups.
   B. Premature infants who survive are constitutionally stronger than full-term infants.
   C. The small intestinal length doubles in the last trimester.
   D. Complications associated with PN are less frequent in the premature infant.
2. A clinical feature associated with enteral autonomy is:
   A. Being a female
   B. Small intestine in continuity with the colon

C. Absent ileocecal valve

D. Having fewer than 10 stools per day

3. PN associated liver disease is caused by:

A. IV lipid

B. Lack of enteral feeding

C. Recurrent infections

D. Multiple factors, including all of the above

4. The best method to provide enteral feeding for children with IF is via:

A. Gastrostomy

B. Nasogastric tube

C. Jejunal feeding

D. Oral feeding

References

1. Goulet O, Ruemmele F, Lacaille F, Colomb V. Irreversible intestinal failure. *J Pediatr Gastroenterol Nutr.* 2004;38(3):250–269.

2. Kocoshis SA, Beath SV, Booth IW, et al; North American Society for Gastroenterology, Hepatology and Nutrition. Intestinal failure and small bowel transplantation, including clinical nutrition: Working Group Report of the Second World Congress of Pediatric Gastroenterology, Hepatology, and Nutrition. *J Pediatr Gastroenterol Nutr.* 2004;39(suppl 2):S655–S661.

3. Squires RH, Duggan C, Teitelbaum DH, Wales PW, Balint J, et al; Pediatric Intestinal Failure Consortium. Natural history of pediatric intestinal failure: initial report from the Pediatric Intestinal Failure Consortium. *J Pediatr.* 2012;161:723–728.

4. Stanger JD, Oliveira C, Blackmore C, Avitzur Y, Wales PW. The impact of multi-disciplinary intestinal rehabilitation programs on the outcome of pediatric patients with intestinal failure: a systematic review and meta-analysis. *J Pediatr Surg.* 2013;48(5):983–92.

5. Andorsky DJ, Lund DP, Lillehei CW, et al. Nutritional and other postoperative management of neonates with short bowel syndrome correlates with clinical outcomes. *J Pediatr.* 2001;139(1):27–33.

6. *Goulet OJ, Revillon Y, Jan D, et al. Neonatal short bowel syndrome. J Pediatr.* 1991;119(1 Pt 1):18–23.

7. Quirós-Teijeira RE, Ament ME, Reyen L, et al. Long-term parenteral nutritional support and intestinal adaptation in children with short bowel syndrome: a 25-year experience. *J Pediatr.* 2004;145(2):157–163.

8. *Spencer AU, Neaga A, West B, et al. Pediatric short bowel syndrome: redefining predictors of success. Ann Surg.* 2005;242(3):403–409; discussion 409–412.

9. Touloukian RJ, Smith GJ. Normal intestinal length in preterm infants. *J Pediatr Surg.* 1983;18(6):720–723.

10. DeLegge M, Alsolaiman MM, Barbour E, et al. Short bowel syndrome: parenteral nutrition versus intestinal transplantation. Where are we today? *Dig Dis Sci.* 2007;52(4):876–892.

11. *Wallander J, Ewald U, Lackgren G, et al. Extreme short bowel syndrome in neonates: an indication for small bowel transplantation? Transplant Proc.* 1992;24(3):1230–1235.

12. Schalamon J, Mayr JM, Hollwarth ME. Mortality and economics in short bowel syndrome. *Best Pract Res Clin Gastroenterol.* 2003;17(6):931–942.

13. Colomb V. Economic aspects of paediatric home parenteral nutrition. *Curr Opin Clin Nutr Metab Care.* 2000;3(3):237–239.

14. Diamond IR, de Silva N, Pencharz PB, Kim JH, Wales PW. Neonatal short bowel syndrome outcomes after the establishment of the first Canadian multidisciplinary intestinal rehabilitation program: preliminary experience. *J Pediatr Surg.* 2007;42:806–811.

15. Ganousse-Mazeron S, Lacaille F, Colomb-Jung V, et al. Assessment and outcome of children with intestinal failure referred for intestinal transplantation. *Clin Nutr.* 2014;pii:S0261-5614(14)00123-X.

16. Hess RA, Welch KB, Brown PI, Teitelbaum DH. Survival outcomes of pediatric intestinal failure patients: analysis of factors contributing to improved survival over the past two decades. *J Surg Res.* 2011;170(1):27–31.

17. Modi BP, Langer M, Ching YA et al. Improved survival in a multidisciplinary short bowel program. *J Pediatr Surg.* 2008;43(1):20–24.

18. Sanchez SE, Javid PJ, Healey PJ, Reyes J, Horslen SP. Ultra-short bowel syndrome in children. *J Pediatr Gastroenterol Nutr.* 2013;56(1):36–39.

19. Sigalet D, Boctor D, Robertson M, et al. Improved outcomes in paediatric intestinal failure with aggressive prevention of liver disease. *Eur J Pediatr Surg.* 2009;19(6):348–353.

20. Tavakkolizadeh A, Whang EE. Understanding and augmenting human intestinal adaptation: a call for more clinical research. *JPEN J Parenter Enteral Nutr.* 2002;26(4):251–255.

21. Drozdowski L, Thomson AB. Intestinal mucosal adaptation. *World J Gastroenterol.* 2006;12(29):4614–4627.

22. Javid P, Kim H, Duggan C, Jaksic T. Serial transverse enteroplasty is associated with successful short-term outcomes in infants with short bowel syndrome. *J Pediatr Surg.* 2005;40(6):1019–1023; discussion 1023–1024.

23. Bianchi A. Intestinal loop lengthening—a technique for increasing small intestinal length. *J Pediatr Surg.* 1980;15(2):145–151.

24. Goulet O, Gobet B, Talbotec C, et al. Outcome and long-term growth after extensive small bowel resection in the neonatal period: a survey of 87 children. *Eur J Pediatr Surg.* 2005;15(2):95–101.

25. Crenn P, Morin MC, Joly F, Penven S, Thuillier F, Messing B. Net digestive absorption and adaptive hyperphagia in adult short bowel patients. *Gut.* 2004;53(9):1279–1286.

26. DiBaise JK, Young RJ, Vanderhoof JA. Intestinal rehabilitation and the short bowel syndrome: part 1. *Am J Gastroenterol.* 2004;99(7):1386–1395.

27. Weser E, Babbitt J, Hoban M, Vandeventer A. Intestinal adaptation. Different growth responses to disaccharides compared with monosaccharides in rat small bowel. *Gastroenterology.* 1986;91(6):1521–1527.

28. Vanderhoof JA, Grandjean CJ, Burkley KT, et al. Effect of casein versus casein hydrolysate on mucosal adaptation following massive bowel resection in infant rats. *J Pediatr Gastroenterol Nutr.* 1984;3(2):262–267.

29. Wasa M, Takagi Y, Sando K, et al. Intestinal adaptation in pediatric patients with short-bowel syndrome. *Eur J Pediatr Surg.* 1999;9(4):207–209.

30. Gambarara M, Ferretti F, Bagolan P. Ultra-short-bowel syndrome is not an absolute indication to small-bowel transplantation in childhood. *Eur J Pediatr Surg.* 1999;9(4):267–270.

31. Jeppesen PB, Mortensen PB. The influence of a preserved colon on the absorption of medium chain fat in patients with small bowel resection. *Gut.* 1998;43(4):478–483.

32. Nightingale JM, Lennard-Jones JE, Gertner DJ, et al. Colonic preservation reduces need for parenteral therapy, increases incidence of renal stones, but does not change high prevalence of gall stones in patients with a short bowel. *Gut.* 1992;33(11):1493–1497.

33. Luo M, Fernández-Estívariz C, Manatunga AK, et al. Are plasma citrulline and glutamine biomarkers of intestinal absorptive function in patients with short bowel syndrome? *JPEN J Parenter Enteral Nutr.* 2007;31(1):1–7.

34. Bernal NP, Stehr W, Zhang Y, Profitt S, Erwin CR, Warner BW. Evidence for active Wnt signaling during postresection intestinal adaptation. *J Pediatr Surg.* 2005;40(6):1025–1029; discussion 1029.

35. Roy CC, Groleau V, Bouthillier L, Pineault M, Thibault M, Marchand V. Short bowel syndrome in infants: the critical role of luminal nutrients in a management program. *Appl Physiol Nutr Metab.* 2014:39(7):745–753.

36. Levy J. Immunonutrition: the pediatric experience. *Nutrition.* 1998;14(7–8):641–647.

37. Vanderhoof JA, Langnas AN. Short-bowel syndrome in children and adults. *Gastroenterology.* 1997;113(5):1767–1778.

38. Gosselin KB, Duggan C. Enteral nutrition in the management of pediatric intestinal failure. *J Pediatr.* 2014;165(6):1085–1090.

39. Ksiazyk J, Piena M, Kierkus J, Lyszkowska M. Hydrolyzed versus nonhydrolyzed protein diet in short bowel syndrome in children. *J Pediatr Gastroenterol Nutr.* 2002;35(5):615–618.

40. Bines J, Francis D, Hill D. Reducing parenteral requirement in children with short bowel syndrome: impact of an amino acid-based complete infant formula. *J Pediatr Gastroenterol Nutr.* 1998;26(2):123–128.

41. Taylor S, Sondheimer J, Sokol R, Silverman A, Wilson H. Noninfectious colitis associated with short gut syndrome in infants. *J Pediatr.* 1991;119(1 Pt 1):24–28.

42. Vanderhoof JA, Grandjean CJ, Kaufman SS, Burkely KT, Antonson DL. Effect of high percentage medium-chain triglyceride diet on mucosal adaptation following massive bowel resection in rats. *JPEN J Parenter Enteral Nutr.* 1984;8(6):685–689.

43. Duro D, Mitchell PD, Mehta NM, et al. Variability of resting energy expenditure in infants and young children with intestinal failure-associated liver disease. *J Pediatr Gastroenterol Nutr.* 2014;589(5):637–641.

44. Blackman JA, Nelson CL. Reinstituting oral feedings in children fed by gastrostomy tube. *Clin Pediatr. (Phila)* 1985;24(8):434–438.

45. Dsilna A, Christensson K, Alfredsson L, et al. Continuous feeding promotes gastrointestinal tolerance and growth in very low birth weight infants. *J Pediatr.* 2005;147(1):43–49.

46. Shulman RJ, Redel CA, Stathos TH. Bolus versus continuous feedings stimulate small-intestinal growth and development in the newborn pig. *J Pediatr Gastroenterol Nutr.* 1994;18(3):350–354.

47. Rhoads JE. The development of TPN: an interview with pioneer surgical nutritionist Jonathan E. Rhoads, MD. [Interview by Carolyn T. Spencer and Charlene Compher]. *J Am Diet Assoc.* 2001;101(7):747–750.

48. Shulman RJ, Phillips S. Parenteral nutrition in infants and children. *J Pediatr Gastroenterol Nutr.* 2003;36(5):587–607.

49. Dudrick SJ, Wilmore DW, Vars HM, Rhoads JE. Long-term total parenteral nutrition with growth, development, and positive nitrogen balance. *Surgery.* 1968;64(1):134–142.

50. Lafeber HN, Sulkers EJ, Chapman TE, et al. Glucose production and oxidation in preterm infants during total parenteral nutrition. *Pediatr Res.* 1990;28(2):153–157.

51. Sheridan RL, Yong-Ming Y, Prelack K, Young VR, Burke JF, Tompkins RG. Maximal parenteral glucose oxidation in hypermetabolic young children: a stable isotope study. *JPEN J Parenter Enteral Nutr.* 1998;22(4):212–216.

52. Kalhan SC, Kilic I. Carbohydrate as nutrient in the infant and child: range of acceptable intake. *Eur J Clin Nutr.* 1999;53(suppl 1):S94–S100.

53. Nose O, Tipton JR, Yabuuchi H. Effect of the energy source on changes in energy expenditure, respiratory quotient, and nitrogen balance during total parenteral nutrition in children. *Pediatr Res.* 1987;21(6):538–541.

54. Safe Practices for Parenteral Nutrition Formulations. National Advisory Group on Standards and Practice Guidelines for Parenteral Nutrition. *JPEN J Parenter Enteral Nutr.* 1998;22(2):49–66.

55. Peters C, Fischer JE. Studies on calorie to nitrogen ratio for total parenteral nutrition. *Surg Gynecol Obstet.* 1980;151(1):1–8.

56. Gutcher GR, Farrell PM. Intravenous infusion of lipid for the prevention of essential fatty acid deficiency in premature infants. *Am J Clin Nutr.* 1991;54(6):1024–1028.

57. Gura KM, Duggan CP, Collier SB, et al. Reversal of parenteral nutrition-associated liver disease in two infants with short bowel syndrome using parenteral fish oil: implications for future management. *Pediatrics.* 2006;118(1):e197–e201.

58. Nehra D, Fallon EM, Potemkin AK, et al. A comparison of 2 intravenous lipid emulsions: interim analysis of a randomized controlled trial. *JPEN J Parenter Enteral Nutr.* 2014;38(6):693–701.

59. Puder M, Valim C, Meisel JA, et al. Parenteral fish oil improves outcomes in patients with parenteral nutrition-associated liver injury. *Ann Surg.* 2009;250:395–402.

60. Mercer DF, Hobson BD, Fischer RT, et al. Hepatic fibrosis persists and progresses despite biochemical improvement in

children treated with intravenous fish oil emulsion. *J Pediatr Gastroenterol Nutr.* 2013;56(4):364–369.

61. Nandivada P, Chang MI, Potemkin AK, et al. The natural history of cirrhosis from parenteral nutrition-associated liver disease after resolution of cholestasis with parenteral fish oil therapy. *Ann Surg.* 2015;261(1):172–179.

62. Soden JS, Lovell MA, Brown K, Patrick DA, Sokol RJ. Failure of resolution of portal fibrosis during omega-3 fatty acid lipid emulsion therapy in two patients with irreversible intestinal failure. *J Pediatr.* 2010;156(2):327–331.

63. Cober MP, Killu G, Brattain A, Welch KB, Kunisaki SM, Teitelbaum DH. Intravenous fat emulsions reduction for patients with parenteral nutrition-associated liver disease. *J Pediatr.* 2012;160(3):421–427.

64. Wozniak LJ, Bechtold HM, Reyen LE, Hall TR, Vargas JH. Vitamin D deficiency in children with intestinal failure receiving home parenteral nutrition [published online ahead of print March 14, 2014]. *JPEN J Parenter Enteral Nutr.*

65. Schwarz K, Ternberg J, Bell M, Keating J. Sodium needs of infants and children with ileostomy. *J Pediatr.* 1983;102(4);509–513.

66. O'Neil M, Teitelbaum DH, Harris MB. Total body sodium depletion and poor weight gain in children and young adults with an ileostomy: a case series. *Nutr Clin Pract.* 2014;29(3):397–401.

67. Gomez R, Fernandez S, Aspirot A, et al. Effect of amoxicillin/clavulanate on gastrointestinal motility in children. *J Pediatr Gastroenterol Nutr.* 2012;54(6):780–784.

68. Schwartz MZ. Novel therapies for the management of short bowel syndrome in children. *Pediatr Surg Int.* 2013;29:967–974.

69. Jeppesen PB. Glucagon-like peptide-2: update of the recent clinical trials. *Gastroenterology.* 2006;130:S127–131.

70. Jeppesen PB, Pertkiewicz M, Messing B, et al. Teduglutide reduces need for parenteral support among patients with short bowel syndrome with intestinal failure. *Gastroenterology.* 2012;143:1473–1481.

71. Thompson JS. Reoperation in patients with the short bowel syndrome. *Am J Surg.* 1992;164(5):453–456; discussion 456–457.

72. Wales PW. Surgical therapy for short bowel syndrome. *Pediatr Surg Int.* 2004;20(9):647–657.

73. Bianchi A. From the cradle to enteral autonomy: the role of autologous gastrointestinal reconstruction. *Gastroenterology.* 2006;130(2 suppl 1):S138–S146.

74. Kim HB, Fauza D, Garza J, Oh JT, Nurko S, Jaksic T. Serial transverse enteroplasty (STEP): a novel bowel lengthening procedure. *J Pediatr Surg.* 2003;38(3):425–429.

75. Modi B, Javid P, Jaksic T, et al; International STEP Data Registry. First report of the international serial transverse enteroplasty data registry: indications, efficacy, and complications. *J Am Coll Surg.* 2007; 204(3):365–371.

76. Garnett GM, Kang KH, Jaksic T, et al. First STEPs: serial transverse enteroplasty as a primary procedure in neonates with congenital short bowel. *J Pediatr Surg.* 2014;49:104–108.

77. Ubesie AC, Kocoshis SA, Mezoff AG, Henderson RJ, Helmrath MA, Cole CR. Multiple micronutrient deficiencies among patients with intestinal failure during and after transition to enteral nutrition. *J Pediatr.* 2013;163:1692–1696.

78. Ohkohchi N, Andoh T, Izumi U, Igarashi Y, Ohi R. Disorder of bile acid metabolism in children with short bowel syndrome. *J Gastroenterol.* 1997;32(4):472–479.

79. Ament ME. Bone mineral content in patients with short bowel syndrome: the impact of parenteral nutrition. *J Pediatr.* 1998;132(3 Pt 1):386–388.

80. Fleming CR, George L, Stoner GL, et al. The importance of urinary magnesium values in patients with gut failure. *Mayo Clin Proc.* 1996;71(1):21–24.

81. Buchman AL. Etiology and initial management of short bowel syndrome. *Gastroenterology.* 2006;130(2 suppl 1):S5–S15.

82. Ziegler TR, Evans ME, Fernández-Estívariz C, Jones DP. Trophic and cytoprotective nutrition for intestinal adaptation, mucosal repair, and barrier function. *Annu Rev Nutr.* 2003;23:229–261.

83. Buxton B. Small bowel resection and gastric acid hypersecretion. *Gut.* 1974;15(3):229–238.

84. Go VL, Poley JR, Hofmann AF, Summerskill WH. Disturbances in fat digestion induced by acidic jejunal pH due to gastric hypersecretion in man. *Gastroenterology.* 1970;58(5):638–646.

85. Williams NS, Evans P, King RF. Gastric acid secretion and gastrin production in the short bowel syndrome. *Gut.* 1985;26(9):914–919.

86. Cortot A, Fleming CR, Malagelada JR. Improved nutrient absorption after cimetidine in short-bowel syndrome with gastric hypersecretion. *N Engl J Med.* 1979;300(2):79–80.

87. Nightingale JM, Walker ER, Farthing MJ, Lennard-Jones JE. Effect of omeprazole on intestinal output in the short bowel syndrome. *Aliment Pharmacol Ther.* 1991;5(4):405–412.

88. Tang SJ, Nieto J, Jenson DM, Ohning GV, Pisegna JR. The novel use of an intravenous proton pump inhibitor in a patient with short bowel syndrome. *J Clin Gastroenterol.* 2002;34(1):62–63.

89. Malagelada JR. Pathophysiological responses to meals in the Zollinger-Ellison syndrome: 2. Gastric emptying and its effect on duodenal function. *Gut.* 1980;21(2):98–104.

90. Chocarro MA, Galindo TF, Ruiz-Irastorza G, et al. Risk factors for esophageal candidiasis. *Eur J Clin Microbiol Infect Dis.* 2000;19(2):96–100.

91. Westergaard H. Bile acid malabsorption. *Curr Treat Options Gastroenterol.* 2007;10(1): 28–33.

92. Nightingale JM, Kamm MA, van der Sijp JR, et al. Disturbed gastric emptying in the short bowel syndrome. Evidence for a 'colonic brake'. *Gut.* 1993;34(9):1171–1176.

93. Reynell PC, Spray GH. Small intestinal function in the rat after massive resections. *Gastroenterology.* 1956;31(4):361–368.

94. Nightingale JM, Lennard-Jones JE, Walker ER. A patient with jejunostomy liberated from home intravenous therapy after 14 years; contribution of balance studies. *Clin Nutr.* 1992;11(2):101–105.

95. Rodrigues CA, Lennard-Jones JE, Thompson DG, et al. The effects of octreotide, soy polysaccharide, codeine and loperamide on nutrient, fluid and electrolyte absorption in the short-bowel syndrome. *Aliment Pharmacol Ther.* 1989;3(2):159–169.

96. Nightingale JM. Hepatobiliary, renal and bone complications of intestinal failure. *Best Pract Res Clin Gastroenterol.* 2003;17(6):907–929.

97. Dibaise JK, Young RJ, Vanderhoof JA. Enteric microbial flora, bacterial overgrowth, and short-bowel syndrome. *Clin Gastroenterol Hepatol.* 2006;4(1):11–20.

98. O'Keefe SJ. Bacterial overgrowth and liver complications in short bowel intestinal failure patients. *Gastroenterology.* 2006;130(2 suppl 1):S67–S69.

99. Puwanant M, Mo-Suwan L, Patrapinyokul S. Recurrent D-lactic acidosis in a child with short bowel syndrome. *Asia Pac J Clin Nutr.* 2005;14(2):195–198.

100. Quigley EM, Quera R. Small intestinal bacterial overgrowth: roles of antibiotics, prebiotics, and probiotics. *Gastroenterology.* 2006;130(2 suppl 1):S78–S90.

101. Perlmutter DH, Boyle JT, Campos JM, Egler JM, Watkins JM. D-Lactic acidosis in children: an unusual metabolic complication of small bowel resection. *J Pediatr.* 1983;102(2):234–238.

102. Mayne AJ, Handy DJ, Pierce MA, George RH, Booth IW. Dietary management of D-lactic acidosis in short bowel syndrome. *Arch Dis Child.* 1990;65(2):229–231.

103. Hosie S, Loff S, Wirth H, Rapp HJ, von Buch C, Waag KL. Experience of 49 longitudinal intestinal lengthening procedures for short bowel syndrome. *Eur J Pediatr Surg.* 2006;16(3):171–175.

104. Coronado BE, Opal SM, Yoburn DC. Antibiotic-induced D-lactic acidosis. *Ann Intern Med.* 1995;122(11):839–842.

105. Goulet O, Ruemmele F. Causes and management of intestinal failure in children. *Gastroenterology.* 2006;130(2 suppl 1):S16–S28.

106. Kelly DA. Liver complications of pediatric parenteral nutrition—epidemiology. *Nutrition.* 1998;14(1):153–157.

107. Teitelbaum DH. Parenteral nutrition-associated cholestasis. *Curr Opin Pediatr.* 1997;9(3):270–275.

108. Kelly DA. Intestinal failure-associated liver disease: what do we know today? *Gastroenterology.* 2006;130(2 suppl 1):S70–S77.

109. Beale EF, Nelson RM, Bucciarelli RL, Donnelly WH, Eitzman DV. Intrahepatic cholestasis associated with parenteral nutrition in premature infants. *Pediatrics.* 1979;64(3):342–347.

110. Günsar C, Melek M, Karaca I, et al. The biochemical and histopathological effects of ursodeoxycholic acid and metronidazole on total parenteral nutrition-associated hepatic dysfunction: an experimental study. *Hepatogastroenterology.* 2002;49(44):497–500.

111. Colomb V, Fabeiro M, Dabbas M, Goulet O, Merckx J, Ricour C. Central venous catheter-related infections in children on long-term home parenteral nutrition: incidence and risk factors. *Clin Nutr.* 2000;19(5):355–359.

112. Burstyne M, Jensen GL. Abnormal liver functions as a result of total parenteral nutrition in a patient with short-bowel syndrome. *Nutrition.* 2000;16(11–12):1090–1092.

113. Cooke RJ, Whitington PF, Kelts D. Effect of taurine supplementation on hepatic function during short-term parenteral nutrition in the premature infant. *J Pediatr Gastroenterol Nutr.* 1984;3(2):234–238.

114. Bresson JL, Narcy P, Putet G, Ricour C, Sachs C, Rey J. Energy substrate utilization in infants receiving total parenteral nutrition with different glucose to fat ratios. *Pediatr Res.* 1989;25(6):645–648.

115. Advenier E, Landry C, Colomb V, et al. Aluminum contamination of parenteral nutrition and aluminum loading in children on long-term parenteral nutrition. *J Pediatr Gastroenterol Nutr.* 2003;36(4):448–453.

116. Kafritsa Y, Fell J, Long S, Bynevelt M, Taylor W, Milla P. Long-term outcome of brain manganese deposition in patients on home parenteral nutrition. *Arch Dis Child.* 1998;79(3):263–265.

117. Goulet O, de Potter S, Antébi H, et al. Long-term efficacy and safety of a new olive oil-based intravenous fat emulsion in pediatric patients: a double-blind randomized study. *Am J Clin Nutr.* 1999;70(3):338–345.

118. Cavicchi M, Crenn P, Beau P, Degott C, Boutron MC, Messing B. Severe liver complications associated with long-term parenteral nutrition are dependent on lipid parenteral input. *Transplant Proc.* 1998;30(6):2547.

119. Kohl M, Wedel T, Entenmann A, et al. Influence of different intravenous lipid emulsions on hepatobiliary dysfunction in a rabbit model. *J Pediatr Gastroenterol Nutr.* 2007;44(2):237–244.

120. Mutanen A, Lohi J, Heikkila P, Koivusalo AI, Rintala RJ, Pakarinen MP. Persistent abnormal liver fibrosis after weaning off parenteral nutrition in pediatric intestinal failure. *Hepatology.* 2013;58:729–738.

121. Wales PW, Allen N, Worthington P, George D, Compher C; the American Society for Parenteral and Enteral Nutrition; Teitelbaum D. A.S.P.E.N. Clinical guidelines: support of pediatric patients with intestinal failure at risk of parenteral nutrition-associated liver disease. *JPEN J Parenter Enteral Nutr.* 2014;38:538–557.

122. Rodrigues AF, Van Mourik IDM, Sharif K, et al. Management of end-stage central venous access in children referred for possible small bowel transplantation. *J Pediatr Gastroenterol Nutr.* 2006;42(4):427–433.

123. Lang EV, Reyes J, Faintuch S, Smith A, Abu-Elmagd K. Central venous recanalization in patients with short gut syndrome: restoration of candidacy for intestinal and multivisceral transplantation. *J Vasc Interv Radiol.* 2005;16(9):1203–1213.

124. Lichtman SN. Translocation of bacteria from gut lumen to mesenteric lymph nodes—and beyond? *J Pediatr Gastroenterol Nutr.* 1991;13(4):433–434.

125. Piedra PA, Dryja DM, LaScolea LJ Jr. Incidence of catheter-associated gram-negative bacteremia in children with short bowel syndrome. *J Clin Microbiol.* 1989;27(6):1317–1319.

126. Kurkchubasche AG, Smith SD, Rowe MI. Catheter sepsis in short-bowel syndrome. *Arch Surg.* 1992;127(1):21–24; discussion 24–25.

127. Weber TR. Enteral feeding increases sepsis in infants with short bowel syndrome. *J Pediatr Surg.* 1995;30(7):1086–1088; discussion 1088–1089.

128. Piper HG, Wales PW. Prevention of catheter-related blood stream infections in children with intestinal failure. *Curr Opin Gastroenterol.* 2013;29:1–6.

129. Oliveira C, Nasr A, Brindle M, Wales PW. Ethanol locks to prevent catheter-related blood stream infections in parenteral nutrition: a meta-analysis. *Pediatrics.* 2012:129:318–329.

130. Baskin KM, Hunnicutt C, Beck ME, Choen ED, Crowley JJ, Fitz CR. Long-term central venous access in pediatric patients at high risk: Conventional versus antibiotic-impregnated catheters. *J Vasc Interv Radiol.* 2014;25:411–418.

131. Moukarzel AA, Haddad I, Ament M, et al. 230 patient years of experience with home long-term parenteral nutrition in childhood: natural history and life of central venous catheters. *J Pediatr Surg.* 1994;29(10):1323–1327.

132. Carlsson E, Bosaeus I, Nordgren S. Quality of life and concerns in patients with short bowel syndrome. *Clin Nutr.* 2003;22(5):445–452.

133. Candusso M, Faraguna D, Sperli D, Dodaro N, et al. Outcome and quality of life in paediatric home parenteral nutrition. *Curr Opin Clin Nutr Metab Care.* 2002;5(3):309–314.

134. Heine RG, Bines, JE. New approaches to parenteral nutrition in infants and children. *J Paediatr Child Health.* 2002;38(5):433–437.

135. Grant D, Abu-Elmagd K, Mazariegos G, et al; Intestinal Transplant Association. Intestinal transplant registry report: global activity and trends. *Am J Transpl.* 2015;15(1):210–219.

136. Botha JF, Grant WJ, Torres C, et al. Isolated liver transplantation in infants with end-stage liver disease due to short bowel syndrome. *Liver Transpl.* 2006;12(7):1062–1066.

137. Diamond IR, Wales PW, Grant DR, Fecteau A. Isolated liver transplantation in pediatric short bowel syndrome: is there a role? *J Pediatr Surg.* 2006;41(5):955–959.

138. Horslen SP, Sudan DL, Iyer KR, et al. Isolated liver transplantation in infants with end-stage liver disease associated with short bowel syndrome. *Ann Surg.* 2002;235(3):435–439.

Test Your Knowledge Answers

1. The correct answer is **C**. The small intestine doubles in length during the last trimester. Therefore, the remaining length of small bowel has a greater inherent capacity to increase in length when the bowel resection occurred earlier in the third trimester.

2. The correct answer is **B**. Features associated with enteral autonomy include absence of cholestasis, an intact ileocecal valve, bowel in continuity, shorter duration of PN, residual intestinal length > 15 cm, and an intact colon. Stool number, by itself, is not a predictor.

3. The correct answer is **D**. The cause of PN–related liver disease is likely multifactorial and not related to just one issue.

4. The correct answer is **D**. Oral feedings not only enable the infant to maintain oral feeding skills and decrease the likelihood of developing oral aversion, but oral feedings will stimulate salivary secretion of hormones such as epidermal growth factor, which is important to the intestinal adaptive process.

28

Pulmonary Disorders

Laura Grande, MS, RD, CSP, LDN; **Allison Mallowe**, MA, RD, LDN; and **Maria Mascarenhas**, MBBS

 Podcast

Learning Objectives

1. Understand the role of nutrition in lung disease.
2. Discuss nutrition as related to complications of cystic fibrosis.
3. List components of nutrition assessment for persons with pulmonary disease.
4. Understand micronutrient abnormalities that can occur in cystic fibrosis.

Cystic Fibrosis

Pathophysiology

Cystic fibrosis (CF) is a autosomal recessive genetic disorder that is most frequently seen in people of northern European descent. In the United States, CF occurs in approximately 1 in 3500 live births and affects approximately 30,000 Americans. The CF gene was isolated in 1989,[1] and since then more than 1800 mutations have been identified. The gene, which is localized on the short arm of chromosome 7, is called the cystic fibrosis transmembrane regulator (*CFTR*) and controls the flow of sodium and chloride ions across the cell membrane. Mutations in the gene result in abnormal epithelial ion transport in multiple organs in the body. Clinical outcomes have been related to the type of mutation. With improved care and the advent of universal newborn screening programs in the United States, it was estimated in 2012 that the median predicted survival age is 41.1 years.[2]

Diagnosis during the neonatal period by newborn screening results in early nutrition intervention and improved nutrition status, which may lead to better quality of life and prolonged survival (see Table 28-1 for clinical features and diagnosis of CF). Historically an abnormal sweat

Table 28-1. Clinical Features and Diagnosis of Cystic Fibrosis

CLINICAL FEATURES MANIFESTED IN INFANTS	CLINICAL FEATURES MANIFESTED IN THE GENERAL CF POPULATION
Meconium ileus	Recurrent cough or wheeze
Meconium peritonitis	Clubbing of fingers and toes
Intestinal atresia	Hyperinflation of chest
Recurrent obstructive respiratory disease/infections	CF-related diabetes
	Chest wall deformities
Rectal prolapse	Nasal polyps
Failure to thrive	Cirrhosis and portal hypertension
Obstructive jaundice	Recurrent pancreatitis
Hyponatremic dehydration	Gallbladder disease
Malabsorption	Focal biliary cirrhosis
Salty taste in sweat	Zinc deficiency and EFAD dermatitis
Zinc deficiency	Fat-soluble vitamin deficiencies
Fat-soluble vitamin deficiency	Sodium depletion without renal disease
	Bronchiectasis
	Bacterial colonization
	DIOS
	Absence of vas deferens

CF, cystic fibrosis; DIOS, distal intestinal obstruction syndrome; EFAD: essential fatty acid deficiency.

Adapted from Gottschlich MM. Pulmonary disease. In: Gottschlich MM, ed. *The Science and Practice of Nutrition Support: A Case-Based Core Curriculum.* Dubuque, IA: Kendall/Hunt Publishing Co; 2001:501–516.

test (chloride values > 60 mEq/L) was considered diagnostic, but it is now recognized that this standard may not always be abnormal. Based on the severity of the mutation, the clinical picture is variable, and gene analysis, nasal potential differences, and sputum cultures, in addition to the clinical features, may be required for the diagnosis of CF.[3]

Because the expression of the *CFTR* gene is limited to epithelial cells, the primarily affected organs are mucus-producing organs such as lungs, gastrointestinal (GI) tract, liver, pancreas, genitourinary system, and sweat glands.[4] The transport of sodium and chloride across cell membranes is regulated by cyclic adenosine monophosphate and calcium, both of which are controlled by CFTR.[5] The respiratory epithelial cells are impermeable to chloride ions, which results in an increase in airway sodium absorption. The movement of sodium into the cells results in the movement of water into the cell, leading to dehydration of the airway mucus and decreased ciliary function. The impaired transport also leads to viscous secretions in the lung, liver, pancreas, and GI tract; duct obstruction in sweat glands; and elevated sweat chloride levels.

Pulmonary involvement is initially associated with infection with *Staphylococcus aureus* and later *Pseudomonas*

aeruginosa. Chronic pulmonary damage, bronchiectasis, fibrosis, and decreasing lung function occur over time. Impaired gas exchange occurs secondary to airflow resistance, hyperinflation, and uneven distribution of ventilation. Both bacterial adherence and colonization result in a sustained host inflammatory response. Stimulated neutrophils release large amounts of oxidants and proteases including elastase, which leads to increased mucus production, bacterial trapping, and further lung damage.[6] Clinical symptoms include cough, production of mucus, air trapping, and ultimately end-stage lung disease requiring lung transplantation.

In the pancreas, thick mucus accumulates in the acinar glands, leading to an obstruction of the ducts. Damage occurs in the glands due to the release of lytic enzymes and subsequent chronic inflammation, fibrosis, fatty infiltration of the pancreas, and pancreatic insufficiency (PI). These changes can occur in utero in patients with severe mutations. PI is seen in about 87% of patients at diagnosis.[2] Patients who have pancreatic sufficiency (PS) may develop PI over time and need to be monitored carefully. Clinical symptoms of PI include steatorrhea, malabsorption, diarrhea, weight loss, poor growth, vitamin deficiencies, increased gas, and abdominal pain. Some patients, including infants, may have a voracious appetite in an effort to ingest sufficient calories to compensate for energy loss in their bowel movements due to maldigestion and malabsorption. Increasing numbers of persons with CF will develop cystic fibrosis–related diabetes (CFRD), and it is expected that this number will increase as life expectancy increases.[7]

Similar to what happens in the lungs, fluid and electrolyte disturbances occur in the GI tract and cause sticky mucus and stool accumulation, which can result in meconium ileus in the newborn and distal intestinal obstruction syndrome (DIOS) in older children and adults. Meconium ileus, or the build-up of meconium in utero, is the earliest manifestation of CF. Infants can be born with meconium plugs, intestinal obstruction, atresias, volvulus, perforations, and meconium pseudocyst. DIOS is the accumulation of sticky stool in the GI tract, primarily in the terminal ileum and cecal area. It may occur in all persons who have CF (PI and less commonly PS). Predisposing factors are decreased fluid and salt intake, fat malabsorption, mucosal inflammation, and dysmotility.[8]

In the liver, CFTR is expressed in the biliary epithelium, and abnormalities of ion transport occur. This results in the decreased flow of bile, with secondary hepatocyte damage, inflammation, fibrosis, and cirrhosis.[9] In males, obstruction of the vas deferens results in infertility, and in patients with mild mutations, infertility may be the presenting feature that leads to the diagnosis of CF later in life.

Nutrition Assessment

A strong correlation exists between pulmonary function and nutrition status. In children, a body mass index (BMI) at or above the 50th percentile has been associated with improved survival and optimal lung function. Associations between deteriorating lung function and worsening nutrition status have been noted.[4,10] Malnutrition results from increased needs (increased metabolic rate,[11] infections, work of breathing, cough); increased losses (malabsorption due to pancreatic, liver, and intestinal disease; intestinal resection; vomiting; and CFRD); and decreased nutrient intake (anorexia, gastroesophageal reflux disease, eating disorders, abdominal pain, constipation, malaise, and medications). Aggressive nutrition intervention is often required to improve nutrition status.

Nutrition assessment is an important component in the care of persons with CF. Factors that affect nutrition status include maldigestion and malabsorption of fat, protein, carbohydrates, and fat-soluble vitamins; decreasing pulmonary function; chronic pulmonary infections and increased oxidative stress; decreased energy intake; increased energy requirements; and CFRD. A comprehensive nutrition assessment must be performed at diagnosis and yearly. This consists of an assessment of (1) growth, including pattern of weight and height based on the growth curve, head circumference (as appropriate), and BMI percentile; (2) biochemical indicators such as vitamin and mineral levels; (3) nutrient intake; (4) eating behavior and family eating patterns; (5) pancreatic enzyme replacement therapy (PERT) management; (6) physical activity; (7) severity of lung disease; (8) presence of any comorbidity such as CFRD, chronic infections, cirrhosis, or bacterial overgrowth; and (9) factors that may impact the patient's ability to meet nutrition goals. Assessment of bone health should be performed yearly, and growth parameters (height, weight, head circumference, weight for length, or BMI percentile) should be assessed and monitored at every visit as indicated. Arm anthropometrics can be measured as well. Based on the above information, caloric requirements are calculated, vitamin and mineral prescriptions adjusted, and anthropometric goals calculated.

A nutrition screen must be performed at every visit to identify inadequate weight gain, weight loss, and faltering of linear growth. When these occur, a nutrition assessment must be performed, causes identified, and appropriate interventions implemented (Table 28-2).

Table 28-2. Nutrition Assessment Parameters for Cystic Fibrosis

PARAMETER	FREQUENCY OF ASSESSMENT AND REASSESSMENT
Anthropometrics	Measured only up to age 2 y
Head circumference	Every 3 mo
Body weight, height, length	
MAMC, TSF	Annually
Nutrition Intake	
24-h recall	Routine care and diagnosis
3-d dietary fat intake and coefficient of fat (<93% or 85% in infants)	Evaluate weight loss, growth, diagnosis
Fecal elastase	
Biochemical	
CBC with differential	Routine care and diagnosis
Iron studies	Diagnose iron-deficiency anemia
Fat-soluble vitamins	Routine care and diagnosis
α-Tocopherol	
Serum plasma retinol	
25-OH vitamin D	
PIVKA II	
Essential fatty acid deficiency	
Ratio of triene to tetraene	Diagnostic
25-OH vitamin D	Yearly

CBC: complete blood count; MAMC, mid-arm muscle circumference; PIVKA II, Proteins Induced by Vitamin K Absence; TSF: triceps skinfold.
Adapted from Gottschlich MM. Pulmonary disease. In: Gottschlich MM, ed. *The Science and Practice of Nutrition Support: A Core-Based Curriculum.* Dubuque, IA: Kendall/Hunt Publishing Co; 2001:501–516.

Nutrition Recommendations

Historically, CF patients and their families have been advised that a high energy intake can be achieved by consuming preferred foods, without consideration of their micronutrients or fiber content. When choosing energy-rich foods, foods that are also nutrient-rich should be encouraged.

Macronutrients

Energy

As previously described, individuals who have CF have increased energy needs. Exact caloric prescriptions and formulas to calculate caloric need are difficult to provide due to individual patient variation[10] but improved weight status has been found at intakes ranging from 110% to 200% of energy needs for the healthy population.[12] Energy needs of each patient should be assessed on an individual basis and reflect the pattern of weight gain and fat stores.[13] An estimation of individual caloric need is based upon nutrition status, growth pattern, fat stores, current dietary intake, degree of fat malabsorption, clinical status (including pulmonary function), level of activity, and incorporation of additional requirements for nutrition repletion, weight gain, and/or catch-up growth.[14]

Fat

The energy goal can be best achieved by consuming a diet that contains 35%–40% of calories as fat.[13] Ongoing research suggests that a diet containing sources of linoleic acid, such as safflower, corn, and soybeans oils, sunflower seeds, and walnuts, may be beneficial for persons who have CF.[15] Historically the amount but not type of fat has been emphasized. Clinicians are encouraged to be aware of the symptoms of essential fatty acid deficiency. Most common symptoms of linoleic acid deficiency are poor growth and scaly skin lesions, confirmed by an increase in triene-tetraene ratio of plasma lipids.[7] Essential fatty acid deficiency can occur not only in patients with severe lung disease, significant malabsorption, and/or cirrhosis but also in patients with normal nutrition status. It is not known whether the deficiency is due to a primary metabolic disorder or due to malabsorption and increased oxidative stress.[15]

Protein

Specific recommendations for protein intake in CF are not available, although some evidence shows that protein needs are met if a higher calorie diet is consumed[13] and 15%–20% of total calories are from protein.[16] In general, patients with CF are thought to consume adequate amounts of protein with their overall high calorie intake.[17] If low protein intake is suspected, oral or enteral supplements can be used to supplement the diet.

Carbohydrate

The diet should contain sufficient carbohydrate to meet energy needs. As with persons who do not have CF, it is best if the source is from foods that contribute to the overall nutrient intake, including fiber.

Infants

Infants require a diet that will promote optimal weight gain and, when indicated, "catch-up" growth. Human milk or standard infant formula is recommended. When necessary, fortified human milk or calorically dense formula may be used to promote and/or maintain weight gain.[18] Infants with CF have specific sodium requirements. To achieve catch-up growth, infants may require 120–150 kcal/kg/d.[13] Hydrolyzed protein formulas containing medium-chain triglycerides are not indicated in the absence of a medical reason, such as bowel surgery with significant bowel resection due to meconium ileus or liver abnormalities. Solids are added to the diet of infants who have CF on the same schedule used for nonaffected infants.[18] Care must be taken when adding solids to avoid replacing nutrient-rich and energy-rich infant milks with low-calorie, low-nutrient foods. Adding oil to commercial jarred infant foods will increase calories; up to 1 teaspoon of oil to every 4 oz of baby food is suggested. Revised guidelines for infant feeding emphasize the safety and benefits of earlier introduction of meat for the energy, protein, zinc, and iron content for all infants.[7] Parents who wish to prepare homemade solids may require instruction. Positive feeding behaviors should be encouraged throughout the feeding experience.[18]

Micronutrients

All persons with CF, both with PI using PERT and with PS, require supplementation with micronutrients.[19] Deficiencies of fat-soluble vitamins[20] and zinc[21] have been demonstrated in infants diagnosed through newborn screening and do not correct without appropriate supplementation and, if indicated, PERT. Children and adolescents are at risk for micronutrient deficiencies due to[14]

- Inadequate intake
- Malabsorption possibly due to suboptimal PERT
- Malabsorption due to incomplete bile salt absorption
- Poor clinical status and poor lung function
- Increased utilization and reduced bioavailability
- Liver disease
- Bowel resection
- Late diagnosis of CF
- Poor adherence to or inappropriate supplementation

Fat-Soluble Vitamins

Multivitamins designed to meet the fat-soluble vitamin needs of persons who have CF (CF–specific multivitamins) are available in North America (Tables 28-3 and 28-4). These vitamins contain fat-soluble and water-soluble vitamins and zinc. The content reflects the recommendations provided in the U.S. Pediatric Nutrition Consensus Report,[13] the European Nutrition Consensus Report,[22] the U.S. Bone Consensus Report,[23] and/or current research. Dosage and form of the CF–specific multivitamin supplementation depends on results of laboratory evaluation of vitamin levels and the patient's age. Patients may require additional single-nutrient supplements (ie, vitamins A, E, D, K) if blood levels cannot be maintained on the CF–specific multivitamins. If the CF–specific multivitamin is unavailable, single-vitamin supplements are necessary to make up the difference in content of traditional multivitamins compared to recommendations. For additional information on the content of CF–specific multivitamins refer to Table 28-3 and 28-4.

VITAMIN A

Vitamin A plays an important role in vision, immunity, lung health, and overall health, yet excessive intake of retinol can cause liver and/or bone complications. Retinol is an acute phase reactant and best measured when the patient is not ill. Liver disease or zinc deficiency can cause low serum retinol levels. A low retinol-binding protein should be corrected before increasing the Vitamin A dose. The total vitamin A content of CF–specific multivitamins is based on both retinol and β-carotene. The risk of toxicity is avoided with a higher concentration of β-carotene.

VITAMIN E

Optimizing serum vitamin E will prevent the neurological complications once seen in people who have CF. More recently the role of vitamin E as an antioxidant in preserving overall health in CF has been investigated.[24] Vitamin E is transported in the body with lipids, including cholesterol. People who have CF often have low cholesterol levels, therefore serum levels should be assessed as a ratio of vitamin E[25] to total lipid[25] or to total cholesterol.[26] The equation used to assess vitamin E status is the ratio of α-tocopherol to total lipids (cholesterol, triacylglycerol, and phospholipid). A ratio of α-tocopherol to total lipids < 0.8 mg/dL or a ratio of α-tocopherol to cholesterol < 2.47 mg/g indicates vitamin E deficiency.[26] Liver disease can cause low vitamin E levels.

VITAMIN D

Persons who have CF are at risk for low serum vitamin D. Serum 25-hydroxyvitamin D [25(OH)D] should be assessed annually, preferably in the late fall and, if necessary, treated daily with vitamin D3-cholecalciferol. Consensus recommendations state that the goal serum level for patients with CF is a minimum of 30 ng/mL. All current CF vitamin brands contain sufficient vitamin D for maintenance therapy for various age groups. If serum vitamin D levels remain low after confirming adherence to regular CF multivitamin therapy, a stepwise approach is recommended to replete low levels.[27] Vitamin D doses should be increased using a vitamin D–only formulation rather than doubling the CF–specific multivitamin and risking excess amounts of other vitamins and minerals. Increases in vitamin D doses are age dependent, and the initial recommendation is to double the total vitamin D dose. If vitamin D levels cannot be corrected to normal after following the step-wise increases, patients should be referred to an endocrinologist for further management of vitamin D deficiency.

VITAMIN K

Vitamin K is essential for normal blood clotting and bone health. Persons who have CF are at risk for vitamin K deficiency due to fat malabsorption and routine use of antibiotics. Additionally, any patient who has CF and liver disease is at greater risk for vitamin K deficiency. Clotting time, or prothrombin time, has been the standard test for assessing overall vitamin K nutrition, but several studies using PIVKA II (Proteins Induced by Vitamin K Absence) provided evidence that in CF, vitamin K deficiency exists in patients with normal prothrombin time.[28-30] Over-the-counter multivitamins contain insufficient vitamin K to meet the needs of persons who have CF. The vitamin K content of CF-specific multivitamins is sufficient for the majority of patients, although some people may require additional supplementation based on laboratory results.

Water-Soluble Vitamins

Deficiency of water-soluble vitamins in CF is rare (riboflavin, vitamin C), but have been reported in patients not receiving multivitamins and/or receiving medications interfering with B vitamins.[31] Patients who have had a resection of the terminal ileum may develop vitamin B12 deficiency requiring supplementation and should be monitored.[14]

Minerals

Sodium Chloride

Persons who have CF lose excessive sodium in their sweat and require supplementation throughout the year, especially in the summer months. Inadequate salt intake can be life threatening and/or result in poor appetite with subsequent poor growth. All infants who have CF and an elevated sweat test are to be supplemented with 12.6 mEq (1/8 teaspoon) of salt daily from birth to 6 months of age, at which time the dose is increased to 25.2 mEq (1/4 teaspoon) daily.[18] The

Table 28-3. Fat-Soluble Vitamin Content of Multivitamins[1,2]

MVW COMPLETE FORMULATION® DROPS CHEWABLES SOFTGELS D3000 SOFTGELS[4]	AQUADEKS® DROPS, CHEWABLES, SOFTGELS	VITAMAX® DROPS, CHEWABLES	CHOICEFUL CHEWABLES, SOFTGELS LABEL DATA	LIBERTAS ABDEK DROPS CHEWABLES, SOFTGELS	POLY-VI-SOL® DROPS CENTRUM® CHEWABLE, TABLET
Total Vitamin A (IU) (Retinol and Beta Carotene)					
4627 / 0.5 ml 75% as beta-carotene	5,751 / 1 ml 87% as beta-carotene	3170 / 1 ml as 100% retinol palmitate	NP	4627 / 1 ml 100% retinol palmitate	1,500 / 1 ml
9254 / 1 ml 75% as beta-carotene	11,502 / 2 ml 87% as beta-carotene	6,340 / 2 ml as 100% retinol palmitate	NP	9254 / 2 ml 100% retinol palmitate	3,000 / 2 ml
16,000 / 1 chewable 88% as beta-carotene	18,167 / 2 chewables 92% as beta-carotene	5,000 / 1 chewable 50% as beta-carotene	13,000 / 1 chewable 88% as beta-carotene	16,000 / 1 chewable 100% as beta-carotene	3,500 / 1 chewable 29% as beta-carotene
32,000 / 2 softgels 88% as beta-carotene	36,334 / 2 softgels 92% as beta-carotene	NP	28,000 / 2 softgels 88% as beta-carotene	32,000 / 2 softgels 88% as beta-carotene	7,000 / 2 tablets 29% as beta-carotene
32,000 / 2 softgels (D3000) 88% as beta-carotene	NP	NP	NP	NP	NP
VITAMIN E (IU)					
50 / 0.5 ml	50 / 1 ml [3]	50 / 1 ml	NP	50 / 1 ml	5 / 1 ml
100 / 1 ml	100 / 2 ml [3]	100 / 2 ml	NP	100 / 2 ml	10 / 2 ml
200 / 1 chewable	100 / 2 chewables[3]	200 / 1 chewable	180 / 1 chewable	200 / 1 chewable	30 / 1 chewable
400 / 2 softgels	300 / 2 softgels[3]	NP	340 / 2 softgels	400 / 2 softgels	60 / 2 tablets
400 / 2 softgels (D3000)	NP	NP	NP	NP	NP
VITAMIN D (IU)					
750 / 0.5 ml	600 / 1 ml	400 / 1 ml	NP	500 / 1 ml	400 / 1 ml
1500 / 1 ml	1200 / 2 ml	800 / 2 ml	NP	1000 / 2 ml	800 / 2 ml
1500/ 1 chewable	1200 / 2 chewables	400 / 1 chewable	800 / 1 chewable	1000 / 1 chewable	400 / 1 chewable
3000 / 2 softgels	2400 / 2 softgels	NP	2000 / 2 softgels	2000 / 2 softgels	800 / 2 tablets
6000 / 2 softgels (D3000)	NP	NP	NP	NP	NP
VITAMIN K (MCG)					
500 / 0.5 ml	400 / 1 ml	300 / 1 ml	NP	400 / 1 ml	0
1000 / 1 ml	800 / 2 ml	600 / 2 ml	NP	800 / 2 ml	0
1000 / 1 chewable	700 / 2 chewables	200 / 1 chewable	600 / 1 chewable	800 / 1 chewable	10 / 1 chewable
1600 / 2 softgels	1400 / 2 softgels	NP	1400 / 2 softgels	1600 / 2 softgels	50 / 2 tablets
1600 / 2 softgels (D3000)	NP	NP	NP	NP	NP

1. The content of this table was confirmed as of May 2014
2. Created by Suzanne H. Michel, MPH, RD, LDN. Please be aware that companies have copied the look and format of this table. Unless the table has Ms. Michel's name on it, she cannot attest to its accuracy.
3. Also contains mixed tocopherols
4. Tangpricha V, Kelly A, Stephenson A, Maguiness K, Enders J, Robinson KA, Marshall BC, Borowitz D, for the Cystic Fibrosis Foundation Vitamin D Evidence-Based Review Committee. An update on the screening, diagnosis, management, and treatment of vitamin D deficiency in individuals with cystic fibrosis: Evidence-based recommendations from the Cystic Fibrosis Foundation. J Clin Endocrinol Metab. 2012;97(4):1082-93.
5. NP = No Equivalent Product
6. AquADEKs® is a registered trademark of Yasoo Health Inc., Vitamax® is a registered trademark of Shear/Kershman Labs. Inc., Poly-Vi-Sol® is a registered trademark of Mead Johnson and Company, Centrum® is a registered trademark of Wyeth Consumer Care, MVW Complete Formulation is a registered trademark of MVW Nutritionals, Inc.

Table 28-4. Water-Soluble Vitamin and Zinc Content of Multivitamins

MVW COMPLETE FORMULATION® DROPS, CHEWABLES, SOFTGELS, D3000 SOFTGELS	AQUADEKS® DROPS, SOFTGELS	VITAMAX® DROPS, CHEWABLES	CHOICEFUL CHEWABLES, SOFTGELS LABEL DATA	LIBERTAS ABDEK DROPS, CHEWABLES, SOFTGELS	POLY-VI-SOL® DROPS CENTRUM® CHEWABLE, TABLET
THIAMIN B1 (MG)					
0.5 / 0.5 ml	0.6 / 1 ml	0.5 / 1 ml	NP	0.5 / 1 ml	0.5 / 1 ml
1 / 1 ml	1.2 / 2 ml	1 / 2 ml	NP	1 / 2 ml	1 / 2 ml
1.5 / 1 chewable	1.5 / 2 chewables	1.5 / 1 chewable	1.2 / 1 chewable	1.5 / 1 chewable	1.5 / 1 chewable
3 / 2 softgels or 2 softgels with D3000	3 / 2 softgels	NP	2 / 2 softgels	3 / 2 softgels	3 / 2 tablets
RIBOFLAVIN B2 (MG)					
0.6 / 0.5 ml	0.6 / 1 ml	0.6 / 1 ml	NP	0.6 / 1 ml	0.6 / 1 ml
1.2 / 1 ml	1.2 / 2 ml	1.2 / 2 ml	NP	1.2 / 2 ml	1.2 / 2 ml
1.7 / 1 chewable	1.7 / 2 chewables	1.7 / 1 chewable	1.4 / 1 chewable	1.7 / 1 chewable	1.7 / 1 chewable
3.4 / 2 softgels or 2 softgels with D3000	3.4 / 2 softgels	NP	3 / 2 softgels	3.4 / 2 softgels	3.4 / 2 tablets
NIACIN (MG)					
6 / 0.5 ml	6 / 1 ml	6 / 1 ml	NP	6 / 1 ml	8 / 1 ml
12 / 1 ml	12 / 2 ml	12 / 2 ml	NP	12 / 2 ml	16 / 2 ml
10 / 1 chewable	10 / 2 chewables	20 / 1 chewable	8 / 1 chewable	10 / 1 chewable	20 / 1 chewable
40 / 2 softgels or 2 softgels with D3000	20 / 2 softgels	NP	36 / 2 softgels	40 / 2 softgels	40 / 2 tablets
PYRIDOXINE B6 (MG)					
0.6 / 0.5 ml	0.6 / 1 ml	0.6 / 1 ml	NP	0.6 / 1 ml	0.4 / 1 ml
1.2 / 1 ml	1.2 / 2 ml	1.2 / 2 ml	NP	1.2 / 2 ml	0.8 / 2 ml
1.9 / 1 chewable	1.9 / 2 chewables	2 / 1 chewable	1.5 / 1 chewable	1.9 / 1 chewable	2 / 1 chewable
3.8 / 2 softgels or 2 softgels with D3000	3.8 / 2 softgels	NP	3.8 / 2 softgels	3.8 / 2 softgels	4 / 2 tablets
B12 (MCG)					
4 / 0.5 ml	0	4 / 1 ml	NP	4 / 1 ml	2 / 1 ml
8 / 1 ml	0	8 / 2 ml	NP	8 / 2 ml	4 / 2 ml
6 / 1 chewable	12 / 2 chewables	6 / 1 chewable	6 / 1 chewable	6 / 1 chewable	6 / 1 chewable
12 / 2 softgels or 2 softgels with D3000	24 / 2 softgels	NP	10 / 2 softgels	12 / 2 softgels	12 / 2 tablets
BIOTIN (MCG)					
15 / 0.5 ml	15 / 1 ml	15 / 1 ml	NP	15 / 1 ml	0
30 / 1 ml	30 / 2 ml	30 / 2 ml	NP	30 / 2 ml	0
100 / 1 chewable	100 / 2 chewables	300 / 1 chewable	80 / 1 chewable	100 / 1 chewable	45 / 1 chewable
200 / 2 softgels or 2 softgels with D3000	200 / 2 softgels	NP	160 / 2 softgels	200 / 2 softgels	60 / 2 tablets
FOLIC ACID (MCG)					
0	0	0	NP	0	0
0	0	0	NP	0	0

Table 28-4. (continued) Water-Soluble Vitamin and Zinc Content of Multivitamins

MVW COMPLETE FORMULATION DROPS, CHEWABLES, SOFTGELS, D3000 SOFTGELS	AQUADEKS DROPS, SOFTGELS	VITAMAX DROPS, CHEWABLES	CHOICEFUL CHEWABLES, SOFTGELS LABEL DATA	LIBERTAS ABDEK DROPS, CHEWABLES, SOFTGELS	POLY-VI-SOL DROPS / CENTRUM CHEWABLE, TABLET
200 / 1 chewable	200 / 2 chewables	200 / 1 chewable	180 / 1 chewable	200 / 1 chewable	400 / 1 chewable
400 / softgels or 2 softgels with D3000	200/2 softgels	NP	360 / 2 softgels	400 / 2 softgels	800 / 2 tablets
ASCORBIC ACID C (MG)					
45 / 0.5 ml	45 / 1 ml	45 / 1 ml	NP	45 / 1 ml	35 / 1 ml
90 / 1 ml	90 / 2 ml	90 / 2 ml	NP	90 / 2 ml	70 / 2 ml
100 / 1 chewable	70 / 2 chewables	60 / 1 chewable	60 / 1 chewable	100 / 1 chewable	60 / 1 chewable
200 / 2 softgels or 2 softgels with D3000	150 / 2 softgels	NP	60 / 2 softgels	200 / 2 softgels	120 / 2 tablets
PANTOTHENIC ACID (MG)					
3 / 0.5 ml	3 / 1 ml	3 / 1 ml	NP	3 / 1 ml	0
6 / 1 ml	6 / 2 ml	6 / 2 ml	NP	6 / 2 ml	0
12 / 1 chewable	12 / 2 chewables	10 / 1 chewable	10 / 1 chewable	12 / 1 chewable	10 / 1 chewable
24 / 2 softgels or 2 softgels with D3000	24 / 2 softgels	NP	16 / 2 softgels	24 / 2 softgels	20 / 2 tablets
ZINC (MG)					
5 / 0.5 ml	5 / 1 ml	7.5 / 1 ml	NP	5 / 1 ml	0
10 / 1 ml	10 / 2 ml	15 / 2 ml	NP	10 / 2 ml	0
15 / 1 chewable	10 / 2 chewables	7.5 / 1 chewable	15 / chewable	15 / 1 chewable	15 / 1 chewable
20 / 2 softgels or 2 softgels with D3000	20 / 2 softgels	NP	30 / 2 softgels	30 / 2 softgels	22 / 2 tablets

salt is added in small, frequent amounts to baby formula or applesauce used to dose PERT until the daily dose is met. Salt supplementation is continued until the child is eating a diet rich in salt and added salt. Children and adolescents are to be counseled to consume salt over and above their usual intake when participating in physical activity. It may be necessary to add salt to sports drinks to meet sodium chloride needs (1/8 teaspoon to 12 oz).[32]

Zinc

Pancreatic insufficient infants, prior to treatment with PERT, lose excessive zinc in their stool. Acrodermatitis enteropathica–like rash, which resembles a severe rash in the diaper area and the perioral area, is a clinical symptom of zinc deficiency and is treated with PERT and zinc supplementation. More subtle symptoms of zinc deficiency that can be seen at any age include lack of appetite, dysgeusia, poor growth, and compromised immunity. Laboratory studies to determine zinc status are generally uninformative.

When zinc deficiency is suspected the usual supplemental dose is 1 mg elemental zinc per kilogram daily for 6 months in addition to that contained in the patient's daily multivitamin. Over-the-counter infant vitamin drops do not contain zinc. Over-the-counter children's chewable vitamins and adult formulations contain zinc as do all of the CF–specific multivitamins. When choosing a zinc preparation, it is important to note which zinc salt is in the chosen product so that the correct dose can be determined. For example, zinc sulfate is 23% elemental zinc but zinc gluconate is only 14% elemental zinc.

Iron

Iron status in the general population is affected by a number of factors, including dietary intake, blood loss, and medications. For persons with CF, all of these factors plus malabsorption, hemoptysis, short bowel syndrome, bacterial overgrowth, liver and renal diseases, and chronic inflammation contribute to altered iron status. Patients can have iron-deficiency anemia, anemia of chronic disease, or a combination of both. Prior to prescribing iron supplementation the form of anemia must be defined.[33] Assessing iron status in CF is complicated by chronic inflammation. Serum ferritin, an acute-phase reactant, may be falsely elevated in CF, thus masking iron-deficiency anemia. Measurement of soluble transferrin receptor levels may be helpful in diagnosis.

Calcium

It is important to optimize the calcium intake of persons who have CF. In lieu of specific calcium recommendations for person who have CF, the registered dietitian should refer to those in the Adequate Intake (AI) for infants <1 year of age and the RDA for patients >1 year of age.[34] The Cystic Fibrosis Foundation Bone Consensus Report may be referred to for more detail regarding bone health and CF.[23]

Magnesium

Patients receiving aminoglycosides may require supplemental magnesium. Blood levels should be monitored.[35]

Fluoride

CF–specific vitamins do not contain fluoride; therefore, the patient's primary care physician may need to prescribe a supplement if local water is not fluoridated.

Assessment

Blood levels of fat-soluble vitamins should be measured at diagnosis for patients diagnosed >1 year of age and annually thereafter.[13] For newly diagnosed infants, it is recommended that levels of vitamins E, A, and D be assessed 1–3 months after starting supplementation and annually thereafter.[18] Prothrombin time is insensitive to vitamin K deficiency in CF.[28] PIVKA II provides a better indicator of vitamin K nutrition and should be measured, if available. Serum electrolytes and complete blood count is measured at 2–3 months of age and annually or as indicated.[18] For children and adolescents, assessment of fat-soluble vitamins, including PIVKA II and complete blood count with differential, is done at diagnosis and annually, unless otherwise indicated. Laboratory studies for individual micronutrients may be necessary when modifying the treatment care plan, such as starting tube feeding.

Pancreatic Enzymes

Persons with PI require PERT. Pancreatic damage and destruction occurs in utero or after birth, resulting in the absence of bicarbonate-rich and enzyme-containing pancre-

atic juice in the duodenum to help digest food. PERT has played a pivotal role in improving the care and outcome of persons with CF.[36] A variety of enzymes are available, with subtle differences among brands and forms. As of this writing, the approved enteric coated products in the United States are Creon by AbbVie, Zenpep by Actavis Pharma, Pertyze by Digestive Care, Pancreaze by Janssen Pharmaceuticals, and Ultresa by Actavis Pharma. The reader is referred to the manufacturers' websites for details regarding enzyme content. A nonenteric coated form of enzyme, such as Viokace by Forest Laboratories, Inc, is subject to destruction by the acidic gastric environment. The enteric coated products consist of microspheres and microtablets. The enteric coating is designed to protect the enzyme from the acidic gastric milieu as well as allowing activation of the enzyme to occur in the alkaline pH of the duodenum, past the acidic gastric contents. If the pancreas is unable to deliver bicarbonate pancreatic juice to the duodenum, gastric acid from the stomach is not neutralized resulting in an acidic duodenal pH. Acidity in the GI tract may prevent or retard dissolution of enteric-coated pancreatic enzymes.[37] If activation does not take place in the small intestine, absorption of macronutrients and micronutrients cannot occur. Additional medications that reduce or block gastric acid production and raise the duodenal pH may be needed to enhance PERT effectiveness. Even so, all nutrients may not be fully absorbed. If fat malabsorption persists, consider lack of bile acids, liver disease, small bowel bacterial overgrowth, and other GI etiologies. Consultation with a pediatric gastroenterologist may be needed.

The PERT products contain lipase, protease, and amylase for digestion of fat, protein, and carbohydrates, respectively. Enzyme activity or potency is based on the amount of lipase per capsule or gel cap. For example, for Creon 6 the 6 refers to 6000 lipase units per capsule. Creon 6 also contains 30,000 amylase units and 19,000 protease units. Refer to the manufacturers' websites for each brand of enzyme and more detail on enzyme contents. PERT starting dose for infants of 2000–4000 units of lipase per 120 mL of formula or breast milk is recommended.[38] Though dosing is best calculated using units of lipase per gram of fat ingested, it is perhaps more practical to use a dosing schedule with weight-adjusted guidelines.[38] For children <4 years of age the recommendation is to begin at 1000 lipase units per kilogram per meal and over 4 years of age 500 lipase units per kilogram per meal. Dosing for snacks is routinely half of the usual meal dose. The recommendations are not to exceed a lipase dose of 2500 units of lipase per kilogram body weight per meal or 10,000 lipase units per kilogram per day and are based on a usual intake of 3 meals plus 2 snacks per day.[38] Enzymes can also be dosed based on grams of fat using the guidelines of 500–4000 units lipase per gram of fat.[38]

Persons with CF should be viewed individually in regard to dosing and response to PERT. Careful monitoring of growth, stool pattern, and specific GI symptoms is necessary to determine the adequacy of therapy. For infants and children unable to swallow enzyme capsules, the enzyme beads are removed from the capsules and mixed with a small amount (1/8 to 1/2 teaspoon for infants, more for children) of applesauce and given at the time of each feeding.[38] To avoid breakdown of the enteric coating, beads should not be added to liquids or acidic foods. PERT is given at the beginning of the feeding or meal. If the meal lasts more than 30 minutes, then it is recommended that the dose be split and given at the beginning and halfway through the meal. For infants, to avoid mucosal erosion, the mouth should be checked for beads following each feeding. The infant's perianal area may require protection against enzyme excreted in the stool. Patients or their caregivers can be instructed to apply a thick layer of barrier cream to protect the skin around the anus.

Persons with CF who receive nasogastric tube, a gastrostomy tube (G tube), or jejunostomy tube feedings need PERT supplementation. The amount and type of enzyme given depends on the type of formula and the ability of the patient to take enzymes orally. In general, a meal dose of PERT is given orally before and after night tube feeds when using an intact formula.[38] Some patients may benefit from an additional dose midway during the feedings at night. This approach is generally not practical and should be done only when other measures such as changing to a lower long-chain of fat formula have not been effective. During the day, PERT is best given before each bolus, and this dose is dependent on the amount and type of fat in the bolus. Currently no enzymes are on the market that are approved for administering via G tube. No evidence-based guidelines are available to guide PERT administration in situations when a patient is unable to swallow by mouth or is intubated and critically ill. The following options have been used. Many CF centers crush Viokace tablets and add the powder directly to the formula approximately 20 minutes prior to tube feed administration.[37] This method allows the nutrients in the formula to be predigested prior to reaching the patient. Another option uses enzyme microspheres mixed in nectar, or thick fruit juice, and administered via a syringe into a 10 French or larger G tube via syringe prior to feedings.[39] Enzyme beads can also be dissolved in a bicarbonate solution and the enzyme/bicarbonate mixture can be administered directly into the feeding tube prior to administering formula, or the mixture can be put directly into the formula. A concern exists about excessive bicarbonate administration resulting in alkalosis. Alternatively, enzyme beads can also be manually crushed into powder and added directly to the formula for predigestion of nutrients.[40] However, the manufacturers do not recommend crushing the beads because crushing the enteric coating would expose the mucosal surfaces of the mouth and esophagus to active enzyme and may cause irritation if taken by mouth. This method is also not recommended by most CF centers. Breaking the enteric coating exposes the enzymes to the acidic environment of the stomach, thus rendering the enzymes inactive. Yet, when beads are crushed and added to tube feed formula, these concerns are negated because digestion of the formula occurs in the container. The discretion of the provider should be used to determine which of these methods is best for the patient and clinical response monitored. With any of the above approaches, the amount of fat in the enteral feeding should be calculated and the appropriate enzyme dose determined. Feeding intolerance and obstruction of feeding tubes have been noted with the above practices.[41]

Eating Behaviors and CF

The importance of nutrition in CF is recognized by the CF care team and by parents of children who have CF. Pressure surrounding the importance of nutrition includes improving and maintaining weight and adherence to PERT and supplemental vitamins and/or minerals. As a result, mealtimes can become challenging. Parents of children with CF commonly report mealtime behavior problems including poor appetite, avoidance of eating by talking, and spitting out food.[42] A negative correlation between the children's caloric intake and the number of problematic mealtime behaviors has been identified.[43]

Young children appear to be particularly at risk for behavioral difficulties at mealtime if their parents feel unusually concerned about their children's health and caloric/food intake.[43] For parents of infants with CF, the transition from formula to solids may present a challenge, and parents may need guidance surrounding positive eating behaviors and high-calorie solids. The toddler stage is typically characterized by changing food interests and neophobia (fear of new foods), which for children with CF may complicate the selection of high-fat foods and food additives.[42] Parents may benefit from guidance to prevent and/or manage food refusal behaviors. Anticipatory guidance might include education centered on avoidance of parental behaviors that may inadvertently reinforce noneating behaviors and advice directed toward reinforcement of desired behaviors through praise and limit setting.[43] As children become adolescents, a struggle for control and independence may ensue. In this period, the challenge may be providing education and direction so that the child/adolescent makes appropriate choices that improve or maintain optimal nutrition status. Birch and Fischer[44] have stated that the foundation for teen and adult eating styles is laid in childhood as the parent and child work through issues of control regarding feeding and eating. CF care teams typically include a social worker and psychologist. These individuals can be very helpful in guiding families to understand feeding difficulties and to help their children.

Nutrition Support

A positive correlation exists between pulmonary function and weight, and a better nutrition status earlier in life is associated with improved lung function and better survival later in life.[12,45] The CF Foundation recommends the following nutrition goals:

- Infants: weight for length at the 50th percentile by 2 years of age
- Children 2–20 years of age: BMI percentile at or above the 50th percentile
- Adults: BMI of 22 for women and 23 for men[12]

Additionally, children are expected to meet their genetic potential for growth. Therefore, nutrition interventions to reach and maintain weight and growth goals are often necessary. Behavioral interventions for parents, caregivers, and patients may also help improve caloric intake, thus allowing weight gain.[42] Weight percentiles are believed to be at their lowest during the first 2 years of life and early adolescence, therefore making aggressive nutrition intervention important during these time periods.[46] For toddlers and older children, initially using high-calorie oral supplements or additives may be indicated. Infant formula can be concentrated or high-calorie modulars added to provide adequate calories. However, in some children this may not be sufficient to sustain a desired weight and growth status, and enteral feeding may be indicated. No specific guidelines exist regarding when to initiate enteral feeding in the pediatric CF population. The Cystic Fibrosis Foundation clinical practice guidelines subcommittee on growth and nutrition has determined that for children with

growth deficits, oral or enteral supplements should be used to improve the rate of weight gain.[12] Enteral tube feeding can be via nasogastric tube, G tube, or jejunostomy tube. The nasogastric tube can be inserted and removed daily for short-term use. Adherence to this intervention may prove difficult. A G tube may be more appropriate and allow for flexibility of feeding. Feeding via the G tube can be intermittent, bolus, or continuous feeds. Continuous feeds generally occur nocturnally. Nighttime feedings allow for regular meal and snack pattern during the day. An intact protein or semi-elemental protein formula may be used. Less pancreatic enzyme may be needed when using a semi-elemental formula because much of the fat is usually in the form of medium chain triglycerides. Enteral tube feeding may be complicated by early morning fullness and vomiting, loss of appetite, poor body image, and self-esteem concerns. The reader is directed to papers related to these concerns.[46–48] It is important to strike a balance between initiation of enteral feeding and severity of lung disease to optimize the benefit of the intervention. Feeding via a jejunostomy tube is infrequent in patients with CF and usually occurs in patients with significant upper GI dysmotility, failure of antireflux procedures, intubated patients, and in some postoperative patients. Parenteral nutrition (PN) is considered a more aggressive intervention and is not routinely used in the daily management of CF.

Nutrition-Related Cystic Fibrosis Complications

CF–Related Bone Disease (CFBD)

CF–related bone disease (CFBD) is increasingly recognized in persons who have CF, and the CF Patient Registry reports an incidence of 11%. This incidence is expected to increase with increased life expectancy.[49] The incidence of osteoporosis and fractures increases with age and is present in adult patients and in those with end-stage lung disease. CFBD is a multifactorial disease, and predisposing factors include malnutrition, increased inflammatory cytokines, vitamin D deficiency, inadequate calcium intake, use of corticosteroids, hypogonadism, short bowel syndrome, male sex, advanced lung disease, liver disease, CFRD, and possible genetic factors (F508del-CFTR is associated with reduced bone density in adults with CF). All patients older than 18 years should have a dual energy X-ray absorptiometry (DXA) scan; if results are normal, then a repeat DXA should be done every 5 years. If the DXA Z-score is between –1 and –2, then the scan should be repeated every 2–4 years. If the

THE A.S.P.E.N. PEDIATRIC NUTRITION SUPPORT CORE CURRICULUM, 2ND EDITION

Z-score is worse than –2, then the scan should be repeated yearly. In addition, children 8 years of age or older with the following risk factors should get a baseline DXA scan: small body size, low weight for height, decreased physical activity, low vitamin D levels, prolonged corticosteroid usage, delayed puberty, low calcium intake, history of fractures, family history of osteoporosis, significant lung disease, or liver disease.[23] Normative data are available for DXA scans for children >3 years of age. Treatment includes optimizing nutrition (calcium, vitamins D and K, and nutrition status), increasing physical activity, controlling underlying inflammation, decreasing use of corticosteroids if possible, treating CFRD, and addressing any hormone deficiencies. In adults, bisphosphonates have been used in patients with osteoporosis and stress fractures, but limited data exist on their safety in children.

CF–Related Diabetes

CFRD is being increasingly recognized in individuals with CF. This may be due in part to increased screening and improved survival. Incidence rates of 2% of children, 19% of adolescents, and 40%–50% of adults have been described from the University of Minnesota where screening is recommended for all children ≥6 years (note: this is different from Cystic Fibrosis Foundation guidelines). In addition, our understanding of the pathophysiology of CFRD has increased significantly. CFRD differs from type 1 and 2 diabetes mellitus; it is seen in patients with severe CF mutations and PI and is considered an insulin-insufficient state.[50] Damage to the islet cells is related to fibrosis and fatty infiltration, which is secondary to obstruction. Mouse models suggest a direct role for CFTR. Delayed and blunted insulin and C-peptide secretion are typically seen on an oral glucose tolerance test (OGTT) in patients with CF even in the absence of CFRD. Abnormalities in glucagon-like peptide-1 and gastric inhibitory polypeptide levels have also been seen.[50] With age, β-cell function declines abnormally, and this decline may be more prominent in patients with CF, leading to the increased incidence of CFRD as patients with CF age. While insulin deficiency is the primary defect, insulin resistance may also play a role during an acute pulmonary exacerbation, chronic severe lung disease, and glucocorticoid therapy and in obese individuals with CF.

A nearly 6-fold increase in mortality rate is seen in patients with CFRD,[50] though improvements in survival with early identification and treatment of CFRD have been reported from the University of Minnesota. BMI and pulmonary function are noted to decrease in the years prior to the diagnosis of CFRD. Improved weight is seen in patients treated with insulin. Complications of CFRD such as retinopathy, microalbuminemia, autonomic neuropathy, gastroparesis, and nephropathy can also occur. Because the onset of CFRD is insidious and is associated with negative outcomes, screening is very important. In CFRD the classic symptoms of polyuria and polydipsia are not often seen. Instead, weight loss, poor growth and a decline in pulmonary function are seen.

The Cystic Fibrosis Foundation offers the following recommendations:[51]

1. OGTT should be done annually at age 10 years and prior to transplant.

2. Fasting and 2-hour postprandial glucose monitoring should be done during hospitalizations and in the outpatient setting during intercurrent illness, intravenous antibiotics, or systemic glucocorticoid use and with enteral feeds.

3. Hemoglobin A_{1C} (HbA$_{1C}$) levels <6.6 do not exclude CFRD. Levels can be falsely low in CF due to accelerated red blood cell turnover.[52]

4. Diagnosis recommendations: Patients need one abnormal OGTT plus a confirmatory test or classic symptoms. The confirmatory tests can include

    a. 2-hour OGTT plasma glucose ≥ 200 mg/dL

    b. fasting plasma glucose ≥ 126 mg/dL

    c. HbA$_{1C}$ ≥ 6.5

    d. classic symptoms of polyuria and polydipsia in the presence of a casual glucose level of ≥ 200 mg/dL

For further details the reader should review the Cystic Fibrosis Foundation guidelines.[51]

Treatment of CFRD is recommended because of the observed benefits noted with treatment. The treatment of choice is insulin, and the regimen is individualized and should be under the direction of an endocrinologist experienced in the care of patients with CF. Oral hypoglycemic agents are currently not recommended. Nutrition therapy is very important. Carbohydrate ingestion is not discouraged; avoidance of foods high in simple sugars (soda, sugary sweets) is helpful in maintaining more stable glucose levels. PERT and their function of fat absorption assist to stabilize glucose levels.[50] Education is very important given the treatment burden from insulin injections, blood glucose, and diet monitoring. In addition to the above, patients need to understand the effects of food intake, stress, illness, and physical activity on insulin needs including the treatment of hypo and hyperglycemia. *Managing Cystic-Fibrosis-Related Diabetes: An Instruction Guide for Parents and Families* is available online from the Cystic Fibrosis Foundation (http://www.cff.org/UploadedFiles/LivingWithCF/StayingHealthy/Diet/Diabetes/CFRD-Manual-5th%20Edition-05-2012.pdf).

Gastrointestinal

GI manifestations are frequently seen in persons with CF and involve all parts of the GI tract.[53] If a gastroenterologist is not on the CF team, a referral should be made for collaborative management in most cases. Gastroesophageal reflux occurs at all ages and the incidence varies between 25% and 100% depending on the study. Complications of gastroesophageal reflux include feeding disorders, decreased caloric intake, failure to thrive, apnea in infants, vomiting, esophagitis, worsening of lung disease, esophageal strictures, and Barrett's esophagus. Reflux can be a significant problem in lung transplant recipients and is associated with rejection in the posttransplant period. Often a fundoplication is recommended in the pretransplant period to prevent bronchiolitis obliterans. Gastroparesis and constipation can be seen in CF, and the latter may be 3 times more frequent than DIOS. Bacterial overgrowth occurs in up to 60% of patients.[54] Predisposing factors include frequent antibiotic use, intestinal dysmotility, history of previous GI surgery, and sticky intestinal secretions that trap bacteria. DIOS is seen in all persons with CF, not just in those with PI. Dehydration of the intestinal secretions, coupled with electrolyte imbalances and sticky mucus, and poor motility lead to the accumulation of stool in the ileocecal junction, resulting in abdominal pain and vomiting. Treatment/prophylaxis consists of optimizing fluid and electrolyte intake, correction of any malabsorption, and the use of laxatives/stool softeners, such as polyethylene glycol. Prevention is vital, and an attempt to find the precipitating factor for every episode should be made. Celiac disease, inflammatory bowel disease, eosinophilic esophagitis, and GI malignancies may also occur in CF.

Patients with PS are at risk for recurrent bouts of pancreatitis. Over time some of these patients may develop PI. The most common liver lesion in patients with CF is fatty liver; hepatitis, hepatic fibrosis, and cirrhosis with portal hypertension are also seen. Gallbladder dysfunction is frequent, and a nonfunctioning gallbladder or gallstones can be seen on ultrasound examination. Biliary dyskinesia can result in right upper quadrant abdominal pain. Some patients with liver disease will progress to end-stage liver disease and develop complications from cirrhosis, portal encephalopathy, and variceal bleeds that may require liver transplantation.[8,9]

Other Chronic Lung Diseases

Overview and Pathophysiology

Chronic lung disease is seen in premature infants who have significant respiratory disease, in infants and children with congenital heart disease who need ventilator support in the neonatal period, in patients with difficult-to-manage asthma or reactive airways disease (RAD), and in patients with chronic respiratory insufficiency requiring ventilator support.

Bronchopulmonary Dysplasia

Bronchopulmonary dysplasia (BPD) is a form of chronic lung disease that develops in preterm infants given positive pressure ventilation and oxygen. The pathophysiology is complex and arises from small airway damage, abnormal alveolar development, and decreased surface area for gas exchange.[55] Additionally, there is damage to small blood vessels in the lungs and secondary damage to the heart and brain. BPD is most commonly seen in preterm infants with a birth weight of more than 1250 g and 30 weeks gestational age. Males tend to be more affected. Surfactant therapy is used soon after birth to prevent lung damage. Energy requirements are increased and range from 140 to 150 kcal/kg/d.[56,57] Vitamin A has been shown in some studies to decrease oxygen support and reduce death; however, vitamin A supplementation has not been widely adopted as a recommendation and remains controversial.[57] Patients with BPD have large insensible water losses and need extra fluid, which may result in opening of the patent ductus arteriosus and further stress on the lungs. Fluid intake of patients with BPD should be monitored closely to ensure adequate hydration and energy intake without causing fluid overload to the lungs. Infants with BPD are also at risk for decreased bone mineralization due to inadequate amounts of calcium in enteral feeds along with limited solubility of calcium in PN. Calcium status should be monitored every 1–2 weeks and an adequate intake of calcium (120–140 mg/kg/d), phosphorus (60–90 mg/kg/d), and vitamin D should be ensured.[57] Adequate intakes of protein (3–3.5 g/kg/d) and antioxidants (copper, zinc, and manganese) are also required, and it is important to avoid excessive carbohydrate intake because it can affect pulmonary function by altering the respiratory quotient. These patients often receive corticosteroids and diuretics for treatment of the lung disease, often with significant consequences: increased sodium, potassium, and magnesium losses; kidney stones; gallstones; and bone disease.

Infants with severe BPD are at high risk for the following problems during the first 2 years of life: pulmonary infections, frequent hospitalizations, RAD, and more frequent visits to the doctor. These patients also may have developmental delay, poor muscular development, poor feeding skills, poor growth, and chronic lung disease. Infants with BPD often have impaired weight for length and problems with oxygen diffusion resulting in a chronic oxygen requirement. Caloric needs are high because catch-up growth is often a goal. The coexistence of reflux and BPD can exacerbate poor oral motor function and can worsen feeding problems in patients with developmental delay. Reflux can also worsen lung disease. Supplemental feeds or calorically dense feedings are often required. For children with BPD, it is best to monitor growth on a regular basis. Anthropometrics provide critical information regarding the growth of the infant or child. In the infant with BPD, factors that may increase caloric requirements include increased basal metabolic rate, increased work of breathing, chronic illness or infections, and respiratory distress or metabolic complications.[56] The infant may struggle with fluid sensitivity, which may limit the intake of calories and nutrients. Infants may have interrupted feeding skill development and therefore may be poor oral feeders.[58] Interprofessional collaboration between team members is indicated, and occupational or speech therapists should provide oral therapy to maximize future feeding potential.

Asthma

Asthma or RAD is the most common cause of hospital admissions in children. This chronic pediatric lung disease involves chronic inflammation of the airways involving eosinophils, mast cells, T lymphocytes, macrophages, neutrophils, and epithelial cells. Additionally variable air flow obstruction is present along with increased bronchial responsiveness to a variety of environmental stimuli. The presence of airway edema and mucus contributes to the obstruction and bronchial reactivity that are seen.[59] Environmental triggers affect the normal development of the respiratory and immune systems in genetically predisposed individuals.[60] Patients often require chronic inhaled corticosteroids or pulses of systemic corticosteroids. Excessive oral corticosteroid use over time can result in growth failure, fluid and sodium retention, a voracious appetite, excessive weight gain, hypertension, glucose intolerance,

and obesity. Chronic corticosteroid can induce decreased bone density.[58] Therefore, adequate calcium and vitamin D supplementation are vital. Determining the adequacy of calcium and vitamin D includes diet assessment, vitamin D level, and DXA scan. Normative data are available for DXA scans for children above 3 years of age.[61] There also appears to be considerable variation in the side effects of inhaled corticosteroids. Growth, puberty, and bone health can be affected depending on the duration and dose.[62] Early data suggest that the use of antioxidants, *Lactobacillus*, and ω-3 fatty acids reduces symptoms and the development of asthma in those with atopy.[62] In children, a linear association between obesity (increased BMI) and asthma has been noted, with a 6% increase in prevalence per unit increase of BMI.[63] Vitamin D has been studied in asthma, and deficiency has been shown to be associated with increased symptoms of asthma, lower lung function, and worsened asthma control. It is important to monitor vitamin D levels in patients with asthma, and supplement with vitamin D if serum levels are low.[64]

Technology Dependent

Children with chronic respiratory failure may require chronic ventilatory support. At-risk children include those with neuromuscular dystrophy, spinal muscular atrophy, Duchenne's muscular dystrophy, spinal cord injuries, BPD, congenital diaphragmatic hernia, severe lung malformations, congenital hypoventilation syndrome, and myelomeningiocoele. Among the patients who require ventilator support, patients with BPD and neuromuscular dystrophy are the most frequent. Respiratory support can be noninvasive bilevel positive airway pressure (BIPAP) or invasive (tracheostomy and ventilator). The pathophysiology includes respiratory insufficiency (seen in BPD and pulmonary hypoplasia), secondary damage to the lungs from severe cardiac disease resulting in decreased surface area, decreased oxygen absorption, increased carbon dioxide retention, poor lung development, small-volume lungs, and insufficient vascular bed. There may also be decreased central drive for respiration as seen in persons with congenital central hypoventilation syndrome. Because these patients have decreased work of breathing, their energy requirements are consequently decreased. If careful attention is not paid to their nutrition regimens, they can have excessive weight gain, which can further impact their respiration status negatively. A commercially available enteral formula is now on the market that offers reduced calories (0.6 cal/mL) in a nutritionally complete formulation for use in circumstances in which calories need to be decreased without changing the volume of the formula. Often, in an attempt to decrease calories, overall nutrient intake, especially protein and mineral intake, suffers. These patients may also be at risk for bone disease due to decreased weight bearing and micronutrient deficiency (vitamin D and calcium).

Lung Transplantation

Lung transplantation remains the most aggressive therapy for end-stage lung disease.[65] Persons with CF and other lung diseases are candidates for lung transplantation when they exhibit severely reduced lung function and progressive deterioration in their health and quality of life.[16] For children and adults, the largest obstacle to long-term survival remains chronic allograft rejection secondary to the development of bronchiolitis obliterans. No level of malnutrition is an absolute contraindication to lung transplantation; however, a BMI > 17 kg/m² or an ideal body weight > 80% is recommended to improve outcomes posttransplant.[66] Enteral feeding tubes are often placed prior to transplant to help improve nutrition status in the malnourished patient. Weight gain is common after transplant, likely as a result of decreased energy needs, long-term steroid use, and overall improved health.[66] There is no pediatric weight criterion for lung transplant; however, one recent study showed no significant negative impact on children with CF who were underweight prior to transplant. Alternatively, children who do not have CF may have poorer outcomes post-transplant if they are underweight. Both groups (CF and non-CF) show decreased survival and worse outcomes after transplant when they are overweight prior to surgery. Further research in the area of weight and nutrition status is needed in the pediatric lung transplant population.[67]

Summary

Nutrition is an important part of the management of the child who has CF and other lung diseases. In general the goal is normal growth and development and correction of nutrition abnormalities that result from the underlying medical condition and the therapies used to treat the disease. Good nutrition status has been associated with improved lung function and outcomes in patients with CF.

Test Your Knowledge Questions

1. Pancreatic enzymes are available in non–enteric-coated and enteric-coated form. How does the enteric coating help with nutrient absorption?
   A. Enteric coating is subject to destruction by the harsh acid–peptic gastric environment.
   B. The coating allows the enzymes to get through the build-up of thick mucus in the pancreatic ducts.
   C. The coating allows for the activation to occur in the alkaline pH of the duodenum, past the gastric contents of the stomach.
2. Which fat-soluble vitamin blood levels should be checked in persons with CF and why?
   A. Vitamins A, D, K, and E and zinc. These are insensitive markers in CF.
   B. Vitamins A, D, and E and PIVKA II, to assure adequacy.
   C. Vitamins A, D, and E and PIVKA II. These are insensitive markers in laboratory tests.
3. A baseline DXA scan is recommended at the age of 8 years, especially if risk factors are present. Which of the following set of risk factors are necessary to be aware of?
   A. Small body size, low weight for height, decreased physical activity, low vitamin D levels, corticosteroid usage, delayed puberty, low calcium intake, history of fractures, family history of osteoporosis, significant lung disease, or liver disease
   B. Increasing physical activity, large body frame, asthma, or low calcium intake
   C. Increasing physical activity, large body frame, low weight for height, history of fractures, corticosteroid use, delayed puberty, or liver disease
4. Patients with asthma often require multiple courses of oral corticosteroids to control symptoms. What is not a nutrition concern in these patients?
   A. Growth failure
   B. Poor weight gain
   C. Glucose intolerance

Acknowledgments

The authors of this chapter for the second edition of this text wish to thank Suzanne Michel, MPH, RD, LDN, for her contributions to the first edition of this text.

References

1. Riordan J, Rommens J, Kerem B, et al. Identification of the cystic fibrosis gene: cloning and characterization of complementary DNA. *Science.* 1989;245(4922):1066–1073.
2. Cystic Fibrosis Foundation Patient Registry. 2012 Annual data report. Bethesda, MD: Cystic Fibrosis Foundation; 2013.
3. Farrell PM, Rosenstein BJ, White TB, et al. Guidelines for diagnosis of cystic fibrosis in newborns through older adults: Cystic Fibrosis Foundation Consensus Report. *J Pediatr.* 2008;153(2):S4–S14.
4. Lubamba B, Dhooghe B, Noel S, Leal T. Cystic fibrosis: Insight into CFTR pathophysiology and pharmacotherapy. *Clin Biochem.* 2012;45(15)1132–1144.

5. Duggan, C, Watkins JB, Walker WA. *Nutrition in Pediatrics: Basic Science and Clinical Applications.* 4th ed. Hamilton, London: BC Decker Inc; 2008.

6. Tiddens H, Rosenfeld M. Respiratory manifestations of cystic fibrosis. In: Taussig LM, Landau LI, eds. *Pediatric Respiratory Medicine.* 2nd ed. Philadelphia, PA: Mosby Elsevier; 2008;871–887.

7. American Academy of Pediatrics, Committee on Nutrition. Kleinman RE, Greer F, eds. *Pediatric Nutrition Handbook.* 7th ed. Elk Grove Village, IL: The American Academy of Pediatrics; 2013.

8. Gelfond D, Borowitz D. Gastrointestinal complications of cystic fibrosis. *Clin Gastroenterol Hepatol.* 2013;11:333–342.

9. Flass T, Narkewicz M. Cirrhosis and other liver disease in cystic fibrosis. *J Cyst Fibros.* 2013;12:116–124.

10. Konstan MW, Butler SM, Wohl MEB, et al. Growth and nutritional indexes in early life predict pulmonary function in cystic fibrosis. *J Pediatr.* 2003;142:624–630.

11. Stallings VA, Tomezsko JL, Schall JI, et al. Adolescent development and energy expenditure in females with CF. *Clin Nutr.* 2005;24:737–745.

12. Stallings VA, Stark LJ, Robinson KA, Feranchk AP, Quinton H; Clinical Practice Guidelines in Growth and Nutrition Subcommittee (Ad Hoc Working Group). Evidence-based practice recommendations for nutrition-related management of children and adults with cystic fibrosis and pancreatic insufficiency: results of a systematic review. *J Am Diet Assoc.* 2008;108:832–839.

13. Borowitz D, Baker RD, Stallings V. Consensus report on nutrition for pediatric patients with cystic fibrosis. *J Pediatr Gastroenterol Nutr.* 2002;35:246–259.

14. Dietitians Association of Australia. Australasian clinical practice guidelines for nutrition and cystic fibrosis, 2006. http://daa.asn.au/wp-content/uploads/2012/09/Guidelines_CF-Final.pdf. Accessed January 2015.

15. Maqbool A, Schall JI, Garcia-Espana JF, et al. Serum linoleic acid status as a clinical indicator of essential fatty acid status in children with cystic fibrosis. *J Pediatr Gastroenterol Nutr.* 2008;47(5):635–644.

16. Gottschlich MM. Pulmonary disease. In: Gottschlich MM, ed. *The Science and Practice of Nutrition Support: A Core-Based Curriculum.* Dubuque, IA: Kendall/Hunt Publishing Co; 2001:501–516.

17. White H, Morton AM, Peckman DG, Conway SG. Dietary intakes in adult patients with cystic fibrosis—do they achieve guidelines? *J Cyst Fibros.* 2004;3:1–7

18. Borowitz D, Robinson KA, Rosenfeld M, et al. Cystic fibrosis evidenced-based guidelines for management of infants with cystic fibrosis. *J Pediatr.* 2009;155:S73–S93.

19. Lancellotti L, D'Orazio C, Mastella G, Lippi U. Deficiency of vitamins E and A in cystic fibrosis is independent of pancreatic function and current enzyme and vitamin supplementation. *Eur J Pediatr.* 1996;155:281–285.

20. Feranchak AP, Sontag MK, Wagerner JS, Hammond KB, Accurso FJ, Sokol RJ. Prospective, long-term study of fat-soluble vitamin status in children with cystic fibrosis identified by newborn screen. *J Pediatr.* 1999;135(5):601–610.

21. Krebs NF, Sontag M, Accurso FJ, Hambidge KM. Low plasma zinc concentrations in young infants with cystic fibrosis. *J Pediatr.* 1998;133(6):761–764.

22. Sinaasappel M, Stern M, Littlewood J, Wolfe S, Steinkamp G, Heijerman HGM. Nutrition in patients with cystic fibrosis: a European consensus. *J Cyst Fibros.* 2002;1:51–75.

23. Aris RM, Merkel PA, Bachrach LK, et al. Consensus statement: guide to bone health and disease in cystic fibrosis. *J Clin Endocrinol Metab.* 2005;90:1888–1896.

24. Wood LG, Fitzgerald DA, Lee AK, et al. Improved antioxidant and fatty acid status of patients with cystic fibrosis after antioxidant supplementation is linked to improved lung function. *Am J Clin Nutr.* 2003;77:150–159.

25. Horwitt MK, Harvey CC, Dahm CH Jr, Searcy MT. Relationship between tocopherol and serum lipid levels for determination of nutritional adequacy. *Ann NY Acad Sci.* 1972;203:223–236.

26. Huang SH, Schall JI, Zemel BS, Stallings VA. Vitamin E status in children with cystic fibrosis and pancreatic insufficiency. *J Pediatr.* 2006;148:556–559.

27. Tangpricha V, Kelly A, Stephenson A, et al. An update on the screening, diagnosis, management, and treatment of vitamin D deficiency in individuals with cystic fibrosis: evidenced-based recommendations from the Cystic Fibrosis Foundation. *J Clin Endocrinol Metab.* 2012;97(4):1082–1093.

28. Beker LT, Ahrens RA, Fink RD, et al. Effect of vitamin K1 supplementation on vitamin K status in cystic fibrosis patients. *J Pediatr Gastroenterol Nutr.* 1997;24:512–517.

29. Wilson DC, Rashid M, Durie PR, et al. Treatment of vitamin K deficiency in cystic fibrosis: effectiveness of a daily fat-soluble vitamin combination. *J Pediatr.* 2001;138:851–855.

30. Conway SP, Wolfe SP, Brownlee KG, et al. Vitamin K status among children with cystic fibrosis and its relationship to bone mineral density and bone turnover. *Pediatrics.* 2005;115:1325–1331.

31. Michel SH, Maqbool A, Hanna MD, Mascarenhas M. Nutrition management of pediatric patients who have cystic fibrosis. *Pediatr Clin N Am.* 2009;56(5):1123–1141.

32. Kriemler S, Wilk B, Schurer W, Wilson W, Bar-Or O. Preventing dehydration in children with cystic fibrosis who exercise in the heat. *Med Sci Sports Exerc.* 1993;31:774–779.

33. Weiss G, Goodnough LT. Anemia of chronic disease. *N Engl J Med.* 2005;352:1011–1023.

34. Ross AC, Manson JE, Abrams SA, et al. The 2011 Dietary Reference Intakes for Calcium and Vitamin D: what dietetics practitioners need to know. *J Am Diet Assoc.* 2011; 111:524-527.

35. von Vigier RO, Truttmann AC, Zindler-Schmocker K, et al. Aminoglycosides and renal magnesium homeostasis in humans. *Nephrol Dial Transplan.* 2000;15:822–826.

36. Littlewood JM, Wolfe SP. Control of malabsorption in cystic fibrosis. *Paediatr Drugs.* 2000;2(3): 205-22.

37. O'Brien CE, Harden H, Com G. A survey of nutrition practices for patients with cystic fibrosis. *Nutr Clin Pract.* 2013;28:237–241.

38. Borowitz DS, Grand RJ, Drurie PR, et al. Use of pancreatic enzyme supplements for patients with cystic fibrosis in the context of fibrosing colonopathy. *J Pediatr.* 1995;127(68):1–4.

39. Ferrie S, Graham C, Hoyle M. Pancreatic enzyme supplementation for patients receiving enteral feeds. *Nutr Clin Pract.* 2011;26:349–351.

40. Berry A. Pancreatic enzyme replacement therapy during pancreatic insufficiency. *Nutr Clin Pract.* 2014;29:312–321.

41. Nicolo M, Stratton K, Rooney W, Boullata J. Pancreatic enzyme replacement therapy for enterally fed patients with cystic fibrosis. 2013;28(4):485–489.

42. Powers SW, Byars KC, Mitchell MJ, Patton SR, Schindler T, Zeller MH. A randomized pilot study of behavioral treatment to increase caloric intake in toddlers with cystic fibrosis. *Children's Health Care.* 2003;32(4):297–311.

43. Crist W, McDonnell P, Beck M, Gillespie CT, Barrett P, Mathews J. Behavior at mealtimes and the young child with cystic fibrosis. *J Dev Behav Pediatr.* 1994;15(3):157–161.

44. Birch LL, Fischer JA. Appetite and eating behavior in children. *Pediatr Clin North Am.* 1995;42(4):931–953.

45. Yen, EH, Quinton H, Borowitz D. Better nutritional status in early childhood is associated with improved clinical outcomes and survival in patients with cystic fibrosis. *J Pediatr.* 2013;162:530–535.

46. Erksine JM, Lingard C, Sontag M. Update on enteral nutrition support for cystic fibrosis. *Nutr Clin Pract.* 2007;22:223–232.

47. Abbott J, Conway S, Etherington C, et al. Perceived body image and eating behavior in young adults with cystic fibrosis and their healthy peers. *J Behav Med.* 2000;23:501–517.

48. Gilchrist FJ, Lenney W. Distorted body image and anorexia complicating cystic fibrosis in an adolescent. *J Cystic Fibros.* 2008;7(5):437–439.

49. Stalvey MS and Clines GA. Cystic fibrosis-related bone disease: insights into a growing problem. *Curr Opin Endocrinol Diabetes Obes.* 2013;20:547–552.

50. Kelly A, Moran A. Update on cystic fibrosis-related diabetes. *J Cyst Fibros.* 2013;12(4):318–331.

51. Moran A, Brunzell C, Cohen RC, et al. Clinical care guidelines for cystic fibrosis-related diabetes. *Diabetes Care.* 2010;33(12):2697–2708.

52. Moran A, Hardin D, Rodman D, et al. Diagnosis, screening and management of cystic fibrosis related diabetes mellitus: a consensus conference report. *Diabetes Res Clin Pract.* 1999;45:61–73.

53. Mascarenhas MR. Treatment of gastrointestinal problems in cystic fibrosis. *Curr Treat Options Gastroenterol.* 2003;6(5):427–441.

54. Fridge JL, Conrad C, Gerson L, Cox K. Risk factors for small bowel bacterial overgrowth in cystic fibrosis. *J Pediatr Gastroenterol Nutr.* 2007;44(2):212–218.

55. Ambalavanan N. Bronchopulmonary dysplasia. http://reference.medscape.com/article/973717-overview. Updated March 28, 2014. Accessed May 2014.

56. Cox JH. Bronchopulmonary dysplasia. In: Groh-Wargo S, Thompson M, Cox JH, eds. *Nutritional Care for High-Risk Newborns.* Chicago, IL: Precept Press Inc; 2000:369-390.

57. Dani C, Poggi C. Nutrition and bronchopulmonary dysplasia. *J Matern Fetal Neonatal Med.* 2012;25(S3):37–40.

58. Redding E, Despino S. Pulmonary diseases. In: Queen Samour P, King K, eds. *Handbook of Pediatric Nutrition.* 4th ed. Sudbury, MA: Jones and Bartlett Publication; 2012:239–271.

59. Morris MJ. Asthma. http://emedicine.medscape.com/article/296301-overview#aw2aab6b2b2. Updated March 27, 2014. Accessed May 2014.

60. Sly PD. Asthma: disease mechanisms and cell biology. In: Taussig LM, Landau LI, eds. *Pediatric Respiratory Medicine.* 2nd ed. Philadelphia, PA: Mosby Elsevier; 2008:791–804.

61. Helba M and Binovitz L. Pediatric body composition analysis with dual-energy X-ray absorptiometry. *Pediatr Radiol.* 2009;39:647–656.

62. Landau LI, Martinez FD. Asthma: treatment. In *Pediatric Respiratory Medicine.* 2nd ed. St. Louis, MO: Mosby Elsevier; 2008:829–844.

63. Sithole F, Douwes J, Burstyn I, et al. Body mass index in childhood: a linear association. *Asthma.* 2008;45(6):473–477.

64. Rance K. The emerging role of vitamin D in asthma management. *J Am Acad Nurse Pract.* 2014;26(5):263–267.

65. Thiou TG, Cahill BC. Pediatric lung transplantation for cystic fibrosis. *Transplantation.* 2008;86(5):636–637.

66. Hadiljiadis D. Special considerations for patients with cystic fibrosis undergoing lung transplantation. *Chest.* 2007;131:1224–1231.

67. Benden C, Ridout DA, Edwards LB, et al. Body mass index and its effect on outcome in children after lung transplantation. *J Heart Lung Transplant.* 2013;32:196–201.

Test Your Knowledge Answers

1. The correct answer is **C**. Acidity in the GI tract may prevent or retard dissolution of enteric-coated pancreatic enzymes. If activation does not occur in the small intestine, then it may be difficult for a person with CF to absorb macronutrients and micronutrients.

2. The correct answer is **B**. Blood levels of fat-soluble vitamins should be measured to assure adequacy (vitamins A, E, D). Prothrombin time is insensitive to vitamin K deficiency in CF. PIVKA II provides a better indicator of vitamin K nutrition.

3. The correct answer is **A**. All risk factors need to be evaluated. Treatment includes optimizing nutrition, increasing physical activity, controlling underlying inflammation, decreased corticosteroid use, and addressing hormone deficiencies.

4. The correct answer is **B**. Nutrition concerns with patients who require oral corticosteroids are growth failure, obesity, glucose intolerance, hypertension, and decreased bone density.

29

Oncology, Hematopoietic Transplant, Gastrointestinal Supportive Care Medications, and Survivorship

Nancy Sacks, MS, RD, LDN; **David Henry**, MS, BCOP, FASHP; **Kristen Bunger**, MS, RD, CNSC; **Kelly Kolp**, RD, CNSC; **Andrea White-Collins**, RN, MS, CPNP; **Britt Olsen**, RN, MSN, CPNP; **Kyrie L. Hospodar**, RN, MSN, CPNP; and **Susan R. Rheingold**, MD

CONTENTS

Learning Objectives

1. The clinician will be able to successfully evaluate the nutrition status of the pediatric oncology patient and determine the caloric, macronutrient, and micronutrient needs of the patient.
2. The clinician will be able to identify the common nutrition issues for children undergoing hematopoietic stem cell transplantation.
3. The clinician will be able to choose the most effective mode of nutrition support and monitor its tolerance in the pediatric oncology population.
4. The clinician will become more knowledgeable regarding types of medication used to alleviate gastrointestinal problems.
5. The clinician will be able to identify the nutrition and activity goals for survivors of childhood cancer.

General Oncology Overview

Pediatric cancer is the leading cause of death by disease in children under the age of 15 years.[1] An estimated 1 in 285 children is diagnosed with cancer before 20 years of age, accounting for over 15,780 new cases a year in the United States.[1] As a result of multimodal therapy, the 5-year survival has improved from < 50% in the 1970s to almost 80% today.[1] Although the cure rate varies by cancer type, 1 in 530 young adults (20–39 years) is a survivor of childhood cancer.[1] The type of cancer and treatments used adversely impact the nutrition status of the child with cancer during and following therapy; therefore, it is essential to maximize nutrition status at diagnosis and throughout therapy and to create healthy lifelong nutrition habits.

Nutrition Aspects: Diagnoses and Malnutrition

The risk of malnutrition is a significant concern during pediatric cancer treatment. Due to the increased nutrition needs for growth and development during childhood, and the metabolic stress of cancer, malnutrition is a frequent treatment complication. Between 6% and 50% of children will present with acute malnutrition at diagnosis.[2–5] A higher incidence of malnutrition may be related to delay in diagnosis, extent of disease, and location of the tumor. During the course of therapy, malnutrition is observed in 8%–32% of children.[6] Younger children may be at higher risk of acute malnutrition due to limited nutrient stores and increased caloric demand for growth. The higher incidences of malnutrition have a di-

rect correlation with more intensive courses of treatment, often including transplant.

Nutrient needs may not be met due to increased metabolic demands, depleted stores, or inadequate intake.[7,8] At diagnosis, nutrition status should not be assessed by weight or appearance alone because large tumor burdens may disguise the loss of adipose and lean muscle mass, therefore making it difficult to assess nutrition status.

Certain diagnoses are more likely to result in nutrition problems due to altered metabolism, physiologic changes, and effects of antineoplastic therapy.[9] Children with sarcomas, neuroblastomas, and brain tumors typically present at diagnosis with protein depletion and weight loss.[10,11] Other diagnoses that are at high risk for nutrition complications include advanced stage Wilms' tumor and acute myelogenous leukemia (AML).

Multimodal Treatment and the Effects on Nutrition

Surgery

Surgical intervention is necessary for most solid tumors. Nausea, vomiting, fatigue, altered bowel motility, and decreased preoperative and postoperative appetite are complications that can impact the ability to meet nutrient requirements. The location of childhood tumors, and the role of surgery in their treatment, are quite different from those seen in adults. Cancers to the head and neck regions are less common, consisting mostly of nasopharyngeal sarcoma, neuroblastoma, and osteogenic sarcoma of the mandible. Surgery for head and neck cancers can lead to difficulty chewing and swallowing.[12] Rhabdomyosarcoma, hepatoblastoma, neuroblastoma, and Burkitt's lymphoma are commonly found in the abdomen and pelvis and can affect the gastrointestinal (GI) tract. Malignancies involving the GI tract can cause changes in absorption and nutrient delivery and affect digestion and absorption prior to surgical resection.[13,14] Postoperative complications from GI tract or intraperitoneal organ surgery can include impaired swallowing function, decreased gastric capacity or emptying, ileus of the small bowel, and altered bowel length and integrity. If children are malnourished at the time of surgery, they have compromised wound healing and an increased risk of morbidity and mortality; whereas well-nourished patients have fewer surgical complications.[15] At the time when energy needs increase because of metabolic changes secondary to surgery, and when optimal wound healing requires good caloric and protein intake, the patient is least likely to consume adequate nutrition orally or even via tube feedings.[16-18] Postoperative pain can also impact nutrition status. Uncontrolled pain, immobility, and narcotic-related sedation or constipation can decrease the patient's interest in, appetite for, wakefulness for, or tolerance of oral intake.

Radiation Therapy

Radiation therapy is a treatment used independently or in conjunction with surgery and chemotherapy. Radiation destroys the genetic material within the cell, thereby killing the malignant cell.[19] Complications arise from radiation therapy because healthy cells within the radiation field are inevitably damaged during treatment. A variety of radiation delivery options now exist, including 3-dimensional conformal radiation, stereotactic radiotherapy, proton therapy, fractionated dosing, and intensity-modulated radiotherapy. Some of the newer modalities decrease radiation exposure to normal healthy cells and decrease toxicity. The choice of therapy is dependent upon diagnosis, location, and the age of the patient, with the goal of therapy being optimal benefit with minimal toxicity.[19-21] The area most susceptible to nutrition effects of radiation is the GI tract.[22] Moderate to severe mucositis, from the mouth to the anus, can result in malabsorption of nutrients, diarrhea, and severe pain both with and without oral intake.

Diarrhea from abdominal/pelvic radiation results in decreased absorption of whatever nutrients the child does manage to consume. Nausea and vomiting are the most common in patients receiving abdominal or cranial radiation. Alterations in salivation and taste buds are seen in patients receiving head and neck radiation, although the potential alterations in dentition generally do not affect short-term nutrition status. Dysphagia and esophagitis can occur with radiation to the chest or upper back. The effect on appetite depends on the involved radiation field, total dose of radiation, and number of fractions received.[21,23] Acute side effects of radiation may begin as early as 1 week from the initiation of radiotherapy and last several weeks after the final fraction. Patients receiving cranial radiation can develop postradiation somnolence syndrome 6–8 weeks after completion of radiation. The syndrome causes severe lethargy and flu-like symptoms, and the associated extended periods of sleep result in the child missing many

Table 29-1. Nutrition-Related Side Effects of Radiation Therapy

LOCATION	ADVERSE REACTION
Central Nervous System Brain and Spinal Cord	Nausea/vomiting Fatigue Loss of appetite Alterations in pituitary functions Growth failure
Head and neck Tongue, larynx, pharynx Oropharynx, tonsils, Salivary glands	Xerostomia Sore mouth/throat Dysphagia Mucositis Altered taste and smell Fatigue Loss of appetite
Abdomen and pelvis Gastrointestinal tract, reproductive organs Rectum, colon, testicles	Nausea/vomiting Diarrhea Abdominal cramping Bloating Gas Enteritis and colitis Lactose intolerance Fatigue Loss of appetite

meals and therefore many calories. Expected nutrition side effects based upon the location of the radiation field are found in Table 29-1.

Chemotherapy

Classic cytotoxic chemotherapy works by inhibiting the division of rapidly dividing cells.[24] Although cancer cells are the main target, rapidly dividing normal cells, including those of the mucosa of the GI tract, taste buds, hair, and bone marrow, are equally affected. The effect of chemotherapy on the patient's nutrition status is associated with the exact medication used, dose, route of administration, and length of treatment. A list of complications of select chemotherapy agents and ranking of emetogenic potential is found in Table 29-2.

The most common nutrition-related side effect of cytotoxic drugs is nausea and vomiting, but with modern antiemetics the degree of emesis is much less severe. Loss of taste buds can make familiar foods unpalatable and cause decreased appetite.[29] Heavy metal agents such as cisplatin are most likely to cause alterations in taste.

Table 29-2. Complications of Select Chemotherapy Agents[24-28]

CHEMOTHERAPY AGENT	NAUSEA/ VOMITING[a]	ANOREXIA	MUCOSITIS	DIARRHEA	CONSTIPATION	ELECTROLYTE DEPLETION	XEROSTOMIA	TASTE ALTERATION
Asparaginase	3	X	X					
Bleomycin	1	X	X					
Carboplatin	4			X				
Cisplatin	5	X	X	X		↓ K, Mg, Zn		
Cyclophosphamide	3	X	X				X	
Cytarabine	4	X	X	X				
Dactinomycin	5	X	X	X			X	X
Daunorubicin	4	X	X	X			X	X
Doxorubicin	3	X	X	X			X	
Etoposide	2	X	X	X				
Fluorouracil	2		X	X				X
Gemcytabine	2		X	X				
Hydroxyurea	1	X	X	X				
Idarubicin	3		X	X				
Ifosfamide	3							
Imatinib	3	X		X				
Irenotecan	4	X		X				
Methotrexate	3	X	X	X		↓ B12, Folate		X
Mitoxantrone	3		X	X				
Procarbizine	2	X	X	X		↓ K, Ca, Phos		
Rituximab	1							
Temozolamide	3	X						
Thioguanine	1	X	X	X				
Topotecan	2	X		X				
Vinblastine	3		X	X	X			
Vincristine	1	X	X	X	X			
Vinorelbine	2	X			X			

[a]Most emetogenic= 5, least emetogenic =1

These side effects, along with anticipatory nausea, lead to anorexia with a loss of interest in eating and subsequent malnutrition. Some chemotherapy agents can cause diarrhea, others constipation, both of which can alter the digestion and absorption of nutrients. Chemotherapy can lead to mucositis due to its effect on epithelial stem cells. The loss of integrity of the oral mucosa makes eating painful,[30] and changes to the lining of the intestine can result in decreased absorption of nutri-

ents.[24,25,31] Nutrition-related side effects of chemotherapy can be found in Table 29-3.

Cancer's Direct Effect on Nutrition Status

Metabolic

Cancer cachexia is defined as a "state of malnutrition characterized by anorexia, weight loss, muscle wasting, asthenia, depression, chronic nausea, and anemia and results in phys-

Table 29-3. Most Commonly Experienced Nutrition-Related Side Effects of Chemotherapy[23-25]

Anorexia	Taste changes
Early satiety	Mucositis/esophagitis
Nausea	Diarrhea
Vomiting	Constipation

iological distress, changes in body composition and alterations in carbohydrate, lipid, and protein metabolism."[26,27] These metabolic alterations result in weight loss from diminished muscle and adipose tissue, which compounds the effects of inadequate intake and anorexia. Cytokines are substances made by the cells of the immune system that mediate cell and tissue function and assist in regulating satiety signals and gastric emptying.[32,33] Elevated cytokine levels are found in patients with cancer, likely contributing to the complex metabolic response of cancer cachexia.[34,35] Table 29-4 outlines the role of select cytokines in nutrition and cachexia. Research has demonstrated that changes in glucose, protein, and lipid metabolism in cancer patients cause weight loss even before the patient experiences decreased appetite and oral intake.[35,38,39]

Energy utilization in the body can range from hypometabolism to hypermetabolism.[40] Tumor cells use glucose as their main energy source, as well as anaerobic metabolism and amino acids for growth.[39,41] Inefficient energy utilization by the tumor causes increased activity of the Cori cycle to produce lactic acid to be converted to glucose. Gluconeogenesis, the production of glucose from the breakdown of fat and protein stores, aids in glucose homeostasis.[28] Muscle protein synthesis is reduced, and acute phase protein production in the liver is increased, leading to the risk of muscle catabolism. Despite the increased demand for glucose, patients frequently exhibit relative glucose intolerance and insulin resistance.[42] An increase in lipolysis and decrease in lipogenesis contributes to promoting large losses in fat mass in oncology patients.

Physiologic

The toxicity of chemotherapy can cause changes in organ function resulting in altered nutrient metabolism and excretion. Cisplatin and cyclophosphamide can cause electrolyte wasting by the kidneys that can last for weeks after the agent is given. Mild to moderate transaminitis and hyperbilirubinemia are common side effects of chemotherapy and reveal change in hepatic function. Tumors of the nasopharynx, neck, mediastinum, and GI tract and organs can cause direct obstruction and lead to decreased oral intake.

Psychosocial

Emotional well-being is essential to achieving and maintaining physical health, including an optimal nutrition status. Depression and anxiety affect up to 20% of all patients diagnosed with cancer and one study in children with cancer found that 59% had mild psychological problems.[43] The specific diagnosis, age and developmental stage of the patient, prognosis, complications of therapy, and support systems (or lack thereof) all impact the psychological response to a cancer diagnosis and treatment.[44] Anxiety appears to affect younger children, and teens can suffer from anxiety as well as depression. Both can lead to inactivity, loss of appetite, self-criticism, and hopelessness. Self-image and self-esteem, including perception of weight status and physical appearance, are important to monitor in the preteen and teenage population. Learned food aversions due to the experience of eating and then vomiting affect toddlers and young children more. Re-establishing normal eating patterns and developing trust that eating can be a successful and even enjoyable process are not likely to occur immediately after completing therapy. A specialized feeding program may be necessary to help overcome food aversions and resume pretreatment eating habits and oral intake.

Table 29-4. Role of Cytokines and Hormones in Cancer Cachexia

CYTOKINE	EFFECT ON NUTRITION
Tumor necrosis factor	Suppresses lipoprotein lipase[27]
	Increases corticotropin-releasing hormone, which suppresses food intake[36]
Interleukin-1	Blocks neuropeptide Y induced feeding; increases corticotropin-releasing hormone[36]
Interleukin-6	Induces cachexia and acute-phase proteins in animal models[27,37]
Interferon (INF)-γ	Induces cachexia; INF-γ antibodies reversed wasting[36]
Peptide YY	Levels increased with greater disease burden; inverse correlation with BMI[24]
Ghrelin	Low values associated with greater disease burden[35]

BMI, body mass index.

Evaluation of Nutrition Status and Determining Nutrient Requirements

Energy and Protein

Determining nutrition status at diagnosis and potential for malnutrition is necessary for good supportive care.[26] Although no specific nutrition protocols exist for pediatric oncology, it is recommended that a patient's nutrition status be categorized using guidelines developed by the Children's Oncology Group, Cancer Control, Nutrition Sub-Committee (Appendix 29-1). The Academy of Nutrition and Dietetics has developed adult nutrition protocols for medical, surgical, and radiation oncology patients that may serve as a resource for the pediatric population, and certainly for the adolescents and young adults frequently treated in pediatric oncology centers.[45,46] Table 29-5 contains components of a nutrition assessment that are commonly used in children with cancer.

Calorie and protein needs are difficult to assess in the pediatric oncology population, and they are affected by current nutrition status, disease state, and therapy protocol. Appendix 29-2 contains formulas to assist in estimation of calorie and protein needs. An activity/stress factor may need to be utilized with these formulas; however, weight loss may be better correlated to decreased oral intake and not increased energy expenditure.[47] Serum albumin and prealbumin values may indicate depleted protein stores, although these values may be inaccurate because they can be influenced by hydration status, stress, and liver function and should be interpreted based on clinical status.

Growth and Development

The goal of nutrition intervention for the child with cancer is to provide adequate nutrients for growth and development and reverse protein calorie malnutrition. Optimal growth and weight gain in pediatric patients are essential for maximizing physical tolerance to treatment and decreasing the amount of treatment delays.[8,48,49] Strategies for nutrition intervention for specific symptoms should be implemented in all patients as outlined in Table 29-6.[50]

Nutrition support should be individualized for each child, with the development of a nutrition plan based upon the patient's nutrition assessment, disease type and stage, treatment, and quality of life considerations. Studies show that pediatric patients who receive intervention from a registered dietitian during active treatment have improved weight status through therapy.[50] Guidelines for nutrition

Table 29-5. Components of Nutrition Assessment

Category	Components
Medical history	Diagnosis stage and date Past medical history Medication history Anticipated therapy protocol
Anthropometics[a]	Weight history BMI/weight-for-age Height-for-age Recent growth trends % Ideal body weight % Usual body weight % Diagnosis weight Mid-arm circumference Triceps skinfold
Dietary intake evaluation	Current intake (amounts, stage, feeding times) Usual intake Feeding behavior Modified oral intake Tube feeds Parenteral nutrition Vitamin/mineral supplementation
Gastrointestinal symptoms/ side effects	Nausea Vomiting Constipation Diarrhea Dry mouth Taste changes Mouth sores Difficulty swallowing Early satiety
Laboratory assessment	Electrolytes Blood glucose Serum proteins Absolute neutrophil count Complete blood count Liver function tests
Quality of life	Activity level Family support system Depression/anxiety Pain Treatment plan Resources

BMI, body mass index.

[a]Refer to Appendix 29-1 and Appendix 29-3.

intervention for pediatric cancer patients have been developed by the American Academy of Pediatrics and modified by Andrassy and Chwals[51] and Mauer et al,[4] and the criteria on nutrition intervention have been outlined by

Table 29-6. Nutrition Strategies for Symptom Management

SYMPTOM	DIETARY INTERVENTION STRATEGIES
Nausea/vomiting	Small frequent meals, high-carbohydrate content, nonacidic beverages, cold clear foods and beverages, avoid extreme temperatures and highly seasoned items, avoid high-fat content items
Anorexia	Small frequent meals, nutrient-dense foods and supplements, carbohydrate and protein modulars, create a pleasant atmosphere, dine with the child, vary colors/flavors/textures of foods
Diarrhea	Low-fat, cold, or room temperature foods, avoid caffeine, encourage adequate fluid intake
Dysgeusia	Herbs, spices, and marinades, cold nonodorous foods, fruit-flavored beverages, good oral hygiene, mint mouthwashes, lemon-flavored beverages, and sour candies
Mucositis	Soft diet, smooth bland moist foods, frozen slushes/ices/ice cream, high-calorie liquid beverages
Xerostomia	Moist foods, encourage liquids with meals, add sauces/gravy/butter/broth, add vinegar and lemons to stimulate saliva, good oral hygiene

the Children's Oncology Group (COG) as described in Appendix 29-1.

Outcome Measures

Biochemical Evaluation

Laboratory tests should be closely monitored from initial nutrition assessment through repletion. One should assess basic electrolytes (sodium, potassium, chloride, bicarbonate), glucose, renal function (creatinine, blood urea nitrogen), minerals (calcium, phosphorus, magnesium), liver function tests (alkaline phosphatase, serum aminotransferase, γ-glutamyltransferase, total bilirubin), and lipids (triglycerides and cholesterol).

Anthropometric

Physical evaluation is an important aspect of a nutrition evaluation. Promoting consistent growth along chart curve percentiles is the goal, so monitoring linear growth is essential for long-term assessment. In addition, z scores are also very important in assessing the status of nutrition-related health and can be a good indicator of identifying malnutrition.[52] Growth should be plotted and monitored for each patient monthly on weight-for-age, length/height for age, body

mass index (BMI) for age (> 2 years), weight-for-length (< 2 years), and head circumference (< 3 years of age). Additionally, weight measurements may be skewed in children with large abdominal tumors (such as heptaoblastoma, Wilms' tumor, or neuroblastoma), prior to tumor resection or those with edema due to corticosteroid use.[31]

Disease Outcome

Though it cannot be used as an independent marker of mortality, more severe malnutrition is frequently related to a worse prognosis.[49,53,54] Several studies in pediatric solid tumors have shown a correlation between outcome and nutrition status.[21,49,53,54] Decreased relapse rates have been correlated with improved nutrition status in children with localized solid tumors and lymphomas, but not with advanced disease at diagnosis.[2]

Similar results have been published associating poor survival outcomes in malnourished and obese children and adolescents with leukemia. Suboptimal nutrition prior to or while receiving therapy for acute lymphoblastic leukemia (ALL) resulted in longer duration of treatment, prolonged hospitalization, higher infection rate, increased mortality during the first 2 phases of treatment, and lower rate of 5-year survival.[55–57] Although it would seem obvious that good nutrition could improve survival rates, while malnutrition could negatively impact outcome, a review of multiple studies does not confirm these expectations. Sala et al[58] suggest that the wide variety of diseases, chemotherapy agents, criteraia used to classify nutrition status, and supportive care measures confound the results of research into nutrition status and outcomes.

Treatment Tolerance

Evidence exists that tolerance of treatment is associated with positive nutrition status, while delays in treatment are seen more often in those with poor nutrition status. The dosing of chemotherapy agents is based upon body surface area, which is affected by weight loss or gain. The metabolism of chemotherapy is also affected by fat and muscle mass, a reflection of nutrition status, which in turn can affect efficacy and tolerance of therapy.[31] Patients treated for stage IV neuroblastoma who were malnourished at diagnosis or who had weight loss early in treatment had more frequent delays in therapy.[48,54] Malnourished patients with ALL or Wilms' tumor were more likely to require a reduction in drug therapy relative to their better-nourished peers.[8,49,59] Patients who developed anthracycline-associated cardiomyopathy were more likely to be malnourished at initiation of therapy.[60] The ability to overcome malnutrition is dependent upon the aggressiveness of the disease state as well as the forcefulness of the efforts at improving nutrition. In a 2004 review of studies on nutrition status and associated morbidities, Sala et al[58] reported that intervention with intravenous (IV) nutrition support and enteral supplementation resulted in better adherence to radiation and chemotherapy treatment schedules.

Selection of Nutrition Support Route

Oral Nutrition

Oral nutrition is important to continue to promote normalized and developmentally appropriate feeding for children and should be encouraged as much as is medically reasonable. Patients and families should be educated on the appropriate strategies to alter nutrient intake using modulars and supplements. Unfortunately many pediatric patients on oral diet alone have significant weight loss and muscle wasting[61,62] and need to be supported by other means.

Enteral Nutrition

Enteral tube feedings (TF) may significantly enhance a child's nutrition status during cancer therapy.[63] Selection of the correct formula must be determined in order to maximize nutrient intake. Though no large clinical trials have been conducted, research suggests that a calorie-concentrated formula may be more beneficial to malnourished patients receiving TF.[64] A pilot study regarding the use of TF to supplement or to provide full calories prior to developing weight loss showed an overall improvement of patient's nutrition status in children who were fed proactively at the end of therapy.[63] Feeds can be provided enterally via nasogastric, nasojejunal, or a percutaneous endoscopy gastrostomy (PEG) tube. Benefits of a PEG tube include a one-time placement in a location that is not apparent, which is especially important for an appearance-conscious adolescent. It also bypasses the issue of tube displacement with emesis and traumatic tube replacement during periods of mucositis. The placement of a prophylactic PEG tube prior to the initiation of radiation for head and neck cancers in adults has resulted in decreased incidence of morbidity related to weight loss.[5] This practice should be considered for pediatric patients because many radiation side effects in adults also appear in children. The downside of PEG tube is the requirement for procedural placement and a risk of cellulitis at the incision site.

Parenteral Nutrition

Parenteral nutrition (PN) support has been documented to increase patient's overall nutrition status, weight, and anthropometric measurements, but it has not improved clinical outcomes.[65,66] Though PN can provide short-term improvement, the effects often subside when the PN is discontinued.[13] PN may be necessary when children are unable to consume adequate calories for many days, such as with uncontrollable vomiting, typhlitis, severe mucositis, or intestinal obstruction.[67] Appendix 29-1 outlines intervention considerations for oral nutrition, enteral nutrition (EN), and PN.

Complementary and Alternative Medicine and Integrative Medicine

Patients and families of patients with chronic diseases often look to resources outside of conventional medicine for treatment. Complementary medicine is used in conjunction with conventional medicine, while alternative medicine replaces the Western approach. Integrative medicine combines standard care with complementary and alternative medicine (CAM) with a holistic focus on wellness rather than on the treatment of disease.[68] The use of CAM in pediatric oncology has been reported in up to 84% of patients in recent years,[68] and CAM has become much more mainstream.[69] In 2008 the American Academy of Pediatrics (AAP) published a policy statement on the use of CAM, noting its increasing popularity, delineating its many components, and identifying areas of concern relative to safety, lack of scientific data, and ethical/legal issues.[70] In 2001 the AAP Committee on Children with Disabilities published a statement on counseling parents who choose CAM therapies.[71]

Limited clinical trials exist on the use of CAM in the pediatric oncology population. Because of differences in metabolism and concerns of drug interactions and toxicity, children should not be placed on adult dosages of nutrition-related supplements. Further evaluation and clinical trials need to be conducted before CAM can be routinely recommended to patients, particularly those who are enrolled in clinical trials. Although mind–body interventions are likely to be low risk, many CAM therapies of interest to this population are ingested agents reputed to boost the immune system, manage treatment-related side effects (such as glutamine for mucositis), fight cancer, or provide nutrition support. The use of antioxidants during chemotherapy is one example of a CAM therapy that seems innocuous enough to parents but may in fact be detrimental for the child receiving certain chemotherapy agents or radiation therapy.[68,72]

Complications of Cancer Treatment

Anorexia or loss of appetite is a common side effect of cytotoxic therapy. Though typically seen as an independent symptom, many variables can cause anorexia. Weight loss, cachexia, dehydration, persistent vomiting, and early satiety can all cause anorexia in children. Anorexia may be perpetuated by multiple cycles of chemotherapy and other treatments.[31,73]

Children receiving chemotherapy are at an increased risk of developing infections. In critically ill adults, malnutrition has been shown to increase the risk of infection by 15%–20%.[33] The association between poor nutrition and infection has also been reported in children with cancer.[30] Nutrient metabolism and absorption can also be altered during infection due to increased production of catecholamines, cortisol, glucagon, and growth hormone.[74]

Mucositis, the inflammation of mucosal membranes lining the digestive tract, is a side effect of many chemotherapy agents and radiation. Mucositis can range in severity from mild erythema to extensive mucosal sloughing causing enteritis-related malabsorption. Oral mucositis can severely impact oral intake and limit the ability to place a nasogastric tube secondary to pain.[21,30] Supplementation with oral glutamine may help to prevent and decrease the severity of mucositis.[68,75,76]

Diarrhea causes a loss of fluids and electrolytes, as well as nutrient malabsorption, and can be linked directly to specific chemotherapies, radiation to the abdominal and pelvic areas, and abdominal surgery.[31,77] Other potential causes for diarrhea during therapy include infections, antibiotics, adverse drug effects, and stress. Malabsorption complicates the use of some nutrition interventions such as oral feeding and TF. When combined with limited nutrient intake, malabsorption can contribute to severe weight loss in a short period of time. Surgery may cause altered nutrient transit time, limiting the opportunity for intestinal absorption. As previously noted, chemotherapy and radiation therapy can lead to suboptimal absorption of nutrients. The decrease in saliva production during and after radiation to the head and neck results in a decrease in oral enzymes, which also exacerbates malabsorption. Late effects of radiation may include mucosal inflammation and intestinal fibrosis for an extended period post therapy that may not be reversible[22]; these conditions may contribute to long-term issues with nutrient malabsorption. Additional oral complications of head and neck radiation and certain chemotherapy agents include dysgeusia, anosmia, and xerostomia, which can significantly alter oral intake because of decreased palatability or decreased tolerance of certain textures. Though these complications generally subside, they can create long-standing food aversions.[17,78]

Gastroesophageal reflux (GER) can be seen in leukemia and lymphoma patients receiving high-dose steroids, patients with GI effects from anthracycline therapy or abdominal radiation, patients with little or no oral intake, and those whose systems are undergoing significant emotional and/or physical stress. The upper epigastric pain, nausea, "burning" or "sour" stomach or reflux can all result in decreased oral intake. Histamine-2 (H2) receptor antagonists or proton pump inhibitors (PPIs) are often used as GI protective agents, and pain medications are utilized as needed. There has been some concern about potential vitamin and mineral deficiency in patients receiving PPIs. While the reduction of gastric acid could limit its valuable role in aiding absorption of vitamins and minerals, children with untreated symptoms of GER are less likely to ingest adequate nutrients in the first place. In addition, most pediatric oncology patients are on PPIs for a relatively limited period of time, far shorter than the years reported in some studies of elderly patients.[79]

Hematopoietic Stem Cell Transplant

Hematopoietic stem cell transplantation (HSCT) is performed to replace diseased and defective bone marrow and restore hematopoietic and immunologic function following ultra-high-dose chemotherapy and/or radiation. HSCT is a broad category that encompasses bone marrow transplantation, peripheral blood stem cell transplantation, and umbilical cord blood transplantation, which are named for the source of hematopoietic stem cells. HSCT is a treatment option for children with a variety of potentially fatal malignant and nonmalignant diseases including certain types of cancers, immunodeficiency syndromes, severe aplastic anemia, Fanconi's anemia, and inherited metabolic disorders like Krabbe's disease and Hurler's syndrome among many others. Pediatric malignancies treated with HSCT include acute myeloid and lymphoblastic leukemia, Hodgkin's and non-Hodgkin's lymphoma, myelodysplastic syndrome, and some solid tumors like high-risk neuroblastoma and brain tumors.

HSCT can be autologous (the patient receives his or her own stem cells), allogeneic (the patient receives cells from another person who may be a sibling, parent [haploidentical], or unrelated donor), or syngeneic (the patient receives cells from his or her identical twin). Donors are selected on the basis of many factors including the level of human leukocyte antigen (HLA) matching. HLAs are genetically defined proteins or antigens that are highly polymorphic and are encoded by the major histocompatibility complex (MHC). Class I HLA (A, B, and C) antigens are expressed on almost all nucleated cells of the body. Class II proteins (DR, DQ, and DP) proteins are mainly expressed on hematopoietic cells (B cells, dendritic cells, and monocytes). HLA typing is currently performed by DNA-based methods. While full HLA matching can reduce the risk of certain types of complications, mismatched donors are appropriate and sometimes preferable in certain situations. Donor availability and clinical circumstances determine the source of the stem cells.[80] Information on types of transplants and their use has been published by the National Cancer Institute.[81]

Transplantation Process

1. *Conditioning:* The purpose of the conditioning regimen is to destroy the defective or diseased marrow, kill cancerous cells, create space for donor cells, and prevent rejection of donor cells by neutralizing the patient's immune system. Conditioning therapy (also known as cytoreduction or preparative regimen) consists of a combination of chemotherapy drugs with or without radiation and is given over a number of days prior to transplant. Two types of conditioning regimens are available: myeloablative and nonmyeloablative. The myeloablative regimen, also known as conventional conditioning, uses high-dose chemotherapy and/or total body irradiation to destroy or "fully ablate" the bone marrow. The high-dose chemotherapy and radiation causes acute and long-term toxicities including severe prolonged mucositis, myelosuppression, nausea, vomiting, and multi-organ toxicity. The nonmyeloablative, or reduced intensity conditioning, uses milder forms of chemotherapy and/or radiation and can be used in patients who would not tolerate or do not require a fully ablative transplant. Reduced-intensity transplants are utilized most frequently in patients with significant comorbidities and/or nonmalignant disorders.[82]

2. *Infusion:* After the completion of conditioning and usually 1 or 2 days of rest, the stem cells are infused via an IV catheter. It can take minutes to several hours to infuse the cells depending on the type of transplant, the donor source, and whether the product was previously frozen or required manipulation.

3. The conditioning regimen results in suppression or ablation of the bone marrow, causing a decrease in white blood cells, platelets, and red blood cells. This period of profound immunosuppression usually lasts for 2–4 weeks depending on the donor source, cell dose, and many other factors. During this period of pancytopenia, patients are at increased risk of infections. Prophylaxis against infections is commonly used. The patients also require frequent blood and platelet transfusions.

4. *Engraftment:* Engraftment is confirmed when absolute neutrophil count is > 500/mm³ for 3 consecutive days. Sometimes, it may take many weeks for cells to engraft. During this process, some patients may develop hyperacute graft-vs-host disease (GVHD), which is also called engraftment syndrome and is characterized by fever, rash, weight gain, and in some cases severe capillary leak and pulmonary edema.

5. *Post engraftment:* In this period of continuing recovery, patients are vulnerable to many complications such as acute GVHD, graft failure, organ toxicity, drug-related adverse reactions, and infections.

6. *Long term:* While most patients recover very well without major complications, they are at a risk of a number of long-term problems including delayed and slow growth and development, organ dysfunction, neurocognitive issues, endocrine problems, chronic GVHD, avascular necrosis, secondary malignancy, and others.

Nutrition Evaluation and Nutrient Requirements

Children undergoing HSCT are at increased risk of malnutrition, and it is critical to assess their needs, anticipate problems, and institute appropriate preventive nutrition support in a timely manner. The toxicity of the conditioning regimen affects the integrity of the GI tract, causing mucositis, nausea, vomiting, and diarrhea. These symptoms may be further exacerbated by post-transplant complications including GVHD, infection, and use of multiple antibiotics and immunosuppressive medications. These and other complexities of HSCT are important to understand. The nutrition status in some patients may be suboptimal due to previous treatments, prolonged hospitalizations, and other problems that have affected their ability to eat or drink well prior to HSCT. This is especially true for children with a diagnosis of AML or high-risk neuroblastoma. Fifty-four percent of pediatric patients undergoing HSCT were reported to have suboptimal nutrition status pretransplant, and impaired pretransplant nutrition status was a negative prognostic factor leading to delayed engraftment.[83] Prevention of malnutrition and preservation of nutrition status is vital for better transplant outcomes. A complete nutrition assessment should be performed at the beginning of transplant consultation and coordination. Many times a long period of time (several weeks to months) may elapse between coordination and admission for transplant, which can be used as an opportunity to prevent any further malnutrition and to prepare the patient for transplant. Nutrition status and nutrient needs continue to change throughout the transplant process, therefore assessment and evaluation are important during the transplant process. Refer to Table 29-5 for Components of Nutrition Assessment in General Oncology section.

Anthropometric Assessment

Weight, height, and BMI are generally a good indicator of nutrition status. These should be measured at the time of admission and throughout the recovery process. As previously discussed, z scores should also be used as an indicator of growth and nutrition status. Serial anthropometric measurements over a period of time are a good measure of long-term nutrition status. Growth charts should be maintained to help assess the growth velocity. However, during the transplant one should be careful about using weight and BMI as the sole criteria to assess changes in nutrition status. Body weight and BMI are affected by hydration, edema, and sinusoidal obstruction syndrome (SOS), which may occur in the early posttransplant period. Cheney et al[84] observed fluid shifts during the first 4 weeks after transplant and concluded that the change in body weight did not correlate with the body cell mass or fluid volume changes.

Calculated arm muscle area correlated well ($P < 0.05$) with changes in body cell mass and is a better reflection of nutrition status. BMI has been reported to be a poor predictor of nutrition status when compared with body cell mass.[83] Despite these limitations, serial height, weight, and BMI measurements combined with assessment of caloric and protein intake and fluid balance are critically important and useful. Weekly measurement of mid-upper arm circumference should be considered.

Energy and Protein Needs

Patients undergoing HSCT show changes in energy requirements throughout the process.[85-87] During the initial period, patients are in a hypermetabolic state with increased catabolism due to mucositis, fever, tissue repair, and marrow regeneration. Increase in the metabolic rate can also be caused by the conditioning regimen, fevers, and post-transplant complications.[85] As a result, the caloric needs of the HSCT patient have been reported to be as high as 150% of the basal

metabolic rate (BMR) of nonstressed, well-nourished patients and 180%–200% of the BMR of the malnourished patient.[88-90] On the other hand, Duro et al[87] observed significant decreases in resting energy expenditure (REE) following allogeneic stem cell transplant in patients with leukemia and aplastic anemia, with return of energy expenditure to pretransplant levels after engraftment. REE decreased by 4%–7% per week post transplant as measured by indirect calorimeter.[87] Duggan et al[86] also reported significant decline in REE after HSCT in pediatric patients, with some of the decrease being attributed to decrease in lean body mass. Studies assessing energy requirement in HSCT are limited, and further studies are needed to better determine the caloric needs of pediatric patients during and post transplant. Based on current literature, using a metabolic cart for assessing caloric requirement is the gold standard. In the absence of a metabolic cart, one should use clinical judgment while using the calorie calculation formula and continue to assess for potential overfeeding or underfeeding. Protein requirements are increased to minimize loss of lean body mass and promote tissue repair. Refer to Table 29-7 for the calorie and protein requirements of HSCT pediatric patient.

Requirements of the HSCT Patient

FLUID NEEDS

In general, daily fluid needs can be assessed using the Holiday Segar method.[91] However, one must take into consideration the various medical factors that impact daily fluid balance. Fluid need is increased with fever, GI losses (eg,

Table 29-7. Calorie and Protein Requirements of Pediatric Patient Undergoing Hematopoietic Stem Cell Transplantation[88,90,93]

AGE	CALORIES[a]	PROTEIN (G/KG/D)
0–12 mo	BMR × 1.6-1.8	3
1–6 y	BMR × 1.6-1.8	2.5–3
7–10 y	BMR × 1.4-1.6	2.4
11–14 y	BMR × 1.4-1.6	2
15–18 y	BMR × 1.5-1.6	1.8
> 19 y	BEE × 1.5	1.5

BEE, basal energy expenditure; BMR, basal metabolic rate; ht, height; wt, weight.

[a]For BMR equation, refer to Appendix 29-2. For the BEE equations:
male, 66 + (13.7 × wt in kg) + (5 × ht) - (6.8 × age);
female, 665 + (9.6 × wt in kg) + (1.7 × ht) - (4.7 × age).

vomiting, diarrhea), mucositis, open skin wounds, and other factors.[88] Liver and kidney dysfunction may lead to fluid retention and may require fluid restriction. In addition to PN and oral or enteral intake, patients can receive significant additional fluid with medications and blood products. Close monitoring of fluid status is very important.

VITAMIN AND MINERAL NEEDS

Vitamin and mineral requirements for patients undergoing HSCT have not been determined. The nutrition support regimen should meet 100% of the dietary reference intake of vitamins and minerals or 100% of the age-appropriate injectable multivitamin for patients receiving PN. If oral intake or EN support does not meet the vitamin and mineral needs, then an iron-free multivitamin and mineral supplement should be provided. Generally, iron supplementation is not required in HSCT patients because they receive frequent blood transfusions and often experience iron overload from these transfusions. The risk of vitamin and mineral deficiency is higher if the patient has diarrhea, vomiting, and malabsorption. Thiamine, vitamin K, vitamin D, calcium, and zinc deficiency have been noted in pediatric HSCT patients. Vitamin K deficiency as determined by Proteins Induced by Vitamin K Absence level (PIVKA-II) was reported in 31% of pediatric patients undergoing HCST and was attributed to use of phenytoin, inadequate intake, or malabsorption.[92] The authors did not find a correlation between prothrombin time and vitamin K status. However, in clinical practice, prolonged prothrombin time may be an indicator of significant vitamin K deficiency, unless liver dysfunction is present, and can guide vitamin K therapy. Antibiotic use has been shown to decrease the production of vitamin K in the body. HSCT patients receive multiple antibiotic treatments post transplant; therefore, vitamin K supplementation of 1 mg/kg should be provided weekly.[88,93] In patients with severe chronic diarrhea, zinc losses may be significant and supplementation may be necessary.

Patients undergoing HSCT often receive multiple agents that alter bone metabolism as part of their treatment. These include methotrexate, steroids, cyclosporine, and total body irradiation. For many patients, physical activity and exposure to sun are very limited and can lead to additional nutrition problems such as osteopenia, vitamin D deficiency, and eventually poor bone health. Therefore serum vitamin D should be routinely monitored as vitamin D 25-OH levels and supplemented. Serum calcium will be maintained by losses from bone so levels may look normal despite bone losses. Supplemental calcium should be encouraged for all patients before, during, and after HSCT. For further information on bone health, refer to the Late Effects of Treatment in Survivorship section.

Provision of Nutrition Support

Oral Route

High-dose chemotherapy and post-transplant complications lead to anorexia, mucositis, nausea, vomiting, taste changes, and diarrhea, causing poor oral intake and malabsorption. Chemotherapy drugs like busulfan, melphalan, cyclophosphamide, methotrexate, carboplatin, and most others can cause taste changes. The etiology of taste changes in HSCT may be multifactorial, including mucositis, hyposalivation, and side effects of medications such as antibiotics and antihypertensive, antidepressant, and many chemotherapeutic agents.[94]

About one-third of patients receiving chemotherapy and/or radiation demonstrate food aversion. Patients learn to avoid foods that remind them of the uncomfortable feeling of nausea and vomiting.[95] Oral intake and appetite in HSCT patient does not return to a normal state until they are 4–6 weeks post-transplant.[96] Severity of oral mucositis and GVHD are the most significant factors affecting return of oral intake.[89] Use of appetite stimulants may be useful to help stimulate appetite in patients who have engrafted and do not have GVHD.

Sometimes even after return of oral intake, nutrition status may be compromised due to malabsorption. A complete GI work-up to rule out fat and carbohydrate malabsorption, pancreatic insufficiency, and bacterial overgrowth may be warranted in infants and toddlers with food aversion. Feeding, speech, and occupational therapy should be considered. Refeeding a child after HSCT is a slow process and needs careful monitoring of symptoms and ongoing assessment of nutrition status.

Diet Restrictions

Many patients become lactose intolerant due to mucositis, therefore a low-lactose diet is recommended. Yogurt is usually well tolerated since some of the lactose is digested by the bacteria in yogurt. Cheese is also well tolerated since the lactose content is reduced. Many lactose-free and lactose-reduced products are available, or patients can take tablets prior to ingesting lactose-containing foods. It is important for patients to gradually increase their lactose intake to stimulate the production of lactase and to avoid problems associated with lactose intolerance such as diarrhea, bloating, and gas.

Studies have shown inconsistent results regarding the effect of dietary modification on the incidence of food-borne illness during HSCT.[97,98] For this reason, some centers use a more liberal approach to dietary restrictions, emphasizing safe food handling, and allowing patients to eat a greater variety of foods (such as well-washed fresh fruits and vegetables) not traditionally included in a neutropenic diet.[99,100] Some institutions still utilize a neutropenic or low bacteria diet in the post-transplant period. The goal of a neutropenic diet is to restrict foods that are believed to contain large amounts of potentially pathogenic bacteria, which can cause infections in the immuno-compromised patient. Such food items include nonpasteurized dairy products; aged cheeses; unwashed fresh fruits and vegetables; deli meats and cheeses; deli-type salads (eg, potato salad, egg salad, tuna salad, and pasta salads); undercooked meat, poultry, egg, fish, and seafood; food with visible mold; salad dressings made with eggs and moldy cheeses; and bakery food products.[90] *Listeria monocytogenes, Escherichia coli, Salmonella* spp., *Cryptosporidium parvum,* and *Campylobacter* spp. are the most common pathogens that cause food-borne illness. Signs and symptoms of a food-borne illness include stomach ache, abdominal pain, diarrhea, nausea, vomiting, headache, fever, and chills.[101]

Enteral Nutrition

Benefits of EN in protecting the gut integrity, preventing bacterial translocation, and being cost effective are well known. However, enteral feeding has not been the norm for most pediatric HSCT patients mainly because of concern for risk of bleeding with tube placement in the presence of pancytopenia and mucositis and due to concerns about delayed gastric emptying and malabsorption of nutrients.[89,102] In 3 small studies involving a total of 138 patients, enteral feeding was found to be not only feasible and cost effective, but also as successful as PN in preserving the nutrition status of children undergoing allogeneic HSCT.[103–105] In an earlier study, Papadopoulou et al[106] reported that EN, when tolerated, is beneficial and prevents the deterioration of nutrition status of pediatric patients undergoing HSCT. EN may be attempted if no active pathology is present in the GI tract and continued if the patient is able to tolerate it. In case of intolerance, it may be possible to modify the formula and tube placement. For example, nasoduodenal or nasojejunal tubes may present a lower risk of vomiting and aspiration.[107] Please refer to

Appendix 29-1 in making decisions regarding type of tube, delivery system, and formula selection.

Parenteral Nutrition

In the setting of GI toxicities leading to poor oral intake and intolerance to EN, PN has been used to support patients after HSCT. Roberts and Thompson[96] reported no difference in length of stay, engraftment time, days to resume oral intake, and rate of infection in patients who received PN vs patients on an oral diet. They concluded that prophylactic use of PN results in improved nutrition status and does not affect time to resume oral intake. Although an older study, Charuhas and Gautier[93] found that patients who were randomized to PN resumed oral intake 6 days later than an IV hydration group. The IV hydration group experienced 1.14% weight loss, and there was no difference observed in readmission, relapse, or survival rates.

Reported benefits of PN include reversal of protein-energy malnutrition, restoration of immune competence, and enhanced tolerance to antineoplastic therapy.[90] However, use of PN is associated with increased risk for several complications including line infections, hyperglycemia, hypertriglyceridemia, and cholestasis.[88] Patients who present with compromised nutrition status prior to transplant are at risk of refeeding syndrome when nutrition support is initiated. If a patient is at high risk for refeeding syndrome, nutrition support should be slowly advanced to meet goal energy requirements.[108,109] As with any patient receiving PN, the patient should be monitored closely and the nutrition support regimen adjusted accordingly. Since most studies have been done on heterogeneous patient populations with regard to type of transplant, diagnosis, type of conditioning regimen, age, and pretransplant nutrition status and had small sample sizes, no established criteria exist as to when PN should be initiated. Based on our clinical experience PN should be initiated after transplant for pediatric patients who receive myeloablative conditioning regimens, who are expected to have severe mucositis, or who had poor nutrition status prior to transplant. However, patients with nonmyeloablative conditioning regimens, with minimal or no mucositis and adequate nutrition status prior to transplant, may be placed on oral nutrition or EN. Clinical judgment about the type of nutrition support should not only include the specifics of patient population but also the risk and benefits of PN.

Nutrition Monitoring During HSCT

Monitoring and evaluating the efficacy of nutrition support in patients undergoing HSCT is very important and involves a complex process. However, data are scarce to support the use of a single specific test or a battery of tests that could be used broadly in most clinical situations. This section will examine the published data on various measures of nutrition assessment.

Fluid and Electrolyte

Multiple factors, including the type and quantity of feeding, impact fluid and electrolyte status. Decisions about the volume and composition of EN or PN must be based on the state of fluid and electrolyte balance, which must be monitored daily in this population. Mucositis, diarrhea, vomiting, excessive salivation, fever, and other factors increase fluid losses. However, fluid retention is commonly seen at the time of engraftment. Other problems, including SOS and renal insufficiency, may also cause fluid retention and electrolyte problems. Severe inflammatory reactions in the posttransplant period may lead to capillary leak and "third-spacing" of fluids. In such a situation the weight may be increased, but the intravascular compartment is depleted. Many drugs such as tacrolimus, cyclosporine, amphotericin, and ifosfamide cause

increased urinary losses of electrolytes requiring increased supplementation. See Table 29-8 for side effects of some of the drugs commonly used in HSCT. In general one should monitor basic biochemical indices like sodium, potassium, chloride, blood urea nitrogen, creatinine, glucose, calcium, phosphorus, and magnesium. See Table 29-9 for the suggested schedule for monitoring of biochemical indices.

Triglycerides and Liver Function Tests

Fasting triglyceride levels should be obtained prior to administration of intravenous fat emulsion (IVFE), and nonfasting levels weekly for the duration of the IVFE therapy. Serum triglyceride levels should be monitored weekly if a patient is receiving cyclosporine, corticosteroids, tacrolimus, or sirolimus, all of which can affect levels.[88,93,102] Liver function tests should also be monitored 2–3 times per week because they may fluctuate significantly during transplant.

Micronutrients

Copper, selenium, and manganese levels should be monitored monthly if a patient has been receiving PN containing

Table 29-8. Side Effects of Some of the Drugs Commonly Used During Hematopoietic Stem Cell Transplantation

DRUG	USAGE	SIDE EFFECT
Steroids	Immunosuppressive	Hyperglycemia, weight gain, osteoporosis, fluid and sodium retention, cardiomyopathy, hypercholesterolemia, hypertriglyceridemia, gut infection
Methotrexate	Immunosuppressive	Mucositis, nausea, vomiting, diarrhea, hepatic and renal toxicities
Cyclosporine	Immunosuppressive	Hypertension, nephrotoxicity, significant hyperkalemia, hypomagnesemia, hepatotoxicity, hyperglycemia, hyperlipidemia, hypercholesterolemia, nausea, vomiting
Tacrolimus	Immunosuppressive	Hypertension, nephrotoxicity, hyperkalemia, hypomagnesemia, hyperbilirubinemia, hypercalcemia, hypercholesterolemia, hyperglycemia, hyperlipidemia, hyperphosphatemia, hypocalcemia, hypokalemia, hypomagnesemia, hyponatremia, hypophosphatemia, elevated hepatic enzymes, nausea/vomiting, anorexia, diarrhea
Sirolimus	Immunosuppressive	Edema, hyperlipidemia, hypercholesterolemia
Cellcept	Immunosuppressive	Nausea, vomiting, diarrhea, anorexia, renal impairment, neutropenia
Antithymocyte globulin (ATG)	Immunosuppressive	Infusion reactions, increased infection risk, hypotension, nausea, vomiting
Acyclovir	Antiviral	Nephrotoxicity, anorexia, nausea, vomiting, diarrhea, elevated hepatic enzymes, hyperbilirubinemia
Cefepime	Antibiotic	Nausea, vomiting, diarrhea
Amikacin	Antibiotic	Nephrotoxicity
Gentamicin	Antibiotic	Nephrotoxicity
Voriconazole	Antifungal	Hepatotoxicity, skin rash, visual problems
Amphotericin	Antifungal	Nephrotoxicity
Micafungin	Antifungal	Hepatotoxic

Data from Clinical Pharmacology [database online]. Tampa, FL: Gold Standard, Inc; 2009. Accessed December 2014.

Table 29-9. Suggested Schedule for Monitoring Blood Biochemical and Other Indices During Early Stages of Hematopoietic Stem Cell Transplantation

LABORATORY TEST	FREQUENCY
Sodium, potassium, chloride, carbonate, BUN, creatinine, calcium, magnesium	Every day until stable on PN, then 3 times per week while on long-term PN
Phosphorus	3 times per week until stable on PN, then weekly
Ionized calcium	With consistent low-serum calcium
LFTs, albumin, total bilirubin	3 times per week until day +30, then weekly while on PN
Prothrombin time	Weekly while on multiple antibiotics
Vitamin D (25 OH D_2 + D_3)	Pretransplant; then every 3 mo until 1 y
Zinc	When increased losses suspected
Manganese, copper, selenium	Monthly when on long-term PN (4–6 wk)
Triglycerides	Weekly while on intravenous lipid emulsion
Weights	Daily while inpatient, then with every outpatient visit
Input/output	Daily while inpatient

BUN, blood urea nitrogen; LFT, liver function tests; PN, parenteral nutrition.

multitrace element solution for more than 1 month, or in the presence of hyperbilirubinemia.[88,93,110] If zinc supplementation is implemented, zinc levels (ie, serum or plasma zinc) should be monitored. However, zinc levels in blood are adversely affected by inflammation or infection so this should be taken into account when interpreting results and should be based on normal ranges for the age and institution. Clinical discretion should be used when evaluating zinc levels, keeping in mind that zinc levels in blood do not reflect tissue stores.

Other Biochemical Indices

While low serum albumin is predictive of an increase in mortality, poor outcome, complication rate, and length of stay and may be low in severe and chronic malnutrition, it is not a good marker of acute nutrition status.[111] Nitrogen balance may be useful to assess protein status, but the accuracy of calculation is compromised in patients with vomiting, diarrhea, and renal insufficiency, and 24-hour urine collections may be difficult. Serum transferrin, prealbumin, and retinol binding protein are also poor indicators of nutrition

status.[111] During inflammatory states, their hepatic synthesis is decreased by as much as 25%, and their intravascular concentration is reduced due to capillary leak.[112] Other factors such as hydration, infection, and liver and renal insufficiency also affect their levels.

Growth

Weight trends should be monitored daily, as well as intake and output, throughout the entire transplant period.[88] Length should be monitored monthly, but one should be mindful that critically ill transplant patients will likely not attain age-expected linear velocity, despite provision of optimal nutrition support. Although weight fluctuates with fluid shifts, one study revealed that weight decreased overall and height increased slowly (1.7 cm/mo) 4 months post transplant.[113] The same study showed that triceps skinfold measurements (TSF) and mid upper arm circumference also decreased. Therefore, TSF should be obtained and monitored. Fluid shifts will not affect skinfold measurement.[113] Bone growth can be monitored by obtaining dual energy X-Ray absorptiometry (DEXA) scan biannually.[114]

HSCT Complications Impacting Nutrition

Pediatric patients undergoing HSCT are at significant risk for developing many complications that may have direct and indirect impacts on the nutrition status. The most important complications are described in the following sections.

Mucositis

Mucositis, or inflammation and breakdown of the mucosal lining of the mouth and gut, may occur in up to 100% of patients undergoing HSCT with high-dose chemotherapy.[115] The severity depends on many factors including the type and dose intensity of chemotherapy and use of concomitant radiation.[116] Mucositis causes severe pain that often necessitates IV narcotics. In the presence of moderate and severe mucositis, oral intake is nearly impossible, and PN is utilized until the GI tract can be used again.

Graft-vs-Host Disease

GVHD is caused by an immunologic reaction in which donor-derived T cells recognize the host cells as foreign and attack them. Generally, acute GVHD occurs before 100 days post-transplant and chronic GVHD develops after more than 100 days from transplant. This definition/classification has been revised by the National Institutes of Health to include late-onset acute GVHD (after day 100) and an overlap syndrome with features of both acute and chronic GVHD.[117,118] Immunosuppressive drug combinations are used to prevent GVHD. Calcineurin inhibitors (cyclosporine, tacrolimus) are generally used with methotrexate, mycophenolate, steroids, or sirolimus. High-dose steroids are used to treat acute GVHD.[119] For treating chronic GVHD, steroids are used with or without calcineurin inhibitors.[120]

Acute GVHD. The organs most commonly affected in acute GVHD are the skin (81%), GI tract (54%), and liver (50%).[121] Skin GVHD usually presents first as a rash. Symptoms of acute GI GVHD include nausea, vomiting, loss of appetite, abdominal pain, and secretory diarrhea, which is voluminous (> 2 L/d) in severe cases.[122] GI GVHD most commonly affects the lower GI tract and causes severe, high-output diarrhea associated with bleeding and cramping abdominal pain.[123] GVHD of the upper GI tract causes decreased appetite, nausea, and vomiting.[102] Continuing GVHD leads to mucosal degeneration, malabsorption, and protein loss. Liver GVHD is characterized by cholestasis. However, it can be difficult to differentiate other causes of liver function impairment, and the differential diagnosis include SOS, infection, sepsis, medication toxicity, hepatic iron overload, or PN–associated cholestasis.[122] Acute GVHD is graded based on the extent of skin, liver, and gut involvement (see Table 29-10 for staging and grading). Five-year survival for patients with grade III GVHD is 25% and grade IV is 5%.[124] Prevalence of acute GVHD varies from 35% to 45% in full-matched sibling donors to 60%–80% in patients with one antigen HLA mismatched transplant.[125] With the same degree of HLA mismatch patients receiving umbilical cord blood transplant have a lower frequency of acute GVHD (35%–65% compared with 60%–80% in patients receiving unrelated donor graft).[126]

Chronic GVHD. Chronic GVHD involves skin, GI tract, liver, lungs, eyes, mouth, and bone marrow. About 22%–29% of pediatric patients undergoing HSCT will develop chronic GVHD.[127] Symptoms of chronic gut GVHD may be similar to those of acute GVHD, or may be more subtle (early satiety, strictures, etc). Risk factors for development of chronic GVHD are multifactorial but include history of acute GVHD. A low-fiber, low-lactose, low-fat, bland diet may be necessary during periods of acute GVHD, but use of this dietary modification is not the norm.[90] PN and sometimes nothing by mouth are warranted when diarrheal output worsens with ingestion of food and EN.

Pancreatic Insufficiency

If diarrhea continues in the absence of GVHD, patients should be evaluated for pancreatic insufficiency.[128] Almost 5% of pediatric patients undergoing HSCT were found to have acute pancreatitis possibly due to prior chemotherapy agents such as asparaginase or use of high dose steroids in transplant.[126]

Table 29-10. Staging and Grading of Acute Graft vs Host Disease (Seattle Criteria)

Stage	Skin*	Liver bilirubin	Gut^#
+	Maculopapular rash < 25% body surface	2–3 mg/dL	Diarrhea, 500–1000 mL/d or persistent nausea
++	Maculopapular rash 25–50% body surface	3–6 mg/dL	Diarrhea, 1000–1500 mL/d
+++	Generalized erythroderma	6–15 mg/dL	Diarrhea, > 1500mL/d
++++	Desquamation and bullae	> 15 mg/dL	Abdominal pain with or without ileus

*Use "rule of nines" or burn chart to determine extent of rash.
^ Diarrhea volumes apply to adults.
# Persistent nausea requires endoscopic biopsy evidence of GVHD histology in the stomach or duodenum.

Overall Grade	Skin	Liver	Gut	Functional Impairment
0 (none)	0	0	0	0
I (mild)	+ to ++	0	0	0
II (moderate)	+ to +++	+	+	+
III (severe)	++ to +++	++ to +++	++ to +++	++
IV (Life threatening)	+ to ++++	++ to ++++	++ to ++++	+++

Reprinted with permission from Sullivan KM. Graft-vs-host disease. In: *Thomas' Hematopoietic Cell Transplantation.* 3rd ed. Blackwell Publishing; 2004:635–664.

Bacterial Overgrowth

Bacterial overgrowth has not been well studied and defined in this group of patients. If diarrhea continues after GVHD and infection and pancreatic insufficiency are ruled out, the patient should be evaluated for bacterial overgrowth. Long-term use of antibiotics and inability to take oral diet for prolonged periods after HSCT can alter the type and quantity of bacterial flora.

Infection

The immunocompromised patient is highly susceptible to bacterial, viral, and fungal infections. *Clostridium difficile* is one of the common infections identified in the transplant population.[129] Some of the viral infections known to cause diarrhea in HSCT patients are adenovirus, cytomegalovirus, and rotavirus.[130] Infections affecting the GI tract can lead to intolerance of oral intake and EN. Antiviral, antifungal, and antibiotic medications can cause loss of appetite, nausea, vomiting, diarrhea, and malabsorption. Antibiotic medications may also decrease the amount of lactase enzyme in the intestine; if symptomatic, these patients may benefit from a low-lactose diet.[131,132]

Hemorrhagic Cystitis

Hemorrhagic cystitis is defined as sustained hematuria and lower urinary tract symptoms such as urgency, frequency, and dysuria in the absence of other causative conditions. The incidence of hemorrhagic cystitis has been reported to be as high as 15% in matched-related donor transplants, 30% in mismatched related donor transplants, and 40% in matched-unrelated or umbilical cord blood donor transplants. Certain types of viral infections, such as human herpes virus 6, and cyclophosphamide and ifosfamide used during the preparative regimen are common causes of cystitis. Hemorrhagic cystitis causes significant morbidity, may lead to renal complications and prolonged hospitalizations, and occasionally contributes to transplant-related mortality. Management tends to consist of hyperhydration, analgesia, transfusions, and treatment of any underlying infection.[133]

Hepatic Sinusoidal Obstructive Syndrome

SOS (formerly called hepatic veno-occlusive disease) typically presents between 1 and 4 weeks post transplant and reflects regimen-related toxicity.[134] Severe SOS leading to liver failure, hepatorenal syndrome, and multiorgan failure is associated with a high mortality rate. Injury to the endothelial cells of the sinusoids, thickening of the hepatic venules due to edema, and deposition of fibrin, factor VII, and blood cell fragments lead to narrowing and increased resistance to the blood flow through the venules. This causes hepatic congestion and portal hypertension.[135] Weight gain, hyperbilirubinemia, ascites, right upper quadrant pain, and hepatomegaly are the clinical symptoms associated with SOS. Preexisting liver dysfunction, prior transplantation, abdominal radiation, and certain types of conditioning regimens are among the factors that increase the risk for SOS.[136] A commonly used agent in the treatment of SOS, Defibrotide, is available at many US transplant centers through an expanded access program overseen by the National Institutes of Health (http://www.clinicaltrials.gov).[137]

HSCT Management

Nutrition assessment, support, and monitoring during the transplant process are a critical part of patient management. These measures are even more important in pediatric patients because of their small size, need for continuing growth and development, and potential for rapid deterioration. Comprehensive assessment may include information about anthropometrics, food intake, appetite, presence of infection, organ dysfunction, wounds, nausea, vomiting, diarrhea, and mucositis as well as other factors. Good clinical judgment is critical, and decision making should be individualized in an effort to provide optimal nutrition management. It is also important to further examine the cost and other factors affecting the nutrition outcomes.

Gastrointestinal Supportive Care Medications

Motility Agents

Motility agents such as metoclopramide and erythromycin have historically had numerous uses, including to aid nasogastric intubations, and for gastroparesis, GER, and intolerance to feedings. Today they are used less frequently but may benefit some patients.

Metoclopramide

Metoclopramide (Reglan) blocks dopamine and at higher doses, 5-hydroxytryptamine-3 (5HT3, serotonin) receptors. Its effects on motility may involve increased release of acetylcholine in the gut. The effect on the gut is increased forward peristalsis in the stomach and duodenum. Metoclopramide has been used for these indications and at higher doses for chemotherapy-induced nausea and vomiting. Data confirming the clinical utility vary with the indication. For chemotherapy-induced nausea and vomiting, combinations of high-dose metoclopramide with dexamethasone and either diphenhydramine or lorazepam were demonstrated to be effective in the 1980s, but serotonin receptor antagonists such as ondansetron have been shown to be superior. Metoclopramide is typically effective in aiding intubations for patients with slow gastric motility and for gastroparesis. Data proving utility in pediatric patients with GER or feeding intolerance are harder to find.[138] However, the value of these potential uses has to be weighed against the potential adverse reactions in children. Children are known to be more sensitive to extrapyramidal side effects of metoclopramide. Diphenhydramine (Benadryl) is effective at preventing or treating dystonias, while lorazepam is often more effective at reducing akathisias.[139] While akathisias and dystonias are generally easily reversed, a few reports describe tardive dyskinesias causing long-term movement disorders.[138] In February of 2009, the Food and Drug Administration (FDA) added a "black box warning" in the labeling regarding the risk of tardive dyskinesia with higher doses or long-term use of metoclopramide. Manufacturers must implement a risk evaluation and mitigation strategy to ensure patients receive a medication guide discussing the risk.[140] The package insert for metoclopramide recommends a maximum of 12 weeks continuous use and does not recommend use in children. The FDA and package insert warnings have greatly reduced any use of metoclopramide in children. The major drug interactions involving metoclopramide relate to its ability to speed transit through the gut. Drugs that are designed for sustained release or that have slow dissolution and absorption may have reduced absorption while a patient is on metoclopramide. Other drugs such as tacrolimus and cyclosporine may have increased absorption when a patient is on metoclopramide.[140] Doses of metoclopramide should be reduced in patients with renal dysfunction.

Erythromycin

Erythromycin is a macrolide antibiotic, but it also is a motilin receptor agonist that increases proximal gut motility.[138,141] Prokinetic effects are evident at doses as low as 4–12 mg/kg/d as compared with the 30–50 mg/kg/d used for antimicrobial effects. Numerous studies suggest activity of erythromycin for improving feeding tolerance in children.[138,141] Typical problems with antimicrobial doses of erythromycin include GI upset, diarrhea, and inhibition of CYP450 (cytochrome P450) 1A2 and 3A4 enzymes causing drug interactions, but these effects are less likely at the lower doses used for motility. Rare ad-

verse effects of erythromycin include hepatotoxicity, ototoxicity, cardiac arrhythmias, and pyloric stenosis.[141] The latter has been reported mostly in infants < 2 weeks old. A theoretical concern is the potential for low-dose antibiotics to result in resistance among bacteria, although this has not been documented with the use of erythromycin at motility dosing.

Acid-Blocker Medications

H2 receptor antagonists and PPIs are commonly used agents for GER disease, gastritis, and ulcer treatment in adults and children. Although antacids or sucralfate may be reasonable for short-term use in pediatrics, the aluminum that can be absorbed from sucralfate and some antacids contraindicates long-term use.

H2 Receptor Antagonists

H2 receptor antagonists (eg, famotidine, rantidine, nizatidine, cimetidine) block histamine-induced acid secretion. Higher doses of H2 receptor antagonists block acid secretion better than lower doses, although PPIs block acid secretion better than high doses of H2 receptor antagonists.[142–144] Adverse effects are uncommon but include headaches, sedation, and GI side effects. Cimetidine may inhibit the metabolism of some drugs, but other H2 receptor antagonists are not likely to affect drug metabolism. Any of these drugs may alter the absorption of other drugs that are sensitive to higher gastric pH (eg, ketoconazole, itraconazole, ampicillin). All 4 H2 receptor antagonists require reduced doses in patients with renal impairment. H2 receptor antagonists are available as nonprescription formulations.

Proton Pump Inhibitors

PPIs (eg, omeprazole, lansoprazole, pantoprazole, esomeprazole, rabeprazole, Dexlansoprazole) block hydrogen/potassium ATPase (the "proton pump"), effectively blocking acid secretion induced by virtually all stimuli. As with H2 receptor antagonists, adverse effects are rare but include headaches and GI effects such as abdominal pain, constipation, or diarrhea. Rare reported side effects of PPIs include bone fractures, increased risk of enteric infections (*Clostridium difficile*), vitamin B12 or iron malabsorption, hypomagnesemia, and rebound hypersecretion of gastric acid.[145] Altered absorption of other drugs can occur due to elevated gastric pH. Before initiating a PPI, interaction with other drugs commonly used in cancer patients should be considered due to their inhibition of CYP450 enzymes.

Competitive inhibition leads to reduced clearance of drugs such as azole class antifungal agents, methotrexate, dasatinib, warfarin, and GVHD prophylaxis medications such as cyclosporine and tacrolimus.[146,147] PPIs work best when administered 30 minutes before a meal.[148] Administration of lansoprazole or omeprazole through an nasogastric tube is best accomplished by either using the lansoprazole oral disintegrating tablets, or mixing the enteric coated granules from the lansoprazole or omeprazole capsule or packet for suspension in 8.4% sodium bicarbonate solution (1 mEq/mL parenteral solutions are generally used for this).[149,150] These formulations are less viscous and appear to flow through tubes better. An alternative is mixing the granules from the capsules with an acidic fruit juice, which preserves the enteric coating until the granules reach the alkaline contents of the small intestine; however, the mixture may not flow through the tube very well. IV formulations are available for pantoprazole, lansoprazole, and esomeprazole. Dosage guidelines are not available, but doses may need to be reduced in patients with significant hepatic impairment. Omeprazole, lansoprazole, and esomeprazole are available as nonprescription drugs.

Antiemetics

Antiemetics in pediatric oncology patients are used primarily for nausea and vomiting due to chemotherapy, radiation, and surgery/anesthesia. Serotonin receptor antagonists and dopamine blockers are generally useful for all 3 etiologies. Other drugs discussed here are mostly used for chemotherapy-induced nausea and vomiting. The most recent American Society of Clinical Oncology antiemetic guidelines include suggestions regarding radiation-induced emesis.[139] The National Comprehensive Cancer Network publishes emesis guidelines (updated annually) on its website,[151] and the Multinational Association of Supportive Care in Cancer (MASCC) also has published guidelines on the Internet.[152] All of these guidelines currently divide chemotherapy drugs into classes that have high, moderate, low, or minimal likelihood of causing emesis. Combinations of a serotonin receptor antagonist with a steroid and aprepitant (Emend) are recommended for highly emetic chemotherapy regimens by all guidelines. Combinations of a serotonin receptor antagonist and a steroid are generally recommended for moderately emetic regimens, a single agent (often steroids or a serotonin receptor antagonist) for low emetogenicity, and antiemetics only "as needed" for minimally emetic regimens. Conditioning regimens for hematopoietic cell transplants are frequently highly emetic.

Serotonin Receptor antagonists

Serotonin receptors (ie, 5HT3) antagonists (ondansetron, granisetron, dolasetron, palonosetron) block the effects of serotonin at the 5HT3 receptors in the GI tract and the chemotherapy receptor trigger zone in the brain. They are generally better at reducing vomiting than at reducing nausea.[153] Used in equivalent doses, these agents do not differ much from each other, although palonosetron has a longer duration of activity, apparently due to its tighter receptor binding and longer half-life. Palonosetron may therefore be better at preventing delayed nausea and vomiting, although most studies have compared it to a single dose of the shorter-acting agents, which are more likely to be used daily. The oral route of administration is equally effective as the IV route, as long as the patient is not actively vomiting. Recently, all antiemetic guidelines have dropped serotonin receptor antagonists from their recommended drugs to treat delayed nausea and vomiting (more than 24 hours after chemotherapy) due to the minimal evidence for their efficacy.[154] The most likely adverse effects with serotonin receptor antagonists are headaches, or constipation with multiple-day use.[153] Prolongation of the QTc interval has been reported with this class of drugs, which is concerning when used with other medication that can prolong QTc. The dolasetron package insert contains a warning regarding use in patients at increased risk of arrhythmias, and dolasetron is not approved for use in children in Canada due to reports of cardiovascular adverse effects (arrhythmias, cardiovascular arrest).[155] Doses of IV ondansetron are also recommended to be given over at least 2–5 minutes to reduce the potential risk of QTc prolongation. Patients who have received therapy with cisplatin, ifosfamide, or anthracyclines (doxorubicin, daunorubicin, idarubicin, epirubicin, mitoxantrone) are at the greatest risk for cardiovascular side effects. Cisplatin and ifosfamide cause electrolyte abnormalities due to renal tubular losses of calcium, magnesium, potassium, phosphate, and bicarbonate, which can impact cardiac function. Oral supplementation of these electrolytes can be challenging due to taste, quantity required, irritation to the stomach, and poor absorption. Anthracyclines and mitoxantrone cause damage to cardiac myofibrils that may result in heart failure for some patients. This is more common at cumulative lifetime doses > 300 mg/m^2 for younger children and 450–550 mg/m^2 for older children and adults. Ondansetron has a prolonged half-life in patients with severe liver impairment and doses should be reduced. Palonosetron, dolasetron, and granisetron do not need dose adjustments in renal or hepatic dysfunction.[155]

Aprepitant

Aprepitant (Emend and fosaprepitant [IV Emend]) is a neurokinin-1 receptor antagonist (its ligand is substance P) that has been found to produce a small reduction in acute nausea and vomiting, but a larger reduction in delayed nausea and vomiting. The FDA-approved oral dosing is for the first 3 days of the chemotherapy regimen, combined with a serotonin receptor antagonist and a steroid, but not as a single agent. Fosaprepitant is the same drug in an IV formulation that can be given to adults as a 150-mg dose only on day 1 of chemotherapy. Until 2008, only the oral formulation was available and therefore the drug was difficult to administer to most children. Although adolescents are often large enough to be dosed as adults, children have been less frequently treated with aprepitant. A potential problem with aprepitant is its ability to inhibit CYP450 microsomal enzymes and reduce metabolism of other drugs. Dexamethasone doses of approximately 12 mg with aprepitant are equivalent to 20 mg without aprepitant. Warfarin doses also require reduction. Theoretical concern exists that some chemotherapy drugs may have reduced clearance when patients take aprepitant, but currently little data suggest clinical problems with this potential interaction. Regardless, it is important to only use aprepitant for highly emetic regimens as indicated in current practice guidelines and to use caution when concomitant chemotherapy agents are known to be metabolized by hepatic CYP450 enzymes.

Glucocorticoids

Steroids have been used as antiemetics since the early 1980s, but it is still not clear how they work. The agents are used mostly in combinations with a serotonin receptor antagonist or metoclopramide, but can be used as single agents for mildly emetic regimens. Steroids are used less frequently in hematologic malignancies for nausea because they are often part of the therapeutic regimen. Glucocorticoids (dexamethasone [Decadron], methylprednisolone sodium succinate [Medrol]) have a long list of adverse effects, but the ones most commonly seen with short-term use are hyperglycemia, GI upset, hypertension, and mental or behavioral changes. Doses should be reduced when used with aprepitant, as previously mentioned.

Phenothiazines

Phenothiazines (eg, prochlorperazine, promethazine, chlorpromazine) and butyrophenones (haloperidol, droperidol) block dopamine receptors in the vomiting center and chemotherapy receptor trigger zone. These agents are currently recommended for acute nausea and vomiting from mildly to moderately emetic chemotherapy regimens or for breakthrough nausea and vomiting. Prochlorperazine and promethazine have been used for delayed nausea and vomiting with some success. Potential side effects include sedation, anticholinergic effects such as urinary retention or constipation, and α-adrenergic blockade effects such as hypotension. However the major adverse effects are extrapyramidal effects: akathisias (restlessness) and dystonias (muscle contraction) such as trismus and torticollis. These effects are more likely in children and many pediatric practitioners limit the use of dopamine blockers due to their side effects. Diphenhydramine (Benadryl) will generally reverse extrapyramidal effects within 30–60 minutes, and has often been used prophylactically to reduce the risk of extrapyramidal reactions. Also of note are specific issues with 2 of these drugs. First, droperidol is either not used or the dose is limited in many institutions due to its ability to lengthen the QTc interval and cause arrhythmias. Second, IV promethazine can be very irritating on injection, and if injected into an artery can cause significant tissue damage. Many institutions are limiting its use to low doses or oral administration. Risk may be minimal if central lines are available for administration, which is commonly the situation in children with cancer.

Cannabinoids

Cannabinoids (dronabinol, nabilone) have been used mostly for patients who have not responded well to more typical antiemetics. These drugs can also be used as appetite stimulants. They are synthetic versions of tetrahydrocannabinol, the psychoactive component of marijuana. Early studies suggested these agents were most effective in younger adult patients, patients who had smoked marijuana, and patients who developed euphoria while taking them. While many pediatric institutions have some experience using these agents in children, little data are published on their use in children, and most of the data relate to nabilone. Recommended doses of dronabinol are very high; some patients tolerate the drug better when lower doses are used and started prior to the chemotherapy. Adverse effects are the same as for marijuana, including euphoria or dysphoria, hypotension, tachycardia, increased appetite, dry mouth, and occasionally hallucinations. In recent years several states have legalized the ability to purchase medical grade marijuana.

Atypical Antipsychotics

Olanzapine is similar to the dopamine blockers discussed above, but it is less likely to cause extrapyramidal side effects. Very few studies have been published, but several case reports and small studies have shown efficacy of olanzapine in adult patients who have not responded well to more standard antiemetics.[153] Adult recommended doses are 5–10 mg/d, with 2.5–5 mg/d being used in case reports in children. Sedation is one of the main short-term side effects, and weight gain and increased risk of metabolic syndrome have been reported with longer use.

Antihistamines and Benzodiazepines

Antihistamines (diphenhydramine) and benzodiazepines (lorazepam) have been used as adjunctive agents for chemotherapy-induced nausea and vomiting. Neither has good activity on its own as an antiemetic for chemotherapy, although the sedation they cause may help the patient sleep through nausea and vomiting. Diphenhydramine has good anticholinergic activity in the brain and is therefore able to reduce and/or treat extrapyramidal reactions from dopamine blockers. Lorazepam is beneficial in reducing or treating akathisias caused by dopamine blockers. Lorazepam's activity as an antianxiety medication and its ability to cause anterograde amnesia in some patients may help reduce anticipatory nausea and vomiting. Some pediatric patients develop paradoxical reactions to these agents, becoming agitated instead of sedated. This appears to be more common in younger patients and with higher doses. Additionally, some pediatric patients become weepy or have hallucinations, limiting the usefulness of lorazepam.

Appetite Stimulants

Weight loss in cancer patients may be due to numerous factors, as described in detail earlier in this chapter. Appetite stimulants have been used in attempts to counter weight loss in cancer patients, but studies have had mixed results. A review of adult studies by Yavuzsen et al[156] suggests that of all the drugs tried, only progestins and glucocorticoids have shown a benefit in cancer-induced anorexia and weight loss. Doubts exist about even these drugs because the weight gain from progestins such as megestrol may consist more of fat and water than lean body mass,[157] and glucocorticoids have negative anabolic effects that result in muscle weakness over time.

Studies have shown at least some increased appetite and weight gain benefit from methylprednisolone, dexa-methasone, and prednisone. In addition to the short-term side effects discussed above in the antiemetic section, glucocorticoids have numerous long-term side effects that include osteoporosis, aseptic necrosis, cataracts, easy tearing of the skin, and loss of muscle strength.

Megestrol and Medroxyprogesterone

Megestrol and medroxyprogesterone are progestins that have an effect of increasing appetite and causing weight gain. A recently published small randomized, double-blind, placebo-controlled trial of megestrol acetate in pediatric patients showed a mean weight gain of 20%; however, the data also suggested that fat body mass increased more reliably than lean body mass.[158] Adrenocortical suppression as measured by morning cortisol was frequent in this study. Potential adverse effects of significance from other studies include thrombophlebitis, photosensitivity, impotence in men, and Cushing's syndrome with adrenocortical suppression and the potential for Addisonian crisis.[155,159]

Dronabinol

Dronabinol (Marinol, but not nabilone) has been studied for weight gain in adults, and is FDA approved for treating anorexia in patients with AIDS. Little data are available on use in cancer patients with anorexia or in pediatrics. While it does stimulate appetite for periods of at least 5 months, minimal evidence exists for efficacy in causing weight gain or reducing weight loss in cancer patients.[155,156,159,160] As noted above in the antiemetic section, many potential adverse effects are associated with dronabinol; however, the doses used for appetite stimulation are lower (2.5 mg twice daily) than those used for nausea/vomiting, so there may be fewer adverse effects. A recent publication suggests the possibility of withdrawal after longer-term therapy; 3 months in an elderly patient.[161]

Cyproheptadine

Cyproheptadine is a serotonin antagonist and antihistamine that has been studied as an appetite stimulant in cancer patients. An early study in adults showed increased appetite but no less weight loss than with a placebo in adults with advanced malignancies.[162] A recent study in children with cancer found that many did respond with weight gain, with drowsiness as the only common side effect.[163] Studies with this agent are ongoing in children. Doses may need to be reduced in patients with hepatic impairment.

Medications for Mucositis

Mucositis occurs inconsistently after chemotherapy regimens outside of the transplant setting, and the time course after chemotherapy generally parallels that of neutropenia. These features make it difficult to study since it occurs erratically and resolves with or without therapy. Medications used for mucositis fit into 2 categories, symptom control or prevention, and most have little if any effect on the healing rate of the mucositis. When mucositis is seen in the mouth, it is presumably occurring throughout the gut, including the stomach. Administration of acid-blocking drugs is commonly thought to help, although data on the value of this treatment are scarce. Medications used to treat symptoms of mucositis include drugs such as "magic mouthwash" combinations, Gelclair, and opioids.

Medications for Treatment of Mucositis Symptoms

Magic mouthwash usually contains viscous lidocaine, diphenhydramine, and an antacid or nystatin. Lidocaine is a strong local anesthetic, diphenhydramine is a weak local anesthetic, and the antacid may help neutralize acid in the stomach, although the dose is probably too low to effectively raise gastric pH. Nystatin is included in these mixtures at some institutions since mucositis may cause or be caused by Candida infections (thrush). Little if any published data exist on the efficacy of these combinations, but they relieve symptoms in some patients. Combinations containing viscous lidocaine have been reported to cause systemic lidocaine toxicity if used in relatively high or frequent doses, especially in small children or infants who swallow it. This is not a problem if used properly and swished and spit out. Gelclair is a polymer-type combination of polyvinylpyrrolidone, hyaluronic acid, and glycyrrhetinic acid. It coats the mucosa of the mouth, protecting it from air and irritants that elicit pain. It is suggested not to eat or drink for an hour or more after using Gelclair. Some patients seem to benefit from this product. Opioids are used when less potent treatments fail, and may allow the patient to maintain oral intake. Opioids can be very helpful, but frequently subject the patient to constipation and sometimes to nausea and vomiting, itching, or when dosed excessively, sedation and respiratory depression.

Medications used to reduce the frequency and severity of mucositis include the following.

Chlorhexidine

Chlorhexidine has antiseptic-type effects, and since mucositis can result from oral infections, this product may the-oretically help. However, minimal evidence demonstrates a benefit in preventing or treating mucositis with chlorhexidine. Recent guidelines from the MASCC[164] do not recommend its use for either prophylaxis or treatment.[165] Since most chlorhexidine-containing products also contain alcohol, they may elicit pain in patients that already have mucositis.

Glutamine

Glutamine is an amino acid that is thought to be especially important to cells of the GI tract. Studies in the past have suggested that it might help maintain the integrity of the gut in patients receiving long-term PN, or may help prevent chemotherapy-induced mucositis. Studies have suggested reduction in mucositis for autologous hematopoietic cell transplant patients, but there also has been a suggestion of increased cancer relapses.[166-168] The most recent MASCC guidelines do not recommend the use of glutamine,[164] but enough interest exists that studies of specialized formulations of glutamine are in clinical trials.

Palifermin

Palifermin is a recombinant human keratinocyte growth factor. It is approved and used for reducing mucositis in patients with hematologic malignancies who are receiving hematopoietic cell transplants. Many practitioners considered its use in solid tumors to be contraindicated because of the potential for stimulating epithelial cells (and perhaps the cancer); however, studies in solid tumors in patients receiving standard chemotherapy are in progress. Palifermin is expensive and does cause some side effects such as "thick tongue," altered taste, and rashes. Palifermin has been demonstrated to reduce the duration and severity of oral mucositis as well as the use of opioids in patients receiving autologous hematopoietic cell transplants for hematologic malignancies. Less data are available for allogeneic transplants.

The MASCC guidelines mention numerous other products (favorably or unfavorably), most of which are not currently used in pediatrics.[164] Slurries or suspensions of sucralfate (Carafate) have been used in children with oral mucositis, but efficacy data are generally lacking, plus several negative studies in adults with radiation-induced oral mucositis.[168] Another product that is being studied currently in children is Traumeel S. It is a homeopathic mixture of approximately a dozen herbals or supplements that are not thought to have side effects, although allergies to ingredients would be a possibility. One study in children and young adults receiving hematopoietic cell transplants showed favorable results, however a larger placebo-controlled study in 181 Children's Oncology Group hematopoietic cell transplant patients did not demonstrate a benefit from Traumeel S mouth rinses.[165]

Late Effects of Treatment for Survivors

The overall 5-year survival rate for childhood cancer is approaching 80% and for some cancer diagnoses the 5-year survival rate is > 95%. Based on these statistics, the United States has approximately 380,000 childhood cancer survivors.[1] Many patients experience late effects or long-term health-related outcomes that can result in organ dysfunction, second malignant neoplasms, and adverse psychological sequelae.[169]

Risk factors for late effects can be due to tumor, tumor treatment, or tumor-induced organ dysfunction, and mechanical effects. The multimodal treatment used during treatment can also be responsible for many late effects. The Children's Oncology Group Long-Term Follow-Up Guidelines for Survivors of Childhood, Adolescent, and Young Adult Cancers (COG-LTFU Guidelines) extensively review late effects of treatments used.[169] Genetic predisposition, capacity for normal tissue repair, organ function not affected by treatment, developmental status, and premorbid state can also influence development of late effects.[170]

Many childhood cancer survivors report unhealthy lifestyle habits. One study evaluated barriers that childhood cancer survivors expressed that prohibited them from adopting a healthier lifestyle including being too tired (57%), being too busy (53%), not belonging to a gym (48%), visual appeal of fatty foods (58%), typical consumption of high-fat foods in social situations (50%), and lack of knowledge about choosing healthier options (a major barrier).[171] A second survey survey found that 79% of childhood cancer survivors did not meet the recommended daily intake for fruits and vegetables, 84% obtained more than 30% of their calories from fat sources, and only 48% met exercise guidelines.[172]

Long-Term Follow-Up Guidelines

The COG-LTFU Guidelines are clinical practice guidelines used in screening and management of late effects that can result from therapy used during treatment for pediatric malignancies.[169] The guidelines are evidence based (utilizing established associations between therapeutic exposures and late effects to identify high-risk categories) and grounded in the collective clinical experience of experts (matching

the magnitude of the risk with the intensity of the screening recommendations). These guidelines are appropriate for survivors of childhood, adolescent, or young adult cancers 2 or more years following the completion of cancer therapy. Given the wide age range, some guidelines may not be applicable (eg, limiting alcohol intake in a 10-year-old), therefore clinicians must be guided by the age of the patient and the relevance of the guidelines. References related to each late effect and patient education materials on a variety of topics are also included in the guidelines.[169]

When determining guidelines for cancer survivors, it is important to use traditional assessments or recommendations, taking into account the age of the survivor and his or her pertinent clinical history. Suggestions are geared toward leading a healthy lifestyle and include nutrition and activity guidelines. Cancer survivors should follow the same guidelines that are used in cancer prevention.

Gastrointestinal Problems in Survivors

Treatment for childhood cancer can result in chronic problems of the intestine or other parts of the GI system including bowel obstruction, gallstones, esophageal stricture, hepatic fibrosis, colorectal cancer, chronic enterocolitis and dental abnormalities.[173]

Treatments that increase risk for having GI late effects include radiation doses of 30 Gy (3000 cGy/rads) or higher to the head, chest, neck, pelvis, or abdomen and surgery in the pelvis or abdomen. Other risk factors include a family history of gallstones or colorectal or esophageal cancer, patient history of bowel adhesions (scarring) or bowel obstruction (blockage), use of tobacco, or chronic GVHD.

Symptoms of GI problems can include chronic nausea, vomiting, acid reflux, constipation or diarrhea, pain (swallowing, abdominal), change in appetite, weight loss, black tarry stools or blood in stool, abdominal distention, and jaundice.

Suggestions for managing GI problems:[174]

1. Eat 5 or more servings of fruits and vegetables
2. Choose a variety of foods from all food groups
3. Include high-fiber foods in the diet (eg, whole grain breads, cereal)
4. Avoid foods high in sugar (eg, candy, soda)
5. Choose low-fat milk and dairy products
6. When eating meats, choose leaner cuts and prepare them by broiling or boiling
7. Decrease high-fat foods (eg, potato chips, french fries)
8. Limit the use of alcohol
9. Do not smoke or use tobacco and avoid secondhand smoke

Endocrine System

Bone Health

Bone is a living growing tissue made up of calcium, phosphorus, magnesium, vitamin D, and fluoride. All of these nutrients are important in the development and maintenance of bone and other calcified tissues. As a consequence of treatment for childhood cancer, survivors may not be able to obtain normal peak bone mass and also may experience an increased loss of calcium from the bones.[175] Survivors are at increased risk for osteopenia and osteoporosis, a result of too little bone formation or too much bone loss; therefore, fractures may occur as bones become weaker. Osteopenia and osteoporosis are diagnosed by DXA scan, which measures bone density or bone mass and takes < 20 minutes to complete.

General risk factors include being female, Caucasian or Asian, or older; having a family history of osteoporosis; having a small/thin frame; smoking; having a diet low in calcium and/or high in salt; drinking increased amounts of alcohol, caffeine, or soda; and lacking weight-bearing exercise. Risk factors in survivors of childhood cancer include anticancer treatment utilizing methotrexate or corticosteroids as well as radiation to weight-bearing bones. Other medical treatments such as anticonvulsants (barbiturates and phenytoin) and medication used to treat early puberty and endometriosis can affect bones. Drugs including aluminum-containing antacids, cholesterol-lowering medication, and high-dose heparin for prolonged periods are risk factors. Suggestions for decreasing risk of osteoporosis include activity with weight-bearing (walking, dancing) and resistance (light weight-lifting) exercises.

General guidelines for calcium requirements are 1000–1500 mg/d (elemental calcium), but may vary based on age, clinical history, and results of DEXA scan. Food sources include dairy products (milk, cheese, yogurt) and nondairy products (salmon, collards, broccoli, white beans, fortified foods such as orange juice and some cereals).

Calcium is found in supplements as a salt bound to carbonate, gluconate, citrate, or lactate. The recommendations are based on elemental calcium: the amount of actual calcium, excluding the salt, in a supplement that is available for absorption. Calcium carbonate is the most prevalent form of calcium supplement on the market and should be taken after meals because it requires stomach acid for better absorption. It provides more elemental calcium (40% elemental) than calcium citrate, therefore not as many tablets are required. Calcium citrate is the best absorbed supplemental calcium. It does not require extra stomach acid for absorption, therefore it may be taken anytime during the day, even on an empty stomach.

Some brands list total weight of calcium salt, not the amount of elemental calcium. Generic brands are less expensive, but they may not meet United States Pharmacopeia standards for quality and purity. It is best to avoid oyster shell, bone meal, or dolomite sources of calcium because they may contain lead, mercury, or arsenic. Nutrition facts label should state percent daily value (%DV) based on 1000 mg of elemental calcium. It is necessary to individualize calcium requirements based on age and clinical history.

Vitamin D is needed to absorb calcium and is generally found in dairy products that are fortified. Although we are able to make vitamin D through sun exposure, most people do not make enough due to the use of sunscreen. In addition, cancer survivors are all at increased risk for the development of secondary skin cancers due to their previous exposure to chemotherapy and/or radiation.[176] Therefore, excessive sun exposure or exposure without sunscreen should be discouraged. The Institute of Medicine panel released new guidelines for vitamin D dosage ranges. The panel raised the safe range for adults to 2000–4000 IU daily and for children over 1 year to 1000–3000 IU daily.[177] The amount of vitamin D prescribed should be individualized based on vitamin D level and adjusted as needed.

Obesity and Metabolic Syndrome

Obesity is a reported late effect in survivors that have been treated for childhood cancer.[178] It most commonly occurs after treatment for acute lymphoblastic leukemia, with and without central nervous system radiation, and brain tumors, which combined account for over 40% of childhood cancer diagnoses.[179] Excessive weight gain can occur during therapy or immediately after treatment and may continue into adulthood.[180]

Metabolic syndrome is a combination of symptoms that include obesity, insulin resistance, hyperglycemia and dyslipidemia and has been seen in survivors, especially those treated with cranial radiation and prolonged corticosteroid use.[181] Metabolic syndrome is often a precursor to the onset of Type 2 diabetes even in young adults. It is therefore extremely important that childhood cancer survivors maintain a healthy weight and participate in aerobic activity.

Heart Health After Treatment for Childhood Cancer[182]

Cardiac disease is the leading noncancer cause of death seen in survivors and occurs in almost 5% of survivors.[183] Risk typically goes up with total cumulative cardiotoxic chemotherapy doses and when combined with radiation to the chest or great vessels.[184] Types of heart problems that can occur after treatment include left ventricular dysfunction, cardiomyopathy, arrhythmias, valvular stenosis or insufficiency, pericardial fibrosis, restrictive pericarditis, conduction disturbances, and coronary artery disease.[185] Risk factors for developing heart problems can be exacerbated by other medical conditions (obesity, high blood pressure, diabetes, elevated cholesterol, or triglycerides). Aerobic exercise is generally safe and healthy for the heart, but some forms of exercise can be stressful to the heart such as wrestling and heavy weight lifting. Survivors who might be at risk for having heart problems should check with their healthcare provider before starting an exercise program or joining a sport team.

Tests that are done to monitor heart function include electrocardiogram, echocardiogram, or multigated acquisition scan and should be recommended by a healthcare provider if appropriate. To prevent problems with the heart, it is best to stay at a healthy body weight, limit fat intake to no more than 30% of calories, exercise moderately for at least 30 minutes on most days, and avoid smoking.

Diet and Physical Activity for Survivors[186]

Once treatment has ended, cancer survivors should adopt the American Institute for Cancer Research Recommendations for Cancer Prevention,[174] which include the following:

1. Be as lean as possible (not underweight)
2. Be physically active (30 minutes on most days)
3. Avoid sugary drinks. Limit intake of processed foods high in fat or added sugar or low in fiber
4. Eat a variety of vegetables, fruits, whole grains, and legumes (beans)
5. Limit consumption of red meat (beef, pork, lamb). Avoid processed meats
6. If consumed, limit alcoholic drinks to 2 for men and 1 for women per day
7. Limit consumption of salty foods and foods processed with salt (sodium)
8. Do not use supplements to protect against cancer
9. Do not smoke or chew tobacco
10. Handle food safely (immune system may be affected in survivors, increasing the risk for food-borne illness)
11. Rethink the pattern of eating in which two-thirds of a meal is vegetables, fruits, whole grains, and beans and one-third comes from cheese or animal foods. Maximize the variety of vegetables and fruits eaten because they contain phytochemicals, which are plant compounds that have antioxidant effects, boost the immune system, promote cellular repair, and have anti-inflammatory, antiviral, and antibacterial activity.

Nutrients should be provided in the diet from a variety of sources. Protein is needed for growth, repair of body tissue, and maintenance of immune function. Carbohydrates and fats are the body's major energy (calorie) sources. Vitamins and minerals are essential for proper growth and development and are needed to utilize the energy in food. Water is important to prevent dehydration, which may cause a person to feel listless or dizzy. Benefits of regular exercise and good nutrition for childhood cancer survivors include promoting healing of tissues/organs damaged by cancer and treatment, building strength and endurance, reducing risk of certain types of adult cancers and diseases (diabetes, heart disease), decreasing stress, and providing a feeling of well-being. Although late effects occur in survivors of pediatric cancer, a healthy lifestyle including a proper diet and adequate exercise is important to decrease the risk of certain types of diseases.

Appendix 29-1. Algorithm for Nutritional Intervention in the Pediatric Oncology Patient

Identify appropriate category: Age > 2 years choose either BMI (Body Mass Index) or IBW (Ideal Body Weight)
Age < 2 years choose WT/LT (Weight for Length) or IBW (Ideal Body Weight)

Categories for Nutritional Status

	Underweight		Normal	Risk of Overweight/Overweight*	
BMI	< 5 th % ile		5 - 85 th % ile	> 85 - 95 th % ile	> 95 th % ile
WT/LT	< 10 th % ile		10 - 90 th % ile		> 90 th % ile
IBW	< 70% Severe	> 70-80% Moderate > 80-90% Mild	> 90 -110 %	>110 - 120%	>120%

*Evaluate for weight gain or loss

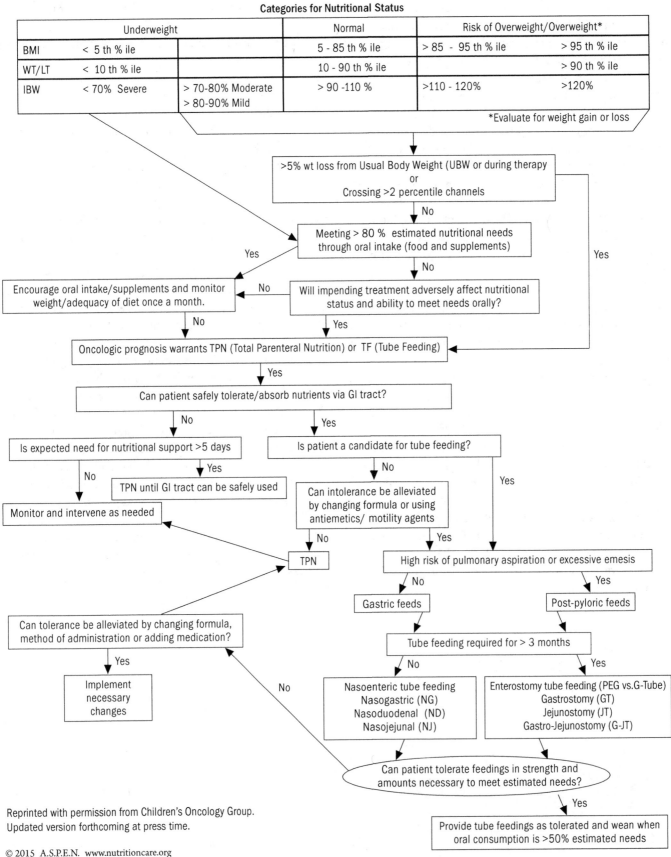

Reprinted with permission from Children's Oncology Group.
Updated version forthcoming at press time.

Appendix 29-2. Algorithm for Nutritional Intervention and Categories of Nutritional Status in the Pediatric Oncology Patient - References and Resources

Definitions:

BMI - Body Mass Index - weight in kilograms divided by height in meters squared (kg/m²)

IBW - Ideal Body Weight for Height or Length - patient's actual weight divided by the ideal weight for height x 100

UBW - Usual Body Weight - weight prior to diagnosis

Methods for Calculating Ideal Body Weight

A. Using the CDC growth charts[1, 2]

0–24 Months of age - IBW is determined from the appropriate growth curve by first identifying the age for which the measured height is on the 50th percentile, then determining the corresponding 50th percentile weight for that height

24 Months - 20 years of age - plot the BMI on the CDC/BMI growth chart. To obtain the IBW, identify the BMI at the 50% ile and convert to kilograms, see example below:

7 YOM   Ht: 124.4 cm   Wt: 21.8 kg

BMI: 14.1 BMI plotted at the 50% = 15.5

15.5 divided by 10,000 × 124.4 cm × 124.4 cm = 24.0 kg IBW

B. Rule of Thumb Method[3] (used in patients who are over 5 feet tall or > 20 years of age):

Females: 100 pounds for five feet and 5 pounds for every inch over five feet

Males: 106 pounds for five feet and 6 pounds for every inch over five feet

C. Using a formula - without using a growth chart

1. patients of 1–18 years of age[4]

a) ht < 60 inches:

IBW = (ht2 × 1.65) / 1000   where ht = cm, IBW = kg

b) ht > 60 inches:

IBW = Females: 42.2 + [2.27 × (ht − 60)] where ht = inches, IBW = kg

Males: 39.0 + [(2.27 × (ht − 60)]

2. patients > 18 years of age[5]

a) Females: IBW = 45.5 + [2.3 × (ht − 60)] where ht = inches, IBW = kg

b) Males: IBW = 50. 0 + [2.3 × (ht − 60)]

Considerations for the overweight population

A. Calculating Adjusted Body Weight[6] - to be used in patients who are > 125% of their IBW

([ABW – IBW] × 0.25) + IBW = wt for use in calculating Basal Energy Expenditure (BEE) and protein requirement

ABW = Actual Body Weight in kg; IBW = ideal body weight for height; 0.25 = 25% of body fat tissue is estimated to be metabolically active

B. Schofield Equations for predicting Resting Energy Expenditure in Children (0–8 years) - more accurately predicts REE in children with altered growth and body composition such as obesity and failure to thrive.[7]

Age (y)	kcal/d	Age (y)	kcal/d
Male		Female	
0–3	0.167 W + 1517.4 H – 617.6	0–3	16.252 W + 1023.2 H – 413.5
3–10	19.59 W + 130.3 H + 414.9	3–10	16.969 W + 161.8 H + 371.2
10–18	16.25 W + 137.2 H – 515.5	10–18	8.365 W + 465 H + 200

W = weight (kg), H = height (cm)

Appendix 29-2 Continued

Appendix 29-2. Algorithm for Nutritional Intervention and Categories of Nutritional Status in the Pediatric Oncology Patient - References and Resources *Continued*

Correction for amputation type and % body weight lost based on segmental weights. Correct weight prior to determining IBW.[8]
AKA - above the knee (9.2%)   BKA - below the knee (5.9%)   HEMI - hemipelvectomy or hip disarticulation (16 %)   ARM - arm disarticulation (5%)

Calculating Protein Needs using Dietary Reference Intakes (DRIs)[9]

Life Stage Group	Age (y)	Protein (g/kg/d)
Infants	0.0-1.0	1.5
Children	1-3 4-13	1.1 0.95
Adolescent	14-18	0.85
Adult	> 18	0.8

Estimating Energy Requirements for children ≥ 1 year of age (W = weight in kilograms) [10] and infants < 1 year of age[11]

	1-3 y	3-10 y	10-18 y	18-30 y
male	60.9W – 54	22.7W + 495	17.5W + 651	15.3W + 679
female	61W – 51	22.5W + 499	12.2W + 746	14.7W + 496

Age	Equation
0-3 mo	(89 × wt (kg) – 100) + 175
4-6 mo	(89 × wt (kg) – 100) + 56
7-12 mo	(89 × wt (kg) – 100) + 22

BMR = _____

Multiply BMR by an activity/stress factor:

      1.3 - for a well-nourished child at bed rest with mild to moderate stress (mild surgery)

      1.5 - for a very active child with mild to moderate stress, an inactive child with severe stress (trauma, sepsis, cancer, extensive surgery), or a child with minimal activity who requires catch-up growth

      1.7 - for an active child requiring catch-up growth or an active child with severe stress

BMR_____ × Factor_____ = _____ kcal/d

References/Resources:

1. St. Jude Children's Research Hospital, Department of Clinical Nutrition. Clinical Practice Guidelines, 2006.
2. Supportive Care of Children with Cancer: Current Therapy and Guidelines from the Children's Oncology Group, third edition, edited by Arnold J. Altman. The Johns Hopkins University Press. 2004.
3. Hamwi, GJ. Therapy changing dietary concepts in diabetes mellitus: Diagnosis and treatment. Volume 1. American Dietetics Association: NY: 73-78, 1964.
4. Traub SL, Johnson CE. Comparison of methods of estimating creatinine clearance in children. American Journal of Hospital Pharmacy: 1980;37:195-201.
5. Devine BJ. Gentamicin therapy. Drug Intelligence and clinical Pharmacy. 1974;8:650-655.
6. American Dietetic Association. Manual of Dietetics. Adjustment in body weight for obese patients. Chicago: Chicago Dietetic Association and South Suburban Dietetic Association. 1989;Appendix 48:622-623.
7. Schofield WN, Human Nutr Clin. 1985;Suppl 1:5-41..
8. Osterkamp, LK. Current perspective on assessment of human body proportions of relevance to amputees. J Am Diet Assoc. 1995; 95:215-218
9. Dietary Reference Intakes for Energy, Carbohydrate, Fiber, Fat, Fatty Acids, cholesterol, Protein, and Amino Acids , 2002.
10. World Health Organization. Energy and protein requirements. Tech. Rep. Ser. 724. Geneva: WHO. 1985.
11. American Dietetic Association. Children with Special Health Care Needs: Nutrition Care Handbook. Lucas, BL, Editor. p. 36; 2004.

Reprinted with permission from Children's Oncology Group. Updated version forthcoming at press time.

Appendix 29-3. Categories of Nutritional Status for the Pediatric Oncology Patient

- Identify appropriate category:

  Age > 2 years - choose either BMI[1] (Body Mass Index)

  or

  IBW[2] (Ideal Body Weight)

  Age < 2 years - choose either WT/LT[3] (Weight for Length)

  or

  IBW2 (Ideal Body Weight)

- Weight loss/gain may or may not be present

Underweight		Normal	Risk of Overweight / Overweight	
BMI < 5th %ile		5th–85th %ile	> 85th-95th %ile	> 95th %ile
WT/LT < 10th %ile		10th–90th %ile	> 90th %ile	
IBW < 70% Severe	> 70-80% Moderate > 80-90% Mild	> 90th-110th %ile	>110th –120th %ile	> 120th %ile

[1]BMI - Body Mass Index (percentile)

Hammer LD, Kraemer HC, Wilson DM, Ritter PL, Dornbusch SM. Standardized percentile curves of body-mass index for children and adolescents. Am J Dis Child. 191;145:259-263.

Pietrobelli A, Faith MS, Allison DB, Gallagher D, Chiumello G, Heymsfield, SB. Body mass index as a measure of adiposity among children and adolescents: a validation study. J Pediatr. 1998;132:204-210.

[2]IBW - Ideal Body Weight for height or length (percentage)

Waterlow JC. Classification and definition of protein-calorie malnutrition. Br Med J 1972;3:566-569.

[3]WT/LT - Weight for Length (percentile)

Motil KJ. Sensititve measures of nutritional status in children in hospital and in the field. Int J Cancer Suppl. 1998;11:2-9.

Reprinted with permission from Children's Oncology Group. Updated version forthcoming at press time.

Test Your Knowledge Questions

1. Mucositis is one of the complications affecting the nutrition status of the pediatric oncology patient. Which chemotherapy agent is most likely to lead to the development of mucositis?
   A. Methotrexate
   B. Cyclophosphamide
   C. Vincristine
   D. Carboplatin

2. The use of EN during HSCT is commonly discouraged because of
   A. The need of frequent tube replacement
   B. Risk of excessive bleeding with tube placement due to mucositis
   C. Dislodgement of the feeding tube
   D. All of the above

3. Which is true regarding agents used to enhance gut motility?
   A. Use of erythromycin to enhance gut motility increases resistance among susceptible bacteria.
   B. Children are more susceptible to the extrapyramidal side effects of both metoclopramide and erythromycin than are adults.
   C. Case reports of tardive dyskinesias with the use of metoclopramide are too infrequent to be considered clinically important.
   D. Motility-enhancing agents may increase or decrease the absorption of other drugs.

4. Survivors of childhood cancer can be at greater risk for osteoporosis due to
   A. History of corticosteroid use
   b. History of methotrexate-containing regimen
   c. Inadequate calcium and vitamin D intake
   d. All of the above

Acknowledgments

The authors of this chapter for the second edition of this text wish to thank Elizabeth Wallace, RD, CNSC, LDN; Seema Desai, MS, RD, LDN, CNSD; Vinod K. Prasad, MD, MRCP; Virginia Guzikowski, MSN, CRNP; Liesje Neiman Carney, RD, CNSD, LDN; and Beth Bogucki Wright, MS, RD, CSP, LDN, for their contributions to the first edition.

References

1. Ward E, DeSantis C, Robbins A, Kohler B, Jemal A. Childhood and adolescent cancer statistics, 2014. *CA Cancer J Clin.* 2014;64(2):83–103.

2. Donaldson SS, Wesley MN, DeWys WD, Suskind RM, Jaffe N, vanEys J. A study of the nutritional status of pediatric cancer patients. *Am J Dis Child.* 1981;135(12):1107–1112.

3. Coates TD, Rickard KA, Grosfeld JL, Weetman RM. Nutritional support of children with neoplastic diseases. *Surg Clin North Am.* 1986;66(6):1197–1212.

4. Mauer AM, Burgess JB, Donaldson SS, et al. Special nutritional needs of children with malignancies: a review. *JPEN J Parenter Enteral Nutr.* 1990;14(3):315–324.

5. Cady J. Nutritional support during radiotherapy for head and neck cancer: the role of prophylactic feeding tube placement. *Clin J Oncol Nurs.* 2007;11(6):875–880.

6. Han-Markey T. Nutritional considerations in pediatric oncology. *Semin Oncol Nurs.* 2000;16(2):146–151.

7. Rickard KA, Grosfeld JL, Kirksey A, Ballantine TV, Baehner RL. Reversal of protein-energy malnutrition in children during treatment of advanced neoplastic disease. *Ann Surg.* 1979;190(6):771–781.

8. Lahorra JM, Ginn-Pease ME, King DR. The prognostic significance of basic anthropometric data in children with advanced solid tumors. *Nutr Cancer.* 1989;12(4):361–369.

9. Cancer Therapy Evaluation Program. Common Terminology Criteria Document for Adverse Events v3.0 (CTCAE). DCTD, NCI, NIH, DHHS; 2008. http://ctep.cancer.gov/protocolDevelopment/electronic_applications/docs/ctcaev3.pdf. Published August 9, 2006. Accessed November 19, 2008.

10. Carter P, Carr D, van Eys J, Coody D. Nutritional parameters in children with cancer. *J Am Diet Assoc.* 1983;82(6):616–622.

11. Smith DE, Stevens MC, Booth IW. Malnutrition at diagnosis of malignancy in childhood: common but mostly missed. *Eur J Pediatr.* 1991;150(5):318–322.

12. Huhmann MB, August DA. Nutrition support in surgical oncology. *Nutr Clin Pract.* 2009;24(4):520–526.

13. Donaldson SS. Effects of therapy on nutritional status of the pediatric cancer patient. *Cancer Res.* 1982;42(2 suppl):729s–736s.

14. Cunningham RS, Herbert V. Nutrition as a component of alternative therapy. *Semin Oncol Nurs.* 2000;16(2):163–169.

15. Barrera R. Nutritional support in cancer patients. *JPEN J Parenter Enteral Nutr.* 2002;26(5 suppl):S63–S71.

16. Children's Oncology Group. Weight gain or loss and nutritional interventions. http://www.childrensoncologygroup. org/index.php/weightgainorweightloss. Accessed December 28, 2014.

17. Ladas EJ, Sacks N, Meacham L, et al. A multidisciplinary review of nutrition considerations in the pediatric oncology population: a perspective from children's oncology group. *Nutr Clin Pract.* 2005;20(4):377–393.

18. National Cancer Institute. Nutrition in Cancer Care (PDQ®). Surgery and nutrition. http://www.cancer.gov/cancertopics/pdq/supportivecare/nutrition/Patient/page4#_284. Updated December 5, 2014. Accessed December 28, 2014.

19. National Cancer Institute. Dictionary of cancer terms. Radiation therapy. http://www.cancer.gov/dictionary?CdrID=44971. Accessed December 28, 2014.

20. National Cancer Institute. Nutrition in Cancer Care (PDQ®). Radiation therapy and nutrition. http://www.cancer.gov/cancertopics/pdq/supportivecare/nutrition/Patient/page4#_286. Updated December 5, 2014. Accessed December 28, 2014.

21. LaFond DA, Bolton RM, et al. In: Baggott C, Foley GV, Fotchman D, Patterson K, eds. *Nursing Care of Children and Adolescents With Cancer and Blood Disorders.* Glenview, IL: Association of Pediatric Hematology/Oncology Nurses; 2011:296–325.

22. Unsal D, Mentes B, Akmansu M, Uner A, Oguz M, Pak Y. Evaluation of nutritional status in cancer patients receiving radiotherapy: a prospective study. *Am J Clin Oncol.* 2006;29(2):183–188.

23. Ogama N, Suzuki S, Umeshita K, et al. Appetite and adverse effects associated with radiation therapy in patients with head and neck cancer. *Eur J Oncol Nurs.* 2010;14(1):3–10.

24. Wilkes C, Ingwersen K, Barton-Burke M. *Oncology Nursing Drug Handbook.* Sudbury, MA: Jones and Bartlett Publishers; 2003.

25. Baltzer CL, Haywood R. *Oncology Pocket Guide to Chemotherapy.* Philadelphia, PA: Mosby Medical Communications, Elsevier Science; 2002.

26. Tyc VL, Vallelunga L, Mahoney S, Smith BF, Mulhern RK. Nutritional and treatment-related characteristics of pediatric oncology patients referred or not referred for nutritional support. *Med Pediatr Oncol.* 1995;25(5):379–388.

27. Barber MD, Ross JA, Fearon KC. Cancer cachexia. *Surg Oncol.* 1999;8(3):133–141.

28. National Cancer Institute. Dictionary of cancer terms. Gluconeogenesis. http://www.cancer.gov/dictionary?CdrID=44111. Accessed December 28, 2014.

29. National Cancer Institute. Nutrition in Cancer Care (PDQ®). Chemotherapy and nutrition. http://www.cancer.gov/cancertopics/pdq/supportivecare/nutrition/Patient/page4#_285. Updated December 5, 2014. Accessed December 28, 2014.

30. Hooke MC, Baggott C, Robinson D, et al. Management of disease and treatment-related complications. In: Baggot C, Foley GV, Fotchman D, Patterson K, eds. *Nursing Care of Children and Adolescents With Cancer and Blood Disorders.* Glenview, IL: Association of Pediatric Hematology/Oncology Nurses; 2011;510–584.

31. Bauer J, Jürgens H, Frühwald MC. Important aspects of nutrition in children with cancer. *Adv Nutr.* 2011;2(2):67–77.

32. National Cancer Institute. Dictionary of cancer terms. Cytokine. http://www.cancer.gov/dictionary?CdrID=46130. Accessed December 28, 2014.

33. Martindale RG, Shikora SA, Nishikawa R, Siepler JK. The metabolic response to stress and alterations in nutrient metabolism. In: Shikora SA, Martindale RG, Schwaitzberg SD, eds. *Nutritional Consideration in the Intensive Care Unit: Science, Rationale and Practice.* Silver Spring, MD: American Society for Parenteral and Enteral Nutrition; 2002:11–19.

34. Jones MO, Pierro A, Hammond P, Lloyd DA. The metabolic response to operative stress in infants. *J Pediatr Surg.* 1993;28(10):1258–1262; discussion 1262–1253.

35. Moschovi M, Trimis G, Vounatsou M, et al. Serial plasma concentrations of PYY and ghrelin during chemotherapy in children with acute lymphoblastic leukemia. *J Pediatr Hematol Oncol.* 2008;30(10):733–737.

36. Argiles JM, Moore-Carrasco R, Busquets S, Lopez-Soriano FJ. Catabolic mediators as targets for cancer cachexia. *Drug Discov Today.* 2003;8(18):838–844.

37. Dunlop RJ, Campbell CW. Cytokines and advanced cancer. *J Pain Symptom Manage.* 2000;20(3):214–232.

38. Ovesen L, Allingstrup L, Hannibal J, Mortensen EL, Hansen OP. Effect of dietary counseling on food intake, body weight, response rate, survival, and quality of life in cancer patients undergoing chemotherapy: a prospective, randomized study. *J Clin Oncol.* 1993;11(10):2043–2049.

39. Cravo ML, Glória LM, Claro I. Metabolic responses to tumour disease and progression: tumour-host interaction. *Clin Nutr.* 2000;19(6):459–465.

40. Bosaeus I, Daneryd P, Lundholm K. Dietary intake, resting energy expenditure, weight loss and survival in cancer patients. *J Nutr.* 2002;132(11 suppl):3465S–3466S.

41. Edén E, Edström S, Bennegård K, Scherstén T, Lundholm K. Glucose flux in relation to energy expenditure in malnourished patients with and without cancer during periods of fasting and feeding. *Cancer Res.* 1984;44(4):1718–1724.

42. Lelbach A, Muzes G, Feher J. Current perspectives of catabolic mediators of cancer cachexia. *Med Sci Monit.* 2007;13(9):RA168–173.

43. National Cancer Institute. Depression (PDQ®). Pediatric considerations for depression. http://www.cancer.gov/cancertopics/pdq/supportivecare/depression/HealthProfessional/page7. Updated August 28, 2014. Accessed December 28, 2014.

44. Hersh SP, Wiener LS. In: Pizzo PA, Poplack DG, eds. *Principles and Practice of Pediatric Oncology.* Philadelphia: Lippincott, Williams & Wilkins; 2002:1365–1391.

45. Gilbreah J, Inman-Felton A, Johnson EQ, et al. *Medical Nutrition Therapy Across the Continuum of Care-Client Protocols.* 2nd ed. Chicago: The American Dietetic Association; 1998.

46. Ladas EJ, Sacks N, Brophy P, Rogers PC. Standards of nutritional care in pediatric oncology: results from a nationwide survey on the standards of practice in pediatric oncology. A Children's Oncology Group study. *Pediatr Blood Cancer.* 2006;46(3):339–344.

47. Green GJ, Weitzman SS, Pencharz PB. Resting energy expenditure in children newly diagnosed with stage IV neuroblastoma. *Pediatr Res.* 2008;63(3):332–336.

48. Rickard KA, Detamore CM, Coates TD, et al. Effect of nutrition staging on treatment delays and outcome in Stage IV neuroblastoma. *Cancer.* 1983;52(4):587–598.

49. Lobato-Mendizábal E, Ruiz-Argüelles GJ, Marín-López A. Leukaemia and nutrition. I: Malnutrition is an adverse prognostic factor in the outcome of treatment of patients with standard-risk acute lymphoblastic leukaemia. *Leuk Res.* 1989;13(10):899–906.

50. Charuhas PM. Introduction to marrow transplant. *American Dietetics Association: Oncology Nutrition Dietetic Practice Group Newsletter* 1994;2–9.

51. Andrassy RJ, Chwals WJ. Nutritional support of the pediatric oncology patient. *Nutrition.* 1998;14(1):124–129.

52. Isanaka S, Villamor E, Shepherd S, Grais RF. Assessing the impact of the introduction of the World Health Organization growth standards and weight-for-height z-score criterion on the response to treatment of severe acute malnutrition in children: secondary data analysis. *Pediatrics.* 2009;123(1):e54–e59.

53. Reilly JJ, Odame I, McColl JH, McAllister PJ, Gibson BE, Wharton BA. Does weight for height have prognostic significance in children with acute lymphoblastic leukemia? *Am J Pediatr Hematol Oncol.* 1994;16(3):225–230.

54. Pedrosa F, Bonilla M, Liu A. Effect of malnutrition at the time of diagnosis on the survival of children treated for cancer in El Salvador and Northern Brazil. *J Pediatr Hematol Oncol.* 2000;22(6):502–505.

55. Viana MB, Murao M, Ramos G, et al. Malnutrition as a prognostic factor in lymphoblastic leukaemia: a multivariate analysis. *Arch Dis Child.* 1994;71(4):304–310.

56. Mejía-Aranguré JM, Fajardo-Gutiérrez A, Reyes-Ruíz NI, et al. Malnutrition in childhood lymphoblastic leukemia: a predictor of early mortality during the induction-to-remission phase of the treatment. *Arch Med Res.* 1999;30(2):150–153.

57. Hafitz MG, Mannan MA. Nutritional status at initial presentation in childhood acute lymphoblastic leukemia and its effect on induction of remission. *Mymensingh Med J.* 2007;17(2 suppl):S46–S51.

58. Sala A, Pencharz P, Barr RD. Children, cancer, and nutrition—a dynamic triangle in review. *Cancer.* 2004;100(4):677–687.

59. Halton JM, Scissons-Fisher CC. Impact of nutritional status on morbidity and dose intensity of chemotherapy during consolidation therapy in children with acute lymphoblastic leukemia (ALL). *J Pediatr Hematol Oncol.* 1999;21(4):317.

60. Obama M, Cangir A, van Eys J. Nutritional status and anthracycline cardiotoxicity in children. *South Med J.* 1983;76(5):577–578.

61. Hays DM, Merritt RJ, White L, Ashley J, Siegel SE. Effect of total parenteral nutrition on marrow recovery during induction therapy for acute nonlymphocytic leukemia in childhood. *Med Pediatr Oncol.* 1983;11(2):134–140.

62. Bakish J, Hargrave D, Tariq N, Laperriere N, Rutka JT, Bouffet E. Evaluation of dietetic intervention in children with me-

dulloblastoma or supratentorial primitive neuroectodermal tumors. *Cancer.* 2003;98(5):1014–1020.

63. Sacks N, Hwang WT, Lange BJ, et al. Proactive enteral tube feeding in pediatric patients undergoing chemotherapy. *Pediatr Blood Cancer.* 2014;61(2):281–285.

64. den Broeder E, Lippens RJ, van 't Hof MA, et al. Nasogastric tube feeding in children with cancer: the effect of two different formulas on weight, body composition, and serum protein concentrations. *JPEN J Parenter Enteral Nutr.* 2000;24(6):351–360.

65. Rickard KA, Foland BB, Detamore CM, et al. Effectiveness of central parenteral nutrition versus peripheral parenteral nutrition plus enteral nutrition in reversing protein-energy malnutrition in children with advanced neuroblastoma and Wilms' tumor: a prospective randomized study. *Am J Clin Nutr.* 1983;38(3):445–456.

66. Rickard KA, Becker MC, Loghmani E, et al. Effectiveness of two methods of parenteral nutrition support in improving muscle mass of children with neuroblastoma or Wilms' tumor. A randomized study. *Cancer.* 1989;64(1):116–125.

67. Bozzetti F. Nutritional support of the oncology patient. *Crit Rev Oncol Hematol.* 2013;87(2):172–200.

68. Post-White J, Ladas E. In: Baggott C, Foley GV, Fotchman D, Patterson K, eds. *Nursing Care of Children and Adolescents With Cancer and Blood Disorders.* Glenview, IL: Association of Pediatric Hematology/Oncology Nurses;2011:612–627.

69. Vickers AJ, Cassileth BR. Unconventional therapies for cancer and cancer-related symptoms. *Lancet Oncol.* 2001;2(4):226–232.

70. Kemper KJ, Vohra S, Walls R; Task Force on Complementary and Alternative Medicine; Provisional Section on Complementary, Holistic, and Integrative Medicine. American Academy of Pediatrics. The use of complementary and alternative medicine in pediatrics. *Pediatrics.* 2008;122(6):1374–1386.

71. American Academy of Pediatrics. Counseling families who choose complementary and alternative medicine for their child with chronic illness or disability. Committee on Children With Disabilities. *Pediatrics.* 2001;107(3):598–601.

72. Sencer SF, Kelly KM. Complementary and alternative therapies in pediatric oncology. *Pediatr Clin North Am.* 2007;54(6):1043-1060; xiii.

73. Bechard LJ, Eshauch AO, Jaksic T, Duggan C. Nutritional Supportive Care. In: Pizzo PA, Poplack DG, eds. *Principles and Practice of Pediatric Oncology.* 4th ed. Philadephia, PA: Lippincott, Williams & Wilkins. 2002:1285–1300.

74. Scrimshaw NS. Effect of infection on nutrition requirements. *JPEN J Parenter Enteral Nutr.* 1991;15(6):589–600.

75. Anderson PM, Schroeder G, Skubitz KM. "Oral glutamine reduces the duration and severity of stomatitis after cytotoxic cancer chemotherapy." Cancer 1998;83(7):1433–1439.

76. Choi K, Lee SS, Oh SJ, et al. The effect of oral glutamine on 5-fluorouracil/leucovorin-induced mucositis/stomatitis assessed by intestinal permeability test. *Clin Nutr.* 2007;26(1):57–62.

77. Cunningham RS, Bell R. Nutrition in cancer: an overview. *Semin Oncol Nurs.* 2000;16(2):90–98.

78. Grant M, Kravits K. Symptoms and their impact on nutrition. *Semin Oncol Nurs.* 2000;16(2):113–121.

79. Heidelbaugh JJ. Proton pump inhibitors and risk of vitamin and mineral deficiency. *Ther Adv Drug Saf.* 2013;4(3):125–133.

80. National Institutes of Health. Stem cell information: hematopoietic stem cells. http://stemcells.nih.gov/info/scireport/pages/chapter5.aspx. Updated January 20, 2011. Accessed December 29, 2014.

81. National Cancer Institute. Bone marrow transplantation and peripheral blood stem cell transplantation. http://www.cancer.gov/cancertopics/factsheet/Therapy/bone-marrow-transplant. Updated August 12, 2013. Accessed December 28, 2014.

82. Abikoff CM, Cairo MS. Reduced intensity conditioning and hematopoietic stem cell transplantation in pediatric nonmalignant disease: a new therapeutic paradigm. *J Pediatr.* 2014;164(5):952–953.e2.

83. White M, Murphy AJ, Hastings Y, et al. Nutritional status and energy expenditure in children pre-bone-marrow-transplant. *Bone Marrow Transplant.* 2005;35(8):775–779.

84. Cheney CL, Abson KG, Aker SN, et al. Body composition changes in marrow transplant recipients receiving total parenteral nutrition. *Cancer.* 1987;59(8):1515–1519.

85. Ringwald-Smith K, Williams R, et al. Determination of energy expenditure in bone marrow transplant patient. *Nutr Clin Pract.* 1998;13(5):215–218.

86. Duggan C, Bechard L, Donovan K, et al. Changes in resting energy expenditure among children undergoing allogeneic stem cell transplantation. *Am J Clin Nutr.* 2003;78(1):104–109.

87. Duro D, Bechard LJ, Feldman HA, et al. Weekly measurements accurately represent trends in resting energy expenditure in children undergoing hematopoietic stem cell transplantation. *JPEN J Parenter Enteral Nutr.* 2008;32(4):427–432.

88. Charuhas PM, Lipkin A, Lessen P, McMillen K. Hematopoietic stem cell transplantation. In: Merritt RJ, DeLegge M, Holcombe B, et al. *The A.S.P.E.N. Nutrition Support Practice Manual.* 2nd ed. Silver Spring, MD: American Society for Parenteral and Enteral Nutrition; 2005:187–199.

89. Bechard LJ. Oncology and stem cell transplantation. In: Baker SS, Baker RD, Davis AM, eds. *Pediatric Nutrition Support.* Sudbury, MD: Jones and Bartlett; 2007:433–445.

90. Charuhas PM. Nutrition management of oncology and marrow/hematopoietic stem cell transplantation. In: Amore-Spalding K, Neiman L. *Pediatric Manual of Clinical Dietetics.* 2nd ed. Chicago: American Dietetic Association; 2008:175–184.

91. Bunting D, D'Souza S. *Pediatric Nutrition Reference Guide.* 8th ed. Houston, TX: Texas Children's Hospital; 2008.

92. Barron MA, Duncan DS, Green GJ, et al. Efficacy and safety of radiologically placed gastrostomy tubes in paediatric haematology/oncology patients. *Med Pediatr Oncol.* 2000;34(3):177–182.

93. Charuhas PM, Gautier ST. Parenteral nutrition in pediatric oncology. In: Chernoff R, Baker RD, Baker SS, Davis AM,

eds. *Pediatric Parenteral Nutrition.* New York: Chapman and Hall; 1997.

94. Wickham RS, Rehwaldt M, Kefer C, et al. Taste changes experienced by patients receiving chemotherapy. *Oncol Nurs Forum.* 1999;26(4):697–706.

95. Capra S, Ferguson M, Ried K. Cancer: impact of nutrition intervention outcome—nutrition issues for patients. *Nutrition.* 2001;17(9):769–772.

96. Roberts S, Thompson J. Graft-vs-host disease: nutrition therapy in a challenging condition. *Nutr Clin Pract.* 2005;20(4):440–450.

97. Moody K, Finlay J, Mancuso C, Charlson M. Feasibility and safety of a pilot randomized trial of infection rate: neutropenic diet versus standard food safety guidelines. *J Pediatr Hematol Oncol.* 2006;28(3):126–133.

98. van Tiel FH, Harbers MM, Terporten PH, et al. Normal hospital and low-bacterial diet in patients with cytopenia after intensive chemotherapy for hematological malignancy: a study of safety. *Ann Oncol.* 2007;18(6):1080–1084.

99. Jubelirer SJ. The benefit of the neutropenic diet: fact or fiction? *Oncologist.* 2011;16(5):704–707.

100. Trifilio S, Helenowski I, Giel M, et al. Questioning the role of a neutropenic diet following hematopoetic stem cell transplantation. *Biol Blood Marrow Transplant.* 2012;18(9):1385–1390.

101. Center for Disease Control and Prevention. Food safety. http://www.cdc.gov/foodsafety/disease.htm. Accessed December 26, 2014.

102. De Santas K, Vlachos A. Care of the hematopoietic stem cell transplant patient after leaving the transplant center. In: Altman AJ, ed. *Supportive Care of Children with Cancer: Current Therapy and Guidelines from the Children's Oncology Group.* 3rd ed. Baltimore, MD: The Johns Hopkins University Press; 2004:286–333.

103. Hopman GD, Peña EG, Le Cessie S, Van Weel MH, Vossen JM, Mearin ML. Tube feeding and bone marrow transplantation. *Med Pediatr Oncol.* 2003;40(6):375–379.

104. Hastings Y, White M, Young J. Enteral nutrition and bone marrow transplantation. *J Pediatr Oncol Nurs.* 2006;23(2):103–110.

105. Garofolo A. Enteral nutrition during bone marrow transplantation in patients with pediatric cancer: a prospective cohort study. *Sao Paulo Med J.* 2012;130(3):159–166.

106. Papadopoulou A, Nathavitharana K, Williams MD, Darbyshire PJ, Booth IW. Diagnosis and clinical associations of zinc depletion following bone marrow transplantation. *Arch Dis Child.* 1996;74(4):328–331.

107. Sefcick A, Anderton D, Byrne JL, Teahon K, Russell NH. Naso-jejunal feeding in allogeneic bone marrow transplant recipients: results of a pilot study. *Bone Marrow Transplant.* 2001;28(12):1135–1139.

108. Dunn RL, Stettler N, Mascarenhas MR. Refeeding syndrome in hospitalized pediatric patients. *Nutr Clin Pract.* 2003;18(4):327–332.

109. Tresley J, Sheean PM. Refeeding syndrome: recognition is the key to prevention and management. *J Am Diet Assoc.* 2008;108(12):2105–2108.

110. Stern JM. Oncology fluid and electrolyte disorders. *Support Line.* 2005;27:19–27.

111. Fuhrman MP, Charney P, Mueller CM. Hepatic proteins and nutrition assessment. *J Am Diet Assoc.* 2004;104(8):1258–1264.

112. Gabay C, Kushner I. Acute-phase proteins and other systemic responses to inflammation. *N Engl J Med.* 1999;340(6):448–454.

113. Rodgers C, Wills-Alcoser P, Monroe R, McDonald L, Trevino M, Hockenberry M. Growth patterns and gastrointestinal symptoms in pediatric patients after hematopoietic stem cell transplantation. *Oncol Nurs Forum.* 2008;35(3):443–448.

114. Wasilewski-Masker K, Kaste SC, Hudson MM, Esiashvili N, Mattano LA, Meacham LR. Bone mineral density deficits in survivors of childhood cancer: long-term follow-up guidelines and review of the literature. *Pediatrics.* 2008;121(3):e705–713.

115. Rubenstein EB, Peterson DE, Schubert M, et al; Mucositis Study Section of the Multinational Association for Supportive Care in Cancer; International Society for Oral Oncology. Clinical practice guidelines for the prevention and treatment of cancer therapy-induced oral and gastrointestinal mucositis. *Cancer.* 2004;100(9 suppl):2026–2046.

116. Bardellini E, Schumacher F, Conti G, Porta F, Campus G, Majorana A. Risk factors for oral mucositis in children receiving hematopoietic cell transplantation for primary immunodeficiencies: a retrospective study. *Pediatr Transplant.* 2013;17(5): 492-497.

117. Filipovich AH, Weisdorf D, Pavletic S, et al. National Institutes of Health consensus development project on criteria for clinical trials in chronic graft-versus-host disease: I. Diagnosis and staging working group report. *Biol Blood Marrow Transplant.* 2005;11(12):945–956.

118. Griffith LM, Pavletic SZ, Lee SJ, Martin PJ, Schultz KR, Vogelsang GB. Chronic graft-versus-host disease—implementation of the National Institutes of Health Consensus Criteria for Clinical Trials. *Biol Blood Marrow Transplant.* 2008;14(4):379–384.

119. MacMillan ML, Weisdorf DJ, Wagner JE, et al. Response of 443 patients to steroids as primary therapy for acute graft-versus-host disease: comparison of grading systems. *Biol Blood Marrow Transplant.* 2002;8(7):387–394.

120. Koc S, Leisenring W, Flowers ME, et al. Therapy for chronic graft-versus-host disease: a randomized trial comparing cyclosporine plus prednisone versus prednisone alone. *Blood.* 2002;100(1):48–51.

121. Martin PJ, Schoch G, Fisher L, et al. A retrospective analysis of therapy for acute graft-versus-host disease: initial treatment. *Blood.* 1990;76(8):1464–1472.

122. Ferrara JL, Levine JE, Reddy P, Holler E. Graft-versus-host disease. *Lancet.* 2009;373(9674):1550–1561.

123. Przepiorka D, Weisdorf D, Martin P, et al. 1994 Consensus Conference on Acute GVHD Grading. *Bone Marrow Transplant.* 1995;15(6):825–828.

124. Cahn JY, Klein JP, Lee SJ, et al; Société Française de Greffe de Moëlle et Thérapie Cellulaire; Dana Farber Cancer Institute; International Bone Marrow Transplant Registry. Pro-

spective evaluation of 2 acute graft-versus-host (GVHD) grading systems: a joint Société Francaise de Greffe de Moëlle et Thérapie Cellulaire (SFGM-TC), Dana Farber Cancer Institute (DFCI), and International Bone Marrow Transplant Registry (IBMTR) prospective study. *Blood.* 2005;106(4):1495–1500.

125. Petersdorf EW, Longton GM, Anasetti C, et al. The significance of HLA-DRB1 matching on clinical outcome after HLA-A, B, DR identical unrelated donor marrow transplantation. *Blood.* 1995;86(4):1606–1613.

126. Barker JN, Wagner JE. Umbilical-cord blood transplantation for the treatment of cancer. *Nat Rev Cancer.* 2003;3(7):526–532.

127. Zecca M, Prete A, Rondelli R, et al; AIEOP-BMT Group. Italian Association for Pediatric Hematology and Oncology-Bone Marrow Transplant. Chronic graft-versus-host disease in children: incidence, risk factors, and impact on outcome. *Blood.* 2002;100(4):1192–1200.

128. Akpek G, Valladares JL, Lee L, Margolis J, Vogelsang GB. Pancreatic insufficiency in patients with chronic graft-versus-host disease. *Bone Marrow Transplant.* 2001;27(2):163–166.

129. Barker CC, Anderson RA, Sauve RS, Butzner JD. GI complications in pediatric patients post-BMT. *Bone Marrow Transplant.* 2005;36(1):51–58.

130. Chakrabarti S, Collingham KE, Stevens RH, Pillay D, Fegan CD, Milligan DW. Isolation of viruses from stools in stem cell transplant recipients: a prospective surveillance study. *Bone Marrow Transplant.* 2000;25(3):277–282.

131. Wingard JR. Opportunistic infections after blood and marrow transplantation. *Transpl Infect Dis.* 1999;1(1):3–20.

132. Burgunder MR, Dickson BJ. Hematopoietic stem cell transplantation. In: Kogut VJ, Luthringer SL, eds. *Nutritional Issues in Cancer Care.* Pittsburgh, PA: Oncology Nursing Society; 2005:253–263.

133. Kloos RQ, Boelens JJ, de Jong TP, Versluys B, Bierings M. Hemorrhagic cystitis in a cohort of pediatric transplantations: incidence, treatment, outcome, and risk factors. *Biol Blood Marrow Transplant.* 2013;19(8):1263–1266.

134. Richardson PG, Elias AD, Krishnan A, et al. Treatment of severe veno-occlusive disease with defibrotide: compassionate use results in response without significant toxicity in a high-risk population. *Blood.* 1998;92(3):737–744.

135. Kumar S, DeLeve L, Kamath P, Tefferi A. Hepatic veno-111. occlusive disease (sinusoidal obstruction syndrome) after hematopoietic stem cell transplantation. *Mayo Clin Proc.* 2003;78:589–598.

136. Cesaro S, Pillon M, Talenti E, et al. A prospective survey on incidence, risk factors and therapy of hepatic veno-occlusive disease in children after hematopoietic stem cell transplantation. *Haematologica.* 2005;90(10):1396–1404.

137. Dignan FL, Wynn RF, Hadzic N, et al; Haemato-oncology Task Force of British Committee for Standards in Haematology; British Society for Blood and Marrow Transplantation. BCSH/BSBMT guideline: Diagnosis and management of veno-occlusive disease (sinusoidal obstruction syndrome) following haematopoietic stem cell transplantation. *Br J Haematol.* 2013;163(4):444–457.

138. Chicella MF, Batres LA, Heesters MS, Dice JE. Prokinetic drug therapy in children: a review of current options. *Ann Pharmacother.* 2005;39(4):706–711.

139. American Society of Clinical Oncology, Kris MG, Hesketh PJ, et al. American Society of Clinical Oncology guideline for antiemetics in oncology: update 2006. *J Clin Oncol.* 2006;24(18):2932–2947.

140. Food and Drug Administration. FDA requires boxed warning and risk mitigation strategy for metoclopramide-containing drugs. http://www.fda.gov/NewsEvents/Newsroom/PressAnnouncements/ucm149533.htm. Accessed October 19, 2014.

141. Curry JI, Lander TD, Stringer MD. Review article: erythromycin as a prokinetic agent in infants and children. *Aliment Pharmacol Ther.* 2001;15(5):595–603.

142. Cuttica CE, Chicella MF, Butler DE, Kaul A. Comparison of pantoprazole, omeprazole and ranitidine in children requiring acid suppression: a prospective pilot study. *J Pediatr Pharmacol Ther.* 2004;9:198–201.

143. Khan S, Shalaby TM, Orenstein SR. The effects of increasing doses of ranitidine on gastric pH in children. *J Pediatr Pharmacol Ther.* 2004;9(4):259–264.

144. Wedlake LJ, Loader G. Cancer therapy-induced mucositis: Where are we now? *Clinical Nutrition Highlights.* 2007;3:2–9.

145. McCarthy DM. Adverse effects of proton pump inhibitor drugs: clues and conclusions. *Curr Opin Gastroenterol.* 2010;26(6):624–631.

146. Whitworth J, Christensen ML. Clinical management of infants and children with gastroesophageal reflux disease. *J Pediatr Pharmacol Ther.* 2004;9(4):243–253.

147. Suzuki K, Doki K, Homma M, et al. Co-administration of proton pump inhibitors delays elimination of plasma methotrexate in high-dose methotrexate therapy. *Br J Clin Pharmacol.* 2009;67(1):44–49.

148. Hatlebakk JG, Katz PO, Camacho-Lobato L, Castell DO. Proton pump inhibitors: better acid suppression when taken before a meal than without a meal. *Aliment Pharmacol Ther.* 2000;14(10):1267–1272.

149. Woods DJ, McClintock AD. Omeprazole administration. *Ann Pharmacother.* 1993;27(5):651.

150. Olabisi A, Chen J, et al. Evaluation of different lansoprazole formulations for nasogastric or orogastric administration. *Hosp Pharm.* 2007;42(6):537–543.

151. National Comprehensive Cancer Network. Antiemesis guidelines. http://www.nccn.org/professionals/physician_gls/f_guidelines.asp#antiemesis. Accessed January 15, 2015.

152. Multinational Association of Supportive Care in Cancer. MASCC antiemetic guidelines. http://www.mascc.org/antiemetic-guidelines. Accessed January 15, 2015.

153. Schwartzberg LS. Chemotherapy-induced nausea and vomiting: which antiemetic for which therapy? *Oncology (Williston Park).* 2007;21(8):946–953; discussion 954, 959, 962 passim.

154. Geling O, Eichler HG. Should 5-hydroxytryptamine-3 receptor antagonists be administered beyond 24 hours after chemotherapy to prevent delayed emesis? Systematic re-eval-

154. uation of clinical evidence and drug cost implications. *J Clin Oncol.* 2005;23:1289- 1294.

155. Taketomo CK, Hodding JH, Kraus DM. *Pediatric Dosage Handbook.* Hudson, OH: Lexicomp; 2007.

156. Yavuzsen T, Davis MP, Walsh D, LeGrand S, Lagman R. Systematic review of the treatment of cancer-associated anorexia and weight loss. *J Clin Oncol.* 2005;23(33):8500–8511.

157. Loprinzi CL, Schaid DJ, Dose AM, Burnham NL, Jensen MD. Body-composition changes in patients who gain weight while receiving megestrol acetate. *J Clin Oncol.* 1993;11(1):152–154.

158. Cuvelier GD, Baker TJ, Peddie EF, et al. A randomized, double-blind, placebo-controlled clinical trial of megestrol acetate as an appetite stimulant in children with weight loss due to cancer and/or cancer therapy. *Pediatr Blood Cancer.* 2014;61(4):672–679.

159. Jatoi A, Windschitl HE, Loprinzi CL, et al. Dronabinol versus megestrol acetate versus combination therapy for cancer-associated anorexia: a North Central Cancer Treatment Group study. *J Clin Oncol.* 2002;20(2):567–573.

160. Cannabis-In-Cachexia-Study-Group, Strasser F, Luftner D, et al. Comparison of orally administered cannabis extract and delta-9-tetrahydrocannabinol in treating patients with cancer-related anorexia-cachexia syndrome: a multicenter, phase III, randomized, double-blind, placebo-controlled clinical trial from the Cannabis-In-Cachexia-Study-Group. *J Clin Oncol.* 2006;24(21):3394–3400.

161. Muramatsu RS, Silva N, Ahmed I. Suspected dronabinol withdrawal in an elderly cannabis-naive medically ill patient. *Am J Psychiatry.* 2013;170(7):804.

162. Kardinal CG, Loprinzi CL, Schaid DJ, et al. A controlled trial of cyproheptadine in cancer patients with anorexia and/or cachexia. *Cancer.* 1990;65(12):2657–2662.

163. Couluris M, Mayer JL, Freyer DR, Sandler E, Xu P, Krischer JP. The effect of cyproheptadine hydrochloride (periactin) and megestrol acetate (megace) on weight in children with cancer/treatment-related cachexia. *J Pediatr Hematol Oncol.* 2008;30(11):791–797.

164. Multinational Association of Supportive Care in Cancer. MASCC/ISOO mucositis guidelines. http://www.mascc.org/mucositis-guidelines. Accessed October 16, 2014.

165. Sencer SF, Zhou T, Freedman LS, et al. Traumeel S in preventing and treating mucositis in young patients undergoing SCT: a report of the Children's Oncology Group. *Bone Marrow Transplant.* 2012;47(11):1409–1414.

166. Anderson PM, Ramsay NK, Shu XO, et al. Effect of low-dose oral glutamine on painful stomatitis during bone marrow transplantation. *Bone Marrow Transplant.* 1998;22(4):339–344.

167. Cockerham MB, Weinberger BB, Lerchie SB. Oral glutamine for the prevention of oral mucositis associated with high-dose paclitaxel and melphalan for autologous bone marrow transplantation. *Ann Pharmacother.* 2000;34(3):300–303.

168. Keefe DM, Schubert MM, et al. Updated clinical practice 141. guidelines for the prevention and treatment of mucositis. *Cancer.* 2007;109(5):820–831.

169. Children's Oncology Group. Long-term follow-up guidelines for survivors of childhood, adolescent and young adult cancer. Version 4.0. http://www.survivorshipguidelines.org/pdf/LTFUGuidelines.pdf. Updated March 2013. Accessed June 17, 2014.

170. Schwartz CL. Late effects of treatment in long-term survivors of cancer. *Cancer Treat Rev.* 1995;21(4):355–366.

171. Arroyave WD, Clipp EC, Miller PE, et al. Childhood cancer survivors' perceived barriers to improving exercise and dietary behaviors. *Oncol Nurs Forum.* 2008;35(1):121–130.

172. Demark-Wahnefried W, Werner C, Clipp EC, et al. Survivors of childhood cancer and their guardians. *Cancer.* 2005;15;103(10):2171–2180.

173. Castellino S. GI Health—Gastrointestinal Health after Childhood Cancer. Health Link—Healthy living after treatment for childhood cancer GI health, Version 3.0 - 10/08. 2008.

174. American Institute for Cancer Research. AICR's Guidelines for Cancer Survivors. Washington DC: American Institute for Cancer Research; 2014. http://www.aicr.org/patients-survivors/aicrs-guidelines-for-cancer.html. Accessed December 26, 2014.

175. Blatt J. Bone Health—Keeping Your Bones Healthy after Childhood Cancer. Health Link—Healthy living after treatment for childhood cancer. Version 3.0 - 10/08. 2008.

176. Kenney LB, Diller L. Childhood cancer survivorship. In: Orkin SH, Fisher DE, eds. *Oncology of Infancy and Childhood.* Philadelphia , PA: WB Saunders & Company; 2009:1255–1289.

177. Institute of Medicine. DRIs for calcium and vitamin D. http://www.iom.edu/Reports/2010/Dietary-Reference-Intakes-for-Calcium-and-Vitamin-D/DRI-Values.aspx. Accessed January 15, 2015.

178. Gleeson HK, Darzy K, Shalet SM. Late endocrine, metabolic and skeletal sequelae following treatment of childhood cancer. *Best Pract Res Clin Endocrinol Metab.* 2002;16(2):335–348.

179. CureSearch for Children's Cancer. Number of diagnoses. http://www.curesearch.org/Number-of-Diagnoses/. Accessed January 15, 2015.

180. Craig F, Leiper AD, Stanhope R, et al. Sexually dimorphic and radiation dose dependent effect of cranial irradiation on body mass index. *Arch Dis Child.* 1999;81(6):500–504.

181. Talvensaari K, Knip M. Childhood cancer and later development of the metabolic syndrome. *Ann Med.* 1997;29(5):353–355.

182. Friedman D, Hudson MM, Landier W. Heart Health—Keeping Your Heart Healthy after Treatment for Childhood Cancer. Health Link—Healthy living after treatment for childhood cancer Version 3.0 - 10/08. 2008.

183. Mertens AC, Yasui Y, Neglia JP, et al. Late mortality experience in five-year survivors of childhood and adolescent cancer: the Childhood Cancer Survivor Study. *J Clin Oncol.* 2001;19(13):3163–3172.

184. Green DM, Grigoriev YA, Nan B, et al. Congestive heart failure after treatment for Wilms' tumor: a report from

the National Wilms' Tumor Study group. *J Clin Oncol.* 2001;19(7):1926- 1934.

185. Stewart JR, Fajardo LF, Gillette SM, Constine LS. Radiation injury to the heart. *Int J Radiat Oncol Biol Phys.* 1995;31(5):1205–1211.

186. Frierdich S. Diet and Physical Activity—Staying healthy through Diet and Physical Activity. Health Link—Healthy living after treatment for childhood cancer Version 3.0 - 10/08. 2008.

Answers

1. The answer is **A**. Methotrexate leads to the development of mucositis which severely compromises oral intake.[144]

2. The answer is **D**. All of the above. EN through the use of feeding tubes is often discouraged in the pediatric hematopoietic transplant population because of the need for frequent tube replacement as a result of vomiting, the risk of bleeding in the presence of thrombocytopenia and pancytopenia with mucositis, dislodgement of the feeding tube, the presence of delayed gastric emptying, and malabsorption of nutrients.[88]

3. The answer is **D**. The absorption of other drugs is increased or decreased.

4. The answer is **D**. All of the factors listed can contribute to osteoporosis in the cancer survivor.

30

Trauma and Burns

Arlet G. Kurkchubasche, MD

CONTENTS

Learning Objectives

1. Understand the components of the stress response and how these contribute to hypermetabolism in trauma and burn patients.
2. Identify childhood conditions that place patients at risk for trauma and child abuse, as well as nutrition impairment.
3. Understand the injury pattern seen in blunt trauma and how it impacts the ability to use enteral nutrition.
4. Understand limitations of methods for predicting energy needs in pediatric patients with significant burn injury.

Nutrition Considerations in the Pediatric Trauma Patient

Trauma, burn injury, and surgery are known stressors resulting in hormonal, metabolic, and immune derangements. The initial physiological response to these events is well studied and is generally described in terms of the hormonal and cytokine responses. These responses include the centrally mediated release of adrenocorticotropic hormone (ACTH), which stimulates cortisol release from the adrenal glands. This augments the action of epinephrine and norepinephrine, which are released from the adrenal medulla via sympathetic stimulation and impact the cardiovascular response. Glucagon is responsible for mobilizing glucose availability via glycogenolysis and gluconeogenesis. During the initial resuscitation, tissue perfusion is reduced and there is an overall (transient) reduction in metabolic rate. This is promptly followed by the hypermetabolic/catabolic phase of injury, which is mediated by the hypothalamic-pituitary axis and the proinflammatory cytokines (ie, tumor necrosis factor, interleukin-6). This phase is characterized by changes in glucose homeostasis, with insulin promoting lipolysis and proteolysis to generate glucose, while relative insulin resistance contributes to elevated serum glucose levels during this acute phase.

Trauma and burn injury have provided good clinical models for studying these responses because they are "quantifiable" injuries in terms of trauma scores and extent of burn injury. The physiological responses in the pediatric patient are fundamentally no different than in the adult. The focus of nutrition management is aligned with the fundamentals of critical care, which attempt to optimize all organ function by ensuring adequate perfusion and tissue oxygenation. Support of this hypermetabolic state, with an aim to control the resultant hyperglycemia and to limit the extent of proteolysis, becomes the focus of nutrition interventions. The specific nutrient requirements and whether certain micronutrients either become conditionally essential or can impact the elaboration of proinflammatory and anti-inflammatory cytokines and other agents such as nitric oxide have been the subject of intense research.

The premise of this chapter on trauma and burns is that the nutrition support of the child in the critical care unit follows clinical guidelines that parallel those of the child presenting with shock and sepsis or respiratory failure. However, what distinguishes this surgical scenario is that appropriate consideration must be given to the actual physical and physiological insult and therapies employed to treat them. Pain management, therefore, plays a significant role in the injured patient. While the use of narcotic and non-narcotic medications contributes to an amelioration of metabolic demands, it also promotes intestinal dysmotility and ileus and thereby impacts enteral feeding tolerance. The use of sedating agents, such as propofol, which are solubilized in a lipid solution, may require consideration when these patients require parenteral nutrition (PN) support to avoid excess dosing of lipids.

In this set of patients, the goals of energy provision are estimated to be 130%–160% of resting energy expenditure (REE) with an expectation to initiate this by day 3 and consistently deliver this by 7 days post injury. Even the route of administration is dependent on patient-specific factors. Particularly in burn injuries, when repeated operative debridement under anesthesia and significant dressing changes may need to be performed under heavy sedation, there has been an impact on nutritional support because of interruptions due to these care needs. This has been well documented in the literature and has prompted the development of algorithms that address these needs. The placement of postpyloric feeding tubes and provision of ongoing enteral feedings have become an accepted intervention to optimize nutrition support, especially since the targets cannot otherwise be achieved.

General Background on Trauma in Childhood

Trauma accounts for significant morbidity, mortality, and long-term disability in children. The patterns of pediatric trauma are both age-related and gender-related. Mechanisms for injury in children in the first 3 years of life include falls, poisoning (including caustic ingestions), transportation-related injuries, foreign body aspiration or ingestion, burn injuries, assault/neglect, and submersion/drowning mechanisms. With the older child, falls and bicycle/pedestrian and transportation-related injuries occur at a greater frequency. These primarily blunt mechanisms are accompanied later in adolescence by an increasing number of penetrating injuries. The specific organ injuries are broadly classified as neurotrauma (closed head injury/traumatic brain injury and spinal cord injury), thoracic trauma (chest wall, pulmonary, and cardiac), abdominal-pelvic trauma (solid and hollow visceral, genitourinary), and musculoskeletal injuries (long bone and pelvic fractures, craniofacial injuries). An anatomical classification system allows for injury severity scoring, which has a strong relationship with outcomes including morbidity, mortality, and length of stay.

While most children are generally healthy prior to their acute injury, others have underlying diagnoses such as neurodevelopmental delay, disorders on the autism spectrum, or attention deficit disorder. These conditions not only modify their risk-taking behaviors and place them at risk for injury but also potentially contribute factors that may result in nutrition depletion over a shorter period of time than expected. On the opposite end of the spectrum, children injured as passive bystanders/occupants of a vehicle may also present with significant issues related to overweight/obesity.[1] These issues may complicate their acute surgical management and impact their nutrition support in the acute phase. The effect of excess weight on outcomes of critically ill children has been evaluated, but not in a specific surgical cohort.[2]

The sections below provide brief descriptions of the most common forms of pediatric trauma and serve to provide a perspective on when, in the course of injury, enteral nutrition is feasible and when there should be an anticipation of prolonged nonenteral nutrition.

Closed Head Injuries/Traumatic Brain Injury

The brain has an inordinately high metabolic demand, and under normal circumstances brain metabolism and cerebral blood flow are generally tightly regulated. When there is a traumatic brain injury, there is frequently a change in cerebral perfusion as a consequence of intracranial pressure changes.[3] Despite this, the brain remains critically dependent on the uninterrupted delivery of both oxygen and glucose. Failure to support the brain adequately during this period likely impacts long-term outcomes. Current brain protective strategies may also affect the actual metabolic demand and alter the extent of caloric support.[4]

Hypothermia protocols in pediatric traumatic brain injury aim to reduce the metabolic needs during periods of relative hypoperfusion. Clearly the nutrition support of such a severely injured patient will require assurance of glucose provision; however, the concomitant use of medications such as glucocorticoids and development of diabetes insipidus (DI) place this patient at risk for hyperglycemia. Furthermore, sodium and water balance are affected by the syndrome of inappropriate antidiuretic hormone secretion (SIADH) and DI, as well as by administration of resuscitative fluids that may include hypertonic saline. These electrolyte and fluid balance issues may impact the ability to provide proteins, which along with lipids remain essential during the catabolic phase. Once neurologic recovery is underway, maintenance of muscular tone for adequate respiratory function and physical rehabilitation is critical. The use of immune-enhancing diets containing omega-3 fatty acids, branched-chain amino acids, and nucleotides has been evaluated in head injury patients and has not shown a benefit over the use of standard nutritional formulations.[5]

With a transition into rehabilitation facilities, nutrition management is still tightly regulated because these patients often have impaired swallowing and airway protection. Estimating caloric needs is difficult, and there are many studies documenting a difference between the calculated needs of the predictive equations and actual needs based on nitrogen balance studies.[6,7] The concern is that overfeeding will lead to hyperglycemia for the reasons mentioned above and an excessive respiratory quotient (RQ) that will impact the patient's ventilatory management.

Spine and Spinal Cord Trauma

This constellation of injuries more often affects the adolescent in the context of sports injuries, diving, and motor vehicle crashes. Injuries to the cervical and thoracolumbar spine are a common concern in the evaluation of the trauma patient, although the incidence is lower than in adults and compromises < 2% of all fractures in children. Options for stabilization are based on the instability of the vertebral column, and these injuries often can be managed nonoperatively. Of primary concern is the protection of the spinal cord and preservation of neurologic function. Secondary concerns relate to the normal ongoing growth and development of the axial skeleton to prevent progressive spinal deformity. Spinal injuries often do not occur in isolation, and there are reciprocal paradigms that ensure full imaging of the thoracolumbar spine when significant abdominal injuries occur that require emergent exploration and, conversely, require spine imaging due to findings such as the "seat belt sign" from lap restraints that can result in Chance fractures (flexion/distraction injury to the lumbar spine), which are associated with small bowel injuries.[8] Both orthopedic surgeons specializing in pediatric spine disorders and neurosurgeons may be involved in the care of these patients. When a spinal cord injury has occurred, particularly in the cervical spine, patient support may require chronic ventilator and nutritional support based on the extent of neurologic deficit.

The peri-injury protection of the spinal cord remains a topic of active research and controversy and includes the acute use of steroids in those with "incomplete" injury as well as hypothermia protocols. The nutrition assessment of these patients becomes a very individualized task due to variability in neuromuscular deficit and metabolic demand despite ongoing perfusion.[9,10]

Blunt Abdominal Trauma/Solid Visceral Injuries

Solid organ injuries are some of the most frequent injuries encountered in the pediatric patient. In contrast to the adult population, these injuries are frequently isolated and can be managed nonoperatively. Despite their prevalence, there has been no universally accepted algorithm for their management. While radiographic parameters permit grading of injuries to indicate severity of injury, it is the hemodynamic response to injury that determines the immediate course of action. Operative intervention is reserved for those with profound or persistent hemodynamic instability. Simple immobilization with bed rest may be sufficient in most patients to permit intrinsic mechanisms for hemostasis to result in the formation of a stable hematoma. Since the stomach is intricately associated with the spleen via the short gastric vessels, it is usually decompressed or enteral feedings are at least withheld for 24 hours to avoid gastric distention and retching. If there has been a significant amount of blood in the abdomen, this not only creates abdominal pain but also is responsible for a transient ileus. The period of observation with bed rest is variable and is generally related to the degree of injury. Hemodynamic instability despite transfusion is the predominant factor in determining whether nonoperative management will be successful. With hemodynamically unstable splenic injuries, splenic salvage can be attempted operatively or splenectomy may become necessary. Given the role of the spleen in the immunocompetency of the child, every effort is made to avoid splenectomy.

Hepatic injuries rarely require operative intervention. In the most severe instances an avulsion of the liver off the retrohepatic vena cava occurs, and these injuries are generally immediately fatal. Parenchymal injuries are best managed nonoperatively, especially if Glisson's capsule is intact. The abdominal wall provides some compression and containment, which is lost with laparotomy. When hemodynamic instability mandates exploration, the liver is packed with laparotomy sponges to compress the injured tissues, arterial inflow can be reduced by occluding the hepatic artery manually, and injured segments can either be compressed with large sutures or resected. Control of hemorrhage is as much a surgical event as it is a medical event in that hypothermia and coagulopathy can rapidly obviate any surgical advances. In the patient who is or becomes stable, postoperative management will assess bilirubin levels, which may become elevated for a number of reasons (shed blood, biloma formation, biliary ascites). Intestinal bleeding may be from hemobilia, in which a fistula forms from the vascular system into the biliary ductal system. Depending on the degree of shock, the liver parenchyma may exhibit some degree of hepatic dysfunction, which should be taken into account when selecting medications. With restoration of adequate perfusion, this is usually only a transient phenomenon. These solid organ injuries are rarely associated with significant gastrointestinal dysfunction, and oral diets are resumed within several days of injury. Depending on the severity of injury and whether there are additional injuries, these patients may benefit from caloric supplementation. This is because these children may not demonstrate a normal appetite and may develop constipation due to the lack of physical activity.

Pancreatic Trauma

The pancreas is typically injured as a consequence of a compression force to the midabdomen. This may be a bicycle handlebar or another object striking the epigastrium, or it can be the consequence of a deceleration injury associated with the use of a seatbelt. Child abuse must always be considered when the mechanism is otherwise not obvious. Complete fractures of the pancreas occur over the neck of the organ where it crosses the spinal column. Initial laboratory assessment in the trauma room has been found to be inadequate for detection of this injury. Amylase and lipase levels rise typically 8 hours after injury. Computed tomography (CT) scanning of the abdomen is a method that often raises concern, and it may not be sufficiently sensitive. While adult trauma protocols would mandate operative exploration, there are case series in pediatric patients in which the injury is managed nonoperatively with the use of endoscopic retrograde cholangiopancreatography (ERCP) for stenting of the ampulla so as to provide a low-pressure system for pancreatic secretions to drain in to the GI tract rather than forming a pseudocyst.[11] These cases are controversial, and the most "conservative" approach may indeed be exploration with resection of the tail of the pancreas, thereby eliminating the ongoing leak of pancreatic enzymes and avoiding prolonged dependency on PN.[12] Resections at this level of the pancreas are not expected to affect glucose homeostasis, although there are some reports of late pancreatic exocrine insufficiency, which present with malabsorption as evidenced by diarrheal stools.

The patient who develops a pancreatic pseudocyst as a consequence of the trauma can be managed with laparoscopic, open, or endoscopic cyst gastrostomy. This is usually delayed for 4–6 weeks to allow the cyst wall to "mature." This allows the cyst content of pancreatic secretions to drain into the intestinal tract with the ultimate expectation that the ductal defect will heal and that the pseudocyst involutes.

The extent of nutrition support depends on the physiologic impact of this traumatic pancreatitis. When jejunal access can be safely established, it is reasonable to use this route once there is evidence of return of intestinal motility. In the most severely injured, with ongoing pancreatitis and perhaps complications such as tissue necrosis and infection, parenteral nutrition is likely essential in the early postinjury period.

Renal Trauma

Injuries to the kidneys are typically unilateral, and assessment must include evaluation of the ureter and bladder. Typically, delayed phase images on CT scans will identify urinary extravasation. In the absence of urine extravasation, renal injuries are primarily managed nonoperatively. Patients remain on bed rest until the hematuria subsides. If urinary extravasation occurs, it is classified as contained or free. The former may permit ongoing nonoperative management, although placement of a ureteral stent or percutaneous drainage would be advised in the latter. In rare cases a primary nephrectomy is performed. Late consequences of renal injury include the development of renovascular hypertension. These patients generally experience a transient ileus and then are able to resume an enteral diet. There are rarely concerns of renal insufficiency that would lead to a consideration of special diets.

Adrenal Hemorrhage

The adrenal glands have an exuberant blood supply from multiple sources. While generally protected in the retroperitoneum, they are at risk for direct injury, but rarely as an isolated organ. Injury is generally evident as adrenal hemorrhage but does not necessarily portend adrenal insufficiency, even when bilateral. When isolated, these injuries have minimal impact on the overall nutrition management of the patient.

Blunt Abdominal Trauma/Hollow Visceral Injuries

Duodenal Injuries

Duodenal hematoma and perforation are not infrequently encountered in pediatric trauma. They occur with blunt force trauma to the epigastrium (ie, bicycle handlebar injury, nonaccidental trauma). While most duodenal hematomas are dealt with nonoperatively, duodenal perforation is a significant injury that demands prompt operative intervention to avoid morbidity and even mortality. Duodenal hematomas become symptomatic when extraluminal blood impacts on the luminal caliber, resulting in gastric outlet obstruction. Passage of a transduodenal feeding tube is almost always possible, either by radiographic guidance or endoscopically. This allows the patient to receive enteral nutrition despite the proximal obstruction, which may require decompression with a concomitant nasogastric tube. Operative intervention is rarely indicated in this injury. Pancreatic injury may be concomitant, so it is wise to check for chemical pancreatitis before initiating feeds. Resolution of the obstruction can occur within 10–14 days of injury as evidenced by improved gastric emptying.

Duodenal perforation is a much more significant injury that, depending on its extent, will require either primary repair with drain placement or sometimes more complicated surgical solutions to protect the duodenal repair from leakage (ie, pyloric exclusion with gastrojejunostomy). Typically, the pyloric channel will open 4–6 weeks later, which prompts the gastrojejunostomy to close spontaneously. These patients will often require PN support in the early postoperative phase until the gastrojejunal anastomosis becomes functional.

Small Intestine and Colon Injuries

Jejunoileal perforations or mesenteric injuries resulting in devascularized segments of small intestine are frequently associated with seatbelt injuries and other mechanisms resulting in deceleration forces on the abdomen. The presence of a Chance fracture, a flexion-distraction fracture of the midlumbar region, was considered a hallmark for potential bowel injury.[13] These may not be evident on initial CT imaging and may present within the first 24 hours, supporting the practice of repeated surgical examination of these patients while *nil per os*. Unless there is an extensive delay in diagnosis (> 24 hours), most of these injuries can be treated with resection and anastomosis and should allow for resumption of oral alimentation within 5 days. Missed injuries are likely the consequence of vascular insufficiency resulting in stricture and may present 4–6 weeks after the traumatic event with symptoms of enteral intolerance.

Injuries to the colon are most likely the consequence of a penetrating rather than blunt mechanism and in the young can involve mechanisms such as falling onto sharp objects, rather than the missile injuries in the teenagers and young adults. Exploration is indicated in hemodynamically unstable patients and those with peritoneal findings. The use of a triple contrast CT involves administration of intravenous, enteral, and rectal contrast and has become a reliable exam in those with a penetrating injury and without the above parameters for exploration. In the absence of massive contamination, primary repair of colon injuries is attempted, in lieu of diversion. A return to oral alimentation should be possible after resolution of postoperative ileus and should not require interval nutritional intervention.

Thoracic Injuries

Thoracic injuries in children may be remarkably unassociated with chest wall signs of trauma. The bony thoracic cage is sufficiently pliable in the young child to permit complete transduction of the impact energy to the lung parenchyma, resulting in pulmonary injury that most often consists of contusion rather than overt tissue disruption. Similarly, the pliability of the intrathoracic vessels results in fewer great vessel injuries than seen in the adult population. Blunt cardiac trauma is also well compensated with the capacity to offset compromised contractility with an increased heart rate response. When intrathoracic injuries occur that require operative intervention, recovery is supported by the generally healthy state of these organs. Often these injuries occur in the setting of multiple trauma and then require mechanical pulmonary support. When in isolation, they are usually of minimal consequence to nutrition management. Notable exceptions include direct esophageal injuries and chylothorax. Esophageal injuries may be the consequence of penetrating trauma, caustic ingestion, or ingestion of batteries. Batteries, particularly disk batteries, are ingested by young children and become lodged in the upper esophagus where they discharge their energy, may leak content, and create pressure-induced mucosal changes from the resultant contraction of the esophagus. With minimal mucosal damage, the patient can frequently return to a normal diet. Depending on the nature and severity of the injury, there may be an indication for gastrostomy or gastrojejunostomy placement for distal enteral feedings.[14] The development of a traumatic chylothorax is most often associated with a diaphragm injury. Depending on the amount of output via chest tubes, this may require initial enteral rest with progression to enteral nutrients with medium-chain triglycerides to reduce lymphatic flow and leak. These injuries may require a prolonged period of nonoperative management and consequent parenteral or enteral nutrition.[15]

Pelvis and Extremity Trauma

When long bone fractures and pelvic fractures occur in multiply injured trauma patients, these injuries contribute to the injury severity score and consequently to the nutrition and metabolic demands of the patient. When these bony injuries are associated with overlying open soft tissue wounds, the risk for infection is increased. Operative management for limiting the extent of contamination and fixation of the fracture are routine measures. Even simple immobilization, whether of a long bone fracture or the pelvis, has metabolic consequences to the patient. The importance of providing adequate vitamin D and calcium is emphasized in the current literature. The focus of the American Academy of Pediatrics consortium on calcium was on prevention to limit the fracture risk for young children and adolescents.[16,17] The prevalence of sports-related injuries in otherwise healthy young adolescents has led to studies of their bone health, including vitamin D status.[18]

In the skeletally immature pediatric patient, the consequences of growth plate fractures, nonunion of fractures, and subsequent growth impairment are critical to address. In the absence of multiple organ injury involving the abdo-

men, these patients rapidly resume enteral intake. Targets for caloric intake should include consideration of level of activity.

Facial trauma constitutes a specific subset of musculoskeletal trauma and is often associated with closed head injury. It has the added concerns for impacting enteral alimentation when the mandible and maxilla are involved. The passage of nasal tubes may be contraindicated in the presence of a basilar skull fracture, and depending on the patient's mental status, alimentation may be accessible via straw through a wire-stabilized jaw, or more extreme measures such as gastrostomy may need to be considered early in the course.

Summary on Pediatric Trauma

While much pediatric trauma is of a minor and ambulatory nature, those children with major single-system injuries or multiply injured pediatric trauma patients require early and intense evaluation for nutrition support. After restoration of vital organ perfusion, consistent nutrition support is a critical intervention to ensure meeting the high metabolic demands imposed by injury.[19]

Pediatric Burns

Burn trauma encompasses injuries that occur as a result of flames, thermal and chemical exposure, inhalation of smoke, and electrical contact. These continue to inflict significant morbidity and mortality on patients at the extremes of age. Young children are particularly vulnerable to both accidental and nonaccidental burn injuries. The management of burns has evolved dramatically in the past 30 years with a centralization of care for the more severely injured patients. This has allowed for more concentrated experiences as well as focused clinical trials. The result of these data has been significantly improved outcomes, with decreased mortality attributable to shock and wound sepsis. These patients, however, require extensive and chronic support from a multidisciplinary team to return to optimal functional status. With a better understanding of the metabolic consequences of burn injury on both the animal research as well as on the clinical research front, the consistent emphasis on the importance of nutrition support has persisted as one of the hallmarks of burn care.[20]

Features Specific to the Pediatric Patient

Children, as compared with adults, will have deeper burn injuries for a given injury mechanism as a consequence of the thinner dermal structure and architecture. In contrast to the older patient, their thermal injury occurs as a consequence of contact with hot liquids in 70% of cases, rather than flame burn. The percent total body surface area (TBSA) involvement by second-degree and third-degree burns remains a critical determinant of mortality. An understanding of individualized burn resuscitation, guided by %TBSA involvement, has led to virtual elimination of burn shock as a cause of immediate death. With injuries involving > 20% of TBSA, there is an associated stress response that leads to the hypermetabolic state that has been well described with burn injury. It is less clear how TBSA impacts the severity of the stress response invoked when greater areas are involved,[21] although TBSA > 30%–40% results in tenfold elevations of urinary catecholamines.[22] Attempts to modulate the severity of this response have been diverse and have included wound management strategies, enteral feeding strategies, and the use of pharmacologic agents. Current therapies that employ early burn wound excision and grafting have had a significant impact in reducing wound infections, reducing transdermal losses of fluid and protein, and achieving earlier healing and rehabilitation. The improved technologies for coverage of burn wounds with reduced frequency of painful dressing changes also will reduce metabolic demands.[23,24]

Use of the intestinal tract for alimentation has been promoted for burn injuries in particular. Concerns about mucosal atrophy and impairment of the gut-associated immune defenses as a consequence of nonuse have been key motivators. While enteral feeding may frequently require administration via nasoenteric tubes, often oral supplementation is well received by young children. At times, simple nighttime supplementation to reach target caloric goals is sufficient. Choice of formula is typically based on calculated caloric needs with special emphasis on protein content. Early enteral feeding has not shown the benefit demonstrated with delayed enteral feeding and risks using an underperfused intestinal tract, thereby subjecting the patient to additional morbidity.[25,26] The use of pharmacologic agents such as growth hormone, oxandrolone (a testosterone analog), and insulin-like growth factor results in decreased catabolism, but it is unclear how this ultimately will affect clinical course and outcomes. The use of low-dose insulin has been described as a useful intervention, which may be a consequence of control of hyperglycemia in a state of relative insulin resistance.[27]

Despite the reluctance to use PN in burn injury, there are reports of the benefits with cautious use with hypocaloric goals.[28]

Inhalation injury also has a greater potential for complications in the young child as a consequence of the decreased luminal diameter of the trachea and bronchi with a propensity for formation of obstructive casts and secretion plugs. Early intubation and respiratory toilet are important, especially in those with associated facial burn injury, given the rapid and dramatic swelling associated with third-space extravasation of resuscitative fluids. These patients remain at risk for prolonged respiratory support and ventilator-associated pneumonias, which further impact their hypermetabolic state.[29] Recent studies document that the highest mortality is encountered in children under 4 years of age with TBSA > 30% and inhalation injury.[30]

Energy Estimates in Burn Injury

Children start off with greater metabolic and specific nutrient demands (greater caloric demand per kilogram) as compared with their adolescent and young adult counterparts, a demand that is amplified by the injury. They generally have lower energy stores, which are more rapidly depleted. Their propensity toward fevers, despite the absence of infection, further compounds their energy demands. Despite the ubiquitous use of the Harris Benedict equation and other variants to estimate caloric needs for these patients, these remain very rudimentary tools and there are data that they do not accurately reflect actual needs as measured by indirect calorimetry.[31] Providing excess calories will not obviate the proteolysis accompanying the hypermetabolic response, but likely contributes to hyperglycemia. How hyperglycemia specifically impacts the incidence of wound infection in burn patients is not known; however, there is enough suggestive evidence from other models of critical illness to avoid blatant overnutrition. On the opposite end, we know that undernutrition negatively impacts wound healing and maintenance of lean body mass. Muscle catabolism, particularly involving the muscles of respiration, leads to functional debilitation that can be measured in terms of prolonged respiratory support; however, physical rehabilitation of the core muscles and extremities is similarly impacted in the later stages of therapy. Despite the consistent recommendation to assess these patients with indirect calorimetry, in general, a target of 120%–130% of REE is believed to be appropriate.[32]

The composition of the energy sources is primarily carbohydrate (up to 60% of calories) but with maximum glucose load limited to 7 mg/kg/min. This is to avoid hyperglycemia and to limit lipogenesis that results in increased oxygen consumption and carbon dioxide elaboration, which raises the RQ. Lipids should initially deliver between 12% and 15% of total nonprotein calories. This lower proportion has been associated with improved clinical outcomes as compared with the higher lipid-containing diets (35% calories from fat) in a randomized clinical trial.[33] The use of omega-3 containing fatty acids is theoretically beneficial from the standpoint of reducing the precursors for prostaglandin E2 and leukotrienes, thereby limiting further immunosuppression. The protein needs are exacerbated in burn patients because of the additional losses via the open wounds in addition to the standard urine losses and the gluconeogenesis as seen in other instances of hypermetabolism. Daily intake of 2.5 g/kg/d and up to 4 g/kg/d may be necessary and is limited by the patient's state of hydration and renal function. Specific "immune-enhancing" diets that contain high protein loads, omega-3 fatty acids, and branched-chain amino acids and nucleotides have not been shown to be superior to standard high-protein diets.[34,35]

The preferred route of nutrition support remains enteral feedings, and these should be instituted as soon as it is deemed safe to use the intestinal tract. In some institutions the early use of postpyloric feedings is encouraged, and techniques have been developed to safely place these devices at the bedside.[36] Although initial studies suggested that early feeding would be beneficial, no clear benefit has been demonstrated in terms of decreased length of stay, morbidity, or mortality.[26] As with any other invasive procedure, the risks and benefits must be considered when initiating enteral feeds. There are case reports of early aggressive enteral feeding leading to luminal obstruction and perforation.[37] PN support retains a critical role in those patients with a prolonged ileus or persistent systemic and visceral hypoperfusion.

Laboratory evaluation using the standard visceral proteins is limited in the immediate/acute injury period and may be more useful as a predictor of outcomes, rather than as a measure of visceral protein status. The degree of hypoalbuminemia observed in early burn injury is attributable to the losses via the burn wound. Further complicating their interpretation is that albumin therapy is prevalent in burn resuscitation and does not reflect intrinsic production. Weight and other anthropometrics are also invalidated in the early resuscitative phase given the rapid expansion of the extravascular space. Trends in prealbumin and other visceral proteins, as well as weight changes once the acute resuscitative phase is complete are reasonable to monitor.

Clinical Example 1

A morbidly obese 14-year-old is transported to the trauma center after being involved in a multivehicle collision as a restrained passenger. Although alert and oriented, she is dyspneic and is found to have a pneumothorax. She has a significant air leak, suggesting a bronchial injury. She is intubated and undergoes bronchoscopy with subsequent thoracotomy for repair of a proximal airway injury. Her initial abdominal exam was unremarkable but limited by obesity. A Focused Assessment with Sonography for Trauma (FAST) exam was not possible, and the urgent intervention for her airway delayed further evaluation. She develops abdominal tenderness, which prompts CT evaluation and subsequent laparotomy for a left hepatic duct avulsion with ischemia to the left lobe of the liver. What are her requirements for energy support in this phase of her acute illness? How are they best met?

Answer/Considerations

The energy assessment of the overweight and morbidly obese teenager who requires critical care support is extraordinarily difficult. In this time of metabolic stress, the goal should not be weight management, but preservation of protein status. Estimates for caloric intake are best derived from assessment of metabolically active tissues, and these are more closely related to ideal body weight than actual. Not only will this patient need to heal her traumatic injuries, but she now has 2 additional wounds (thoracotomy and laparotomy) to heal. Indirect calorimetry will likely provide the best guidance in this scenario. Given the intra-abdominal injuries, one would expect a period of ileus to follow, and thus provision of nutrients should not be delayed and initially can occur by parenteral route.

Clinical Example 2

A 12-year-old equestrian sustained a kick to her stomach while grooming her horse. Her initial abdominal CT shows a hematoma over the neck of the pancreas. There is no free fluid in the abdomen. She is nauseated and a nasogastric tube evacuates bilious fluid. Over the next 24 hours she continues to complain of abdominal pain and her amylase rises to 950. Do you advise nutritional supplementation at this point?

It is now 5 days later, an ERCP has been done, and there is no major ductal injury. Her abdominal pain is improved and amylase is 200. What do you expect her ability to eat will be within the next 48 hours?

Answer/Considerations

Pancreatic injuries, despite nonoperative management, can lead to significant metabolic stress as a consequence of the inflammatory nature of the retroperitoneal injury (hematoma), which is further exacerbated by release of pancreatic enzymes. While we can expect this patient to have been active and healthy from a nutrition standpoint, we would anticipate a return to GI function within perhaps 5 days. The information related to the ERCP would suggest that cautious introduction of enteral feeds would be acceptable and that her response to enteral stimulation of pancreatic secretions must be monitored. Should she develop recurrent pain and pancreatitis with oral intake, institution of PN until such time as a jejunal feeding tube can be placed would be appropriate.

Clinical Example 3

A 2-year-old is brought to the trauma/burn unit with 35% TBSA injury from a hot oil burn to his face, trunk, and lower extremities. Within 24 hours, he has developed anasarca, but is hemodynamically stable and making urine at 1 mL/kg/h. He is scheduled to undergo burn wound excision on the following day. When do you consider starting nutrition support? How do you best determine his caloric needs? How do you initiate caloric intake?

Answer/Considerations

This child has sustained a significant injury and is expected to exhibit a stress response leading to catabolism. Nutrition support will become essential for re-establishing a positive nitrogen balance. Given the extent of injury, this child will likely have central venous access and provision of glucose and protein can be started early via this route. At the time of operation it would be ideal to have a nasoenteral tube placed for subsequent enteral feeding access. Energy requirements are notoriously difficult to predict, and indirect calorimetry remains the most accurate tool.

Test Your Knowledge Questions

1. Blunt abdominal trauma with injury to the liver:
   A. Requires prolonged support on PN
   B. Requires specialized formulas to account for hepatic insufficiency
   C. Rarely requires operative intervention
   D. Is rare in the pediatric patient
2. Pancreatic trauma may result in all except:
   A. Chemical pancreatitis
   B. Prolonged intestinal ileus
   C. Clinical features of pancreatic insufficiency
   D. Diabetes mellitus
3. Closed head injury patients unequivocally benefit from provision of immunonutrients.
   A. True
   B. False
4. Total burn surface area (TBSA) is most predictive of:
   A. Mortality
   B. Metabolic stress
   C. Energy needs
   D. None of the above

References

1. Rana AR, Michalsky MP, Teich S, Groner JI, Caniano DA, Schuster DP. Childhood obesity: A risk factor for injuries observed at a level-1 trauma center. *J Pediatr Surg.* 2009;44(8):1601–1605.
2. Goh VL, Wakeham MK, Brazauskas R, Mikhailov TA, Goday PS. Obesity is not associated with increased mortality and morbidity in critically ill children. *JPEN J Parenter Enteral Nutr.* 2013;37(1):102–108.
3. Philip S, Udomphorn Y, Kirkham F, Vavilala M. Cerebrovascular pathophysiology in pediatric traumatic brain injury. *J Trauma.* 2009;67(2 Suppl):S128.
4. Mtaweh H, Smith R, Kochanek PM, et al. Energy expenditure in children after severe traumatic brain injury. *Pediatr Crit Care Med.* 2014;15(3):242–249.
5. Briassoulis G, Filippou O, Kanariou M, Papassotiriou I, Hatzis T. Temporal nutritional and inflammatory changes in children with severe head injury fed a regular or an immune-enhancing diet: a randomized, controlled trial. *Pediatr Crit Care Med.* 2006;7(1):56.
6. Havalad S, Quaid M, Sapiega V. Energy expenditure in children with severe head injury: lack of agreement between measured and estimated energy expenditure. *Nutr Clin Pract.* 2006;21(2):175.
7. Joffe A, Anton N, Lequier L, et al. Nutritional support for critically ill children. *Cochrane Database Syst Rev.* 2009(2):CD005144.
8. Daniels AH, Sobel AD, Eberson CP. Pediatric thoracolumbar spine trauma, *J Am Acad Orthop Surg.* 2013;21:707–716.
9. Patt P, Agena S, Vogel L, Foley S, Anderson C. Estimation of resting energy expenditure in children with spinal cord injuries. *J Spinal Cord Med.* 2007;30(Suppl 1):S83.
10. Brown RL, Brunn MA, Garcia VF. Cervical spine injuries in children: A review of 103 patients treated consecutively at a level 1 pediatric trauma center. *J Pediatr Surg.* 2001;36(8):1107.

11. Maeda K, Ono S, Baba K, Kawahara I. Management of blunt pancreatic trauma in children. *Pediatr Surg Int.* 2013;29(10):1019–1022.

12. Beres AL, Wales PW, Christison-Lagay ER, McClure ME, Fallat ME, Brindle ME. Non-operative management of high-grade pancreatic trauma: is it worth the wait? *Pediatr Surg.* 2013;48(5):1060–1064.

13. Achildi O, Betz RR, Grewal H. Lapbelt injuries and the seatbelt syndrome in pediatric spinal cord injury. *J Spinal Cord Med.* 2007;30:S21–S24.

14. Fuentes S, Cano I, Benavent MI, Gomez A. Severe esophageal injuries caused by accidental ingestion of button batteries in children. *J Emerg Trauma Shock.* 2014;7(4):316–321.

15. Seitelman E, Arellano JJ, Takabe K, Barrett L, Faust G, George Angus LD. Chylothorax after blunt trauma. *J Thorac Dis.* 2012;4(3):327–330.

16. Baker SS, Cochran WJ, Flores CA, et al. American Academy of Pediatrics. Committee on Nutrition. Calcium requirements of infants, children, and adolescents. *Pediatrics.* 1999;104(5):1152.

17. Goulding A. Risk factors for fractures in normally active children and adolescents. *Med Sport Sci.* 2007;51:102.

18. James JR, Massey PA, Hollister AM, Greber EM. Prevalence of hypovitaminosis D among children with upper extremity fractures. *J Pediatr Orthop.* 2013;33(2):159–162.

19. Hasenboehler E, Williams A, Leinhase I, et al. Metabolic changes after polytrauma: an imperative for early nutritional support. *World J Emerg Surg.* 2006;1:29.

20. Purdue G. American Burn Association presidential address 2006 on nutrition: yesterday, today, and tomorrow. *J Burn Care Res.* 2007;28(1):1.

21. Atiyeh B, Gunn SWA, Dibo S. Metabolic implications of severe burn injuries and their management: a systematic review of the literature. *World J Surg.* 2008;32(8):1857.

22. Chan M, Chan G. Nutritional therapy for burns in children and adults. *Nutrition.* 2009;25(3):261.

23. Saba S, Tsai R, Glat P. Clinical evaluation comparing the efficacy of aquacel ag hydrofiber dressing versus petrolatum gauze with antibiotic ointment in partial-thickness burns in a pediatric burn center. *J Burn Care Res.* 2009;30(3):380.

24. Saffle JR. Closure of the excised burn wound: temporary skin substitutes. *Clin Plast Surg.* 2009;10;36(4):627–641.

25. Venter M, Rode H, Sive A, Visser M. Enteral resuscitation and early enteral feeding in children with major burns—effect on McFarlane response to stress. *Burns.* 2007;33(4):464–471.

26. Peck M, Kessler M, Cairns B, Chang Y, Ivanova A, Schooler W. Early enteral nutrition does not decrease hypermetabolism associated with burn injury. *J Trauma.* 2004;57(6):1143.

27. Schulman C, Ivascu F. Nutritional and metabolic consequences in the pediatric burn patient. *J Craniofac Surg.* 2008;19(4):891.

28. Dylewksi ML, Baker M, Prelack K, et al. The safety and efficacy of parenteral nutrition among pediatric patients with burn injuries. *Pediatr Crit Care Med.* 2013;14(3):e120–e125.

29. Palmieri T, Warner P, Mlcak R, et al. Inhalation injury in children: a 10 year experience at Shriners Hospitals for children. *J Burn Care Res.* 2009;30(1):206.

30. Sheridan RL, Schnitzer JJ. Management of the high-risk pediatric burn patient. *J Pediatr Surg.* 2001;36(8):1308–1312.

31. Suman OE, Mlcak RP, Chinkes DL, Herndon DN. Resting energy expenditure in severely burned children: analysis of agreement between indirect calorimetry and prediction equations using the Bland-Altman method. *Burns.* 2006;32(3):335–342.

32. Chan MM, Chan GM. Nutritional therapy for burns in children and adults. *Nutrition.* 2009;25(3):261–269.

33. Garrel DR, Razi M, Larivire F, et al. Improved clinical status and length of care with low-fat nutrition support in burn patients. *JPEN J Parenter Enteral Nutr.* 1995;19(6):482.

34. Saffle JR, Wiebke G, Jennings K, Morris SE, Barton RG. Randomized trial of immune-enhancing enteral nutrition in burn patients. *J Trauma.* 1997;42(5):793–800.

35. Marin V, Rodriguez-Osiac L, Schlessinger L, Villegas J, Lopez M, Castillo-Duran C. Controlled study of enteral arginine supplementation in burned children: impact on immunologic and metabolic status. *Nutrition.* 2006;22(7–8):705.

36. Cone L, Gilligan M, Kagan R, Mayes T, Gottschlich M. Enhancing patient safety: the effect of process improvement on bedside fluoroscopy time related to nasoduodenal feeding tube placement in pediatric burn patients. *J Burn Care Res.* 2009;30(4):606.

37. Scaife CL, Saffle JR, Morris SE. Intestinal obstruction secondary to enteral feedings in burn trauma patients. *J Trauma.* 1999;47(5):859.

Test Your Knowledge Answers

1. The correct answer is **C**. Solid organ injuries are common in the child due to the exposure of the liver and spleen in the upper abdomen. Unless there is hemody-

namic instability, these rarely require operative intervention and can be managed with physical limitations. Nutrition support generally consists of resumption of an age-appropriate diet with caloric supplementation, when caloric intake is inadequate.

2. The correct answer is **D**. While the extent of pancreatic trauma is quite variable, it is often accompanied by chemical pancreatitis and ileus. When resection occurs, it is usually over the neck of the pancreas and leaves sufficient endocrine tissue for normal glucose control, but may impact exocrine function as evidenced by steatorrhea.

3. The correct answer is **B**. While the concept of immunonutrition is appealing in this population of patients, randomized clinical studies have failed to show benefit.

4. The correct answer is **A**. TBSA remains a predictor of mortality. In children under 4 years of age, inhalation injury combined with a TBSA injury of > 30% defines the highest mortality risk group. It is not clearly proportional to the extent of the stress response, which is mediated by multiple additional factors. Estimates of energy needs based on TBSA are consistently inaccurate in their targets.

31

Surgery

Arlet G. Kurkchubasche, MD

Learning Objectives

1. Identify factors that impact nutrition requirements associated with acute metabolic changes in the neonatal and pediatric surgical patient.
2. Identify methods for optimizing nutrition support throughout the perioperative period by using clinical assessment, laboratory analysis, and bedside calorimetry.
3. Provide a basis for determining when to initiate and progress enteral feeding in a core group of neonatal surgical conditions.
4. Delineate strategies to limit the progression of cholestatic jaundice in the postoperative infant with intestinal dysfunction.

General Nutrition Considerations in Pediatric Surgery

The metabolic consequences of surgical stress have been extensively studied and show a characteristic/stereotypic response in terms of hormone and cytokine elaboration. The resultant hypermetabolic state during the phase of injury and recovery has been the focus of nutrition support. In pediatrics, the challenge is not only to provide nutrients to support immediate metabolic needs, but also to avert catabolism of limited protein and fat stores while providing substrate for growth and development.

Wound failure, infection, and mortality are primary outcome measures related to perioperative nutritional status. The discipline of surgical nutrition progressed at a time when critical care advancements allowed us to support infants with more complex conditions, and the institution of parenteral nutrition (PN) changed the face of postoperative care for this subset of patients. With time, however, an awareness of its potential for adverse effects has become apparent, specifically the unique problem of cholestasis in the pediatric population.

With further advances in the science of intestinal physiology, the complexity of the intestinal tract and its role in fluid, electrolyte, and nutrient assimilation, as well as in immune sampling functions, became evident. Provision of appropriate nutrition held the promise of enhanced immune function, fewer complications related to catabolism, and overall improved outcomes. Studies on immunomodulatory agents provided either parenterally or enterally in clinical sepsis have been conducted on adults and pediatric patients alike. In the pediatric literature, the focus came to rest on the components of breast milk, which appeared to be beneficial in averting gut-derived sepsis.[1]

The limitations of clinical research in pediatrics are evident when it comes to studies requiring repeated blood sampling and invasive procedures; however, there is reason to believe that the findings from adult clinical trials can be applied to pediatric patients. There is a wealth of knowledge from observational studies in pediatrics about growth needs for all age groups and for many with congenital conditions, but these studies are generally careful to exclude more complex surgical patients. The best quantitative neonatal and pediatric data related to the metabolic response to stress are derived from studies of a relatively homogeneous group of infants who undergo cardiopulmonary bypass for repair of congenital cardiac disease or who require extracorporeal membrane oxygenation (ECMO) for pulmonary support.[2,3] These infants, however, cannot represent the entire spectrum of pediatric surgical conditions, and much work remains to be done.

Nutrition assessment and support of the pediatric surgical patient requires consideration of the acute impact of the surgical intervention and the more chronic consequences of intestinal resection or reconstruction. Potential postoperative complications and underlying congenital disorders may further contribute to persistent impairment of intestinal function. Cholestasis, regardless of etiology, is an additional morbidity that may impact recovery. While hyperbilirubinemia associated with a primary disorder may not be preventable, efforts should be made to limit cholestasis related to PN.[4]

The first section of this chapter will focus on perioperative nutrition support and the general concept of adjustments in nutrition considerations for the neonatal and pediatric patient in response to altered metabolic demands as a consequence of surgery. Recent publications also

indicate the complex relationship between patients with underlying intestinal problems who are on PN and their propensity for a systemic inflammatory response syndrome–like reaction affecting their morbidity and mortality.[5] Patients who experience stresses as a consequence of trauma or burn injury are discussed elsewhere (Chapter 30). The second section focuses on nutrition support strategies specific to some of the congenital gastrointestinal (GI) disorders encountered in the neonatal pediatric surgery patient.

Pediatric surgical care, from the newborn infant to the mature adolescent, requires a fundamental knowledge of the physiological changes that occur with growth and maturation. Depending on the underlying condition, patients will have variable impairments of GI function that may be related to intestinal motility, mucosal absorptive capacity, and immune function. The perioperative state is a dynamic period; as the patient's clinical status evolves, reassessment and redirection of nutrition care must occur. Because these patients also represent a spectrum of acute and chronic disease, a uniform set of standards for nutrition care can be difficult to generate.

The principles upon which guidelines are established should focus on and correspond to the general American Society for Parenteral and Enteral Nutrition guidelines for nutrition assessment in pediatrics. These include:

1. Individualized assessment of nutrition status to determine the urgency and extent of patient support needs.
2. Consideration of the timing of onset of postoperative nutrition support and the appropriate use of PN when the alimentary tract is compromised, with consideration for provision of either enteral nutrition (EN) or PN support within 3 days of hospitalization.
3. Provision of nutrition in a manner (enteral or parenteral) most consistent with safe clinical practice.
4. Avoidance of potential complications by continuous reassessment of individual risk/benefit ratios, including optimal timing for alimentary tract challenge.
5. Methods for determining the adequacy of nutrition support.

General Nutrition Considerations in Neonatal Surgery

Neonatal Assessment, Nutrient Composition, and Targets for Nutrition Support in the Early Postoperative Period
Infants with congenital disorders of the abdomen and especially the intestinal tract have fluid and nutrition needs that require frequent reassessment in the immediate periopera-

tive period. The excess fluids required to restore or maintain vital organ perfusion are not necessarily accompanied by a greater demand for caloric provision.[6-8] It is important to consider these requirements separately and avoid the potential for overfeeding and hyperglycemia. Many factors in the postoperative patient impact energy estimates, including the use of mechanical ventilation, the provision of external heat support, and the use of sedating agents and neuromuscular blockers. Pain control has a tremendous impact on perioperative hormonal stress response. Preemptive analgesia using local and regional anesthesia helps to reduce the stress response and is part of current surgical practice; for instance, in infants undergoing patent ductus arteriosus ligation, a fentanyl anesthetic resulted in improved protein metabolism.[9,10]

The assessment of intravascular volume status can be quantified using weight, fluid balance records, and occasional invasive monitoring with central venous pressure. Assessment of metabolic demands is not as straightforward. Unless nitrogen balance studies are readily accessible, the best estimates for caloric provision are made on the basis of the infant's gestational age and formulas for resting energy expenditure in the acute and recovery phases, which are best modified with estimated stress factors.

Anthropometric parameters remain the mainstay of nutritional assessment in the neonate, so feedback on nutrition interventions is not immediate in nature. Ideally, one would be able to assess parameters in real time and make the necessary adjustments to assure a positive nitrogen balance along with anticipated weight gain. In the absence of this technology, the focus remains on maintaining euglycemia and avoiding hyperlipidemia and azotemia/uremia, while providing an escalating amount of balanced macronutrients in the form of carbohydrates, lipids, and protein.

Laboratory parameters may be used to assess nutrition status; however, in infants these must be used as trends rather than absolute measures, because there are often no gestationally appropriate controls.[11] Principal laboratory markers include total protein, albumin, prealbumin (evaluated in the context of a normal C-reactive protein [CRP]), and retinol-binding protein. These function as measures of protein anabolism after the acute phase of injury and are difficult to interpret early in the postoperative state, but they are valuable as preoperative assessment tools. Often, non-protein calories in an amount of 60–80 kcal/kg/d, perhaps even less, are sufficient to meet initial goals in the neonate.[12]

It has been documented that preterm neonates often require a generous protein supply, perhaps as high as 4 g/ kg/d, which primarily serves to provide substrate for tissue repair but does not independently prevent catabolism of the existing muscle mass. Counting this protein delivery as energy-yielding caloric intake may result in inadequate caloric provision; this is the basis for calculating and targeting nonprotein calories in the acute perioperative setting. To provide an optimal substrate for nutrient assimilation, a nonprotein calorie:nitrogen ratio of 130:1 to 210:1 is generally recommended as the target PN solution. In practice, we aim for a target of 180:1. However, while the calculation of caloric targets in terms of nonprotein calories may be important in the early perioperative phase, targets should revert to total caloric intake once the acute wound-healing demands return toward baseline. The time for this transition is perhaps best estimated by normalization of CRP and should correspond to clinical indicators such as wound status, return of intestinal function, and lack of infectious complications.

Cholestasis: PN–Associated and Other Origins

Cholestasis is a significant problem in pediatric surgical patients, who frequently require prolonged PN support and are at further risk for hepatic injury by virtue of their underlying diagnosis, nonenteral feeding status, and susceptibility to sepsis. Newborn infants may have transient indirect hyperbilirubinemia; the marker of significant cholestasis is a direct bilirubin exceeding 2 mg/dL. This is often accompanied by elevation of the serum transaminases; gamma-glutamyl transpeptidase is the most sensitive to ongoing inflammation. The alkaline phosphatase level must be interpreted cautiously, as much of this enzyme may be derived from bone rather than liver and fractionated evaluation may be necessary. With the onset of jaundice, some key interventions must occur before ascribing the finding to PN–associated liver disease (PNALD). An ultrasound evaluation of the liver and gallbladder must be used to document the absence of gallstones, sludge, and ductal dilation. Cholelithiasis is a known consequence of massive enteral resection. Ultrasound also serves to document the direction of portal venous blood flow, which should be toward the liver parenchyma. Hemolysis should also be excluded prior to a PNALD diagnosis.

For patients who are anticipated to have a prolonged dependence on PN (> 1 month), several hepatoprotective strategies are generally instituted. The initiation of enteral feeds is the single most important intervention in limiting cholestasis.[13] *Cycling* refers to delivering the PN solution over a limited number of hours per day. The primary limiting factor in establishing this therapy is the ability of the infant to tolerate extended periods without access to glucose, given limited glycogen stores. Seizures as a consequence of hypoglycemia carry the most profound risk for neurological devastation. The initiation of this strategy in term infants usually corresponds to the onset of a baseline enteral feeding regimen to support euglycemia. The procedure for cycling involves reducing the rate of the PN infusion to 50% for 1 hour prior to discontinuing the infusion and reinitiating the next PN solution at 50% of the goal rate for 1 hour before increasing to the goal rate (see Figure 31-1). Determining the target number of hours off PN also involves calculating the consequent glucose infusion rate (GIR) in the limited period of infusion and not blindly exceeding standards. While infants are hospitalized, they continue to receive lipid infusions over 24 hours to help minimize the use of additional carrier fluids for medication administration and avoid repeated entry into saline-locked or heparin-locked lines. Once on home PN, lipids are infused over the same time interval as the dextrose and amino acid solution, allowing the line to be heparin-locked once daily.

Another hepatoprotective strategy involves maintaining specific relative ratios between macronutrients. Examples of this include targeting a nonprotein calorie:nitrogen ratio of approximately 180:1, and ensuring that lipid calories do not exceed 30% of total nonprotein calories. The specific role of lipids in preventing and potentially reversing cholestasis has been the subject of much investigation. Lipids are a dense source of calories and have been particularly useful in the fluid-restricted preterm infant. The commercially available formulation of lipids is an omega 6–rich soy-based substrate with intrinsically proinflammatory properties. The use of a fish oil–based omega 3–rich emulsion has been associated with reversal of cholestasis and even avoidance of cholestasis when used pre-emptively,[14] although the same effect has been achieved by restricting the infusion of commercially available agents to 1 g/kg/day.[15,16] The future promises to provide us with more complex balanced lipid emulsions that may be used with less impact on the GIR (as high as 15 mg/kg/min)—a necessary consequence of lipid restriction.[17]

Recurrent infections are another source of strain on the liver and may contribute to progressive dysfunction. While the care and maintenance of central venous access is not generally considered a specifically hepatoprotective strategy, the avoidance of central line–associated bloodstream infections is an important goal. Any infection further compounds the potential for progressive cholestasis. Many bloodstream infections originate from enteric organisms that breach the mucosal barrier and enter first the portal and then the system circulation. Management of the intestinal microflora may require the use of antibiotics and probiotics when recurrent Gram-negative and fungal infections occur. When stenosis or stricture result in segmental regions of dilation and stasis, resection or stricturoplasty may be required, followed by tapering enteroplasty for autologous reconstruction. These issues are also discussed in Chapter 27.

As the infant enters the recovery phase without any infectious or wound-healing complications, the focus changes toward the more typical pediatric goals of nutrition support covering both acute needs and those for growth and development. At this point, documentation of weight gain, normalization of acute-phase reactants (eg, CRP), and establishment of increasing prealbumin values become the primary outcome measures. As mentioned above, the focus on providing protein purely for wound-related anabolism is reduced at this point, and caloric provision should include protein-derived calories to avoid the complications of overfeeding.

Initiation and Choice of Enteral Alimentation

EN is incrementally introduced when there is evidence of GI tract motility (onset of stooling or stoma output) and assurance that newly created anastomoses have achieved satisfactory healing. General principles in managing postoperative patients include a conceptual understanding of normal postoperative events such as paralytic ileus, delayed gastric emptying, the effect of narcotic analgesics, and the peri-anastomotic edema that may impede transit during the first 48 hours after surgery. Guidelines for determining the ability to initiate feeding include an assessment of gastric output in terms of volume and nature (bilious/nonbilious); physical examination for abdominal distention and the presence of bowel sounds; and assessment of output, whether by stoma or per rectum. It is important to remember that motility recovers first in the distal intestine, so an isolated stool does not indicate recovery of overall GI motility. The recognition of potential intestinal complications such as anastomotic leak, intra-abdominal sepsis, wound failure at the level of the abdominal wall closure, and even stoma-related problems (eg, stomal stenosis or prolapse), is critical.

The timing of feeding initiation therefore depends on an assessment of the risks and benefits of providing enteral nutrients. Choice and mode of feeding are often determined by the infant's gestational maturity, the history of mucosal injury/disruption, the effectiveness of motility, the urgency to transition off PN, and the presence of

Figure 31-1. Cycling Rates for PN
D15, 15% dextrose; D20, 20% dextrose; GIR, glucose infusion rate; IV, intravenous.

Formula to determine goal rate

Determine the PN total volume to be delivered over next 24 hours

Determine time off PN – that will be "Y"

Total volume divided by [24 – (Y + 1)] = goal rate

The first hour of the new bag will run at 50% of the goal rate.

Goal rate will run 24 – Y – 2 hours = X hours

The last hour's worth of PN will again run at 50% of the goal rate.

PN will then be off for Y hours.

Note: Lipid solution runs over 24 hours unless patient is on 3-in-1 PN or the period of infusion can be limited to 12 hours (ie, at home).

Schematic to illustrate calculation of cycling rates

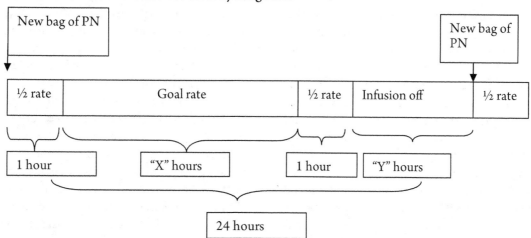

	240 mL PN	Max GIR (assume D20 and 2.5 kg infant)	450 mL PN	Max GIR (assume D20 and 4 kg infant)	Max GIR (assume D15 and 4 kg infant)
Continuous	10 mL/h x 24 h	13.3	18.75 mL/h	15.65	11.74
2 hours off	5.7 mL/h x 1 h 11.4 mL/h x 20 h 5.7 mL/h x 1 h Off x 2 h	15.2	10.7 mL/h x 1 h 21.4 mL/h x 20 h 10.7 mL/h x 1h Off x 2 h	17.8	13.4
4 hours off	6.3 mL/h x 1 h 12.6 mL/h x 18 h 6.3 mL/h x 1 h Off x 4 h	16.8	11.8. mL/h x 1 h 23.7 mL/h x 18 h 11.8 mL/h x 1 h Off x 4 h	19.7	14.8
6 hours off	7.1 mL/h x 1 h 14.1 mL/h x 16 h 7.1 mL/h x 1 h Off 6 h	18.8	13.2 mL/h x 1 h 26.5 mL/h x 16 h 13.2 mL/h x 1 h Off x 6 h	22.1	16.6

Note: As PN is consolidated over time, GIR limits may be approached; this must also be considered when cycling PN.

$$\text{GIR (mg/kg/min)} = \frac{\text{IV rate (mL/h) x dextrose concentration (g/dL) x 0.167}}{\text{Weight (kg)}}$$

gastroesophageal reflux (GER). In general, breast milk should remain the first choice for all of its qualities related to optimizing gut mucosal function and immunity. Although donor breast milk lacks some of the immune benefits, it remains a desirable nutrient source. When commercial formulas are necessary, infants who have no history of a compromised intestinal wall (mucosal damage, transmural edema/fibrosis) can be started on standard hydrolyzed whey-based formulas for gestational age; infants with a positive history should be started on a more elemental substrate to optimize absorption in the presence of a compromised mucosal barrier. Casein hydrolysates (Pregestimil, Alimentum) are common options for the infant surgical patient; the choice of a specific formula is often based on fat composition and osmotic load. However, these specialized formulas provide only a fraction of the calcium and phosphorus needs for a preterm infant, and this must be taken into consideration with supplementation when possible. Elemental formulas that consist of amino acids and were designed to obviate protein allergies (Neocate, EleCare) may in some instances be better tolerated in those with compromised motility as well. Theoretically, they reduce the luminal content of nutrients that reach the distal intestine. In addition, hydrolyzed formulas limit bacterial overgrowth and carbohydrate fermentation, both of which result in excess reducing substances being excreted along with luminal fluids in the form of diarrhea or frequent loose stools. As the patient's intestinal tract recovers, transition to a more complex and age-appropriate formula can be accomplished in a gradual manner. Infants with congenital disorders that do not affect the intestine itself, such as omphalocele, congenital diaphragmatic hernia (CDH), malrotation without volvulus, pyloric stenosis, and thoracic conditions, should be able to tolerate standard formulas.

Guidelines for caloric estimates in critically ill surgical infants requiring respiratory support are difficult to establish, but are best assessed using a metabolic cart.[7] The acutely ventilated patient probably does not require a major revision in energy provision, but infants who are chemically relaxed, actively ventilated, and not participating in the work of breathing may benefit from an objective assessment. Most recent publications have focused on a subset of neonatal cardiac surgery patients[2,3] who can be analyzed as a reasonably cohesive group. Outside this group are infants with CDH who are intubated but variably assisted with ventilation and require attention to avoid an inappropriate respiratory quotient, which might adversely impact their ability to eliminate CO_2. Each of these patients is unique; generic formulas cannot be applied to them.

The goal is to have a patient who is in optimal nutritional shape. This is a multifactorial evaluation: the surgeon hopes to see that the infant has an appropriate weight gain of 1% to 2% of body weight per day and is demonstrating appropriate somatic growth in length, head circumference, and triceps skinfold measurement. For patients who will require another surgical intervention, the progressive increase of serum albumin toward the normal range is also a reassuring parameter. To achieve these goals, one can ideally provide a balanced enteral and parenteral regimen. Sufficient EN (trophic or greater) should be provided to stimulate the mucosa, maintain mucosal health, and promote motility. The limits of "tolerance" are probably best defined by evaluating the volume and nature of the output. Stool output per rectum is difficult to quantify other than by frequency; stools in excess of 8 per day would be indicative of feeding intolerance. Stoma output, on the other hand, is easier to quantify: outputs are evaluated in the context of total enteral intake and should not exceed 30% by volume.

Other formulas for assessment of normal stoma output are based on weight, with expected output estimated at 1 mL/kg/h and tolerable amounts to allow progression of enteral feeds set at either 30 mL/kg/d or 2 mL/kg/h.[18] Excess output serves as an indicator of inadequate absorptive capacity and osmotic fluid loss and should be further evaluated by assay or measurement of stool-reducing substances, stool pH, and fecal fat. Reducing substances will shed light on carbohydrate malabsorption: contents of 1% or greater in the presence of loose stools constitute an indication for intervention, depending on the type of enteral intake. Stool pH reflects whether there are organic acids generated by unabsorbed sugars; this can happen independent of the presence of reducing substances. The percentage of unabsorbed dietary fat can be estimated by quantifying the amount of fat in the stool sample.

Ideally, a target caloric goal is established for each patient, and EN is pushed to the limit of tolerance, with PN providing the balance of calories necessary to achieve weight gain and laboratory goals. Aggressive advancement of EN needs to be balanced with concerns about surpassing tolerance and induction of intestinal diseases such as necrotizing enterocolitis (NEC). The use of distal refeeding provides a valuable adjunct in situations where ostomies and mucous fistulas have been created, at least contributing to the restoration of a complete enterohepatic pathway for bile if the distal ileum has been retained.[19] However, the benefits of distal refeeding are counterbalanced by the often complex contraptions that have to be created to collect and reinfuse stoma output. There is also a risk of perforating the distal intestine with repeated catheterization. The decisions involved in these complicated cases require that all care providers reach a consensus on short-term and long-term plans for the patient. Only then can the ideal nutrition support plan be instituted.

All surgical patients must be monitored carefully for the onset of jaundice. Often the default reason for the onset of direct hyperbilirubinemia is the use of PN; however, surgical patients can develop intestinal obstruction at the level of an anastomosis, at the level of a proximal stoma, or at a random site due to peritoneal adhesions or previous ischemia resulting in stricture formation. These conditions must remain in the foreground as correctable causes of obstructive jaundice. Others conditions include drug-related cholestasis (seen with cephalosporins), low-grade sepsis, and even secondary disorders such as biliary tract disease (gallstones and sludge).

Surgical Considerations for Nutrition Support in Infants with Specific Congenital Disorders

Proximal Intestinal Obstruction

A congenital proximal intestinal obstruction is usually recognized antenatally or in the immediate postnatal period and typically prompts urgent operative intervention. While surgery can be temporized with effective nasogastric suction, delay of operation is reserved for those infants with suspected congenital heart disease who will require further evaluation (ie, patients with esophageal atresia and duodenal atresia) or who would benefit from stabilization of their transitional circulation changes before undergoing anesthesia and operative stress. Although unusual, concerns about the presence of an underlying nonsurvivable metabolic disorder or lethal chromosomal disorder constitutes another justification for delaying surgical intervention.

Esophageal Atresia

The most complex decision-making involves infants who have esophageal atresia and are significantly preterm and/or have low birth weight. Surgery may safely be delayed 1–2 days while postnatal circulation stabilizes and the infant undergoes screening for disorders in the VACTERL association (vertebral, anorectal, cardiac, tracheo-esophageal, renal, and limb). During this time, most neonates will be started on at least peripheral PN, with a plan to escalate to central PN once appropriate venous access has been established via a temporary umbilical venous catheter, a peripherally inserted central catheter (PICC) line, or a surgically placed central venous line inserted at the time of operative repair. The expectation is that the infant will not be able to use the intestinal tract until approximately 7 days after surgery, when the esophageal anastomosis is evaluated for patency and the absence of leaks.

Transanastomotic tubes are not routinely placed at the time of operation. Their association with anastomotic complications remains speculative but unsubstantiated in the literature.[20] When there is a leak, the period of nonenteral alimentation may extend for another 5–7 days, since there is no safe esophageal access to the stomach or beyond. Even in the presence of a transanastomotic tube, feeding is not initiated because of concerns about GER with gastric feeding. The use of gastrostomy tubes (G-tubes) has generally been limited to infants with long-gap atresia who will undergo esophageal reconstruction/repair at a later date, or to infants who are expected to have poor oral-motor skills or other feeding dysfunction based on concomitant disorders (trisomy, retrognathia, etc.). Given the reliance on PN for 7 days or more, most neonatal centers will place central venous access preoperatively (PICC line) or at the time of reconstruction. Because these considerations for alimentation are not based on technique, there is no difference in the postoperative management of thoracoscopic or open repair.

After the esophageal anastomosis is verified to be free of leaks using a contrast esophagram, the contrast is often followed through the duodenum, primarily to establish the absence of malrotation. Duodenal stenosis due to annular pancreas and duodenal atresia can coexist with esophageal atresia. This will not be apparent at surgery because the abdominal cavity is not entered. Enteral feeds can be commenced, preferably by mouth, to avoid repeated instrumentation of the esophagus. Esophageal dysmotility is common and has been manometrically documented as an interruption of the progression of the peristaltic wave at the level of the anastomosis.

The more capacious proximal pouch initially requires time for emptying into the narrower distal segment. As the infant grows, the 2 segments will become more consistent in caliber in the absence of stricture formation at the anastomosis. Delayed emptying of the proximal pouch will result in oral regurgitation and tracheal compression, which becomes clinically evident as desaturation with feeds. These behaviors are anticipated in the early course, and any exacerbation should be considered a symptom of a progressive anastomotic stricture. Infants must have the head of their bed elevated and should be fed upright. The goal of oral feeding should be to allow the infant to practice frequently with low-volume amounts (5–10 mL every 3 hours). Once small amounts are tolerated, gradual progression may occur. Since GER will likely be the next hurdle to progression of feeds, it is more effective to provide more frequent lower-volume feeds every 3 hours. When breastfeeding is initiated, it should be limited similarly in time and the feeding interval progressed as the infant tolerates it. Although it is difficult to measure breastfeeding intake, reports indicate that weighing the infant pre-feed and post-feed may be a useful method. Alternatively, lactating mothers who know the typical volume generated on a given schedule can express a measured quantity of breast milk before nursing the infant.

These infants are prone to acid reflux, which is detrimental to the anastomosis and can result in stricture formation. Acid reduction therapy should be started in the immediate postoperative period and maintained for 6–12 months. Metoclopramide may be helpful when feeds are first initiated to promote gastric emptying, although this medication comes with a risk for dystonia, and parents must be aware of the risk/benefit relationship. Optimally, the infant will progress to full feeds over a period of 5–7 days. Infants with symptomatic tracheomalacia may have delayed progression. They may require repeated intubation for mechanical ventilatory support, or they may require support with high-flow nasal cannula oxygen, which compromises their ability to tolerate gastric feeds. In these instances, it may be advisable to place a transpyloric feeding tube to enable the infant to take EN and be weaned off PN while his or her airway disability is being addressed. Severe cases may require placement of a G-tube. The reluctance to place a gastrostomy is based on the potential for further affecting the abnormal angle of His (at the gastroesophageal junction) and potentiating reflux. Surgical therapy for GER, while necessary in a subset of infants, is avoided where possible due to (1) the inherent dysmotility of the esophagus, which may not be able to overcome any degree of distal obstruction; and (2) the shortened length of the esophagus. While these concerns may be considered surgically with a performance of a "floppy" or looser fundoplication and/or esophageal lengthening procedures such as the Collis gastroplasty, these are best avoided unless a recalcitrant esophageal stricture forms.[21]

During infancy, the choice of formula should be based on gestational age. There are no specific intestinal absorptive defects to prompt the use of more elemental formulas.

Caloric concentration of infant formulas is often necessary and advisable to accomplish nutrition goals, given the propensity for GER. Long-term nutrition problems in esophageal atresia relate to ongoing issues with GER and proximal strictures. Surveillance esophagrams are sometimes indicated, and mechanical or hydrostatic fluoroscopic dilatation is usually effective in treating strictures. With progression to solid foods, these children must be coached to chew well and consume liquids with their meals to overcome any potential residual esophageal dysmotility. It is not unusual for overly large pieces of food to become lodged at the level of the anastomosis and result in esophageal obstruction. This problem tends to resolve with age, maturity, and increasing esophageal caliber.

Duodenal Atresia

Duodenal atresia can be identified antenatally, providing an opportunity for prenatal counseling. This section focuses on the concern for potential associated anomalies (cardiac and chromosomal) and the timing and strategy for operative repair. While most infants can undergo this reconstructive operation within 48 hours of birth, there are some in whom the management of prematurity and congenital heart disease will delay the timing of operation and prolong the need for PN. Based on the specific functional cardiac defect, a decision can be made with the cardiologists to proceed early with abdominal surgery before pulmonary pressures rise significantly and impact perioperative fluid and cardiac management. This can reduce the cholestatic consequences of the anatomic obstruction and prolonged PN, a combination that may become detrimental with time.

For anatomic reasons, the repair of duodenal atresia involves no resection; instead, it involves creating an anastomosis that joins the dilated proximal segment to a segment of the much smaller distal duodenum. During surgery, an assessment is made of the distal bowel to ensure that there are no further sites of atresia. The proximal duodenum is assessed in terms of its caliber for possible tapering duodenoplasty. Furthermore, the overall situation is assessed to determine the potential need for prolonged gastric decompression via gastrostomy. With a satisfactory anastomosis, the stomach remains decompressed for an average of 5 days. The pylorus remains incompetent in the immediate perioperative period, so the resolution of bilious output is not a reliable indicator of improved gastric emptying. Because a duodenal leak can be a catastrophic complication, a contrast study for anatomic and functional evaluation is obtained in infants before commencing feeds. In the absence of a contrast study, progressive decrease in output indicates forward peristalsis through the anastomosis and is the best indication that it is safe to start enteral feeds.

When breast milk is not available, the choice of infant formula is based on gestational age. There are no predictable associated absorption disorders to require specialized formulas. The mode of feeding depends on the child's anatomic and functional considerations. While intermittent oral feeds may be a successful strategy, often a more rapid transition from PN to EN is achieved with continuous gastric feeds that are then transitioned to bolus and oral feeds. Certainly, oral feeds can be added on top of continuous feeds to allow the infant to acquire oral motor skills. The more complicated infants have greater duodenal dysmotility and may have required a tapering enteroplasty; they often have a G-tube inserted to facilitate gastric decompression, thereby protecting the anastomosis and allowing the infant greater success in extubating from mechanical ventilation without a nasogastric tube in place. Given the potentially complex and prolonged postoperative course in this disorder, PN is started routinely and converted to central formulation once central venous access has been established.

Jejunoileal Atresia

As the anatomic site of obstruction extends further distally, the immediate postoperative problems related to the provision of EN are generally less frequent and less severe. These proximal obstructions can occur in isolation or in various constellations of increasing complexity.

In the simple mucosal web or single transmural atresia, operative considerations are relatively simple if the infant has normal overall intestinal length. A resection of the abnormally dilated jejunal segment and primary anastomosis to the distal unused bowel results in the least size discrepancy between adjacent limbs of intestine and has the highest success rate for recovery of bowel function. These infants would be anticipated to tolerate the onset of enteral feedings after bilious nasogastric output has resolved and volumes have decreased in concert with the passage of bile-pigmented stool output. This can occur 5–10 days after surgery and mandates use of PN in the interim.

Infants with multiple intestinal atresias have reduced overall bowel length. Operative methods to salvage length must be considered in relation to the infant's gestational age and how it relates to ongoing longitudinal growth of the intestine. Infants delivered at term and diagnosed with multiple intestinal atresias have less opportunity to compensate for lost intestinal length. The most proximal segment of

intestine will be the only segment dilated, and length can be preserved by performing a standard longitudinal tapering enteroplasty. Only in the event of severe congenital short bowel should more novel techniques such as the serial transverse enteroplasty procedure or Bianchi be considered to optimize the salvage of mucosal surface area and promote intestinal contractility.[22] As many as possible of the subsequent atretic portions of intestine should be salvaged using a "shish kebab" technique, in which continuity is created over a silastic catheter.[23] Surgical clinical judgment will dictate which segments are reasonable to salvage, as leaking or obstructed anastomoses will only compromise recovery.[24,25]

In the most complex variant of jejunoileal atresia, the "apple peel deformity," there is a complicated malformation of the proximal intestine along with preservation of the distal ileum on a vascular pedicle that provides retrograde perfusion for a variable length of intestine. The particular anatomic appearance of the twisted intestine, "maypoled" around the single vascular trunk originating from the distal ileal arcade, is important to recognize so that inadvertent further vascular compromise is avoided by torque from a poorly aligned enteric anastomosis. Furthermore, careful perioperative fluid management is essential to preserve adequate perfusion to the distal-most intestine. Hypotension will result in splanchnic vasoconstriction, compromising mucosal flow to this vulnerable section of bowel.

Nutrition considerations in these infants focus on the provision of adequate PN calories via central access, with early contemplation of techniques to limit cholestatic disorders. This is necessary since the process to complete conversion to enteral feeds may be prolonged by dysmotility and complications such as NEC. With the intent to gradually stimulate the bowel for adaptation, continuous feeds are most often initiated, and the infants, who often have G-tubes to facilitate this, are allowed to sham-feed by mouth and eventually later converted to full bolus feeds by mouth or G-tube.[26]

Distal Intestinal Obstruction

Distal intestinal obstruction usually involves the distal ileum and beyond. These infants will present with abdominal distention that is not relieved with nasogastric decompression. Distal ileal atresia or obstruction from inspissated meconium can result in volvulus of the distended, fluid-filled segment and cause ischemic necrosis of more extensive regions of the intestine. In the absence of significant intestinal loss, these conditions are unlikely to require more than conventional perioperative nutrition support. Resection of the right colon, including the ileocecal valve, is usually well tolerated. The need for replacement of vitamin B$_{12}$ must be considered at a later time (age 2 years) if a significant portion of terminal ileum accompanies the resection. More extensive colon resections, as might be encountered in Hirschsprung's disease, have more significant effects on resorption of water and electrolytes. Patients with Hirschsprung's disease and anorectal malformations require long-term dietary management, with the focus on achieving optimal evacuation of stool.

Colon Atresia

Colon atresia is a rare condition, accounting for only 10% of all intestinal atresia. Most common is a vascular defect at the level of the middle colic artery, resulting in an interruption of continuity at the mid-transverse colon. The right colon becomes massively distended since a competent ileocecal valve may not allow for distribution of the enteric contents into the terminal ileum.

Operatively, there are several solutions for this condition. An extended right hemicolectomy with anastomosis of the ileum to the transverse colon results in permanent loss of a significant surface area for nutrient and water absorption. Fortunately, the left colon can compensate for the water absorption with adaptation, and the patient should not have persistent watery stools. More complicated solutions focus on preserving the right colon with a proximal diverting stoma in the hopes that it will decompress and regain its normal caliber and motility. Nutrition considerations in these patients are generally simple and are impacted by whether a second reconstructive operation is necessary.

Meconium Ileus and Variants

This is the earliest clinical presentation of cystic fibrosis and early recognition may be protective of pulmonary disease because therapy can be undertaken pre-emptively. Clinically, it presents as distal ileal obstruction due to inspissated luminal contents. Meconium ileus may be complicated further by either (1) perforation of the obstructed bowel, resulting in meconium peritonitis; or (2) volvulus of the distended bowel, resulting in ischemia and stricture formation that may appear identical to an atresia. Simple meconium ileus in which there is only luminal inspissation can often be decompressed with sequential retrograde gastrograffin enemas, but surgery is sometimes necessary. In the process of attempting to decompress the obstructed segment with saline or N-acetylcysteine irrigation, it is possible to perforate or excessively traumatize the intestine. Often the safest choice is placement of a T-tube that provides access for con-

tinued postoperative irrigation and gradual resolution of the obstruction. In the event of complicated meconium ileus due to luminal discontinuity, a resection and primary anastomosis may be possible, but because of the risk of recurrent distal obstruction, creating a "vented" anastomosis (Bishop Koop or Santulli stoma) provides the greatest assurance of success. This allows the enteric contents to evacuate via stoma should distal obstruction reoccur and provides direct access to the distal bowel to treat with 3% N-acetylcysteine solution. The most difficult variant to deal with operatively is meconium peritonitis, in which it may not be possible to identify the site of perforation or mobilize it to create a stoma. If possible, a proximal diverting stoma becomes necessary, with staged exploration and restoration of continuity at a later date. If the distal end of the bowel can be identified, this is helpful in trying to prepare it for the subsequent operation and for consideration of distal refeeding of proximal stoma output. In rare cases, all of the bowel may be extensively entrapped by the leaked meconium, with no bowel visible. Wide drainage of the meconium-covered peritoneal surfaces for a few weeks while maintaining the infant on PN is an option that allows for slow separation of the inflamed intestines from the meconium surface and may avoid injury to the initially hidden intestinal mass.

Nutrition management of these infants requires consideration of a likely underlying diagnosis of cystic fibrosis, which must be verified by testing. While in the past it was taught that EN with a protein hydrolysate formula or breast milk did not require provision of pancreatic enzymes, common practice now is to provide these enzymes to optimize whatever enteral intake is available for absorption. This practice has to be balanced with past concerns about mucosal damage from specific formulations of enzyme dosing. The infant with a diverting stoma is a classic example of the nutrition decision-making involved with a child who will require a second complicated operation 6 weeks or more in the future. Cholestatic jaundice is based not only on PN exposure but also on possible underlying liver disease associated with cystic fibrosis. Once intestinal continuity to a stoma or the rectum is established postoperatively, the goal is to wean PN support expeditiously while recognizing that these infants tend to have higher-than-usual caloric requirements.

Hirschsprung's Disease

Hirschsprung's disease is a consequence of the absence of the ganglion cells from the rectum and distal-most colon, typically involving the rectosigmoid. The enteric ganglion cells are essential for relaxation of the intestine, and their absence results in a functional obstruction of the colon where the ganglion cells are absent (aganglionosis). With this obstruction, there is dilation of the normal colon proximal to the transition zone beyond which the infant's neural crest cells failed to migrate during the embryonic period. Hirschsprung's disease most often affects term or near-term infants; it is unusual in preterm infants. The newborn who is diagnosed and promptly undergoes reconstructive surgery—whether open, laparoscopic-assisted, or transanal—is likely to be able to start normal EN within 5 days of the operation. Therefore, the provision of even peripheral PN during the first few days of life, once the child has been diagnosed, is probably sufficient. This scenario, however, changes with a late diagnosis of Hirschsprung's disease, which is often associated with significant failure to thrive, enterocolitis, and long-segment disease. These situations are independent predictors of a difficult postoperative course; surgeons will often choose not to operate immediately and instead manage these patients medically (with irrigations if the transition zone is distal) or perform a stoma at the point where ganglion cells are present. Failure of the initial reconstruction potentially leads to a lifetime of anorectal disability. Once diverted or established on an effective irrigation program, the alimentary tract can again be challenged with nutrients and should be able to function appropriately, allowing the infant to thrive. The infant with total colon aganglionosis is essentially diverted at the level of the terminal ileum and may require PN support transiently until adaptation has occurred. The rare infant with aganglionosis extending into the small intestine will often have severe short bowel syndrome (SBS) and must be managed accordingly. These are some of the most challenging patients to manage in terms of their fluid needs.

Anorectal Malformations

Children with isolated anorectal malformations generally have no specific nutrition requirements. Their anorectal defect will either respond to progressive dilation, allowing for a delayed operative intervention, or will require a diverting colostomy. These children grow and develop normally in the absence of associated disorders.

After reconstruction, children with Hirschsprung's disease and low variants of imperforate anus will have issues related to stooling, with some developing severe functional constipation that may progress to overflow incontinence. Children with high imperforate anus tend to have problems with fecal incontinence, either due to absence of the sphinc-

ter complex or deficient innervation. Appropriate dietary management, along with a supervised bowel management program, is essential to the well-being of children with this spectrum of disease. Dietary considerations include provision of sufficient nonabsorbable fiber intake, along with sufficient liquid intake to assure daily evacuation.

Abdominal Wall and Diaphragm

Omphalocele

Omphalocele and gastroschisis are 2 very distinct congenital disorders with completely different considerations in terms of their postnatal GI function. While both conditions involve the presence of an abdominal wall defect, the intestine is protected within a membrane in patients with omphalocele and is not subject to the fascial constriction and amniotic exposure encountered in gastroschisis. Omphalocele can be associated with genetic disorders as well as renal and cardiac defects, and these conditions typically determine outcomes in these patients. Beckwith-Wiedemann syndrome is diagnosed when the omphalocele is associated with macroglossia, hypoglycemia, and hemihypertrophy. The hypoglycemia is a transient metabolic condition with no long-term implications for glycemic control, but the syndrome places the patient at risk for solid organ tumors. Associated congenital heart disease may involve various intracardiac defects or a constellation of defects involving the heart, pericardium diaphragm, and sternum, which are referred to as the pentalogy of Cantrell. Depending on the size of the abdominal wall defect, the liver and intestine are typically extraabdominal, and reconstruction can be accomplished in one stage rather than several.

A small omphalocele can be closed within days after birth once associated anomalies have been excluded. The child is typically kept *nil per os* (NPO) preoperatively; this may not be strictly necessary, but it is convenient for preoperative evaluations. Once a small omphalocele is closed, enteral alimentation can be commenced as soon as there is evidence of GI motility/function. While there are no predictable GI problems, extrinsic gastric compression from the oversized liver and GER are not uncommon and may require transient postpyloric feeding.

In the more complicated giant omphaloceles, PN is commonly started to bridge the child's nutrition needs while multiple operative procedures interfere with consistent EN. Ethical considerations arise when an infant with omphalocele is diagnosed with a lethal chromosomal disorder such as trisomy 18. Often the surgical condition can be managed in a nonoperative manner and EN can be delivered in a relatively noninvasive manner via a nasogastric feeding tube if the child will not feed by mouth.

The outcomes of omphalocele should be excellent except for the most complex disorders.

Gastroschisis

Gastroschisis is frequently the more complex abdominal wall defect from the standpoint of operative interventions and nutrition support. This abdominal wall defect is typically a relatively small, full-thickness aperture to the right of the umbilical cord insertion. Much of the GI tract is extruded through this defect and is bathed in amniotic fluid throughout pregnancy. The exposed intestine is at risk for torsion and vascular impairment from a tight fascial defect (which remains fixed as the intestine and its mesentery enlarge), and is subject to serosal irritation and trauma by virtue of its extraperitoneal location.

Immediate postnatal coverage of the intestine is accomplished by either primary abdominal closure or more commonly by placement of a temporary "silo." This is a sterile, transparent plastic bag that is oblong in shape and has a flexible ring at the open end. It is placed over the intestines, accommodating them vertically, and the ring is placed through the fascial opening and rests on the undersurface of the abdominal wall. Gradual compression of the silo, from the top down, forces the intestine into the gradually expanding abdominal space and ultimately allows for abdominal wall closure. Although there are multiple variations in technique to achieve reduction and closure, there do not appear to be any remarkable differences in outcomes with respect to time to full feeds and hospital discharge.[27] Nonoperative bedside closure with simple coverage using the umbilical remnant has also been described and is being evaluated for its long-term outcomes.

The most important predictor of outcomes appears to be the original condition of the intestine.[28] The intestinal surface in gastroschisis has a variable appearance and ranges from nonedematous, pliable, and virtually normal intestine without surface adhesions to stiff, edematous bowel whose contour and continuity cannot be assessed visually or even by palpation. Further complicating the presenting features is the tendency for these children to have a shorter-than-normal length of intestine. Fortunately, some of these changes resolve with time; however, the period of time to normal intestinal peristalsis can be quite variable. After an extended period of observation of 4–6 weeks without evidence of bowel continuity, contrast studies are indicated to evaluate whether an intestinal atresia is present. Evaluation much earlier is without benefit, as the abdomen will be quite hostile to exploration secondary to adhesions.

An interesting situation arises when an atretic segment is recognized at birth. Although the intuitive response would be to divert at that level to allow for some enteral stimulation, this is not generally advisable. There is limited abdominal wall surface area for a stoma, and the edema of the intestine rarely allows it to reach the abdominal wall in an orientation that is feasible for creation of a stoma. It is currently considered best practice to close the abdomen and correct the atresia in a second operation.[29,30]

Given the primary dysfunction of the intestine on multiple levels, these infants may require an extended period of PN support. During the initial few weeks, the infant remains decompressed with a nasogastric tube. Again, in contrast to other children who may require prolonged decompression, there is a reluctance to perform any visceral procedure, even a gastrostomy, due to abdominal wall constraints and the altered surface characteristics of the GI tract. Unless these children are substantially preterm, they usually have an uneventful perioperative course with a short duration of mechanical ventilation. There are no known interventions that lead to a more rapid resolution of intestinal edema. In general, these infants require up to 180–200 cc/kg/d of intravenous fluid support in the first few days, as they are projected to be relatively volume-depleted on presentation and continue to require good vascular perfusion of the intestine. The peripheral edema that may appear occurs on a different basis than that of the intestine, which likely happens as a consequence of vascular and lymphatic congestion at the fascial ring defect. In contrast to the peripheral edema, it is unlikely that diuresis would affect this visceral edema in the early phases.

The onset of intestinal feeding must coincide with evidence of effective full intestinal peristaltic activity as indicated by decreasing nasogastric output and onset of stooling. Early feeding into a dysmotile and transmurally altered intestine likely accounts for the higher incidence of NEC in gastroschisis than in any other gestational age–matched infant population. The mode of feeding has been long debated. Bolus feeds offer the theoretic advantage of optimally stimulating pancreatobiliary secretions, while continuous feedings are likely to advance more rapidly to full volumes, obviating the need for prolonged PN support. Continuous feedings can certainly be augmented by interval bolus feeds, allowing the child to develop the necessary oral feeding skills and possibly stimulating GI hormones. Vigilance is essential as the enteral component is advanced. Guidelines for advancement of feeds should take into account the frequency of stools as well as the pH and reducing substances, as these may indicate poor absorption and/or an excessive osmotic load. Because of the perceived fragility of the intestine, this author's practice is generally to use a more elemental formula and limit the osmolality, trying not to increase the caloric density of feeds until the child is almost fully established on EN.

Setbacks relate to septic events concerning the central line, which are usually Gram-negative in etiology and reflect the ongoing reduced mucosal barrier defense in the intestine. Given the combination of cholestasis and poor motility, these patients are excellent candidates for cycled enteral antibiotics to obviate bacterial overgrowth and its complications. Gastroschisis is one of the more common causes of neonatal SBS. The etiologies involve congenital torsion or ischemic necrosis of entire segments of intestine, simple atresias, and postnatal loss of intestine due to poor perfusion, NEC, or surgical catastrophes. Caloric estimates for the needs of these infants depend on their phase of recovery. In the initial postnatal period, there appears to be an intense inflammatory state as evidenced by elevated CRP, which resolves as the bowel recovers. The incidence of cholestatic jaundice is likely multifactorial in this population.[30]

Congenital Diaphragmatic Hernia

Congenital diaphragmatic hernia (CDH) involves a heterotopic location for the viscera within either chest cavity, as well as associated defects in lung and pulmonary vascular development and maturation. While the former is a surgically correctable defect, the second component determines the child's clinical course and ultimate prognosis. Infants with CDH, therefore, fall into several categories. There are those with a diaphragmatic defect, usually first detected postnatally, in whom there is little hemodynamic and pulmonary compromise; they tolerate surgery well and can be transitioned relatively quickly to enteral feedings. Infants in whom the defect was identified early in gestation tend to have a greater degree of pulmonary hypoplasia and more difficulty with pulmonary hypertension; they may require cardiac and pulmonary support via ECMO. As a result, nutrition support in this disorder spans the whole spectrum and must be individualized.

The GI tract, although displaced initially, is fundamentally normal in terms of its motility and absorption capacity. As such, there are no specific recommendations for the type of enteral alimentation. Consideration needs to be given to the fact that total fluid provision will likely be restricted in the postoperative patient as he or she is weaned off ventila-

tory support. While it is enticing to provide highly concentrated formulas, this has to be balanced with the potential for mucosal damage leading to enteric-derived sepsis in vulnerable infants who likely have multiple vascular access points. Provision of adequate calories is likely best accomplished with highly concentrated formula once the infant has tolerated enteral feedings and becomes limited in the amount of volume that can be delivered for reasons of gastric capacity and emptying. All children with CDH have some degree of foregut dysmotility, which renders them at risk for GER.[31,32] The risk of reflux with aspiration is particularly pronounced in these patients, who already have a compromised pulmonary system, given the nature of the congenital defect. This risk forms the basis for providing continuous feeds initially to fulfill enteral needs and then transitioning them to bolus feeds. Again, the provision of continuous enteral feedings should not be a disincentive for oral feeds. Feeding can be structured to deliver the targeted volume of feeds over 1 hour or even more as the child tolerates.

Infants with CDH and severe cardiopulmonary compromise who require maximal medical support for control of pulmonary hypertension are often severely fluid-restricted, and this further limits the ability to provide adequate nutrition support. The assessment of caloric needs is especially difficult because there are so many confounding factors, such as level of sedation, possible chemical muscular relaxation, degree of mechanical respiratory support, and level of temperature support. During this phase, the goal of nutrition support is to provide the essential components to allow for basic metabolic needs and repair of tissues. Calories earmarked for growth and development become priorities as the infant's clinical condition improves. When these patients required cardiopulmonary support on ECMO, it was assumed that as the lungs were being "rested," the metabolic demands would decrease. This assumption, however, has been shown to be incorrect; these patients continue to exhibit a hypermetabolic response, and this persists after decannulation.[33,34] In the past there has been debate as to the safety of administering lipids to an infant on ECMO. The consensus now is that lipids can safely be administered via a central line separate from the ECMO circuit. In contrast, the dextrose and amino acid solution is typically administered via the cannulae. This allows for safe delivery of dextrose concentrations greater than 20%, since there are sufficiently high flow rates directly into the atrium. Provision of high glucose loads along with insulin therapy has been shown to be beneficial in this population to limit protein catabolism.[35,36]

Hepatobiliary Disorders

Biliary Atresia

Infants presenting with direct hyperbilirubinemia are promptly evaluated for surgically correctable biliary tract disorders such as biliary atresia and choledochal cyst. While other conditions such as neonatal hepatitis also lead to similar laboratory presentations, they (as well as a host of infectious disorders and enzymatic defects) require medical support only. Biliary atresia most often becomes evident at 1 month of age, and the infant may have experienced failure to thrive of unknown etiology. Hallmarks of clinical diagnosis include jaundice, acholic stools, and dark urine. Ultrasound, HIDA scan, and percutaneous liver biopsy should confirm the diagnosis. Once established, preoperative administration of vitamin K is one of the standard recommendations to optimize coagulation parameters. The diagnosis is further confirmed intraoperatively by demonstrating a lack of an extrahepatic ductular system.

Reconstruction involves creation of a jejunal limb that is anastomosed to the portal plate, the region of the liver where the hepatic ducts would be presumed to originate from the liver parenchyma. In fortunate situations, there is early evidence of bile flow with resolution of the hyperbilirubinemia. Postoperative steroids are frequently used as a choleretic and to reduce parenchymal inflammation in the liver. This postoperative course is typically a period of 5 days of non-enteral alimentation to allow for healing of the intestinal anastomosis, with subsequent initiation of enteral feedings. Unfortunately, with a frequent delay in diagnosis to 2 months of age, some infants will be in very poor nutritional condition. On preoperative assessment, some surgeons will opt to place central venous access at the time of operation to provide the debilitated child with some interim nutrition to optimize healing and prevent further weight loss.

There is no indication for preoperative nutrition repletion, because decompression of the obstructed biliary tract is the most important goal. Postoperative feedings are generally breast milk if available or a protein hydrolysate formula with approximately 50% medium-chain triglyceride oil, because medium-chain triglycerides are more easily absorbed by infants with liver disease. These children have an impaired ability to digest fats and require supplementation with fat-soluble vitamins A, D, E, and K. There are reports of these infants requiring a disproportionately larger caloric intake than others their size.

More on the nutrition support of the child with surgically non-correctable liver disease is discussed elsewhere.[37,38]

Choledochal Cyst

Infants with choledochal cyst may present during the neonatal period or later, but generally before 5 years of age. The acute presentation may include pancreatitis in addition to hyperbilirubinemia. These children rarely have chronic malnutrition despite complaints of abdominal pain. Subsequent to resection of the choledochal cyst, which involves variable portions of the extrahepatic ductal system and reconstruction of biliary outflow with a standard Roux-en-Y hepaticojejunostomy, these patients will be able to consume a normal diet and in the absence of significant underlying liver disease do not need special nutritional formulations.

Other (Non-GI) Malformations

Thoracic Disorders

Children who require thoracic operations for congenital lung lesions or even foregut duplications can be treated by routine postoperative guidelines and have no special nutritional considerations other than those imposed by virtue of prolonged ventilatory support and concern for reflux with aspiration. Many of these operations can now safely be achieved with minimally invasive techniques, further reducing surgical stress and postoperative pain response, and minimizing wounds to heal. Infants born with chylothorax, or those who develop it as a consequence of perioperative complications, can be managed depending on the amount of daily chylous output with gut rest and PN support, and the subsequent introduction of enteral feeds with high concentration of medium-chain triglyceride oil.

Urologic, Neurosurgical, and Orthopedic Disorders

Infants born with complex urological defects such as bladder exstrophy and cloacal exstrophy will require a number of staged surgical interventions by various specialists. The intestinal tract is intact and generally normal in bladder exstrophy, but there is imperforate anus with exteriorization of the hindgut between the 2 bladder halves in cloacal exstrophy. This portion of the hindgut will need to be tubularized to create a distal stoma or require proximal diversion. Hydronephrosis, prune belly syndrome, and other congenital renal anomalies may have evidence of renal insufficiency or failure that will require adjustments to the infant's nutrient intake as discussed in other chapters. Congenital neurosurgical and orthopedic interventions generally do not involve the peritoneal cavity or even the retroperitoneum and, therefore, do not impact enteral feeding status. Depending on the extent of operation and metabolic stress, adjustments primarily affect caloric goals and will need to be individualized.

Neonatal Airway Disorders

Infants who require interventions to their airway frequently have associated aerodigestive disorders that may extend to foregut dysmotility syndromes. Reconstructive interventions for laryngomalacia, subglottic stenosis, and tracheomalacia require protection of the airway from GER. Often tracheostomy can be averted by appropriate management of enteral feedings, along with pharmacologic interventions to limit exposure of the glottic structures to acid gastric contents. This may require insertion of a postpyloric feeding tube to ensure continued nutrition support without the risk of reflux. If the reflux is chronic in nature, early consideration for a Nissen fundoplication is appropriate.

Infants with airway compromise have an increased work of breathing and may exhibit failure to thrive despite mechanical feeding. Once supported with a tracheostomy, the infant will often show rapid catch-up growth and can sustain a reduction in caloric goals. It is important to remember that despite the presence of a tracheostomy, the airway is not completely protected from either GER or aspiration of salivary secretions, because the pediatric airway often does not require a cuffed tracheostomy, and every conscious effort is made to preserve some airflow past the cords to prevent progressive subglottic stenosis.

Nutrition Support in Infants with Acute GI-Related Disorders

Necrotizing Enterocolitis

NEC remains one of the most frequent indications for emergency surgery on preterm neonates. Although mortality has decreased over time and management of intestinal dysfunction has improved, NEC remains a diagnosis with significant morbidity and mortality. Although this is not intended to be an exhaustive summary of the pathophysiology of NEC, it is important to understand some of the mechanisms thought to be responsible for its development, as they influence the way surgeons treat infants who have experienced mucosal injury and may be at further risk.

NEC is best considered as a consequence of the exposure of an immature and naïve intestinal tract with potentially compromised perfusion to pathogenic organisms that traverse the intestinal barrier and initiate the gut-derived sepsis syndrome. The gut mucosal barrier is compromised on several levels in the premature infant.[39] The normally acidic environment of the stomach serves as an initial barrier to microbes, but acid production is often immature and is often altered iatrogenically with acid-suppressing medications in the hopes of avoiding gastritis and ulceration. Other factors include the limited supply of luminal protective factors such as the lectins and immunoglobulin A provided by maternal milk. Structurally, the mucosal surface provides opportunities for the attachment of bacteria via a decreased mucus barrier, tight junctions that may not be as tight in older, full-term infants, and active translocation mechanisms that are suited for sampling a safer environment than that provided in a neonatal intensive care unit. Mucosal integrity may become further compromised with decreased visceral perfusion. The mucosa are at greatest risk with hypoperfusion, and mucosal sloughing, as evidenced by bloody stools, is an early indication of potential NEC (Bell stage 1 NEC). Altered perfusion may be the consequence of primary cardiac events (congenital heart disease, patent ductus arteriosus), pulmonary compromise with consequent hypoxia and resultant shunting away from the viscera, and other events, such as hemorrhage (pulmonary, intraventricular). Beyond the mucosal border, the immaturity of the host immune system is overcome due to the limited phagocytic and bactericidal activity of neutrophils and other components of the gut-associated lymphoid tissue. These speculated factors may all contribute to facilitating an enteric source of sepsis.

Needless to say, the etiology of NEC is manifold and complex. The radiographic hallmarks are pneumatosis intestinalis and portal venous gas, both of which portend that there has been transgression of the mucosa by gas-producing organisms. If the sepsis can be controlled and the intestine is able to maintain its integrity, no operative intervention is necessary (Bell stage 2 NEC). However, if evidence of perforation occurs or the abdominal sepsis fails to come under control, operative intervention becomes necessary (Bell stage 3 NEC). The options are often dictated by the infant's size and degree of clinical instability. In the smallest and most unstable infant, placement of a peritoneal drain may be all that can be safely offered, while in larger or more stable infants a limited laparotomy at the bedside or in the operating room may allow for more definitive therapy. A current multi-institutional trial is underway through the Neonatal Network to provide some randomized, controlled data.

At surgery, the extent of intestinal involvement becomes apparent. In the least severe circumstances, a limited segment of intestine has transmural gangrene or has perforated. A choice between resection and diversion with stoma versus primary anastomosis is made based on the patient's overall condition and the condition of the intestine. In infants with more extensive and even skip involvement, proximal diversion and excision of only those areas of definite gangrene become the guiding principles so as to preserve as much intestinal length as possible. Despite optimal management, these affected areas may progress to full-thickness gangrene or heal as fibrotic strictures, further compromising residual length and potentially resulting in SBS. Survival is only possible if the sepsis is controlled.[40]

Acute management focuses on providing adequate perfusion to the residual intestine in order to allow it to recover from the initial insult. This results in the generous provision of intravenous fluids early on and the restriction of fluids upon resolution of the sepsis in order to optimize pulmonary function. However, this approach compromises the ability to provide optimal nutrition in a consistent manner. Enteral feeding would be considered no earlier than 7 days after surgery. As in other complex GI disorders, a coherent plan must be generated by the managing teams to best use a combination of EN and PN. Recurrent sepsis and progressive cholestatic jaundice are the predictors of mortality. All techniques available should be use to limit these complications in these patients. Reconstitution of the full GI tract is accomplished after 6 weeks to limit operative complications and to give sufficient time for strictures to form and be identified so that they can be treated in the same operation.[41] Even in infants managed without operative intervention, clinicians must maintain suspicion for developing strictures, particularly if the colon was involved, which can be difficult to tell nonoperatively. Fluoroscopic studies can be used in antegrade and/or retrograde fashion prior to reconnection or in early difficulties with the reinstitution of feeds to identify or rule out stricture formation. Aggressive feeding of an infant with a distal bowel obstruction will only lead to a recurrence of NEC.[42] While the specific amino acid composition of neonatal PN is addressed in other sections, much attention had been focused on the utility of providing glutamine to this population with a compromised gut mucosal barrier; however, this does not appear to be an effective strategy.[43,44]

Infants who survive the early postoperative course associated with NEC are among those at highest risk for intestinal dysfunction, SBS, and cholestasis. All nutrition techniques described earlier in relation to the initiation of trophic feedings, enteral antibiotics, and cycling of PN should be applied in this context. The optimal timing of refeeding and stoma closure remains a topic of controversy is often determined individually or according to institutional preferences rather than by evidence-based protocols.

Isolated Intestinal Perforation

Isolated intestinal perforation closely mimics NEC in that it presents with evidence of visceral perforation (usually pneumoperitoneum in the absence of pneumatosis) or portal venous gas and thus requires some surgical intervention. Infants with this disorder usually have extremely low birth weight (< 750 g), are in their first week of life, and may never have been fed. Often the diagnosis remains speculative, since many are treated with peritoneal drainage only and isolated involvement of a small intestinal segment cannot be verified without surgery. These infants are generally thought to have a better prognosis because of limited colonization of the GI tract during the first week of life, better source control of sepsis once the abdomen has been drained, a self-sealing perforation site, and consequently a less profound sepsis syndrome. The initiating events remain elusive, but may be related to focal perfusion defects or focal luminal injury by medications such as indomethacin.

The same concerns about indications for laparotomy, length of NPO status, and length of antibiotic therapy apply as for infants with NEC. From a nutrition standpoint, one assumption is that the remainder of the GI tract will not have experienced the same generalized mucosal insult as encountered in NEC, and that enteral feedings and rehabilitation should be achievable with greater success rates.

Intestinal Malrotation and Midgut Volvulus

Midgut volvulus as a consequence of intestinal malrotation can occur at any age, having been described both prenatally and in adult patients. The first month of life is, however, the most common time of presentation. The infant who is born with intestinal malrotation and experiences a midgut volvulus can be severely compromised. With timely diagnosis and intervention, the midgut (proximal jejunum to mid-transverse colon) should be salvageable. At surgery, the abdomen may be filled with chylous ascites as a consequence of obstruction and rupture of the mesenteric lymphatics. Untwisting of the mesenteric pedicle will restore venous drainage and allow for improved arterial inflow. Resection is considered only if there are regions of complete necrosis. Any intestinal segment with borderline perfusion is retained and reassessed at 24 hours with a second-look laparotomy to avoid unnecessary resection leading to SBS.

Depending on the extent of the intestinal injury, these infants must initially be fed cautiously to avoid a "second hit" to a compromised bowel. The perioperative nutrition support team must target metabolic needs as well as protein substrate for tissue repair. In the absence of any significant intestinal resection, there should be no ongoing considerations. The management of the child who suffers massive intestinal loss is covered in the chapter on intestinal failure (Chapter 27). As with NEC, infants with midgut volvulus and necrosis are the most likely to have lost the terminal ileum and will likely require vitamin B_{12} supplementation in the future.

Pyloric Stenosis

Infants with pyloric stenosis primarily require rehydration and correction of electrolytes preoperatively but then can resume a normal infant diet. How this is initiated varies by institution. In general, no postoperative feeding tubes are placed, as they put the exposed pyloric channel mucosa at risk of perforation. These infants are typically hungry and have good feeding skills. In this author's institution, our feeding protocol was developed to provide a consistent algorithm that allows the vast majority of infants to be discharged home within 24 hours of surgery. We hold oral feeds for 6 hours and then test the stomach with 2 small-volume (15 mL) Pedialyte feeds 2 hours apart. If the child experiences no vomiting, then formula or breast milk is offered at 30 mL volumes every 3 hours and advanced by 15 mL every second feed to a maximum of 60 mL, providing the necessary volumes for the average 3 to 3.5 kg infant with pyloric stenosis. At this point, the infant can be discharged home and feedings advanced by the parents as tolerated, with the proviso that individual volumes should not be excessive to minimize reflux.

Recurrent vomiting will always raise the spectre of recurrent stenosis or an incomplete operation, both of which are rare events in experienced hands. The infant's stomach is capacious given the preoperative obstruction, but more frequent limited volume feeds will assure retention of feeds and optimal absorption. All parents are amazed by the infant's persistent need to feed within the first month postsurgery. This resolves spontaneously as the child achieves "catch-up" growth. Persistent vomiting should prompt consideration of GER, which can be ameliorated with antacid therapy, including a dose of sodium bicarbonate, which may also act to help disintegrate a mucus plug in the pyloric channel. More serious considerations should include the potential for an intraoperative bowel injury or wound/fascial dehiscence, but typically these infants will have other symptoms in addition to persistent vomiting. If ranitidine was provided perioperatively, it can usually be discontinued at the follow-up visit 3–4 weeks later. Most of these infants have undergone multiple formula changes prior to their diagnosis; we reas-

sure parents that the formula is now less important and that they should use what they have at home and what is most accessible.[45]

The technique (laparoscopic or open) of pyloromyotomy does not have an impact on tolerance of feeds or time to discharge.

Nutrition Support in Children and Adolescents Requiring Surgery

General Principles

In the older child and adolescent, many of the surgical interventions for GI problems are of an acute nature (ie, appendicitis, Meckel's diverticulum, duplications of the GI tract, and intestinal obstruction due to hernia) where there are typically no premorbid nutrition impairment concerns. Children presenting with more chronic disorders, such as inflammatory bowel disease, polyposis syndromes, and chronic GER require a closer evaluation of their nutrition status before elective surgery is contemplated. Despite these logical considerations, there is a paucity of data to correlate preoperative nutritional assessment with postoperative outcomes.[46] Some of these chronic conditions can be the consequence of neonatal interventions with adapted SBS, late stenosis, and dysmotility in atresia (duodenal and jejunoileal) patients. Malignancies affecting the GI tract are generally rare and most frequently involve lymphomas, although carcinoid tumors, desmoid tumors, and other solid visceral tumors will impact the GI tract. Abdominal visceral transplantation is yet another surgical intervention in which specialized focus on nutrition management must occur,[47] but these more complex topics of inflammatory bowel disease, malignancy, and transplantation are addressed in the chapters for these individual topics.

Nutrition management of the acutely ill surgical patient is generally focused on resumption of enteral intake; when this becomes delayed beyond 5–7 days, consideration is given to PN support. There is evidence from the critical care literature to indicate that many of these acutely ill patients are significantly undernourished while in the intensive care unit. There is also evidence that simple calculation of resting energy expenditure without accounting for physical activity underestimates caloric requirements.[48,49] While there is a consistent attempt to provide early enteral feedings to medical patients and trauma patients in the intensive care unit setting , these principles cannot be applied to the surgical patient, who likely is at higher risk for anastomotic breakdown, abdominal sepsis, and the development of complications such as surgical site infections, fascial dehiscence, and enterocutaneous fistulae, which then further complicate clinical and nutrition management. Despite these surgical concerns, the initiation of enteral feedings should be a clinical goal to allow transition off PN support at the earliest feasible time. The ability to handle complex wound failure has been markedly improved with advances in enterostomal care and with the use of negative pressure wound devices that contribute to more rapid closure of open wounds and even enterocutaneous fistulae. The earlier control of fluid and protein losses from these wounds should impact overall protein balance in a favorable manner.

The subset of children who present the highest risk for emergency operation are those with chronic malnutrition. Examples include children with failure to thrive on the basis of congenital heart disease or developmental delay resulting in inadequate oral intake, and children with spine deformities (severe kyphosis and scoliosis) who are at risk for the superior mesenteric artery syndrome, in which there is duodenal obstruction as a consequence of extrinsic compression of the third portion of the duodenum between the superior mesenteric artery and the vertebral column. Children with spastic quadriplegia and seizure disorders may have a limited gastric capacity and poor gastric emptying with a tendency to reflux, limiting their enteral intake. Children with malignancies are often nutritionally depleted as a consequence not only of the disease process, but also the therapies applied. At children's hospitals we have become much more attuned to the preoperative nutrition evaluation of these patients in an effort to optimize outcomes from often extensive surgical interventions. Much of the focus, therefore, is on the provision of feeding access for nutrition support.

Feeding Access in Pediatrics

Many children are referred for placement of enteral feeding devices. If access is required for more than a temporary situation, the options include the various techniques of gastrostomy placement (percutaneous endoscopic gastrostomy, laparoscopic G-tube, open G-tube), insertion of a gastrojejunal device, and direct jejunal feeding tubes. Despite their seemingly simple and innocuous nature, these interventions have the potential for complications and morbidity.[50,51]

When placing a gastrostomy, consideration should be given to the potential for promoting increased reflux on the basis of anatomic alterations. Children who have typically only consumed small amounts of food may not have evidence of reflux until larger volumes are directly administered into the gastric lumen. A preoperative evaluation should be conducted to assess the risks, particularly when these children are developmentally delayed and at risk for aspiration. Anatomic evaluation with an upper GI fluoroscopy study will determine whether there are impediments to proper gastric emptying that may be amenable to correction in the same operation. The principal diagnosis to be considered is malrotation with partial duodenal obstruction on the basis of Ladd's bands. Typically a pH study or impedance study is conducted to address whether GER is present, and to what extent . If consideration is given to an antireflux operation, a nuclear medicine gastric emptying scan can be useful. A gastric emptying scan can also provide information about reflux, although it is less quantifiable than the tests noted above. Gastric outlet procedures (eg, pyloromyotomy and pyloroplasty) are occasionally considered in patients at increased concern for early failure of a fundoplication.

Insertion of Gastrostomy Tube

When a G-tube is inserted for the sole purpose of providing enteral access, enteral feedings can be commenced within 24 hours of operation. With open and laparoscopic techniques, there may be some initial postoperative ileus; however, the main reason for decompressing the stomach or at least avoiding exogenous input is to allow a seal to form between the gastrostomy and the abdominal wall so that with retching and vomiting there is no extravasation between these structures into the peritoneal cavity.

How enteral feedings are provided depends on the child's underlying situation. If the feedings are for supplementation of oral feeds, then oral intake can be started and G-tube feeds given as small bolus volumes, which are increased according to tolerance. In children with neurological deficits or developmental delay, initiation of G-tube feeds may be best assessed by open vented feeds. Rapid egress of formula from the feeding bag into the stomach with no regurgitation into the tube suggests a large-capacity stomach that will accommodate additional volumes, whereas slow evacuation into the stomach suggests a smaller stomach capacity or increased resistance because of abdominal wall contraction, possibly due to pain or spasticity. In this latter situation, it may be more efficient to provide initial feeds as slow continuous drips rather than as bolus volumes. Closed infusion of feeds is the least cumbersome method, but risks GER with the potential for aspiration or requires communication from the patient that the stomach is full. This may be exhibited as retching or visceral pain initiated by overdistention.

In some children with significant reflux there may be concerns about proceeding with a fundoplication. The child may be so nutritionally depleted that the risks are not in favor of proceeding with a major operation. In this situation, a gastrostomy tract can become the conduit for a gastrojejunostomy tube, which allows for gastric decompression and jejunal feedings. The disadvantage to the commercially available button gastrojejunostomy tubes is that they have a minimum size of 16 French and are excessively large and stiff for infants, but they become usable at a patient size of about 10 kg. In smaller patients, other devices can be jury-rigged to achieve the same tasks. However, these tubes are meant as transient feeding support devices, and repeated insertion by required fluoroscopy is not ideal in the pediatric patient. The author's institution uses them as a bridge to help the patient achieve an improved nutrition state and become a better candidate for fundoplication.

Children with neurodevelopmental impairment, spasticity, and seizures often have a higher risk for disruption of their fundoplication and avoiding this operation with the use of jejunal tubes is often enticing. Discussions with the family and caretakers should evaluate not only the child's operative risk but also whether continuous feeding via a gastrojejunostomy tube or jejunostomy tube will interfere with their daily activity schedule. These tubes do not allow for bolus feedings other than through the gastrostomy limb. Often the ability to provide intermittent bolus feeds provides significant improvement in quality of life for both the child and the family.[52] With the advent of the laparoscopic fundoplication, there is less surgical impact in terms of abdominal wall wound healing and pain, although early studies showed that surgical stress in terms of hormone release was not altered. With excellent short-term results, this operation has gained favor; however, its long-term efficacy, especially in higher-risk populations, is still under evaluation.[53]

Primary jejunostomy tubes have been avoided in all but the most chronic and perhaps institutionalized patients, since they represent a long-term commitment to continuous enteral feedings. Operatively, a tract is developed through the abdominal wall and an imbricated jejunal limb before the tube enters the jejunal lumen. This establishes a relatively long tract for reliable replacement of the tube in the correct orientation and minimizes risk of leakage. These tubes have a role in the management of complex surgical patients.

When preoperative nutrition repletion is not feasible before an urgent surgical intervention, the focus must then be on providing early nutrition support, which may require the placement of central venous access or reliable enteral access for this purpose at the time of operation.

Test Your Knowledge Questions

1. Which of the following strategies is considered beneficial in reducing cholestasis?
   A. Provision of > 40% of calories as lipid emulsion
   B. Maintaining GIR > 15 mg/kg/min
   C. Continuous provision of PN
   D. Initiation of enteral feedings

2. Which is a contraindication to commencing enteral feedings?
   A. Bilious nasogastric output in jejunoileal atresia
   B. Contrast extravasation on postoperative day 7 after esophageal atresia repair
   C. Abdominal distention with lack of stoma output
   D. All of the above

3. On a 3 kg infant status poststoma closure after resection for NEC, when should enteral feedings be limited?
   A. Number of bowel movements exceeds 8 over a 24-hour period
   B. Reducing substances < ½%
   C. Fecal pH > 7
   D. Mucoid stools

4. Which clinical diagnosis is expected to have impairment of intestinal motility and may require prolonged PN support?
   A. Gastroschisis
   B. Omphalocele
   C. Hirschsprung's disease
   D. Malrotation without midgut volvulus

References

1. Barlow B, Santulli T, Heird W, Pitt J, Blanc W, Schullinger J. An experimental study of acute necrotizing enterocolitis—the importance of breast milk. *J Pediatr Surg.* 1974;9(5):587–595.
2. Nydegger A, Bines JE. Energy metabolism in infants with congenital heart disease. *Nutrition.* 2006;22(7–8):697–704.
3. Owens J, Musa N. Nutrition support after neonatal cardiac surgery. *Nutr Clin Pract.* 2009;24(2):242–249.
4. Vaidyanathan B, Radhakrishnan R, Sarala D, Sundaram K, Kumar R. What determines nutritional recovery in malnourished children after correction of congenital heart defects? *Pediatrics.* 2009;124(2):e294–e299.
5. Chawla BK, Teitelbaum DH. Profound systemic inflammatory response syndrome following non-emergent intestinal surgery in children. *J Pediatr Surg.* 2013;48:1936–1940.
6. Jaksic T, Shew SB, Keshen TH, Dzakovic A, Jahoor F. Do critically ill surgical neonates have increased energy expenditure? *J Pediatr Surg.* 2001;36(1):63–67.
7. Garza JJ, Shew SB, Keshen TH, Dzakovic A, Jahoor F, Jaksic T. Energy expenditure in ill premature neonates. *J Pediatr Surg.* 2002;37(3):289–293.

8. Pierro A, Eaton S. Metabolism and nutrition in the surgical neonate. *Semin Pediatr Surg.* 2008;17(4):276–284.

9. Gruber EM, Laussen PC, Casta A, et al. Stress response in infants undergoing cardiac surgery: a randomized study of fentanyl bolus, fentanyl infusion, and fentanyl-midazolam infusion. *Anesth Analg.* 2001;92(4):882–890.

10. Shew SB, Keshen TH, Glass NL, Jahoor F, Jaksic T. Ligation of a patent ductus arteriosus under fentanyl anesthesia improves protein metabolism in premature neonates. *J Pediatr Surg.* 2000;35(9):1277–1281.

11. Hulst JM, van Goudoever JB, Zimmermann LJI, Tibboel D, Joosten KFM. The role of initial monitoring of routine biochemical nutritional markers in critically ill children. *J Nutr Biochem.* 2006;17(1):57–62.

12. Reynolds RM, Bass KD, Thureen PJ. Achieving positive protein balance in the immediate postoperative period in neonates undergoing abdominal surgery. *J Pediatr.* 2008;152(1):63–67.

13. Javid PJ, Collier S, Richardson D, et al. The role of enteral nutrition in the reversal of parenteral nutrition-associated liver dysfunction in infants. *J Pediatr Surg.* 2005;40(6):1015–1018.

14. Gura K, Duggan C, Puder M, et al. Reversal of parenteral nutrition- associated liver disease in two infants with short bowel syndrome using parenteral fish oil: implications for future management. *Pediatrics.* 2006;118:e197–201.

15. de Meijer VE, Gura KM, Le HD, Meisel JA, Puder M. Fish oil-based lipid emulsions prevent and reverse parenteral nutrition-associated liver disease: the Boston experience. *JPEN J Parenter Enteral Nutr.* 2009;33(5):541–547.

16. Lee SI, Valim C, Johnston P, et al. The impact of fish oil-based lipid emulsion on serum triglyceride, bilirubin, and albumin levels in children with parenteral nutrition-associated liver disease. *Pediatr Res.* 2009;66(6):698–703.

17. Blackmer A, Warschausky S, Siddiqui S, et al. Preliminary findings of long-term neurodevelopmental outcomes of infants treated with intravenous fat emulsion reduction for the management of parenteral nutrition associated cholestasis. *JPEN J Parenter Enteral Nutr.* 2015;39(1):34–46.

18. Boarini JH. Principles of stoma care for infants. *J Enterostomal Ther.* 1989;16(1):21–25.

19. Al-Harbi K, Walton JM, Gardner V, Chessell L, Fitzgerald PG. Mucous fistula refeeding in neonates with short bowel syndrome. *J Pediatr Surg.* 1999;34(7):1100–1103.

20. Alabbad SI, Ryckman J, Puligandla PS, Shaw K, Nguyen LT, Laberge J. Use of transanastomotic feeding tubes during esophageal atresia repair. *J Pediatr Surg.* 2009;44(5):902–905.

21. Goyal A, Jones MO, Couriel JM, Losty PD. Oesophageal atresia and tracheo-oesophageal fistula. *Arch Dis Child Fetal Neonatal Ed.* 2006;91(5):F381–F384.

22. Ching YA, Fitzgibbons S, Valim C, et al. Long-term nutritional and clinical outcomes after serial transverse enteroplasty at a single institution. *J Pediatr Surg.* 2009;44(5):939–943.

23. Yardley I, Khalil B, Minford J, Morabito A. Multiple jejunoileal atresia and colonic atresia managed by multiple primary anastomosis with a single gastroperineal transanastomotic tube without stomas. *J Pediatr Surg.* 2008;43(11):e45–e46.

24. Piper HG, Alesbury J, Waterford SD, Zurakowski D, Jaksic T. Intestinal atresias: factors affecting clinical outcomes. *J Pediatr Surg.* 2008;43(7):1244–1248.

25. Wales PW, Dutta S. Serial transverse enteroplasty as primary therapy for neonates with proximal jejunal atresia. *J Pediatr Surg.* 2005;40(3):E31–E34.

26. Stollman TH, de Blaauw I, Wijnen MHWA, et al. Decreased mortality but increased morbidity in neonates with jejunoileal atresia: a study of 114 cases over a 34-year period. *J Pediatr Surg.* 2009;44(1):217–221.

27. Pastor AC, Phillips JD, Fenton SJ, et al. Routine use of a SILASTIC spring-loaded silo for infants with gastroschisis: a multicenter randomized controlled trial. *J Pediatr Surg.* 2008;43(10):1807–1812.

28. Bergholz R, Boettcher M, Reinshagen K, Wenke K. Complex gastroschisis is a different entity to simple gastroschisis affecting morbidity and mortality—a systematic review and meta analysis. *J Pediatr Surg.* 2014;49:1527–1532.

29. Phillips JD, Raval MV, Redden C, Weiner TM. Gastroschisis, atresia, dysmotility: surgical treatment strategies for a distinct clinical entity. *J Pediatr Surg.* 2008;43(12):2208–2212.

30. Walter-Nicolet E, Rousseau V, Kieffer F, et al. Neonatal outcome of gastroschisis is mainly influenced by nutritional management. *J Pediatr Gastroenterol Nutr.* 2009;48(5):612–617.

31. Diamond I, Sterescu A, Pencharz P, Kim J, Wales P. Changing the paradigm: omegaven for the treatment of liver failure in pediatric short bowel syndrome. *J Pediatr Gastroenterol Nutr.* 2009;48(2):209–215.

32. Muratore CS, Utter S, Jaksic T, Lund DP, Wilson JM. Nutritional morbidity in survivors of congenital diaphragmatic hernia. *J Pediatr Surg.* 2001 8;36(8):1171–1176.

33. Keshen TH, Miller RG, Jahoor F, Jaksic T. Stable isotopic quantitation of protein metabolism and energy expenditure in neonates on- and post-extracorporeal life support. *J Pediatr Surg.* 1997;32(7):958–962.

34. Shew SB, Keshen TH, Jahoor F, Jaksic T. The determinants of protein catabolism in neonates on extracorporeal membrane oxygenation. *J Pediatr Surg.* 1999;34(7):1086–1090.

35. Agus MSD, Javid PJ, Ryan DP, Jaksic T. Intravenous insulin decreases protein breakdown in infants on extracorporeal membrane oxygenation. *J Pediatr Surg.* 2004;39(6):839–844.

36. Hulst JM, van Goudoever JB, Zimmermann LJ, et al. Adequate feeding and the usefulness of the respiratory quotient in critically ill children. *Nutrition.* 2005;21(2):192–198.

37. Willot S, Uhlen S, Michaud L, et al. Effect of ursodeoxycholic acid on liver function in children after successful surgery for biliary atresia. *Pediatrics.* 2008;122(6):e1236–1241.

38. DeRusso P, Ye W, Shepherd R, et al. Growth failure and outcomes in infants with biliary atresia: a report from the biliary atresia research consortium. *Hepatology.* 2007;46(5):1632–1638.

39. Petrosyan M, Guner Y, Williams M, Grishin A, Ford H. Current concepts regarding the pathogenesis of necrotizing enterocolitis. *Pediatr Surg Int.* 2009;25(4):309–318.

40. Hall NJ, Peters M, Eaton S, Pierro A. Hyperglycemia is associated with increased morbidity and mortality rates

in neonates with necrotizing enterocolitis. *J Pediatr Surg.* 2004;39(6):898–901.

41. Al-Hudhaif J, Phillips S, Gholum S, Puligandla PP, Flageole H. The timing of enterostomy reversal after necrotizing enterocolitis. *J Pediatr Surg.* 2009;44(5):924–927.

42. Bohnhorst B, Müller S, Dördelmann M, Peter CS, Petersen C, Poets CF. Early feeding after necrotizing enterocolitis in preterm infants. *J Pediatr.* 2003;143(4):484–487.

43. Albers MJIJ, Steyerberg E, Hazebroek FWJ, et al. Glutamine supplementation of parenteral nutrition does not improve intestinal permeability, nitrogen balance, or outcome in newborns and infants undergoing digestive-tract surgery: results from a double-blind, randomized, controlled trial. *Ann Surg.* 2005;241(4):599–606.

44. Calder P. Immunonutrition in surgical and critically ill patients. *Br J Nutr.* 2007;98(suppl 1):S133–S139.

45. St. Peter SD, Tsao K, Sharp SW, Holcomb III GW, Ostlie DJ. Predictors of emesis and time to goal intake after pyloromyotomy: analysis from a prospective trial. *J Pediatr Surg.* 2008;43(11):2038–2041.

46. Wessner S, Burjonrappa S. Review of nutritional assessment and clinical outcomes in pediatric surgical patients: does preoperative nutritional assessment impact clinical outcomes? *J Pediatr Surg.* 2014;49:823–830.

47. Asfaw M, Mingle J, Hendricks J, Pharis M, Nucci A. Nutrition management after pediatric solid organ transplantation. *Nutr Clin Pract.* 2014;29:192–200.

48. van der Kuip M, de Meer K, Westerterp KR, Gemke RJ. Physical activity as a determinant of total energy expenditure in critically ill children. *Clin Nutr.* 2007;26(6):744–751.

49. Singer P, Berger MM, Van den Berghe G, et al. ESPEN guidelines on parenteral nutrition: intensive care. *Clin Nutr.* 2009;28(4):387–400.

50. Vervloessem D, van Leersum F, Boer D, et al. Percutaneous endoscopic gastrostomy (PEG) in children is not a minor procedure: risk factors for major complications. *Semin Pediatr Surg.* 2009;18(2):93–97.

51. Beres A, Bratu I, Laberge J. Attention to small details: big deal for gastrostomies. *Semin Pediatr Surg.* 2009;18(2):87–92.

52. Veenker E. Enteral feeding in neurologically impaired children with gastroesophageal reflux: Nissen fundoplication and gastrostomy tube placement versus percutaneous gastrojejunostomy. *J Pediatr Nurs.* 2008;23(5):400–404.

53. Kane TD. Laparoscopic Nissen fundoplication. *Minerva Chir.* 2009;64(2):147–157.

Test Your Knowledge Answers

1. The correct answer is **D**. The initiation of enteral feedings is the most effective intervention to stimulate hepatobiliary secretions and lead to resolution of cholestasis. Excessive lipid and carbohydrate calories are considered to be provocateurs of cholestasis. Cycling of PN has been touted to reduce cholestasis.

2. The correct answer is **D**. Persistent bilious drainage from the stomach implies distal obstruction. The exception to this rule is congenital duodenal atresia as a result of congenital dilation and incompetence of the pyloric channel. Despite evacuation of duodenal content in a prograde manner, there may be some retrograde flow into the stomach. Contrast extravasation in esophageal atresia should initially be managed with continued NPO to allow the leak to seal without exogenous contamination of the mediastinum. Passage of a transpyloric feeding tube would require excessive manipulation. Abdominal distention with lack of stoma output is indicative of ileus or intestinal obstruction.

3. The correct answer is **A**. Advancement of enteral feedings is safe when there is no evidence of diarrhea or malabsorption. Reducing substances < ½% and fecal pH > 7 are indicative of appropriate absorption. Mucoid stools are a nonspecific finding that only become concerning if they contain gross blood. Increased frequency of bowel movements is a generic indicator for feeding intolerance; however, consideration must also be given to the quantity and nature of the stool. Small smears should not be considered as bowel movements, whereas large-volume watery output is of concern.

4. The correct answer is **A**. The hallmark of gastroschisis is that in the majority of patients there is intestinal wall edema and serositis, resulting in the inability to determine whether there is continuity or an atresia present. This is further compounded by the fact that the intestine returns to normal morphology over a variable period that ranges from 4–10 weeks. The intestine in omphalocele is normal other than its covered extra-abdominal location. In the absence of other disorders, these infants tolerate enteral feedings promptly. Patients with Hirschsprung's disease have impaired motility, but once they are diagnosed they undergo a primary reconstruction or diverting colostomy and should have no extended dependence on PN. The intestine in congenital malrotation is functionally normal, although there may be some delayed gastric emptying associated with Ladd's bands. If midgut volvulus occurs, the patient is at risk for loss of the entire midgut intestine.

PART IV

NUTRITION CARE OF THE PEDIATRIC PATIENT

32

Assessment of Nutrition Status by Age and Determining Nutrient Needs

Timothy Sentongo, MD, ABPNS

 Video

CONTENTS

Learning Objectives

1. Identify the important components of pediatric nutrition assessment ranging from growth measurements to using reference data and standard deviation scores.
2. Describe the domains of nutrition assessment in pediatrics.
3. Recognize the potential nutrition deficiencies and excesses commonly found among the pediatric population.
4. Understand how to determine nutrient requirements.

Background

Effective pediatric nutrition support involves accurate assessment of nutrition status and provision of appropriate nutrients to optimize growth and functional development and to mitigate any negative nutrition effects of disease on organ and cellular function. Severe deviation in growth measurements is one of the major clinical manifestations of malnutrition. Malnutrition encompasses excess growth

Table 32-1. Key Domains to Be Encompassed During Nutrition Assessment

DOMAIN	ASSESSMENT	VARIABLES
A	Anthropometric variables	Weight (kg), length (cm), height (cm), head circumference (cm) Weight-for-length, BMI (kg/m²) Mid-arm circumference (cm) Triceps skinfold thickness (mm) Percentile growth charts: Fenton, WHO growth standard, CDC growth reference Use of z scores Frisancho skinfold reference data
B	Dynamism of growth	Change in growth z score
C	Duration of nutrition abnormalities	Acute (< 3-mo duration) vs chronic (> 3-mo duration)
D	Etiology/pathogenesis of nutrition abnormalities	Dietary intakes and mechanism of nutrition imbalance
E	Impact of nutrition abnormalities on the patient's function and development	

BMI, body mass index; CDC, Centers for Disease Control and Prevention; WHO, World Health Organization.

(overweight/obesity) and inadequate growth (underweight/weight loss), and both are associated with increased morbidity, impaired functional capacity, and decreased survival. The rates of growth and nutrition related risks for morbidity vary by childhood phase; that is, infancy, midchildhood, and adolescence. During infancy, rapid gains in weight and length are normal. However, persistence of rapid weight gain into midchildhood is a predictor of progression to obesity.[1] Also, significant underweight (severe malnutrition) during infancy and midchildhood is associated with a > 9-fold risk of death from intercurrent illness compared with lesser degrees of malnutrition.[2,3] Sufficient dietary intake of calcium during childhood and adolescence is important for achieving an adulthood bone mass that protects against later morbidity.[1] Therefore, nutrition assessment of infants, children, and adolescents is crucial for enabling practitioners to identify individuals at risk for weight loss, poor growth, obesity, and nutrition deficits or excesses. The five domains of an in-depth nutrition assessment are presented in Table 32-1 and described in this chapter. They include anthropometric measurements with comparison to reference standards; reviewing growth dynamism (change in growth z scores); establishing whether growth and/or nutrient deficits are acute vs chronic; obtaining detailed diet history, monitoring biochemical indices, and determining

the etiology/pathogenesis of nutrition imbalances; and assessing the impact of nutrition abnormalities on the child's functional capacity and development.[4] The protein, energy, and micronutrient requirements for healthy children and adolescents are based on dietary reference intakes for their age, weight, and sex established by the Institute of Medicine.[5] During illness and in patients with abnormalities in growth and body composition, the energy requirements may need to be directly measured or estimated using prediction equations.

Domain A: Anthropometric Variables

The anthropometric variables commonly used for nutrition assessment and monitoring growth are weight (kg), length/height (cm), head circumference (cm), mid-upper arm circumference (MUAC, cm), and triceps skinfold (mm). These parameters are measured longitudinally to monitor adequacy of growth and establish the effectiveness of nutrition therapy. Weight and length/height may be combined to compute weight-for-length and body mass index (BMI, kg/m²), which are indices used for comparing appropriateness of the child's weight for their length/height (ie, normal vs overweight vs leanness/wasting). All anthropometric measurements and indices must be compared with the appropriate reference data to enable interpretation of growth and nutrition status. The recommended frequency for obtaining anthropometric measurements is presented in Table 32-2.

Table 32-2. Longitudinal Measurement Schedule for Children Born at Term

WEIGHT, LENGTH, WEIGHT-FOR-LENGTH, HEAD CIRCUMFERENCE	
Birth	Once
2–6 wk	Every 2 wk
2–12 mo	Monthly
14–24 mo	Every 2 mo
WEIGHT, HEIGHT, BMI	
2–5 y	Every 6 mo
6–18 y	Every 12 mo
ARM CIRCUMFERENCE, TRICEPS SKINFOLD	
3–12 mo	Monthly
14–24 mo	Every 2 mo
2–5 y	Every 6 mo
6–18 y	Every 12 mo

BMI, body mass index.

Newborns and Preterm Infants

The Fenton[6] 2003 sex-neutral weight, length, and head circumference growth charts for newborns post conception age 22–50 weeks are the most widely used growth references for newborn preterm infants. They assume that the ideal velocity of weight gain should be equivalent to fetal growth, and the curves from 40 to 50 weeks correspond with the average male and female World Health Organization (WHO) 2006 growth standards.[7] Revised sex-specific Fenton growth charts with a smoothed transition to WHO growth standards became available in 2013 (see Appendix 32-1).[8] The alternative newborn and preterm infant growth charts from Olsen et al[9] in 2010 are sex-specific growth charts for weight, length, and head circumference for infants at postconception age 22–42 weeks. The Olsen growth curves were generated from a compilation of a very large racially diverse group of infants and are considered more reflective of current advances in prenatal care.

Newborn term and preterm infants are classified based on their birth weight (See Table 32-3) and estimated gestational age based on last menstrual period, prenatal ultrasound, or the Dubowitz et al[10] newborn maturational exam. Thereafter, longitudinal measurements of weight, length, and head circumference compose the main method for assessing nutrition status and monitoring adequacy of growth. Infants with birth weight < 2500 g regardless of gestational age are referred to as having low birth weight (LBW). Small for gestational age (SGA) or intrauterine growth restriction (IUGR) refers to newborns with birth weight < 10th percentile for gestational age. LBW and SGA are caused by preterm birth, retarded intrauterine growth, or a combination of both factors.[11] Infants who are born SGA but with proportional reductions in weight, length, and head circumference may be categorized as "symmetrical IUGR" or "proportional" or "stunted" IUGR. "Asymmetrical" or "disproportional" or "wasted" IUGR refers to SGA infants with LBW but relatively normal length and head circumference. The management distinction is that "symmetrical IUGR" usually reflects a fetal problem with onset during the first few months of pregnancy with a high likelihood of impaired long-term growth potential. In contrast, asymmetrical IUGR develops during the second half of pregnancy from impaired fetal nutrition and/or oxygen supply secondary to a placental problem. Infants with asymmetrical IUGR typically exhibit greater postnatal catch-up growth and less severe cognitive deficits compared with those with symmetrical IUGR.[11] Large for gestational age (LGA) refers to newborns with a birth weight > 90th percentile for gestational age. The major causes of LGA include maternal diabetes, Beckwith-Wiedeman syndrome, and other genetic disorders.

Table 32-3. Classification of Preterm and Newborn Infants by Birth Weight and Growth Percentile

CATEGORY	BIRTH WEIGHT
Term, large for gestational age	> 4500 g
Term, normal for gestational age	2500–4499 g
Low birth weight	< 2500 g
Very low birth weight	< 1500 g
Extremely low birth weight	< 1000 g
Micronate	< 750 g
CLASSIFICATION	**BIRTH WEIGHT PERCENTILE**
Large for gestational age	Birth weight > 90th percentile
Small for gestational age; intra-uterine growth restriction	Birth weight < 10th percentile

Term Infants to Age 20 Years

Growth in children aged < 24 months should be analyzed using the WHO international growth standards for weight, length, weight-for-length, and head circumference regardless of type of feeding.[7] The WHO growth charts are based on the premise that growth of the healthy breastfed infant is the standard against which all infants should be compared (see Appendix 32-2). Healthy breastfed infants have similar growth in head circumference and length as their formula-fed counterparts; however, the patterns of weight gain differ. Healthy breastfed infants typically gain weight faster than formula-fed infants during the first 3–4 months of life then gain weight more slowly for the remainder of infancy.[7] Therefore, children age > 4 months identified as having low weight for age on the WHO growth standard are more likely to have a substantial deficiency. Growth in children and young adults aged 2–20 years should be analyzed using the Centers for Disease Control and Prevention (CDC) growth reference charts published in 2000.[12] These growth charts may be accessed at http://www.cdc.gov/growthcharts/cdc_charts.htm.

Use of Z Scores vs Percentiles

Percentiles are adequate for assessing growth when anthropometric measurements fall within the 3rd to 97th percentiles (2 standard deviations). However, in situations in which growth measurements are outside the range of normal (ie, < 3rd or > 97th percentile), percentiles are very inconvenient for quantifying the severity of malnutrition.

Table 32-4. Comparison of Percentiles, Z Scores, and Definitions of Growth Status

PERCENTILE	Z SCORE	HEIGHT	WEIGHT	WEIGHT-FOR-LENGTH	BMI
≥ 97th	≥ 2.0	Tall stature	Overweight	Overweight	Obesity
85th–97th	1.0 to 2.0	Normal	Normal	Risk for overweight	Overweight
3rd–97th	−2.0 to 2.0	Normal	Normal	Normal	—
3rd–16th	−2.0 to 1.0	Normal	Risk for underweight	Mild malnutrition	Risk for underweight
< 3rd	−2.0 to −3.0	Short stature	Moderate underweight	Moderate malnutrition	Moderate underweight
< 3rd	< −3.0	Stunted	Severe underweight	Severe malnutrition (wasting)	Severe underweight

BMI, body mass index.

Therefore, the WHO recommends using standard deviation scores (z scores) to define growth in individuals and groups of children. The scores are computed as (observed value − population median)/standard deviation, where the median and standard deviation are age and sex specific. Therefore, a growth z score represents the number of standard deviations a growth measurement is above or below the median value. The z-score values of −2.0, 0, and +2.0 correspond to the 3rd, 50th, and 97th percentiles, respectively. The z-score values that fall between −2.0 and −1.0 (3rd to 16th percentile) correspond with mild malnutrition; z scores > −3.0 but < −2.0 represent moderate malnutrition; and z scores ≤ −3.0 indicate severe malnutrition (Table 32-4).[13] The WHO has defined severe malnutrition in children as a weight-for-height z score < −3.0 and/or the presence of edema (see Table 32-5).[14] Children with a weight-for-height z score < −3 have a >9-fold increased risk of death from intercurrent illness compared with children with a weight-for-height z score > −2,[2,3] and therefore need immediate attention for nutrition rehabilitation and monitoring for refeeding syndrome. The software listed in Appendix 32-3 may be used to computer z scores.

Weight

Weight in infants (age < 12 months) should be measured without clothing or diapers to the nearest 0.01 kg. Older children should be measured to the nearest 0.1 kg while wearing little or no outer clothing and no shoes.[15] Weight

Table 32-5. World Health Organization Diagnostic Criteria for Severe Acute Malnutrition[14]

INDICATOR[a]	MEASURE	CUTOFF
Severe wasting	Weight-for-height	z score < −3.0
Severe wasting	Mid-upper arm circumference	< 115 mm
Bilateral edema	Clinical sign	

[a]Severe wasting and bilateral edema are independent indicators of severe acute malnutrition that require urgent action.

is a composite measure and therefore does not differentiate the specific contributions of muscle, fat tissue, bone mass, or excess fluid (eg, edema or ascites). Tall thin children may weigh the same as similarly aged children who are short and overweight. Therefore, weight measurements alone are inadequate for interpreting growth and nutrition status.

Length/Height

Linear growth in children aged < 24 months and in older children unable to stand erect unsupported is assessed with the child lying supine on a "length board." Linear growth in children aged > 2 years is based on standing height measured using a wall-mounted stadiometer. The child's heels, buttocks, and back should be against the stadiometer, and the head positioned with the Frankfurt plane (an imaginary line extending from the lower margin of the orbit to upper margin of the auditory meatus) parallel to the floor.[15] Height is greatly influenced by hereditary factors; therefore, interpretation of growth status in children age 2–9 years is improved by making comparisons with the with the "midparental height." The midparental height may be estimated using the Tanner-Goldstein-Whitehouse[16] approach as follows: for girls, subtract 13 cm from father's height and calculate the average with the mother's height and for boys, add 13 cm to the mother's height and then average with the father's height. Thereafter, plot the value at the end of the height line; that is, age 20 years on the 2–20 years growth percentile chart. The child's expected height should fall within the range of 8.5 cm above (97th centile) and 8.5 cm below (3rd centile) the value obtained for midparental height. Children with height percentiles that are extrapolated to fall outside the 17 cm range should be considered for evaluation of abnormal linear growth.

Weight-for-Length and BMI

Weight-for-length and BMI are important for assessing appropriateness of the child's weight for their stature. The measures are useful for identifying wasting (thinness, inappropriately low weight for stature), overweight, and obesity. Weight-for-length is used in children aged < 24 months, and BMI used in children aged > 2 years. Interpretation of weight-for-length and BMI percentiles and z scores is presented in Table 32-4. Weight-for-length z score < –3.0 represents severe malnutrition. Children with severe malnutrition have a 9-fold risk of death from intercurrent illness compared with those with mild or moderate malnutrition.[2,3] Acute malnutrition may develop secondary to an illness that negatively impacts food/energy intake or balance, environmentally induced nutrition restrictions or deprivation, or both. Children with acute malnutrition usually rapidly regain their weight following nutrition intervention and treatment or recovery from the inciting disease.[17] Chronic food restriction, multiple episodes of acute malnutrition without adequate interval recovery, or both may lead to retarded linear growth (stunting), which is the hallmark of chronic malnutrition.[18]

The range of normal BMI changes during growth from infancy through childhood and adolescence. Therefore, BMI-for-age percentiles or z scores, but not the actual BMI, should be the basis for interpreting body weight-for-height status. BMI-for-age is the recommended screening tool for overweight and obesity in children aged 2–20 years. Overweight is defined as BMI-for-age ≥ 85th and < 95th percentile, and obesity is BMI-for-age ≥ 95th percentile.[12,19] Obesity is characterized by excess body fat. BMI is inadequate for differentiating between increased weight from excess fat mass (adiposity) vs lean tissue vs both; however, values >95th percentile are highly correlated with increased body fat and comorbidities of cardiovascular disease.[20,21] BMI values in the intermediate range (85th–95th percentile) may result in a missed diagnosis of excess adiposity because there racial differences in body composition. For example, non-Hispanic black girls aged 8–19 years were found to have slightly higher fat mass but considerably higher lean mass than non-Hispanic white girls, resulting in higher body weight but lower percentage body fat.[21] Morbidity and cardiovascular risk are linked to the excess adiposity and not lean tissue. Dual-energy X-ray absorptiometry (DXA) is one of the most accurate methods available for measuring total body fat mass (kg) and lean soft tissue mass (kg) directly. Percent body fat (%BF) percentile charts based on DXA measurements in U.S. children and adolescents aged 8–19 years have been published by the CDC.[22] Age-specific and sex-specific %BF > 75th percentile is associated with a higher risk of dyslipidemia and has also been used as the

cutoff to define excess adiposity.[21,23] However, %BF percentile charts may still underestimate obesity because children with both high fat mass and lean body mass may have normal %BF. Likewise, %BF may be normal or increased (ie, cachectic obesity or sarcopenic obesity) in patients with chronic disorders that disproportionately deplete lean tissue; for example, juvenile rheumatoid arthritis, Crohn's disease, and end-stage renal disease.[24] Therefore, measuring tissue-specific indices, such as fat mass index (FMI) and lean body mass index (LBMI), has been suggested as an alternative to overcome the inadequacies of BMI and %BF. FMI (kg/m^2) and LBMI (kg/m^2) may be calculated using DXA-derived fat mass (kg) and lean body mass (kg) divided by the child's height in meters squared (m^2). Reference data, with 5th to 95th percentile age-based growth charts for FMI and LBMI in children age 8–20 years, are now also available.[25]

Evaluation of overweight and obesity should be individualized to the child's clinical presentation and family history (see Table 32-6). The history and physical and laboratory examinations should screen for medical conditions associated with obesity as well as adiposity-related comorbidities, such as acanthosis nigricans (indicative of insulin resistance), hypertension, dyslipidemia, glucose intolerance, and increased hepatic transaminases (indicative of fatty liver).[26] The importance of obtaining precise measurements of body composition lies in loss of lean tissue being closely related to impaired clinical outcomes, decreased survival, and increased medication toxicity in patients with cancer.[24] Therefore, the future of nutrition assessment will be to increasingly incorporate data from repeated evaluations of fat mass and lean body mass into routine clinical care.

Head Circumference

Brain growth occurs most rapidly from birth to age 3 years and thereafter slows down. Head circumference (cm) is measured using a nonstretchable measuring tape[15] and plotted using the WHO international growth charts. Decreased head circumference is among the sequelae of severe chronic malnutrition and predicts delays in learning and psychomotor development.[27]

MUAC and Triceps Skinfold

MUAC and triceps skinfold measurements are useful for assessing the body composition (fat mass and fat-free mass) especially in children with growth measurements (weight, length/height, and BMI) that plot at extreme ends (< 3rd or > 97th percentile) on the standard growth charts. Soft tissue anthropometry requires a well-trained anthropometrist for

Table 32-6. Evaluation of Overweight and Obesity Individualized to the Child's Clinical Presentation and Family History

FINDINGS	POTENTIAL CONDITIONS
History	
Developmental delay	Genetic disorders
Poor linear growth	Hypothyroidism, Cushing's syndrome, Prader-Willi syndrome
Headaches	Pseudotumor cerebri
Nighttime breathing difficulty and/or daytime somnolence	Sleep apnea, obesity, hypoventilation syndrome
Abdominal pain	Gall bladder disease, GERD
Hip or knee pain	Slipped capital femoral epiphysis
Oligomenorrhea or amenorrhea	Polycystic ovary syndrome
Physical examination	
Dysmorphic features	Genetic disorders, including Prader-Willi syndrome
Moon facies	Cushing's syndrome, primary vs. secondary (corticosteroid medication induced)
Blurred optic discs	Pseudotumor cerebri
Hirsutism	Polycystic ovary syndrome; Cushing's syndrome (primary or secondary)
Acanthosis nigricans	Insulin resistance, NIDDM
Truncal obesity	Risk of cardiovascular disease; Cushing's syndrome; steroids
Abdominal skin striae	Cushing syndrome, primary or secondary
Undescended testicle	Prader-Willi syndrome
Limited hip range of motion	Prader-Willi syndrome
Lower leg bowing	Blount's disease
Laboratory findings	
Dyslipidemia	
Increased hepatic transaminases	Fatty liver
Increase serum glucose, hemoglobin A_{1c}	Insulin resistance, NIDDM

GERD, gastroesophageal reflux disease; NIDDM, non–insulin-dependent diabetes mellitus.

reliable and reproducible measurements.[15] Detailed instructions concerning technique and appropriate tools for measuring circumferences, skinfolds, and extremity lengths are presented by Lohman et al.[28]

MUAC is a composite measure of muscle, fat, and bone at the mid upper arm.[15] MUAC is relatively stable in children from 6 to 59 months. MUAC measurements < 125 to 130 mm in children age 6–59 months or a MUAC z score < −2.0 indicates moderate malnutrition.[29] A MUAC value < 110 mm (z score < −3.0) regardless of age[29] indicates severe malnutrition with increased risk of death. Therefore, MUAC < 110 mm has been recommended as a screening tool to identify children that need to be immediately hospitalized for nutrition intervention.[30]

MUAC is measured with the subject's arm bent to a 90° angle at the elbow, with the upper arm parallel to the body. The distance between the acromion, the bony protrusion on the posterior of the upper shoulder, and the olecranon (ie, the tip) of the elbow is measured, and the midpoint between these 2 landmarks is marked. Thereafter, the subject's arm should be allowed to relax and hang loosely by the side of the body. A nonstretchable measuring tape is then positioned at the marked mid-point, snugly but not pinching the skin, and used to measure the circumference in millimeters. Refer to Appendix 32-4 for the reference data and percentiles for MUAC by Frisancho.[31] MUAC z scores may be computed using the nutrition calculator program in Epi Info version 3.5.3 (http://wwwn.cdc.gov/epiinfo/html/prevVersion.htm). Also refer to Appendix 32-5 for combined MUAC z scores and growth curves for children aged 6–59 months.[29]

Triceps skinfold thickness is a measure of subcutaneous fat at the mid-arm. Fat mass is an indicator of the body's energy reserves. Fat stores at the mid-arm get depleted during nutrition restriction and replenished after nutrition intervention.[32] Therefore, measuring triceps skinfold thickness is useful during initial assessment and monitoring response to nutrition intervention. Triceps skinfold is also the best single anthropometric indicator of %BF in children aged 6–12 years.[33] Thereafter, correlations between triceps skinfold and %BF becomes poor because of pubertal growth and sex-related changes in the body's composition of fat and lean tissue.[25,33] Estimations of whole body fat mass (kg) using triceps skinfold combined with the biceps, subscapular, and suprailiac skinfold measurements correlates well with fat mass obtained using DEXA and ADP.[34] Accurate measurement of skinfold thicknesses is much more difficult to obtain in obese compared with normal-weight and underweight children.[34]

Triceps skinfold thickness is measured with a skinfold caliper. Triceps skinfold is measured at the midpoint upper arm circumference (refer to MUAC measurement above). The child's arm should hang loosely at the side and the examiner should grasp a vertical pinch of skin and subcutaneous fat between the thumb and forefinger, about 1 cm above the previously marked midpoint. The skinfold is pulled away from the muscle and the caliper is placed on the marked midsection. Three readings should be taken, and the average of the 3 is recorded in millimeters. The reading is measured as the calipers come in contact with the skin and the dial reading stabilizes.[28] Reference data and percentiles for triceps skinfold measurements are presented in Appendix 32-6.[31] The frequency for measuring triceps skinfold is presented in Table 32-2.

Growth Velocity Charts

WHO gender-specific growth velocity charts for weight at 1, 2, 3, 4, and 6 months and for length or head circumference increments conditional on age are available for children aged term birth to 24 months. The growth velocities of individual children are characterized by high variability in consecutive growth intervals. Alternating or irregular patterns of high and low growth velocities may occur in successive periods even in the absence of illness or other morbidity. It is not unusual for a child to grow at the 95th velocity percentile one month and then at the 20th the next month while continuing to track on the attained weight-for-age chart. Weight losses or slow gains (related to acute illness or otherwise) in a given period are normally followed by higher velocities, likely indicating catch-up growth. Weight, length, and head circumference increment velocity standards are available at http://www.who.int/childgrowth/standards/en/.

Disease-Specific Growth Reference Charts

Cerebral Palsy

Growth charts for children with cerebral palsy categorized according to the level of motor disability and feeding ability (with or without feeding tube) are available at: http://www.LifeExpectancy.org/articles/GrowthCharts.shtml. The classification system for motor disability in children with cerebral palsy is the 5-level Gross Motor Function Classification System (GMF-CS) presented in Table 32-7. The growth goals and expectations for children with cerebral palsy are influenced by the severity of disability. Children with GMF-CS levels I and II weigh more than those with GMF-CS levels III through V. Therefore, growth curves stratified by severity of gross motor dysfunction appear to be more appropriate.[35,36] Growth curves are also available for upper arm length and lower leg lengths of children with quadriplegic cerebral palsy.[37] However, the use of weight, which is simple and reliable to measure, combined with the appropriate growth reference may have more practical ben-

Table 32-7. Gross Motor Function Classification System (GMF-CS)

GMF-CS	FUNCTION
I	Walks without limitation
II	Walks with limitations
III	Walks using a handheld mobility device
IV	Self-mobility with limitations, may use powered mobility
V	Transported in a manual wheelchair

efits over other more detailed but potentially inaccurately obtained anthropometric measurements.[36]

Genetic Disorders

Disease-specific growth reference charts for several genetic disorders including Down's syndrome, achondroplasia, Marfan's syndrome, William's syndrome, Fragile X, and so forth have been compiled in a virtual issue of the *American Journal of Medical Genetics* Part A, which is online and freely accessible on the Wiley Blackwell Interscience web page of the journal at http://www.interscience.wiley.com/ajmg.[38]

Domain B: Dynamism of Growth

Growth in healthy children is expected to be sustained at stable rates; that is, remain in the same percentile or z score range throughout childhood and adolescence. Accelerated vs decelerated growth is an increase or decline in z score of > 1 standard deviation (SD), respectively, compared to a previous measurement. A change in z score of 1 SD is equivalent to crossing over 1 major percentile curve (3rd, 15th, 50th, 85th, or 97th) on the WHO or CDC growth monitoring charts.[39] Accelerated weight gain or a change in z score of +0.67 between birth and 2 years in children born at term with low or normal birth weight age is associated with increased risk for future obesity and associated morbidities.[1,40] Catch-up growth or compensatory growth is when children with history of weight loss or linear growth retardation because of an illness, inadequate nutrition, or a hormonal deficiency state experience a period of increased growth velocity after treatment and correction of the impediment.

Domain C: Duration of Nutrition Abnormalities

Duration of Abnormal Growth, Illness, or Injury

An acute medical condition is an illness or injury that ordinarily lasts < 3 months or was first noticed < 3 months before the reference date of interview. Medical conditions with a duration > 3 months may be defined as chronic.[41] Malnutrition should be defined as acute or chronic depending on whether the duration is shorter or longer than 3 months.[4] Acute malnutrition negatively impacts weight more than length/height, resulting in anthropometric measurements that show wasting (ie, decreased weight-for-length, BMI, or both). Chronic undernutrition negatively impacts both weight and linear growth, resulting in stunting (height/length z score < –2.0). If the nutrition insult is prolonged or remains untreated, decreased brain growth and head circumference may also occur.[42] Acute malnutrition responds very well to therapy of the underlying illness and nutritional supplements. However, stunted linear growth is less likely to be fully compensated following treatment especially after age 2–5 years.[43]

Puberty Status

Determination of pubertal status is a vital component of nutrition assessment and interpretation of growth status. Puberty is a period of intense hormonal activity and the final phase of rapid linear growth and maturation prior to adulthood. Both forms of malnutrition (obesity and underweight) may affect the onset and duration of the pubertal growth spurt. Childhood obesity is associated with earlier onset of pubertal growth, while malnutrition from deficiency of nutrients may delay puberty. The age at entry into Tanner stages may be used to classify children as early or late onset pubertal growth for purposes of assessing growth velocities during adolescence. Onset of a chronic illness prior to the age of peak growth velocity may negatively impact final height.[44] In addition to the increased linear growth, puberty is marked by rapid progression through the different developmental stages of secondary sexual characteristics. These include the Tanner stages for growth of pubic hair in both sexes, breast development in females, genital development in males, and increase in testicular volume in boys and onset of menarche in girls. The pubertal stage may be determined by physical exam and also reliably by a patient's self-assessment using a pictograph (Appendix 32-7).[45,46] The mean timing for onset of peak velocity in height gain and growth of secondary sexual characteristics is during Tanner stage 3. The first secondary sexual characteristic to reach peak growth velocity in boys is genital stage (age 13 years), closely followed by testis volume, pubic hair stage, and then height. In girls the sequence is height (11.9 years) followed by breast stage (12 years), pubic hair, and then onset of menarche (mean age 13.1 years). Peak growth velocity for height approaches 10 cm/y for boys and 8 cm/y for girls.[47]

Domain D: Determining Etiology and Pathogenesis of Nutrition Abnormalities

The strongest predicator of malnutrition is the presence of an underlying disease.[4] Growth abnormalities and nutrient deficiencies may develop as a consequence of inadequate dietary intake, increased requirements, nutrient malabsorption, or altered nutrient utilization. Inflammatory conditions may induce decreased appetite and poor food intake while increasing calorie requirements and promoting catabolism and nutrient-wasting (eg, cytokine-driven anorexia and skeletal muscle breakdown).[48] Malnutrition in inflammatory disorders may be refractory to mere provision of nutrients[49] until adequate treatment of the underlying disorder. Therefore, nutrition assessment should include a description of the mechanisms leading to nutrient imbalance. Serum concentrations of several of nutrition biomarkers, including transthyretin (prealbumin), retinol-binding protein, zinc, selenium, and vitamins A, D, B6, and C, may be transiently decreased during the first 3–5 days of a systemic inflammatory response.[50,51] Therefore, serum concentration of C-reactive protein should also be measured as a biomarker of inflammation status[4] to provide context for interpretation of nutrition labs.

Domain E: Impact of Nutrition Abnormalities on the Patient's Function and Development

Functional capacity and neurocognitive development are negatively impacted by malnutrition. Functional capacity depends on lean body mass and muscle strength. Chronic malnutrition is associated with decreased muscle mass and delayed development of important motor skills and thus delays the child's opportunities for actions independent of a caregiver.[52] Stunting is independently associated with delayed sitting, standing, walking, and learning compared to children with normal growth.[53] Likewise, nutrition therapy combined with participation in early intervention therapies and psychosocial stimulation yields significantly better long-term improvements in growth, development, and cognitive development compared to nutrition supplementation without psychosocial stimulation.[54,55] Hypothermia and slow heart rate result from generalized slowing of homeostatic functions as an adaptation process in patients with severe nutrition deprivation.[56,57] The triad of encephalopathy, high output heart failure, and severe lactic acidosis is pathognomonic of thiamine deficiency (acute beri beri).[58,59] Other commonly encountered functional impediments related to severe malnutrition are listed in Table 32-8.

Table 32-8. Nutrition Concerns Based on Physical Examination[86,88-90]

SITE	PHYSICAL EXAMINATION	POTENTIAL NUTRITION/METABOLIC STATUS
Skin	Pallor	Iron, folate, vitamin B12, riboflavin deficiency
	Dry scaly skin	Essential fatty acid and biotin deficiency; vitamin A excess or deficiency
	Necklace distribution dermatitis, rough skin	Niacin deficiency
	Acral distribution dermatitis	Zinc deficiency
	Peri-orifice (oral, vulval/perianal) distribution dermatitis	Biotin deficiency
	Acanthosis	Obesity/metabolic syndrome
	Edema: swollen feet, ankles, indentation of skin with application of pressure	Hypoproteinemia, edematous malnutrition
Nails	Koilonychia (spoon-shaped nails)	Iron deficiency. Also deficiency of riboflavin, vitamin C, and niacin (pellagra)
	Transverse leukonychia (opaque white band affecting multiple nails)	PEM, zinc deficiency, pellagra (niacin), and inadequate dietary calcium
	Haplonychia (soft nails)	Deficiency of vitamins A, B6, C, D and inadequate dietary calcium
	Beau's lines (transverse grooves or depression)	Period of severe illness: PEM, pellagra
Neck	Enlarged thyroid	Iodine deficiency
Face	Moon face	Edematous PEM (kwashiorkor)
	Bilateral temporal wasting	Severe PEM
	Apathy	Chronic PEM
Mouth	Oral mucocutaneous rash, angular stomatitis, cheilosis	Deficiency of vitamin B complex (riboflavin, niacin, B6, biotin), iron deficiency
	Bleeding gums	Vitamin C deficiency
Tongue	Atrophic glossitis (burning tongue)	Deficiency of iron, riboflavin, B6, niacin, vitamin B12
	Diminished taste	Zinc deficiency
Eyes	Night blindness, Bitot's spots, corneal keratosis, keratomalacia	Vitamin A deficiency
Hair	Dull, easily pluckable, hypopigmented	PEM (kwashiorkor)
	Increased lanugo body hair	History of significant weight loss
	Hypopigmented hair	PEM, copper deficiency
	Brittle easily breakable hair	Zinc deficiency
	Hair loss, alopecia	Biotin deficiency, low ferritin; vitamin A toxicity
Dentition	Excessive dental carries	Inadequate fluoride; night-time bottle; increased consumption of sweet liquids
Abdomen	Distension: hepatomegaly	Fatty liver from severe malnutrition
	Distension: ascites	Hypoproteinemia; edematous malnutrition
Bones	Tibial bowing/genu varum	Rickets, vitamin D deficiency
Musculoskeletal	Muscle twitching: face vs. carpal muscles, Chvostek vs Trosseau signs	Vitamin D deficiency with hypocalcemia
Temperature	Hypothermia	Severe PEM, global malnutrition
Heart rate	Low heart rate/bradycardia	Severe PEM, global malnutrition
	Tachycardia, lactic acidosis	Beri beri (thiamine deficiency)

PEM, protein energy malnutrition.

Example

You are asked to evaluate a 5-month-old female infant with a history of birth weight 3100 g being re-admitted to the hospital because of persistent poor growth. She initially presented at age 2 months with feeding difficulty prompting hospitalization and a work-up that showed aspiration risk. She was managed for dysphagia with poor per oral intake. She has intermittently been on nasogastric feeds since age 2 months. She has also been admitted multiple times to other hospitals. Her history reveals that she gains weight whenever hospitalized but is unable to maintain at home. The history is negative for vomiting or diarrhea. The newborn screen is negative for cystic fibrosis, thyroid disease, and metabolic disorders. She is not yet rolling from prone to supine. Her anthropometric parameters at age 5 months are weight 4910 g (< 3rd%; z score −2.79); length 60.8 cm (7th%; z score −1.46); weight-for-length < 3rd%; z score −2.28; head circumference 40.3 cm (18th%; z score −0.90). She is not dysmorphic. The current laboratory tests show prealbumin of 19 mg/dL (normal level > 21).

Nutrition Assessment

Growth assessment (Domains A, B, and C): 5-month-old female infant with moderate acute malnutrition.

Pathogenesis (Domain D): i) Feeding dysfunction with inadequate calorie intake, and ii) suspected inconsistent administration of supplemental feeds by caregivers, resulting in nutrition failure to thrive.

Functional impact (Domain E): Delays in motor development (not yet rolling over).

Determination of Nutrient Needs[60]

The normal nutrition requirements for infants, children, and adolescents is the level of energy, protein, and micronutrient intake from food that balances expenditure and losses and is associated with growth and deposition of tissue at rates consistent with good health.[61] In premature infants, the requirements are defined by the level of protein, energy, fluid, and micronutrient intake that will support growth and composition of body weight at rates similar to a normal fetus of same postconceptional age.[26]

Protein and Energy Requirements of the Premature Infant

Preterm birth interrupts the rich supply of nutrients that support normal growth and development of the fetus. Inadequate postnatal nutrition and acute neonatal illnesses (eg, respiratory distress syndrome, bronchopulmonary dysplasia, necrotizing enterocolitis) are major causes of restricted growth in preterm and LBW infants. The preterm infant should be weighed nude, at the same time of day and on the same scale, on a daily basis to monitor nutrition status. The average daily weight gain is compared in grams per kilogram per day or grams per day to the expected fetal growth rate (Table 32-9), and weekly growth is assessed by plotting measurements on the Fenton growth charts. Extreme weight changes may be due to fluid shifts or medical conditions, and these factors should be considered before modifying an infant's nutrition support regimen. Poor early postnatal growth is associated with impaired neurocognitive development.[62] The goals for nutrition management of preterm infants are early implementation of nutrient intakes at levels that support growth similar to intrauterine rates and stimulation of the gastrointestinal tract to gradually assume full responsibility for digestion and absorption of nutrients.[63] The estimated average energy and protein requirements for preterm infants to achieve fetal rates of weight gain are displayed in Table 32-9.[62] Therefore, parenteral nutrition should be promptly initiated within 24–36 hours of birth and enteral feeds introduced at trophic rates (10–20 mL/kg/d) for 1–5 days depending on illness severity and degree of prematurity. Thereafter, the enteral feeds can be advanced at about 20–35 mL/d as the parenteral nutrition is gradually reduced.[64] Human milk is the preferred enteral feeding because of its multiple benefits, including reduced risk of necrotizing enterocolitis, trophic effects on the immature gastrointestinal tract, enhanced gastric emptying, immunological benefits, and earlier achievement of full enteral feedings.[26] Human milk alone has inadequate protein and calories for meeting the nutrition needs of the preterm infant. Therefore, when intakes reach 100–150 mL/kg/d, fortification is recommended.[64]

Calcium and Phosphorous Requirements

The last trimester of pregnancy is the period of greatest bone mineral accretion; therefore, infants born prematurely (<28 weeks gestation) and/or LBW infants (< 2500 g) have a high risk for low bone mass and developing metabolic bone disease (osteopenia of prematurity or rickets of prematurity). Furthermore, adequate intake of calcium/phosphorous within the first few weeks of life is limited by inability to tolerate full enteral feeds and incompatibility-related restrictions in parenteral solutions. Metabolic bone disease may be diagnosed by appearance of demineralized bone and fractures on plain x-ray; however, this is a late finding. DEXA is the gold standard for detecting and monitoring metabolic bone disease, but it involves exposure to some degree of ionizing radiation; therefore, it is not yet routinely used in preterm infants.[65] Serum alkaline phosphatase concentrations increase if there is high bone turnover or deficiency of mineral substrate (cal-

Table 32-9. Protein and Energy Intakes Needed to Achieve Fetal Rates of Weight Gain[62]

	BODY WEIGHT, g					
	500–700	700–900	900–1200	1200–1500	1500–1800	1800–2200
Fetal weight gain, g/d	13	16	20	24	26	29
Fetal weight gain, g/kg/d	21	20	19	18	16	14
Protein, g/kg/d						
Inevitable loss	1.0	1.0	1.0	1.0	1.0	1.0
Growth	2.5	2.5	2.5	2.4	2.2	2.0
Required protein intake						
Parenteral	3.5	3.5	3.5	3.4	3.2	3.0
Enteral	4.0	4.0	4.0	3.9	3.6	3.4
Energy, kcal/kg/d						
Loss (expenditure)	60	60	65	70	70	70
Resting expenditure	45	45	50	50	50	50
Other expenditure	15	15	15	20	20	20
Growth (accretion)	29	32	36	38	39	41
Required intake						
Parenteral	89	92	101	108	109	111
Enteral	105	118	119	127	128	131
Protein/energy, g/100 kcal						
Parenteral	3.9	3.8	3.5	3.1	2.9	2.7
Enteral	3.8	3.7	3.4	3.1	2.8	2.6

cium, phosphorous, vitamin D). A high serum alkaline phosphatase level is inversely correlated with low serum phosphorous. A combination of serum alkaline phosphatase >900 U/L and serum inorganic phosphate < 1.8 mmol/L has high sensitivity and specificity for reduced bone mineral content measured by DEXA.[66] Providing adequate calcium and phosphorous to maintain normal serum phosphorous concentrations optimizes bone mineralization. Commercial preterm infant formulas with increased protein, calories, calcium, and phosphorous are available. All preterm infants with postconception age < 34 weeks and/or severe illness have immature suck and swallow, and enteral feeds must therefore be administered via nasogastric tube. Parenteral nutrition should not be discontinued until the enteral feeds provide at least 90% of the required fluid intake.[62]

Protein and Energy Requirements of Full-Term Infants and Children

The components of energy expenditure are basal metabolism, thermic effect of food, energy cost of growth, energy expended for physical activity, and energy utilized in for temperature regulation.[60] Protein is essential to maintain cellular integrity and function, wound healing, health, and reproduction. Sufficient nonprotein calories (ie, carbohydrates, fats) must be consumed so that the carbon skeletons of amino acids are not diverted to metabolic pathways for generation of energy.[67]

Nutrition Requirements by Age Category

Energy and Protein Requirements for Infants Age Birth to 6 Months

Infants double their birth weight by age 6 months and triple it by age 12 months.[68] For infants age birth to 6 months, the recommended protein, energy, and micronutrient intakes are based on an adequate intake (AI) level derived from the average daily intake by full-term infants who are born to healthy, well-nourished mothers and exclusively breastfed. For infants age 7–12 months, the AI is based on nutrients provided by 0.6 L/d of human milk, which is the average volume consumed in this age category and the usual intake of complementary weaning foods consumed by infants in this age category.[60]

Protein and Energy Requirements After Age > 6 Months

During nutrition support, sufficient nonprotein calories (ie, carbohydrates, fats) must be provided so that the carbon skeletons of amino acids are not used to meet energy needs.[67] Protein intake for children age 7–12 months and age 14–18 years is based on an estimated average requirement (EAR) value. The EAR for protein is the average daily protein intake level estimated to meet the requirement of half the healthy individuals at a particular life stage, with values differing based on sex. The recommended protein intake for children age 1–13 years is based on a recommended dietary allowance (RDA) value. The RDA is average daily dietary intake level sufficient to meet the nutrient requirement of nearly all (97%–98%) healthy individuals at a particular life stage or for their sex.

The components of energy expenditure are basal metabolism, thermic effect of food, energy cost of growth, energy expended for physical activity, and energy utilized for temperature regulation.[60] Basal energy expenditure (also referred to as resting energy expenditure [REE]) is the biggest contributor to total daily energy requirements (65%–70%); diet-induced thermogenesis constitutes 5%–10%, and physical activity 25%–30%. The energy cost of growth is too small to measure except in rapidly growing infants.[69] It is estimated to be approximately 5–8 kcal/g of weight gain (see Table 32-10).[70–72] Weight is the best predictor of energy requirements. Estimation of energy requirements in healthy children aged birth to 18 years with normal growth, body composition, and physical activity levels are calculated using the 2005 Dietary Reference Intake/Institute of Medicine (IOM) equations based on age, weight, and physical activity level (Appendix 32-8).

Estimating Energy Requirements During Illness

Indirect Calorimetry

Reliance on RDA to guide energy intake is inappropriate during illness because several factors may impact energy expenditure, such as fever, sepsis, inflammation, sedation, decreased physical activity, mechanical ventilation, surgery, and medications.[73] Therefore, actual measurement of energy expenditure using indirect calorimetry is the best available method to accurately determine the calorie needs for achieving weight maintenance, gain, or loss and to avoid hypofeeding or hyperfeeding.[73] REE is measured with a computerized metabolic cart, preferably in a thermoneutral room with the patient rested. The principle is to measure oxygen consumption and carbon dioxide production at steady state. Thereafter, the Weir equation[74] is used to calculate energy equivalency from the oxygen consumption and carbon dioxide production. The measured REE may then be compared with REE values obtained using the WHO[61] and/or Schofield[75] energy prediction equations to determine whether the patient is hypermetabolic, hypometabolic, or eumetabolic. Patients with a measured REE within 90%–110% of predicted values are considered eumetabolic.[76] Total energy expenditure (TEE), which is the clinically required information, is estimated by multiplying measured REE with a coefficient based on the patient's physical activity level and illness severity, especially in disorders associated with malabsorption or pulmonary disease (eg, cystic fibrosis). Physical activity and stress level coefficients are presented in Table 32-11. The WHO REE prediction equations are based on age, sex, and weight, while the Schofield REE equations also include height in the calculation, which appears to improve accuracy in patients with altered body composition (eg, overweight/obesity or failure to thrive).[77,78] The WHO and Schofield REE prediction equations are presented in Appendix 32-8.

Example

A 16-kg, normally active, internationally adopted 6-year-old boy with history of moderate underweight presents because of failure of catch-up growth. His REE was measured to determine metabolic rate and serve as a basis to calculate his energy needs,

Table 32-10. Components of Energy Expenditure[69]

COMPONENT	% TOTAL DAILY ENERGY EXPENDITURE
Resting energy expenditure[a]	60–70
Diet induced thermogenesis	5–10
Physical activity	25–30
Growth	< 5

[a]Approximately equivalent to basal metabolic rate.

Table 32-11. Activity and Stress Factors[14]

ACTIVITY/STRESS ADJUSTMENT FACTORS	DEFINITION
REE × 1.3	For a well-nourished child on bedrest with mild-to-moderate stress
REE × 1.5	For a normally active child with mild-to-moderate stress; an inactive child with severe stress (ie, trauma, stress, cancer), or a child with minimal activity and malnutrition requiring catch-up growth
REE × 1.7	For an active child requiring catch-up growth or an active child with severe stress

REE, resting energy expenditure.

including a goal to gain 1 kg weight in the next 30 days. The energy cost of growth is estimated to be approximately 5–8 kcal/g of weight gain.[70-72] His measured REE was 900 kcal/d (eumetabolic) and physical activity coefficient 1.5 (normally active). Therefore, the child's daily TEE (kcal/d) at his current rate of growth and level of physical activity is 900 × 1.5 = 1350 kcal/d. The energy cost of 1 kg weight gain at rate of ~7 kcal/g is 7 kcal/g × 1000 g (ie, 7000 kcal). To achieve the 1-kg weight gain in 30 days: 7000/30 = 233 kcal/d × 30 days is needed in addition to his TEE. Therefore, the daily energy intake required to achieve a 1-kg weight gain at the current level of physical activity is 1350 + 233 = 1583 kcal/d.

Prediction Equations

When indirect calorimetry is not available, REE can be estimated using either WHO or Schofield energy prediction equation, and then TEE, which is the clinically required information, may then be calculated as the product of REE (kcal) and a coefficient based on disease severity and/or level of physical activity.

Refeeding Syndrome

Refeeding syndrome is a feeding-induced metabolic syndrome occurring in previously starved or severely malnourished patients. Refeeding syndrome is characterized by shift from starvation-related fat and protein catabolism to carbohydrate metabolism and resultant anabolic effects from increased secretion of insulin. The anabolic effects of insulin include increased cellular uptake of glucose, potassium, magnesium, and phosphate. The hallmark of refeeding syndrome is hypophosphatemia. Other deficiencies occur including hypokalemia and hypomagnesemia with potential sequelae of arrhythmia, edema, congestive heart failure, and death within a few days of implementing aggressive nutrition therapy. Insulin also exerts a natriuretic effect on the kidneys, resulting in sodium and fluid retention. The anabolism may unveil other nutrient deficiencies (eg, thiamine deficiency/beriberi) further leading to life-threatening circumstances.[79] The risk for developing refeeding syndrome is highest in patients underfed for at least 10–14 days (regardless of therapy with crystalloid intravenous fluids); patients with a history of acute weight loss of >10% in the preceding 1–2 months, severe malnutrition (< 80% ideal body weight or weight-for-length/height z score <–3),[3,14] decreased prealbumin,[80] anorexia nervosa, marasmus, and edematous malnutrition (kwashiorkor); and in children with malnutrition secondary to neglect, cerebral palsy, and dysphagia.[79] The metabolic derangements underlying

refeeding syndrome can be avoided by initiating feeds at a calorie intake of 50%–75% of the measured or predicted REE and appropriate monitoring and supplementation with phosphorus, potassium, and magnesium. The calorie intake is then gradually increased by 10%–20% per day until the goal is reached, while closely monitoring and correcting any biochemical abnormalities.[81]

Vitamin and Mineral Needs

Calcium

According to the American Academy of Pediatrics (AAP), the primary need for dietary calcium in otherwise healthy infants, children, and adolescents is to enhance bone mineralization.[26] Maintaining adequate calcium intake during childhood is necessary for maximizing peak bone mass and decreasing the risk of osteoporosis later in adulthood.[26] Exercise, in addition to calcium intake, is important for achieving peak bone mass. Wyshak and Frisch[82] reported a positive relationship between cola consumption and bone fractures. However, it is uncertain if this finding may be attributed to the potential excess phosphorus content found in colas or due to the diminished calcium intake related to decreased consumption of dairy products (specifically milk). Currently, dual-energy radiograph absorptiometry (ie, DEXA scan) is the method used in many studies to measure bone mineral content and bone mineral density of specific areas or the entire skeleton, with notably negligible levels of radiation exposure.[26]

According to the AAP,[26] "the optimal primary nutritional source during the first year of life is human milk." Preterm infant formulas are fortified with calcium and phosphorous in a 2:1 ratio to optimize absorption and bone mineralization. The bioavailability of calcium in human milk is greater than that found in infant formulas and cow's milk. Therefore, standard infant formulas contain increased concentrations of calcium content to increase their comparability to human milk.

According to the AAP, calcium retention is relatively low in toddlers and increases as puberty approaches.[26] The majority of bone formation and the efficiency of calcium absorption are highest during puberty. Data from balance studies suggest that maximal net calcium balance is achieved with intakes of 1200–1500 mg daily in most healthy adolescents.[26] Calcium intakes on food labels are indicated as a percentage of the daily value in each serving. The daily value is currently set at 1000 mg daily. Calcium supplementation should be considered for children who are

Table 32-12. Recommendations for Adequate Dietary Calcium Intake in the United States[26]

AGE	CALCIUM INTAKE, mg/d (mmol/d)
0–6 mo	210 (5.3)
7–12 mo	270 (6.8)
1–3 y	500 (12.5)
4–8 y	800 (20.0)
9–18 y	1300 (32.5)
19–50 y	1000 (25)
50 to >70 y	1200 (30)

on dairy-restricted diets or prolonged therapy with medications that inhibit calcium absorption or enhance its excretion (eg, glucocorticoids and diuretics).[26] The AI levels for calcium are presented in Table 32-12.

Iron

Iron deficiency is the most common nutrition deficiency in the world.[26] The major adverse effect of iron deficiency is onset of cognitive and motor developmental delays. Furthermore, during iron-deficiency states there is enhanced absorption and brain accretion of other divalent cations, including lead and manganese, that are detrimental to health.[26] Iron deficiency is associated with physical findings of pallor, koilonychia, and glossitis (see Table 32-8). Decreased serum ferritin with or without iron deficiency has been associated with hair loss.[83] The incidence of iron-deficiency anemia peaks in children between the ages of 6 and 20 months, or earlier with premature infants, with a second peak around puberty. Additionally, toddlers are often at risk for iron-deficiency anemia due to transitioning from iron-fortified formula to cow's milk. Individuals at risk for developing iron deficiency include premature and LBW infants, overweight children, children with caregivers of low socioeconomic status, adolescent females with increased menstrual losses, athletes, and patients with malabsorption disorders affecting the duodenum/jejunum, occult gastrointestinal bleeding, and/or history of chronic inflammatory diseases. During active inflammation, cytokine-induced malabsorption of dietary iron occurs.[84] This is mediated through up-regulation of hepatic synthesis of hepcidin, which in the presence of tumor necrosis factor-α causes degradation of ferroportin, the enteric iron exporter.[84,85] Adequate intake of riboflavin is also essential for optimized absorption and utilization of iron.[85] The hallmark of iron deficiency is microcytic anemia. The recommended screening test for iron deficiency is measuring hemoglobin or hematocrit; however, anemia represents the most severe end of the iron-deficiency spectrum (see Table 32-13). Serum concentrations of ferritin may be spuriously elevated in patients with active inflammation. In addition, microcytic anemia must be differentiated from anemia of chronic disease and thalassemia traits that should not be treated with iron supplements.

More than 80% of the iron stores of the term infant are accrued during the third trimester of pregnancy. Therefore, infants born prematurely require more iron postnatally during the first year of life to catch up to infants born at term.[26] Iron intake requirements for premature infants range from 2 mg/kg/d for infants with birth weights between 1500 and 2500 g to 4 mg/kg/d for infants weighing < 1500 g at birth.[26] Adequate iron stores are needed for optimal growth and development. According to the AAP, "Infants who are not breastfed or who are partially breastfed should receive an iron-fortified formula (containing between 4 to 12 mg of iron per liter) from birth to 12 months."[26]

The recommended treatment dose for iron-deficiency anemia is 3–6 mg/kg or elemental iron administered daily in 3 divided doses for at least 4 weeks with concomitant intake of vitamin C to enhance the iron absorption. Prophylactic iron supplementation is recommended for those identified at an increased risk of iron-deficiency anemia.[26]

Vitamin D

Cases of rickets caused by nutrient deficiency continue to be reported in the United States and other Western countries. Vitamin D deficiency in exclusively breastfed infants is attributed to breast milk's low vitamin D content; it may also be caused by an inadequate conversion of the inactive form of vitamin D within the body to the active form due to decreased sun exposure. As a result, the AAP recently issued updated

Table 32-13. Progression of Biochemical Markers of Iron Deficiency

BIOCHEMICAL MARKER	EARLY PHASE IRON DEFICIENCY	MIDPHASE WITH COMPENSATION	LATE PHASE: ESTABLISHED IRON DEFICIENCY
Serum iron	↓	↓↓	↓↓↓
% Saturation	↓	↓↓	↓↓↓
Ferritin	↓	↓↓	↓↓↓
Total iron-binding capacity	Normal	↑	↑↑
Mean corpuscular volume	Normal	↓	↓↓
Red blood cell distribution width	Normal	Normal	↓
Hemoglobin	Normal	Normal	↓

Table 32-14. Level of Fluoride in Community Drinking Water and Recommended Fluoride Supplementation

	MEASURED LEVELS, ppm[a]		
Age	< 0.3	<0.3–0.6	> 0.6
0–6 mo	None	None	None
6 mo–3 y	0.25 mg/d	None	None
3–6 y	0.5 mg/d	0.25 mg/d	None
6–16 y	1 mg/d	0.5 mg/d	None

[a]1 ppm = 1 mg/L.[31]

guidelines for vitamin D intake for infants, children, and adolescents to prevent vitamin D deficiency, which in turn will reduce the incidence of rickets. The 2008 guidelines recommend a daily intake of 400 IU of vitamin D for all infants, children, and adolescents starting from the first few days of life.[26]

Fluoride

According to the CDC, dental caries may be the most prevalent of infectious diseases in children. Primary tooth decay can affect children's growth, lead to malocclusion, and cause lifelong oral health problems.[86] Fluoride use is considered the most important tool in preventing and controlling caries. Fluoride prevents caries by reducing tooth enamel solubility, which diminishes the effects of plaque-forming pathogens, and promoting remineralization of demineralized areas.[87] Recommendations to aid in the prevention of dental caries include the establishing and maintaining good oral hygiene, optimizing systemic and topical fluoride exposure, eliminating bedtime bottles and sweet liquids, and limiting sugar consumption and frequent snacking.[86] The American Academy of Pediatric Dentistry (AAPD) reports that the adjustment of fluoride levels in community water to the optimal concentration is the most beneficial and inexpensive method of reducing the incidence of dental caries. However, when drinking water fluoridation is not possible, the AAPD supports the intake of daily fluoride supplements and the use of fluoride-containing preparations (eg, toothpastes, gels, and mouth rinses). Caution is needed with topical fluoride use in children due to the risk of excessive exposure to fluoride.[26] Table 32-14 details recommendations for fluoride supplementation based on levels found in community drinking water.[26]

Acknowledgments

The authors of this chapter for the second edition of this text wish to thank Liesje Neiman Carney, RD, CNSD, LDN; and Jennifer Blair, MA, RD, CSP, LDN, for their contributions to the first edition of this text.

Test Your Knowledge Questions

1. A 21-month-old boy with biliary atresia status post Kasai portoenterostomy currently on supplemental nasogastric feeds presents for pre–liver transplant follow-up. His growth measurements are 8.3 kg for weight and 81 cm for length. His growth measurements at age 13 months were 7.3 kg and 73 cm for weight and length, respectively. What is your assessment of his nutrition status?
    A. Normal growth on current feeding regimen
    B. Underweight but growing steadily on his curve
    C. Stunted growth on the current feeding regimen
    D. Wasting and increased risk for mortality
2. Review the statements and indicate whether they are *true* or *false*.
    A. Obesity may be defined as weight-for-length or BMI > 85th percentile.
    B. The risk of mortality in children with moderate malnutrition is very similar to that of children with mild malnutrition.
    C. A MUAC measurement of 125 mm corresponds to severe malnutrition.
    D. A height *z* score of 1.0 (85th percentile) corresponds to tall stature.
3. Link the following nutrients with deficiency or toxicity symptoms. Select each nutrient only once.

    1. Niacin; 2. Iron; 3. Copper; 4. Zinc; 5. Biotin; 6. Calcium; 7. Pyridoxine; 8. Riboflavin
    A. Peri-orifice distributed dermatitis, glossitis, alopecia
    B. Glossitis, cheilosis, pallor, koilonychia
    C. Dysphagia, microcytosis, vegan diet, menorrhagia
    D. Transverse leukonychia, alopecia, dermatitis, dysgeusia
    E. Anemia, hypopigmented hair, osteopenia
    F. Diarrhea, dermatitis, dementia, death
4. You are asked to evaluate the growth status of 5-year-old girl with cerebral palsy and a history of dysphagia and feeding tube; she wears ankle braces and ambulates independently. What is the appropriate reference to use?
    A. WHO growth charts for children age birth to 60 months
    B. CDC growth charts for children age 2–20 years
    C. Cerebral palsy GMF-CS I chart for tube-fed children
    D. Cerebral palsy GMF-CS II chart for tube-fed children

   E. Cerebral palsy GMF-CS III chart for tube-fed children

   F. None of the above

5. Which of the following methods is the most reliable for estimating body fat and lean tissue?

   A. Skinfold anthropometry

   B. Bioelectrical impedance analysis

   C. BMI

   D. Dual x-ray absorptiometry (DXA)

6. Answer *true* or *false* to the following:

   A. Reference data are available for percent body fat (%BF).

   B. Malnourished patients may have increased %BF.

   C. BMI is strongly correlated with %BF.

References

1. Cameron N, Demerath EW. Critical periods in human growth and their relationship to diseases of aging. *Am J Phys Anthropol.* 2002;Suppl 35:159–184.

2. Black RE, Cousens S, Johnson HL, et al; Child Health Epidemiology Reference Group of WHO and UNICEF. Global, regional, and national causes of child mortality in 2008: a systematic analysis. *Lancet.* 2010;375(9730):1969–1987.

3. Olofin I, McDonald CM, Ezzati M, et al; Nutrition Impact Model Study (anthropometry cohort pooling). Associations of suboptimal growth with all-cause and cause-specific mortality in children under five years: a pooled analysis of ten prospective studies. *PLoS One.* 2013;8(5):e64636.

4. Mehta NM, Corkins MR, Lyman B, et al; American Society for Parenteral and Enteral Nutrition Board of Directors. Defining pediatric malnutrition: a paradigm shift toward etiology-related definitions. *JPEN J Parenter Enteral Nutr.* 2013;37(4):460–481.

5. Food and Nutrition Board, Institute of Medicine. Panel on Macronutrients, Panel on the Definition of Dietary Fiber, Subcommittee on Upper Reference Levels of Nutrients, Subcommittee on Interpretation and Uses of Dietary Reference Intakes, and the Standing Committee on the Scientific Evaluation of Dietary Reference Intakes, Food and Nutrition Board. Protein and amino acids. In: *Dietary Reference Intakes for Energy, Carbohydrate, Fiber, Fat, Fatty Acids, Cholesterol, Protein and Amino Acids.* Washington, DC: National Academies Press; 2005:589–768.

6. Fenton TR. A new growth chart for preterm babies: Babson and Benda's chart updated with recent data and a new format. *BMC Pediatr.* 2003;3:13.

7. Grummer-Strawn LM, Reinold C, Krebs NF; Centers for Disease Control and Prevention (CDC). Use of World Health Organization and CDC growth charts for children aged 0–59 months in the United States. *MMWR Recomm Rep.* 2010;59(RR-9):1–15.

8. Fenton TR, Kim JH. A systematic review and meta-analysis to revise the Fenton growth chart for preterm infants. *BMC Pediatr.* 2013;13:59.

9. Olsen IE, Groveman SA, Lawson ML, Clark RH, Zemel BS. New intrauterine growth curves based on United States data. *Pediatrics.* 2010;125(2):e214–e224.

10. Dubowitz LM, Dubowitz V, Goldberg C. Clinical assessment of gestational age in the newborn infant. *J Pediatr.* 1970;77(1):1–10.

11. Kramer MS. Determinants of low birth weight: methodological assessment and meta-analysis. *Bull World Health Organ.* 1987;65(5):663–737.

12. Kuczmarski RJ, Ogden CL, Grummer-Strawn LM, et al. CDC growth charts: United States. *Adv Data.* 2000;(314):1–27.

13. Use and interpretation of anthropometric indicators of nutritional status. WHO Working Group. *Bull World Health Organ.* 1986;64(6):929–941.

14. *WHO Child Growth Standards and the Identification of Severe Acute Malnutrition in Infants and Children: A Joint Statement by the World Health Organization and the United Nations Children's Fund.* Geneva: World Health Organization, 2009.

15. Zemel BS, Riley EM, Stallings VA, Evaluation of methodology for nutritional assessment in children: anthropometry, body composition, and energy expenditure. *Annu Rev Nutr.* 1997;17:211–235.

16. Tanner JM, Goldstein H, Whitehouse RH. Standards for children's height at ages 2–9 years allowing for heights of parents. *Arch Dis Child.* 1970;45(244):755–762.

17. Gorstein J, Sullivan K, Yip R, et al. Issues in the assessment of nutritional status using anthropometry. *Bull World Health Organ.* 1994;72(2):273–283.

18. Richard SA, Black RE, Gilman RH, et al; Childhood Infection and Malnutrition Network. Wasting is associated with stunting in early childhood. *J Nutr.* 2012;142(7):1291–1296.

19. Reilly JJ. Diagnostic accuracy of the BMI for age in paediatrics. *Int J Obes (Lond).* 2006;30(4):595–597.

20. Krebs NF, Jacobson MS. Prevention of pediatric overweight and obesity. *Pediatrics.* 2003;112(2):424–30.

21. Flegal KM, Ogden CL, Yanovski JA, et al. High adiposity and high body mass index-for-age in US children and adolescents overall and by race-ethnic group. *Am J Clin Nutr.* 2010;91(4):1020–1026.

22. Ogden CL, Li Y, Freedman DS, Borrud LG, Flegal KM. Smoothed percentage body fat percentiles for US children and adolescents, 1999–2004. *Natl Health Stat Rep.* 2011;(43):1–7.

23. Lamb MM, Ogden CL, Carroll MD, Lacher DA, Flegal KM. Association of body fat percentage with lipid concentrations in children and adolescents: United States, 1999–2004. *Am J Clin Nutr.* 2011;94(3):877–883.

24. Thibault R, Pichard C. The evaluation of body composition: a useful tool for clinical practice. *Ann Nutr Metab.* 2012;60(1):6–16.

25. Weber DR, Moore RH, Leonard MB, Zemel BS. Fat and lean BMI reference curves in children and adolescents and their utility in identifying excess adiposity compared with BMI and percentage body fat. *Am J Clin Nutr.* 2013;98(1):49–56.

26. Kleinman R, ed. *Pediatric Nutrition Handbook.* 6th ed. Elk Grove Village, IL: American Academy of Pediatrics; 2009.

27. Park H, Bothe D, Holsinger E, Kirchner HL, Olness K, Mandalakas A. The impact of nutritional status and longitudinal recovery of motor and cognitive milestones in internationally adopted children. *Int J Environ Res Public Health.* 2011;8(1):105–116.

28. Lohman TG, Roche AF, Martorell R. *Anthropometric Standardization Reference Manual.* Champaign, IL: Human Kinetics Books; 1988.

29. de Onis M, Yip R, Mei Z. The development of MUAC-for-age reference data recommended by a WHO Expert Committee. *Bull World Health Organ.* 1997;75(1):11–18.

30. Myatt M, Khara T, Collins S. A review of methods to detect cases of severely malnourished children in the community for their admission into community-based therapeutic care programs. *Food Nutr Bull.* 2006;27(3 suppl):S7–S23.

31. Frisancho AR. New norms of upper limb fat and muscle areas for assessment of nutritional status. *Am J Clin Nutr.* 1981;34(11):2540–2545.

32. Mascarenhas MR, Zemel B, Stallings VA. Nutritional assessment in pediatrics. *Nutrition.* 1998;14(1):105–115.

33. Roche AF, Sievogel RM, Chumlea WC, Webb P. Grading body fatness from limited anthropometric data. *Am J Clin Nutr.* 1981;34(12):2831–2838.

34. Buison AM, Ittenbach RF, Stallings VA, Zemel BS. Methodological agreement between two-compartment body-composition methods in children. *Am J Hum Biol.* 2006;18(4):470–480.

35. Day SM, Strauss DJ, Vachon PJ, Rosenbloom L, Shavelle RM, Wu YW. Growth patterns in a population of children and adolescents with cerebral palsy. *Dev Med Child Neurol.* 2007;49(3):167–171.

36. Brooks J, Day S, Shavelle R, Strauss D. Low weight, morbidity, and mortality in children with cerebral palsy: new clinical growth charts. *Pediatrics.* 2011;128(2):e299–e307.

37. Spender QW, Cronk CE, Charney EB, Stallings VA. Assessment of linear growth of children with cerebral palsy: use of alternative measures to height or length. [erratum in *Dev Med Child Neurol.* 1990;32(11):1032]. *Dev Med Child Neurol.* 1989;31(2):206–214.

38. Hall JG, Allanson JE, Gripp KW, Slavotinek AM. Special section. Syndrome-specific growth charts. *Am J Med Genet A.* 2012;158A(11):2645–2646.

39. Nash A, Dunn M, Asztalos E, Corey M, Mulvihill-Jory B, O'Connor DL. Pattern of growth of very low birth weight preterm infants, assessed using the WHO Growth Standards, is associated with neurodevelopment. *Appl Physiol Nutr Metab.* 2011;36(4):562–569.

40. Ong KK, Ahmed ML, Emmett PM, Preece MA, Dunger DB. Association between postnatal catch-up growth and obesity in childhood: prospective cohort study. *BMJ.* 2000;320(7240):967–971.

41. Adams PF, Hendershot GE, Marano MA. *Current Estimates from the National Health Interview Survey, 1996.* Atlanta, GA: National Center for Health Statistics; 1999. Vital and Health Statistics 10(200).

42. Engsner G, Habte D, Sjögren I, Vahlquist B. Brain growth in children with kwashiorkor. A study using head circumference measurement, transillumination and ultrasonic echo ventriculography. *Acta Paediatr Scand.* 1974;63(5):687–694.

43. Physical status: the use and interpretation of anthropometry. Report of a WHO Expert Committee. *World Health Organ Tech Rep Ser.* 1995;854:1–452.

44. Sentongo TA, Semeao EJ, Piccoli DA, Stallings VA, Zemel BS. Growth, body composition, and nutritional status in children and adolescents with Crohn's disease. *J Pediatr Gastroenterol Nutr.* 2000;31(1):33–40.

45. Morris NM, Udry JR. Validation of a self-administered instrument to assess stage of adolescent development. *J Youth Adolesc.* 1980;9(3):271–280.

46. Schall JI, Semeao EJ, Stallings VA, Zemel BS. Self-assessment of sexual maturity status in children with Crohn's disease. *J Pediatr.* 2002;141(2):223–229.

47. Cole TJ, Pan H, Butler GE. A mixed effects model to estimate timing and intensity of pubertal growth from height and secondary sexual characteristics. *Ann Hum Biol.* 2014;41(1):76–83.

48. Delano MJ, Moldawer LL. The origins of cachexia in acute and chronic inflammatory diseases. *Nutr Clin Pract.* 2006;21(1):68–81.

49. Jensen GL, Bistrian B, Roubenoff R, Heimburger DC. Malnutrition syndromes: a conundrum vs continuum. *JPEN J Parenter Enteral Nutr.* 2009;33(6):710–716.

50. Duncan A, Talwar D, McMillan DC, Stefanowicz F, O'Reilly DS. Quantitative data on the magnitude of the systemic inflammatory response and its effect on micronutrient status based on plasma measurements. *Am J Clin Nutr.* 2012;95(1):64–71.

51. Ingenbleek Y, Young V. Transthyretin (prealbumin) in health and disease: nutritional implications. *Annu Rev Nutr.* 1994;14:495–533.

52. Groos AD. Delayed motor development in relation to nutritional status among children under two years of age in two districts of Simbu Province. *P N G Med J.* 1991;34(4):238–245.

53. Wu L, Katz J, Mullany LC, et al. Association between nutritional status and positive childhood disability screening using the ten questions plus tool in Sarlahi, Nepal. *J Health Popul Nutr.* 2010;28(6):585–594.

54. Walker SP, Chang SM, Powell CA, Baker-Henningham H. Building human capacity through early childhood intervention: the Child Development Research Programme at the Tropical Medicine Research Institute, the University of the West Indies, Kingston, Jamaica. *West Indian Med J.* 2012;61(4):316–322.

55. McCormick MC, Brooks-Gunn J, Buka SL, et al. Early intervention in low birth weight premature infants: results at 18 years of age for the Infant Health and Development Program. *Pediatrics.* 2006;117(3):771–780.

56. Maitland K, Berkley JA, Shebbe M, Peshu N, English M, Newton CR. Children with severe malnutrition: can those at highest risk of death be identified with the WHO protocol? *PLoS Med.* 2006;3(12):e500.

57. Williams PM, Goodie J, Motsinger CD. Treating eating disorders in primary care. *Am Fam Physician.* 2008;77(2):187–195.

58. Sriram K, Manzanares W, Joseph K. Thiamine in nutrition therapy. *Nutr Clin Pract.* 2012;27(1):41–50.

59. Centers for Disease Control and Prevention (CDC). Lactic acidosis traced to thiamine deficiency related to nationwide shortage of multivitamins for total parenteral nutrition—United States, 1997. *MMWR Morb Mortal Wkly Rep.* 1997;46(23):523–528.

60. Food and Nutrition Board, Institute of Medicine. *Dietary Reference Intakes for Energy, Carbohydrate, Fiber, Fat, Fatty Acids, Cholesterol, Protein and Amino Acids (Macronutrients).* A Report of the Panel on Macronutrients, Subcommittees on Upper Reference Levels of Nutrients and Interpretation and Uses of Dietary References, and the Standing Committee on the Scientific Evaluation of Dietary Reference Intakes. Washington, DC: National Academies Press; 2005.

61. Energy and protein requirements. Report of a joint FAO/WHO/UNU Expert Consultation. *World Health Organ Tech Rep Ser.* 1985;724:1–206.

62. Ziegler EE. Meeting the nutritional needs of the low-birth-weight infant. *Ann Nutr Metab.* 2011;58(suppl 1):8–18.

63. Ziegler EE, Carlson SJ, Early nutrition of very low birth weight infants. *J Matern Fetal Neonatal Med.* 2009;22(3):191–197.

64. Groh-Wargo S, Sapsford A. Enteral nutrition support of the preterm infant in the neonatal intensive care unit. *Nutr Clin Pract.* 2009;24(3):363–376.

65. Tinnion RJ, Embleton ND. How to use... alkaline phosphatase in neonatology. *Arch Dis Child Educ Pract Ed.* 2012;97(4):157–163.

66. Backström MC, Kouri T, Kuusela AL, et al. Bone isoenzyme of serum alkaline phosphatase and serum inorganic phosphate in metabolic bone disease of prematurity. *Acta Paediatr.* 2000;89(7):867–873.

67. Duffy B, Gunn T, Collinge J, Pencharz P. The effect of varying protein quality and energy intake on the nitrogen metabolism of parenterally fed very low birthweight (less than 1600 g) infants. *Pediatr Res.* 1981;15(7):1040–1044.

68. Butte NF, Hopkinson JM, Wong WW, Smith EO, Ellis KJ. Body composition during the first 2 years of life: an updated reference. *Pediatr Res.* 2000;47(5):578–585.

69. Pencharz PB, Azcue MP. Measuring resting energy expenditure in clinical practice. *J Pediatr.* 1995;127(2):269–271.

70. Forbes GB, Kreipe RE, Lipinski BA, Hodgman CH. Body composition changes during recovery from anorexia nervosa: comparison of two dietary regimes. *Am J Clin Nutr.* 1984;40(6):1137–1145.

71. Spady DW, Payne PR, Picou D, Waterlow JC. Energy balance during recovery from malnutrition. *Am J Clin Nutr.* 1976;29(10):1073–1088.

72. Forbes GB, Brown MR, Welle SL, Lipinski BA. Deliberate overfeeding in women and men: energy cost and composition of the weight gain. *Br J Nutr.* 1986;56(1):1–9.

73. Mehta NM, Compher C. A.S.P.E.N. Clinical Guidelines: nutrition support of the critically ill child. *JPEN J Parenter Enteral Nutr.* 2009;33(3):260–276.

74. Weir JB. New methods for calculating metabolic rate with special reference to protein metabolism. *J Physiol.* 1949;109(1–2):1–9.

75. Schofield WN. Predicting basal metabolic rate, new standards and review of previous work. *Hum Nutr Clin Nutr.* 1985;39(suppl 1):5–41.

76. Firouzbakhsh S, Mathis RK, Dorchester WL, et al. Measured resting energy expenditure in children. *J Pediatr Gastroenterol Nutr.* 1993;16(2):136–142.

77. Sentongo TA, Tershakovec AM, Mascarenhas MR, Watson MH, Stallings VA. Resting energy expenditure and prediction equations in young children with failure to thrive. *J Pediatr.* 2000;136(3):345–350.

78. Kaplan AS, Zemel BS, Neiswender KM, Stallings VA. Resting energy expenditure in clinical pediatrics: measured versus prediction equations. *J Pediatr.* 1995;127(2):200–205.

79. Fuentebella J, Kerner JA. Refeeding syndrome. *Pediatr Clin North Am.* 2009;56(5):1201–1210.

80. Gaudiani JL, Sabel AL, Mehler PS. Low prealbumin is a significant predictor of medical complications in severe anorexia nervosa. *Int J Eat Disord.* 2014;47(2):148–156.

81. Dunn RL, Stettler N, Mascarenhas MR. Refeeding syndrome in hospitalized pediatric patients. *Nutr Clin Pract.* 2003;18(4):327–332.

82. Wyshak G, Frisch RE. Carbonated beverages, dietary calcium, the dietary calcium/phosphorus ratio, and bone fractures in girls and boys. *J Adolesc Health.* 1994;15(3):210–215.

83. Kantor J, Kessler LJ, Brooks DG, Cotsarelis G. Decreased serum ferritin is associated with alopecia in women. *J Invest Dermatol.* 2003;121(5):985–988.

84. Semrin G, Fishman DS, Bousvaros A, et al. Impaired intestinal iron absorption in Crohn's disease correlates with disease activity and markers of inflammation. *Inflamm Bowel Dis.* 2006;12(12):1101–1106.

85. Lynch S. Influence of infection/inflammation, thalassemia and nutritional status on iron absorption. *Int J Vitam Nutr Res.* 2007;77(3):217–223.

86. Nield LS, Stenger JP, Kamat D. Common pediatric dental dilemmas. *Clin Pediatr (Phila).* 2008;47(2):99–105.

87. Ananian A, Solomowitz BH, Dowrich IA. Fluoride: a controversy revisited. *N Y State Dent J.* 2006;72(3):14–18.

88. Mock DM. Skin manifestations of biotin deficiency. *Semin Dermatol.* 1991;10(4):296–302.

89. Cashman MW, Sloan SB. Nutrition and nail disease. *Clin Dermatol.* 2010;28(4):420–425.

90. Finner AM. Nutrition and hair: deficiencies and supplements. *Dermatol Clin.* 2013;31(1):167–172.

Test Your Knowledge Question answers

1. Response: Growth of children age < 24 months is assessed using the WHO growth standard. Patients with growth measurements > 97th or < 3rd percentile should have z scores computed. At age 13 months the growth status was weight 7.3 kg (< 3rd percentile), z score –2.7; length 73 cm (5th percentile), z score –1.62; and weight-for-length < 3rd percentile, z score –2.75. At age 21 months the growth status was weight 8.3 kg (< 3rd percentile), z score –2.93; length 81 cm (7th percentile),

z score −1.44; and weight-for-length < 3rd percentile, z score −3.12. Therefore, even though there have been gains in length (cm) and weight (kg), this child's growth has *actually worsened*. The growth pattern is most consistent with wasting. Weight-for-length z score < −3.0 is associated with a > 9-fold risk of mortality. The correct response is **D**.

2. Response (A): **False**. Obesity is BMI percentile > 97th percentile. Weight-for-length and BMI are not equivalent. Increased weight-for-length corresponds to overweight. Response (B): **True**. The risk of mortality in children with moderate malnutrition is relatively similar to that in children with mild malnutrition.[2,14] Response (C): **False**. Mid-arm circumference of 125 mm corresponds to moderate wasting. A mid-arm circumference of 115 mm corresponds with severe wasting and increased risk of death. This measure has been used as screening tool to quickly identify children with severe malnutrition and those requiring comprehensive nutrition rehabilitation.[14] Response (D): **False**. Tall stature is height z score > 2.0 (97th percentile).

3. Response: 1) **F**; 2) **C**; 3) **E**; 4) **D**; 5) **A**; 8) **B**

4. Correct response: **D**. This child with cerebral palsy wears braces but ambulates independently (GMF-CS II). The child has a G-tube, which indicates some degree of major disability. The appropriate age and sex growth reference is cerebral palsy age birth to 25 years growth chart for girls with GMF-CS II who are tube fed. The chart can be accessed at www.LifeExpectancy.org/articles/GrowthCharts.shtml.

5. Correct response: **D**. DXA is the gold standard.

6. Response (A): **True**. CDC percentage body fat percentile charts are available (see Ogden et al[22]). Response (B): **True**. Malnourished patients may have increased %BF. This demonstrates the limitations of using %BF to diagnosis adiposity. Patients with chronic diseases that disproportionately depleted lean tissue without necessarily increased fat tissue (eg, juvenile rheumatoid arthritis, Crohn's disease, and end-stage renal disease). This phenomenon is also referred to as cachectic obesity. Therefore, interpretation of %BF should also consider BMI. Increased %BF in patients with BMI > 95th percentile represents adiposity. Response (C): **False**. BMI is only correlated with %BF in patients with BMI percentile > 95th%.

Appendix 32-1. Fenton 2013 Growth Charts for Preterm Girls

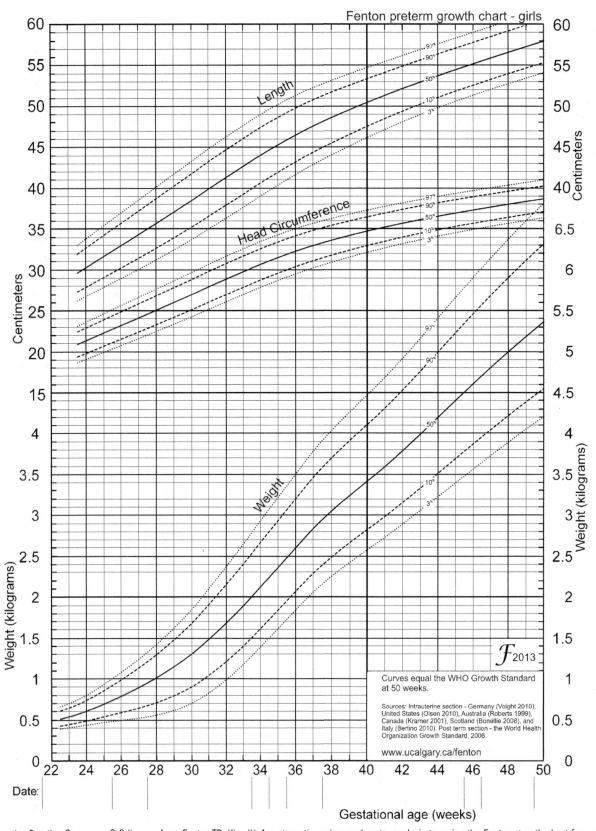

Reprinted under Creative Commons 2.0 license from Fenton TR, Kim JH. A systematic review and meta-analysis to revise the Fenton growth chart for preterm infants. *BMC Pediatrics*. 2013;13:59.

Appendix 32-1. (continued) Fenton 2013 Gender-Specific Growth Charts for Preterm Boys

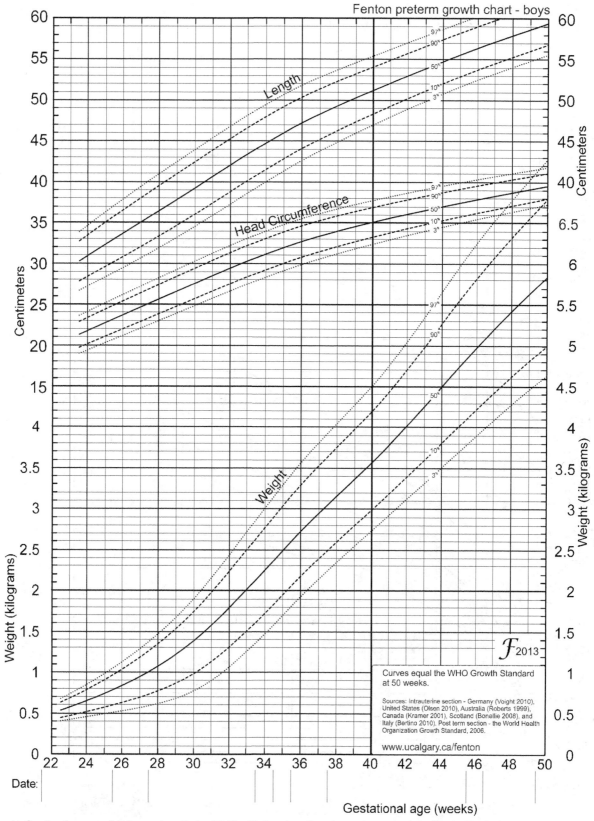

Fenton preterm growth chart - boys

Curves equal the WHO Growth Standard at 50 weeks.

Sources: Intrauterine section - Germany (Voight 2010), United States (Olsen 2010), Australia (Roberts 1999), Canada (Kramer 2001), Scotland (Bonellie 2008), and Italy (Bertino 2010). Post term section - the World Health Organization Growth Standard, 2006.

www.ucalgary.ca/fenton

Gestational age (weeks)

Date:

Reprinted under Creative Commons 2.0 license from Fenton TR, Kim JH. A systematic review and meta-analysis to revise the Fenton growth chart for preterm infants. *BMC Pediatrics.* 2013;13:59.

Appendix 32-2.

Birth to 24 months: Girls
Length-for-age and Weight-for-age percentiles

NAME _____

RECORD # _____

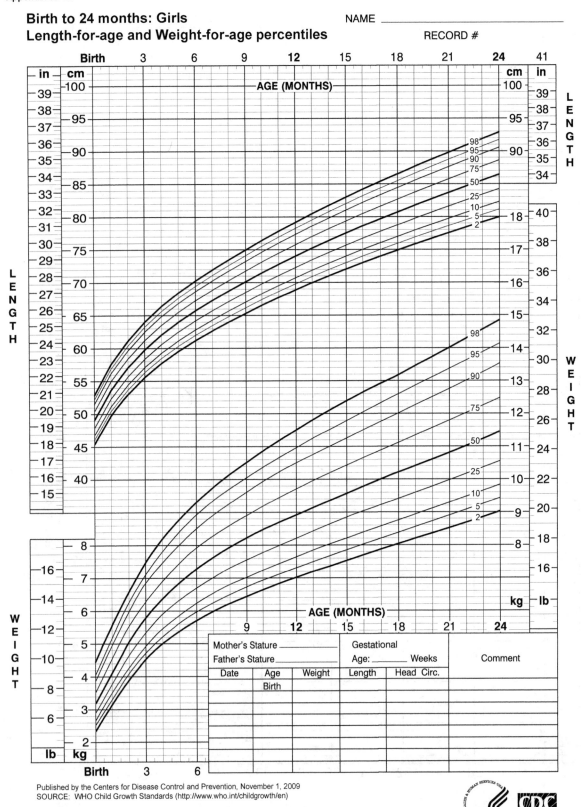

Published by the Centers for Disease Control and Prevention, November 1, 2009
SOURCE: WHO Child Growth Standards (http://www.who.int/childgrowth/en)

Appendix 32-2. (continued)

Birth to 24 months: Girls
Head circumference-for-age and
Weight-for-length percentiles

NAME _____

RECORD # _____

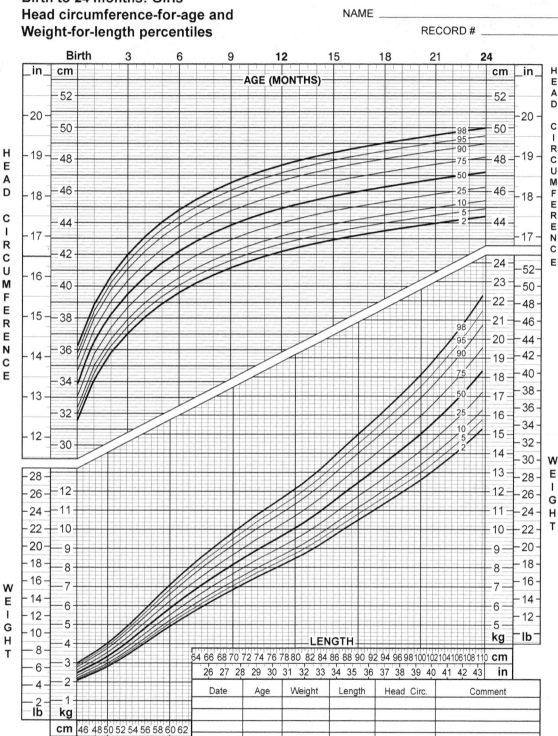

Published by the Centers for Disease Control and Prevention, November 1, 2009
SOURCE: WHO Child Growth Standards (http://www.who.int/childgrowth/en)

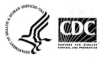

Appendix 32-2. (continued)

Birth to 24 months: Boys
Length-for-age and Weight-for-age percentiles

NAME _____

RECORD # _____

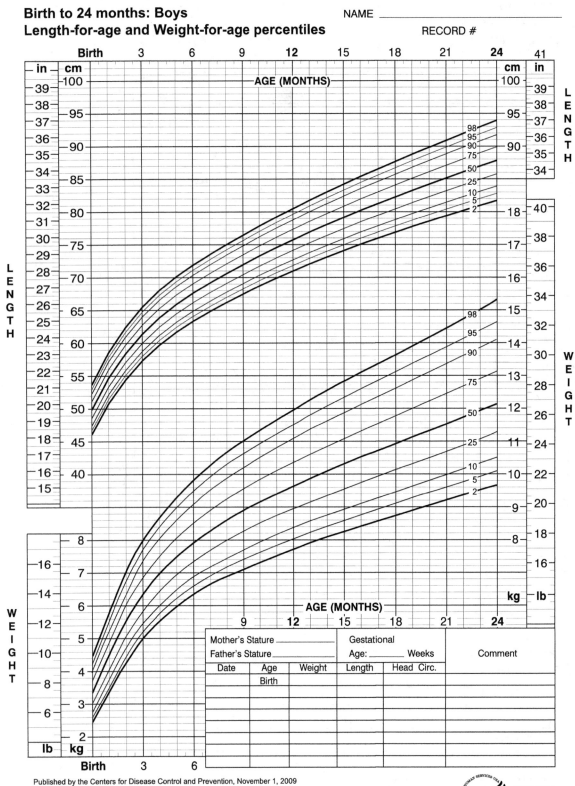

Published by the Centers for Disease Control and Prevention, November 1, 2009
SOURCE: WHO Child Growth Standards (http://www.who.int/childgrowth/en)

SAFER · HEALTHIER · PEOPLE™

Appendix 32-2. (continued)

Birth to 24 months: Boys
Head circumference-for-age and
Weight-for-length percentiles

NAME _____

RECORD # _____

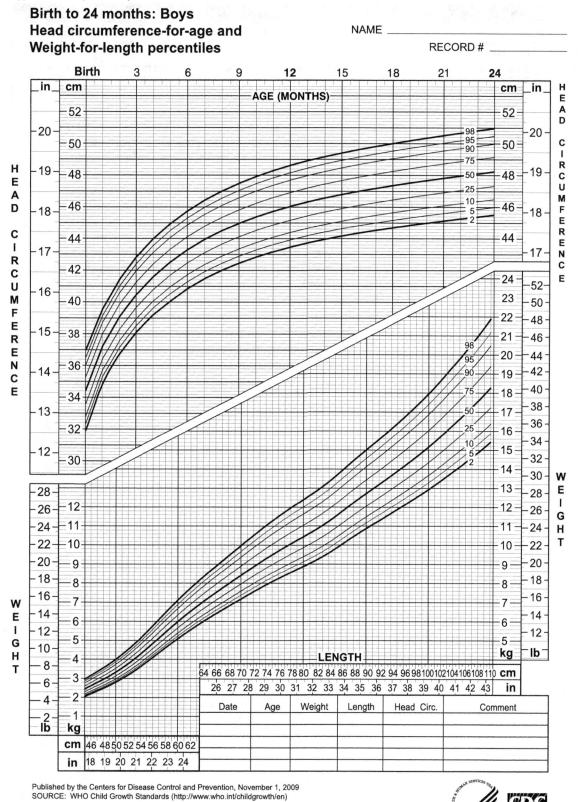

Date	Age	Weight	Length	Head Circ.	Comment

Published by the Centers for Disease Control and Prevention, November 1, 2009
SOURCE: WHO Child Growth Standards (http://www.who.int/childgrowth/en)

Appendix 32-3. Resources for Calculating *Z* Scores of Anthropometric Parameters

CDC GROWTH CHARTS	WHO GROWTH CHARTS
STAT GrowthCharts (compatible with iPod Touch, iPhone, iPad)	STAT GrowthCharts WHO (compatible with iPod Touch, iPhone, iPad)
Epi Info NutStat: (available for download) http://www.cdc.gov/growthcharts/computer_programs.htm	WHO *z* score charts: http://www.who.int/childgrowth/standards/chart_catalogue/en/index.html
CDC website: *z* score data files available as tables http://www.cdc.gov/growthcharts/zscore.htm	WHO Multicentre Growth Study website: http://www.who.int/childgrowth/software/en
	All 4 macros (SAS, S-Plus, SPSS, and STATA) calculate the indicators of the attained growth standards

Appendix 32-4. Percentiles of Upper Arm Circumference

Percentiles of upper arm circmference (mm) and estimated upper arm muscle circumference (mm) for whites of the United States Health and Nutrition Examination Survey I of 1971 to 1974

Age group	Arm circumference (mm)							Arm muscle circumference (mm)						
	5	10	25	50	75	90	95	5	10	25	50	75	90	95
Males														
1–1.9	142	146	150	159	170	176	183	110	113	119	127	135	144	147
2–2.9	141	145	153	162	170	178	185	111	114	122	130	140	146	150
3–3.9	150	153	160	167	175	184	190	117	123	131	137	143	148	153
4–4.9	149	154	162	171	180	186	192	123	126	133	141	148	156	159
5–5.9	153	160	167	175	185	195	204	128	133	140	147	154	162	169
6–6.9	155	159	167	179	188	209	228	131	135	142	151	161	170	177
7–7.9	162	167	177	187	201	223	230	137	139	151	160	168	177	190
8–8.9	162	170	177	190	202	220	245	140	145	154	162	170	182	187
9–9.9	175	178	187	200	217	249	257	151	154	161	170	183	196	202
10–10.9	181	184	196	210	231	262	274	156	160	166	180	191	209	221
11–11.9	186	190	202	223	244	261	280	159	165	173	183	195	205	230
12–12.9	193	200	214	232	254	282	303	167	171	182	195	210	223	241
13–13.9	194	211	228	247	263	286	301	172	179	196	211	226	238	245
14–14.9	220	226	237	253	283	303	322	189	199	212	223	240	260	264
15–15.9	222	229	244	264	284	311	320	199	204	218	237	254	266	272
16–16.9	244	248	262	278	303	324	343	213	225	234	249	269	287	296
17–17.9	246	253	267	285	308	336	347	224	231	245	258	273	294	312
18–18.9	245	260	276	297	321	353	379	226	237	252	264	283	298	324
19–24.9	262	272	288	308	331	355	372	238	245	257	273	289	309	321
25–34.9	271	282	300	319	342	362	375	243	250	264	279	298	314	326
35–44.9	278	287	305	326	345	363	374	247	255	269	286	302	318	327
45–54.9	267	281	301	322	342	362	376	239	249	265	281	300	315	326
55–64.9	258	273	296	317	336	355	369	236	245	260	278	295	310	320
65–74.9	248	263	285	307	325	344	355	223	235	251	268	284	298	306
Females														
1–1.9	138	142	148	156	164	172	177	105	111	117	124	132	139	143
2–2.9	142	145	152	160	167	176	184	111	114	119	126	133	142	147
3–3.9	143	150	158	167	175	183	189	113	119	124	132	140	146	152
4–4.9	149	154	160	169	177	184	191	115	121	128	136	144	152	157
5–5.9	153	157	165	175	185	203	211	125	128	134	142	151	159	165
6–6.9	156	162	170	176	187	204	211	130	133	138	145	154	166	171
7–7.9	164	167	174	183	199	216	231	129	135	142	151	160	171	176
8–8.9	168	172	183	195	214	247	261	138	140	151	160	171	183	194
9–9.9	178	182	194	211	224	251	260	147	150	158	167	180	194	198
10–10.9	174	182	193	210	228	251	265	148	150	159	170	180	190	197
11–11.9	185	194	208	224	248	276	303	150	158	171	181	196	217	223
12–12.9	194	203	216	237	256	282	294	162	166	180	191	201	214	220
13–13.9	202	211	223	243	271	301	338	169	175	183	198	211	226	240
14–14.9	214	223	237	252	272	304	322	174	179	190	201	216	232	247
15–15.9	208	221	239	254	279	300	322	175	178	189	202	215	228	244
16–16.9	218	224	241	258	283	318	334	170	180	190	202	216	234	249
17–17.9	220	227	241	264	295	324	350	175	183	194	205	221	239	257
18–18.9	222	227	241	258	281	312	325	174	179	191	202	215	237	245
19–24.9	221	230	247	265	290	319	345	179	185	195	207	221	236	249
25–34.9	233	240	256	277	304	342	368	183	188	199	212	228	246	264
35–44.9	241	251	267	290	317	356	378	186	192	205	218	236	257	272
45–54.9	242	256	274	299	328	362	384	187	193	206	220	238	260	274
55–64.9	243	257	280	303	335	367	385	187	196	209	225	244	266	280
65–74.9	240	252	274	299	326	356	373	185	195	208	225	244	264	279

Reprinted with permission from Frisancho AR. New norms of upper limb fat and muscle areas for assessment of nutritional status. *Am J Clin Nutr.* 1981;34:2540-2545.

Appendix 32-5. Combined MUAC-Age Reference Data for Boys and Girls Age 6–59 Months

Age (months)	−4 SD	−3 SD	−2 SD	−1 SD	Mean	+1 SD	+2 SD	+3 SD
6	9.7	10.9	12.0	13.2	14.3	15.5	16.7	17.8
7	9.9	11.0	12.2	13.4	14.6	15.7	16.9	18.1
8	10.0	11.2	12.4	13.6	14.8	16.0	17.2	18.3
9	10.1	11.3	12.5	13.7	14.9	16.2	17.4	18.6
10	10.2	11.5	12.7	13.9	15.1	16.3	17.5	18.8
11	10.3	11.6	12.8	14.0	15.2	16.5	17.7	18.9
12	10.4	11.7	12.9	14.1	15.4	16.6	17.9	19.1
13	10.5	11.7	13.0	14.2	15.5	16.7	18.0	19.2
14	10.5	11.8	13.1	14.3	15.6	16.8	18.1	19.4
15	10.6	11.9	13.1	14.4	15.7	16.9	18.2	19.5
16	10.6	11.9	13.2	14.5	15.8	17.0	18.3	19.6
17	10.7	12.0	13.2	14.5	15.8	17.1	18.4	19.7
18	10.7	12.0	13.3	14.6	15.9	17.2	18.5	19.8
19	10.7	12.0	13.3	14.6	15.9	17.2	18.5	19.8
20	10.7	12.1	13.4	14.7	16.0	17.3	18.6	19.9
21	10.8	12.1	13.4	14.7	16.0	17.3	18.7	20.0
22	10.8	12.1	13.4	14.7	16.1	17.4	18.7	20.0
23	10.8	12.1	13.4	14.8	16.1	17.4	18.8	20.1
24	10.8	12.1	13.5	14.8	16.1	17.5	18.8	20.1
25	10.8	12.2	13.5	14.8	16.2	17.5	18.8	20.2
26	10.8	12.2	13.5	14.9	16.2	17.5	18.9	20.2
27	10.8	12.2	13.5	14.9	16.2	17.6	18.9	20.3
28	10.8	12.2	13.5	14.9	16.3	17.6	19.0	20.3
29	10.8	12.2	13.6	14.9	16.3	17.6	19.0	20.4
30	10.9	12.2	13.6	14.9	16.3	17.7	19.0	20.4
31	10.9	12.2	13.6	15.0	16.3	17.7	19.1	20.4
32	10.9	12.2	13.6	15.0	16.4	17.7	19.1	20.5
33	10.9	12.3	13.6	15.0	16.4	17.8	19.1	20.5
34	10.9	12.3	13.7	15.0	16.4	17.8	19.2	20.6
35	10.9	12.3	13.7	15.1	16.4	17.8	19.2	20.6
36	10.9	12.3	13.7	15.1	16.5	17.9	19.3	20.6
37	10.9	12.3	13.7	15.1	16.5	17.9	19.3	20.7
38	10.9	12.3	13.7	15.1	16.5	17.9	19.3	20.7
39	11.0	12.4	13.8	15.2	16.6	18.0	19.4	20.8
40	11.0	12.4	13.8	15.2	16.6	18.0	19.4	20.8
41	11.0	12.4	13.8	15.2	16.6	18.1	19.5	20.9
42	11.0	12.4	13.8	15.3	16.7	18.1	19.5	20.9
43	11.0	12.4	13.9	15.3	16.7	18.1	19.6	21.0
44	11.0	12.5	13.9	15.3	16.8	18.2	19.6	21.1
45	11.0	12.5	13.9	15.4	16.8	18.2	19.7	21.1
46	11.1	12.5	13.9	15.4	16.8	18.3	19.7	21.2
47	11.1	12.5	14.0	15.4	16.9	18.3	19.8	21.2
48	11.1	12.5	14.0	15.5	16.9	18.4	19.8	21.3
49	11.1	12.5	14.0	15.5	17.0	18.4	19.9	21.4
50	11.1	12.6	14.0	15.5	17.0	18.5	20.0	21.4
51	11.1	12.6	14.1	15.5	17.0	18.5	20.0	21.5
52	11.1	12.6	14.1	15.6	17.1	18.6	20.1	21.6
53	11.1	12.6	14.1	15.6	17.1	18.6	20.1	21.6
54	11.1	12.6	14.1	15.6	17.2	18.7	20.2	21.7
55	11.1	12.6	14.1	15.7	17.2	18.7	20.3	21.8
56	11.1	12.6	14.1	15.7	17.2	18.8	20.3	21.9
57	11.1	12.6	14.1	15.7	17.3	18.8	20.4	21.9
58	11.1	12.6	14.2	15.7	17.3	18.9	20.5	22.0
59	11.1	12.6	14.2	15.8	17.3	18.9	20.5	22.1

Reprinted with permission from Frisancho AR. New norms of upper limb fat and muscle areas for assessment of nutritional status. *Am J Clin Nutr.* 1981;34:2540–2545.

Appendix 32-5. (continued) Combined MUAC-for-Age Growth Reference Curve for Boys and Girls Aged 6–59 Months

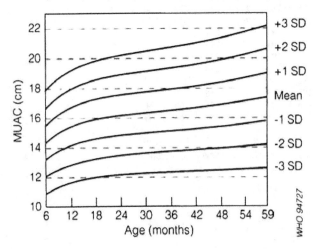

Appendix 32-6. Triceps Skinfold Percentiles

Percentiles for triceps skinfold for whites of the United States
Health and Nutrition Examination Survey I of 1971 to 1974

Age group	Triceps skinfold percentiles (mm²)															
	n	5	10	25	50	75	90	95	n	5	10	25	50	75	90	95
	Males								Females							
1–1.9	228	6	7	8	10	12	14	16	204	6	7	8	10	12	14	16
2–2.9	223	6	7	8	10	12	14	15	208	6	8	9	10	12	15	16
3–3.9	220	6	7	8	10	11	14	15	208	7	8	9	11	12	14	15
4–4.9	230	6	6	8	9	11	12	14	208	7	8	8	10	12	14	16
5–5.9	214	6	6	8	9	11	14	15	219	6	7	8	10	12	15	18
6–6.9	117	5	6	7	8	10	13	16	118	6	6	8	10	12	14	16
7–7.9	122	5	6	7	9	12	15	17	126	6	7	9	11	13	16	18
8–8.9	117	5	6	7	8	10	13	16	118	6	8	9	12	15	18	24
9–9.9	121	6	6	7	10	13	17	18	125	8	8	10	13	16	20	22
10–10.9	146	6	6	8	10	14	18	21	152	7	8	10	12	17	23	27
11–11.9	122	6	6	8	11	16	20	24	117	7	8	10	13	18	24	28
12–12.9	153	6	6	8	11	14	22	28	129	8	9	11	14	18	23	27
13–13.9	134	5	5	7	10	14	22	26	151	8	8	12	15	21	26	30
14–14.9	131	4	5	7	9	14	21	24	141	9	10	13	16	21	26	28
15–15.9	128	4	5	6	8	11	18	24	117	8	10	12	17	21	25	32
16–16.9	131	4	5	6	8	12	16	22	142	10	12	15	18	22	26	31
17–17.9	133	5	5	6	8	12	16	19	114	10	12	13	19	24	30	37
18–18.9	91	4	5	6	9	13	20	24	109	10	12	15	18	22	26	30
19–24.9	531	4	5	7	10	15	20	22	1060	10	11	14	18	24	30	34
25–34.9	971	5	6	8	12	16	20	24	1987	10	12	16	21	27	34	37
35–44.9	806	5	6	8	12	16	20	23	1614	12	14	18	23	29	35	38
45–54.9	898	6	6	8	12	15	20	25	1047	12	16	20	25	30	36	40
55–64.9	734	5	6	8	11	14	19	22	809	12	16	20	25	31	36	38
65–74.9	1503	4	6	8	11	15	19	22	1670	12	14	18	24	29	34	36

Reprinted with permission from Frisancho AR. New norms of upper limb fat and muscle areas for assessment of nutritional status. *Am J Clin Nutr.* 1981;34:2540–2545.

Appendix 32-7.

GIRLS   SELECT ONE FROM EACH SET OF DRAWINGS BELOW.

SET ONE: The drawings below show 5 <u>different stages of how the breasts grow</u>. A girl can go through each of the 5 stages as shown. Please look at each drawing and read the sentences that match the drawings. Then, mark an "X" in the box above the drawing that you think is <u>closest</u> to your stage of breast growth.

Name _____

D.O.B. _____   Age _____

Medical Record No. _____

Stage 1	Stage 2	Stage 3	Stage 4	Stage 5

| The nipple is raised a little. The rest of the breast is still flat. | This is the breast bud stage. In this stage, the nipple is raised more than in stage 1. The breast is a small mound. The areola is larger than stage 1. | The breast and areola are both larger than in stage 2. The areola does not stick out away from the breast. | The areola and the nipple make up a mound that sticks up above the shape of the breast. NOTE: This stage may not happen at all for some girls. Some girls develop from stage 3 to stage 5 with no stage 4. | This is the mature adult stage. The breasts are fully developed. Only the nipple sticks out in this stage. The areola has moved back in the general shape of the breast. |

SET TWO: The drawings below show 5 <u>different stages of female pubic hair growth</u>. A girl goes through each of the 5 stages as shown. Please look at each drawing and read the sentences below that match each drawing. Then, mark an "X" in the box above the drawing that you think is <u>closest</u> to the amount of your pubic hair growth.

Stage 1	Stage 2	Stage 3	Stage 4	Stage 5

| There is no pubic hair at all. | There is a little soft, long, lightly-colored hair. This hair may be straight or a little curly. | The hair is darker in this stage. It is coarser and more curled. It has spread out and thinly covers a bigger area. | The hair is now as dark, curly, and coarse as that of an adult female. The area that the hair covers is not as big as that of an adult female. The hair has NOT spread out to the legs. | The hair is now like that of an adult female. It covers the same area as that of an adult female. The hair usually forms a triangular (∇) pattern as it spreads out to the legs. |

Adapted from: Morris, N.M., and Udry, J.R., (1980), Validation of a Self-Administered Instrument to Assess Stage of Adolescent Development. *Journal of Youth and Adolescence, Vol. 9 No. 3: 271-280.*

Reprinted with kind permission from Springer Science and Business Media.

Appendix 32-7. (continued)

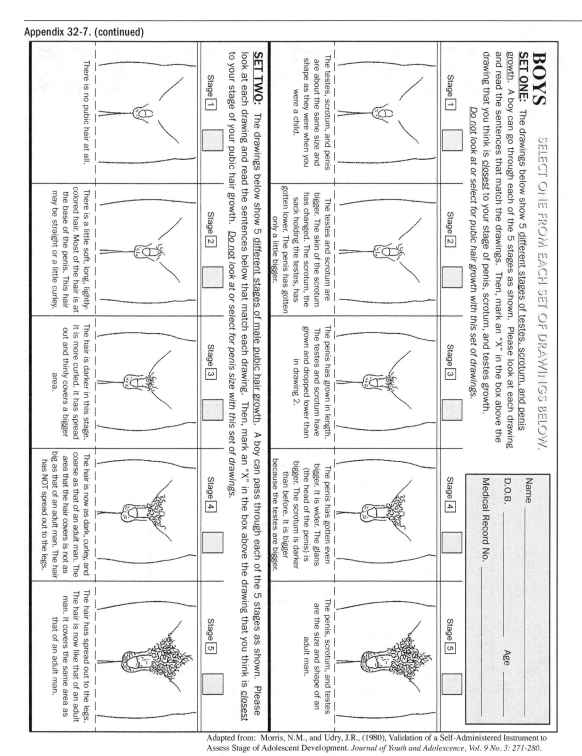

Adapted from: Morris, N.M., and Udry, J.R., (1980), Validation of a Self-Administered Instrument to Assess Stage of Adolescent Development. *Journal of Youth and Adolescence, Vol. 9 No. 3: 271-280.*

Appendix 32-8. Estimating Nutrient Needs

NAME OF EQUATION OR FORMULA	DESCRIPTION	CALCULATIONS FOR THE EQUATION OR FORMULA	APPLICABLE TO WHICH PATIENT POPULATIONS?	SOURCE
ENERGY				
1989 Recommended Daily Allowance (RDA)	Based on the median energy intakes of children followed in longitudinal growth studies. It can overestimate needs in non-active populations (eg, bedridden) and does not provide a range of energy needs. Though an outdated reference, still widely used.	**Infants:** 0–0.5 y: 108 x wt (kg) 0.5–1 y: 98 x wt **Children:** 1–3 y: 102 x wt 4–6 y: 90 x wt 7–10 y: 70 x wt **Males:** 11–14 y: 55 x wt 15–18 y: 45 x wt **Females:** 11–14 y: 47 x wt 15–18 y: 40 x wt	Most often used for healthy infants and children	Committee in Dietary Allowances, Food and Nutrition Board, National Research Council. *Recommended Dietary Allowances.* 10th ed. Washington, DC: National Academy Press; 1989.
Estimated Energy Requirements (EER) (new DRI/ IOM equation) & Physical Activity (PA) Co-Efficients	Replaces the 1989 Recommended Dietary Allowances (RDA). Energy needs were determined from children with normal growth, body composition, and activity, and who are also metabolically normal.	EER = TEE + energy deposition **Ages 0-36 mo:** 0–3 mo: (89 x wt [kg] – 100) + 175 4–6 mo: (89 x wt [kg] – 100) + 56 7–12 mo: (89 x wt [kg] – 100) + 22 13–36 mo: (89 x wt [kg] –100) + 20 **Ages 3–8 y—Boys:** EER = 88.5 – (61.9 x age [y]) + PA x (26.7 x wt [kg] + 903 x ht[m]) + 20 kcal PA = 1 if PAL is estimated to be > 1 < 1.4 (sedentary) PA = 1.13 if PAL is estimated to be > 1.4 < 1.6 (low active) PA = 1.26 if PAL is estimated to be > 1.6 < 1.9 (active) PA = 1.42 if PAL is estimated to be > 1.9 < 2.5 (very active) **Ages 3–8 y—Girls:** EER = 135.3 – (30.8 x age [y]) + PA x (10 x wt [kg] + 934 x ht [m]) + 20 kcal PA = 1 if PAL is estimated to be > 1 < 1.4 (sedentary) PA = 1.16 if PAL is estimated to be > 1.4 < 1.6 (low active) PA = 1.31 if PAL is estimated to be > 1.6 < 1.9 (active) PA = 1.56 if PAL is estimated to be > 1.9 < 2.5 (very active) **Ages 9–18 y—Boys:** EER = 88.5 – (61.9 x age [y]) + PA x (26.7 x wt [kg] + 903 x ht [m]) + 25 kcal PA = 1 if PAL is estimated to be > 1 < 1.4 (sedentary) PA = 1.13 if PAL is estimated to be > 1.4 < 1.6 (low active) PA = 1.26 if PAL is estimated to be > 1.6 < 1.9 (active) PA = 1.42 if PAL is estimated to be > 1.9 < 2.5 (very active) **Ages 9–18 y—Girls:** EER = 135.3 – (30.8 x age [y]) + PA x (10 x wt [kg] + 934 x ht [m]) + 25 kcal PA = 1 if PAL is estimated to be > 1 < 1.4 (sedentary) PA = 1.16 if PAL is estimated to be > 1.4 < 1.6 (low active) PA = 1.31 if PAL is estimated to be > 1.6 < 1.9 (active) PA = 1.56 if PAL is estimated to be > 1.9 < 2.5 (very active)	Children with normal growth, body composition, and activity, and who are also metabolically normal	National Academy of Sciences, Institute of Medicine, Food and Nutrition Board. *Dietary Reference Intakes for Energy, Carbohydrate, Fiber, Fat, Fatty Acids, Cholesterol, Protein, and Amino Acids (Macronutrients) (2005).*

Appendix 32-8. (continued) Estimating Nutrient Needs

NAME OF EQUATION OR FORMULA	DESCRIPTION	CALCULATIONS FOR THE EQUATION OR FORMULA	APPLICABLE TO WHICH PATIENT POPULATIONS?	SOURCE
EER (new DRI/IOM equation) & obesity co-efficients/factors		**Weight Maintenance TEE in Overweight Boys Ages 3–18 y:** TEE = 114 – (50.9 x age [y]) + PA x (19.5 x weight [kg] + 1161.4 x height [m]) PA = 1 if PAL is estimated to be > 1 < 1.4 (sedentary) PA = 1.12 if PAL is estimated to be > 1.4 < 1.6 (low active) PA = 1.24 if PAL is estimated to be > 1.6 < 1.9 (active) PA = 1.45 if PAL is estimated to be > 1.9 < 2.5 (very active) **Weight Maintenance TEE in Overweight Girls Ages 3–18 y:** TEE = 389 - (41.2 x age [y]) + PA x (15 x weight [kg] + 701.6 x height [m]) PA = 1 if PAL is estimated to be > 1 < 1.4 (sedentary) PA = 1.18 if PAL is estimated to be > 1.4 < 1.6 (low active) PA = 1.35 if PAL is estimated to be > 1.6 < 1.9 (active) PA = 1.6 if PAL is estimated to be > 1.9 < 2.5 (very active)	Overweight children who are metabolically normal	National Academy of Sciences, Institute of Medicine, Food and Nutrition Board. *Dietary Reference Intakes for Energy, Carbohydrate, Fiber, Fat, Fatty Acids, Cholesterol, Protein, and Amino Acids (Macronutrients) (2005).*
Schofield	A predictive equation for calculating basal metabolic rate (BMR) in healthy children that was developed by analysis of Fritz Talbot tables.	**Males:** 0–3 y: (0.167 x wt [kg]) + (15.174 x ht [cm]) - 617.6 3–10 y: (19.59 x wt [kg]) + (1.303 x ht [cm]) + 414.9 10–18 y: (16.25 x wt [kg]) + (1.372 x ht [cm]) + 515.5 > 18 y: (15.057 x wt [kg]) + (1.0004 x ht [cm]) + 705.8 **Females:** 0–3 y: (16.252 x wt[kg]) + (10.232 x ht [cm]) - 413.5 3–10 y: (16.969 x wt [kg]) + (1.618 x ht [cm]) + 371.2 10–18 y: (8.365 x wt [kg]) + (4.65 x ht [cm]) + 200 >18 y: (13.623 x wt [kg]) + (23.8 x ht [cm]) + 98.2	Healthy children, acutely ill patients in the hospital setting	Schofield WN. Predicting basal metabolism rate, new standards and review of previous work. *Hum Nutr Clin Nutr.* 1985;39C:5–91.
FAO/WHO	The "WHO equation" was developed for use in healthy children; however, it is commonly used to predict resting energy expenditure (REE) of acutely ill patients in the hospital setting.	**Males:** 0–3 y: (60.9 x wt [kg])– 54 3–10 y: (22.7 x wt [kg]) + 495 10–18 y: (17.5 xwt [kg]) + 651 **Females:** 0–3 y: (61 x wt [kg]) – 51 3–10 y: (22.5 x wt [kg]) + 499 10–18 y: (12.2 x wt [kg]) + 746	Healthy children who are acutely ill patients in the hospital setting	World Health Organization. *Energy and Protein Requirements. Report of a Joint FAO/WHO/UNU Expert Consultation.* Technical Report Series 724. World Health Organization, Geneva, 1985.
Estimating calorie needs for developmental disabilities	Children with developmental disabilities (DD) may have a slower basal energy need due to a decreased muscle tone, growth rate, and motor activity. The recommendation to calculate energy needs in children with DD per cm of height is based on the fact that they tend to have a shorter height when compared to children with normal growth.	**Cerebral palsy (age 5–11 y*):** Mild-moderate activity: 13.9 kcal/cm height Severe physical restrictions: 11.1 kcal/cm height Severe restricted activity: 10 kcal/cm height Athetoid Cerebral Palsy: Up to 6000 kcal/day (adolescence) **Down Syndrome (5 – 12 y*):** Boys 16.1 kcal/cm height Girls 14.3 kcal/cm height Prader-Willi Syndrome (for all children and adolescents): 10 – 11 kcal/cm height for maintenance 8.5 kcal/cm height for weight loss Myelomeningocele (Spina bifida) (over 8 years of age and minimally active): 9 – 11 kcal/cm height for maintenance 7 kcal/cm height for weight loss Approximately 50% RDA for age after infancy	Children with developmental disabilities *This reference applies to the specific ages listed. Please refer to another equation for ages outside of the referenced ages, and apply an appropriate activity/stress factor.	Rokusek C, Heindicles E. *Nutrition and Feeding of the Developmentally Disabled.* Brookings, SD: South Dakota University Affiliated Program, Interdisciplinary Center for Disablities; 1985.

Appendix 32-8. (continued) Estimating Nutrient Needs

NAME OF EQUATION OR FORMULA	DESCRIPTION	CALCULATIONS FOR THE EQUATION OR FORMULA	APPLICABLE TO WHICH PATIENT POPULATIONS?	SOURCE
Peterson's Failure to Thrive (FTT)	This calculates nutrients in excess of the requirements of the RDA. Concerns with using this equation include refeeding syndrome.	[RDA for weight age (kcal/kg) x Ideal body weight for height] ÷ Actual weight	Infants and children who present underweight and need to achieve catch-up growth	Peterson KE, Washington J, Rathbun JM. Team management of failure to thrive. *J Am Diet Assoc.* 1984;84:810–815.
FAO/WHO/UNU (aka "Dietz equation")	Food and Agriculture Organization, World Health Organization, United Nations University	Boys 10–18 y BMR = 16.6 weight (kg) + 77 height (m) + 572; Girls 10–18 y BMR = 7.4 weight (kg) + 482 height (m) + 217	Overweight/ obese adolescents in an outpatient setting	Dietz WH, Brandini LG, Schoeller DA. Estimates of metabolic rate in obese and non-obese adolecents. *J Pediatr.* 1991;118:146–149.
White equation	Developed for use in the pediatric critical care population by including temperature as a gauge of the body's inflammatory response. It is not commonly used in clinical practice, and recent studies have shown decreased accuracy especially in smaller, younger patients. This equation should not be used in patients less than 2 months of age.	EE (kJ/day) = (17 × age [mo]) + (48 × weight [kg]) + (292 × body temperature [C]) – 9677	Pediatric critical care population	White MS, Shepherd RW, McEniery JA. Energy expenditure in 100 ventilated, critically ill children: improving the accuracy of predictive equations. *Crit Care Med.* 2000;28(7):2307–2312.
STRESS FACTORS FOR ENERGY				
Stress Factors	The use of stress factors along with predictive energy equations should be considered for use in hospitalized children whose energy requirements may be altered due to metabolic stress.	Starvation 0.70–0.85; Surgery 1.05–1.5; Sepsis 1.2–1.6; Closed head injury 1.3; Trauma 1.1–1.8; Growth failure 1.5–2; Burn 1.5–2.5	Pediatric hospitalized population	Leonberg B. ADA *Pocket Guide to Pediatric Nutrition Assessment.* Chicago, IL: American Dietetic Association; 2007. Table 8.10
PROTEIN				
A.S.P.E.N. Clinical Guidelines: Nutrition Support of the Critically Ill Child	Metabolic stress increases catabolism and breakdown of lean body mass. To meet the increased demands of metabolic stress and spare the use of endogenous protein stores, a greater amount of protein is needed in this population until the underlying stress has been overcome. Recommendations are based on limited data.	0–2 y: 2–3 g/kg/d; 2–13 y: 1.5–2 g/kg/d; 13–18 y: 1.5 g/kg/d	Pediatric critical care population	Mehta NM, Compher C, A.S.P.E.N. Board of Directors. A.S.P.E.N. Clinical Guidelines: Nutrition Support of the Critically Ill Child. *JPEN J Parenter Enteral Nutr.* 2009;33(3):260–276.

Appendix 32-8. (continued) Estimating Nutrient Needs

NAME OF EQUATION OR FORMULA	DESCRIPTION	CALCULATIONS FOR THE EQUATION OR FORMULA	APPLICABLE TO WHICH PATIENT POPULATIONS?	SOURCE
For the injured child	Metabolic stress increases catabolism and breakdown of lean body mass. To meet the increased demands of metabolic stress and spare the use of endogenous protein stores, a greater amount of protein is needed in this population until the underlying stress has been overcome.	0–2 y: 2–3 g/kg/d 2–13 y: 1.5–2 g/kg/d Adolescents: 1.5 g/kg/d	Pediatric critical/surgical care population	Jaksic T. Effective and efficient nutritional support for the injured child. *Surg Clin North Am.* 2002;82(2):379–391, vii.
Dietary Reference Intake (DRI)	Replaces the 1989 Recommended Dietary Allowances (RDA). Protein needs were determined from children with normal growth, body composition, and activity, and who are also metabolically normal.	0–6 mo: 1.52 g/kg/d *This is an Adequate Intake recommendation, not enough research has been conducted to establish an RDA for this age group. 6–12 mo: 1.2 g/kg/d; 12–36 mo: 1.05 g/kg/d; 4–13 y: 0.95 g/kg/d; 14–18 y: 0.85 g/kg/d; >18 y: 0.8 g/kg/d	Children with normal growth, body composition, and activity, and who are also metabolically normal	National Academy of Sciences, Institute of Medicine, Food and Nutrition Board. *Dietary Reference Intakes for Energy, Carbohydrate, Fiber, Fat, Fatty Acids, Cholesterol, Protein, and Amino Acids (Macronutrients) (2005).*
1989 Recommended Dietary Allowance (RDA)	Based on the median nutrient intakes of children followed in longitudinal growth studies It can overestimate needs in non-active populations (eg, bedridden) and does not provide a range of energy needs. Though an outdated reference, still widely used.	0–6 mo: 2.2 g/kg/d; 6–12 mo: 1.6 g/kg/d; 1–3 y: 1.2 g/kg/d; 4–6 y: 1.1 g/kg/d; 7–14 y: 1 g/kg/d; 15–18 y (males): 0.9 g/kg/d; 15–18 y (females): 0.8 g/kg/d	Children with normal growth, body composition, and activity, and who are also metabolically normal	Committee in Dietary Allowances, Food and Nutrition Board, National Research Council. *Recommended Dietary Allowances.* 10th ed. Washington, DC: National Academy Press; 1989.
Peterson's Failure to Thrive (FTT)	This calculates nutrients in excess of the requirements of the RDA. Concerns with using this equation include refeeding syndrome. It can be calculated using a method similar to the one for calories above.	[Protein Required for Weight Age (g/kg/d) x Ideal Weight for Age (kg)] ÷ Actual Weight (kg)	Infants and children who present underweight and need to achieve catch-up growth	Peterson KE, Washington J, Rathbun JM. Team management of failure to thrive. *J Am Diet Assoc.* 1984;84:810–815.

Source: Ludlow V, Randall R, Burritt E, Rago D. Estimating Nutrient Needs, Pediatric Module. A.S.P.E.N. Enteral Nutrition Practitioner Tutorial Project. In press.

33

Nutrition Access

Beth Lyman, RN, MSN, CNSC; and Sohail R. Shah, MD, MSHA, FAAP

 Video

Learning Objectives

1. Describe the indications for use and appropriate management of nutrition access devices, including enteral and venous access devices.
2. Relate the key components of nutrition access management that caregivers need to be taught.
3. Formulate an evidence-based plan of care for nutrition access devices to guide clinical interventions that are age-appropriate and patient-specific.

Background

Nutrition access devices allow nutrition support clinicians to deliver parenteral and enteral nutrition formulas to patients. These devices include temporary and longer-term or permanent products for both enteral and parenteral formula delivery. It is within the scope of medical and nutrition support practice to select the appropriate device(s) and then insert and maintain these devices, but it is the patients and their families who live with them. Therefore, decisions about if and when to place a feeding tube or venous access device (VAD) for nutrition support begins with the family and continues to involve them throughout the process of addressing the child's nutritional issues.

Nutrition support clinicians must be able to teach healthcare professionals and families how to care for these devices, as failure to do so can have dire consequences for the patient. Often a vascular access team is used to assist with such tasks as peripherally inserted central catheter (PICC) placement and complication management. In a similar manner, enteral access teams are formed to address the insertion and management of various enteral access devices. Both vascular and enteral access teams can assist nutrition support clinicians with complication management and the education of parents or caregivers. All types of caregiver education need to take into consideration the health literacy of the individual(s) being taught. Using a teach-back approach to assess the understanding of the caregiver is a good way to gauge comprehension of the information presented. This chapter addresses indications for use, care, and management of complications related to nutrition access devices.

Types of Tubes

Nasogastric Tube

Nasogastric (NG) tubes are indicated for children who have an intact and functional gastrointestinal tract and will require enteral formula for less than 12 weeks. An exception to this would be an older child who self-inserts an NG tube at night for overnight enteral feeding. NG tubes are indicated for patients who have minimal gastroesophageal reflux, normal gastric emptying, and low risk of aspiration.[1] NG tubes are soft, flexible tubes made of silicone or polyurethane, and the typical size range used in pediatric practice is from 5 to 12 French (Fr). The tube diameter (Fr) is chosen based on the patient's age, body size, nare size, and type of formula needed. Small-diameter tubes are more comfortable for the patient but can become clogged, particularly if the patient receives a fiber-containing formula or if there are additives to the formula.

NG tubes can be easily placed by the family. Self-insertion by a child as young as 10 years of age can allow that child to be more active in his/her own care. The use of a rewards and consequences system for children old enough to understand is a good approach for when tubes are replaced. Teaching for caregivers needs to cover the following topics: age-appropriate comfort positioning, correct position of the head, blowing into the face to elicit a startle reflex and immediate swallowing, use or avoidance of water to drink during the procedure, how far to place the new tube, and

how to secure the tube. Confirmation of placement of NG tubes in the home is a topic ripe for research, because there is no standard recommendation. Institutional policy on this should be followed. Written instructions should be provided in the family's language of preference, and caregivers should be supervised performing this task prior to discharge. Always provide contact information for the family in case they need help, and outline what would indicate a life-threatening complication. Tubes can become dislodged as well, especially by an active or agitated child. NG tubes should be replaced or changed according to manufacturer's recommendations. Children with NG tubes can be encouraged to eat orally while receiving NG tube feedings if it is clinically appropriate.

Orogastric Tube

Orogastric (OG) tubes are not used as frequently because they restrict oral feedings. OG tubes are most useful in infants to avoid nasal obstruction or in children in whom an NG tube cannot be passed (ie, choanal atresia). A small study published in 2011 saw no differences in aspiration when a child had an OG tube and received an oral diet.[2] Another study looking at hypoxemia and bradycardia for neonates who were crossed over to receive enteral feeds via OG and then NG or vice versa found no difference in primary outcome measures using either tube.[3]

Gastrostomy Tube

Gastrostomy (G) tubes are a method of administering enteral nutrition for any child who requires it over the long term (> 3 months). These tubes allow direct access to the stomach through the anterior abdominal wall and allow for direct enteral administration, similar to an NG tube. The benefits of a G tube over a nasoenteral tube (NG or nasojejunal [NJ]) are added comfort, decreased likelihood of displacement, and the fact that it is less noticeable to others.

Gastrostomies can be placed surgically or endoscopically and come in a variety of sizes and types.[4,5] Surgically placed gastrostomies can be placed laparoscopically or through an upper midline incision. The initial gastrostomy placement may be a G tube or a G button, which is a low-profile device that sits at skin level. The endoscopically placed gastrostomy is referred to as a percutaneous endoscopic gastrostomy (PEG) tube. After placement, the G tube or G button may be used immediately; however, each of these gastrostomy tracts must mature (usually 8 to 12 weeks) prior to replacement.[6] After that time, caregivers can be taught how to change the device themselves.

Gastrojejunostomy Tube

Gastrojejunostomy (GJ) tubes are meant for long-term use and are inserted into the wall of the stomach, similar to a G tube. There are 2 ports: 1 into the stomach for fluids, medications, feedings, or venting and the other into the jejunum for continuous drip-feeding administration. GJ tubes are recommended for patients who require long-term enteral nutrition and have demonstrated intolerance to gastric feedings due to delayed gastric emptying, gastroesophageal reflux, or risk of aspiration.[7] The most common reasons for GJ tube replacement include accidental dislodgement, clogging, coiling back into the stomach, or a broken tube.[13]

Jejunostomy Tube

Jejunostomy (J) tubes are surgically or endoscopically placed into the jejunum. J tubes are typically not placed unless a child is going to need the tube for 6 months or longer.[14] The negative aspects of J tubes include mandatory continuous feedings and surgical emergencies (volvulus) around the tube or the need for urgent surgical replacement. Caregiver education for NJ, GJ, and J tubes must cover prevention of clogging by flushing with 10 mL to 20 mL of water every 4 hours during the day; avoiding medications down the tube or careful flushing with medications; and avoiding fiber-containing or high-caloric-density formulas in smaller-bore tubes. Education must also cover what to do and whom to contact if the tube is accidentally removed or dislodged.

Tube Insertion

Most NG tubes are placed at the bedside. Attempts are made to make the child as comfortable as possible. Infants or young children should be swaddled for comfort and to prevent their arms from flailing about during insertion. Accurate measurement to estimate how far the NG tube needs to be placed can be done using the NEMU method, which involves placing the tip of the NG tube from the **nare** to the **earlobe**, to the xiphoid process, to the umbilicus, and then finding the **midpoint** between the xiphoid process and **umbilicus**. NEMU compared favorably with an age-related, height-based equation developed by Cigrin-Ellett.[9] Either method is recommended, especially for neonates.

The cervical spine of the child should be slightly flexed and not hyperextended.[10] A small amount of lubricant or water can be used at the tip of the tube for ease of insertion. The tip is inserted into the nare and then slid carefully down the nasopharynx, orpharynx, esophagus, and into the stomach. It is then secured to the cheek near the nare. Parents are

taught the technique for NG tube insertion when it will be used in the home.

NJ tubes are inserted in a similar manner, but they require fluoroscopy or an abdominal x-ray for accurate placement or to confirm placement. The only exception is when the Cortak™ system is used (see Electromagnetic Tube Placement, below). Bedside placement of these tubes is becoming a more common nursing procedure. Placement mimics that of NG tubes, except that the child may be turned onto his or her right side. Use of sterile water or oral electrolyte solution instilled slowly via syringe helps float the tube postpylorus once the nurse knows he/she is in the stomach. A prompt vacuum effect when trying to aspirate contents using an empty syringe is suggestive of postpyloric tube placement. These tubes cannot be replaced at home. If the tube migrates back into the stomach, it must be replaced.

G, GJ, and J tubes are placed endoscopically or surgically by a pediatric gastroenterologist, radiologist, or surgeon. If a tube is dislodged, families should be instructed to insert a replacement tube or temporary tube of the same diameter into the tract immediately to avoid premature closure until a more permanent tube can be placed.

Verification of Placement

Verifying correct placement of an enteral tube is imperative prior to administering enteral formula. A retrospective study looking at 326 x-rays compared to NG tube placement and intragastric air done in a neonatal intensive care unit found half to be malpositioned.[11] Malpositioned tubes were defined as in the esophagus, curled upward in the stomach, or postpylorus. Another retrospective study using x-rays to assess NG tube placement in neonates found a 59% incidence of malpositioned tubes.[12] In both of these studies, 6% to 7% of tubes were in the esophagus. A tube accidentally inserted into the respiratory tract would certainly have disastrous or even deadly consequences for the patient and could be life-altering for the individual who placed the tube.[13]

Radiology

A chest or abdominal x-ray that identifies the tip of the tube is the gold standard for confirming placement of gastric or postpyloric tubes. However, a survey of critical care nurses by Metheny documented poor compliance with national organization recommendations to confirm placement of an NG tube using an x-ray.[14] There is concern for pediatric patients about increased radiation exposure from x-rays, and alternative methods have been used to confirm placement, but each has its own set of limitations.[15]

Air Insufflation With Auscultation

This method for verifying NG tube placement involves instilling air into the tube using a syringe while using a stethoscope to listen for the sound of moving air over the stomach or left upper quadrant. This method is inexpensive and relatively easy to do, but it is the least accurate of all methods. Air instilled into a feeding tube that is mistakenly placed in the lung can be heard in the abdomen. Many case reports in the literature describe the inability of clinicians to determine gastric versus respiratory placement. In 2012, the Child Health Patient Safety Organization recommended that this method no longer be used to verify NG tube placement.[16]

Gastric Aspirate/pH Testing

Aspirating gastric contents and confirming pH is an alternative to the gold standard radiograph and is the recommended bedside method to confirm NG placement.[15] A large study by Gilbertson found endotracheal pH aspirate to be ≥ 6 and misplaced tubes to have a pH of ≥ 5.5. She recommended a pH of ≤ 5 as the cutoff for confirming NG placement.[17] This study did not use a neonatal population. Confounding variables in the use of pH measurements to confirm NG tube placement are the use of continuous enteral feedings, acid-suppressing medications, and time of the last bolus feeding. Also, sterile water used to lubricate the inside of the NG tube to allow for easy removal of the stylet has a pH of 6. This water must be removed prior to checking the pH of the gastric contents. If the gastric pH is > 5, if gastric aspirate cannot be obtained, if the patient clinically deteriorates during placement, or if the patient develops low oxygen saturation, an x-ray is necessary to confirm placement.[18]

Electromagnetic Tube Placement

The Cortrak System™ assists with feeding tube placement by displaying the approximate location of the feeding tube during real-time placement. This system uses feeding tubes with a specialized stylet that has an electromagnetic transmitter. A receiver unit is placed on the patient's chest at the xiphoid process and acquires the signal from the stylet. It tracks the course of the stylet in the tube as it is advanced and displays it on a monitor. Pediatric patients who can tolerate a feeding tube of 8 Fr or larger are candidates for this device. Research using this product in pediatric patients has been conflicting, however. Powers compared the use of the Cortrak machine and x-rays to verify placement and found the Cortrak method to be 100% accurate in the 18 children studied.[19] However, another study comparing Cortrak to blind placement of postpyloric tubes in a population of critically ill children found the Cortrak system took longer to place the tube.[20] This later study did require an x-ray to verify placement, which is not needed with the Cortrak system.

Reverification of Placement

For NG and OG tubes, aspiration of fluid from the tube can be used if the child has been fed recently. Obtaining enteral formula is often used to reverify placement. For NJ or J tubes, aspiration of formula from the tube or a prompt vacuum effect with an empty syringe is suggestive of appropriate placement.

Nursing Care Related to Feeding Tubes

Aspiration Precautions

Infants and children lying flat are at increased risk of reflux and aspirating formula. It is important to position the infant or child to prevent aspiration episodes, with the head of the child elevated at least 30^0 while receiving a feeding.[1,10] It may also be necessary to feed the child at risk for aspiration via a postpyloric tube.

Securing the Tube

NG, NJ, and OG tubes can easily be pulled out by an infant or child tugging on the tube, sneezing, or vomiting. To prevent dislodgement, the tube is secured on the child's face. Every effort should be used to use hypoallergenic adhesive products to avoid skin reactions or tearing of the facial skin. An apple pectin thin wafer (Duoderm™) on the cheek near the nare can be used as a base to lay the external portion of the NG or OG tube, and then it can be covered with a transparent dressing. It is recommended that the excess tubing be fixed to the back of the infant or child's shirt using tape. This helps to keep the tube out of sight and prevents the child from grabbing it.

J tubes and G tubes, including low-profile devices, can also be pulled out, but this is less likely. Most of the permanent feeding devices have an internal retaining bolster or water-filled balloon. If 1 of these tubes is accidentally dislodged with the bolster or balloon intact, the family should know to expect some bleeding and local stomal trauma. To prevent loss of patency, the ostomy should be cannulated with either the same tube (with the balloon deflated and then reinflated after insertion) or a temporary tube. Many permanent feeding tubes have an external bolster to prevent migration of the tube into the stomach and possible blockage of the pylorus. G or J tubes can be secured to the abdomen with various commercially available products. The cost of the product, size of the child, and bulkiness of the device should be factored into how to best secure the tube to the abdomen. For a comparison of nursing care for feeding tubes, see Table 33-1.

Site Care

Keeping the site clean and dry is the most important aspect of caring for an enteral feeding tube. Washing the nose and face with a mild soap and water daily is enough to keep nasoenteric tubes clean.

Ostomy sites should be monitored daily for cleanliness. Mild soap and water is enough to keep these sites clean, gently scrubbing off any crusted areas. A slit absorbent pad can be placed between the device and the skin to keep the ostomy site dry if there is some leakage. For the most part, a dressing is not required. An over-the-counter antibiotic ointment may be needed if the site becomes erythematous and tender; families should be advised to use the ointment for 3 days, and if the site is not better, to contact their provider. If there is improvement, the ointment can be applied 2 to 3 times daily for a total of 10 days.

Checking Residual Volumes

It is not recommended to check residual volumes routinely, as there is much debate over their significance. Intolerance to feedings is demonstrated by mood (fussiness), vomiting, retching, or abdominal distention. Residual volumes are influenced by the enteral formula used, gastric emptying, gastroesophageal reflux, respiratory compromise, timing of the measurement in relation to the feed, and delivery method. In general, residuals that are collected should be re-fed to the patient, as this can be a significant source of calorie loss.

Flushing the Tube

Small-bore temporary feeding tubes may clog from enteral formula and medication incompatibility. A retrospective study looking at the use of pancreatic enzymes activated with sodium bicarbonate documented a 48% success rate in 53 of 110 occluded tubes. This study involved adult and pediatric patients and used Creon™ 12 000 units and 650 mg of sodium bicarbonate dissolved in sterile water.[21] In general, routine flushing of enteral tubes after each bolus feeding or interrupting continuous feeding for water flushes is not recommended in children.[10] If a tube becomes clogged, water is readily available and is the preferred flushing solution. Sterile or purified water is preferred over tap water in a hospitalized population.[10]

It is important to take the child's age into account when flushing an enteral feeding tube with water. Immature kid-

neys cannot remove excess water, and too much free water can dilute sodium levels, causing seizures related to hyponatremia in worst-case scenarios. For most NG and OG tubes, 3 to 5 mL of water will suffice to flush a feeding tube. Smaller volumes may be used in premature or small infants.

Medication Administration

Enteral feeding tubes of all types are often used for medication administration. Some medications can be easily given via enteral tube, such as liquid suspensions or solutions, crushed solid tablets, and capsules. More complex formulations, such as extended- or sustained-release products, are problematic.

Liquid forms of medication are preferred. Some solutions and suspensions may be too viscous to put safely through a small-bore feeding tube; these medications must be diluted with sterile water. Suspensions must be shaken thoroughly prior to administration.[10] Improper medication administration can lead to inaccurate medication provision.

Medications in solid form, such as tablets or capsules, must be crushed or opened and mixed with water prior to administering through an enteral feeding tube. It is important to mix the medication well to prevent underdosing due to adherence of the medication to the syringe barrel.

After medications are administered through an enteral feeding tube, the tube should be flushed with purified water to prevent clogging and ensure the entire dose is delivered to the child. When formula and medications are given concurrently, flushing with water before and between medications (as well as after) prevents mixing of medications.[11]

In the case of GJ tubes, caregivers should be taught about what medication is being given, why it is being given, and where it is to be administered. Certain medications, including vitamins and minerals, require activation in the stomach or are predominantly absorbed in the small intestine. Medications that alter pH may also affect the activity of concomitant medications. A consultation with a pharmacist is warranted when deciding to give medications via jejunal or gastric tube. A pharmacist will also provide information about medication compatibility if the decision is made to add it directly to an enteral formula.[10]

Feeding Pumps

Enteral feeding pumps are useful for delivering continuous enteral formula or for a regulated rate for bolus feedings. Some feeding pumps are small enough to be worn in a small backpack for ease of mobility and flexibility of schedules. The ideal pediatric pump is not position-sen-

Table 33-1. Comparison of Feeding Tubes and Troubleshooting Issues

	GASTROSTOMY	GASTROJEJUNOSTOMY	COMMENTS
Type of Feeding	Bolus, gravity or continuous drip	Continuous drip via pump only	Pay attention to where the port for feeding is located
Medication Administration	• Give medications first if patient receives bolus feeds • Avoid giving high volumes of liquid medications at one time	• Use GJ if gastric emptying is known to be poor • Avoid giving high volumes of liquid medications via the J port, as this can cause cramping and diarrhea	• Check with pharmacist or Lexi-comp to see if medications need to be given via stomach • Medications are often given via the G port even when we feed into the J port • Liquid medications are hyperosmolar
Flushes	Can give water after bolus feeds	• Flush with no more than 20 mL of water for small children • Flush the J port every 4 h while the child is awake to prevent clogging	• The smaller the child, the smaller the water bolus should be • For children with a cardiac history, check with the provider about water flushes • For developmentally delayed children, water flushes may be liberalized to provide free water
Site Care	• Wash with soap and water • Rotate once or twice daily	• Wash with soap and water • NEVER ROTATE	Rotating the GJ tube can twist it out of the small bowel and into the stomach
Replacement	• Done by caregivers after first 8 weeks post-insertion • Verify proper placement by aspirating gastric contents	• Done by IR • For infants, it may need to be done within a few hours of dislodgement to prevent hypoglycemia	When in doubt about placement, obtain a dye study
When to Get Worried	• Pain with feeds could indicate an infection or misplaced G tube • Black drainage could indicate gastric mucosal erosion at the stoma • Erosion of the epithelial skin layer • Increase in abdominal distention • Signs of increasing reflux • No weight gain with feedings • Respiratory distress during feedings	• Pain with feeds could indicate an infection or misplaced G tube • Black drainage could indicate gastric mucosal erosion at the stoma • Erosion of the epithelial skin layer • Vomiting of formula could indicate J port has migrated back into the stomach	• Anything you don't like about how the patient is tolerating feeds • Be sure to resize both tubes periodically as the child gains weight to avoid pain, gastric ulceration, and epithelial layer erosion • Vent the G tube or gastric port to allow air to come out if the patient has distention • Try postpyloric feeds for an infant with reflux who is not gaining weight. Do this for a short time and reassess • Instruct caregivers to call 911 for respiratory problems • Consider admission for poor or no weight gain when the patient should be receiving adequate calories
Granulation Tissue	Caused by movement of the tube	Caused by movement of the tube	• Abnormal tissue must be treated to prevent local site infection and bleeding • Treat with steroid cream, silver nitrate, or other topical product that will shrink the tissue

	NASOGASTRIC	POSTPYLORIC	COMMENTS
Type of Feeding	Bolus, gravity, or continuous drip	Continuous drip via pump only	Avoid fiber-containing or highly viscous formulas in small-bore tubes
Medication Administration	If able give orally	• If able give orally • Flush with 3–5 mL of water after medications • Avoid crushed pills if possible	—

Table 33-1. Comparison of Feeding Tubes and Troubleshooting Issues (continued)

	NASOGASTRIC	POSTPYLORIC	COMMENTS
Flushes	Not typically necessary unless giving bolus feeds	Flush every 4 h while the child is awake to prevent clogging	• The smaller the child, the smaller the water bolus should be • For children with a cardiac history, check with the provider about water flushes • For developmentally delayed children, water flushes may be liberalized to provide free water
Skin Care	Secure with hypoallergenic products	Secure with hypoallergenic products	For infants, a Steri-Strip™ mustache may be helpful; watch the pacifier and make sure it does not catch in securement products
Replacement	May be done in the hospital, outpatient clinic, or home depending on institutional policy	Replaced in a healthcare facility by a healthcare provider	For infants, it may need to be done within a few hours of dislodgement to prevent hypoglycemia
When to Get Worried	• Vomiting with feedings • Increase in abdominal distention • Yellow drainage from the nare • Signs of increasing reflux • No weight gain with feedings • Respiratory distress during feedings	• Vomiting with feedings that looks like formula, which could indicate the tube has migrated into the stomach • Increase in abdominal distention • Yellow drainage from the nare • Signs of increasing reflux • No weight gain with feedings • Respiratory distress during feedings	• Try to vent the tube for abdominal distention • Move the tube to the opposite nare if there is yellow drainage, and assess for sinusitis • For any signs of clinical deterioration or lack of progress related to the nutrition access device, re-evaluate patient • Instruct caregivers to call 911 for respiratory problems

G, gastrostomy; GJ, gastrojejunostomy; IR, intestinal rehabilitation; J, jejunostomy.

sitive, can be increased in increments of 0.1 mL up to 5 mL/h, and is relatively lightweight. Providers and caregivers need to be aware that enteral feeding pumps are not free of malfunctions. Most manufacturers of feeding equipment and pumps have safeguards in place to prevent flow errors. Pumps should accurately administer formula within 5% of the ordered amount. Periodic calibration of the pump is important to ensure the accuracy of the delivery system.[10] Clinicians need to be aware of special limitations imposed by manufacturers. An alert was sent out regarding the use of 1 pump that strongly recommended it not be used to deliver homemade blenderized diets.[23] When such an alert is sent out, healthcare providers, families, and durable medical equipment companies need to be made aware so they can act accordingly.

Vascular Access Devices

When an infant or child requires parenteral nutrition (PN), consideration of the most appropriate VAD includes goals of therapy, anticipated length of therapy, and patient-specific considerations, such as peripheral venous access options or the need for intermittent rather than daily PN. Other considerations, such as psychosocial concerns, are also part of the decision-making process when longer-term PN is

anticipated. In pediatrics, the use of peripheral parenteral nutrition (PPN) may be the initial nutrition intervention. Regardless of the type of VAD used, meticulous care of the skin, device, and catheter hub have been reported to decrease complications related to the use of the device.[24,25]

Peripheral Intravenous Catheters

Neonatal and pediatric patients may receive a short course of PPN prior to the initiation of PN. Selection of the most appropriate peripheral intravenous (IV) site involves avoidance of antecubital fossa veins in case a PICC is needed and scalp veins in case of accidental catheter dislodgement or infiltration. After appropriate hand hygiene, the use of clean gloves is recommended when inserting a peripheral IV catheter.[26] If the IV catheter becomes dislodged into surrounding tissue, the infiltration should be graded and treated according to severity, including removal of the catheter, elevation of the extremity, and possible antidote administration.[27] PPN-related tissue necrosis from an infiltration-related event is caused by IV calcium and requires a cold compress to assist in sequestering the calcium. An osmolarity of no greater than 900 mOsm is suggested for PPN solutions to prevent irritation or of the vein or phlebitis.[28]

Peripherally Inserted Central Catheters

If PN is required for greater than 5 to 7 days, a PICC is often placed, with the tip of the catheter located in the superior vena cava just above the veno-atrial junction. A PICC that is in place prior to initiation of PN may need to have tip placement verified prior to its use for PN, as PICCs are associated with a higher rate of malposition than other types of VADs.[27] Case reports in the literature document intracranial malpositioning resulting in seizures and stroke in pediatric patients who had a PICC for PN.[28,29] One report in the literature looked at complication rates when PICCs were used for children with intestinal failure. Investigators reported 95 PICCs were placed in 45 infants, with a central line–associated bloodstream infection (CLABSI) rate of 5.3 per 1000 days and a thrombosis rate of 2 per 1000 patient days.[30] It was felt that the lack of need for anesthesia and smaller-bore catheters were advantageous.

As PICCs are the preferred VAD for neonates receiving PN, it is important to discern the best practices related to PICC placement and use. The use of chlorhexidine for bathing neonates with a birth weight of ≥ 1000 g but less than 28 days old was found to result in a CLABSI rate of 1.92 per 1000 patient days compared to infants who were bathed with mild soap, who had a CLABSI rate of 6 per 1000 patient days.[31] Axillary PICC placement has been associated with a 12-fold decrease in inflammation, blockage, edema, and infection compared to PICCs placed in other sites.[32] A multicenter cohort study of 3967 neonates who had 4797 PICCs reported an increased risk of CLABSI during the first 2 weeks after PICC placement, with this increase being sustained thereafter.[33] Investigators cautioned daily evaluation of the ongoing need for a PICC.

PICCs should be secured to the skin.[25] The use of sutures has been documented to result in less migration, occlusion, and leakage when compared to the use of tape.[34] However, sutures can become inflamed, requiring removal. The use of an adhesive securement device has been shown to be easier to place and associated with fewer complications than sutures in pediatric patients.[35] PICCs may be used for home PN administration, particularly for short-term needs (less than 6 weeks), but they are also often used successfully for longer.

Temporary VADs

Critically ill children who require PN will typically have a single-lumen or multi-lumen temporary VAD via the subclavian, internal jugular, or femoral vein. Reduction of CLABSIs continues to be an ongoing focus in all healthcare settings, including critical care units. One approach has been to use antibiotic-impregnated VADs. This approach is controversial in pediatrics due to concerns about sensitization and the development of drug resistance. One study using antibiotic-impregnated VADs saw comparable infection rates, but the antibiotic VADs were in place an average of 18 days before infection occurred, compared to 5 days for the nonantibiotic VADs.[11] While it is often thought that femoral VAD placement is more likely to lead to CLABSI due to proximity to fecal contamination, a study by Reyes et al found that this was not the case. In a retrospective study, they looked at 4512 pediatric intensive care unit patients and found no association between site of temporary VAD and CLABSI.[37] A report looking at placement of femoral VADs found the left femoral vein to be most commonly medial to the femoral artery, compared to the right femoral vein, where there can be some overlap.[38] Investigators recommend use of the left femoral vein where possible.

Tunneled VADs

When it is apparent that long-term PN is needed for a patient, plans for the most appropriate VAD need to be made. A patient who will go home for up to 6 weeks of PN can often use the same PICC already in place. A tunneled, cuffed catheter is most often used for infants and children who require home PN for an extended or indefinite period. Tunneled catheters can vary by size, number of lumens, and material. The size and number of lumens may be selected based on the patient's age and indications for catheter placement. However, the minimum number of lumens and smallest-diameter catheter to meet the patient's needs should be selected to minimize complications, including thrombosis and venous stenosis. The material of the catheter (polyurethane versus silicone) has not been shown to affect the duration of function, although fracture rates may be different.[39] However, a polyurethane tunneled VAD cannot be used for ethanol lock therapy. Prior to discharge, families need to be educated on the care of the tunneled VAD, including dressing changes, flushes, and emergency measures.

Implanted VADs

Implantable VADs are used when prolonged vascular access is necessary. They come in multiple French sizes, single- or double-lumen, and can be either polyurethane or silicone. They are generally best suited for intermittent therapies given over an extended period of time. Benefits of implantable devices include patients' ability to participate in most daily activities, less perception of altered body image, decreased dressing changes, and a lower risk of infection. The location of the subcutaneous implantable VAD is often provider-dependent; however, some data demonstrate decreased complications with placement below the clavicle rather than in the inframammary line.[40] Implanted VADs may be accessed immediately after placement without any increased risk of complications.[41] These implantable devices may develop catheter-associated or subcutaneous pocket infections. Pocket infections require removal of the catheter and device, along with appropriate antibiotic treatment. Since implanted VADs requires a needle through the skin to access the device, they are not commonly used for daily long-term PN administration.

Nursing Care Related to VADs

Obtaining Laboratory Specimens From a VAD

The VAD is often used to obtain laboratory specimens to avoid venipuncture. Approaches to obtaining laboratory specimens are compared in Table 33-2. Two studies in the literature document the safe and reliable method of blood sampling, which involves repeated pushing and pulling of blood into an empty syringe before obtaining a specimen in a new syringe.[42,43] Nursing should have options for specimen collection based on what is best for that patient. It is important for nursing staff to stop all infusions when using a multi-lumen catheter to assure accurate laboratory sample results. When the waste approach is used, 1 study has validated the safety of 3 mL versus 5 mL of waste when blood samples are obtained from a tunneled or implanted VAD.[44] Other sources recommend a discard volume of 1 mL to 3 mL, or twice the priming volume.

VAD Site Care

Meticulous and routine site care is essential for the prevention of CLABSI. The 2011 Centers for Disease Control and Prevention (CDC) Guidelines for the Prevention of Intravascular Catheter-Related Infections recommends the use of chlorhexidine for skin antisepsis in children over 2 months of age.[25] Transparent dressings are changed every 7 days, or when nonocclusive or soiled.[25] For children who have a history of CLABSI or have a temporary VAD and are over the age of 2 months, it is recommended that a chlorhexidine-impregnated sponge be placed over the VAD insertion site.[25] This makes it impossible to inspect the insertion site, but it can still be palpated for tenderness. It is also important to protect the VAD using the dressing to help secure the line. Tunneled VADs often have a long external segment that can be looped under the transparent dressing as a stress loop to prevent accidental dislodgement.

Hub Care

Again, meticulous attention to clean or aseptic technique is recommended when the hub of the VAD or the needleless

Table 33-2. Comparison of Techniques Used to Obtain Blood Samples from a VAD

TYPE OF TECHNIQUE	DESCRIPTION	PROS	CONS
Traditional	1. Stop infusion 2. Flush VAD with NS 3. Obtain a waste specimen of 3–5 mL 4. Obtain blood needed for labs ordered 5. Flush VAD with NS 6. Restart infusion	"Gold standard" procedure at this time When done properly, low risk of infection associated with obtaining labs.	Increases blood loss when doing frequent blood sampling Increases exposure of staff to blood Potential for confusing the waste syringe with the sample syringe
Return the Waste	1. Fill a syringe with heparin and remove it 2. Stop infusion 3. Flush VAD with NS 4. Obtain a waste specimen of 3–5 mL 5. Have a nurse rotate the waste specimen 6. Obtain blood needed for labs ordered 7. Return the waste specimen to the patient 8. Flush VAD with NS 9. Restart infusion	Decreases the blood loss for the patient	Potential for reinfusion of blood clots Potential for contamination of blood being reinfused
Push-Pull Method	1. Stop infusion 2. Aspirate 3–5 mL of blood into a syringe 3. Reinfuse that blood and repeat the aspiration/reinfuse procedure a total of 3 times 4. Place a new syringe on the VAD and obtain blood needed for ordered labs	Limits patient blood loss from blood sampling	Potential for hemolysis due to turbulence created by the pushing and pulling May not be feasible for some VADs that are difficult to draw from

cap is accessed.[25] Doing a 15-second scrub with either 70% alcohol or chlorhexidine prior to accessing the catheter or adapter is recommended. The CDC recommends changing the needleless adapter when IV fluids are changed or every 72 hours. An additional layer of protection can be obtained by adding an alcohol-impregnated sponge cap over the needleless adapter. One study done at North Shore Hospital in the Chicago area documented a reduction in CLABSI from 4.2 per 1000 patient days to 0.94 per 1000 patient days after implementing this cap.[45] Hub care is part of a bundle of practices done in an effort to prevent CLABSIs.

Routine Flushing

Traditionally, the VAD has been flushed with normal saline and then with heparin of varying concentrations based on the weight of the child, the number of times the line will be accessed intermittently, and the lumen diameter. Increasingly, normal saline alone is being used to maintain the patency of a VAD when used intermittently. A study done in Italy using pediatric oncology patients aged infant to 17 years reported occlusion rates of 4% complete and 23% partial. Investigators found that smaller tunneled catheters (4.2 Fr) were more likely to occlude.[46] Use of normal saline alone to maintain patency of a VAD is appropriate for children who are cycled off PN for a few hours per day when the lumen of the VAD is larger.

Safety Issues

All caregivers of children with a VAD need to be aware of the safety issues associated with the current age of the child, as well as those to be anticipated as the child grows. For example, babies who are teething need to have a pacifier to prevent them from sucking or chewing on their IV tubing. The IV tubing can also be taped over the shoulder to keep it out of easy reach. "Out of sight, out of mind" works for many infants and toddlers to protect the line. This method will also benefit children with ostomies, who should have the VAD dressing and tubing as far away from the ostomy as possible.

One of the many reports in the literature describes the use of a VAD by parents with Munchausen syndrome by proxy.[47] This term is now referred to as pediatric condition falsification, and is a form of child abuse in which the caregiver is the perpetrator by insisting on invasive and painful procedures for his/her child. Because this condition can be life-threatening for the child, any suspicion of this condition needs to be addressed prior to placement of a VAD for PN. While this form of abuse is difficult to prove, certain typical behaviors seen in caregivers include "doctor shopping"

to different healthcare providers and facilities, discrepancy between reported symptoms and what is observed, caregiver reluctance to leave the child while at the hospital, and overzealous attachment to certain healthcare providers.[47] Parents or caregivers should not be allowed to access or care for a VAD unless specifically trained to do so, and then only with the permission of the nurse.

Administration Set Changes

Controversy exists about when to change IV tubing that has been used to administer PN and lipids. Also, the A.S.P.E.N. Parenteral Nutrition Safety Consensus Recommendations suggest that IV administration sets be completely changed every 24 hours, as lipids are typically co-infused.[26] The newest CDC Guidelines for the Prevention of Intravascular Catheter-Related Infections does recommend changing IV administration sets for 3-in-1 PN every 24 hours.[25] It is also recommended that needleless systems be used to access IV administration sets, and to change the system no more often than every 72 hours.[25] All IV administration sets should be di-2-ethylehxyl phthalate (DEHP)–free.[26] Hospital performance improvement projects or larger multicenter collaborative projects focusing on bundling of care around VADs and competency validation of nursing practice are recommended to reduce CLABSI risk (see Table 33-3 for a summary of such practices).[25]

Central Line–Associated Bloodstream Infection

Two therapies often discussed to prevent and treat CLABSI are the use of ethanol or antibiotic locks. Ethanol lock therapy involves filling and closing a catheter lumen with 70% ethanol for a minimum of 2 hours, using the fill volume for the VAD. Ethanol locks alone have been shown to be effective in reducing CLABSI, and when used in conjunction with standard antibiotic therapy, are effective in clearing CLABSI.[48–50] Criteria for starting ethanol lock therapy include the following: more than 1 previous CLABSI, > 5 kg weight, silicone VAD, and the ability of the family to appropriately perform the task, with no concerns about the psychosocial situation in the home.

Similarly, antibiotic lock therapy consists of instilling an antibiotic solution into a catheter hub for a specified period of time. Several antibiotic formulations have been proven to be effective in clearing and reducing the incidence of CLABSI, but the most promising research is using taurolidine, which is not available in the United States.[23,51–53]

Table 33-3. Prevention of CLABSIs

ASPECT OF CARE	ACTION
Hand Hygiene	• Use an antiseptic skin soap to wash hands before placing or accessing a VAD, or use an alcohol-based hand sanitizer
Catheter Insertion	• Staff involved in central line placement must be competent to do this procedure • Use maximal sterile barriers, including masks, gowns, drapes, sterile gloves, and a kit with all needed supplies • Allow nursing to call a "time out" for an observed break in sterile technique • Avoid placement of a central line in a febrile patient • Avoid guidewire replacement of a central line
Catheter Access	• Vigorously clean the hub of the catheter with 70% alcohol or chlorhexidine wipes before entering the line, or use a passive disinfection device • Have a policy on routine injection cap changes • Avoid stopcocks on central lines • Use sterile, prefilled syringes for central line flushing • Limit accessing for labs to 1 time per day if possible
Catheter Dressing Change	• Use a kit with all supplies needed • Use Chloraprep™ as the preferred skin disinfectant • Use a mask and gown for PICC dressings • Prefer a transparent dressing over a gauze-and-tape dressing to allow the site to be assessed • Restrain the patient as needed to prevent accidental dislodgement • Place a stress loop in the VAD tubing or extension tubing
Diagnosis of Bloodstream Infection	• Obtain a peripheral and central blood culture • Staff obtaining blood cultures should be specially trained and competent to avoid contamination • Draw a minimum of 1 mL for a blood culture • Use clinical and other labs to validate diagnosis • Do not necessarily remove the central line
IV Tubing Changes	• Lipids: every 24 h • PN: every 96 h unless a 3:1 solution, then every 24 h or if cycled off a few hours per day per CDC • recommendations
Other	• Evaluate all supplies used on CVCs for defects that could lead to infection • When using outside pharmacies, surveillance of possible IV fluid–related infections is needed • Have a surveillance plan within the institution to trend infections and look for a root cause

CDC, Centers for Disease Control and Prevention; CLABSI, central line–associated bloodstream infection; IV, intravenous; PICC, peripherally inserted central catheter; PN, parenteral nutrition; VAD, venous access device.

Thrombosis

VAD-related thrombosis has a variable incidence dependent upon the type of catheter, duration of therapy, and patient- and disease-related factors. The majority of VAD-related thrombosis remains asymptomatic in children, but a common question is the role of prophylaxis and surveillance. Routine prophylaxis for thrombosis after placement of a VAD is unnecessary and may be reserved for children at a higher risk for thromboembolism based on patient- and disease-related factors (ie, history of deep venous thrombosis or known hypercoagulable state).[54] Similarly, routine surveillance for VAD-related thrombosis is not recommended due to its significant costs and the infrequency with which it results in changes to patient management.[55]

Anticipatory Guidance

Some children literally grow up with a VAD or an enteral access device. As they progress through the various stages of childhood to adolescence, it is important that parents and caregivers be aware of age-appropriate actions to keep the device and child safe. See Table 33-4 for a summary of issues to consider. This table also stresses the importance of raising the child in a loving yet structured environment where appropriate behavior is expected and discipline is commensurate with the infraction.

Table 33-4. Intestinal Failure Anticipatory Guidance Sheet

AGE/STAGE	VAD	FEEDING TUBE	DEVELOPMENT	SOCIAL/SCHOOL	VILLAGE
Infancy	Tunneled Prevent ostomy drainage onto hub of catheter Prevent ostomy getting pulled as infant discovers fingers Watch for sucking on the VAD or IV tubing Be prepared for possible hospitalization for infections in VAD	NG tube: prevent frequent removal by using washcloths as arm splints as needed Tape securely G tube: watch for granulation tissue as infant starts to crawl Promote tummy time Watch tapes and skin cleansers; be gentle with the little ones	Cognitive: usually age-appropriate to advanced Fine motor: often age-appropriate Gross motor: delayed in sitting up, turning over, crawling, and walking Oral feeding skill development needs to be worked on: very important	Usually very social and interactive Usually happy, so pay attention to when infant is not very responsive and interactive Make sure siblings do not feel neglected Get grandparents involved if possible	IR team: physician, dietitian, nurse, pharmacist OT PT Social worker Check out the Oley Foundation or other parent/patient support groups Access only reputable websites
Toddlers	Prevent accidental pulling as child runs while on PN	Get a very small backpack for the enteral pump, or put it in a toddler play shopping cart so the toddler can push it	Cognitive: can still be quite advanced Fine motor: child will want to feed self Gross motor: allow and encourage development, but keep safety in mind; play dates with peers need to be monitored closely Oral: picky eaters can have IF, too! If an oral aversion exists, this is the time to address it with an inpatient stay if no progress is being made on an outpatient basis Watch child at family events—may get into food that he/she cannot tolerate Watch what siblings offer child	Early childhood education is appropriate so the child learns rules are for everyone; this also identifies gaps in learning At this point, parenting needs to focus on normal discipline so the toddler does not become manipulative and poorly behaved Use a reward/consequence system for controlling behavior that really matters, like staying still for a VAD dressing change	Same IR team OT may or may not be involved; typically not as involved once oral feeding skills are age-appropriate PT may not be needed Social worker is quite important Parents: don't neglect your marriage Friends and relatives start to step up and become more involved as the toddler gets older (and cuter!)
Early School Years	Protect VAD while at school Carefully consider what physical activities your child will be allowed to participate in: soccer? dance? gymnastics? T-ball/baseball? What about swim lessons?	By this age, a low-profile G tube will most likely have been inserted if enteral feeds are still needed School lunch issues will need to be addressed with the school and child. Expect some cheating. Also, make sure the teacher knows what special treats your child can have during parties. Provide them yourself if you need to	Cognitive: some learning issues may surface depending on the early hospital course in the NICU. This may not relate to IF issues at all. Work on self-esteem: get your child in something he/she enjoys and is good at, such as music lessons, Scouts, church group, etc. Fine motor: not typically a problem for these kids Gross motor: watch what playground and sports activities your child enjoys. Soccer is not recommended if a VAD is in place. Gymnastics/tumbling could be problematic if the VAD is in place, as it can come out of place with flips. Dance could be fine Oral: oral aversions may remain to a limited extent. Mealtimes need to include the child	Social: get your child a "circle of friends." Encourage normal social outings, but make sure parents of friends are aware of your child's special needs re: diet and VAD/G tube School: have a section 504 plan to address toilet issues, ostomy issues, special food issues, activities, etc. Meet with the teacher at the beginning of each school year. Make a rule about school attendance that sets a clear message that school is mandatory. No blood, no fever, no doctor's appointment—school must be attended	Besides healthcare providers and relatives, the village expands to teachers, school aides, school nurses, coaches, and parents of friends Keep a wide circle of close acquaintances, including church members and neighbors Parents are still the most important members of the village, and you will transition to the role of care coordinator as time goes on

Table 33-4. Intestinal Failure Anticipatory Guidance Sheet (continued)

AGE/STAGE	VAD	FEEDING TUBE	DEVELOPMENT	SOCIAL/SCHOOL	VILLAGE
Tweens	Often the VAD is out or not used nightly. Think about a port-a-cath if using only 3–4 nights per week	Deal with issues of swimming, etc. based on your healthcare provider's recommendations. Still avoid lakes, oceans, and dirty water if possible. Focus on what the child can do with the G tube in place. Your child will be hooking and unhooking the feeding delivery set tubing by now. Encourage more and more self-care	Cognitive: should be same as early school years. If your child is hospitalized, set aside time every day to do homework once he/she is medically stable. This sets up a routine that allows for a smoother transition back to school. It also sends a message that the hospital is not a place to dodge homework and slack off

Fine motor: encourage building of model airplanes, cars, or making jewelry to help a child who cannot be as physically active as peers to feel accomplished

Gross motor: discuss team sports, more involved dance, or gymnastics with your healthcare provider, especially if a VAD is still in place. Encourage bike riding and physically taxing activities to the level your child is challenged but not exhausted

Oral: expect cheating, expect your child to tolerate foods that are not on the approved list. Pick your battles carefully

This is the time when children start becoming a bit noncompliant with medications | Social: what about over-nights with friends? Can the tube feeding be skipped for a night? This needs to be discussed with the healthcare provider. Do you like your child's friends? Do they treat your child with respect? If not, try to find some kids you know are nice and work very hard to get friendships going that you know will bring out the best in your child. Self-esteem issues in this age and with these kids can lead to kids accepting ridicule from friends just to avoid being lonely

School: same as above—attendance is mandatory, good grades are the goal, participation in after-school activities should be at the level your child can tolerate. While school attendance is mandatory, school activities are not. Some kids in this age group want to do it all but may not be physically able to do so | The village becomes wider and the influence of parents begins to wane. This is hard for all parents to see and deal with. Testing boundaries within a safe village with teachers and neighbors keeping an eye out can prevent serious accidents or unsafe behaviors

While trying not to be alarmist, make sure people who have your child in their home know the limits and will honor them |
| Adolescents | Expect more risk-taking behaviors. Discuss with your healthcare provider when and how much responsibility your child should take for flushing the VAD, starting home PN, doing dressing changes, etc.

Expect the child to want the VAD out and to work more diligently on enteral feeds and oral diet to accomplish this | Some adolescents opt for night-time NG tubes at this age due to body-image issues. This is especially true if IF happens during the adolescent years. Allow your child to make these choices. The child will place the tube and often prepare the formula, load the pump, and run it themselves. You still need to make sure this is done.

Expect negotiations to do tube feeds 5–6 nights per week to get 1–2 nights off | Cognitive: often these kids excel academically if parents have set expectations in early years

Fine motor: same as above

Gross motor: expect kids to test limits and engage in risk-taking behaviors. Competitions involving no physical contact tend to be popular, such as cross-country running

Oral: expect some experimentation with alcohol. Avoid soft drinks. Encourage healthy eating habits and make sure supplements like vitamins, calcium, etc. are taken (if ordered) | Social: friends and school activities take center stage. Encourage as much involvement in school activities as your child can tolerate. Set limits and have a curfew just as if your child did not have IF. Focus on normal teen behaviors and have consequences for breaking rules. Being lenient with rules in this age group is a mistake

Watch out for friends who indulge in risk-taking behaviors. Your child may end up in the hospital for something that just gives a friend a headache

School: as above. Start a dialogue about college | The village has parents playing a different role—more of an observer, advisor, clarifier of expectations. Grandparents can often be more influential than parents

Start a dialogue about transitioning to adult providers if appropriate. Consider college location into the mix of proximity to healthcare providers, and the medical stability and maturity of the adolescent |

G, gastrostomy; IF, intestinal failure; IR, intestinal rehabilitation; IV, intravenous; NG, nasogastric; NICU, neonatal intensive care unit; OT, occupational therapist; PN, parenteral nutrition; PT, physiotherapist; VAD, venous access device.

Test Your Knowledge Questions

1. An infant who presents with a 3-day history of gastro-enteritis with both vomiting and diarrhea is most likely to be started on PN using:
    A. Peripheral vein
    B. Femoral PICC
    C. Tunneled catheter
    D. PN is not warranted in this child

2. An 8-month-old, 4 kg baby with intestinal failure receives PN via a silicone tunneled VAD. The decision is made to start an ethanol lock due to repeated CLABSIs. This decision is:
    A. Not wise because the catheter has to be polyure-thane.
    B. Worrisome due to exposure to ethanol at such a young age.
    C. Appropriate standard of care at this point in time.
    D. Not wise due to the weight of the child.

3. A 4-year-old with a low-profile balloon G tube inserted 1 week ago accidentally pulls it out with the balloon inflated. Prior to discharge, the family should:
    A. Have been instructed to place a temporary catheter in the site immediately.
    B. Go to the emergency department for replacement.
    C. Do nothing and contact the surgeon on call.
    D. A and B

4. The most appropriate method for bedside verification of the placement of an NG tube is:
    A. pH
    B. Air insufflations and auscultation
    C. Inspection of gastric contents
    D. X-ray

References

1. Baker SS, Baker RD, Davis AM. *Pediatric Nutrition Support.* Sudbury, MA: Jones and Bartlett Publishers; 2007.
2. Leder SB, Lazarus CL, Suiter DM, Acton LM. Effect of orogastric tubes on aspiration status and recommendations for oral feeding. *Otolaryngol Head Neck Surg.* 2011;144(3):372–375.
3. Bohnhorst B, Cech K, Peter C, Doerdelmann M. Oral versus nasal for placing feeding tubes: no effect on hypoxemia and bradycardia in infants. *Neonatology.* 2010;98(2):143–149.
4. Akay B, Capizzani TR, Lee AM, et al. Gastrostomy tube placement in infants and children: is there a preferred technique. *J Pediatr Surg.* 2010;54(6):1147–1152.
5. Buderus S, Adenaeuer M, Dueker G, Bindl L, Lentze MJ. Balloon gastrostomy buttons in pediatric patients: evaluation with respect to size, lifetime in patients, and parent acceptance. *Klin Padiatr.* 2009;221(2):65–68.
6. Islek A, Sayari E, Yilmaz A, Artan R. Percutaneous gastrostomy in children: is early feeding safe? *J Pediatr Gastrenteol Nutr.* 2013;57(5):659–662.
7. Egnell C, Eksborg S, Grahnquist L. Jejunostomy enteral feeding in children: outcome and safety. *JPEN J Parenter Enteral Nutr.* 2013;38(5):631–636.
8. Al-Zubeidi D, Demir H, Bishop WP, Rahhal RM. Gastrojejunal feeding tube use by gastroenterologists in a pediatric academic center. *J Pediatr Gastrenteol Nutr.* 2013;56(5):523–527.
9. Cirgin Ellett ML, Cohen MD, Perkins SM, Smith CE, Lane KA, Austin JK. Predicting the insertion length for gastric tube placement in neonates. *J Obstet Gynecol Neonatal Nurs.* 2011;40(4):412–421.
10. Bankhead R, Boullata J, Brantley S, et al. Enteral nutrition practice recommendations. *JPEN J Parenter Enteral Nutr.* 2009;33(2):122–167.
11. Fisher C. Clogged feeding tubes: a clinician's thorn. *Pract Gastroenterol.* 2014;127: 16–22.
12. deBoer JC, Smit BJ, Mainous RO. Nasogastric tube position and intragastric air collection in a neonatal intensive care population. *Adv Neonatal Care.* 2009;9(6):293–298.
13. Quandt D, Schraner T, Bucher HU, Mieth RA. Malposition of feeding tubes in neonates: is it an issue? *J Pediatr Gastrenteol Nutr.* 2009;48(5):608–611.
14. Kemper C, Northington L, Wilder K, Visscher D. A call to action: the development of enteral access safety teams. *Nutr Clin Pract.* 2014;29(3):264–266.
15. Metheny NA, Stewart BJ, Mills AC. Blind insertion of feeding tubes in intensive care units: a national survey. *Am J Crit Care.* 2012;21:352–360.
16. Irving SY, Lyman B, Northington L, Bartlett JA, Kemper C, and the NOVEL Project Work Group. Nasogastric tube placement and verification in children: review of the current literature. *Nutr Clin Pract.* 2014;29(3):267–276.
17. National Association of Childrens Hosptials (NACH), ECRI Institute. *Blind Pediatric NG Tube Placements Continue to Cause Harm.* Overland Park, KS: Child Health Patient Safety Organization, Inc; 2012.
18. Gilbertson HR, Rogers EJ, Ukoumunne OC. Determination of a practical pH cutoff level for reliable confirmation of nasogastric tube placement. *JPEN J Parenter Enteral Nutr.* 2011;35(4):540–544.
19. Richardson DS, Branowicki PA, Zeidman-Rogers L, Mahoney J, MacPhee M. An evidence-based approach to nasogastric tube management: special considerations. *J Pediatr Nurs.* 2006;21(5):288–292.
20. Powers J, Luebbehusen M, Spitzer T, et al. Verification of an electromagnetic placement device compared with abdominal radiograph to predict accuracy of feeding tube placement. *JPEN J Parenter Enteral Nutr.* 2011;35(4):535–539.
21. Kline AM, Sorce L, Sullivan C, Weishaar J, Steinhorn DM. Use of a noninvasive electromagnetic device to place transpyloric feeding tubes in critically ill children. *Am J Crit Care.* 2011;20(6):453–459.
22. Stumpf JL, Kurian RM, Vuong J, Dang K, Kraft MD. Efficacy of a creon delayed-release pancreatic enzyme protocol for

clearing occluded enteral feeding tubes. *Ann Pharmacother.* 2014;48(4):483–487.

23. *Enteralite™ Infinity™ Ambulatory Feeding Pumps.* Salt Lake City, UT: Moog Medical Devices Group; February 3, 2014.

24. Huang EY, Chen C, Abdullah F, et al. Strategies for the prevention of central venous catheter infections: an American pediatric surgical association outcomes and clinical trials committee systematic review. *J Pediatr Surg.* 2011;46(10):2000–2011.

25. Miller-Hoover S. Pediatric central line: bundle implementation and outcomes. *J Infus Nurs.* 2011;34(1):36–48.

26. O'Grady NP, Alexander M, Burns LA, et al. *Guidelines for the Prevention of Intravascular Catheter-Related Infections.* Atlanta, GA: Centers for Disease Control and Prevention; 2011.

27. Ayers P, Adams S, Boullata J, et al. A.S.P.E.N. parenteral nutrition safety consensus recommendations. *JPEN J Parenter Enteral Nutr.* 2014;38(3):296–333.

28. DiChicco R, Seidner DL, Brun C. Tip position of long-term central venous catheter devices used for parenteral nutrition. *JPEN J Parenter Enteral Nutr.* 2007;31(5):382–387.

29. Anderson C, Graupman PC, Hall WA. Pediatric intracranial complications of central venous catheter placement. *Pediatr Neurosurg.* 2004;40:28–31.

30. Parikh S, Narayann V. Misplaced peripherally inserted central catheter: an unusual cause of stroke. *Pediatr Neurol.* 2004;30(3):210–212.

31. Piper HG, deSilva NT, Amaral JG, Wales PW. Peripherally inserted central catheters for long-term parenteral nutrition in infants with intestinal failure. *J Pediatr Gastrenterol Nutr.* 2013;56(5):578–581.

32. Quach C, Milstone AM, Perpete C, Bonenfant M, Moorer DL, Perreault T. Chlorhexidine bathing in a tertiary care neonatal intensive care unit: impact on central line-associated bloodstream infections. *Infect Control Hosp Epidemiol.* 2014;35(2):158–163.

33. Panagiotounakou P, Antonogeorgos G, Gounari E, Papakakis S, Labadaridis J, Gounaris AK. Peripherally inserted central venous catheters: frequency of complications in premature newborn depends on the insertion site. *J Perinatol.* 2014;34(6):461–463.

34. Milstone AM, Reich NG, Advani S, et al. Catheter dwell time and CLABSIs in neonates with PICCs: a multicenter cohort study. *Pediatrics.* 2013;132(6):1609–1615.

35. Graf JM, Newman CD, McPherson ML. Sutured securement of peripherally inserted central catheters yields fewer complications in pediatric patients. *JPEN J Parenter Enteral Nutr.* 2006;30(6):532–535.

36. Frey AM, Shears GJ. Why are we stuck on tape and suture? *J Infus Nurs.* 2006;29(1):34–38.

37. Chelliah A, Heydon KH, Zaoutis TE. Observational trial of antibiotic-coated central venous catheters in critically ill pediatric patients. *Pediatr Infect Dis.* 2007;26(9):816–820.

38. Reyes JA, Habash ML, Taylor RP. Femoral central venous catheters are not associated with higher rates of infection in the pediatric critical care population. *Am J Infect Control.* 2012;40(1):43–47.

39. Ozbek S, Avdin BK, Apiliogullari S, et al. Left femoral vein is a better choice for cannulation in children: a computed tomography study. *Pediatr Anaesth.* 2013;23(6):524–528.

40. Cohen AB, Dagli M, Stavropoulos SW, et al. Silicone and polyurethane tunneled infusion catheters: a comparison of durability and breakage rates. *J Vasc Interv Radiol.* 2011;22(5):638–641.

41. Fallon SC, Larimer EL, Gwilliam NR, et al. Increased complication rates associated with port-a-cath placement in pediatric patients: location matters. *J Ped Surg.* 2013;48(6):1263–1268.

42. Hanley C, Nagel K, Odame I, Fitzgerald P, Husain M. Immediate versus delayed access of implantable venous access devices: does the timing of access make a difference to the frequency of complications? *J Pediatr Hematol Oncol.* 2003;25(8):613–615.

43. Barton SJ, Chase T, Latham B. Comparing two methods to obtain blood specimens from pediatric central venous catheters. *J Pediatr Oncol Nurs.* 2004;21(6):320–326.

44. Adlard K. Examining the push-pull method of blood sampling from central venous access devices. *J Pediatr Oncol Nurs.* 2008;25(4);200–207.

45. Cole M, Price L, Parry A. A study to determine the minimum volume of blood necessary to be discarded from a central venous catheter before a valid sample is obtained in children. *Pediatr Blood Cancer.* 2007;48:687–695.

46. New research shows effectiveness of SwabCap. *Infection Control Today.* September 20, 2010. http://www.infectioncontroltoday.com/news/2010/09/new-research-shows-effectiveness-of-swabcap.aspx. Accessed May 28, 2014.

47. Buchini S, Scarsini S, Montico M, Buzzetti R, Ronfani L, Decorti C. Management of central venous catheters in pediatric onco-hematology using 0.9% sodium chloride and positive-pressure-valve needleless connector. *Eur J Oncol Nurs.* 2014;18(4):393–396.

48. Feldman KW, Hickman RO. The central venous catheter as a source of medical chaos in Munchausen syndrome by proxy. *Pediatr Surg.* 1998;334:623–627.

49. Peroni KP, Nespor C, Ng M, et al. Evaluation of ethanol lock therapy in pediatric patients on long-term parenteral nutrition. *Nutr Clin Pract.* 2013;28(2):226–231.

50. Jones BA, Hull MA, Richardson DS, et al. Efficacy of ethanol locks in reducing central venous catheter infections in pediatric patients with intestinal failure. *J Pediatr Surg.* 2010;45(6):1287–1293.

51. Valentine KM. Ethanol lock therapy for catheter-associated blood stream infections in a pediatric intensive care unit. *Pediatr Crit Care Med.* 2011;12(6):292–296.

52. Hndrup MM, Moller JK, Schroder H. Central venous catheters and catheter locks in children with cancer: a prospective randomized trial of taurolidine versus heparin. *Pediatr Blood Cancer.* 2013;60(8):1292–1298.

53. Chu HP, Brind J, Tomar R, Hill S. Significant reduction in central venous catheter-related bloodstream infections in children on HPN after starting treatment with taurolidine line lock. *J Pediatr Gastrenterol Nutr.* 2012;55(4):403–407.

54. Denaburg M, Patel S. Salvage antibiotic-lock therapy in critically ill pediatric patients: a pharmacological review for pediatric intensive care unit nurses. *Adv Crit Care.* 2013;24(3):233–238.

55. Gasior AC, Marty Knott E, St. Peter SD. Management of peripherally inserted central catheter associated deep vein thrombosis in children. *Pediatr Surg Int.* 2013;29(5):445–449.

56. Haddad H, Lee KS, Higgins A, McMillan D, Price V, El-Naggar W. Routine surveillance ultrasound for the management of central venous catheters in neonates. *J Pediatr.* 2014;164(1):118–122.

Test Your Knowledge Answers

1. The correct answer is **A**. The peripheral vein is the most appropriate venous access option for an infant who cannot seemingly tolerate anything enterally but should turn around in just a few days.

2. The correct answer is **D**. This child is under the recommended weight of > 5 kg.

3. The correct answer is **D**. Families should receive a temporary catheter prior to discharge, along with written instructions for what to do in case the G tube comes out in the first 8 weeks post-insertion.

4. The correct answer is **A** or **D**. Ideally pH is used, but in some patients an x-ray may be indicated, so either answer would be acceptable and certainly superior to the other options.

34

Enteral Nutrition Support: Determining the Best Way to Feed

Jessica Monczka, RD, LDN, CNSC

CONTENTS

Learning Objectives

1. Define indications for enteral nutrition support in infants and children.
2. Explain the options for the delivery of enteral nutrition including route of tube placement, site of feeding delivery, and schedule of feeding regimen, considering the benefits and risks of each option.
3. Identify complications associated with enteral nutrition, as well as monitoring parameters for tube-fed patients.

Introduction

Enteral nutrition (EN), the process of providing nutrients via the gastrointestinal tract (GIT), is the preferred method of providing nutrition support to pediatric patients who cannot meet their nutrient needs via oral intake alone. EN can be provided by mouth or by feeding tube; for the purposes of this chapter, EN will refer to nonoral feeding via the GIT.

In patients with a functional and safely accessible GIT, EN is preferred over parenteral nutrition (PN) support for a number of reasons including the following:[1-4]

- Supports normal endocrine, paracrine, and neural function
- Improves mesenteric blood flow
- Decreases GIT permeability and prevents structural and functional alterations of the gut barrier
- Promotes pancreatic and biliary secretions
- Lowers the risk of metabolic complications (glucose and electrolyte disturbances, aluminum toxicity) compared to PN
- Reduces infection risk

- Lowers cost
- Maintains gut-related immune system function

It has been well established that EN is preferred over the parenteral route whenever possible. Unfortunately, randomized, controlled trials are lacking, and recommendations have been made using lower quality evidence. In addition to the moral implications of withholding nutrition support for pediatric patients, blinding a study to examine the outcomes of EN versus PN would likely not be possible. Despite the lack of randomized, controlled trials, EN is associated with improved outcomes and should be the preferred mode of delivery when nutrition support is indicated. In the pediatric intensive care unit, a protocolized EN regimen, including promoting early EN and minimizing interruptions, may increase enteral nutrient delivery and positive outcomes.[5-7]

Indications for EN

EN may be the appropriate therapy for infants and children with a variety of diagnoses, for short- or long-term support. If the GIT is functional, EN is indicated and would be the preferred mode of nutritional support. In situations where the GIT is not fully functional, EN supplemented by PN may be indicated. The indications for EN generally fall into the following categories:[8]

Inadequate Oral Intake

Some medical conditions make it difficult to consume adequate food and hydration by mouth. Intake may be inadequate for several different reasons: developmental (eg, preterm infants), behavioral (eg, feeding aversions, fatigue), or anatomical (eg, cancer, burns, mucositis, etc).

Increased nutritional need is a frequent etiology for inadequate oral intake in children. Infants with congenital heart disease (CHD), for example, experience high metabolic demand coupled with reduced splanchnic blood flow leading to difficulty achieving optimal growth with oral intake alone. Allowing oral feeding attempts of short duration (dictated by the level of tachypnea and tachycardia with feeding) supplemented with EN is common practice for CHD infants who are experiencing failure to thrive.

Children with cystic fibrosis (CF) can have nutrient needs 150%–200% of healthy age-matched peers due to increased work of breathing and malabsorption. Body mass index for age correlates directly with pulmonary function tests and positive outcomes for these patients; therefore, meeting elevated nutrient needs is imperative. Greater than 90% of CF patients also have difficulty absorbing nutrients due to pancreatic insufficiency. Children with CF may bene-

fit from a percutaneous endoscopic gastrostomy (PEG) tube placement for long-term EN supplementation.[9]

Airway Protection

In some situations, it may not be safe for children to take nutrients orally. Infants born prematurely have immature suck-swallow-breathe coordination until approximately 34 weeks gestation and will require EN for safe administration of enteral nutrients. Following open heart surgery, infants can develop a paralyzed vocal cord and may have aspiration with attempts to take oral fluid. In these infants, a speech or occupational therapy consult and an oropharyngeal motility study may be indicated to evaluate safety of oral intake. Similarly, older children who have had an extended airway intubation may be unable to safely take oral nutrients and require short- or long-term EN support.

Inadequate Intestinal Function

Children with gastrointestinal dysfunction may require EN. Slow continuous drip feedings may improve nutrient absorption in a child who is unable to meet needs by mouth due to suboptimal bolus assimilation. Specialty formulas with peptide or amino acid–based protein sources, which are less palatable for oral consumption but can be delivered via enteral feeding tube, may be required in children with poor digestion and absorption. EN may be used as primary therapy in certain conditions including inborn errors of metabolism, eosinophilic esophagitis, and Crohn's disease (Table 34-1).

Contraindications to EN Support

In some situations, providing nutrition support via the GIT is not the best choice. If the GIT cannot be reached safely, EN may be contraindicated. Severe mucositis or severe thrombocytopenia in an oncology patient could lead to further damage with enteral feeding tube placement. Facial or esophageal injuries or burns could also preclude safe access to the GIT. Signs and symptoms that the gut is not functioning properly, such as gastrointestinal bleeding, ileus, free air, or pneumotosis on abdominal imaging, should be considered carefully and may be signs of an unsafe situation for EN support. During episodes of hemodynamic instability, mesenteric blood flow is diminished and the potential for ischemic bowel damage needs to be considered.

Critically ill children may be unable to tolerate EN due to hemodynamic instability, vasopressor medications (eg, dopamine, dobutamine, epinephrine), or extracorporeal membrane oxygenation (ECMO), although this remains an

Table 34-1. Indications for Enteral Nutrition

Inadequate Oral Intake		
Increased nutrient needs	Cystic fibrosis Bronchopulmonary dysplasia CHD Renal disease Infection Surgery Burn Trauma Failure to thrive	Unable to meet needs via PN due to elevated nutrient requirements
Developmental	Preterm birth Prolonged intubation in a neonate or infant Neuromuscular disorders Neurological impairment	Immature suck-swallow-breathe coordination until ~34 weeks
Behavioral	Feeding aversions Unpalatable diet Anorexia nervosa or other feeding disorder	Multiple or traumatic intubations Chronic illness Prolonged EN requirement Metabolic or GI disorder requiring unpalatable EN formula
Anatomical	Cancer, burns, mucositis Congenital malformation Tracheoesophageal fistula Oral intubation	Can interfere with adequate intake if oral/esophageal involvement
Airway Protection		
Anatomical	Tracheoesophageal fistula Paralyzed vocal cord Severe reflux requiring postpyloric EN route	Congenital malformation Laryngeal nerve damage during open heart surgery can lead to aspiration with oral fluid attempts
Developmental	Neurodevelopmental delay Cerebral palsy	Unable to safely swallow
Inadequate Intestinal Function		
Malabsorption	Short bowel syndrome High output ostomy Crohn's disease Pancreatic insufficiency	Continuous EN infusion may be required to ensure maximum nutrient absorption

area of controversy.[10] In periods of hemodynamic instability, clinicians may be hesitant to feed enterally due to risk of bowel ischemia. However, critically ill pediatric patients have been shown to tolerate full-strength, continuous EN while receiving ECMO[10] and tolerate goal EN while receiving cardiovascular medication support (continuous infusion of dopamine, dobutamine, epinephrine, norepineph-

rine, or phenylephrine).[11] Once clinically stable, the ECMO patient may tolerate and perhaps benefit from EN, provided the medical team is vigilant in monitoring for any signs of feeding intolerance.[10,12,13] If less than goal rate EN is tolerated, a combination of EN and PN support to fully meet nutritional needs may be warranted. It can be difficult to determine which child will tolerate EN, and feeding decisions must be made on a case-by-case basis.

Determining the Appropriate EN Route and Regimen

When initiating EN in hospitalized children, the route of tube introduction, as well as the site of nutrient administration, are considerations that need to be made by the multidisciplinary team.

Site of Delivery: Gastric Versus Postpyloric

Gastric feeding tubes are easier to place and provide a more physiologic feeding method than postpyloric delivery. The gastric route also allows for bolus feeding methods and a more hyperosmolar formula. When it is safe to do so, gastric provision of EN is recommended. In premature infants receiving human milk, bolus feedings may reduce losses of fat, calcium, and phosphorus from the milk.[14] In some situations, it may not be possible to administer adequate formula into the stomach. Gastroparesis or gastric outlet obstruction may restrict gastric emptying, requiring a postpyloric route to provide adequate nutrients. If the child is at high risk for aspiration, postpyloric feeding may be the safer method.

Hospitalized infants and children at high risk for aspiration include those with:

- Neurologic dysfunction
- Vocal cord paralysis
- Swallowing dysfunction
- Anatomic problems—cleft palate, laryngeal cleft, esophageal atresia, tracheoesophageal fistula, duodenal obstruction, malrotation
- Gastroparesis
- Gastric outlet obstruction
- Previous surgical interventions to the GIT

In children receiving mechanical ventilation, postpyloric nutrient delivery may improve the percentage of goal volume delivered.[15] There is insufficient evidence to make a practice recommendation, however, and the site of formula administration in this population should be determined on a case-by-case basis.[16] As the critically ill child requiring postpyloric feeds begins to stabilize, EN should be transitioned to a more physiologic gastric bolus feeding method as tolerated. If long-term EN is in the child's nutrition plan, they should transition to a practical home EN regimen as soon as possible.

Difficulties associated with postpyloric tube placement need to be considered when deciding about tube placement. Postpyloric positioning requires experienced personnel and careful technique, and complications such as pneumothorax and malpositioning need to be included in the decision-making process.

There are no clear recommendations for preterm infants regarding the site of EN delivery. A 2013 Cochrane review of premature infants given gastric or posypyloric feedings found no beneficial effect of postpyloric delivery. In fact, an increased rate of gastrointestinal disturbance and mortality was seen in preterm infants with postpyloric feeding tubes.[17] The authors recommended cautious interpretation of the results, however, as the postpylorically fed infants tended to be a sicker and more premature group.

Route of Tube Placement: Nasoenteric Versus Semipermanent

The tube that will physically deliver the EN can be placed in various locations depending on the desired route of administration, and the type of feeding tube will be different depending on the route.

While length of therapy has the most influence, some clinical scenarios may dictate one route over another. For instance, trauma or surgery to the upper GIT may cause a child to require transabdominal tube placement, even if for shorter-term enteral access. In the opposite scenario, congenital malformations or abdominal surgery may cause a child to require a nasoenteric feeding route, even in the setting of long-term EN.

Nasal or oroenterically placed feeding tubes can be done at the bedside by trained personnel. Correct placement should be confirmed before each use. This route is relatively simple, does not require sedation, and leaves no permanent scarring. Fine bore feeding tubes (silicone and polyurethane) are flexible and less likely to cause erosions, inflammation, or strictures. Fine bore tubes can be left in place for up to 8 weeks, depending on the manufacturer. However, nasally or orally placed feeding tubes may significantly contribute to oral feeding aversion for chronically ill infants and young children.

When long-term EN is anticipated (greater than 6–12 weeks), semipermanent access via the transabdominal route (gastrostomy tube) should be considered by the multidisciplinary team. These tubes require a sedated procedure for

placement and when removed will leave a small abdominal scar. Caregiver input should be included in the decision-making process.

Semipermanent feeding tube placement techniques are as follows:

- Endoscopically (percutaneous endoscopic gastrostomy or PEG)
- Radiologically
- Surgically

PEG insertion is the most common technique due to the decreased complication rate and cost. Patients can receive a PEG feeding tube and be discharged home within 1–2 days if there are no complications or problems with formula tolerance. Despite historical data showing no major complications when EN resumed 6 hours post-PEG placement,[18] the practice varies widely, with EN generally started 4–24 hours post-PEG. More recent studies have shown no increased complications when EN started 3–4 hours post-PEG.[19,20] See Chapter 33 for a more in-depth discussion on placement techniques.

Initiation and Advancement

When initiating EN, the first step to consider is which method of feeding would best fit the current clinical picture. Intermittent or bolus feeding more closely matches what a normal oral diet would entail and may therefore be more physiological. Bolus feeds should not be given in a shorter period of time than a child would be expected to consume if given an oral feeding and should not be spaced out beyond their normal between-meal times. For example, infants are generally given feedings every 3–4 hours for a total of 6–8 feedings per day, while older children may tolerate their full daily volume with 4 bolus feedings per day. Maximum volumes for continuous and bolus feedings are determined by the child's response to the regimen, weight gain and growth, and overall GI status.[21-23]

In some situations, such as severe diarrhea and malabsorption, or reduced splanchnic blood flow in the setting of CHD, continuous feeding may increase absorption of enteral nutrients and improve growth.[24] For a critically ill child with labile hemodynamics requiring multiple drips, continuous feeds would provide the lowest possible infusion rates and may be the best option to achieve successful enteral feeding.

Initiation and advancement is dependent on the patient's age, underlying disease, risk of refeeding syndrome or other complications, and current clinical condition. In some cases the child may be too unstable to tolerate more than a small trophic rate of EN; however, providing a combination of EN and PN support will provide some positive gastrointestinal benefit while providing the remainder of nutrient needs parenterally.

Complications and Monitoring

Successful delivery of the EN prescription can be complicated by a number of mechanical and metabolic abnormalities.[21] For the developing infant or young child, lack of oral stimulation during prolonged periods of EN support can have profound effects on feeding success after the child recovers and has been deemed ready to safely attempt an oral diet. Early therapy with speech and occupational therapists is paramount to inducing optimal oral recovery. Infectious, gastrointestinal, pulmonary, metabolic, or tube-related mechanical complications can occur. Prior to starting an EN regimen, the child's medical and nutritional history should be considered, including the period of nil per os (NPO) status prior to initiating EN as well as any preexisting physical or biochemical abnormalities.

Mechanical

Although generally less severe than the complications associated with the parenteral route, enteral tube–related problems are common.

Nasoenteric Tubes: Modern feeding tubes are smaller and more flexible and are associated with fewer problems than their predecessors. Correct placement should be confirmed before initial feeding, although the optimal safe method is not well agreed upon. Tubes can migrate from their intended position; for instance, a postpyloric tube may be inadvertently pulled back into the stomach, putting a child at risk for aspiration. Tubes should be monitored for correct position (monitoring is covered in more detail in Chapter 36). Tube occlusion can occur when medications are given without adequate water flushes or when added directly to the enteral formula causing viscous or curdled formula.

Gastric Tubes: Semipermanent gastric tubes can be fitted too loose or too tight causing chronic inflammation at the stoma site or leakage of gastric contents. Tubes can be placed improperly with the bumper or balloon inflated inside the abdominal cavity, with subsequent EN infusion into the peritoneum. Chronic irritation at the stoma site can lead to granulation tissue. Excessive pain at the tube site and inability to twist the tube in its tract can indicate buried bumper syndrome, which is a rarer but fairly serious late complication of gastric tube placement.

For more detailed information regarding feeding tube problems and troubleshooting ideas, see Table 33-1 in Chapter 33.

Gastrointestinal

Abdominal distension, cramping, nausea, vomiting, and diarrhea can occur with EN. Symptoms may be associated with an acute gastroenteritis, side effects of medications, rapid administration of bolus feedings, formula intolerance, or malabsorption. Liquid formulations of pediatric medications often contain sugar or sugar substitutes that can contribute to loose stools. Antibiotics diminish healthy gut flora and can cause diarrhea.

Constipation is also common among infants and children. Inadequate fluid intake, limited mobility, and narcotic administration can contribute to constipation, as well as an underlying medical condition, gastric dysmotility, or small bowel obstruction. Monitoring stooling patterns in hospitalized children and prescribing adequate softeners or motility agents can help prevent constipation-related intolerance of EN.

Hypertonic feeds delivered postpylorically or rapid gastric emptying can lead to dumping syndrome. For the latter, cornstarch is sometimes included with the feeding regimen to try to minimize hypoglycemia that can be associated with dumping.

Stool studies checking for reducing substances, inflammatory markers, guaiac, or bacterial cultures can help differentiate the cause of gastrointestinal distress. Careful evaluation of the tube location, formula prescription, and medication regimen can help identify potential problems. Small bowel bacterial overgrowth should be considered in the differential diagnosis in patients with a history of gastrointestinal problems.

Oral Motor Deficit

Pediatric patients receiving EN for an extended period of time may have difficulty resuming oral feeding. Infants who are kept NPO for prolonged periods of time do not receive normal oral motor stimulation and cannot achieve their developmental milestones for feeding. Preterm infants should receive oral stimulation therapy throughout their hospitalization, with nonnutritive sucking encouraged at approximately 30 weeks gestation. They should begin to develop coordinated suck-swallow-breathe patterns between 32 and 34 weeks gestation. Older children should be evaluated for safe swallowing function, with appropriate ongoing oral motor interventions to minimize declines during EN therapy. Involving the speech-language or occupational therapist early and prioritizing oral skills throughout the duration of EN therapy will help achieve successful reintroduction of oral nourishment in children able to wean off EN.

Refeeding Syndrome

Malnourished patients at risk for refeeding syndrome should be monitored closely when initiating and advancing EN. During starvation, total body electrolyte stores are depleted. This may not be evident in laboratory testing as intracellular minerals are not measured in serum samples. As glucose supplied by nutrition support (enteral or parenteral) is infused, insulin stimulates the sodium-potassium ATPase channel to transport glucose into the cell. Serum levels of phosphorus, potassium, and magnesium are depleted as they are taken up by the cell. Additional information pertaining to refeeding syndrome can be found in chapters 19 and 29.

Drug-Nutrient Interactions

It is important to keep medication compatibility in mind when creating a nutrition plan for initiation, advancement, and goal feeds. The EN regimen may need to be adjusted to account for nutrient-medication incompatibilities. Certain medications may require EN to be held for a predetermined time around each dose. Working with the multidisciplinary team to develop the EN plan will ensure medication compatibility is taken into consideration.

Micronutrient Deficiency

Many pediatric diagnoses will alter the energy needs of children, causing them to require much more or much less formula than the standard reference child of the same age and size. The majority of available EN products are formulated in a fixed ratio to meet energy needs in a predetermined volume. Since feeds are primarily ordered to meet energy needs, children with very high or very low energy needs may not have their needs met by a single enteral formula product. Children with severe developmental delays may require significantly less energy than the recommended dietary reference intake for age and, therefore, will receive considerably less formula than another child of the same size. This can lead to deficiencies in micronutrients, protein, and fluid. Specific micronutrient intake provided by the nutrition prescription should be calculated and supplements provided to ensure nutrient needs are met. Close monitoring for biochemical or clinical signs of micronutrient alterations will help identify problems and guide treatment. Special attention should be paid to providing adequate sodium and fluid intake, with supplements included in the feeding regimen as needed.[25,26] Free water flushes should be added to the EN regimen to ensure fluid needs are met. Chronically ill children are often vitamin D deficient and 25-hydroxyvitamin D [25(OH)D] levels should be checked in patients deemed at risk. Risk factors for vitamin D deficiency are as follows:[27-29]

- Antiepileptic medication use
- Antiretroviral medication use
- Obesity
- Malabsorption syndromes (eg, CF, inflammatory bowel disease, Crohn's disease)
- Nonambulatory status
- Breastfed infants

In summary, patients receiving EN should be monitored for complications. GI complications may manifest clinically as abdominal distension, vomiting, or diarrhea. Tube-related mechanical problems should be evaluated and treated appropriately to avoid serious complications. Biochemical indices should be monitored to avoid micronutrient deficiencies or refeeding syndrome in patients deemed at risk. If respiratory symptoms occur with feeds, aspiration should be ruled out. EN regimens should be frequently reassessed to ensure complications are addressed, macronutrient and micronutrient needs are met, and the optimal nutrition plan is in place.

EN Formula Selection

Human milk and infant and pediatric formulas are covered in detail in Chapters 11, 12, and 13. Age-appropriate enteral formulas should be chosen, with options for condition- or disease-specific formulations as indicated. Although in the past adult formulas have been diluted for use in children greater than 1 year of age, there are now a variety of appropriate products available for ages 1 to 10, which avoids problems with inadequate micronutrient provision from diluted formulas.

The American Academy of Pediatrics recommends that all premature infants should receive human milk, using pasteurized donor human milk if the mother's own milk is not available.[30] For any infant weighing less than 1.5 kg, human milk fortification should be used to ensure adequacy of macronutrients and micronutrients for optimal growth.[31,32]

EN Formula Safety

Microbial contamination of EN formulas is common.[33-37] Powdered formulas are not sterile and have been implicated in infections leading to meningitis and necrotizing enterocolitis.[38] When clinically acceptable sterile liquid formulations are commercially available, they should be used in lieu of powdered formula. More recently, closed system enteral products have become commercially available. Closed system containers can be directly spiked to the tube feeding line rather than opening containers of formula and pouring into a feeding bag. With the introduction of closed enteral feeding systems, EN safety has improved for adolescent patients and adults, and the safe hang time has increased. However, closed enteral feeding systems are generally 1 liter and larger, so for infants and young children, small feeding volumes preclude the use of these safer closed EN systems.

Formula manipulation with powdered products is common in pediatrics and can be another source of contamination. For hospitalized infants, formula should be prepared by specialized personnel using aseptic technique to minimize contamination. For home EN, parents and caregivers should be instructed on good hand washing and clean technique to minimize contamination risk (Table 34-2).

Administration sets for open system EN should be changed at least every 24 hours. More information is available as part of the A.S.P.E.N. Enteral Nutrition Practice Recommendations.[21]

Preparing for Home EN

Pediatric patients dependent on EN, who are otherwise stable for discharge, can receive their continuous or intermittent feeds at home via pump or syringe. The responsibility of providing safe EN shifts from well-trained medical staff to inexperienced parents or caregivers at discharge. Thorough education and training must be provided by qualified members of the healthcare team. The home caregiver must demonstrate competence in the safe and effective preparation and administration of home EN.

Home EN discharge teaching should include:[39]
- Knowledge of the type of formula
- Method of administration and feeding schedule
- Route of administration and duration of therapy
- Proper care of the enteral access device
- Product safety information including hang time and stability at room temperature
- Clean technique
- Monitoring and identification of potential complications

Home EN education should also include information about outpatient resources and peer support groups including The Oley Foundation (www.oley.org), a national, independent, nonprofit organization that provides up-to-date information, outreach services, conference activities, and emotional support for home EN patients and families.

Conclusion

Every child should be evaluated individually when determining the best way to provide optimal nutrition to promote growth and development. Nutritional needs should be reevaluated on a regular basis to ensure appropriate nutrient delivery and optimal growth and development. Pediatric data may not be rigorous, and more clinical trials are needed to determine the best way to feed hospitalized infants and children. When determining the nutrition plan for home, the entire family must be taken into consideration. What works for one child and caregiver may not work for another. Factors to consider may include the patient's baseline nutrition status, the functionality of the GIT, access options, administration schedule, and modality. It is essential to be flexible and supportive when working with caregivers to develop a nutrition plan of care that is best for their child and their lives.

Test Your Knowledge Questions

1. DB is a 9-year-old boy with CF admitted with pulmonary exacerbation. His BMI for age plots below the 10th percentile. He takes a high-calorie, high-protein diet and takes pancreatic enzymes with every meal and snack. He has undergone RD counseling during previous visits and has incorporated liquid supplements by mouth. Your recommendations include:
   a. Encourage a high-calorie, high-protein diet with snacks between each meal.
   b. Evaluate the pancreatic enzyme dosing to determine if he is receiving optimal replacement therapy

Table 34-2. Room Temperature Formula Stability[21]

4 Hour Hang Time
Sterile Formula in an Open System (Neonate)
Nonsterile Powdered Formula
Nonsterile Powdered Additives
Human Milk
8 Hour Hang Time
Sterile Formula in an Open System for Inpatient Administration
12 Hour Hang Time
Sterile Formula in an Open System for Home Administration
24–48 Hour Hang Time
Sterile Formula in a Closed System

and ask about the stooling pattern to evaluate for malabsorption.

   c. Encourage liquid-nutrition supplements at least 3 times daily.

   d. Recommend a PEG tube for supplemental EN.

   e. Check vitamin levels and adjust supplements as needed.

2. You are rounding in the pediatric cardiac intensive care unit on a 15-day-old boy with hypoplastic left heart syndrome s/p palliative surgery, tolerating a small amount of human milk given via nasogastric feeding tube but unable to advance to goal rate and wean off PN due to worsening tachypnea, tachycardia, and cool extremities. The medical team would like your input on the nutrition plan. You would recommend to:

   a. Advance the EN and wean the PN off because double-blinded, randomized controlled trials have shown clear benefits of EN over PN in pediatric patients.

   b. Continue the EN plus PN combination nutrition support to ensure 100% of the infant's estimated nutritional needs are met.

   c. Hold the EN and increase PN back to goal rate since the child does not seem to be tolerating enteral feeds.

   d. Change to elemental formula, which is better tolerated in hemodynamically unstable infants.

3. This patient may be unable to tolerate adequate nutrient intake by mouth:

   a. Preterm infant at 30 weeks gestation.

   b. Term infant with Pierre Robin syndrome.

   c. 9-year-old male with severe autism.

   d. All of the above.

4. A 10-year-old child with cerebral palsy is admitted from home with respiratory illness. The child has very low energy needs as evidenced by being overweight despite receiving 50% of the dietary reference intake for age from the home EN regimen. Your nutrition plan includes:

   a. Calculating the maintenance fluid needs and adjusting the fluid boluses if needed.

   b. Adding sodium chloride to maintain at least 1–2 mEq per kg per day from the daily nutrition prescription.

   c. Checking vitamin and mineral levels and supplementing as needed.

   d. All of the above.

Acknowledgments

The author of this chapter for the second edition of this text wishes to thank Liesje Nieman Carney, RD, CNSD, LDN; Andrea Nepa, MS, RD, CSP, LDN; Sherri Shubin Cohen, MD, MPH; Amy Dean, MPH, RD, LDN; Colleen Yanni, MS, RD, LDN; and Goldie Markowitz, MSN, CRNP, for their contributions to the first edition of this text.

References

1. Baker S, Baker R, Davis A. *Pediatric Nutrition Support*. Boston, MA: Jones & Bartlett; 2007.

2. Mehesh C, Sriram K, Lakshmiprabha V. Extended indications for enteral nutritional support. *Nutrition*. 2000;16:129–130.

3. McClave SA, Heyland DK. The physiologic response and associated clinical benefits from provision of early enteral nutrition. *Nutr Clin Pract*. 2009;24(3):305–315.

4. Matarese LE, Mullin GE, Raymond JL. Enteral nutrition. In: *The Health Professional's Guide to Gastrointestinal Nutrition*. Chicago, IL: Academy of Nutrition and Dietetics; 2014:235–257.

5. Mehta NM, Compher C. A.S.P.E.N. clinical guidelines: nutrition support of the critically ill child. *JPEN J Parenter Enteral Nutr*. 2009;33(3):260–276.

6. Martinez EE, Bechard LJ, Mehta NM. Nutrition algorithms and bedside nutrient delivery practices in pediatric intensive care units: an international multicenter cohort study. *Nutr Clin Prac*. 2014;29(3):360–367.

7. Mehta NM. Approach to enteral feeding in the PICU. *Nutr Clin Prac*. 2009;24:377–387.

8. Braegger C, Decsi T, Dias JA, et al. Practical approach to paediatric enteral nutrition: a comment by the ESPGHAN committee on nutrition. *JPEN J Pediatr Gastroenterol Nutr*. 2010;51:110–122.

9. Woestenenk JW, Castelijns SF, van der Ent CK, Houwen RH. Nutritional intervention in patients with Cystic Fibrosis: a systematic review. *J Cyst Fibros*. 2013;12(2):102–115.

10. Pettignano R, Heard M, Davis R, Labuz M, Hart M. Total enteral nutrition versus total parenteral nutrition during pediatric extracorporeal membrane oxygenation. *Crit Care Med*. 1998;26(2):358–363.

11. King W, Petrillo T, Pettignano R. Enteral nutrition and cardiovascular medications in the pediatric intensive care unit. *JPEN J Parenter Enteral Nutr*. 2004;28:334–338.

12. Jaksic T, Hull MA, Modi BP, Ching YA, George D, Compher C; American Society for Parenteral and Enteral Nutrition (A.S.P.E.N.) Board of Directors. Nutrition support of neonates supported with extracorporeal membrane oxygenation (ECMO). *JPEN Parenter Enteral Nutr*. 2010;34(3):247–253.

13. Cilley, RE, Wesley, JR, Zwischenberger, JB, Bartlett, RH. Gas exchange measurements in neonates treated with extracorporeal membrane oxygenation. *J Pediatr Surg*. 1988;23(4):306–311.

14. Rogers SP, Hicks, PD, Abrams SA. Continuous feedings of fortified human milk lead to nutrient losses of fat, calcium and phosphorous. *Nutrients*. 2010;2(3):230–240.

15. Meert KL, Daphtary KM, Metheny NA. Gastric vs small-bowel feeding in critically ill children receiving mechanical ventilation: a randomized controlled trial. *Chest*. 2004;126:872–878.

16. Mehta NM, Compher C. A.S.P.E.N. clinical guidelines: nutrition support of the critically ill child. *JPEN Parenter Enteral Nutr*. 2009;33(3):260–276.

17. Watson J, McGuire W. Transpyloric versus gastric tube feeding for preterm infants. *Cochrane Database Syst Rev*. 2013;(2):CD003487. doi:10.1002/14651858.CD003487.pub3.

18. Werlin S, Glicklich M, Cohen R. Early feeding after percutaneous endoscopic gastrostomy is safe in children. *Gastrointest Endosc*. 1994;40:692–693.

19. Corkins MR, Fitzgerald JF, Gupta SK. Feeding after percutaneous endoscopic gastrostomy in children: early feeding trial. *J Pediatr Gastroenterol Nutr*. 2010;50(6):625–627.

20. Islek A, Sayar E, Yilmaz A, Artan R. Percutaneous endoscopic gastrostomy in children: is early feeding safe? *J Pediatr Gastroenterol Nutr*. 2013;57(5):659–662.

21. Bankhead R, Boullata J, Brantley S, et al. Enteral nutrition practice recommendations. *JPEN J Parenter Enteral Nutr*. 2009;33(2):122–167.

22. Koletzko B, Goulet O, Hunt J, et al. Guidelines on paediatric parenteral nutrition of the European Society of Paediatric Gastroenterology, Hepatology, and Nutrition (ESPGHAN) and the European Society for Clinical Nutrition and Metabolism (ESPEN), supported by the European Society of Paediatric Research (ESPR). *J Pediatr Gastroenterol Nutr*. 2005;41;S28–S32.

23. Lord L, Harrington M. Enteral nutrition implementation and management. In: Merritt R, ed. *The A.S.P.E.N. Nutrition Support Practice Manual*. 2nd ed. Silver Spring, MD: American Society for Parenteral and Enteral Nutrition; 2005:76–89.

24. Axelrod D, Kazmerski K, Iyer K. Pediatric enteral nutrition. *JPEN Parenter Enteral Nutr*. 2006;30(1):S21–S26.

25. McGowan JE, Fenton TR, Wade AW, Branton JL, Robertson M. An exploratory study of sodium, potassium, and fluid nutrition status of tube-fed nonambulatory children with severe cerebral palsy. *Appl Physiol Nutr Metab*. 2012;37(4):715–723.

26. National Research Council. *Dietary Reference Intakes for Water, Potassium, Sodium, Chloride, and Sulfate*. Washington, DC: The National Academies Press; 2005.

27. Sentongo TA, Semaeo EJ, Stettler N, Piccoli DA, Stallings VA, Zemel BS. Vitamin D status in children, adolescents, and young adults with Crohn disease. *Am J Clin Nutr*. 2002;76(5):1077.

28. Pappa HM, Langereis EJ, Grand RJ, Gordon CM. Prevalence and risk factors for hypovitaminosis D in young patients with inflammatory bowel disease. *J Pediatr Gastroenterol Nutr*. 2011;53(4):361.

29. Shellhaas RA, Joshi SM. Vitamin D and bone health among children with epilepsy. *Pediatr Neurol*. 2010;42(6):385–393.

30. Johnston M, Landers S, Noble L, Szucs K, Viehmann L. Breastfeeding and the use of human milk. *Pediatrics*. 2012;129(3):827–841.

31. Sullivan S, Schanler RJ, Kim JH, et al. An exclusively human milk-based diet is associated with a lower rate of necrotizing enterocolitis than a diet of human milk and bovine milk-based products. *J Pediatr*. 2010;156:562–567.

32. Quigley MA, Henderson G, Anthony MY, McGuire W. Formula milk versus donor breast milk for feeding preterm or low birth weight infants. *Cochrane Database Syst Rev*. 2007;(4):CD002971.

33. Patchell CJ, Anderton A, MacDonald A, et al. Bacterial contamination of enteral feeds. *Arch Dis Child*. 1994;70:327–330.

34. Roy S, Rigal M, Doit C, et al. Bacterial contamination of enteral nutrition in a pediatric hospital. *J Hosp Infect*. 2005;59:311–316.

35. Kim H, Ryu JH, Beuchat LR. Attachment of and biofilm formation by *Enterobacter sakazakii* on stainless steel and enteral feeding tubes. *Appl Environ Microbiol*. 2006;72:5846–5856.

36. Anderton A, Nwoguh CE, McKune I, Morrison L, Grieg M, Clark B. A comparative study of the numbers of bacteria present in enteral feeds prepared and administered in hospital and the home. *J Hosp Inf*. 1993;23:43–49.

37. Bott L, Husson MO, Guimber D, et al. Contamination of gastrostomy feeding systems in children in a home-based enteral nutrition program. *J Pediatr Gastroenterol Nutr*. 2001;33:266–270.

38. Centers for Disease Control and Prevention. *Enterobacter sakazakii* infections associated with the use of powdered infant formula—Tennessee, 2001. *MMWR*. 2002;51:297–300.

39. Kovacevich DS, Frederick A, Kelly D, Nishikawa R, Young L; American Society for Parenteral and Enteral Nutrition Board of Directors; Standards for Specialized Nutrition Support Task Force. Standards for specialized nutrition support: home care patients. *Nutr Clin Prac*. 2005;20:579–590.

Test Your Knowledge Answers

1. The best answer in this clinical scenario is **D**. All choices are possible interventions that could be made, but this child is in nutritional failure and at this point a PEG feeding tube would be recommended to supplement his oral diet. Intermittent nocturnal feeds could provide additional nutrients while the child sleeps.

2. The best answer is **B**. While EN is certainly preferred if the GIT is functional, hemodynamically unstable infants may not tolerate goal EN. There is a lack of high-quality evidence comparing EN to PN, particularly in pediatric patients, so you would not be able to state this as a reason to wean off PN. If the infant is able to tolerate a small amount of enteral human milk, giving a combination of EN and PN support would be preferred over withholding EN altogether. Elemental formula would not be indicated over human milk in this patient.

3. The best answer is **D**. Preterm infants will not develop the suck-swallow-breathe mechanism until approximately 34 weeks gestation. Approximately 50% of infants born with Pierre Robin syndrome will require EN

support. Children with severe autism can have significant feeding aversions, making them unable to meet nutrient needs via oral intake alone.

4. The best answer is **D**. Fluids should be evaluated in children with low energy needs as they are at high risk for constipation. If receiving standard enteral formula in a fixed ratio dosed for energy needs, they will not meet their fluid needs via formula alone. Electrolytes may also be deficient. Sodium and potassium should be evaluated to ensure minimum needs are met. In addition to electrolytes, vitamin and mineral needs may not be met by the low volume of enteral formula. Vitamin D in particular is often deficient in chronically ill children due to medications (antiseizure therapies), inadequate supply in the enteral formula, poor sunlight exposure with chronic illness, and malabsorption.

35

Parenteral Nutrition Support

Catherine M. Crill, PharmD, FCCP, BCPS, BCNSP; and **Kathleen M. Gura**, PharmD, BCNSP, FASHP, FPPAG

CONTENTS

Learning Objectives

1. Determine the appropriateness for beginning parenteral nutrition therapy in a given pediatric patient.
2. Describe the typical macronutrient and micronutrient makeup of both central and peripheral parenteral nutrition formulations for neonates (preterm and term), infants, children, and adolescents.
3. Identify common complications with pediatric parenteral nutrition and describe how they are assessed and can be prevented and/or managed.
4. Identify ways to increase the safety of the parenteral nutrition process in institutions and at home, from order prescribing to administration.

Introduction

The practice of parenteral nutrition (PN) has been lifesaving in pediatric patients, such as premature neonates and patients with short bowel syndrome (SBS), who would otherwise not have been able to sustain themselves on an enteral diet alone. PN is a complex solution of macronutrients, micronutrients, fluid, electrolytes, and additives. The clinician's role in providing safe and effective PN support to pediatric patients requires knowledge of appropriate indications and access for PN, optimal macronutrient and micronutrient provision, and assessment for and management of complications. Safety in PN support must be ensured throughout the PN process, from prescribing to compounding and administration of PN, and to the transition to home PN support.

Indications for Parenteral Nutrition

PN is indicated in patients when the gastrointestinal (GI) tract is not functional or cannot be accessed, or when nutrient needs exceed what can be provided through enteral nutrition (EN).[1] PN is routinely used in premature neonates and patients with congenital heart disease, congenital anomalies of the GI tract, necrotizing enterocolitis (NEC), SBS, and other GI conditions. It is also routinely used in critically ill patients and patients receiving extracorporeal membrane oxygenation (ECMO).

Prematurity

Premature and low birth weight infants need a source of nutrition immediately after birth due to low nutrient reserves, increased energy expenditure, and immaturity of the GI tract, as well as their increased propensity for acute and chronic illness.[2,3] Premature infants may be unable to digest nutrients enterally due to immature intestinal development and low digestive enzyme production.[4] Early PN administration in low birth weight premature neonates results in improved outcomes in growth.[2,3,5] Thus, PN should be initiated in these patients within the first 24–48 hours of life and continued until adequate EN is tolerated. Starter PN solutions are often used in institutions with newborn intensive care units to provide early protein provision until an individual PN solution can be prescribed, compounded, and available for administration. These starter solutions contain dextrose and amino acids and may also contain a minimum amount of additives such as calcium and heparin. Premature infants, particularly those weighing < 1500 g, are also prone to reflux, generalized GI dysmotility, and delayed gastric emptying.[6] "Organized" gut motility does not begin until 32–34 weeks of gestation.[7] PN is weaned slowly as EN intake, oral intake, or both increase, so that overall the nutrient intake remains optimal during this transition.

Other neonates and infants should receive PN if it is anticipated that they will be unable to receive enteral feedings for more than 2–3 days. Infants have limited fat and glycogen stores, and when these are depleted, infants begin to catabolize protein stores for energy. EN is commonly withheld if the following conditions are present: severe respiratory failure associated with hypoxia and acidosis; hypotension treated with vasopressors; perinatal asphyxia with signs of organ involvement; clinical signs of NEC or intestinal obstruction; congenital heart disease with decreased left-sided outflow; patent ductus arteriosus with left to right shunt or requiring indomethacin or surgical ligation; or sepsis-associated paralytic ileus. In addition, red blood cell transfusion has been associated with decreased tissue perfusion in preterm infants receiving enteral feedings.[8] Due to concerns for development of NEC, some clinicians will hold enteral feedings and give PN support for 24–48 hours in preterm infants receiving blood transfusions.

Gastrointestinal Conditions

Several congenital anomalies of the GI tract (esophageal or intestinal atresias, tracheoesophageal fistula, malrotation with volvulus, Hirschsprung's disease, anorectal malformations, and abdominal wall defects) generally require PN support for a period of time while the patient is on bowel rest before and after surgical correction. In addition, children who develop GI disorders that temporarily prohibit the use of EN (appendicitis, chronic or intractable diarrhea or vomiting, malrotation, intussusception, severe inflammatory bowel disease, acute pancreatitis, obstruction, pseudoobstruction, motility disorders, or severe gastroesophageal reflux disease) are given PN support in order to maintain nutrition status during illness while the GI tract is inaccessible.

NEC, a condition primarily affecting premature infants, is characterized by GI ischemia and necrosis. NEC is managed with bowel decompression and rest, systemic antibiotic therapy, and potential surgical resection of necrotic bowel. NEC in infants requires PN because enteral feedings are withheld for 10 days to 3 weeks to support bowel healing and recovery.[9]

PN support is required in patients following major small bowel resection resulting in SBS. Common causes for SBS in pediatric patients are intestinal atresias, gastroschisis, NEC, Hirschsprung's disease, and volvulus.[10] Functional SBS may occur without resection and is the result of obstruction, dysmotility, or disease-associated loss of absorptive capacity. PN is always indicated for SBS in the immediate postoperative period; however, many individuals with SBS can adapt to enteral feeds and be successfully weaned from PN over time.[10,11] Individuals with intestinal failure, as defined by the inability to maintain protein-energy, fluid, electrolyte, or micronutrient balance, usually require PN long term.[12]

Critical Illness

Critically ill patients are at risk for malnutrition primarily due to protein catabolism that is directly related to the severity of their illness or injury.[13] While EN is the preferred method of feeding critically ill pediatric patients with a functioning GI tract, clinical factors such as hemodynamic instability and feeding intolerance often necessitate the use of PN support in these patients.[13] In infants and children with congenital heart disease, PN may be used until tolerance to

EN is established, especially preoperatively and postoperatively due to increased nutrient needs to support recovery. In patients who are receiving vasopressor medications (eg, dopamine, dobutamine, epinephrine), EN may be withheld due to concerns about bowel ischemia and the potential risk for NEC. PN is occasionally needed to treat individuals with chyle leaks (ie, chylothorax, chylous effusion, chylous ascites, or chylopericardium) who do not respond to enteral diets restricted in long-chain triglycerides (LCTs) and high in medium-chain triglycerides (MCTs).[14] Because intravenous (IV) fat emulsion (IVFE) is infused directly into the bloodstream and bypasses the lymph system, it does not affect the volume of chyle produced.

Extracorporeal Membrane Oxygenation

Treatment with ECMO and the use of vasopressor support may not be absolute contraindications to enteral feedings; however, many clinicians are hesitant to enterally feed these patients. Concerns about the possible effect of hypoxia on the gut during ECMO have led to the use of PN as the main source of nutrition support. A study in infants on ECMO receiving vasopressors compared PN to full-strength, continuous EN via either nasogastric or postpyloric feeding tubes.[15] No cases of NEC or intestinal perforation were documented. Although the PN group achieved goal calories more rapidly (3.07 ± 2.1 days vs 4.25 ± 2.6 days for the EN group), the benefits of EN outweighed the risks of PN. The authors concluded that vasoactive drug infusions should not be considered a contraindication to enteral feeding.[15] American Society for Parenteral and Enteral Nutrition (A.S.P.E.N.) guidelines recommend that nutrition support be initiated expeditiously in pediatric patients on ECMO. Generally, this is accomplished with PN initiation within 24 hours of ECMO cannulation; EN may be initiated when patients have stabilized clinically.[16]

Other Indications

Patients with failure to thrive, especially those with diarrheal losses, are commonly given PN to allow bowel rest and promote weight gain until the reason for the failure to thrive can be determined and adequate tolerance of EN can be established. Other indications for PN support in pediatric patients include high output fistulas, graft-vs-host disease, severe GI side effects of chemotherapy including radiation enteritis, cancer cachexia, diaphragmatic hernia, meconium aspiration, and organ failure (liver, renal, pulmonary, pancreas) when EN is contraindicated and the child is catabolic or in preparation for organ transplant in malnourished patients.[17,18] While severely malnourished patients with anorexia nervosa who require urgent nutrition rehabilitation may more readily accept PN rather than EN support, PN should be considered a last resort therapy with eating disorders.[19]

Parenteral Access

Vascular access is not defined by the initial point of entry, but by the position of the catheter tip. With central venous access devices (CVADs), the catheter tip should be in the distal portion of the superior vena cava or at the junction of the superior vena cava and the right atrium.[1] In the event that central access is not obtained, PN can be administered through a peripheral vein; however, the final osmolarity is limited to 900 mOsm/L to minimize risk of phlebitis and infiltration.[20] The PN components that impart the greatest osmolarity to a solution are protein (100 mOsm/%), dextrose (50 mOsm/%), and sodium and potassium salts (2–3 mOsm/mEq). With peripheral PN (PPN) solutions, dextrose concentration is limited to 10%–12.5%. This limitation means that the PPN requires a relatively large volume to adequately administer nutrients. In the critically ill infant or child, nutrient requirements often cannot be met with PPN due to fluid restriction. If PN support is expected to be needed for more than 7–10 days, central access should be obtained.[1] Adequate PN support requires a CVAD and allows for administration of a solution with a high osmolarity (ie, > 900 mOsm/L).

Macronutrients

See Table 35-1 for recommendations for macronutrient initiation and advancement in PN for pediatric patients.[17,20–23]

Protein

Protein is administered as a crystalline amino acid solution, which provides 4 kcal/g. Specialized amino acid solutions (see Table 35-2) are available for infants and children; these include TrophAmine 6% and 10% (B. Braun), Premasol 6% and 10% (Baxter Healthcare), and Aminosyn-PF 7% and 10% (Hospira). These specialized solutions contain increased concentrations of essential amino acids, including histidine and tyrosine, and low concentrations of phenylalanine, methionine, and glycine. They also contain glutamic acid, aspartic acid, taurine, and N-acetyl-L-tyrosine (TrophAmine, Premasol), which are not present in standard amino acid products. The pediatric amino acid products have a lower pH, which allows higher concentrations of calcium and phosphorus to be added to the solution. The addition of cysteine lowers the pH further, thereby optimizing calcium and phosphorus solubility within PN solutions.

Table 35-1. Recommendations for Initiation and Advancement of Macronutrients in Parenteral Nutrition[17,20-23]

	INITIATION		ADVANCE BY		GOALS	
INFANTS (< 1 y)	PRETERM	TERM	PRETERM	TERM	PRETERM	TERM
Protein (g/kg/day)[a]	3–4	2.5–3	–	–	3–4	2.5–3
Dextrose (mg/kg/min)	6–8	6–8	1–2	3.5	10–14 (max 14–18)	10–14 (max 14–18)
Fat (g/kg/day)	0.5–1	0.5–1	0.5–1	0.5–1	3 (max 0.15 g/kg/h)	2.5–3 (max 0.15 g/kg/h)
CHILDREN (1-10 y)						
Protein (g/kg/day)	1.5–2.5		–		1.5–2.5	
Dextrose (mg/kg/min)	3–6		2–3		8–10	
Fat (g/kg/day)	1–2		0.5–1		2–2.5	
ADOLESCENTS						
Protein (g/kg/day)	0.8–2		–		0.8–2	
Dextrose (mg/kg/min)	2.5–3		1–2		5–6	
Fat (g/kg/day)	1		1		1–2	

Glucose infusion rate (mg/kg/min) = [dextrose (g/day) × 1000] / [24 (h/day) × 60 (min/h) × weight (kg)].
[a]Protein does not need to be titrated; protein needs will be increased with critical illness.

TrophAmine and Aminosyn PF were designed to replicate plasma amino acid patterns of breastfed infants. Premasol, introduced in 2003, was formulated to be similar to TrophAmine; the only difference is that TrophAmine contains sodium metabisulfite as an antioxidant. Premasol and Aminosyn PF do not contain sulfites and may be used in patients with sulfite allergy. The use of TrophAmine compared with Aminosyn PF has been associated with a decrease in PN–associated liver disease (PNALD).[24]

Dextrose

Carbohydrate calories are supplied in PN through the use of dextrose, which provides 3.4 kcal/g. Final concentrations of dextrose in PN solutions used in pediatric patients range from 10% to 12.5% for PPN and up to 25% or higher for central PN. In general, the dextrose content in PN should not exceed the maximum glucose oxidation rate (see Table 35-1). Exceeding the glucose oxidation or glucose infusion rate results in fat production, a consequence that may be desired in the short term for some patients, such as very low birth weight preterm neonates.[25] However, excess glucose provision has been associated with hepatic steatosis and should be avoided in long-term PN patients at risk for PNALD.[23,25,26]

Intravenous Fat Emulsion

The availability of IVFE products in the United States has changed over the last several years (see Table 35-3).[27-29] While products containing soybean oil or a combination of safflower and soybean oils were once available, only the soybean oil emulsions are currently available. In addition, a 10% soybean oil emulsion is either no longer available (Intralipid product) or out of stock per the manufacturer (Liposyn III). In an effort to address IVFE product shortages, the U.S. Food and Drug Administration (FDA) has recently approved marketing for 2 additional IVFE products. Clinolipid 20% (Baxter Healthcare), an olive oil/soybean oil emulsion, received FDA approval in October 2013, but was still not available in the U.S. as of January 2015. Nutrilipid 20% (B. Braun), a soybean oil emulsion, received approval in August 2014 and became available in December 2014. The 10% IVFE products have a higher phospholipid to triglyceride ratio; higher phospholipids are associated with decreased triglyceride clearance in neonates and infants.[21] The 20% products are preferred when infusing IVFE with a 2-in-1 PN solution; 30% products should be reserved for use in total nutrient admixtures (TNAs). While a gram of fat provides 9 kcal, the caloric content of IVFE is slightly greater per gram (2 kcal/mL for 20% IVFE products) due to the additional calories from the egg phospholipids (emulsifier) and glycerin. The labeling for IVFE products contains a warning about pulmonary fat accumulation and deaths in preterm infants associated with IVFE infusion; infusion rate should be as slow as possible and should not exceed 0.25 g/kg/h.[28,29] Other sources recommend a lower maximum infusion rate of 0.15 g/kg/h.[30] The use of TNAs in neonates and infants is not recommended.[20]

Table 35-2. Chart Comparing the Commercially Available Pediatric Amino Acid Products[a]

COMPANY	B. BRAUN (MCGAW), BETHLEHEM, PA	HOSPIRA (ABBOTT), ABBOTT PARK, IL	BAXTER, DEERFIELD, IL
PRODUCT Introduction date (FDA approval date)	TROPHAMINE July 20, 1984	AMINOSYN PF Sept. 6, 1985	PREMASOL June 23, 2003
Amino acid content (g/100 mL)			
Essential amino acids			
Isoleucine	0.820	0.760	0.820
Leucine	1.400	1.200	1.400
Lysine	0.820	0.677	0.820
(added as lysine acetate)	1.200	–	–
Methionine	0.340	0.180	0.340
Phenylalanine	0.480	0.427	0.480
Threonine	0.420	0.512	0.420
Tryptophan	0.200	0.180	0.200
Valine	0.780	0.673	0.780
Cysteine	< 0.016	–	< 0.016
(as cysteine HCl H_2O)	< 0.024	–	–
Histidine	0.480	0.312	0.480
Tyrosine	0.240	0.044	0.240
(added as tyrosine	0.044	–	–
and N-acetyl-L-tyrosine)	0.240	–	–
Nonessential amino acids			
Alanine	0.540	0.698	0.540
Arginine	1.200	1.227	1.200
Proline	0.680	0.812	0.680
Serine	0.380	0.495	0.380
Glycine	0.360	0.385	0.360
L-Aspartic acid	0.320	0.527	0.320
L-Glutamic acid	0.500	0.820	0.500
Taurine	0.025	0.070	0.025
Sodium metabisulfite NF (as an antioxidant)	< 0.050	0	0
pH adjusted with glacial acetic acid USP			
Average pH (range)	5.5 (5.0–6.0)	5.5 (5.0–6.5)	5.5 (5.0–6.0)
Calculated osmolarity (mOsmol/L)	875	788	865
Total amino acids (g/L)	100	100	100
Total nitrogen (g/L)	15.5	15.2	15.5
Protein equivalent (g/L)	97	100	—
Electrolytes (mEq/L)			
Sodium	5	None	—
Acetate	97	46	94
Chloride	< 3	None	< 3

Source: FDA, U.S. Food and Drug Administration.
[a]Ten percent pediatric amino acid formulations.

Table 35-3. Comparison of Commercially Available[a] Intravenous Fat Emulsions[27-29]

PRODUCT	INTRALIPID	LIPOSYN III	NUTRILIPID
Manufacturer	Fresenius Kabi (through Baxter)	Hospira	B. Braun[b]
Concentrations	20%, 30%	10%, 20%, 30%	20%
Lipid source	Soybean oil	Soybean oil	Soybean oil
Availability	Available	Out of stock	Available
Fatty acid content, %			
Linoleic	44–62	54.5	48–58
Oleic	19–30	22.4	17–30
Palmitic	7–14	10.5	9–13
Linolenic	4–11	8.3	4–11
Stearic	1.4–5.5	4.2	2.5–5
Calories, kcal/mL			
10%	–	1.1	-
20%	2	2	2
30%	3	2.9	-
Egg yolk phospho-lipids, %			
10%	–	1.8	-
20%	1.2	1.2	1.2
30%	1.2	1.2	-
Phosphorus, mmol/100 mL	1.5	NA	
Glycerin, %			
10%	–	2.5	-
20%	2.25	2.5	2.5
30%	1.7	2.5	-
pH			
10%	–	8.3 (6–9)	-
20%	8 (6–8.9)	8.3 (6–9)	6.8 (6–8.9)
30%	8 (6–8.9)	8.4 (6–9)	-
Osmolarity, mOsm/L			
10%	–	284	-
20%	260	292	390
30%	200	293	-
Phytosterols, mg/L	348 ± 33	NA	NA
α-Tocopherol (mg/L)	38	NA	NA

NA, content not available.

[a]Commercially available within the United States.

[b]Package insert information for B. Braun Nutrilipid available at http://www.bbraunusa.com/documents/Nutrilipid_PI_-final_.pdf.

Administration of IVFE in pediatric patients presents challenges to clinicians. Since IVFE products are not manufactured in units smaller than 100 mL, they are commonly repackaged into syringes to provide smaller unit volumes (consistent with daily doses of IVFE for neonates and infants) via syringe pump technology.[31] While this practice decreases risk for inadvertent administration of large amounts of IVFE to small patients,[32,33] repackaged IVFE has resulted in bacterial and fungal contamination during compounding or infusion.[31,34–37] Shorter hang times for repackaged IVFE (eg, 12 hours) should be considered to decrease the potential for infusing contaminated IVFE into small patients.[31,38,39]

IVFE not only supplies a concentrated source of calories but also provides essential fatty acids for cell membrane integrity and brain development. The lower osmolarity of IVFE also helps prolong the integrity of peripheral lines. It is crucial to provide infants and children a minimum amount of lipids (0.5–1 g/kg/day) to prevent essential fatty acid deficiency (EFAD).[21,30] While EFAD has historically been defined as a triene to tetraene ratio ≥ 0.4,[40] individual laboratories may have different criteria for determining deficiency. For example, Mayo Clinical Laboratories has developed a new set of standards for assessing the triene to tetraene ratio for various age groups. Clinicians should refer to the individual laboratory's reference ranges when assessing for EFAD.

Micronutrients

Electrolytes

Close monitoring of electrolyte status is essential. In newborns, the addition of electrolytes to PN may be deferred until the second day of life in some cases. Potassium is generally added once normal kidney status and good urine output are established, and sodium is often added once diuresis begins. Daily adjustments to electrolyte intake are often necessary. Electrolyte requirements of preterm and term infants are generally similar, with the exception of calcium and phosphorus. Prescribing electrolytes as amount per kilogram per day is recommended in pediatric patients (see Table 35-4).[39]

Calcium and Phosphorus

The provision of adequate calcium and phosphorus in an optimal ratio is important for bone mineralization in neonates and infants, particularly those born preterm since maximum calcium and phosphorus accretion rates occur over the

Table 35-4. Parenteral Nutrition Electrolyte and Mineral Dosing Guidelines[a]

ELECTROLYTE	PRETERM NEONATES	INFANTS/CHILDREN	ADOLESCENTS AND CHILDREN > 50 kg
Sodium	2-5 mEq/kg	2-5 mEq/kg	1-2 mEq/kg
Potassium	2-4 mEq/kg	2-4 mEq/kg	1-2 mEq/kg
Calcium	2-4 mEq/kg	0.5-4 mEq/kg	10-20 mEq/day
Phosphorus	1-2 mmol/kg	0.5-2 mmol/kg	10-40 mmol/day
Magnesium	0.3-0.5 mEq/kg	0.3-0.5 mEq/kg	10-30 mEq/day
Acetate	As needed to maintain acid base-balance		
Chloride	As needed to maintain acid base-balance		

[a]Assumes normal organ function and losses.
Reprinted with permission from Mirtallo J, Canada T, Johnson D, et al. Safe practices for parenteral nutrition. *JPEN J Parenter Enteral Nutr.* 2004;28(6):S39-S70.

last 6 weeks of gestation. While solubility limits within PN solutions prohibit the supply of minerals that is provided in utero during the last trimester (6–7.5 mEq/kg/day calcium and 2.3–2.7 mmol/kg/day phosphorus), providing calcium and phosphorus in a ratio of 1.7 mg calcium to 1 mg phosphorus optimizes bone accretion of both minerals and minimizes urinary losses.[38,41] When dosing in milliequivalents per kilogram per day and millimoles per kilogram per day in a premature neonate, this ratio would be consistent with giving 3.5 mEq/kg/day calcium gluconate and 1.4 mmol/kg/day phosphorus (as either sodium or potassium phosphate).

Calcium and phosphorus solubility is enhanced by an acidic solution pH and decreased solution temperature. Solution pH is decreased by the use of pediatric amino acid products, addition of cysteine, and higher amino acid and dextrose concentrations. Calcium gluconate is the preferred salt for use in PN solutions since it is more stable and disassociates less rapidly than calcium chloride. While visual assessment of the solution will detect macroprecipitates, calcium phosphate microprecipitates can form that cannot be seen by the naked eye. To prevent potentially fatal pulmonary emboli from systemic infusion of calcium phosphate precipitates, the recommendation is to calculate the amount of calcium and phosphate in PN solutions, utilize solubility checks during compounding, and filter PN solutions with a 0.2 micron filter during administration. In addition, the use of TNAs is not recommended in neonates and infants.

Vitamins

Parenteral multivitamin products are available for pediatric patients (< 11 years of age) and are dosed based on weight (see Table 35-5).[42-44] In children and adolescents > 11 years,

the adult parenteral multivitamin product (dose = 10 mL) should be used. Since the adult product is available with and without vitamin K, it is important to make sure that the multivitamin product with vitamin K is used in pediatric patients unless a reason exists for vitamin K restriction (eg, warfarin therapy). While Greene et al[42] explored the need for changes to parenteral vitamin and trace element products in 1988, parenteral multivitamin or trace element products for infants and children (< 11 years of age) have not been reformulated since their inception.[45] A.S.P.E.N. convened the Novel Nutrient Task Force in 2009 to recommend what changes, if any, were needed in the currently available multivitamin and trace elements products. With respect to vitamins, the Task Force noted the need for potentially increased daily vitamin D supplementation, in addition to daily carnitine and choline supplementation. The Task Force also recommended the need for a parenteral choline product (either as a single entity or incorporated into a multivitamin product), as well as a parenteral cholecalciferol or ergocalciferol product (for PN–dependent patients with vitamin D deficiency unresponsive to enteral supplementation).[45]

Trace Elements

The Nutrition Advisory Group of the American Medical Association has recommended that 5 trace elements (chromium, copper, manganese, selenium, and zinc) be supplemented in patients receiving PN.[42] Two of these trace elements, chromium and manganese, have been found to accumulate in patients receiving prolonged PN.[46,47] Chromium is a contaminant of large and small volume parenteral products used in PN compounding; thus, deficiency is rare in PN patients.[45,46] Chromium is eliminated renally and may also accumulate in patients with renal failure.[46] If deficiency occurs, it may present as glucose intolerance, hyperlipidemia, peripheral neuropathy, or encephalopathy.[46,48] Manganese is a cofactor for a number of enzymatic processes; it is eliminated via the

Table 35-5. Dosing Recommendations[a] for Pediatric Parenteral Multivitamins[42-44]

MANUFACTURER RECOMMENDATIONS[B]		NAG-AMA RECOMMENDATIONS	
Weight, kg	Dose, mL	Weight, kg	Dose, mL
< 1	1.5	< 2.5	2 mL/kg
≥ 1 to < 3	3.25	≥ 2.5	5 mL
≥ 3	5		

NAG-AMA, Nutrition Advisory Group-American Medical Association.
[a]Assumes normal organ function.
[b]Infuvite Pediatric (Baxter) and MVI-Pediatric (Hospira).

biliary system.[47,49] It has also been found to accumulate in patients with or without liver disease receiving long-term PN, which raises concerns about neurotoxicity.[45,47,50] Manganese deficiency in PN patients is not common; deficiency has only been reported in a single child with SBS.[47]

Serious micronutrient deficiencies have been documented when copper, selenium, and zinc have not been supplemented in patients receiving PN; recent reports have surfaced during times of PN product shortages.[42,45,50–57] Copper is an important component for hemoglobin synthesis, neurologic development, and bone and connective tissue function.[51,58] Clinical manifestations of copper deficiency include hypochromic, microcytic anemia that is unresponsive to iron therapy, neutropenia, leukopenia, bone demineralization or osteoporosis, loss of hair and skin pigmentation, and cardiac and nervous system abnormalities.[51,58] Preterm infants may be at greater risk for deficiency.[51,58] Conditions requiring higher copper intake include increased biliary losses due to jejunostomy output or via external biliary drainage and persistent diarrhea or GI fluid losses.[51] Since copper undergoes biliary elimination, it is has been withheld from PN in patients with cholestasis; however, cases of copper deficiency have been reported.[54] In patients with cholestasis, it is recommended to reduce supplementation by 50% of the amount typically provided for age, monitor serum copper levels and ceruloplasmin, and adjust supplementation accordingly.[51,59]

Selenium is critical for antioxidant capacity, primarily through glutathione peroxidase, for immune function, and as a cofactor for thyroid hormone production and regulation; needs may be increased with critical illness and thermal injury.[52,60] Selenium deficiency may present as cardiomyopathy (ie, Keshan disease), myalgias, myositis, hemolysis, and impaired cellular immunity.[52,60]

Zinc offers antioxidant properties, has been associated with immune competence and wound healing, and is critical for growth in infants and children.[53,61] In addition, zinc is primarily eliminated via the GI tract and adequate supplementation becomes increasingly more important in patients with excessive fluid losses from wounds, stool, and ostomy output.[53,61] Patients with severe burn injuries have greater zinc needs due to losses from skin.[45] Zinc deficiency may result in dermatitis, alopecia, anorexia, growth failure, delayed sexual maturation, reduced taste, poor night vision, immune compromise, and impaired wound healing.[53,61] Some conditions that require additional zinc intake include elevated urinary zinc excretion (eg, high-output renal failure) and increased GI excretion (eg, high-volume stool loss and fistula/stoma losses).

Parenteral multitrace element products that contain zinc, copper, chromium, and manganese with or without selenium are available (see Table 35-6); single-entity products exist for copper, chromium, iodine, manganese, molybdenum, selenium, and zinc.[62,63] Dosing of pediatric multitrace element products is problematic in that the weight-based dosage recommendations underestimate the recommended daily intake for some trace elements such as zinc, while intake is excessive for others like chromium and manganese that are contaminants in PN solutions and can accumulate in patients receiving long-term PN support (see Table 35-7). In addition, none of the currently available neonatal and pediatric multitrace element products contain selenium; it must be supplemented using a single-entity product. Important trace elements may also be neglected in the currently available products. Iodine, fluoride, and molybdenum are routinely supplemented in multitrace element preparations available outside the United States. Although iodine supplementation is not needed in patients on short-term PN, deficiency may occur in patients receiving chronic therapy.[64] Deficiency of molybdenum has not been reported in pediatrics; however, one adult case of deficiency has been documented.[45] Revised recommendations for multitrace element products have been made multiple times, primarily advocating for increased selenium, decreased copper and chromium, and decreased or no manganese in commercially available products.[20,50] Despite these recommendations, no substantial changes have been made to the product formulations during the last 3 decades. The A.S.P.E.N. Novel Nutrient Task Force most recently recommended decreased manganese to 1 mcg/kg/day in neonates, and no chromium and the addition of selenium at 2 mcg/kg/day in all pediatric products.[45] Until an optimal multitrace element product is marketed, one mechanism for dose-adjusting trace elements based on age-specific or disease-specific needs is to supplement PN solutions with copper, selenium, and zinc using the single-entity products instead of the multitrace element products. Thus, accumulation with chromium and manganese can be avoided. For institutions using the multitrace element products, supplemental selenium is necessary and additional zinc may be required in certain patients, such as preterm infants and those with increased GI losses. In addition, routine monitoring of copper in patients with cholestasis and of chromium and manganese in all patients is advised.

Table 35-6. Comparison of Multitrace Element Products[62,63]

	MULTITRACE-4 NEONATAL	MULTITRACE-4 PEDIATRIC	TRACE ELEMENTS INJECTION 4-PEDIATRIC	PEDITRACE	MULTITRACE-5 CONCENTRATE	ADDAMEL N
Manufacturer	American Regent	American Regent	American Regent	Fresenius Kabi (imported)[a]	American Regent	Fresenius Kabi (imported)[a]
Preservative	None	None	0.9% benzyl alcohol	None	0.9% benzyl alcohol and preservative free	None
Minerals (per 1 mL)[b]						
Zinc, mg	1.5	1	0.5	0.25	5	0.65
Copper, mcg	100	100	100	20	1000	130
Manganese, mcg	25	25	30	1	500	27
Chromium, mcg	0.85	1	1	–	10	1
Selenium, mcg	–	–	–	2	60	3.2
Fluorine, mcg	–	–	–	57	–	95
Iodine, mcg	–	–	–	1	–	13
Molybdenum, mcg	–	–	–	–	–	1.9
Iron, mg	–	–	–	–	–	0.11

[a]Fresenius Kabi USA is coordinating (effective May 2013) with the U.S. Food and Drug Administration to provide alternative trace elements products during trace element product shortages
[b]Product salt forms as follows:
American Regent products: zinc, copper, manganese (sulfate), chromium chloride, selenious acid.
Peditrace: zinc, copper, manganese (chloride), sodium selenite, sodium fluoride, potassium iodide.
Addamel N: zinc, copper, manganese, chromic, ferric (chloride), sodium selenite, sodium molybdate, sodium fluoride, potassium iodide.

Parenteral Nutrition Additives

Medications

Heparin is commonly added to PN solutions to reduce central line–associated bloodstream infections (CLAB-

Table 35-7. Trace Element Requirements[a] in Pediatric Patients

TRACE ELEMENT	PRETERM NEONATES < 3 kg	TERM NEONATES 3–10 kg	CHILDREN 10–40 kg	ADOLES-CENTS > 40 kg
	mcg/kg/day	mcg/kg/day	mcg/kg/day	(Per day)
Zinc	400[b]	50–250	50–125	2–5 mg
Copper	20	20	5–20	200–500 mcg
Manganese	1	1	1	40–100 mcg
Chromium	0.05–0.2	0.2	0.14–0.2	5–15 mcg
Selenium[b]	1.5–2	2	1.0–2	40–60 mcg

[a]Assumes normal organ function and losses.
[b]Commercially available multitrace element products will not meet needs; additional supplementation required with single entity products.
Reprinted with permission from Mirtallo J, Canada T, Johnson D, et al. Safe practices for parenteral nutrition. *JPEN J Parenter Enteral Nutr.* 2004;28(6):S39-S70.

SIs), catheter thrombus, or central vein thrombosis, as well as to maintain or increase longevity of a peripheral access device.[38,65] In addition, heparin has been proposed to improve lipid clearance by activation of lipoprotein lipase.[17] Typical heparin doses used are 0.5 units or 1 unit per mL PN solution.[17,38,65] Recent A.S.P.E.N. clinical guidelines do not support adding heparin to PN solutions for decreasing the risk of central vein thrombosis.[38] Heparin is also a high-alert medication; the Institute for Safe Medication Practices (ISMP) recommends avoiding using heparin as an additive to PN solutions to decrease the potential for adverse events.[66] While heparin is compatible in dextrose/amino acid solutions, its addition to TNAs has been found to destabilize the formulation.[38,67] Other medications that may be added to PN solutions include histamine-2 receptor antagonists (eg, ranitidine) and regular human insulin.

Carnitine

Carnitine is responsible for the transport of long-chain fatty acids into the mitochondria for oxidation and energy production.[68] Carnitine may be considered a conditionally essential nutrient in premature neonates and infants receiving

PN due to the lack of placental carnitine transfer in the third trimester and enzymatic immaturity in the biosynthetic pathway of carnitine from lysine and methionine.[68] Decreased carnitine concentrations have been reported in infants and children on PN without supplemental carnitine.[68] In addition, patients with SBS or other GI conditions affecting absorption may not be carnitine sufficient despite significant enteral intake.[68] Potential benefits of carnitine supplementation include improved fatty acid oxidation, improved lipid tolerance, and positive nitrogen balance and weight gain.[68] Carnitor (Sigma-Tau Pharmaceuticals) is available for supplementation via PN. Recommended doses in PN have ranged from 10 to 20 mg/kg/day[68]; however, a study in preterm neonates receiving 20 mg/kg/day found carnitine concentrations that exceeded the reference range.[69] Lower starting doses of 10–15 mg/kg/day and assessing carnitine status periodically in long-term PN patients seem prudent. The A.S.P.E.N. Novel Nutrient Task Force recently recommended routine carnitine supplementation of 2–5 mg/kg/day to neonatal PN if no enteral source was provided.[45]

Cysteine

Cysteine has been considered a conditionally essential amino acid in neonates and infants due to the enzymatic immaturity of the transsulfuration pathway responsible for the conversion of methionine to cysteine and ultimately to taurine.[70] Cysteine is not a component of crystalline amino acid solutions because it is unstable and will form an insoluble precipitate.[21] Common dosing for L-cysteine hydrochloride is 30–40 mg per gram of pediatric amino acids; however, 20 mg/g may be adequate.[71] In general, current practice suggests supplementation with L-cysteine hydrochloride for the first year of life, although actual practice varies widely.[20] Riedijk et al[72] have suggested that cysteine requirements are satisfied in 1-month-old preterm infants born at 32 weeks of gestation or older who are on a full enteral diet. In addition, the A.S.P.E.N. Cysteine Product Shortage Considerations[71] state that cysteine supplementation is not needed under normal feeding and growth situations if patients are receiving a minimum of 3 g/kg/day protein. It is important to note that a benefit of the addition of L-cysteine hydrochloride to PN is decreased solution pH, which increases the solubility of calcium and phosphorus.

Monitoring

Prior to initiation of PN support, checking the following biochemical indices is recommended: serum electrolytes (sodium, potassium, chloride, bicarbonate, calcium, magnesium, phosphorus), serum glucose, liver function (ie, alkaline phosphatase, alanine aminotransferase, aspartate aminotransferase, gamma-glutamyl transferase), total bilirubin, conjugated or direct bilirubin, prealbumin, albumin, triglyceride, renal function (blood urea nitrogen, serum creatinine), and complete blood count. In addition, weight and height, fluid status, and clinical status should be assessed. Following the initiation of PN, patients require close biochemical monitoring (serum electrolytes, glucose, triglyceride) in addition to assessment of growth (daily for neonates and infants) and clinical status. The monitoring is then slowly decreased in frequency depending on the patient's clinical status and demonstration of stable parameters. In addition to routine comprehensive chemistry, liver function, and complete blood count assessment, patients on long-term PN, such as those with SBS, require continual assessment for growth (weight/height, body mass index at ≥ 2 years of age) to include plotting on Centers for Disease Control and Prevention/World Health Organization growth charts, and periodic assessment of micronutrient status (iron studies, trace elements, vitamins), carnitine status, thyroid studies, fatty acid panel (if receiving intermittent or low-dose IVFE), vitamin D, and bone density (every 5 years). For a more detailed discussion on monitoring and assessment of PN patients, see Chapter 36.

Complications

The provision of PN to pediatric patients is associated with unique potential risks and calls for a diligent inter-professional team approach to prevent, monitor for, and manage complications effectively. Initiating EN as soon as medically appropriate is the key to minimizing the potential adverse effects of PN. Complications of PN can be mechanical (issues with infusion devices or PN bags or administration sets, catheter leaks or breaks, catheter tip migration, pneumothorax), infectious (CLABSIs), metabolic (hyperglycemia, hypertriglyceridemia, fluid and electrolyte abnormalities, acid-base disorders, PNALD, metabolic bone disease, refeeding syndrome, EFAD), and nutritional (micronutrient toxicity or deficiency). Many of these complications are discussed in greater detail elsewhere in this text (see chapters 7, 8, 9, 26, 27, and 33). In addition, trace element (chromium, copper, manganese, selenium, and zinc) toxicity and deficiency have been reviewed in the micronutrient section of this chapter. The discussion in the following text will focus on assessment and management of metabolic bone disease, CLABSIs, aluminum toxicity, and iron deficiency.

Metabolic Bone Disease

Bone disease in patients receiving PN is multifactorial; however, the use of PN and aluminum contamination are predisposing risk factors.[73] Preterm neonates and infants are at greatest risk due to rapidly growing bone and inability to give similar amounts of calcium and phosphorus that are provided in utero. Routine assessment for bone disease should include serum calcium and phosphorus and alkaline phosphatase. Normal serum calcium concentrations do not equate with adequate bone mineralization; the body's homeostatic mechanisms maintain normal serum calcium in the calcium-deprived state via renal calcium conservation, increased intestinal calcium absorption, and pulling calcium from bone. Metabolic bone disease may present with hypercalcemia or hyperphosphatemia. Other assessment methods include radiographs (ordered for other purposes) that can be reviewed for signs of demineralization, and parathyroid hormone and vitamin D assessment. In patients on long-term PN, bone density testing should be conducted periodically. Prevention and management of metabolic bone disease centers around optimizing adequate minerals via PN; decreasing aluminum exposure; supplementing additional calcium, phosphorus, and vitamin D enterally (when indicated); encouraging weight bearing exercise; and instituting pharmacotherapy when bone disease is unresponsive to additional mineral and vitamin D supplementation. In preterm neonates receiving PN, decreased bone disease was seen with high-dose (75 mg/kg/day calcium and 44.1 mg/kg/day phosphorus) compared with low-dose (45 mg/kg/day calcium and 26.5 mg/kg/day phosphorus) calcium and phosphorus in PN.[74]

Central Line–Associated Bloodstream Infections

CLABSIs are a common complication in patients receiving PN. Risk factors include poor central line care, use of the central line for blood draws, bacterial overgrowth, and contamination of the central line with ostomy or stool output. Preventing initial and repeat CLABSIs is important to improve patient morbidity and decrease the risk of developing PNALD. Assessment for CLABSIs is conducted when a patient receiving PN has documented fever; blood cultures are drawn from the periphery and the central line. Systemic antibiotics are initiated empirically after blood cultures are drawn and then adjusted based on microorganism growth and pathogen identified. In patients receiving long-term PN, catheter salvage is desired to preserve access sites; however, this is not always possible. Retention or removal of the catheter is determined by the patient's clinical status, pathogen

identified, and type of access device. Antimicrobial lock therapy has offered additional support to the armamentarium of systemic antibiotics in assisting with clearance of identified pathogens from catheters, as well as catheter salvage. Lock therapy involves having an antibiotic, typically vancomycin or gentamicin, or ethanol (70% solution) dwell in the catheter for a period of time. Ethanol lock therapy has been found to effectively prevent catheter-related infections in PN patients as well.[75] A.S.P.E.N. guidelines suggest using ethanol lock in pediatric intestinal failure patients to prevent CLABSIs and to reduce catheter replacements.[76]

Typical ethanol lock protocols utilize at least once weekly (and up to daily) locks for a minimum period of 2 hours up to the entire period that the patient is cycled off PN. Protocols also differ on whether the ethanol is flushed through or withdrawn after dwell time is complete. Ideally, the ethanol would be flushed through the catheter to avoid coating the catheter with proteins from blood; however, little is known about the effects of chronic ethanol exposure in small patients. Research is needed to determine the best approach with respect to number of days per week, length of dwell time, and whether the ethanol should be instilled or withdrawn.[76] Of note, ethanol is incompatible with heparin. Catheters should be flushed well with normal saline before and after ethanol locks. In addition, ethanol administration with metronidazole can result in a disulfiram-like reaction. Until more information is available about the likelihood of reactions in patients receiving concomitant ethanol lock and metronidazole therapies, withdrawal of ethanol from the catheter in patients on metronidazole is advised.

Aluminum Toxicity

Large and small volume parenteral products utilized during PN compounding are commonly contaminated with aluminum, which can be especially dangerous for infants and children. Preterm infants are extremely vulnerable to aluminum toxicity due to immature renal function and the likelihood for long-term PN.[20]

The FDA mandated in 2004 that products used in compounding PN should state the aluminum content at the end of the product's shelf life on the label. The FDA identified 5 mcg/kg/day as the maximum amount of aluminum that can be safely tolerated; amounts exceeding this limit may be associated with central nervous system or bone toxicity.[20] The mandate has resulted in decreased aluminum contamination in marketed products. While aluminum content can be reduced by using products with the least amount of contamination and using them earlier in their shelf lives, it is still difficult to achieve the recommended maximum limit set by the FDA in pediatric PN.[77-79] Clinicians should attempt to lower aluminum doses by choosing products with the least contamination when feasible and safe for patients. An acceptable substitution would be to use the least contaminated product when multiple manufacturers produce the same product. An unsafe substitution would be to use calcium chloride instead of calcium gluconate. Despite its higher aluminum content, calcium gluconate remains the preferred calcium salt for PN compounding since it is considerably more stable and poses significantly lower risk for calcium phosphate precipitation.[20,80]

Iron Deficiency

Iron is an essential nutrient for numerous body processes (neurotransmitter production, cell replication, oxidative metabolism). Iron-deficiency anemia is characterized by progressive depletion of iron stores resulting in a microcytic hypochromic anemia.[81] Blood loss (including phlebotomy), iron intake, and erythropoiesis (including erythropoietin use) can influence iron stores. When routine complete blood count monitoring suggests iron-deficiency anemia, assessment of serum ferritin concentrations reveals the body's iron stores. Low serum ferritin concentrations are an accurate reflection of iron deficiency; however, inflammatory states, iron overload, or a recent red blood cell transfusion can result in elevated serum ferritin concentrations. Iron sufficiency can also be determined by measuring the zinc protoporphyrin to heme ratios, which reflect the availability of iron that can be incorporated into the protoporphyrin molecule to form heme. In states of iron deficiency, zinc is incorporated instead. An elevated ratio suggests iron deficiency, although it may also be seen in patients receiving erythropoietin due to increased erythropoiesis.

Since parenteral multivitamin products do not contain iron, patients on PN must receive an exogenous source of iron to prevent deficiency. Patients who receive frequent blood transfusions will often not require additional iron because a typical transfusion will provide approximately 3 months' worth of iron.[82] Oral iron is the preferred route of supplementation in patients who can tolerate and absorb enteral therapy; however, parenteral iron supplementation is warranted in patients with severe iron-deficiency anemia who fail to respond to oral therapy. Children with intestinal failure who initially require parenteral iron may eventually be transitioned to enteral iron as their bowel adapts. The oral iron absorption test is used to assess GI iron absorption. A low dose of 5–20 mg (elemental) of ferrous sulfate is given

to detect mild iron deficiency.[83] A minimal rise in serum iron will occur in iron sufficient patients, while a 100 mcg/dL rise in serum iron can be seen within 1–2 hours after administration in patients with iron deficiency.[84]

Parenteral iron preparations include iron dextran, sodium ferric gluconate, iron sucrose, and ferumoxytol. Table 35-8 summarizes dosing, administration, safety, and adverse effects for each of these products.[85-90] Due to reports of anaphylactic and other adverse reactions associated with high molecular weight (HMW) iron dextran, practitioners have been reluctant to use it. However, a benefit of iron dextran is that it can be given as a total dose infusion (TDI) or as intermittent infusions. While some adverse reactions appear to be dose related, studies have demonstrated the overall safety and efficacy of larger TDIs.[91-93] These results, along with the convenience and cost effectiveness of a single infusion, have made TDI the preferred method of administration of iron dextran.

Life-threatening hypersensitivity reactions are characterized by acute respiratory failure and cardiovascular collapse, including hypotension, bronchospasm, oral or pharyngeal edema, loss of consciousness, severe pain, and muscle spasms. This response appears to be due to both the toxic effects of and the high antigenicity of free dextran molecules, similar to the types of reactions seen with contrast media or opiates.[94] In some cases, the acute onset of chest and back pain or tightness without hypotension, tachypnea, tachycardia, wheezing, stridor, or periorbital edema can occur. The immunologic basis of allergic hypersensitivity to parenteral iron is still not known although both antibody-mediated and nonantibody-mediated, dose-dependent mechanisms have been observed in patients after an anaphylactic event.[95,96] Based on information in the FDA's adverse events reporting database, adverse events are greatest with HMW iron dextran formulations and less with the newer iron products.[97] Other experts, including representatives from the FDA, have cautioned that it is not possible to draw conclusions about the comparative risks from the different iron products using this database.[98,99]

Of the various parenteral iron products, only the iron dextran products carry boxed warnings in the product labeling about the risk for anaphylactic-type reactions. Reports of patients reacting to subsequent doses of iron dextran despite tolerating test doses prompted the expansion of the box warning in September 2009.[100] This modified warning cautioned prescribers that fatal reactions have occurred even after the test dose was tolerated; the reactions may be delayed in onset. The warning also states that patients with a

Table 35-8. Comparison of Parenteral Iron Products[85-90]

		IRON DEXTRAN (INFED) LMW	IRON DEXTRAN (DEXFERRUM) HMW	SODIUM FERRIC GLUCONATE (FERRLECIT)	IRON SUCROSE (VENOFER)	FERUMOXYTOL (FERAHEME)
FDA-approved indications	Adults	IDA when oral therapy failed	IDA when oral therapy failed	IDA (HD + EPO)	IDA in CKD (nondialysis ± EPO; dialysis + EPO)	IDA in CKD
	Pediatrics	IDA when oral therapy failed	IDA when oral therapy failed	Children ≥ 6 y: IDA (HD + EPO)	Children ≥ 2 y: IDA in CKD (nondialysis ± EPO; dialysis + EPO)	No
Dosage (replacement)		TDI: dose in milliliters [50 mg/mL] = 0.0442 × LBW [kg] × (desired Hgb – observed Hgb) + (0.26 × LBW [kg]). Dilute dose in 250–1000 mL NS and infuse over 4–6 h (max rate 50 mg/min) Or Sequential daily doses up to the total replacement dose as individual, undiluted injections: Infants < 5 kg: 25 mg Children 5–10 kg: 50 mg Children > 10 kg and adults: 100 mg (max rate 50 mg/min)			Adult: cumulative dose of 1000 mg Nondialysis: 200 mg on 5 different occasions HD: 100 mg during consecutive dialysis sessions (up to 1000 mg total) PD: 3 doses, each 14 days apart, totaling 1000 mg (300 mg day 1, 300 mg day 14, 400 mg day 28) Pediatric: 0.5 mg/kg slow IV injection or infusion	Adult: 510 mg (17 mL) as a single dose, followed by a second 510 mg dose 3–8 days after initial dose Recommended doses may be re-administered with persistent or recurrent IDA Pediatric: no dosing recommendations available
Dosage (maintenance) when enteral not an option						
	Neonate	Serum ferritin < 40 mg/L: 2 mg/kg, 3 times per week Serum ferritin 40–100 mg/L: 2 mg/kg twice per week Serum ferritin 100–400 mg/L: 1.5 mg/kg twice per week; if serum ferritin remains low, increase dose to 2 mg/kg twice per week		Contraindicated	AOP: 1 mg/kg/day infused over 2 h Serum ferritin < 40 mg/L: 2 mg/kg, 3 times per week Serum ferritin 40–100 mg/L: 2 mg/kg twice per week Serum ferritin 100–400 mg/L: 1.5 mg/kg twice per week; if serum ferritin remains low, increase dose to 2 mg/kg twice per week	
	Child			Children ≥ 6 y: 8 doses of 1.5 mg/kg (0.12 mL/kg) repeated at sequential dialysis sessions	Children > 2 y: 0.5 mg/kg, not to exceed 100 mg per dose, every 2 wk for 12 wk; may be repeated if necessary Or Children ≥ 2 y and adolescents < 15 y: 1 mg/kg/dialysis	

Table 35-8.(Continued) Comparison of Parenteral Iron Products[85-90]

		IRON DEXTRAN (INFED) LMW	IRON DEXTRAN (DEXFERRUM) HMW	SODIUM FERRIC GLUCONATE (FERRLECIT)	IRON SUCROSE (VENOFER)	FERUMOXYTOL (FERAHEME)
	Adult			Adults may receive up to 125 mg (10 mL) per dose during HD to achieve a cumulative dose of 1 g over 8 sequential sessions		
Administration	IV push	Yes, 50 mg/min	Yes, 50 mg/min	Yes, 12.5 mg/min (ie, a typical adult dose of 125 mg can be infused over 10 min)	Yes, 20–50 mg/min or 40–100 mg/min (indication dependent)	Yes, 1 mL/s (30 mg/s), repeat 3–8 days later
	IV infusion	See above for TDI Neonates: Dilute dose in 10 mL D10W and infuse over hours	No	125 mg/100mL NS over 1 h	Yes, 100 mg/100mL NS over 15 min; 300 mg/250 mL NS over 1.5 h; 400 mg/250 mL NS over 2.5 h or give undiluted by slow IV injection over 5 min or diluted in 25 mL NS and administered over 5–60 min	No
	IM injection	Yes, ≤ 100 mg by Z-Track technique	No	No	No	No
Safety	Anaphylaxis warning	Yes (boxed)	Yes (boxed)	Yes	Yes	Yes
	Test dose	Yes, over 30 s followed by 1 h observation	Yes, over 5 min followed by 1 h observation	No	No	No
		Recommended test dose: Infants < 10 kg: 10 mg Children 10–20 kg: 15 mg Children > 20 kg/adults: 25 mg				
	PN compatibility	Yes, nonlipid PN only	Yes, nonlipid PN only	No	No	No
Common adverse reactions	CV	Hypotension, flushing, chest pain	Hypotension, flushing, chest pain	Hypotension, chest pain	Hypotension, hypertension, chest pain	Hypotension, hypertension, chest pain
	CNS	Headache, weakness, dizziness	Headache, weakness, dizziness	Syncope, dizziness, headache	Headache, dizziness, fatigue	Headache, dizziness
	GI	NVD	NVD	NVD	NVD	NVD
	MSK	Arthralgia	Arthralgia	Muscle cramps	Muscle cramps	Back pain
	Other	Malaise	Malaise	Edema	Edema	Edema
Other	Preservative	No	No	Benzyl alcohol	No	No

AOP, anemia of prematurity; CKD, chronic kidney disease; CNS, central nervous system; CV, cardiovascular; D10W, 10% dextrose in water; EPO, erythropoietin; FDA, U.S. Food and Drug Administration; GI, gastrointestinal; HD, hemodialysis; Hgb, hemoglobin; HMW, high molecular weight; IDA, iron-deficiency anemia; IM, intramuscular; IV, intravenous; LMW, low molecular weight; MSK, musculoskeletal; NS, normal saline; NVD, nausea, vomiting, diarrhea; PD, peritoneal dialysis; TDI, total dose infusion.

history of drug allergy are more susceptible, especially with large doses. There does not appear to be cross-reactivity between the parenteral iron formulations because large studies have shown that patients who have experienced anaphylactic-type reactions to iron dextran have been subsequently able to tolerate other iron preparations.[101,102] However, the rate of ferric gluconate intolerance was noted to be higher in patients who had a prior history of iron dextran intolerance.[101] Moreover, patients with multiple drug allergies may similarly be at an increased risk of hypersensitivity reactions.[94,103] Despite the lack of a boxed warning, anaphylactic reactions are still a risk with the newer parenteral iron products since reports of adverse events have emerged during postmarketing surveillance. When any of the parenteral iron preparations are being administered, a system should be in place for patient monitoring and emergency equipment, and rescue medications should be readily available. Hypotension has been reported with the administration of iron sucrose and may be linked to rate of infusion or total dose given. In comparison with other parenteral iron products, ferumoxytol has negligible free iron release; this may account for the decreased incidence of free iron–like reactions such as GI symptoms and hypotension.[104]

Iron dextran is the only formulation with extensive compatibility in nonlipid-containing PN. Iron dextran has been shown to be physically compatible when added to a nonlipid-containing PN at a concentration of 100 mg/L for 18 hours at room temperature, or at 10 mg/L for 48 hours when the amino acid concentration is ≥ 2%.[105] Adding iron preparations to lipid-containing PN is not recommended because of the potential for coalescence of small lipid particles due to destabilization of negative surface charges by the iron cations. The labeling for iron sucrose warns that the product should not be mixed with other medications, nor should it be added to PN. However, one study found that iron sucrose at concentrations up to 0.25 mg/dL in nonlipid-containing PN (using neonatal amino acid and cysteine doses) were chemically and physically stable for 24 hours.[106] Iron sucrose concentrations ≥ 1 mg/dL were found to be chemically, but not physically stable and therefore not compatible with PN.[106]

For years, practitioners have been cautious about using parenteral iron in septic patients, citing its potential to fuel bacterial growth. Bacteria require iron to replicate. High intake of parenteral iron can lead to transferrin oversaturation resulting in the formation of catalytically active iron within 3.5 hours after an IV injection. Given that catalytically active iron can be potentially toxic and may promote bacte-

rial growth, lower doses should be used so as not to cause transferrin oversaturation.[107] In one pediatric study, the incidence of neonatal sepsis was greater in a group of infants who received intramuscular (IM) iron dextran injections in comparison to those who did not.[108] It was thought that IM iron dextran impaired the immunity of the treated infants, thus making them more susceptible to *Escherichia coli* sepsis. Another prospective, multicenter, cohort-controlled observational trial conducted in dialysis patients suggested there might be a slightly increased risk of bacteremia in patients given high-frequency, high-dose IV iron.[109] Based on these findings, it may be prudent to hold doses of parenteral iron in septic patients, especially those with gram-negative bacteremia, until the sepsis has resolved. This precaution is also noted in the package insert for HMW iron dextran products.

Parenteral Nutrition Safety

PN is considered a high-alert medication by the ISMP. Ensuring the safe provision of PN within healthcare institutions and at home requires knowledgeable and skilled clinicians involved in the practice of nutrition support and the development and continual review of policies, protocols, and procedures that support practice that minimizes errors with PN therapy. The increased incidence of PN product shortages has further affected the safety of the PN process and has negatively impacted patient care.[110] While the examples of adverse outcomes related to PN product shortages have been numerous, the most dramatic example to date has been multiple patient deaths associated with contaminated PN solutions that were traced back to amino acids made from powders during an amino acid product shortage.[110] It is imperative that clinicians work together to adequately address PN product supply issues, have protocols in place to manage shortages of PN products, and develop safeguards within the system to prevent patient injury. The A.S.P.E.N. PN Safety Consensus Recommendations were published in 2014 and review practices that minimize errors throughout the PN process (prescribing, order review and verification, compounding, and administration) and include recommendations on PN product shortages and when providing PN support at home.[39,111] Table 35-9 provides a summary of key recommendations from this document. In addition to the consensus recommendations, A.S.P.E.N. has developed a PN safety toolkit (www.nutritioncare.org/pnsafety) that offers clinicians and institutions safety checklists for prescribing, order review and verification, compounding and administration of PN, materials to improve PN safety within institutions (PN Safety Preparation Checklist, "Improving Parenteral Nutrition (PN) Safety: Prescribing and Labeling in Our Facility" PowerPoint presentation, example order and label templates), current information on PN product shortages, and links to educational opportunities on PN Safety, related publications, and the PN adverse event reporting program (collaboration between A.S.P.E.N. and ISMP).[112]

Home Parenteral Nutrition Therapy

Many pediatric patients on long-term PN support, particularly those with SBS or intestinal failure, will eventually require home PN therapy. Patients should be receiving cyclic PN prior to consideration for home PN discharge. Overnight cyclic PN allows patients time away from infusion pumps during the day to attend school and participate in typical children's activities. The process of discharge on home PN is a complex one that requires the collaboration of the patient and caregivers and an interprofessional team of clinicians from both the discharging

institution and the accepting home care company. In order to ensure a smooth and safe transition to home PN for all patients, institutions should develop policies and procedures to be followed when sending patients home on PN support. Procedures to be incorporated include initial and follow-up care conferences, home assessment, orders for PN and supplies in the home (to include review and verification of home PN order/label), patient and caregiver education and training (PN preparation and additives, CVAD care, infusion pump technology, ethanol lock, monitoring for adverse events, emergency care plan), and follow-up after discharge.[113-115] The A.S.P.E.N. PN Safety Consensus guidelines include recommendations specific to home PN support.[39] In addition, A.S.P.E.N. standards have been published for the provision of nutrition support in home care.[115] Home PN patients should ideally be followed in the outpatient setting by an interprofessional team (physician, pharmacist, dietitian, nurse) that will review laboratory and make changes to PN and other nutrition orders as needed based on clinical

Table 35-9. Recommendations from American Society for Parenteral and Enteral Nutrition Parenteral Nutrition Safety Consensus[39,111]

GENERAL	PRESCRIPTION	ORDER REVIEW/VERIFICATION	LABELING
• Clinicians (interprofessional) with expertise in nutrition support, annual competencies • Develop policies and procedures for all parts of PN process • Education to nonnutrition clinicians on policies and procedures • Perform PN process during daylight hours • Avoid distractions • QI programs to report, track, analyze errors in PN process	• Standardized PN order format and review process for all patients within institution • Educate prescribers on PN prescribing and monitoring • Confirm access • Ideally, CPOE with current patient information (eg, laboratory) displayed, clinical decision support, and limits • When CPOE not available, PN should be prescribed using a standardized order template as an editable electronic document (avoid handwritten) • Follow A.S.P.E.N. guidelines for inclusion on PN order form • Avoid handwritten, verbal, telephone orders • Order in amount per kilogram per day for neonatal and pediatric orders (amount per day for adults) • Order electrolytes as complete salt form • Use full generic names • Abbreviations consistent with ISMP • Include nutrition-related orders • Avoid prescribing with nonnutrient medications • Reorder PN in its entirety	• Order review by skilled and knowledgeable pharmacists • Ideally, CPOE fully integrated with ACD • When CPOE to ACD integration not possible, standardized editable electronic order form • Avoid verbal and telephone orders • Avoid manually transcribing into ACD; if must be done, use pharmacist double-check • Pharmacist double-check after PN transcribed and before compounding • When compounding outsourced, electronically transmit PN orders to avoid transcription errors • Perform clinical review of order, compare order to previous day, double check calculations and conversions • Perform safety review (compatibility, calcium phosphate precipitation risk, stability) • Modifications communicated to prescriber and documented	• Standardized labeling for PN formulations • Follow A.S.P.E.N. guidelines for inclusion on PN label • Sequence of order templates and PN labels should match

Table 35-9. Recommendations from American Society for Parenteral and Enteral Nutrition Parenteral Nutrition Safety Consensus[39,111] (continued)

COMPOUNDING	ADMINISTRATION	PN SHORTAGES	HOME
• Operate/comply with USP <797> • Consider outsourcing or using standardized, commercially available PN when USP <797> compliance not possible • Conduct in-depth education/ training on CSPs and ACD for all staff participating in compounding process with ongoing competency assessment/verification • Certify pharmacy technicians involved in making CSPs/PNs • Have policy and procedures for use of standardized commercially available PNs No additions outside pharmacy ACD • Use hard/soft limits • Use weight-based limits • Limit access to ACD database • Permit only pharmacists to override alerts; double-check by another pharmacy staff (ideally pharmacist) • Have appropriate additive sequence • Have a checklist for new product entry • Use barcode technology • Have independent double-check process for initial daily ACD setup • Trace tubing sets daily and with each change in source container • Limit manual compounding • If multiple containers used for single additive, present all containers to pharmacist for verification • Verify manual additives by including inspection of actual vials and syringes, not proxy methods (eg, syringe pullback) • Use a verification process: after order entry, before manually injecting into PN, after PN compounded	• Conduct education and ongoing validation of competency in PN administration • Ensure hand hygiene • Use sterile technique/CVAD care • Inspect PN container/formulation • Verify PN label against PN order • Verify patient identity • Trace administration tubing at initiation and handoff • Double-check process of infusion pump settings before PN infusion • Filter PN • Maintain prescribed rate (double check) • Institute monitoring protocol • Avoid verbal orders • Institute administration safeguards • Have policy and procedure for PN extravasation • Have a protocol for safe operation of infusion pumps • Review compatibility and stability by pharmacist prior to co-infusion of meds with PN • Discontinue inpatient PNs prior to discharge to home or transfer to another facility	• Institute conservation, allocation, and substitution strategies/protocols for PN product shortages • Communicate shortages and management strategies to prescribers and staff • Have processes to evaluate compounding pharmacies and product compounded by compounding pharmacies • Modify PN order/label/ACD software to reflect shortages • Report, track, evaluate errors associated with shortages • Monitor patients for nutrient deficiencies during product shortages • Seek out other sources of PN components • Develop drug conservation policy on handling and disposition of PN components (while maintaining sterility and integrity)	• Create a home PN process • Create a separate standardized home PN order template and label • Have a standardized pharmacy review and verification process • Ensure that home PN labels and materials are patient-centered, emphasize patient instructions, use simple language, give explicit instructions, include purpose, limit auxiliary information, address limited English proficiency, improve readability • Do not use home PNs in acute care facilities • Print copy of initial PN order and any changes to patient/ caregiver for review with formulation label

ACD, automated compounding device; A.S.P.E.N., American Society for Parenteral and Enteral Nutrition; CPOE, computerized physician order entry; CSP, compounding sterile products; CVAD, central venous access device; ISMP, Institute for Safe Medication Practices; PN, parenteral nutrition; QI, quality improvement; USP, United States Pharmacopeia.

status. Long-term monitoring and assessment for PN complications and micronutrient deficiency and toxicity is critical in these patients. For more detailed discussion, please see recommendations for monitoring for long-term PN patients reviewed earlier in this chapter as well as Chapter 36.

Test Your Knowledge Questions

1. A 30 weeks gestation preterm neonate is admitted to the neonatal intensive care unit after delivery. A starter PN solution is ordered to infuse until an individual PN solution can be prescribed and compounded. When considering bone mineralization needs, which of the following represents the optimal ratio of calcium to phosphorus (mg:mg) to provide this patient?
   A. 1:1
   B. 1.3:1
   C. 1.7:1
   D. 2:1

2. A 3-month-old preterm infant (26 weeks gestation) has SBS due to NEC. The patient has remaining an intact duodenum, 50-cm jejunum, and 15-cm proximal ileum in continuity with the colon. The patient has had 2 CLABSIs and enteral feedings are currently only providing 20 kcal/kg/day. The patient also has evidence of PNALD. A care conference is scheduled to discuss the long-term management of this patient and the potential for discharge home on PN support. Which of the following recommendations would be best to address this patient's recurrent CLABSIs?
   A. Ethanol lock therapy
   B. Cyclic oral antibiotic therapy
   C. Permanent removal of central access
   D. Addition of heparin 1 unit per mL PN

3. The nutrition support team is revising its PN ordering procedures to prepare for the implementation of computerized order entry and electronic medical record at their institution. The best way to order nutrients for pediatric PN patients is:
   A. Amount per day
   B. Amount per kg per day
   C. Amount per liter
   D. Percent concentration

Acknowledgments

The authors of this chapter for the second edition of this text wish to thank Liesje Nieman Carney, RD, CNSD, LDN; Andrea Nepa, MS, RD, CSP, LDN; Sherri Shubin Cohen, MD, MPH; Amy Dean, MPH, RD, LDN; Colleen Yanni, MS, RD, LDN; and Goldie Markowitz, MSN, CRNP, for their contributions to the first edition of this text.

References

1. Corkins MR, Griggs KC, Groh-Wargo S, et al; Task Force on Standards for Nutrition Support: Pediatric Hospitalized Patients; American Society for Parenteral and Enteral Nutrition Board of Directors; American Society for Parenteral and Enteral Nutrition. Standards for nutrition support: pediatric hospitalized patients. *Nutr Clin Pract*. 2013;28:263–276.
2. Hay WW Jr. Strategies for feeding the preterm infant. *Neonatology*. 2008;94:245–254.
3. Ehrenkranz RA. Early, aggressive nutritional management for very low birth weight infants: what is the evidence? *Semin Perinatol*. 2007;31:48–55.
4. Commare CE, Tappenden KA. Development of the infant intestine: implications for nutrition support. *Nutr Clin Pract*. 2007;22:159–173.
5. Moyses HE, Johnson MJ, Leaf AA, Cornelius VR. Early parenteral nutrition and growth outcomes in preterm infants: a systematic review and meta-analysis. *Am J Clin Nutr*. 2013;97:816–826.
6. Berseth CL. Gastrointestinal motility in the neonate. *Clin Perinatol*. 1996;23:179–190.
7. American Academy of Pediatrics Committee on Nutrition. Nutritional needs of the preterm infant. In: Kleinman RE, ed. *Pediatric Nutrition Handbook*. 6th ed. Elk Grove, IL: American Academy of Pediatrics; 2009:79–112.
8. Marin T, Josephson CD, Kosmetatos N, Higgins M, Moore JE. Feeding preterm infants during red blood cell transfusion is associated with a decline in postprandial mesenteric oxygenation. *J Pediatr*. 2014;165:464–471.
9. Fallon EM, Nehra D, Potemkin AK, et al; American Society for Parenteral and Enteral Nutrition (A.S.P.E.N.) Board of Directors. A.S.P.E.N. clinical guidelines: nutrition support of neonatal patients at risk for necrotizing enterocolitis. *JPEN J Parenter Enteral Nutr*. 2012;36:506–523.
10. Peterson J, Kerner JA. New advances in the management of children with intestinal failure. *JPEN J Parenter Enteral Nutr*. 2012;36(suppl):36S–42S.
11. Tappenden KA. Intestinal adaptation following resection. *JPEN J Parenter Enteral Nutr*. 2014;38(suppl):23S–31S.
12. O'Keefe SJD, Buchman AL, Fishbein TM, Jeejeebhoy KN, Jeppeson PB, Shaffer J. Short bowel syndrome and intestinal failure: consensus definitions and overview. *Clin Gastroenterol Hepatol*. 2006;4:6–10.
13. Mehta NM, Compher C; A.S.P.E.N. Board of Directors. A.S.P.E.N. clinical guidelines: nutrition support of the critically ill child. *JPEN J Parenter Enteral Nutr*. 2009;33:260–276.
14. Tutor JD. Chylothorax in infants and children. *Pediatrics*. 2014;133:722–733.
15. Pettignano R, Heard M, Hart M, Davis R. Total enteral nutrition versus total parenteral nutrition during pediatric extracorporeal membrane oxygenation. *Crit Care Med*. 1998;26(2):358–363.
16. Jaksic T, Hull MA, Modi BP, Ching YA, George D, Compher C; American Society for Parenteral and Enteral Nutrition (A.S.P.E.N.) Board of Directors. A.S.P.E.N. clinical guide-

lines: nutrition support of neonates supported with extracorporeal membrane oxygenation. *JPEN J Parenter Enteral Nutr.* 2010;34:247–253.

17. A.S.P.E.N. Board of Directors and the Clinical Guidelines Taskforce. Administration of specialized nutrition support—issues unique to pediatrics. *JPEN J Parenter Enteral Nutr.* 2002;26:97SA–110SA.

18. A.S.P.E.N. Board of Directors and the Clinical Guidelines Taskforce. Specific guidelines for disease—pediatrics. *JPEN J Parenter Enteral Nutr.* 2002;26:111SA–138SA.

19. A.S.P.E.N. Board of Directors and the Clinical Guidelines Taskforce. Psychiatric disorders: eating disorders. *JPEN J Parenter Enteral Nutr.* 2002;26:94SA–95SA.

20. Mirtallo J, Canada T, Johnson D, et al; Task Force for the Revision of Safe Practices for Parenteral Nutrition. Safe practices for parenteral nutrition [erratum in *JPEN J Parenter Enteral Nutr.* 2006;30:177]. *JPEN J Parenter Enteral Nutr.* 2004;28:S39–S70.

21. American Academy of Pediatrics Committee on Nutrition. Parenteral nutrition. In: Kleinman RE, ed. *Pediatric Nutrition Handbook.* 6th ed. Elk Grove, IL: American Academy of Pediatrics; 2009:519–540.

22. A.S.P.E.N. Board of Directors and the Clinical Guidelines Taskforce. Normal requirements—pediatrics. *JPEN J Parenter Enteral Nutr.* 2002;26:25SA–32SA.

23. Bresson JL, Narcy P, Putet G, Ricour C, Sachs C, Rey J. Energy substrate utilization in infants receiving total parenteral nutrition with different glucose to fat ratios. *Pediatr Res.* 1989;25:645–648.

24. Wright K, Ernst KD, Gaylord MS, Dawson JP, Burnette TM. Increased incidence of parenteral nutrition-associated cholestasis with Aminosyn PF compared to Trophamine. *J Perinatol.* 2003;23(6):444–450.

25. Shulman RJ, Phillips S. Parenteral nutrition in infants and children. *J Pediatr Gastroenterol Nutr.* 2003;36:587–607.

26. Cole CR, Kocoshis SA. Management of infants with short bowel syndrome and intestinal failure. *Nutr Clin Pract.* 2013;28:421–428.

27. Vanek VW, Seidner DL, Allen P, et al; Novel Nutrient Task Force, Intravenous Fat Emulsions Workgroup and American Society for Parenteral and Enteral Nutrition (A.S.P.E.N.) Board of Directors. A.S.P.E.N. position paper: clinical role for alternative intravenous fat emulsions. *Nutr Clin Pract.* 2012;27:150–192.

28. Intralipid [package insert]. Uppsala, Sweden: Fresenius Kabi (manufactured for Baxter Healthcare Corporation); 2012.

29. Liposyn III [package insert]. Lake Forest, IL: Hospira, Inc; 2005.

30. Kerner JA, Poole RL. The use of IV fat in neonates. *Nutr Clin Pract.* 2006;21:374–380.

31. Crill CM, Hak EB, Robinson LA, Helms RA. Evaluation of microbial contamination associated with different preparation methods for neonatal intravenous fat emulsion infusion. *Am J Health Syst Pharm.* 2010;67:914–918.

32. Chuo J, Lambert G, Hicks RW. Intralipid medication errors in the neonatal intensive care unit. *Jt Comm J Qual Patient Saf.* 2007;33:104–111.

33. Hicks RW, Becker SC, Chuo J. A summary of NICU fat emulsion medication errors and nursing services. Data from MEDMARX. *Adv Neonatal Care.* 2007;7:299–310.

34. McKee KT Jr, Melly MA, Greene HL, Schaffner W. Gram-negative bacillary sepsis associated with use of lipid emulsion in parenteral nutrition. *Am J Dis Child.* 1979;133:649–650.

35. Jarvis WR, Highsmith AK, Allen JR, Haley RW. Polymicrobial bacteremia associated with lipid emulsion in a neonatal intensive care unit. *Pediatr Infect Dis.* 1983;2:203–208.

36. de Beaufort AJ, Bernards AT, Dijkshoorn L, van Boven CPA. *Acinetobacter junii* causes life-threatening sepsis in preterm infants. *Acta Paediatr.* 1999;88:772–775.

37. Reiter PD. Sterility of intravenous fat emulsion in plastic syringes. *Am J Health Syst Pharm.* 2002;598:1857–1859.

38. Boullata JI, Gilbert K, Sacks G, et al; American Society for Parenteral and Enteral Nutrition. A.S.P.E.N. clinical guidelines: parenteral nutrition ordering, order review, compounding, labeling, and dispensing. *JPEN J Parenter Enteral Nutr.* 2014;38:334–377.

39. Ayers P, Adams S, Boullata J, et al; American Society for Parenteral and Enteral Nutrition. A.S.P.E.N. parenteral nutrition safety consensus recommendations. *JPEN J Parenter Enteral Nutr.* 2014;38:296–333.

40. Chessman KH, Kumpf VJ. Assessment of nutrition status and nutrition requirements. In: Dipiro JT, Talbert RL, Yee GC, Matzke GR, Wells BG, Posey LM, eds. *Pharmacotherapy. A Pathophysiologic Approach.* 9th ed. New York, NY: McGraw-Hill; 2014:2385–2404.

41. Pelegano JF, Rowe JC, Carey DE, et al. Effect of calcium/phosphorus ratio on mineral retention in parenterally fed premature infants. *J Pediatr Gastroenterol Nutr.* 1991;12:351–355.

42. Greene HL, Hambidge M, Schanler R, Tsang R. Guidelines for the use of vitamins, trace elements, calcium, magnesium, and phosphorus in infant and children receiving total parenteral nutrition: report of the Subcommittee on Pediatric Parenteral Nutrient Requirements from the Committee on Clinical Practice Issues of the American Society for Clinical Nutrition. *Am J Clin Nutr.* 1988;48:1324–1342.

43. Infuvite Pediatric [package insert]. Boucherville, QC, Canada: Sandoz Canada (distributed by Baxter Healthcare Corporation); 2007.

44. MVI-Pediatric [package insert]. Lake Forest, IL: Hospira, Inc.; 2007.

45. Vanek VW, Borum P, Buchman A, et al; Novel Nutrient Task Force, Parenteral Multi-Vitamin and Multi–Trace Element Working Group; American Society for Parenteral and Enteral Nutrition (A.S.P.E.N.) Board of Directors. A.S.P.E.N. position paper: recommendations for changes in commercially available parenteral multivitamin and multi-trace element products. *Nutr Clin Pract.* 2012;27:440–491.

46. Moukarzel A. Chromium in parenteral nutrition: too little or too much? *Gastroenterology.* 2009;137(5 suppl):S18–S28.

47. Hardy G. Manganese in parenteral nutrition: who, when, and why should we supplement? *Gastroenterology.* 2009;137(5 suppl):S29–S35.

48. Solomons NW. Chromium. In: Baumgartner TG, ed. *Clinical Guide to Parenteral Micronutrition*. 3rd ed. Deerfield, IL: Fujisawa, USA, Inc; 1997:327–339.

49. Solomons NW. Manganese. In: Baumgartner TG, ed. *Clinical Guide to Parenteral Micronutrition*. 3rd ed. Deerfield, IL: Fujisawa, USA, Inc.; 1997:341–350.

50. Buchman AL, Howard LJ, Guenter P, Nishikawa RA, Compher CW, Tappenden KA. Micronutrients in parenteral nutrition: too little or too much? The past, present, and recommendations for the future. *Gastroenterology*. 2009;137(5 suppl):S1–S6.

51. Shike M. Copper in parenteral nutrition. *Gastroenterology*. 2009;137(5 suppl):S13–S17.

52. Shenkin A. Selenium in intravenous nutrition. *Gastroenterology*. 2009;137(5 suppl):S61–S69.

53. Jeejeebhoy K. Zinc: an essential trace element for parenteral nutrition. *Gastroenterology*. 2009;137(5 suppl);S7–S12.

54. Hurwitz M, Garcia MG, Poole RL, Kerner JA. Copper deficiency during parenteral nutrition: a report of four pediatric cases. *Nutr Clin Pract*. 2004;19:305–308.

55. Pramyothin P, Kim DW, Young LS, Wichanswaakun S, Apovian CM. Anemia and leucopenia in a long-term parenteral nutrition patient during a shortage of parenteral trace element products in the United States. *JPEN J Parenter Enteral Nutr*. 2013;37(3):425–429.

56. Oguri T, Hattori M, Yamawaki T, et al. Neurological deficits in a patient with selenium deficiency due to long-term total parenteral nutrition. *J Neurol*. 2012;259:1734–1735.

57. Centers for Disease Control and Prevention. Notes from the field: zinc deficiency dermatitis in cholestatic extremely premature infants after a nationwide shortage of injectable zinc—Washington, DC, December 2012. *MMWR Morb Mortal Wkly Rep*. 2013;62:136–137.

58. Solomons NW. Copper. In: Baumgartner TG, ed. *Clinical Guide to Parenteral Micronutrition*. 3rd ed. Deerfield, IL: Fujisawa, USA, Inc; 1997:311–322.

59. Corkins MR, Martin VA, Szeszycki. Copper levels in cholestatic infants on parenteral nutrition. *JPEN J Parenter Enteral Nutr*. 2013;37:92–96.

60. Nichoalds GE. Selenium. In: Baumgartner TG, ed. *Clinical Guide to Parenteral Micronutrition*. 3rd ed. Deerfield, IL: Fujisawa, USA, Inc.; 1997:387–400.

61. Solomons NW. Zinc. In: Baumgartner TG, ed. *Clinical Guide to Parenteral Micronutrition*. 3rd ed. Deerfield, IL: Fujisawa, USA, Inc.; 1997:293–307.

62. American Regent. Trace element products. http://www.americanregent.com/MultipleTraceElementAdditives.aspx. Accessed July 10, 2014.

63. American Society of Health-System Pharmacists. Trace elements injection (July 3, 2014) shortage information. http://www.ashp.org/menu/DrugShortages/CurrentShortages/Bulletin.aspx?id=785. Updated July 3, 2014. Accessed July 10, 2014.

64. Zimmermann MB, Crill CM. Iodine in enteral and parenteral nutrition. *Best Pract Res Clin Endocrinol Metab*. 2010;24:143–158.

65. Kerner JA Jr, Garcia-Careaga MG, Fisher AA, Poole RL. Treatment of catheter occlusion in pediatric patients. *JPEN J Parenter Enteral Nutr*. 2006;30:S73–S81.

66. Institute for Safe Medication Practices. Action needed to prevent dangerous heparin–insulin confusion. ISMP Medication Safety Alert. Horsham, PA: Institute for Safe Medication Practices. May 3, 2007.

67. Johnson OL, Washington C, Davis SS, Schaupp K. The destabilization of parenteral feeding emulsions by heparin. *Int J Pharm*. 1989;53:237–240.

68. Crill CM, Helms RA. The use of carnitine in pediatric nutrition. *Nutr Clin Pract*. 2007;22:204–213.

69. Crill CM, Storm MC, Christensen ML, Hankins CT, Jenkins MB, Helms RA. Carnitine supplementation in premature neonates: effect on plasma and red blood cell total carnitine concentrations, nutrition parameters and morbidity. *Clin Nutr*. 2006;25:886–896.

70. Helms RA, Chesney RW, Storm MC. Sulfur amino acid metabolism in infants on parenteral nutrition. *Clin Nutr*. 1995;14:381–387.

71. American Society for Parenteral and Enteral Nutrition. Parenteral nutrition cysteine product shortage considerations, September 2011. http://www.nutritioncare.org/Professional_Resources/Guidelines_and_Standards/Guidelines/PN_Cysteine_Product_Shortage_Considerations/. Accessed July 7, 2014.

72. Riedijk MA, van Beek RHT, Voortman G, de Bie HMA, Dassel ACM, van Goudoever JB. Cysteine: a conditionally essential amino acid in low-birth-weight preterm infants? *Am J Clin Nutr*. 2007;86:1120–1125.

73. Nehra D, Carlson SJ, Fallon EM, et al; American Society for Parenteral and Enteral Nutrition (A.S.P.E.N.) Board of Directors. A.S.P.E.N. clinical guidelines: nutrition support of neonatal patients at risk for metabolic bone disease. *JPEN J Parenter Enteral Nutr*. 2013;37:570–598.

74. Pereira-da-Silva L, Costa A, Pereira L, et al. Early high calcium and phosphorus intake by parenteral nutrition prevents short-term bone strength decline in preterm infants. *J Pediatr Gastroenterol Nutr*. 2011;52(2):203–209.

75. Oliveira C, Nasr A, Brindle M, Wales PW. Ethanol locks to prevent catheter-related bloodstream infections in parenteral nutrition: a meta-analysis. *Pediatrics*. 2012;129:318–329.

76. Wales PW, Allen N, Worthington P, George D, Compher C, American Society for Parenteral and Enteral Nutrition; Teitelbaum D. A.S.P.E.N. clinical guidelines: support of pediatric patients with intestinal failure at risk of parenteral nutrition-associated liver disease. *JPEN J Parenter Enteral Nutr*. 2014;38(5):538–557.

77. Poole RL, Pieroni KP, Gaskari S, Dixon T, Kerner JA. Aluminum exposure in neonatal patients using the least contaminated parenteral nutrition solution products. *Nutrients*. 2012;4:1566–1574.

78. Poole RL, Pieroni KP, Gaskari S, Dixon T, Kerner JA. Aluminum in pediatric parenteral nutrition products: measured versus labeled content. *J Pediatr Pharmacol Ther*. 2011;16:92–97.

79. Speerhas RA, Seidner DL. Measure versus estimated aluminum content of parenteral nutrient solutions. *Am J Health Syst Pharm*. 2007;64:740–746.

80. Driscoll DF, Newton DW, Bistrian BR. Potential hazards of precipitation associated with calcium chloride in parenteral

nutrition admixtures: response to Migaki et al. *JPEN J Parenter Enteral Nutr.* 2012;36(5):497–498.

81. Clark S.F. Iron deficiency anemia. *Nutr Clin Pract.* 2008;23:128–141.

82. Muñoz M, Breymann C, García-Erce JA, Gómez-Ramírez S, Comin J, Bisbe E. Efficacy and safety of intravenous iron therapy as an alternative/adjunct to allogeneic blood transfusion. *Vox Sang.* 2008;94(3):172–183.

83. Crosby WH, O'Neil-Cutting MA. A small-dose iron tolerance test as an indicator of mild iron deficiency. *JAMA.* 1984;251(15):1986–1987.

84. Josephs HW. Absorption of iron as a problem in human physiology; a critical review. *Blood.* 1958;13(1):1–54.

85. INFeD (iron dextran) injection [package insert]. Morristown, NJ: Watson Pharma, Inc; 2009.

86. Dexferrum (iron dextran) injection [package insert]. Shirley, NY: American Regent, Inc; 2010.

87. Venofer (iron sucrose) injection [package insert]. Shirley, NY: American Regent Inc; 2008.

88. Ferrlecit (sodium ferric gluconate) injection [package insert]. Bridgewater, NJ: Sanofi-Aventis US LLC; 2014.

89. Feraheme (ferumoxytol) injection [package insert]. Lexington, MA: AMAG Pharmaceuticals; 2009.

90. Ohls RK, Ehrenkranz RA, Wright LL, et al. Effects of early erythropoietin therapy on the transfusion requirements of preterm infants below 1250 grams birth weight: a multicenter, randomized, controlled trial. *Pediatrics.* 2001;108(4):934–942.

91. Mamula P, Piccoli DA, Peck SN, et al. Total dose intravenous infusion of iron dextran for iron-deficiency anemia in children with inflammatory bowel disease. *J Pediatr Gastroenterol Nutr.* 2002;34:286–290.

92. Auerbach M, Witt D, Toler W, et al. Clinical use of the total dose intravenous infusion of iron dextran. *J Lab Clin Med.* 1988;111:566–570.

93. Halpin TC Jr, Bertino JS, Rothstein FC, et al. Iron-deficiency anemia in childhood inflammatory bowel disease: treatment with intravenous iron-dextran. *JPEN J Parenter Enteral Nutr.* 1982;6:9–11.

94. Fishbane S, Kowalski EA. The comparative safety of intravenous iron dextran, iron saccharate, and sodium ferric gluconate. *Semin Dialysis.* 2000;13:381–384.

95. Monaghan MS, Glasco G, St John G, Bradsher RW, Olsen KM. Safe administration of iron dextran to a patient who reacted to the test dose. *South Med J.* 1994;87:1010–1012.

96. Novey HS, Pahl M, Haydik I, Vaziri ND. Immunologic studies of anaphylaxis to iron dextran in patients on renal dialysis. *Ann Allergy.* 1994;72:224–228.

97. Bailie GR. Comparison of rates of reported adverse events associated with IV iron products in the United States. *Am J Health Syst Pharm.* 2012;69:310–320.

98. Wysowski DK, Swartz LB, Borders-Hemphill BV, Goulding MR, Dormitzer C. Use of parenteral iron products and serious anaphylactic-type reactions. *Am J Hematol.* 2010;85:650–654.

99. Auerbach M, Kane RC. Caution in making inferences from FDA's adverse event reporting system. *Am J Health Syst Pharm.* 2012;69:922–923.

100. MedWatch: The FDA Safety Information and Adverse Event Reporting Program. Dexferrum (iron dextran injection)—labeling change. http://www.fda.gov/downloads/Safety/MedWatch/SafetyInformation/SafetyAlertsforHumanMedicalProducts/UCM186900.pdf. Updated October 16, 2009. Accessed July 11, 2014.

101. Coyne DW, Adkinson NF, Nissenson AR, et al. Sodium ferric gluconate complex in hemodialysis patients. II. Adverse reactions in iron dextran-sensitive and dextran-tolerant patients. *Kidney Int.* 2003;63:217–224.

102. Van Wyck DB, Danielson BG, Aronoff GR. Safety and efficacy of iron sucrose in patients sensitive to iron dextran: North American clinical trial. *Am J Kidney Dis.* 2000;36:88–97.

103. Silverstein SB, Rodgers GM. Parenteral iron therapy options. *Am J Hematol.* 2004;76:74–78.

104. Balakrishnan VS, Rao M, Kausz AT, et al. Physicochemical properties of ferumoxytol, a new intravenous iron preparation. *Eur J Clin Invest.* 2009;39(6):489–496.

105. Mayhew SL, Quick MW. Compatibility of iron dextran with neonatal parenteral nutrient solutions. *Am J Health Syst Pharm.* 1997;54:570–571.

106. MacKay M, Rusho W, Jackson D, McMillin G, Winther B. Physical and chemical stability of iron sucrose in parenteral nutrition. *Nutr Clin Pract.* 2009;24:733–737.

107. Parkkinen J, von Bonsdorff L, Peltonen S, et al. Catalytically active iron and bacterial growth in serum of haemodialysis patients after i.v. iron-saccharate administration. *Nephrol Dial Transplant.* 2000;15:1827–1834.

108. Barry DM, Reeve AW. Increased incidence of gram-negative neonatal sepsis with intramuscular iron administration. *Pediatrics.* 1977;60:908–912.

109. Hoen B, Paul-Dauphin A, Kessler M. Intravenous iron administration does not significantly increase the risk of bacteremia in chronic hemodialysis patients. *Clin Nephrol.* 2002;57:457–461.

110. Holcombe B. Parenteral nutrition product shortages: impact on safety. *JPEN J Parenter Enteral Nutr.* 2012;36(2 suppl):44S–47S.

111. Ayers P, Adams S, Boullata J, et al. A.S.P.E.N. parenteral nutrition safety consensus recommendations: translation into practice. *Nutr Clin Pract.* 2014;29(3):277–282.

112. American Society for Parenteral and Enteral Nutrition. Parenteral nutrition safety toolkit. https://www.nutritioncare.org/Guidelines_and_Clinical_Practice/Toolkits/Parenteral_Nutrition_Safety_Toolkit/. Accessed January 7, 2015

113. Norman JL, Crill CM. Optimizing the transition to home parenteral nutrition in pediatric patients. *Nutr Clin Pract.* 2011;26:273–285.

114. Kumpf VJ, Tillman EM. Home parenteral nutrition: safe transition from hospital to home. *Nutr Clin Pract.* 2012;27:749–757.

115. Durfee SM, Adams SC, Arthur E, et al; Home and Alternate Care Standards Task Force; American Society for Parenteral and Enteral Nutrition. A.S.P.E.N. standards for nutrition support: home and alternate site care [published online ahead of print June 25, 2014]. *Nutr Clin Pract.* 2014;29(4):542–555.

Test Your Knowledge Answers.

1. Answer: **C**. The provision of adequate calcium and phosphorus in an optimal ratio is important for bone mineralization in neonates and infants, particularly those born preterm since maximum calcium and phosphorus accretion rates occur over the last 6 weeks of gestation. Providing calcium and phosphorus in a ratio of 1.7 mg calcium to 1 mg phosphorus optimizes bone accretion of both minerals and minimizes urinary losses.

2. Answer: **A**. Ethanol lock therapy has been found to be effective in the prevention of catheter related infections in PN patients. A.S.P.E.N. guidelines suggest using ethanol lock in pediatric intestinal failure patients to prevent CLABSIs and reduce catheter replacements. Cyclic oral antibiotics may be appropriate for patients with bacterial overgrowth. While catheters occasionally must be removed due to infection, the goal in patients with SBS is catheter retention in order to preserve long-term access sites. While heparin has been added to PN solutions to reduce CLABSIs, recent A.S.P.E.N. clinical guidelines and ISMP recommendations do not support the use of heparin addition to PN solutions.

3. Answer: **B**. According to the A.S.P.E.N. PN Safety Consensus Recommendations, PN ingredients shall be ordered in amount per kilogram per day for pediatric and neonatal patients. In adult patients, PN ingredients shall be ordered as amount per day. It is not recommended to order ingredients as amount per liter, percent concentration, or volume.

36

Evaluation and Monitoring of Pediatric Patients Receiving Specialized Nutrition Support

Elaina Szeszycki, PharmD, BCNSP; **Wendy Cruse,** MMSc, CLS, RD; and **Michelle Beitzel,** PharmD

 Video

Learning Objectives

1. Determine patient-specific objective and subjective criteria for reassessment of stated nutrition goals.
2. Assess gastrointestinal tolerance of enteral nutrition based on defined parameters.
3. Assess tolerance to parenteral nutrition based on defined parameters.
4. Evaluate the appropriateness of parenteral nutrition solutions in regards to solubility and stability.
5. Discuss the laboratory monitoring required for patients receiving specialized nutrition support.

Management of Pediatric Patients Receiving Nutrition Support Therapy

Nutrition therapy is a component of medical treatment that includes oral, enteral, and parenteral nutrition (PN). Management of pediatric patients receiving nutrition support is complex and requires continuous monitoring of tolerance and the efficacy of the nutrition intervention. The nutrition care plan must consist of nutrition goals that are both short term and long term. Monitoring parameters are established based on the patient's initial nutrition status and route of nutrition therapy.[1] These parameters are then used to determine if the patient-specific set of goals are being met and whether the goals and nutrition care plan need to be reevaluated as suggested in Figure 36-1.

Nutrition Monitoring and Evaluation

Complications associated with the delivery of enteral nutrition (EN) and PN may be prevented or reduced with monitoring and timely formula adjustments based on the patient's growth and tolerance to nutrition therapy. Development of enteral and parenteral monitoring guidelines is critical to ensure all parameters are being assessed and should be included in each individualized nutrition care plan.[1] Institutions should follow individualized monitoring guidelines for inpatients and outpatients based on their patient population. The nutrition care plan is determined based on the patient's baseline nutrition status, need for correction of nu-

---

Figure 36-1. Continuous Evaluation and Assessment of Nutrition Care Plan for Patients Receiving Nutrition Support

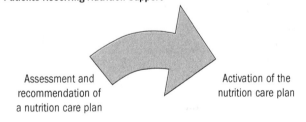

Assessment and recommendation of a nutrition care plan

Activation of the nutrition care plan

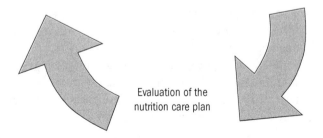

Evaluation of the nutrition care plan

---

tritional deficiencies, and achievement of optimal growth.[1] See Chapter 32 for initial nutrition assessment guidelines. Monitoring parameters are also based on nutrition goals set in the nutrition care plan, specific disease process, clinical status, and patient tolerance.[1]

Nutrition monitoring includes the patient's growth, fluid status, physical assessment, clinical status, tolerance to EN and PN, medication changes, and laboratory values. Frequency of monitoring depends on the age, severity of illness, tolerance of specialized nutrition support (SNS), comorbid diseases, and degree of malnutrition.[1] Preterm neonates, infants, critically ill patients, and severely malnourished children at risk for refeeding syndrome and during transition periods between PN, EN, and oral diet may require more frequent monitoring as discussed later in the chapter. Indirect calorimetry may be used to more precisely determine a patient's calorie needs especially in the critically ill patient.[2]

Baseline and serial anthropometric measurements are monitored closely in children. Weight, height or length, head circumference, weight for length, and body mass index (BMI) should be plotted on age-appropriate growth curves.[1,3] Baseline and serial skinfold thickness and mid-arm circumference may be used to assess patient's lean body mass, especially in patients with edema or ascites.[3] See Chapter 32 for further details. In addition to growth curve percentiles, z scores should also be used because they are more sensitive and provide a more exact identification of growth deviation, especially when growth parameters plot > 97th–98th percentile and < 2nd–3rd percentile. Both are used to determine nutritional status, adequacy of nutrition support, and nutrition goals.[3] See Chapter 32 for details regarding growth assessment and monitoring.

Refeeding Syndrome

When any form of nutrition support is initiated in a severely malnourished child, careful monitoring must take place to avoid refeeding syndrome.[4,5] Refeeding syndrome occurs when nutrition support is provided to a patient with depleted stores of nitrogen and electrolytes, as in the state of malnutrition. When nourishing the body tissue with these nutrients, a sudden decrease in electrolyte and mineral serum levels, particularly potassium, phosphorus, and magnesium, can occur. These decreased levels can potentially result in muscle weakness, impaired cardiac function, and ultimately death. Hypophosphatemia is associated with malnutrition in children within the first 10 days of intensive care hospitalization, thus putting them at risk for refeeding syndrome.[6]

Thus, careful monitoring of phosphorus as well as potassium and magnesium is critical when initiating nutrition support in severely malnourished patients.[6] Baseline electrolyte levels should be obtained, and depleted minerals and electrolytes should be replaced before initiation of nutrition therapy.[4] Electrolyte levels should initially be monitored every 6–12 hours for the first 3 days until levels are stable, and daily thereafter.[7,8] Daily monitoring of serum electrolytes, minerals, and vital signs during advancement of nutrition support would be a minimum expectation in malnourished patients. Supplements may be administered by mouth, in patients with safe airway, or feeding tube, when patients are being fed enterally, as tolerated. Intravenous (IV) electrolytes may be provided when patients are receiving primarily PN. Should the child experience diarrhea and/or vomiting when receiving oral/enteral therapy or if serum levels are moderately to severely depleted, electrolyte replacement may be given via IV infusion. This is also discussed in Chapter 34.

Calorie Provision

It is essential to avoid providing excess or suboptimal calories to children receiving EN and/or PN because they are not utilizing hunger and satiety cues and do not have the ability to choose more or fewer calories as their growth and nutrition needs change. It is important to utilize growth charts and calculate rate of weight gain to evaluate growth velocity over various time frequencies.[9,10] In a hospital setting, growth velocity may be calculated every 3–7 days and in an outpatient setting weekly, monthly, or yearly assessment is beneficial. Excessive calories from PN may contribute to cholestatic liver disease. Maximal dextrose infusion varies according to age, and information is increasing about the maximal glucose infusion rate (GIR) range for differing age groups.[11] This should allow for more appropriate dextrose ordering and potentially decrease complications associated with excess carbohydrate intake (eg, hyperglycemia, elevated liver enzymes, cholestasis, and ultimately fatty liver).[12,13]

Feeding Route

The route of nutrition support needs to be reevaluated frequently. When adequate intake cannot be achieved orally, > 60%–80% for > 10 days, EN is the preferred route when the child has a partially functional gut.[14] EN preserves gastrointestinal (GI) function, is less costly, and is associated with less risk compared with PN. PN should be used when the GI tract is not functional or if inadequate absorption is apparent and thus adequate nutrition support is not possible via the enteral route.[1] If PN is indicated, consider the provision of an oral diet as well as trophic enteral feedings or combined EN and PN. Adequacy and appropriateness of the route for specialized nutrition support must be reassessed frequently and adjusted as needed. It is important to continually reevaluate if the child can tolerate increasing amounts of nutrition via enteral or oral route. See Chapter 33 for guidelines on determining the best feeding route.

Enteral Nutrition

Monitoring

Many parameters may be used to monitor patients receiving EN. During the initiation and advancement of EN, monitoring will initially be more frequent and then become less frequent as the child becomes more stable. A proposed monitoring protocol for infants and children receiving EN initially and then when stable, both while in hospital and at home, is provided in Table 36-1.[15,16]

Evaluation of Growth and Nutrition Adequacy

Monitoring serial anthropometric data, with corresponding percentiles and z scores, as well as growth velocity allows the clinician to determine appropriateness of the nutrition therapy to support optimal growth. Calculating calorie, protein, vitamin, mineral, and fluid delivery is initially done to determine if the nutrition plan meets the child's nutritional needs and to determine if additional free-water, vitamin, or mineral supplement is needed. Periodic reevaluation of nutrient delivery compared to age-based guidelines is essential to determine if the nutrition care plan continues to be adequate. Fluid status may be assessed by balancing total fluid intake/delivery with fluid output including urine, stool, or ostomy output, emesis, wound losses, and tube drainage.

Evaluation of Formula Tolerance

Assessing tolerance to EN consists of monitoring GI symptoms.[14] These include nausea, vomiting, diarrhea, constipation, and abdominal pain or distention. Identification of other causes of these symptoms such as infection, bacterial overgrowth, or medications should be considered before strategies are taken to alter the type of formula or feeding delivery.[17] Care should be taken in the preparation, storage, and delivery of formulas and human milk to prevent bacterial contamination to the patient. Slowing the rate of formula administration or selecting a lower calorie concentration formula are options to improve formula tolerance. Stool

Table 36-1. Suggested Parameters to Monitor for Infants and Children Receiving Enteral Nutrition

	INITIAL WEEK	DURING HOSPITALIZATION	OUTPATIENT EN ONLY PATIENT	OUTPATIENT EN WITH PN PATIENT
GROWTH PARAMETERS				
Weight				
NICU	Daily	Daily	Weekly to monthly	Weekly
Infants	Daily	Daily	Weekly to monthly	Weekly
Children	Daily	Daily to twice weekly	Weekly or at clinic	Weekly
Length				
NICU	Baseline	Weekly	Monthly or at clinic	Monthly or at clinic
Infants	Baseline	Monthly		
Children	Baseline	Monthly		
Height (> 24 mo)	Baseline	Monthly		
Head circumference (< 24 mo)	Baseline	Weekly to monthly	Monthly or at clinic	Monthly or at clinic
Weight gain	Daily to weekly	Daily to weekly	Weekly to monthly	Weekly
Linear/OFC gain				
NICU	Weekly	Weekly	Monthly	Monthly
Infants	Weekly	Weekly to monthly		
INTAKE PARAMETERS				
Intake Calories Protein Vitamins Minerals Fluid balance	Daily	Weekly	Monthly	Weekly
GI TOLERANCE				
Abdominal girth	As indicated	As indicated	As indicated	As indicated
Gastric residuals	As ordered or reported	As ordered or reported	As ordered or reported	As ordered or reported
Emesis	As reported	As reported	As reported	As reported
Stool (volume, frequency, consistency, color) Ostomy (volume, consistency)	Daily as reported	Daily as reported	Report changes in stool pattern	Report changes in stool pattern
PHYSICAL				
Temperature	Per nursing policy	Per nursing policy	Report when > 101°F (38.5°C)	Report when > 101°F (38.5°C)
Tube placement	Prior to each feeding	Prior to each feeding	Prior to each feeding	Prior to each feeding
Tube site care	Daily	Daily	Daily	Daily

EN, enteral nutrition; GI, gastrointestinal; NICU, neonatal intensive care unit; OFC, occipital frontal circumference; PN, parenteral nutrition;

frequency, consistency, color, and presence of blood or fat should be noted. If a patient has an ostomy, it is essential to record volume of ostomy output daily. Ostomy volume goal may be ≤ 40 mL/kg/d or ≤ 30% of formula volume deliv-

ered.[18] Color and consistency may also provide additional insight when evaluating ostomy output. Large amounts of stool or ostomy output may indicate the need to reduce or avoid advancement of formula volume or caloric concentration. Large stool volume or ostomy output or excessive vomiting may require transitioning to an elemental formula that will allow for more passive digestion and absorption. If feeding tolerance cannot be achieved by these strategies and excessive diarrhea, ostomy, or vomiting continues, the initiation of IV fluids or PN may be required to avoid dehydration or nutritional deficiencies.

Various stool studies can also assist in identifying causes of enteral therapy intolerance. Fecal fat is used to measure the amount of fat present in the stool to identify fat malabsorption. The presence of reducing substances and acidic stools indicate carbohydrate malabsorption. The presence of α-1 antitrypsin is a marker for a protein-losing enteropathy or an indicator of enteral protein loss. Stool osmolarity with electrolytes may help distinguish between an osmotic or secretory diarrhea. Stool elastase can aid in the diagnosis of exocrine pancreatic insufficiency and potential need for pancreatic enzyme replacement.[19] Macronutrient malabsorption prompts the clinician to change the patient's formula to improve tolerance. The presence of blood in the stool may indicate cow-milk protein allergy.[20] A formula-fed infant may require changing to an extensively hydrolyzed protein-based formula or, in extreme cases, an amino acid–based formula. When a cow-milk protein allergy is suspected, an elimination diet is indicated in a breastfeeding mother. Therefore, evaluating the cause of the GI symptoms will determine therapy.

Gastric residuals have been monitored in pediatric intensive care unit (ICU) patients due to risk of ventilator-associated pneumonia and in the neonatal intensive care unit (NICU) population due to risk of developing necrotizing enterocolitis while receiving EN. However, recent literature does not support this practice.[21] Consider providing continuous enteral feeding instead of intermittent or postpyloric feedings for feeding intolerance. Changing formulas based on qualities such as osmolality and total content and type of fat, carbohydrate, protein, and fiber should be considered for feeding intolerance. Feeding intolerance may require consultation of a pediatric GI or surgical physician to evaluate for conditions such as an intestinal inflammatory process, necrotizing enterocolitis, small bowel bacterial overgrowth, bowel obstruction, or intestinal strictures. Feeding intolerance interrupts the advancement and provision of EN, thus resulting in the patient not receiving their nutritional needs.[21]

Monitoring Laboratory Values

Routine monitoring of laboratory values is not indicated for medically stable pediatric patients receiving EN at ad-

vised levels and achieving adequate growth.[15]Serum zinc and fat-soluble vitamins are monitored in the presence of fat malabsorption, and additional laboratory monitoring may be necessary based on concurrent disease states. Please see the related chapters. Physical assessment including clinical signs of nutrient excess or deficiency must be assessed periodically and may prompt further testing. See Chapter 32 for details of physical findings and related nutrition concerns.

Oral Feeding

Introduction to oral feeding is critical in all infants receiving EN. Allowing the infant to take a minimal volume of formula orally may reduce the tendency toward oral aversion so commonly seen in these children. When an infant is unable to feed orally, holding the infant during a feeding and allowing them to experience nonnutritive sucking on a pacifier is important for development and promotes the feeling of satiety. It is also critical in older children receiving tube feeding to be allowed to eat and drink once safety has been established either via observation or oximetry-swallow study. Speech-language pathologists work to reduce the occurrence of oral aversion or poor development of oral-motor skills that are commonly seen in infants and children receiving EN. EN can be transitioned to oral diet should the child be able to tolerate and safely consume an oral diet.

Revision of Enteral Plan

Revision of the EN care plan will be based on patient's tolerance of the EN regimen and achievement of goals. If goals are not being met, the nutrition care plan must be adjusted according to the patient's tolerance. As a child ages, the formula type and volume will need to be adjusted based on the child's needs, recommended daily allowance (RDA), and dietary reference intake. Vitamin and mineral supplementation may allow for the feeding plan to be nutritionally adequate. If a patient consistently consumes > 80% of nutritional needs orally and maintains adequate growth, consider discontinuing EN.[22] Once a patient demonstrates adequate growth solely on an oral diet, consider removal of the feeding device. Special care is needed for children requiring extremely low calorie levels. Additional evaluation for the nutritional adequacy of the plan as well as monitoring nutritional status of any suboptimal nutrient is warranted. If the EN plan is not supporting appropriate growth and making adjustments to the EN plan does not support the nutrition goals, then supplementation with PN or a transition to all PN may be required

Parenteral Nutrition

Once the decision has been made to initiate PN, vascular access is evaluated. If deemed appropriate based on nutrition goals, a PN solution is formulated accordingly. IV access is continuously monitored for mechanical complications along with metabolic and infectious complications related to PN as discussed in following text. As with EN, patient allergy information or any history of infusion-related incidents should be evaluated prior to the initiation of PN.

Evaluation of Growth and Nutrition Adequacy

Evaluation and monitoring of growth and nutrition in PN dependent patients is similar to those receiving EN with regards to z scores, anthropometrics, and growth velocity. The difference lies in the provision of calories and protein, whereas patients will require 5%–10% less due to circumventing any digestion or absorption issues with direct administration of the solution into the venous system.

Evaluation of Vascular Access

Monitor for Mechanical Complications

The decision to order peripheral parenteral nutrition (PPN) vs central parenteral nutrition (CPN) is based on nutrition needs, anticipated length of therapy, and patency of peripheral veins. PPN is limited based on osmolarity due to the vesicant properties of PN ingredients. Institutions generally set osmolarity limits for neonatal PPN at 900–1200 mOsm/L and pediatric PPN at 600–900 mOsm/L.[16] Maximum dextrose concentration for pediatric and neonatal PPN is 12.5%, but ultimately the osmolarity of the solution dictates the amount of nutrients, electrolytes, and minerals that can be ordered.[23] Lower concentrations of dextrose may be necessary in children with poor peripheral access, or PPN may need to be avoided completely depending on the fragility of their veins as seen in chronically ill children. Amino acids, dextrose, calcium, sodium, and potassium are the main determinants of osmolarity. If PPN is utilized, the IV site needs to be monitored closely (every 3–4 hours) for early signs of infiltration, which include erythema, swelling, pain, and streaking. It is difficult to provide 100% of nutrition goals with a peripheral solution but may be effective for a short period of time. While a patient is on PPN and EN is not a viable option within 5–7 days, serious consideration should be given to placement of a catheter for central venous access.[16]

If central access is obtained it is helpful to note the date of insertion, location, type of catheter, and number of lumens. These initial data will be useful when monitoring for catheter-related complications such as dislodgement, thrombosis, and embolism. Heparin is routinely added to neonatal and pediatric PN solutions to maintain patency of the central venous catheter.[24] Low flow volumes, smaller catheters, and frequent interruptions of PN solutions may play a role in increased incidence of catheter clotting in pediatric patients compared to adults.[25] Data suggest that a heparin concentration of 0.5 units/mL in neonatal PN solutions may be as effective for maintaining catheter patency as 1 unit/mL.[26] Please see Chapter 33 for additional information.

Monitor for Infectious Complications

Catheter-related bloodstream infections (CRBSIs) are a well-known complication of vascular access devices. By monitoring for fever and changes in the complete blood count (CBC), potential infections can be identified and treated promptly.[27] The most recent Center for Disease Control (CDC) guidelines for catheter maintenance were published in 2011.[28] The replacement of the infected catheter is recommended in most CRBSIs. However, continual replacement of the catheter can lead to the loss of venous access sites. This can be problematic for many PN patients due to their long-term need for a vascular access device. One strategy used to prevent CRBSIs has been the use of agents to sterilize the catheter lumen. The first of these was antibiotic lock therapy (ALT), which has been studied since the late 1980s.[29] This method involves using concentrated antibiotic solutions and dwelling the solution in the catheter lumen for a period of time. Problems associated with ALT are the development of antibiotic resistance with long-term use, lack of documented stability, and expense.[30]

Another agent that has been shown to reduce CRBSI is ethanol. Opilla et al specifically studied the use of ethanol for the home PN patient and showed a statistically significant reduction in CRBSIs and catheter exchanges.[31] The use of ethanol lock therapy (ELT) has been shown to be safe for the pediatric patient.[32-34] Currently, no standardized dose, concentration, frequency, or dwell time exists for the use of ethanol lock therapy. Factors that must be considered when choosing to utilize an ethanol lock include catheter material, catheter age, and compliance.[35] Recently a review evaluating the evidence for prophylaxis of CRBSI with ELT suggest that this therapy does decrease the incidence of infections and catheter removal and may be efficacious in combination with systemic antibiotics for the treatment of CRBSI. The regimens utilized still varied among institutions regarding volume of lock, flush vs withdraw, catheter type, frequency, and dwell time.[36]

Bacterial overgrowth can be a complication in patients with intestinal failure receiving PN and requires treatment when identified. Abdominal discomfort, bloating, cramps, gas, changes in stool color, consistency, and odor are common signs and symptoms. When the preceding signs and symptoms are identified, the patient should be treated. Due to the difficulty in diagnosing small bowel bacterial overgrowth, treatment centers around symptomatic improvement with cyclical antibiotics covering enteric aerobic and anaerobic bacteria or probiotics.[37] If a fever is also present, the patient should be evaluated for bacteremia due to possible translocation from the GI tract.[27] (See Chapter 27.)

Evaluation of PN Solution Tolerance

Monitor PN Volume

Generally PN volume is based on a patient's maintenance volume requirement (refer to Chapter 9). Fluid volume may be restricted or increased depending on disease processes and clinical condition. Multiple subjective and objective factors can be evaluated to aid in determining if the volume of PN or total fluid intake is appropriate. Weight, intake from all sources, output from all sources, laboratory results , vital signs, and physical assessment should be evaluated on a daily basis initially when PN is started (Table 36-2). Frequency of routine weights and laboratory results can be decreased as the patient stabilizes. If a patient is going home on PN or has limited access, total fluid requirement may be incorporated into the PN solution as possible.

Monitor for Metabolic Complications of Macronutrients

Blood urea nitrogen (BUN) is used as a monitoring tool for hydration status, and it may also indicate excessive amino acid administration.[38] An elevated BUN in the neonate more likely reflects immature renal function rather than excessive amino acid intake. If an elevated BUN cannot be explained by changes in renal function, medications (eg, high-dose steroids, amphotericin, aminoglycosides, and diuretics), bleeding, or dehydration then the nonprotein calorie to nitrogen (NPC:N) ratio needs to be evaluated. The ideal NPC:N ratio in stable patients is 150–250:1.[39] The ratio may be less in critically ill patients or higher in renal failure patients. If the ratio is low and BUN is elevated, it may be necessary to decrease the amino acid and adjust PN accordingly to maintain adequate caloric intake. Conversely, a low BUN level may indicate suboptimal amino acid administration. Ammonia levels and mental status are monitored in liver disease patients. Please refer to Chapter 26.

Table 36-2. Parameters to Evaluate Adequacy of PN Volume

PARAMETER	DEHYDRATION	FLUID OVERLOAD
Weight change: real vs fluid	Rapid ↓ weight	Rapid ↑ weight
Intake: intravenous fluids, PN, blood products, medications, EN	Total intake < total output	Total intake > total output
Output: urine, gastric, stool, bile, chest tube, wound, skin	Decreased urine output, dark urine	Increased urine output in patients with normal renal and liver function
Laboratory	↑ Blood urea nitrogen, ↑ sodium, ↑ serum osmolality, ↑ urine specific gravity, ↑ albumin or Hgb	↓ Sodium, ↓ serum osmolality, ↓ urine specific gravity, ↓ albumin or Hgb
Vitals	↑ Heart rate, ↑ losses with fever	↑ Respiratory rate
Medications	Addition of diuretic or change in frequency	Fluid retention with steroids or excessive sodium intake
Physical examination	Thirst, dry lips, dry mucous membranes, dry skin, headache, dizziness	Peripheral, facial, and orbital edema, ↑ abdominal girth, shortness of breath

EN, enteral nutrition; Hgb, hemoglobin; PN, parenteral nutrition.

Dextrose is best monitored by venous blood glucose and capillary glucose. The frequency of venous or capillary glucose monitoring depends on history of glucose intolerance, presence of diabetes, or concurrent medications affecting blood glucose control. The frequency may vary from every 2 hours to every 24 hours depending on factors listed above. Capillary glucose monitoring is useful for frequent monitoring so that the central line does not have to be accessed an inordinate number of times during the day or when verifying an abnormal glucose level from a venous sample. The frequency of monitoring can be modified to 1 or 2 times weekly once the patient has established good blood glucose control on the goal PN formula.

Unexplained hyperglycemia should prompt the calculation of the GIR from the PN solution and other dextrose-containing solutions. Pediatric patients receiving PN for > 2 weeks on a stable regimen may be cycled 12–22 hours per day in an effort to ease daily activities and decrease hepatic complications related to PN.[40] Initially, blood glucose levels should be obtained during the high rate of cyclic PN infusion and 1–2 hours after cycle completion to evaluate for hyperglycemia and hypoglycemia. Levels > 150 mg/dL will require a decrease in dextrose amount or lengthening of cyclic infusion to decrease the GIR. In the NICU setting, maximum tolerated serum glucose level may be as high as 180 mg/dL to achieve adequate nutrition. Levels < 60 mg/dL or any symptoms of hypoglycemia will require a longer taper period off of the cyclic PN or adjustment of regular insulin if present in PN solution.[41]

Triglyceride levels are monitored daily as lipid intake is increased and then weekly once the dose is stable and levels are adequate. Maximal lipid infusion for adults is 0.125 g/kg/h.[42] Information regarding maximal infusion rate for pediatrics is limited, but it is well-documented that longer infusion rates, 12–24 hours, improve tolerance to lipid infusions.[43] Decreasing the lipid dose or infusing lipids every other day or 3–5 times a week instead of daily in long-term PN patients will allow for further clearance of the lipid and possibly avoid triglyceride levels > 200 mg/dL. It is recommended to reduce or hold at current lipid infusion when levels are > 250 mg/dL. Limiting the dose and therefore decreasing phytosterol intake may also reduce the cholestasis commonly noted in pediatric patients receiving long-term PN.[44] Even though an hourly dose limit in pediatrics has not been published, calculating the lipid infusion rate in grams per kilograms per hour and comparing to the adult limit can still be helpful if hypertriglyceridemia is an issue.

Patients with a true egg allergy may require a test dose of lipid emulsion to better evaluate for any hypersensitivity reaction that may result in anaphylaxis, hives, rash, or itching.[45] The emulsifier in currently marketed long-chain triglyceride lipid emulsions contains egg phospholipid. Even though reactions to PN components are rare, some case reports suggest that multivitamins, lipid emulsions, iron dextran, or preservatives may be causative agents.[46,47] If a reaction does occur and PN is suspected, eliminating 1 agent at a time helps to determine the causative ingredient. If PN is required for more than a week with no EN then alternate routes may need to be identified to provide the particular causative agent. Vitamins may be administered orally or via a feeding tube or topical safflower oil in the case of lipid intolerance.

Monitoring the Integrity of PN Solutions

A number of factors influence the solubility of minerals such as calcium and phosphorus, the compatibility of PN solutions, and the integrity of total nutrient admixtures (TNA). Factors that influence calcium and phosphorus solubility are listed in Table 36-3. The pH of the amino acid solution drives the pH of the PN solution. The ideal pH for calcium and phosphorus solubility is ~ 5–6.[48] Solubility will decrease as the pH becomes more acidic or alkaline. Higher concentrations of amino acid allow for higher calcium and phosphorus doses to be admixed in a 2-n-1 or 3-n-1 solution. Some clinicians feel that the amount of lipid emulsion can influence how much calcium and phosphorus can be admixed in PN solutions, but the concentration of lipid emulsion is not a variable evaluated in calcium/phosphorus solubility graphs.

Solubility graphs in Trissel's and King's reference texts have been a primary source for determining adequacy of calcium and phosphorus amounts ordered in various PN solutions.[49,48] Today, some of the order-entry software utilized with the automated compounding hardware has incorporated the calcium/phosphorus solubility graphs into alerts. The order entry pharmacist is alerted when the solubility graphs are exceeded. This feature eliminates manual plotting of concentration points but still requires critical evaluation of all graphs to determine if each individual solution is appropriate for compounding. Changes in any of the PN ingredients may affect the stability or solubility of the formulation and thus warrants constant surveillance during compounding and administration.

Practitioners were reminded in a tragic fashion how important order of mixing is when compounding PN solutions. At least 2 deaths have been associated with calcium-phosphorus precipitation in PN solutions.[50] Temperature and lighting also play a role and need to be investigated when precipitation occurs, PN solutions look abnormal or become discolored, PN filters occlude, and when the solution otherwise meets all solubility and stability limits. Neonatal PN solutions are particularly at risk for stability issues due to bilirubin lights, heat from the extensive amount of equipment utilized in these units, and frequent co-infusion of medications with limited IV access.

Table 36-3. Factors Negatively Affecting Calcium and Phosphorus Solubility

Increased temperature
Increased concentrations of calcium and phosphorus
Type of amino acid product and decreased concentration
Decreased dextrose concentration
pH of final solution < 5 and > 7
Omission of cysteine
Bright lighting
Order of mixing without significant separation of calcium and phosphorus

TNAs are complex solutions that require additional scrutiny and compounding limits due to their opaque nature. Factors involved for ensuring the integrity of the emulsion are listed in Table 36-4. Minimum concentrations of the macronutrients should be determined, especially for TNA, to maintain the integrity of the emulsion.[51,52] A minimum amount of IV lipid is required to provide adequate emulsifier for a TNA.[53] It is yet to be determined how product packaging of current lipid formulations will affect the integrity of TNA.[54] Refer to Appendix 36-1 for an example of institutional-derived dosing and stability limits.

Comparison of 3-n-1 and 2-n-1 Solutions

When PN is compounded with amino acids and dextrose it is referred to as 2-n-1. TNA, or 3-n-1, refers to PN solutions compounded with amino acids, dextrose, and lipids. The opaque nature of a TNA or 3-n-1 is considered a disadvantage due to the inability to see obvious precipitates. Calcium and phosphorus intakes are felt to be less with TNA, but again lipid is not a limiting factor in the solubility of these 2 minerals. Divalent cations such as calcium, magnesium, and zinc may be somewhat limited in TNA due to the anionic nature of the lipid emulsions.[52] It may be difficult to provide higher doses of these divalent cations in low-volume solutions or for patients receiving magnesium-wasting medications.

As with calcium and phosphorus solubility, higher concentrations of amino acid and dextrose provide a protective

effect on the emulsion. The amino acids form a protective layer around the lipid globules, while the hypertonicity of the dextrose prohibits excessive movement and possible coalescence of globules.[55] The most problematic TNAs are the initial neonatal formulations for extremely low birth weight infants with low dextrose and lipid concentrations. Centers that compound TNAs or 3-n-1 formulations must invest in automated compounding systems that interface with advanced order-entry software containing multiple manufacturer and institutional limits. These dosing and stability limits will aid in identifying solutions potentially unsafe for patient administration.

Although TNAs require rigorous review, they do allow for all nutrients to be in one bag and therefore only one infusion pump. Nursing time is less compared with the time needed when lipids are administered separately in syringes every 12 hours and co-infused with a 2-n-1 solution. Some institutions infuse lipids in syringes over 24 hours, but the Centers for Disease Control and Prevention (CDC) recommendation states IV lipids should not be infused longer than 12 hours to avoid microbial growth.[56] Crill et al[57] reported no contamination of IV lipids when administered from the original container either as a drawn-down or non–drawn-down and infused over 24 hours. In a small study conducted by DeDonato and colleagues,[58] no difference was observed in microbial growth between 12-hour and 24-hour separate lipid infusion. Concern exists for increase in lipid peroxidation once lipids are transferred from their original container.[59] Clinical consequence is not known at this time, and it is not clear whether peroxidation occurs at a quicker rate in TNA or lipids administered via syringe. Another advantage of TNA is 24-hour infusion of lipid and decreased risk of microbial growth compared to lipid alone.[56] Table 36-5 outlines the advantages and disadvantages of 3-n-1 or TNA over 2-n-1 solutions. Each institution needs to determine which mode of PN ordering works best for its patient populations.

Metabolic Bone Disease

Metabolic bone disease (MBD) is a complication that may result from long-term PN. It may present as osteomalacia, osteopenia, or osteoporosis. Several factors may increase the incidence of MBD. Those include medications, calcium and vitamin D malabsorption, metabolic acidosis, high aluminum concentrations in PN, and other nutrient deficiencies. In addition to the presence of bone pain or nontraumatic fracture, the following laboratory tests may indicate suspicion of MBD: low to normal parathyroid hormone (PTH),

Table 36-4. Factors Affecting Total Nutrient Admixture Stability

Final pH (5–6)	Optimal pH for stability
Divalent cation concentration (calcium, magnesium, zinc)	Maximum concentration limits required
Trivalent cations (iron dextran)	Not stable in TNA
Type of amino acid and concentration	Higher concentrations improve stability
Dextrose concentration	Lower concentrations will limit stability
Anionic emulsifier	Protects emulsion integrity
Multivitamin products	Protects emulsion integrity
Temperature	Avoid administration in warm areas
Order of mixing	Critical to avoid precipitation and instability
Product packaging	Lipids in plastic: effect on stability?

TNA, total nutrient admixtures.

Table 36-5. Advantages and Disadvantages of Total Nutrient Admixtures

ADVANTAGES	DISADVANTAGES
Allows for 24-h lipid infusion	Prohibits visual inspection
Decrease labor costs	Limited compatibility information
Decreased equipment and supply cost	Minimum macronutrient amount required for stability
Decreases microbial growth opportunity	

elevated alkaline phosphatase, suboptimal vitamin D levels, changes in serum calcium levels, and hypercalciuria.[60-62] Therefore, monitoring a yearly PTH along with vitamin D (25-hydroxy and 1,25-dihydroxy) and bone-density measurements may be indicated in long-term PN patients.[13] It is recommended to maximize calcium and phosphorus intake in neonatal PN solutions while providing parenteral vitamin D (included in parenteral multivitamin products).[63]

Guidelines for Monitoring Nutrition Laboratory Values in Children Receiving EN and PN

The goals for monitoring patients receiving SNS are to ensure the efficacy of the regimen and to identify and prevent potential complications. It is important that the nutrition support team (physician, nurse, pharmacist, and dietitian) establish goals for the patient prior to initiating SNS. The monitoring of patients requiring EN and/or PN must include both clinical data and laboratory testing. Sample patient data sheets are included (Appendices 36-2 to 36-4). Appendix 36-2 may be utilized for patients started on PN or a combination of PN/EN. Appendix 36-3 can be utilized in addition to Appendix 36-2 for those patients receiving PN for greater than 3 months. Appendix 36-4 can be used for pediatric patients > 40 kg with PN units listed as grams, milliequivalents, or millimoles per day. Every patient must have documented baseline data in order for appropriate evaluation and monitoring to take place.

It is important to note that it is impossible to create a "one size fits all" set of monitoring guidelines. Each patient's monitoring regimen must be created based on the specific disease state and individualized long-term goals. New patients will require the most frequent monitoring, while stable long-term SNS patients may require less intense monitoring. EN-only patients will require less laboratory monitoring, while those on PN will require regular laboratory testing. The following information should be used as a general guideline and can be customized to the specific patient needs. Please refer to disease-specific chapters in this

book for additional monitoring that may be required. Tables 36-6 and 36-7, which appear at the end of this chapter, are examples of suggested monitoring for short-term and long-term laboratory testing.

Physical Data

A number of objective physical pieces of data can be collected to aid in evaluating adequacy and tolerance to SNS. Developing standards of practice, order sets, policies, and procedures in all institutions caring for patients requiring SNS can assist those individuals responsible for monitoring these complex patients. Table 36-1 delineates some general guidelines, but individual patient needs and clinical situation should dictate specific monitoring parameters and the frequency.

Table 36-6. Frequency of Short- and Long-Term Metabolic Monitoring

PARAMETER	INITIAL	FOLLOW-UP
BMP	Daily	Included in CMP
CMP	Weekly	Every 1–4 wk
Magnesium	Daily to weekly	Every 1–4 wk
Phosphorous	Daily to weekly	Every 1–4 wk
Prealbumin	Weekly	Monthly
Triglycerides	Daily to weekly	Monthly
PT/INR	Weekly	Monthly
CBC differential/ platelets	Weekly	Every 1–4 wk
GGTP	Baseline if indicated	Monthly

BMP, basic metabolic panel; CBC, complete blood count; CMP, comprehensive metabolic panel; GGTP, γ-glutamyl transpeptidase; INR, international normalized ratio; PT, prothrombin time.

Table 36-7. Frequency of Long-Term Nutrition-Related Monitoring

PARAMETER	INITIAL	FOLLOW-UP
Iron studies	3 mo	Every 3–6 mo
Zinc	3 mo	Every 3–6 mo
Selenium	3 mo	Every 3–6 mo
Manganese	3 mo	Every 3–6 mo
Copper	3 mo	Every 3–6 mo
Chromium	3 mo	Every 3–6 mo
Vitamin D	3–6 mo	Every 12 mo
Vitamins A and E	6 mo	Every 12 mo
Vitamin B_{12} and folate	6 mo	Every 12 mo
Carnitine	3 mo	Every 3–12 mo
Thyrotropin	Baseline if indicated	Every 12 mo

Chemistry Profile Monitoring[27,60,64-67]

The monitoring of electrolytes, minerals, renal function, glucose, and acid-base balance is essential in PN. When initiating a patient on PN, a baseline basic metabolic panel (BMP), magnesium, phosphorous, and triglyceride level should be ordered and monitored daily until the patient has reached the caloric goal established at initial assessment. The frequency may be decreased to twice weekly in which one day includes the comprehensive metabolic panel (CMP), which encompasses the hepatic function along with the BMP. As the patient stabilizes, laboratory tests may be decreased to weekly. Finally, these tests may be reduced to every 2–4 weeks when the PN formula is stable and if appropriate goals are being met for the current condition and growth needs.

Nutrition-Related Laboratory Tests

Prealbumin can be used to monitor protein status due to its shorter half-life of 2–3 days in comparison to albumin.[68] However, other factors can influence prealbumin levels such as inflammatory states, end-stage liver disease, untreated thyroid disease, renal disease, and zinc deficiency. These limitations should be considered when interpreting a patient's prealbumin level.[69-71] Monitoring of prealbumin and albumin levels may be helpful in long-term stable patients for identifying resolution of acute illness or readiness for surgery.[72]

Changes in triglyceride levels can be influenced by a variety of factors including disease state, organ function, medications, nutrition status, and current nutrient intake. They should be monitored daily when SNS is initially started, followed by a weekly level, and then decreased to monthly.[27,38,43,73]

Carnitine is often added to the PN solution because it is not a standard ingredient, the patient is not receiving EN, or a deficiency has been documented. A patient who has a deficiency may present with increased triglyceride levels, hypoglycemia, hyperbilirubinemia, or decreased weight gain along with a multitude of other clinical symptoms.[74-76] Currently a carnitine dose of 10–20 mg/kg/d is recommended for IV or oral supplementation and should be initiated in any patient receiving PN for > 7 days.[77] Data support dosages of 5–10 mg/kg/day when started in PN from day 1 of therapy to prevent development of deficiency.[78] Although most EN formulas contain adequate dietary carnitine, supplementation can be considered in EN patients with malabsorption or bowel resection if deficiency is suspected or confirmed by laboratory testing. A carnitine profile, including ester/free ratio, should be monitored every 3–6 months if the patient is being supplemented. A yearly carnitine profile is sufficient for patients not receiving the RDA.

Linoleic and α-linolenic acid, known as essential fatty acids (EFAs), must be obtained orally, enterally, or parenterally in all patients since the body cannot synthesize them. If inadequate amounts are provided, an essential fatty acid deficiency (EFAD) may eventually occur. If reduced or lipid-free PN is provided for a significant amount of time or a clinical manifestation of an EFAD occurs, it is recommended to order an EFA profile. The resulting triene to tetraene ratio can determine if an EFAD exists.[43,79-81]

Liver Enzymes and Bilirubin

Hepatic and biliary complications are a well-documented adverse effect of PN in children.[82-85] It is necessary to monitor liver enzymes, which generally include alkaline phosphatase, aspartate aminotransferase, and alanine aminotransferase, on a weekly basis when initiating PN. A total bilirubin should also be followed. If prolonged PN is anticipated or the patient becomes jaundiced, a direct or conjugated bilirubin level is helpful to monitor for cholestasis.[40] A direct bilirubin > 2 mg/dL may prompt earlier monitoring of the trace elements copper, and manganese due to the biliary tract being the primary excretory pathway for copper and manganese.[86] Liver enzymes and total bilirubin are included when ordering the CMP as previously discussed. Once stabilized these laboratory tests can be monitored every 2–4 weeks.

γ-Glutamyl transpeptidase (GGTP) is another liver enzyme that is more specific for liver and biliary tract problems.[41] GGTP is the most sensitive liver enzyme for detecting biliary obstruction, cholangitis, or cholecystitis.[68] It can be ordered for further diagnosis when the traditional liver enzymes are elevated or as a regularly monitored monthly test if the patient is at risk for biliary complications.

If a patient on long-term PN has a significantly increased alkaline phosphatase level, it may be advisable to request an alkaline phosphatase isoenzyme test. This test will give the clinician a breakdown of the source of the alkaline phosphatase, which can be liver, bone, or intestinal. This is clinically useful if liver dysfunction or metabolic bone disease due to PN therapy is suspected.[87]

The prothrombin time (PT) and international normalized ratio (INR) can be utilized in long-term monitoring of PN. The PT can be elevated in a patient who is developing hepatocellular disease or obstructive biliary disease or more rarely a vitamin K deficiency.[41,88,89] Vitamin K or phytonadione content in injectable adult and pediatric multivitamin should provide the recommended daily amount parenterally, but patients with malabsorption and liver disease may require additional supplementation via PN. These same patients on EN may also require additional supplementation enterally. A baseline and then monthly check of the PT/INR is adequate.

Trace Elements (See Also Chapter 6)

A patient's initial PN usually contains a trace element package that has a manufacturer-determined dose of zinc, copper, manganese, chromium, and/or selenium (see Chapter 35).[90] When a patient is receiving PN for several months or has developed cholestasis, it is important to assess the status of those trace elements. After 3 consecutive months on PN (unless clinically indicated earlier),[91] a patient should be assessed for zinc, selenium, manganese, copper, and chromium.[27] Long-term use of standard multitrace products can result in both excessive and deficient concentrations, especially in patients who have abnormalities in the GI tract. Although measuring blood concentrations of these trace elements is not necessarily the most accurate due to the body's ability to store these elements, it is generally the easiest and least costly way to monitor.[92] It is also important to note that these elements should not be checked in times of acute inflammatory conditions due to the body's sequestration of some elements during this time. Levels may be falsely decreased in these types of situations.[93]

Assessment of these elements should occur every 3–12 months while receiving PN.[27,92] If a patient is found to have an elevated level of any standard element, the multitrace element of the PN can be omitted and separate elements added. Additionally, if any element is found to be deficient, it can be added in addition to the standard multitrace. It is important to be familiar with the content of both pediatric and adult trace minerals solutions so that you can adjust supplementation accordingly when switching to individual trace minerals. There are limits to concentrations of trace elements in PN so this must be considered,[49,94] and in that situation, oral supplementation may be an option (see Table 36-8). After altering the dosage of any element it should be rechecked in approximately 1–3 months. If a patient's condition has completely stabilized, it is reasonable to monitor only once per year.

Aluminum, considered an ultratrace element, is a known contaminant of PN products. It is important to monitor due to the patient's continued exposure and risk for toxicity, especially for high-risk populations such as premature neonates, infants receiving long-term PN, and hemodialysis patients on PN. It is reasonable to check an aluminum level each year during PN therapy. If the aluminum is elevated, the PN pharmacist can look at the current PN components and make adjustments if possible since aluminum contamination varies between different PN product manufacturers.[95] One example would be to omit cysteine from a neonatal PN order if the infant is > 3 months of age and PN dependent.

Molybdenum deficiency is rare but can occur in a PN patient, especially those with decreased intestinal absorption.[96,97] If desired, a molybdenum level may be checked yearly unless otherwise clinically indicated. If a deficiency is detected, molybdenum may be supplemented via PN in the form of ammonium molybdate.

Iodine is an element not supplied by standard multitrace products in PN. Therefore, it is possible, although unlikely, for a SNS patient to become deficient.[98,99] This can routinely be assessed with a yearly thyrotropin and triiodothyronine test or urine iodine concentration.

Table 36-8 lists suggested enteral doses[100] for trace mineral supplementation if parenteral options are not available or a patient is on EN. Compounding of liquid preparations may be required for a suitable concentration and administration via

Table 36-8. Enteral Options for Trace Metals[a]

	PRETERM[1]	TERM < 6 mo	PEDIATRIC 7 mo–3 y	PEDIATRIC 4–8 y	PEDIATRIC 9–13 y	PEDIATRIC 14–18 y, ADULTS
Zinc	1000–3000 mcg/kg/d	2000 mcg/d[b]	3000 mcg/d[c]	5000 mcg/d[c]	8000 mcg/d[c]	M, 11,000 mcg/d[c] F, 9000 mcg/d[c]
Copper	120–150 mcg/kg/d	200 mcg/d[b]	220 mcg/d[b] (7 mo–1 y) 340 mcg/d[c] (1–3 y)	440 mcg/d[c]	700 mcg/d[c]	890 mcg/d
Selenium	1.3–4.5 mcg/kg/d	15 mcg/d[b]	20 mcg/d[b,c]	30 mcg/d[c]	40 mcg/d[c]	55 mcg/d[c]

[a]Doses listed as elemental.
[b]Adequate intake.
[c]Recommended dietary allowance.

feeding tubes. Consult your multivitamin formulary because some of these preparations may contain the desired minerals.

Iron Studies and Anemia

When patients are dependent on EN and/or PN, the potential exists for them to become anemic. The 4 nutrients that are most likely to be the reason for anemia are iron, copper, vitamin B_{12}, and folic acid. Standard PN contains 3 of the previous nutrients with the exception being iron due to its incompatibility with lipid emulsion.[94] Enterally fed patients typically are provided with all 4 nutrients. However, the standard quantities provided may not always be adequate for the specific disease process that is being treated. For example, a patient who has shortened bowel will generally have less absorption of the nutrients from EN and may become deficient over time.

Iron deficiency can be recognized by abnormalities in the CBC. In general a decrease in hemoglobin and mean corpuscular volume (MCV) are present.[27] It may take some time for the deficiency to occur so a routine CBC (at least monthly) is recommended to monitor for these changes.[60,64,65] When these abnormalities are present, an iron panel can be ordered if indicated to confirm the deficiency. An iron panel should include serum iron, ferritin, transferrin saturation, and iron-binding capacity. In a deficient patient, the serum iron and ferritin may be reduced and the binding capacity elevated. It is best to draw this panel in the absence of acute infectious or inflammatory processes because they can lower serum iron since iron can be bound to proteins and elevate ferritin, an acute phase reactant, as listed in Table 36-9.[101] After confirming the deficiency, the iron may be supplemented orally. If the patient does not respond to oral iron, parenteral iron may be used as a separate infusion or added to the PN. The only parenteral iron that may be used in PN is iron dextran (refer to Chapter 35), and it can only be added in the absence of lipids in the formulation for stability reasons.[102] Monitoring of iron status should occur every 3–6 months in a deficient patient or a patient receiving supplementation.

Copper deficiency can also present with anemia and neutropenia.[103,104] This can result from decreased absorption or increased losses from the intestinal tract. Copper deficiency can also occur due to high zinc, vitamin C, or iron supplementation or from the use of gastric acid–suppressing medications.[105] Iatrogenic copper deficiency may occur with inadequate amounts in PN due to concern for accumulation in patients with cholestasis. Measuring serum copper or serum cerulosplasmin levels can assess the patient's copper

Table 36-9. Factors That May Influence Iron Panel Assessment

IRON PANEL	INCREASED LEVELS	DECREASED LEVELS
Iron	More than adequate iron	Infection, inflammation, iron deficiency
TIBC	Iron deficiency	Infection, inflammation
Ferritin	Infection, inflammation	Iron deficiency
% Transferrin saturation	More than adequate iron	Iron deficiency

TIBC, total iron binding capacity.

status.[92] This test can be performed with the other multi-trace elements levels as previously discussed.

Both vitamin B_{12} and folic acid deficiencies can present as a macrocytic anemia with an elevated MCV. Because these 2 nutrients have an intertwined relationship in the body, it is recommended to assess the status of both whenever either is measured. Patients without an ileocecal valve are particularly at risk for the development of vitamin B_{12} deficiency since this is a site for absorption. It is possible for the body to maintain serum vitamin B_{12} levels even though storages have been depleted. Therefore, it can also be beneficial to check methylmalonic acid and homocysteine levels when vitamin B_{12} deficiency is truly suspected. These 2 tests will be elevated in most patients even with a minimal vitamin B_{12} deficiency.[106] However, homocysteine levels may also be elevated in the presence of folic acid and vitamin B_6 deficiency, therefore it is not a specific indicator of vitamin B_{12} deficiency.[107] A yearly measure of these vitamins is normally sufficient unless deficiency is suspected[91] or in evaluating after increased supplementation. Also see chapters 6–8.

Vitamins

Fat-soluble vitamins A, D, E, and K are standard components of most parenteral multivitamin products and EN products. It is possible for a patient to accumulate excessive amounts due to the body's storage of these vitamins, but it is also possible for deficiency to occur with certain disease states. Monitoring the levels of vitamins A, D, and E once yearly is recommended unless otherwise clinically indicated.[27] Obtaining vitamin D levels every 3–6 months may be necessary in patients malnourished prior to initiation of SNS, patients with malabsorption, and patients with reduced sun exposure.[108] Vitamin K status is more commonly assessed by the PT or INR as previously discussed.

The water-soluble vitamins including B_1, B_2, B_6, B_{12}, niacin, folic acid, pantothenic acid, biotin, and vitamin C are also components of parenteral multivitamins and EN. Routine monitoring of these vitamins is not indicated (except for B_{12} and folic acid as previously discussed) unless a clinical reason exists to believe that a deficiency or toxicity is occurring; for example, when a patient receives loop diuretic therapy, which has been associated with thiamine deficiency.[91,109] Also see chapters 7 and 8.

Pharmacotherapy Issues Related to Evaluation and Monitoring

Medication and PN Ingredient Shortage

Chronic medication and PN shortages have created many challenges for ensuring adequate therapy for patients receiving SNS. Shortages have forced many practitioners involved with these therapies to be creative with the available supply, even resorting to utilizing very small amounts of adult trace element solution in neonates so that selenium can be provided. Increased utilization of enteral supplementation and increased laboratory draws for monitoring has also been a result of the PN ingredient shortages. This is not ideal and raises the question of risk vs benefit for each individual patient. The American Society for Parenteral and Enteral Nutrition provides a number of documents to assist the practitioner in making decisions regarding managing available supply.[110] It is crucial to bring inventory specialists, buyers, managers, operation supervisors, and nutrition support experts together on a routine basis to discuss current shortages, anticipated shortages, and restriction criteria in the event of critical shortages. Dissemination of information and education regarding the shortages is of the utmost importance as well.

Evaluate Drug and Nutrient Interactions

The process of evaluating for drug-nutrient interactions begins with the patient medication profile and nutrition regimen. A number of excellent published resources and pharmacy computer databases can be utilized to identify drug-nutrient interactions.[111,112] Pharmacy order entry systems can provide alerts for particular medications (eg, fluoroquinolones and phenytoin) when patients are receiving enteral feedings. Once an interaction is identified, the severity along with the source of the interaction needs to be evaluated closely to determine a course of action. A number of interactions may be avoided by administering the drug and the particular nutrient, vitamin, or mineral at separate times

during the day. If enteral formula ingredients interfere with drug absorption, consultation with a pharmacist and dietitian can aid in developing a revised enteral regimen for the patient that will allow for improved drug absorption.

Particular medications may induce certain electrolyte and mineral wasting or retention. Oral, enteral, or parenteral electrolyte and mineral supplementation may be required while a patient is receiving these offending agents. PN is not meant to be a vehicle for acute electrolyte and mineral replacement but can aid in supplementing patients with chronic electrolyte and mineral abnormalities. Electrolyte and mineral supplementation should not be added directly to enteral formulas due to the potential for instability but should be diluted and given orally or flushed via a feeding tube. Table 36-10 lists some common drug-induced metabolic disorders.[113,114] Patients on these particular medications require at least weekly laboratory monitoring. Frequency of monitoring is dependent on renal and hepatic function as well.

Compatibility of Medications

Nutrition support practitioners rely on critical review of available PN stability literature, parenteral product manufacturer studies, and in-house stability studies to determine maximum concentrations for micronutrients and compatible medications that can be safely added to PN solutions. Certain medications may be co-infused with PN or TNA if no other access is available. A number of published compatibility charts exist, but it is still a good practice to compare your own institution's PN solutions against published charts and studies.[102,115] A range of PN solutions and TNA have been tested, but testing each individual solution that may be prescribed in clinical practice for stability is impossible. In general, it is best to avoid admixing or co-administering medications with PN and EN unless absolutely necessary

Table 36-10. Drug-Induced Metabolic Disorders

Loop Diuretics: hyponatremia, hypokalemia, hypocalcemia, metabolic alkalosis
H2 antagonists: hyponatremia
Corticosteroids: hypokalemia, hypocalcemia, hypophosphatemia, metabolic alkalosis
Amphotericin B: hypokalemia, hypomagnesemia, metabolic acidosis
Cyclosporine, Tacrolimus: hypomagnesemia, hyperkalemia, hypertriglyceridemia
Aminoglycosides: metabolic acidosis
Citrate: hypocalcemia

and after consultation with a pharmacist due to the limited amount of data available.

Summary

In summary, the numerous subjective and objective data obtained from the patient needs to be evaluated to determine the efficacy, tolerance, or any complications of the SNS. The frequency of evaluating and monitoring the data is dependent on the type of SNS provided, the stability of the patient, any concurrent medical diagnoses, and progression to nutrition goals. This is a constant process throughout the growth and development of the pediatric patient. This chapter should serve as a guide for developing the evaluation and monitoring plan for pediatric patients receiving SNS.

Appendix 36-1. Parenteral Nutrition Limits

	Adult	Pediatric	NICU		Stability	Usual Dose	Comments
Na	180	180	180	mEq/L			Osmolarity
		0–6	0–6	mEq/kg		X	
K	150	150	150	mEq/L	X		
		0–6	0–5	mEq/kg		X	
Ca	30	30	30	mEq/L	X		
		0–2	0–4.5	mEq/kg		X	
PO$_4$	35	30	30	mmol/L	X		
		0–2	0–2	mmol/kg		X	
Mg	24	24	13	mEq/L	X		
		0–0.5	0–1	mEq/kg		X	
Cl	300	250	250	mEq/L			
		0–8	0–10	mEq/kg		X	
Ac	300	250	250	mEq/L			
		0–8	0–10	mEq/kg		X	
Zn	10	5	5	mg/L	X		Total zinc
		300	400	mcg/kg		X	or DC fat
Cysteine			120	mg/kg		X	
Vitamin K	10	10	n/a	***mg***		X	mg/day
Ranitidine	n/a	100	100	mg/L	X		
		0–6	2	mg/kg		X	
Famotidine	40	n/a	n/a	mg/L	X		
				mg/kg			
Folic acid		2.5	2.5	***mg***			Not mg/L
		10	10	mg/d	X		
Heparin	1000	1000	1000	units/L		X	
Vitamin C	500	700	700	mg/d	X		Total dose
Carnitine	50	50	50	mg/kg/d	X	X	
Amino acid	Min 20 g/L	Min 10 g/L or DC lipids	Min 10 g/L or DC lipids		X		Need 20 g/L if dextrose < 10% or DC lipids
Dextrose	Min 50 g/L	Min 50 g/L	Min 50 g/L		X		DC lipids if < 50 g/L
Lipid	Min 5 g/L	Min 5 g/L	Min 5 g/L		X		DC lipids if < 5 g/L

Appendix 36-2. Neonatal and Pediatric Nutrition Monitoring Form

Name:_____	MRN:_____	Admit Date:_____	MD:_____			
DOB:_____	Age:___y___m___d	DX:_____	Date:_____	wt_____:___%ile	WA_____	
Goals: Calories (kcal/d):_____		kcal/kg:_____		ht/lt_____:___%ile	HA_____	
Protein (g/d):_____		g/kg:_____		wt/ht_____%ile	BMI_____	
Fluid (mL/d):_____		mL/kg:_____		dry wt_____	IBW_____	

LABS								
Date								
Weight (kg)								
Sodium / Potassium	/	/	/	/	/	/	/	/
Chloride / Carbon Dioxide	/	/	/	/	/	/	/	/
BUN / Creatine	/	/	/	/	/	/	/	/
Glucose / Calcium	/	/	/	/	/	/	/	/
Phosphorous / Magnesium	/	/	/	/	/	/	/	/
Total/conj. Bilirubin	/	/	/	/	/	/	/	/
Cholesterol / Triglyceride	/	/	/	/	/	/	/	/
AST / ALT	/	/	/	/	/	/	/	/
AlkPhos / GGT	/	/	/	/	/	/	/	/
Hgb / Hct	/	/	/	/	/	/	/	/
WBC / platelets	/	/	/	/	/	/	/	/
INR								
Zinc								
Albumin / Prealbumin	/	/	/	/	/	/	/	/

PN SCRIPT																
AA/Dex/lipid (gm/kg/d)	/	/	/	/	/	/	/	/	/	/	/	/	/	/	/	/
Na (mEq/kg)																
K (mEq/kg)																
Cl (mEq/kg)																
Anions (A,C)																
Ca (mEq/kg)																
P (mmol/kg)																
Mg (mEq/kg)																
Heparin																
MVI:Peds/Adult																
TMS:Peds/Adult																
Zinc (mcg/kg)																
Copper (mcg/kg)																
Manganese (mcg/kg)																
Chromium (mcg/kg)																
Selenium (mcg/kg)																
Carnitine (mg/kg)																
Rate/Cycle																
Total Volume/d																
Total Calories/d																
Kcal/kg																
GIR																
NPC:N																
Wt used for script																
kcal/mL																

ENTERAL								
Formula								
Rate/Cycle	/	/	/	/	/	/	/	/
Route								

TOTALS								
mL PN/EN	/	/	/	/	/	/	/	/
kcal								
kcal/kg								
Protein (g)								
Protein (g/kg)								

OUTPUT								
UOP mL/kg/h	/	/	/	/	/	/	/	/
Emesis								
Stool								
Ostomy mL/d / mL/kg	/	/	/	/	/	/	/	/
Total mL								

Appendix 36-3. Long-Term Lab Tracking Sheet

Patient:	D.O.B.	Physician:	Diagnosis:
Medical Record Number:		Fax:	Phone:	Home Health Care:
PN start date:		Pager:		Lab Location / Phone:
Enteral Formula:		Other Contact:		Family Contact:

Lab Location:																							
Date:																							
Every Month																							
Pre-Albumin																							
Triglyceride																							
GGT																							
MCV																							
Every 3 Months																							
Selenium																							
Manganese																							
Copper																							
Chromium																							
Zinc																							
Ferritin																							
Iron Serum																							
TIBC																							
Transferrin Saturation																							
Carnitine Total																							
Carnitine Free																							
Carnitine Ratio																							
Every 12 Months																							
Vitamin A																							
Vitamin D																							
Vitamin E																							
Vitamin B-12																							
RBC Folate																							
TSH																							
Free T4																							
Aluminum																							
Recorded By:																							
Reviewed By:																							
Date Faxed to Physician:																							

Appendix 36-4. Pediatric Patient > 40 kg PN Monitoring Form

Pediatric Patients > 40 kg - Riley Children's Hospital at IU Health						

Name: _____ MRN: _____ DOB: _____ Age: ____y____m____d Admit Date: _____
Allergies: _____ Dx: _____
Actual Body Wt.: _____ IBW: _____ Adjusted Body Weight: _____ Wt. for Calc.: _____ BMI: _____

Goals

LABS							
Date							
Daily weight (kg)							
Na (135–145 mmol/L)							
K (3.5–5.5 mmol/L)							
Cl (98–108 mmol/L)							
CO$_2$ (22–29 mmol/L)							
BUN/Cr (5–20 / 0.3–1)							
Gluc (70–99 mg/dL)							
Ca (8.5–10.5 mg/dL)							
PO$_4$ (2.6–5 mg/dL)							
Mg (1.6–2.9 mg/dL)							
Total / Conj. Bilirubin	/	/	/	/	/	/	/
Cholesterol / TG	/	/	/	/	/	/	/
AST / ALT	/	/	/	/	/	/	/
AlkPhos / GGT	/	/	/	/	/	/	/
Hgb / Hct	/	/	/	/	/	/	/
WBC / Platelets	/	/	/	/	/	/	/
INR							
Zinc (60–150 mcg/dL)							
Albumin (3.5–5 g/dL)							
Pre-Alb (10–40 mg/dL)							

PN ORDER							
AA/Dex/Lipid (g/d)	//	//	//	//	//	//	//
NaCl (mEq/d)							
Na Acetate (mEq/d)							
Na Phos (mmol/d)							
KCl (mEq/d)							
K Acetate (mEq/d)							
K Phos (mmol/d)							
Mg Sulfate (mEq/d)							
Ca Gluconate (mEq/d)							
Reg Insulin (units/d)							
Heparin (units/d)							
MVI	Y N	Y N	Y N	Y N	Y N	Y N	Y N
TMS	Y N	Y N	Y N	Y N	Y N	Y N	Y N
Selenium (mcg/d)							
Zinc (mg/d)							
Copper (mg/d)							
Thiamine (mg/d)							
Folic Acid (mg/d)							
Rate or Cycle (mL/time)							
TOTAL Volume (daily)							
TOTAL Calories (daily)							
kcal/kg kcal/mL							
GIR (mg/kg/min)							
NPC:Nitrogen (150-250:1)							
Wt. Used for Order							

Appendix 36-4. Pediatric Patient > 40 kg PN Monitoring Form (Continued)

DAILY I/O							
INPUT							
IVF (mL)							
PN (mL)							
IV/EN Liquid Meds (mL)							
EN Formula / Liquids							
EN Route(s)							
Total EN Fluid Volume							
TOTAL INPUT (mL)							
OUTPUT							
Urine (mL |mL/kg/h |#)							
Mixed Urine/Stool |mL	Y N	Y N	Y N	Y N	Y N	Y N	Y N
Stool (mL |#)							
Emesis (mL |#)							
Drains/G Tube/Misc. (mL)							
Ostomy (mL/d)							
TOTAL OUTPUT (mL)							
I/O Difference (± mL)							

Home Diet:

Home Medications / Supplements:

Procedures:

Scope Results

Endoscopy:

Colonoscopy:

Progress Notes:

Periodic Lab Monitoring of Trace Elements								
Date:								
Copper								
Manganese								
Chromium								
Selenium								
Carnitine								
Aluminum								
Zinc								

Test Your Knowledge Questions

1. You are following a former 28-week gestation child who is now 2 years old. She receives bolus G-tube feedings due to history of failure to thrive and severe oral motor feeding aversion. Appropriate growth parameters have been achieved on current feeding plan. She has a recent history of aspiration pneumonia and received antibiotics. She is admitted with acute onset of diarrhea. All of the following options should initially be considered except:

    A. Screen for bacterial overgrowth
    B. Review current medications with pharmacist to identify any that could cause diarrhea
    C. Transition to an elemental formula
    D. Rule out infectious causes of diarrhea such as *Clostridium difficile*

2. A once stable patient on cyclic PN is now experiencing hyperglycemia, all below are acceptable responses except:

    A. Decrease GIR
    B. Increase PN cycle
    C. Consider work-up for infection
    D. Start subcutaneous long-acting insulin

3. A PN order is being evaluated for adequate calcium and phosphorus solubility at order entry, which factor negatively affects solubility?

    A. Decreased calcium concentration
    B. Increased dextrose concentration
    C. Decreased amino acid concentration
    D. Addition of cysteine

4. Which of the following nutritional components cannot be added to a 3-n-1 PN solution?

    A. Essential fatty acids
    B. Iron
    C. Vitamin K
    D. Carnitine

5. An infant dependent on PN has developed cholestasis with a direct bilirubin > 2 mg/dL. Which of the following trace minerals should be monitored for adjustment in supplementation?

    A. Selenium
    B. Copper
    C. Zinc
    D. Chromium

References

1. Corkins MR, Griggs KC, Groh-Wargo S, et al; Task Force on Standards for Nutrition Support: Pediatric Hospitalized Patients; American Society for Parenteral and Enteral Nutrition Board of Directors; American Society for Parenteral and Enteral Nutrition. Standards for nutrition support: pediatric hospitalized patients. *Nutr Clin Pract.* 2013;28(2):263–276.

2. Mehta NM, Smallwood CD, Graham RJ. Current applications of metabolic monitoring in the pediatric intensive care unit. *Nutr Clin Pract.* 2014:29:338–347.

3. Mehta NM, Corkins MR, Lyman B, et al; American Society for Parenteral and Enteral Nutrition Board of Directors. Defining pediatric malnutrition: a paradigm shift toward etiology-related definitions. *JPEN J Parenter Enteral Nutr.* 2013;37(4):460–481.

4. Bankhead R, Boullata J, Brantley S, et al; A.S.P.E.N. Board of Directors. Enteral nutrition practice recommendations. *JPEN J Parenter Enteral Nutr.* 2009;33(2):122–167.

5. Kraft MD, Btaiche IF, Sacks GS. Review of the re-feeding syndrome. *Nutr Clin Pract.* 2005;20:625–633.

6. Santanan e Meneses JF, Leite HP, de Carvalho WB, Lopes E Jr. Hypophosphatemia in critically ill children: prevalence and associated risk factors. *Pediatr Crit Care Med.* 2009;10:234–238.

7. Parrish CR. The refeeding syndrome in 2009: prevention is the key to treatment. *J Support Oncol.* 2009;7:20–21.

8. McCray S, Walker S, Parrish CR. Much ado about refeeding. *Practical Gastroenterol.* 2005;30(1):26–44.

9. Danner E, Joeckel R, Michalak S, Phillips S, Goday PS. Weight velocity in infants and children. *Nutr Clin Pract.* 2009;24:76–79.

10. Guo S, Roche AF, Fomon SJ, et al. Reference data on gains in weight and length during the first two years of life. *J Pediatr.* 1991;119:355–362.

11. Koletzko B, Goulet O, Hunt J, Krohn K, Shamir R; Parenteral Nutrition Guidelines Working Group; European Society for Clinical Nutrition and Metabolism; European Society of Paediatric Gastroenterology, Hepatology and Nutrition (ESPGHAN); European Society of Paediatric Research (ESPR). 1. Guidelines on paediatric parenteral nutrition of the European Society of Paediatric Gastroenterology, Hepatology and Nutrition (ESPGHAN) and the European Society for Clinical Nutrition and Metabolism (ESPEN), supported by the European Society of Paediatric Research (ESPR). *J Pediatr Gastroenterol Nutr.* 2005;41:S28–S32.

12. Burke JF, Wolfe RR, Mullany CJ, Mathews DE, Bier DM, et al. Glucose requirements following burn injury. Parameters of optimal glucose infusion and possible hepatic and respiratory abnormalities following excessive glucose intake. *Ann Surg.* 1979;190(3):274–285.

13. Btaiche IF, Khalidi N. Metabolic complications of parenteral nutrition in adults, part 2 [erratum in *Am J Health Syst Pharm.* 2004;61(24):2616]. *Am J Health Syst Pharm.* 2004;61:2050–2059.

14. Braegger C, Decsi T, Dias JA, et al; ESPGHAN Committee on Nutrition. Practical approach to paediatric enteral nutrition: a comment by the ESPGHAN Committee on Nutrition. *J Pediatr Gastroenterol Nutr.* 2010;51(1):110–122.

15. Moyer-Mileur L. Anthropometric and laboratory assessment of very low birth weight infants: the most helpful measurements and why. *Semin Perinatol.* 2007;31:96–103.

16. A.S.P.E.N. Board of Directors and the Clinical Guidelines Task Force. Guidelines for the use of parenteral and enteral nutrition in adult and pediatric patients. *JPEN J Parenter Enteral Nutr.* 2002;1SA–138SA.

17. Barrett JS, Shepherd SJ, Gibson PR. Strategies to manage gastrointestinal symptoms complicating enteral feeding. *JPEN J Parenter Enteral Nutr.* 2009;33:21–26.

18. Wessel JJ, Kocoshis SA. Nutritional management of infants with short bowel syndrome. *Semin Perinatol.* 2007;31:104–111.

19. Zella GC, Israel EJ. Chronic diarrhea in children. *Pediatr Rev.* 2012;33(5):207–218.

20. Koletzko S, Niggemann B, Arato A, et al; European Society of Pediatric Gastroenterology, Hepatology, and Nutrition. Diagnostic approach and management of cow's-milk protein allergy in infants and children: ESPGHAN GI Committee practical guidelines *J Pediatr Gastroenterol Nutr.* 2012;55:221–229.

21. Martinez EE, Bechard LJ, Mehta NM. Nutrition algorithms and bedside nutrient delivery practices in pediatric intensive care units: an international multicenter cohort study. *Nutr Clin Pract.* 2014;29:360–367.

22. Axelrod D, Kazmerski K, Iyer K. Pediatric enteral nutrition. *JPEN J Pediatr Enteral Nutr.* 2006;30:S21–S26.

23. Seashore JH, Hoffman M. Use and abuse of peripheral parenteral nutrition in children. *Nutr Support Serv.* 1983;3(10):8–13.

24. Imperial J, Bistrain BR, Bothe A Jr, Bern M, Blackburn GL. Limitation of central vein thrombosis in total parenteral nutrition by continuous infusion of low-dose heparin. *J Am Coll Nutr.* 1983;2:63–73.

25. Kakzanov V, Monagle P, Chan A. Thromboembolism in infants and children with gastrointestinal failure receiving long-term parenteral nutrition. *JPEN J Parenter Enteral Nutr.* 2008;32:88–93.

26. Szeszycki E, Kastner A, Mobley L, Gervasio J. A comparison of the efficacy of 0.5 units/ml versus 1 unit/ml of heparin in neonatal parenteral nutrition. Abstract presented at: A.S.P.E.N. Nutrition Week; February 1–4, 2009; New Orleans, Louisiana.

27. Siepler J. Principles and strategies for monitoring home parenteral nutrition. *Nutr Clin Pract.* 2007;22:340–350.

28. O'Grady NP, Alexander M, Burns LA, et al; the Healthcare Infection Control Practices Advisory Committee (HICPAC). Guidelines for the Prevention of Intravascular Catheter-Related Infections. Atlanta, GA: Centers for Disease Control and Prevention; 2011:1–83.

29. Messing B, Peitra-Cohen S, Debure A, Bernier J. Antibiotic-lock technique: a new approach to optimal therapy for catheter-related sepsis in home-parenteral nutrition patients. *JPEN J Parenter Enteral Nutr.* 1988;12:185–189.

30. Bestul MB, VandenBussche HL. Antibiotic lock technique: review of the literature. *Pharmacotherapy.* 2005;25:211–227.

31. Opilla MT, Kirby DF, Edmond MB. Use of ethanol lock therapy to reduce the incidence of catheter-related bloodstream infections in home parenteral nutrition patients. *JPEN J Parenter Enteral Nutr.* 2007;31(4):302–305.

32. Mouw E, Chessman K, Lesher A, Tagge E. Use of an ethanol lock to prevent catheter-related infections in children with short bowel syndrome. *J Pediatr Surg.* 2008;43(6):1025–1029.

33. Onland W, Shin CE, Fustar S, Rushing T, Wong WY. Ethanol-lock technique for persistent bacteremia of long–term intravascular devices in pediatric patients. *Arch Pediatr Adolesc Med.* 2006;160(10):1049–1053.

34. Dannenberg C, Bierbach U, Rothe A, Beer J, Korholz D. Ethanol-lock technique in the treatment of bloodstream infections in pediatric oncology patients with broviac catheter. *J Pediatr Hematol Oncol.* 2003;25(8):616–621.

35. Crnich CJ, Halfmann JA, Crone WC, Maki DG. The effects of prolonged ethanol exposure on the mechanical properties of polyurethane and silicone catheters used for intravascular access. *Infect Control Hosp Epidemiol.* 2005;26:708–714.

36. Tan M, Lau J, Guglielmo BJ. Ethanol locks in the prevention and treatment of catheter-related bloodstream infections. *Ann Pharmacother.* 2014;48(5):607–615.

37. Grace E, Shaw C, Whelan K, Andreyev HJ. Review article: small intestinal bacterial overgrowth—prevalence, clinical features, current and developing diagnostic tests, and treatment. *Aliment Pharmacol Ther.* 2013;38:674–688.

38. Shulman RJ, Phillips S. Parenteral nutrition in infants and children. *J Pediatr Gastroenterol Nutr.* 2003;36(5):588–607.

39. Wesley JR, Coran AG. Intravenous nutrition for the pediatric patient. *Semin Pediatr Surg.* 1992;1:212–230.

40. Jensen AR, Goldin AB, Koopmeiners JS, Stevens J, Waldhausen JH, Kim SS. The association of cyclic parenteral nutrition and decreased incidence of cholestatic liver disease in patients with gastroschisis. *J Pediatr Surg.* 2009;44(1):183–189.

41. Btaiche IF, Khalidi N. Parenteral nutrition-associated liver complications in children. *Pharmacotherapy.* 2002;22:188–211.

42. Mirtallo J, Canada T, Johnson D, et al; Task Force for the Revision of Safe Practices for Parenteral Nutrition. Safe practices for parenteral nutrition [Erratum in *JPEN J Parenter Enteral Nutr.* 2006;30(2):177]. *JPEN J Parenter Enteral Nutr.* 2004;28(6):S39–S70.

43. Kerner JA, Poole RL. The use of IV fats in neonates. *Nutr Clin Pract.* 2006;21:374–380.

44. Pianese P, Salvia G, Campanozzi A, et al. Sterol profiling in red blood cell membranes and plasma of newborns receiving total parenteral nutrition. *J Pediatr Gastroenterol Nutr.* 2008;47(5):645–651.

45. Intralipid 20% A 20% I.V. Fat emulsion [package insert]. Clayton, NC: Kabi Pharmacia; 1991.

46. Bullock L, Etchason E, Fitzgerald JF, McGuire WA. Case report of an allergic reaction to parenteral nutrition in a pediatric patient. *JPEN J Parenter Enteral Nutr.* 1990;14:98–100.

47. Market AD, Lew DB, Schropp KP, Hak EB. Parenteral nutrition-associated anaphylaxis in a 4-year-old child. *J Pediatr Gastroenterol Nutr.* 1998;26(2):229–231.

48. Trissel LA, ed. Handbook on Injectable Drugs. 16th ed. Bethesda, MD: American Society of Health-System Pharmacists; 2011:47-90.

49. Trissel LA, ed. *Handbook on Injectable Drugs.* 11th ed. Bethesda, MD: American Society of Health–System Pharmacists; 2001:195–205.

50. Food and Drug Administration. Safety alert: hazards of precipitation associated with parenteral nutrition. *Am J Hosp Pharm.* 1994;51:1427–1428.

51. Bullock L, Fitzgerald JF, Walter WV. Emulsion stability in total nutrient admixtures containing a pediatric amino acid formulation. *JPEN J Parenter Enteral Nutr.* 1992;16:64–68.

52. Driscoll DF, Bhargava HN, Li L, Zaim RH, Babayan VK, Bistrian BR. Physicochemical stability of total nutrient admixtures. *Am J Health Syst Pharm.* 1995;52:623–634.

53. Driscoll DF, Giampietro K, Wichelhaus DP, et al. Physicochemical stability assessments of lipid emulsions of varying oil composition. *Clin Nutr.* 2001;20:151–157.

54. Driscoll DF, Ling PR, Bistrain BR. Physical stability of 20% lipid injectable emulsions via simulated syringe infusion: effects of glass vs. plastic product packaging. *JPEN J Parenter Enteral Nutr.* 2007;31:148–153.

55. Warshawsky, KY. Intravenous fat emulsions in clinical practice. *Nutr Clin Pract.* 1992;7(4):187–196.

56. O'Grady NP, Alexander M, Dellinger EP, et al; Healthcare Infection Control Practices Advisory Committee. Guidelines for the prevention of intravascular catheter–related infections. *Infect Control Hosp Epidemiol.* 2002;23:759–769.

57. Crill CM, Hak EB, Robinson LA, Helms RA. Evaluation of microbial contamination associated with different preparation methods for neonatal intravenous fat emulsion infusions. *Am J Health Syst Pharm.* 2010;67(11):914–918.

58. DeDonato BM, Bickford LI, Gates RJ. Microbial growth in neonatal intravenous fat emulsion administered over 12 hours versus 24 hours. *J Pediatr Pharmacol Ther.* 2013;18:298–302.

59. Neuzil J, Darlow BA, Inder TE, Sluis KB, Winterbourn CC, Stocker R. Oxidation of parenteral lipid emulsion by ambient and phototherapy lights: potential toxicity of routine parenteral feeding. *J Pediatr.* 1995;126:785–790.

60. Ireton-Jones C, DeLegge MH, Epperson LA, Alexander J. Management of the home parenteral nutrition patient. *Nutr Clin Pract.* 2003;18:310–317.

61. Ferrone M, Geraci M. A review of the relationship between parenteral nutrition and metabolic bone disease. *Nutr Clin Pract.* 2007;22:329–339.

62. Klein GL. Metabolic bone disease of total parenteral nutrition. *Nutrition.* 1998;14:149–152.

63. Nehra D, Carlson SJ, Fallon EM, et al; American Society for Parenteral and Enteral Nutrition. A.S.P.E.N. clinical guidelines: nutrition support of neonatal patients at risk for metabolic bone disease. *JPEN J Parenter Enteral Nutr.* 2013;37:570–598.

64. Kovacevish D, Canada T, Lown D. Monitoring home and other alternate site nutrition support. In: Gottschlich M, Fuhrman M, Hammond KA, Holcombe BJ, eds. *The Science and Practice of Nutrition Support.* Dubuque, IA: Kendall/Hunt Publishing Co; 2000:731–756.

65. Vanderhoof J, Young R. Overview of considerations for the pediatric patient receiving home parenteral and enteral nutrition. *Nutr Clin Pract.* 2003;18:221–226.

66. Sacks G, Mayhew S, Johnson D. Parenteral nutrition implementation and management. In: Merritt R, ed. *The A.S.P.E.N. Nutrition Support Practice Manual.* 2nd ed. Silver Spring, MD: American Society for Parenteral and Enteral Nutrition; 2005:108–117.

67. Kovacevich DS, Frederick A, Kelly D, Reid N, Young L; American Society for Parenteral and Enteral Nutrition Board of Directors and the Standards for Specialized Nutrition Support Task Force. Standards for specialized nutrition support: home care patients. *Nutr Clin Pract.* 2005;20:579–590.

68. Pagana KD, Pagana TJ, eds. *Mosby's Diagnostic and Laboratory Test Reference.* 8th ed. St. Louis, MO: Mosby; 2007:755–756.

69. Fuhrman MP, Charney P, Mueller CM. Hepatic proteins and nutrition assessment. *J Am Diet Assoc.* 2004;104:1258–1264.

70. Marshall WJ. Nutritional assessment: its role in the provision of nutrition support. *J Clin Pathol.* 2008;61:1083–1088.

71. Myron Johnson A, Merlini G, Sheldon J, Ichihara K; Scientific Division Committee on Plasma Proteins (C-PP), International Federation of Clinical Chemistry and Laboratory Medicine (IFCC). Clinical indications for plasma protein assays: transthyretin (prealbumin) in inflammation and malnutrition. *Clin Chem Lab Med.* 2007;45:419–426.

72. Yang HT, Yim H, Cho YS, et al. Prediction of clinical outcomes for massively-burned patients via serum transthyretin levels in the early postburn period [Erratum in *J Trauma Acute Care Surg.* 2012;73(2):534]. *J Trauma Acute Care Surg.* 2012;72:999–1005.

73. Crook MA. Lipid clearance and total parenteral nutrition: the importance of monitoring plasma lipids. *Nutrition.* 2000;16:774–775.

74. Borum PR. Carnitine in neonatal nutrition. *J Child Neurol.* 1995;10(suppl):2S25–2S31.

75. Winter SC, Szabo-Aczel S, Curry CJ, Hutchinson HT, Hogue R, Shug A. Plasma carnitine deficiency: clinical observations in 51 pediatric patients. *Am J Dis Child.* 1987;141:660–665.

76. Tao RC, Yoshimura NN. Carnitine metabolism and its application in parenteral nutrition. *JPEN J Parenter Enteral Nutr.* 1980;4:469–486.

77. Crill CM, Helms RA. The use of carnitine in pediatric nutrition. *Nutr Clin Pract.* 2007;22:204–213.

78. Vanek VW, Borum P, Buchman A, et al; Novel Nutrient Task Force, Parenteral Multi-Vitamin and Multi–Trace Element Working Group; American Society for Parenteral and Enteral Nutrition (A.S.P.E.N.) Board of Directors. A.S.P.E.N. position paper: recommendations for changes in commercially available parenteral multivitamin and multi-trace element products. *Nutr Clin Pract.* 2012;27:440–491.

79. Hamilton C, Austin T, Seidner DL. Essential fatty acid deficiency in human adults during parenteral nutrition. *Nutr Clin Pract.* 2006;21:387–394.

80. Postuma R, Pease PW, Watts R, Taylor S, McEvoy FA. Essential fatty acid deficiency in infants receiving parenteral nutrition. *J Pediatr Surg.* 1978;13:393–398.

81. Panel on Macronutrients, Panel on the Definition of Dietary Fiber, Subcommittee on Upper Reference Levels of Nutrients, Subcommittee on Interpretation and Uses of Dietary

Reference Intakes, and the Standing Committee on the Scientific Evaluation of Dietary Reference Intakes. *Dietary Reference Intakes for Energy, Carbohydrate, Fat, Fatty Acids, Cholesterol, Protein, and Amino Acids.* Washington DC: The National Academies Press; 2005:422–541.

82. Postuma R, Trevenen CL. Liver disease in infants receiving parenteral nutrition. *Pediatrics.* 1979;63:110–115.

83. Kelly DA. Liver complications of pediatric parenteral nutrition-epidemiology. *Nutrition.* 1998;14:153–157.

84. Quigley EM, Marsh MN, Shaffer JL, Markin RS. Hepatobiliary complications of total parenteral nutrition. *Gastroenterology.* 1993;104:286–301.

85. Payne-James JJ, Silk DB. Hepatobiliary dysfunction associated with total parenteral nutrition. *Dig Dis.* 1991;9:106–124.

86. McMillan NB, Mulroy C, MacKay MW, McDonald CM, Jackson WD. Correlation of cholestasis with serum copper and whole-blood manganese levels in pediatric patients. *Nutr Clin Pract.* 2008;23:161–165.

87. Litmanovitz I, Eliakim A, Arnon S, et al. Enriched post-discharge formula versus term formula for bone strength in very low birth weight infants: A longitudinal pilot study. *J Perinat Med.* 2007;35(5):431–435.

88. Duerksen DR, Papineau N. The prevalence of coagulation abnormalities in hospitalized patients receiving lipid-based parenteral nutrition. *JPEN J Parenter Enteral Nutr.* 2004;28:30–33.

89. Deitcher SR. Interpretation of the international normalized ratio in patients with liver disease. *Lancet.* 2002;359:47–48.

90. Pluhator-Murton MM, Fedorak RN, Audette RJ, Marriage BJ, Yatscoff RW, Gramlich LM. Trace element contamination of total parenteral nutrition. 1. Contribution of component solutions. *JPEN J Parenter Enteral Nutr.* 1999;23:222–227.

91. Jensen GL, Binkley J. Clinical manifestations of nutrient deficiency. *JPEN J Parenter Enteral Nutr.* 2002;26:S29–S33.

92. Fuhrman MP. Micronutrient assessment in long–term home parenteral nutrition patients. *Nutr Clin Pract.* 2006;21:566–575.

93. Prelack K, Sheridan RL. Micronutrient supplementation in the critically ill patient: strategies for clinical practice. *J Trauma.* 2001;51:601–620.

94. Clintec Nutrition Company in cooperation with Wagner DR and Atkins J. *Total Nutrient Admixtures: Clinical and Practical Guidelines.* Newport Beach, CA: Clintec Nutrition Co; 1992.

95. Poole RL, Hintz SR, Mackenzie NI, et al. Aluminum exposure from pediatric parenteral nutrition: meeting the new FDA regulation. *JPEN J Parenter Enteral Nutr.* 2008;32(3):242–246.

96. Heimburger DC, McLaren DS, Shils M. Clinical manifestations of nutrient deficiencies and toxicities: a resume. In: Shils ME, Shike M, Ross AC, Caballero B, Cousins RJ, eds. *Modern Nutrition in Health and Disease.* 10th ed. Philadelphia, PA: Lippincott Williams & Wilkins; 2006:595–612.

97. Nielsen FH. Boron, manganese, molybdenum, and other trace elements. In: Bowman BA, Russel RM, eds. *Present Knowledge in Nutrition.* 8th ed. Washington, DC: ILSI Press; 2001:384–400.

98. Ibrahim M, Morreale de Escobar GM, Visser TJ, et al. Iodine deficiency associated with parenteral nutrition in extreme preterm infants. *Arch Dis Child Fetal Neonatal Ed.* 2003;88:F56–F57.

99. Moukarzel AA, Buchman AL, Salas JS, et al. Iodine supplementation in children receiving long-term parenteral nutrition. *J Pediatr.* 1992;121:252–254.

100. Otten JJ, Pitzi-Hellwig J, Meyers LD, eds. *Dietary Reference Intakes: The Essential Guide to Nutrient Requirements.* Washington, DC: National Academies Press; 2006.

101. Northrop-Clewes CA. Interpreting indicators of iron status during an acute phase response—lessons from malaria and human immunodeficiency. *Ann Clin Biochem.* 2008;45(1):18–32.

102. Trissel LA. Compatibility of medications with 3-in-1 parenteral nutrient admixtures. *JPEN J Parenter Enteral Nutr.* 1999;23:67–74.

103. Nagano T, Toyoda T, Tanabe H, et al. Clinical features of hematological disorders caused by copper deficiency during long-term enteral nutrition. *Intern Med.* 2005;44:554–559.

104. Fuhrman MP, Herrmann V, Masidonski P, Eby C. Pancytopenia after removal of copper from total parenteral nutrition. *JPEN J Parenter Enteral Nutr.* 2000;24:361–366.

105. Beshgetoor D, Hambidge M. Clinical conditions altering copper metabolism in humans. *Am J Clin Nutr.* 1998;67:1017–1021S.

106. Oberly MJ and Yang DT. Laboratory testing for cobalamin deficiency in megaloblastic anemia. *Am J Hematol.* 2013;88:522–526.

107. Clark SF. Vitamins and trace elements. In: Gottschlich MM, DeLegge, MH, Mattox T, Mueller C, Worthington P, eds. *The A.S.P.E.N. Nutrition Support Core Curriculum: A Case-Based Approach—The Adult Patient.* Silver Spring, MD: American Society for Parenteral and Enteral Nutrition; 2007:129–159.

108. Misra M, Pacaud D, Petryk A, et al. Vitamin D deficiency in children and its management: Review of current knowledge and recommendations. *Pediatrics.* 2008;122:398–417.

109. Sica DA. Loop diuretic therapy, thiamine balance, and heart failure. *Congest Heart Fail* 2007;13(4):244–247.

110. A.S.P.E.N. Clinical Practice Committee Shortage Subcommittee. A.S.P.E.N. parenteral nutrition trace element product shortage considerations. *Nutr Clin Pract.* 2014;29(2):249–251.

111. Nyffeler MS, Frankel E, Hayes E, et al. Drug-nutrient interactions. In: Merritt R, DeLegge MH, Holcombe B, et al., eds. *The A.S.P.E.N. Nutrition Support Practice Manual.* 2nd ed. Silver Spring, MD: American Society for Parenteral and Enteral Nutrition; 2005:118–136.

112. Drug Interactions Search. Truven Health Analytics. Greenwood Village, CO. http://www.micromedexsolutions.com. Accessed January 2015.

113. Navaneethan SD, Sankarasubbaiyan SG, Jeevanantham VM. Tacrolimus-associated hypomagnesemia in renal transplant recipients. *Transplantation Proc.* 2006;38(5):1320–1322

114. Brown RO. Drug-nutrient interactions. In: Cresci G, ed. *Nutrition Support for the Critically Ill Patient: A Guide to Practice.* Boca Raton, FL: CRC Press; 2005:341–355.

115. Robinson CA, Lee JE. Y-site compatibility of medications with parenteral nutrition. In: Phelps SJ, Hak EB, Crill CM, eds. *Teddy Bear Book: Pediatric Injectable Drugs.* 8th ed. Bethesda, MD: American Society of Health-System Pharmacists; 2007:459–463.

Test Your Knowledge Answers

1. The correct answer is **C**. In light of recent antibiotic therapy, it would be possible that she has developed bacterial overgrowth, resulting in diarrhea. Therefore, it would be practical to screen and treat if indicated. It is reasonable to review the medications with the pharmacist. It is possible that the recent antibiotic therapy caused the acute diarrhea event. Since the current tube-feeding regimen has promoted appropriate growth and has otherwise been well tolerated, it is recommended to review the other options before trialing a new formula. She could have developed *Clostridium difficile* as a result of the antibiotic therapy. It would be reasonable to test for an infectious cause of the diarrhea and treat accordingly.

2. The correct answer is **D**. Hyperglycemia in a stable patient usually indicates an acute issue with high likelihood of infection so a work-up may be warranted depending on other clinical parameters. Initially decreasing the GIR or extending the PN cycle are the easiest and safest interventions while the etiology of hyperglycemia is being determined. If the hyperglycemia persists with modifications in PN then regular insulin may be added to PN. A subcutaneous long-term insulin product could result in hypoglycemia if PN is discontinued or solution modified.

3. The correct answer is **C**. Decreased calcium concentrations, increased dextrose concentrations, and addition of cysteine provide a favorable environment for calcium and phosphorus solubility. Decreased amino acid concentrations can be a limiting factor to the calcium and phosphorus solubility curve and so the concentration may need to be increased if possible so that the calcium and phosphorus doses do not have to be decreased.

4. The correct answer is **B**. Iron products cannot be added to a PN that contain lipids due to incompatibility. Essential fatty acids are contained in the lipid emulsions so are therefore provided in a 3-n-1. Vitamin K is a component of some injectable multivitamin products and can also be added separately if desired. Carnitine is compatible with PN and can be ordered if needed.

5. The correct answer is **B**. Copper and manganese are excreted via the biliary system and thus require laboratory monitoring to better evaluate supplementation. Omission of copper is not routinely recommended without monitoring to avoid deficiency. Selenium and chromium are excreted in the urine and zinc is excreted in urine, stool, and skin.

37

Ethical Issues in Providing Nutrition

Kelly Cronin Komatz, MD, MPH, FAAP, FAAHPM

CONTENTS

Learning Objectives

1. Define "natural" vs "medical" provision of nutrition.
2. Review the importance of determining goals of treatment.
3. Introduce a clinical ethical decision-making approach and tool.

Case Study

Mary is a 12-year-old girl who was diagnosed soon after birth with congenital toxoplasmosis. Mary has been cared for by her parents and younger brother in her home with the assistance of nurses throughout her life. She is unable to walk or care for herself, but she is interactive with her family through vocalizations, smiles, grimaces, and laughs.

The family has made several difficult decisions over Mary's 12 years of life, including not having surgery for her scoliosis or tendon releases for her hip contractures and not having a tracheostomy placed when she was admitted for aspiration pneumonia last year. The family has always known that Mary's life expectancy was limited and has made medical decisions for Mary based on her quality of life and comfort.

Mary is now demonstrating signs and symptoms of not being able to tolerate her gastrostomy tube feedings. The palliative care team has been making home visits to assess Mary and has prescribed different treatment options to try to keep Mary comfortable. These treatments have included medications, changes in her enteral formula, attempts at changing the rate of her feedings, and eventually attempting clear fluids only. However, each time Mary's feedings approach the goal for volume and/or calories, she demonstrates pain within an hour of starting the feeding.

The family sees that the enteral feedings are causing Mary pain and distress. The father is struggling with withdrawing her medically provided enteral nutrition and "starving Mary to death." The father also expresses concern that if they do choose to withhold her nutrition, the local news channel will be on their front lawn because they are "starving" their daughter.

This family's struggle to withdraw medically provided nutrition is commonplace for any caregiver whose loved one is nearing the end of life, whether from a lifelong medical condition or from an acute illness.

"Natural" vs "Medical" Provision of Nutrition

It is important when discussing ethical issues that the terms and phrases being used are understood by all parties involved in the patient's care. An important difference exists between the "natural" provision of nutrition compared with the "medical" provision of nutrients. These terms can be used in various manners, but for the purpose of this chapter the definition put forth by Nicolas Porta and Joel Frader[1] is helpful because they describe their typical usage in the clinical and bioethical literature. The natural provision of nutrition refers to all feedings that do not require medical intervention—specifically breast, bottle, cup, and other oral feedings. Medical provision of nutrition refers to nutrition that requires a special physician order; for example, the use of a nasogastric or orogastric tube, central intravenous (IV) catheter, or the placement of a gastrostomy or jejunostomy feeding tube.

Determining the Goals of Nutrition

When ethical questions arise in healthcare decision making, using a framework of goals is important when discussing the use or disuse of a particular medical intervention. For example, a child who is placed on a ventilator after a sudden acute event affecting their ability to appropriately breathe has normal oxygenation and ventilation as the goal. Another example would be the child who has undergone cardiac surgery to correct a congenital heart defect. That child is likely to be maintained on a ventilator and to receive infusions of blood pressure–sustaining medications as well as nutrition provided through a central line during the immediate postoperative period. Therefore, the goal in both cases is sustaining the child until the time their healing begins.[2]

However, when discussing the ethics of providing nutrition, it is important to expand the discussion related to overall goals of treatment. In its basic form, the goal of providing pediatric patients with nutrition is to provide them with the calories, protein, vitamins, and minerals needed to meet basic metabolic demands for appropriate growth and development. It is important to recognize that goals of treatment can change with time and often do. For example, providing medical nutrition through a central line to a child awaiting an organ transplant can undergo change if the patient experiences severe complications that preclude receipt of a transplant. The discussion related to continuing the parenteral nutrition might change to new goals related to improved quality of life and allow for "de-medicalization" of the child and his/her nutrition.[2]

Do We Tend to See Medical Feeding in a Different Light From Other Medical Interventions?

The provision of nutrition to a pediatric patient often has values assigned to it that make the provision of medical nutrition unique from other forms of life-sustaining medical interventions. Rarely is the removal of a ventilator described as "suffocating the patient to death." However, when the decision is made to withhold or withdraw medical nutrition, it is often described as "starving the patient to death." The tendency to use this language demonstrates that certain value is placed upon the provision of medical "feedings" that is inherently related to the value of providing a patient nutrition.[3]

An example of this perspective of value assigned to feeding and nutrition is demonstrated in a pair of surveys done with pediatric healthcare providers.[2] The Pediatric Section of the Society of Critical Care Medicine found that 98% of physicians were likely to withhold cardiopulmonary resuscitation, 86% withdraw ventilators, but only 42% would withdraw tube feedings.[4] Another survey of pediatric residents in their third year of training demonstrated that 100% would withhold cardiopulmonary resuscitation (CPR) and vasoactive medicines, 97% would withdraw ventilator support, but only 45% would withdraw artificial hydration and nutrition.[5]

Why Is Unique Value Assigned to Feeding vs Nutrition?

Ethical issues involving the provision of withholding or withdrawing nutrition often take place in a unique and complex social dynamic and are charged with emotions. What is it about feeding that makes it more likely to have additional value ascribed to it as opposed to other medical interventions? Language and terminology are always important in conversations, but especially so when discussions related to end-of-life decision making are taking place. The term "food" elicits images of eating, chewing, tasting, and swallowing along with the pleasures and social connotations that accompany those actions. Failing to distinguish between "food" and the technical process of delivering hydration and nutrition through medical devices will make discussions surrounding end-of-life decisions more difficult. Receiving fluids and nutrition through a tube or IV catheter is not the same as eating a meal. This point is discussed further in the American Academy of Pediatrics Clinical Report on Forgoing Artificial Hydration and Nutrition.[6]

The clinical report from the American Academy of Pediatrics outlines several general principles when considering withholding or withdrawing medical hydration and nutrition[6]:

> Medically provided fluids and nutrition constitute a medical intervention that may be withheld or withdrawn for the same types of reasons that justify the medical withholding or with drawing of other medical treatments.

> Medically provided fluids and nutrition can be withdrawn from children when such measures only prolong and add morbidity to the process of dying.

Dr. Carter wrote about the unique value assigned to feeding in the first edition of this book.[2] Why does feeding have more value ascribed to it than other medical interventions to sustain other organ systems? A possibility is that providing nutrition to a child is a fundamental responsibility of the caregiver. Children are born unable to provide themselves with nutrition, and several years of development must take place before they are able to independently obtain and consume nutrition. This responsibility is so ingrained in the caregiver's being, that limiting its provision, no matter how beneficent the motives, causes feelings of guilt and/or neglect in attending to these basic care-giving duties.

Ethical Principles in Decision Making

Ethical theories are broad based and reflect a philosophical commitment to moral reasoning and decision making that may apply to many situations throughout all types of human interactions, not just medically based issues. Bioethics reflects the adaptation of ethical considerations with an emphasis on how best to support quality of life with changing advances in medicine and biological sciences. The basic bioethical principles include:

1. Autonomy—Respect the ability of individuals to make informed decisions affecting health. Parents are the decision-makers for infants and children who cannot make their own decisions.

2. Nonmaleficence—Avoid doing harm.
3. Beneficence—Do good.
4. Justice—Distribute goods and resources fairly.

Decision making in pediatrics is unique because in most situations the parents are the decision-makers. It is understood then that they are the "surrogate decision-makers." In adult medicine, competent adults are able to make their own decisions, thereby exercising their own autonomy. However, a child cannot participate in most decision-making discussions, and therefore a triad relationship exists between the parents/caregivers, the physician, and the child patient. It is accepted in pediatrics that parents will be making decisions with their child's best interest in mind.

The principles of avoiding harm (nonmaleficence) and doing good (beneficence) are more heavily weighted when making decisions related to hydration and nutrition. How can it be harmful to provide nutrition and hydration to a child? Is it not good when a child is fed and thriving? Professionals are obligated to report to child protection agencies when a child is "failing to thrive" due to lack of adequate of nutrition. So how can it be okay to withhold adequate nutrition in a child?[7]

Determining Goals of Care and Introduction of the 4 Topics Approach

Ethical dilemmas often occur because of uncertainty, lack of clarity, or conflict regarding the medical facts, goals of treatment, or different value systems. The use of a systematic framework for identifying and negotiating these differences can assist in resolving clinical ethical problems. The 4 topics model proposed by Jonsen and his colleagues[8] is adaptable to clinical problems in medicine, especially in pediatrics, and discussions related to withholding and withdrawing of life-sustaining treatments including medical hydration and nutrition. The following case will introduce the 4 topics approach applied to withdrawing life-sustaining treatments.

Case Study

Lisa is a 3-year-old girl admitted to the pediatric intensive care unit (PICU) after being found in a neighbor's swimming pool. Her time of submersion is unknown; however, emergency medical technicians were able to resuscitate her after several minutes of CPR and medications. Lisa has been in the PICU for 5 days, and her physical examination demonstrates decorticate posturing, no gag reflex, and no spontaneous respirations over the ventilator. Magnetic resonance imaging of Lisa's brain demonstrates changes consistent with severe anoxic brain injury. Her electroencephalogram shows marked slowing and abnormalities consistent with anoxic encephalopathy.

Lisa's family has had several long discussions with the medical team, including the palliative care team, and has discussed what Lisa's life would be like with this degree of brain injury. The family has elected to allow her to be withdrawn from the ventilator and "to allow for a natural death."

The medical team is in agreement with the withdrawal of the ventilator or "life support"; however, not all members of the medical team agree to allow the family to stop Lisa's IV fluids and nasogastric tube feedings because "this would be the same as committing physician-assisted suicide."

The 4 topics approach is an extremely useful tool when faced with this type of ethical challenge. The 4 topics method provides a framework for sorting through and focusing on specific aspects of each individual case (Table 37-1). The 4 topics include medical indications, patient preferences, quality of life, and contextual features.[9]

In Lisa's case, the medical indications focused on beneficence and nonmaleficence include: What is her prognosis and is her condition reversible? For patient preferences, although Lisa is a minor, it is accepted that Lisa's parents will act in her best interest and consider her quality of life. The topic of quality of life includes the basic principles related to beneficence, nonmaleficence, and respect for patient autonomy. In Lisa's case: Is there the likelihood of return to a normal life? What are the plans to forgo treatment, and are there plans for comfort and palliative care? The decision to withdraw life-sustaining treatment in Lisa's case also needs to be viewed in the contextual feature of loyalty and fairness (justice). Are there family issues that might influence the treatment decisions? Are there financial, economic, re-ligious, or cultural factors? Are there medical providers' issues that might influence treatment decisions?

Medical Futility

Medical futility is often referred to when discussing life-sustaining treatment, including artificial hydration and nutrition, in complex medical situations. It is important to realize as healthcare professionals that there is no single agreed upon definition for "medical futility." Some bioethicists avoid the term completely in discussing difficult situations like withholding or withdrawing of artificial hydration and nutrition.

It is important to recognize goals of care when discussing medical futility, and these cross several domains including biological, ethical, legal, societal, and financial considerations as discussed by Swetz et al.[10]

Hospital ethics committees are a resource for medical providers and families when wrestling with these difficult questions about life-sustaining medical treatments. Most hospitals' ethics committees can be consulted by anyone on the treatment team, including nurses, ancillary staff, and family members. The ethics committee can only make recommendations to the treating team members and often are able to bring the team and family to an agreement about plans of care. Situations regarding withholding or withdrawal of artificial hydration and nutrition should only rarely go to the legal system.

Palliative Care

Ethical challenges in nutrition management for pediatric patients always need to be evaluated in the context of goals and values, which warrants open communication and a collaborative approach within the medical team. Over the past decade, the subject of palliative and end-of-life care has received increased attention in the United States. Most major hospitals, including pediatric hospitals, have dedicated palliative care teams. These teams are crucial in assisting the medical team and parents/caregivers when making difficult medical decisions. Intentions at the end-of-life change focus from life-sustaining or life-prolonging treatments to comfort measures. When this decision has been made, the palliative care is invaluable to the patient and the rest of the family during the dying process.[2]

Hellmann et al[11] surveyed parents who made the decision to withdraw medical hydration and nutrition while their infant was in the neonatal intensive care unit. Their study concentrated on only the parents who decided to withdraw medical hydration and nutrition independent of a decision

Table 37-1. The 4 Topics Approach

MEDICAL INDICATIONS	PATIENT PREFERENCES
Medical history	Personal history
Accurate diagnosis	Religious and personal values
Accurate prognosis	Expressed preferences
Treatment options	Advance directives
	Self-assessment of quality of life
	Ability to make & communicate decisions

QUALITY OF LIFE	CONTEXTUAL FEATURES
External assessment of benefits and burdens	Economic—insurance, availability, cost
Subjective judgment	Family preferences
Who should decide when the patient cannot?	Legal issues
	Burdens on caregivers

to withdraw mechanical ventilator support. In other words, they excluded parents of patients for whom withdrawal of ventilator support and cessation of feeding were undertaken at the same time, with death occurring within 23 hours; this situation did not constitute a conscious elective decision solely about withdrawing medical hydration and nutrition.

The study[11] identified 3 themes regarding the decision to withdraw medical hydration and nutrition: communication, decision making, and the dying experience. The authors further identified subthemes within these categories. In the communication category, parents' responses consistently identified subthemes of the virtues of good communication, the importance of relationship building, admitting the uncertainty of prognoses, and ways of sharing information.

The decision-making domain encompassed subthemes of the parents as decision-makers, their reluctance to have to make the decision, the actual decision itself, and the process of getting to that decision. As expected, parents struggled the most with the domain of decision making. In the dying experience, subthemes included the myriad of parent emotions, achieving the best in a bad situation, receiving encouragement and support, and making a life after death. In this study the median time between the actual withdrawal of medical hydration and nutrition and the child's death was 16 days.

After the decision has been made to withhold or withdraw medically provided hydration and nutrition, the medical team needs to continue to support the parents/caregivers in their decision. The physical changes that a person undergoes are often times distressing to observe. The person's body starts to show signs of dehydration, with decreased urine output and dry lips/skin, which can be treated with optimum mouth care. The person also demonstrates weight loss as the body utilizes muscle stores to sustain itself. For families who are caring for a child who is no longer receiving hydration and/or nutrition, the visual appearance and the prolonged time course to death is very difficult to endure regardless of all the "right" decisions being made.

Dr. Joel Frader[12] expands upon the importance of being present for the families during the decision-making process but also emphasizes the need to be available for continuing support after the actual withdrawal of medical hydration and nutrition. The family needs continuing support through a child's dying process to have ready access to the medical team and have questions answered, to ensure the child is not suffering, and to receive continued support that the decision was in the child's best interest. Watching a child die from the disease process while medical fluids and nutrition are

withheld generates very strong emotions. Young children depend on us to feed them. We obsess about babies' weight gain, wanting them round and healthy. Not feeding our loved ones is a difficult concept, particularly if it causes pain and harm to the dying child. Moreover, dying this way may take some time, between 1 and 3 weeks, depending on the child's age and the state of the child's cardiovascular system. The waiting takes a toll.

As Dr. Frader states further in his perspective piece in the Hastings Center Report[12]:

> I believe candor, acknowledgement of uncertainty about the child's experience, and a solemn promise to respond quickly and unhesitatingly to signs of distress or discomfort make a difference. I believe clinicians need to spend all available time at the bedside during the child's dying because we clinicians need to stay connect to the reality of death.

Nutrition Support Teams

Most hospitals have nutrition support teams to assess patients receiving parenteral and enteral nutrition. The team includes a physician, dietitian, nurse, and pharmacist, and it provides the unique perspectives and skill sets needed to deliver safe and appropriate nutrition support therapy. The team can become an important resource for parents, caregivers, and others on the medical care team when withholding and withdrawing medical hydration and nutrition are being discussed. This is especially true in the acute care setting, home health, or palliative and hospice care.

The American Society for Parenteral and Enteral Nutrition Board of Directors has issued a statement regarding the ethics of withholding and/or withdrawing nutrition support therapy.[13] The statement includes the following points, specifically as they relate to this chapter.

1. Legally and ethically, nutrition support therapy should be considered a medical therapy.
2. The decision to receive or refuse nutrition support therapy should reflect the autonomy and wishes of the patient. The benefits and burdens of nutrition support therapy, and the intervention required to deliver it, should be considered before offering this therapy.

At this point of the overall statement, it is important to recognize that nutrition support can sometimes be a burden. Nutrition is not often thought of in this way; however, when a patient is unable to receive enteral nutrition without the placement of a gastrostomy tube or when a patient who was already receiving enteral nutrition is now having abdominal pain related to his or her gastrostomy tube feedings due to disease progression, it is ethical to look at withholding these feedings.

Nutrition support therapy should be modified or discontinued when disproportionate burdens exist or when benefit can no longer be demonstrated.

Summary

The provision of medically provided hydration and nutrition has become readily accepted within the practice of medicine and is often overlooked as being a "medical" therapy that is essentially life-prolonging. This includes enteral feedings through oro/nasal or gastrostomy tubes as well as parenteral nutrition. Ethical challenges present themselves when families have to decide to forgo these treatment options, and the challenge is best met with open dialogue, respectful listening, and clarity of communication and sensitivity between the patient, family, and medical team. The dietitian has an integral role to play in these matters and is a valued interdisciplinary team member across diverse diagnostic categories, care environments, and the age continuum of pediatrics.[2]

Test Your Knowledge Questions

1. How do Porta and Frader distinguish between "natural" and "medical" nutrition?
   A. Natural nutrition is a mandatory act.
   B. Medical nutrition is a mandatory act.
   C. Natural nutrition is always optional.
   D. Medical nutrition is always optional.
   E. None of the above.
2. Which of the following actions is **not** recommended as a way to help reach an ethical decision regarding the provision of nutrition?
   A. Make sure everyone on the team is using the same definition for commonly used medical and ethical terms.
   B. Avoid talking to the family or the patient until a decision is made so that the team does not appear uncertain.
   C. Define the long-term goal of providing nutrition to the patient.
   D. Discuss with the family their views and beliefs regarding feeding and/or the provision of nutrition.
   E. Carefully examine the context (goals, values, burdens, and benefits) of the nutrition dilemma.

Acknowledgments

The author of this chapter for the second edition of this text wishes to thank Patrick Jones, MD; MA, and Brian Carter, MD, for their contributions to the first edition of this text.

References

1. Porta N, Frader J. Withholding hydration and nutrition in newborns. *Theor Med Bioeth.* 2007;28:443–451.
2. Jones PM, Carter B. Ethical issues in the provision of nutrition. In: Corkins M, Balint J, eds. *A.S.P.E.N. Pediatric Nutrition Support Core Curriculum.* 1st ed. Silver Spring, MD: American Society for Parenteral and Enteral Nutrition; 2010:477–486.
3. Carter BS, Leuthner SR. The ethics of withholding/withdrawing nutrition in the newborn. *Semin Perinatol.* 2003;27(6):480–487.
4. Society of Critical Care Medicine, Task Force on Ethics. Consensus report on the ethics of forgoing life-sustaining treatments in the critically ill. *Crit Care Med.* 1990;18(12);1435–1439.
5. Rubenstein JS, Unti SM, Winter RJ. Pediatric resident attitudes about technologic support of vegetative patients and the effect of parental input—a longitudinal study. *Pediatrics.* 1994;94(1):8–12.
6. Diekema DS, Botkin JR. Forgoing medically provided nutrition and hydration in children. *Pediatrics.* 2009;124:813–822.
7. Truog RD. Withholding and withdrawing life-sustaining treatments. In: Quill TE, Miller FG, eds. *Palliative Care and Ethics.* New York, NY: Oxford University Press; 2014:187–198.
8. Jonsen AR, Siegler M, Winslade WJ. *Clinical Ethics.* 4th ed. New York, NY: McGraw-Hill; 1998.
9. Schumann JH, Alfandre D. Clinical ethical decision making: the four topics approach. *Semin Med Pract.* 2008;11:36–42.
10. Swetz KM, Burkle CM, Berge KH, Lanier WL. Ten common questions (and their answers) on medical futility. *Mayo Clin Proc.* 2014;89:943–959.
11. Hellmann J, Williams C, Ives-Baine, L, Shah PS. Withdrawal of artificial nutrition and hydration in the neonatal intensive care unit: parental perspectives. *Arch Dis Child Fetal Neonatal Ed.* 2013;98:F21–F25.
12. Frader JE. Discontinuing artificial fluids and nutrition: discussions with children's families. *Hastings Cent Rep.* 2007;37(1):49.
13. Tappenden KA. The ethics of nutrition support—ripped from the headlines. *Nutr Clin Pract.* 2008;23:579–580.

Test Your Knowledge Answers

1. The correct answer is **E**.
2. The correct answer is **B**.

Index

Page numbers followed by *f* or *t* indicate figures or tables, respectively.

A

Abbott Nutrition, 187*t*
Abdomen
    physical examination, 539*t*
    surgery, 517–519
ABPM. *See* Ambulatory blood pressure monitoring
Academy of Breastfeeding Medicine, 154
Academy of Nutrition and Dietetics Association (AND), 160
Acanthosis nigricans, 207
ACE. *See* American College of Endocrinology
Acid-blocker medications, 476
Acute kidney injury (AKI), 352–353, 368–369
    general management of, 374*t*
    neonatal issues, 369–371
ADA. *See* American Diabetes Association
Added rice starch infant formulas, 172
Adenosine triphosphate (ATP), 284, 415
ADH. *See* Antidiuretic hormone
Adipose tissue, 33
Adrenal hemorrhage, 499
Adverse food reaction, 290*t*
AHA. *See* American Heart Association
Air insufflation with auscultation, 570
Airway disorders, 521

AKI. *See* Acute kidney injury
Alagille syndrome, 413
Alcohol, 72
Allergen, 280*t*. *See also* Food allergies
α-linolenic acid, 33
Aluminum, 362
    toxicity, 603–604
Ambulatory blood pressure monitoring (ABPM), 365
American Academy of Pediatrics, 348
American College of Endocrinology (ACE), 200
American Diabetes Association (ADA), 310
American Heart Association (AHA), 200, 347, 365
Amino acids, 45
    commercially available, 597*t*
    conditionally essential, 46–48
    essential, 46*t*
    functions of, 50, 51*t*
    infant formulas, 174–175, 176*t*
    kidney in metabolism of, 49–50
    large neutral, 322
    liver in metabolism of, 49–50
    plasma, 52
    in pregnancy nutrition, 132
    sulfur, 46
    transport of, 44*f*
    of urea cycle, 48
Amylase
    pancreatic, 24*f*

    salivary, 24*f*
Amylose, 24
Anaphylaxis, 290*t*
    food allergy, 292
AND. *See* Academy of Nutrition and Dietetics Association
Anemia, 627
Animal models
    dietary manipulation, 142–143
    endocrine mechanisms, 144
    maternal iron deficiency, 144
    maternal obesogenic, 143–144
    maternal protein restriction, 143
    paracrine mechanisms, 144
    surgical manipulation, 144
Anorectal malformations, 517
Anorexia nervosa, 276*t*
Anthropometric measurements
    growth and
        BMI, 264
        growth charts, 264–265
        height, 264
        length, 264
        neurological impairment and, 264–265
        triceps skinfold, 264
        upper arm anthropometrics, 264
        weight, 264
    nutrition assessment, 532
        to age 20 years, 533
        BMI, 534–535